Herbal and Traditional Medicine

Molecular Aspects of Health

OXIDATIVE STRESS AND DISEASE

Series Editors

LESTER PACKER, PH.D.
ENRIQUE CADENAS, M.D., PH.D.

University of Southern California School of Pharmacy
Los Angeles, California

1. Oxidative Stress in Cancer, AIDS, and Neurodegenerative Diseases, *edited by Luc Montagnier, René Olivier, and Catherine Pasquier*
2. Understanding the Process of Aging: The Roles of Mitochondria, Free Radicals, and Antioxidants, *edited by Enrique Cadenas and Lester Packer*
3. Redox Regulation of Cell Signaling and Its Clinical Application, *edited by Lester Packer and Junji Yodoi*
4. Antioxidants in Diabetes Management, *edited by Lester Packer, Peter Rösen, Hans J. Tritschler, George L. King, and Angelo Azzi*
5. Free Radicals in Brain Pathophysiology, *edited by Giuseppe Poli, Enrique Cadenas, and Lester Packer*
6. Nutraceuticals in Health and Disease Prevention, *edited by Klaus Krämer, Peter-Paul Hoppe, and Lester Packer*
7. Environmental Stressors in Health and Disease, *edited by Jürgen Fuchs and Lester Packer*
8. Handbook of Antioxidants: Second Edition, Revised and Expanded, *edited by Enrique Cadenas and Lester Packer*
9. Flavonoids in Health and Disease: Second Edition, Revised and Expanded, *edited by Catherine A. Rice-Evans and Lester Packer*
10. Redox–Genome Interactions in Health and Disease, *edited by Jürgen Fuchs, Maurizio Podda, and Lester Packer*
11. Thiamine: Catalytic Mechanisms in Normal and Disease States, *edited by Frank Jordan and Mulchand S. Patel*

Related Volumes

Vitamin E in Health and Disease: Biochemistry and Clinical Applications, *edited by Lester Packer and Jürgen Fuchs*

Vitamin A in Health and Disease, *edited by Rune Blomhoff*

Free Radicals and Oxidation Phenomena in Biological Systems, *edited by Marcel Roberfroid and Pedro Buc Calderon*

Biothiols in Health and Disease, *edited by Lester Packer and Enrique Cadenas*

Handbook of Antioxidants, *edited by Enrique Cadenas and Lester Packer*

Handbook of Synthetic Antioxidants, *edited by Lester Packer and Enrique Cadenas*

Vitamin C in Health and Disease, *edited by Lester Packer and Jürgen Fuchs*

Lipoic Acid in Health and Disease, *edited by Jürgen Fuchs, Lester Packer, and Guido Zimmer*

Flavonoids in Health and Disease, *edited by Catherine Rice-Evans and Lester Packer*

Additional Volumes in Preparation

Phytochemicals in Health and Disease, *edited by Yongping Bao and Roger Fenwick*

Herbal and Traditional Medicine

Molecular Aspects of Health

edited by
Lester Packer
Choon Nam Ong
Barry Halliwell

MARCEL DEKKER   NEW YORK

Library of Congress Cataloging-in-Publication Data
A catalog record for this book is available from the Library of Congress.

ISBN: 0-8247-5436-0

This book is printed on acid-free paper.

Headquarters
Marcel Dekker, 270 Madison Avenue, New York, NY 10016, U.S.A.
tel: 212-696-9000; fax: 212-685-4540

Distribution and Customer Service
Marcel Dekker, Cimarron Road, Monticello, New York 12701, U.S.A.
tel: 800-228-1160; fax: 845-796-1772

World Wide Web
http://www.dekker.com

Current printing (last digit):

10 9 8 7 6 5 4 3 2

PRINTED IN THE UNITED STATES OF AMERICA

Series Introduction

Oxygen is a dangerous friend. Overwhelming evidence indicates that oxidative stress can lead to cell and tissue injury. However, the same free radicals that are generated during oxidative stress are produced during normal metabolism and thus are involved in both human health and disease.

- Free radicals are molecules with an odd number of electrons. The odd, or unpaired, electron is highly reactive as it seeks to pair with another free electron.
- Free radicals are generated during oxidative metabolism and energy production in the body.
- Free radicals are involved in:
  - Enzyme-catalyzed reactions
  - Electron transport in mitochondria
  - Signal transduction and gene expression
  - Activation of nuclear transcription factors
  - Oxidative damage to molecules, cells, and tissues
  - Antimicrobial action of neutrophils and macrophages
  - Aging and disease

Normal metabolism is dependent on oxygen, a free radical. Through evolution, oxygen was chosen as the terminal electron acceptor for respiration. The two unpaired electrons of oxygen spin in the same direction; thus, oxygen is a biradical, but is not a very dangerous free radical. Other oxygen-derived free radical species, such as superoxide or hydroxyl radicals, formed during metabolism or by ionizing radiation are stronger oxidants and are therefore more dangerous.

In addition to research on the biological effects of these reactive oxygen species, research on reactive nitrogen species has been gathering momentum. NO, or nitrogen monoxide (nitric oxide), is a free radical generated by NO synthase (NOS). This enzyme modulates physiological responses such as vasodilation or signaling in the brain. However, during inflammation, synthesis of NOS (iNOS) is induced. This iNOS can result in the overproduction of NO, causing damage. More worrisome, however, is the fact that excess NO can react with superoxide to produce the very toxic product peroxynitrite. Oxidation of lipids, proteins, and DNA can result, thereby increasing the likelihood of tissue injury.

Both reactive oxygen and nitrogen species are involved in normal cell regulation in which oxidants and redox status are important in signal transduction. Oxidative stress is increasingly seen as a major upstream component in the signaling cascade involved in inflammatory responses, stimulating adhesion molecule and chemoattractant production. Hydrogen peroxide, which breaks down to produce hydroxyl radicals, can also activate NF-κB, a transcription factor involved in stimulating inflammatory responses. Excess production of these reactive species is toxic, exerting cytostatic effects, causing membrane damage, and activating pathways of cell death (apoptosis and/or necrosis).

Virtually all diseases thus far examined involve free radicals. In most cases, free radicals are secondary to the disease process, but in some instances free radicals are causal. Thus, there is a delicate balance between oxidants and antioxidants in health and disease. Their proper balance is essential for ensuring healthy aging.

The term oxidative stress indicates that the antioxidant status of cells and tissues is altered by exposure to oxidants. The redox status is thus dependent on the degree to which a cell's components are in the oxidized state. In general, the reducing environment inside cells helps to prevent oxidative damage. In this reducing environment, disulfide bonds (S—S) do not spontaneously form because sulfhydryl groups kept in the reduced state (SH) prevent protein misfolding or aggregation. This reducing environment is maintained by oxidative metabolism and by the action of antioxidant enzymes and substances, such as glutathione, thioredoxin, vitamins E and

C, and enzymes such as superoxide dismutase (SOD), catalase, and the selenium-dependent glutathione and thioredoxin hydroperoxidases, which serve to remove reactive oxygen species.

Changes in the redox status and depletion of antioxidants occur during oxidative stress. The thiol redox status is a useful index of oxidative stress mainly because metabolism and NADPH-dependent enzymes maintain cell glutathione (GSH) almost completely in its reduced state. Oxidized glutathione (glutathione disulfide, GSSG) accumulates under conditions of oxidant exposure, and this changes the ratio of oxidized to reduced glutathione; an increased ratio indicates oxidative stress. Many tissues contain large amounts of glutathione, 2–4 mM in erythrocytes or neural tissues and up to 8 mM in hepatic tissues. Reactive oxygen and nitrogen species can directly react with glutathione to lower the levels of this substance, the cell's primary preventative antioxidant.

Current hypotheses favor the idea that lowering oxidative stress can have a clinical benefit. Free radicals can be overproduced or the natural antioxidant system defenses weakened, first resulting in oxidative stress, and then leading to oxidative injury and disease. Examples of this process include heart disease and cancer. Oxidation of human low-density lipoproteins is considered the first step in the progression and eventual development of atherosclerosis, leading to cardiovascular disease. Oxidative DNA damage initiates carcinogenesis.

Compelling support for the involvement of free radicals in disease development comes from epidemiological studies showing that an enhanced antioxidant status is associated with reduced risk of several diseases. Vitamin E and prevention of cardiovascular disease is a notable example. Elevated antioxidant status is also associated with decreased incidence of cataracts and cancer, and some recent reports have suggested an inverse correlation between antioxidant status and occurrence of rheumatoid arthritis and diabetes mellitus. Indeed, the number of indications in which antioxidants may be useful in the prevention and/or the treatment of disease is increasing.

Oxidative stress, rather than being the primary cause of disease, is more often a secondary complication in many disorders. Oxidative stress diseases include inflammatory bowel diseases, retinal ischemia, cardiovascular disease and restenosis, AIDS, ARDS, and neurodegenerative diseases such as stroke, Parkinson's disease, and Alzheimer's disease. Such indications may prove amenable to antioxidant treatment because there is a clear involvement of oxidative injury in these disorders.

In this series of books, the importance of oxidative stress in diseases associated with organ systems of the body is highlighted by exploring the scientific evidence and the medical applications of this knowledge. The series also highlights the major natural antioxidant enzymes and antioxidant substances such as vitamins E, A, and C, flavonoids, polyphenols, carotenoids, lipoic acid, and other nutrients present in food and beverages.

Oxidative stress is an underlying factor in health and disease. More and more evidence indicates that a proper balance between oxidants and antioxidants is involved in maintaining health and longevity and that altering this balance in favor of oxidants may result in pathological responses causing functional disorders and disease. This series is intended for researchers in the basic biomedical sciences and clinicians. The potential for healthy aging and disease prevention necessitates gaining further knowledge about how oxidants and antioxidants affect biological systems.

Lester Packer
Enrique Cadenas

Preface

The concept for this book arose during a visit by Lester Packer to the National University of Singapore (NUS) as a distinguished visiting Professor in the Medical School's Department of Biochemistry during August/September 2001.

This volume seeks to highlight traditional and herbal medicines with emphasis on both the molecular basis of their biological activity and their health effects. It is timely because there is now unprecedented interest throughout the world in bringing to light the molecular basis of the biological activity of traditional remedies used for centuries and in some cases for thousands of years. Many of these traditional medicines (TMs) are derived from plants and herbs (phytomedicines) or from products that are often readily available as herbal supplements. These herbal supplements are experiencing enormous popularity in Western countries. They are administered both orally and by topical application.

Recognition of the rise in interest in alternative and complementary forms of medicine has been reflected by governmental and nongovernmental changes. For example, the United States has established new programs within the National Institutes of Health by the Office of Dietary Supplements and the

National Center for Complementary and Alternative Medicine (NCCAM), which seeks to support basic and clinical research programs to verify health claims and to determine the molecular basis of the biological activity, an aim closely aligned with the concept of this book. Western and traditional medicine is now at a crossroads and the future holds great promise from merging and appropriately coordinating medical research and practice, bringing together the best of both biomedical worlds for management of health and disease.

There have been literally thousands of traditional medicines described with origins in the Chinese and Indian subcontinent, Singapore, Malaysia, Japan, Korea, and tribal cultures in all continents throughout the world. Indeed, knowledge about some of these remedies is being lost in developing countries through urbanization. The list of herbal remedies is staggering, and many books, pharmacopoeias, and an extensive literature have documented their existence and reported on their beneficial effects toward health and well-being, disease prevention, and treatment. However, for most TMs the active principles and basic mechanisms of action are not well known.

Some herbal remedies are widely used by people or medical practitioners throughout the world. We decided that it would be important to review and critically evaluate the issues involved in the wider use of traditional and herbal products for health maintenance and treatment of disease: the drawbacks in their continuing and further use, issues regarding their chemistry and methods of preparation, the proper design to conduct clinical trials to evaluate their efficacy, their potential adverse affects, the challenges that lie ahead in combining traditional and western medicines, and their role in national health care and public policy issues.

We attempted to select from some of the best-case scenarios and from among the most widely used and known herbal remedies to report on their alleged effects on health and disease in the light of the current knowledge concerning their basic biological mechanisms of action and to point out directions for future fundamental and clinical studies.

We would like to acknowledge the valuable technical assistance of Ma Hnin Hnin Aung of the National Institute of Education, Nanyang Technological University, Singapore, for her skills in communicating with the authors and coeditors to help bring about the successful completion of this book.

Lester Packer
Choon Nam Ong
Barry Halliwell

Contents

Contributors

Bharat B. Aggarwal, Ph.D. Professor of Cancer Medicine, Department of Bioimmunotherapy, The University of Texas M.D. Anderson Cancer Center, Houston, Texas, U.S.A.

Hooi Hoon Ang, B.Pharm.(Hons), Ph.D. Associate Professor, School of Pharmaceutical Sciences, University Science Malaysia, Minden, Penang, Malaysia

Bimal H. Ashar, M.D. Department of Medicine, Johns Hopkins University School of Medicine, Baltimore, Maryland, U.S.A.

Michael Aviram, D.Sc. Head, Lipid Research Laboratory, Rambam Medical Center, Faculty of Medicine, Technion-Israel Institute of Technology, Haifa, Israel

Yongping Bao, M.D., Ph.D. Department of Nutrition, Institute of Food Research, Norwich, England

Iris F. F. Benzie, D.Phil., F.I.B.M.S. Professor, Ageing and Health Section, Faculty of Health and Social Sciences, The Hong Kong Polytechnic University, Hong Kong, China

Alok Chandra Bharti, Ph.D. Institute of Cytology and Preventive Oncology (ICMR), Uttar Pradesh, India

Emily Bilbow Department of Biology, Wilkes University, Wilkes-Barre, Pennsylvania, U.S.A.

Ann M. Bode, Ph.D. Research Associate Professor, Hormel Institute, University of Minnesota, Austin, Minnesota, U.S.A.

Gerard Bodeker, M.Psych., Ed.D. Department of Clinical Medicine, University of Oxford Medical School, Oxford, England

Peter Bucheli, Ph.D. Project Manager, Nutrition, Nestlé Red Centre Shanghai Ltd., Shanghai, China

John A. Buswell, Ph.D. Edible Fungi Institute, Shanghai Academy of Agricultural Sciences, Shanghai, People's Republic of China

Paul Pui-Hay But, Ph.D. Department of Biology and Institute of Chinese Medicine, Chinese University of Hong Kong, Shatin, Hong Kong, China

Maria C. Carles, Ph.D. Postdoctoral Fellow, Department of Molecular and Experimental Medicine, The Scripps Research Institute, La Jolla, California, U.S.A.

Sui-Yung Chan, Ph.D., M.B.A., B.Sc.(Pharm)(Hons) Associate Professor, Department of Pharmacy, National University of Singapore, Singapore, Republic of Singapore

Keli Chen, M.B.B.S. Professor, Department of Pharmacy, Hubei College of Chinese Traditional Medicine, Wuhan City, People's Republic of China

Zhen Yu Chen, Ph.D. Professor, Department of Biochemistry, Chinese University of Hong Kong, Shatin, Hong Kong, China

George W. Cherry, D.Phil.(Oxon) Director, Wound Healing Institute, Department of Dermatology, Oxford University, Oxford, England

Kyung-Joo Cho, Ph.D. Department of Biological Sciences, Korea Advanced Institute of Science and Technology, Daejeon, South Korea

Yves Christen, Ph.D. Vice President, Research Department, Ipsen, Paris, France

Henry Hin-Chung Chu Department of Medicine and Therapeutics, Chinese University of Hong Kong, Shatin, Hong Kong, China

An-Sik Chung, Ph.D. Professor, Department of Biological Sciences, Korea Advanced Institute of Science and Technology, Daejeon, South Korea

Raymond Cooper, Ph.D. Executive Director, Scientific Affairs, Pharmanex, LLC, Provo, Utah, U.S.A.

Adrian S. Dobs, M.D., M.H.S. Department of Medicine, Johns Hopkins University School of Medicine, Baltimore, Maryland, U.S.A

Zigang Dong, M.D., Dr.PH. Professor, Hormel Institute, University of Minnesota, Austin, Minnesota, U.S.A.

Edzard Ernst, M.D., Ph.D., F.R.C.P., F.R.C.P.Ed. Professor, Department of Complementary Medicine, Peninsula Medical School, Universities of Exeter & Plymouth, Devon, England

Bianca Fuhrman, Ph.D. The Lipid Research Laboratory, Rambam Medical Center, Haifa, Israel

David Grasso Department of Biology, Wilkes University, Wilkes-Barre, Pennsylvania, U.S.A.

Renée J. Grayer, Ph.D. Jodrell Laboratory, Royal Botanic Gardens, Kew, Richmond, Surrey, England

Christine A. Haller, M.D. Assistant Adjunct Professor and Chief, Toxicology Service, Departments of Medicine and Laboratory Medicine, University of California, San Francisco, and San Francisco General Hospital, San Francisco, California, U.S.A.

Barry Halliwell, Ph.D., D.Sc. Head, Department of Biochemistry, National University of Singapore, Singapore, Republic of Singapore

Walter K. K. Ho, Ph.D. Professor, Department of Biochemistry, Chinese University of Hong Kong, Shatin, Hong Kong, China

Yu Huang, Ph.D. Professor, Department of Physiology, Chinese University of Hong Kong, Shatin, Hong Kong, China

Margaret A. Hughes, Ph.D. Clinical Scientist, Department of Dermatology, Oxford Wound Healing Institute, and Churchill Hospital, Oxford, England

Haruyo Ichikawa, Ph.D. Department of Pharmacy, Niigata University of Pharmacy and Applied Life Sciences, Niigata, Japan

Nancy Y. Ip, Ph.D. Professor, Department of Biochemistry, Hong Kong University of Science and Technology, Hong Kong, China

Kristen Jones Department of Biology, Wilkes University, Wilkes-Barre, Pennsylvania, U.S.A.

Kenneth M. Klemow, Ph.D. Professor, Department of Biology, Wilkes University, Wilkes-Barre, Pennsylvania, U.S.A.

Robert Kam-Ming Ko, Ph.D. Associate Professor, Department of Biochemistry, Hong Kong University of Science and Technology, Hong Kong, China

Ling Dong Kong, Ph.D. Associate Professor, School of Life Sciences, Nanjing University, Nanjing, Jiangsu, People's Republic of China

Tetsuya Konishi, Ph.D. Professor, Functional Food Sciences, Niigata University of Pharmacy and Applied Life Sciences, Niigata, Japan

Anushree Kumar Department of Bioimmunotherapy, University of Texas M.D. Anderson Cancer Center, Houston, Texas, U.S.A.

Wei Lan, Ph.D. Medical Manager, Medical Department, Roche Hong Kong Limited, Tsuen Wan, Hong Kong, China

The-Trung Le, M.D., Ph.D., D.Sc. Professor of Surgery, National Institute of Burns, Military Academy of Medicine, Hanoi, Vietnam

Seng-Teik Lee, M.D., F.R.C.S., F.A.M.S. Senior Consultant and Clinical Professor, Department of Surgery, National University of Singapore, and Singapore General Hospital, Singapore, Republic of Singapore

Ping Chung Leung, D.Soc.S.(Hon), D.Sc., F.R.C.S., M.B.B.S., F.H.K.A.M. (Orth) Professor, Institute of Chinese Medicine, Chinese University of Hong Kong, Shatin, Hong Kong, China

Shaoping Li, Ph.D. Assistant Professor, Institute of Chinese Medical Sciences, University of Macau, Macau, China

Lis Sa Elissa Lim, M.Phil. Research Scholar, Department of Obstetrics and Gynecology, National University of Singapore, Singapore, Republic of Singapore

Jin Liu, Ph.D. Postdoctoral Scholar, Department of Oncological Sciences, Huntsman Cancer Institute, University of Utah, Salt Lake City, Utah, U.S.A.

Maria A. Livrea, Ph.D. Professor, Department of Pharmaceutical, Toxicological and Biological Chemistry, University of Palermo, Palermo, Italy

Yin Sze Loh, M.B.B.S.(Singapore) Research Clinician-Scientist, Department of Obstetrics and Gynecology, National University Hospital, Singapore, Republic of Singapore

Duncan H. F. Mak, M.Phil. Visiting Scholar, Department of Chemistry, Hong Kong University of Science and Technology, Hong Kong, China

Jason McDermott Department of Biology, Wilkes University, Wilkes-Barre, Pennsylvania, U.S.A.

Lester A. Mitscher, Ph.D. Kansas University Distinguished Professor, Department of Medicinal Chemistry, The University of Kansas, Lawrence, Kansas, U.S.A.

Mah-Lee Ng, Ph.D. Associate Professor, Department of Microbiology, National University of Singapore, Singapore, Republic of Singapore

Hiroshi Nishida, Ph.D. Assistant Professor, Department of Pharmacy, Niigata University of Pharmacy and Applied Life Sciences, Niigata, Japan

Elizabeth Offord, Ph.D. Department of Nutrition, Nestlé Research Center, Lausanne, Switzerland

Choon Nam Ong, Ph.D. Department of Community, Occupational and Family Medicine, National University of Singapore, Singapore, Republic of Singapore

Eric Pape Department of Biology, Wilkes University, Wilkes-Barre, Pennsylvania, U.S.A.

Jong Dae Park, Ph.D. Head, Ginseng Efficacy Laboratory, Division of Ginseng Research, KT & G Central Research Institute, Daejeon, South Korea

Shazib Pervaiz, M.B.B.S., Ph.D. Associate Professor, Department of Physiology, National University of Singapore, Singapore, Republic of Singapore

Manh-Hung Pham, M.D., Ph.D., D.Sc. Professor of Immunology, National Institute of Burns, Military Academy of Medicine, Hanoi, Vietnam

Thang T. Phan, M.D., Ph.D. Assistant Professor, Departments of Surgery and Bioengineering, National University of Singapore, and Singapore General Hospital, Republic of Singapore

Peter Natesan Pushparaj, M.Sc.(Biochem), M.Sc.(Zoology), B.Ed., Ph.D. Department of Biochemistry, Faculty of Medicine, National University of Singapore, Singapore, Republic of Singapore

Peter Rose, Ph.D. Department of Community, Occupational and Family Medicine, National University of Singapore, Singapore, Republic of Singapore

Han-Ming Shen, Ph.D. Assistant Professor, Department of Community, Occupational and Family Medicine, National University of Singapore, Singapore, Republic of Singapore

Ranxin Shi, M.Sc. Department of Community, Occupational and Family Medicine, National University of Singapore, Singapore, Republic of Singapore

Ichiro Shimizu, M.D., Ph.D. Associate Professor, Department of Digestive and Cardiovascular Medicine, Tokushima University School of Medicine, Tokushima, Japan

Subramanian Sivakami, Ph.D. Professor, Department of Life Sciences, University of Mumbai, Mumbai, India

Dalia Somjen, Ph.D. Vice Manager, Endocrine Laboratory, Institute of Endocrinology, The Tel-Aviv Sourasky Medical Center, Tel-Aviv, Israel

Snait Tamir, Ph.D. Head, Department of Nutrition Science, Tel-Hai Academic College, Upper Galilee, Israel

Benny Kwong-Huat Tan, M.B.B.S., Ph.D. Associate Professor, Department of Pharmacology, National University of Singapore, Singapore, Republic of Singapore

Chee-Hong Tan, B.Sc., M.Sc., Ph.D. Associate Professor, Department of Biochemistry, National University of Singapore, Singapore, Republic of Singapore

Ren Xiang Tan, Ph.D. Professor, Institute of Functional Biomolecules, State Key Laboratory of Pharmaceutical Biotechnology, Nanjing University, Nanjing, Jiangsu, People's Republic of China

Luisa Tesoriere, M.D. Associate Professor, Department of Pharmaceutical, Department of Toxicological and Biological Chemistry, University of Palermo, Palermo, Italy

G. Neil Thomas, Ph.D. Department of Community Medicine, University of Hong Kong, Pokfulam, Hong Kong, China

Brian Tomlinson, M.D., F.R.C.P. Professor, Department of Medicine and Therapeutics, Chinese University of Hong Kong, Shatin, Hong Kong, China

Karl W. K. Tsim, Ph.D. Associate Professor, Department of Biology, Hong Kong University of Science and Technology, Hong Kong, China

Jacob Vaya, Ph.D. Head, Department of Biotechnology and Environmental Science, Tel-Hai Academic College, and Laboratory of Natural Medicinal Compounds, MIGAL-Galilee Technology Center, Kiryat Shmona, Israel

Sissi Wachtel-Galor, B.Sc., M.Sc. Ageing and Health Section, Faculty of Health and Social Sciences, The Hong Kong Polytechnic University, Hong Kong, China

XueJiang Wang, M.D. Professor, College of Traditional Chinese Medicine and Pharmacology, Capital University of Medical Sciences, Beijing, China

John H. Weisburger, Ph.D. Senior Member and Director Emeritus, Institute for Cancer Prevention, American Health Foundation, Valhalla, New York, U.S.A.

Matthew Whiteman, Ph.D. Department of Biochemistry, National University of Singapore, Singapore, Republic of Singapore

Gary Williamson, Ph.D. Professor, Nutrient Bioavailability Group, Nestlé Research Center, Lausanne, Switzerland

Chi-Hao Wu, M.S. Department of Food Science, National Chung Hsing University, Taichung, Taiwan

Ann-Teck Yap, B.Sc.(Hong) Postgraduate Student, Department of Microbiology, National University of Singapore, Singapore, Republic of Singapore

Sook Peng Yap, B.Sc.(Hons) Department of Obstetrics and Gynecology, National University of Singapore, Singapore, Republic of Singapore

Gow-Chin Yen, Ph.D. Professor, Department of Food Sciences, National Chung Hsing University, Taichung, Taiwan

Eu Leong Yong, M.D., Ph.D. Associate Professor and Senior Consultant, Department of Obstetrics and Gynecology, National University of Singapore, Singapore, Republic of Singapore

Amy C. Y. Zhang, Ph.D. Research and Development, Epitomics, Inc., Burlingame, California, U.S.A.

1

Integrating Traditional and Complementary Medicine into National Health Care*

Learning from the International Experience

Gerard Bodeker
University of Oxford Medical School
Oxford, England

I. INTRODUCTION

As the global public's use of traditional and complementary medicine increases, governments are being challenged to develop sound policies, regulations, and trade standards (Bodeker, 2001). Public access to their health care system of choice and public safety are both important dimensions of the policy challenge.

---

*This paper draws on work reported in two previous papers: "Planning for Cost-effective Traditional Health Services," WHO Kobe, Japan, for which support was received from WHO Kobe Center; and Noller et al., 2001, for which support was received in part from the Commonwealth Foundation.

In this chapter, an attempt is made to survey salient issues relevant to policy, as so many countries are now grappling with the policy dimensions of the ever-increasing demand from the public.

II. TRADITIONAL ORIGINS

In most developing countries, traditional health systems are grounded in long-standing cultural and spiritual values and it is important that policy reflect and support this rather than attempt to replace tradition with science alone.

Traditional health knowledge extends to an appreciation of both the material and nonmaterial properties of plants, animals, and minerals. Its classificatory systems range in scope from the cosmological to the particular in addressing the physiological makeup of individuals and the specific categories of materia medica—the materials used for therapeutic purposes in traditional health systems—needed to enhance health and well-being. Mental, social, spiritual, physical, and ecological factors are all taken into account.

A fundamental concept found in many systems is that of balance—the balance between mind and body, between different dimensions of individual bodily functioning and need, between individual and community, individual/community and environment, and individual and the universe. The breaking of this interconnectedness of life is a fundamental source of *dis-ease*, which can progress to stages of illness and epidemic. Treatments, therefore, are designed not only to address the locus of the disease but also to restore a state of systemic balance to the individual and his or her inner and outer environment (Bodeker, 2000).

The cosmologies of traditional health systems ascribe life, spiritual value, and interconnectedness among all life forms to the aspects of the natural world used in the process of promoting human health and well-being.

In establishing policy it is important that these fundamental theoretical underpinnings of traditional health systems be respected and perpetuated to ensure their continuity in an intact form.

III. WHO POLICY

The May 2002, WHO Traditional Medicines Strategy 2002–2005 focuses on four areas identified as requiring action if the potential of traditional and complementary medicine (T/CAM) to play a role in public health is to be maximized. These areas are: policy; safety, efficacy, and quality; access; and rational use. Within these areas, WHO 2002–2005 identifies respective challenges for action.

A. National Policy and Regulation

Lack of official recognition of T/CAM and T/CAM providers
Lack of regulatory and legal mechanisms
T/CAM not integrated into national health care systems
Equitable distribution of benefits in indigenous knowledge and products
Inadequate allocation of resources for T/CAM development and capacity building

B. Safety, Efficacy, and Quality

Inadequate evidence-base for T/CAM therapies and products
Lack of international and national standards for ensuring safety, efficacy, and quality control
Lack of adequate regulation of herbal medicines
Lack of registration of T/CAM providers
Inadequate support of research
Lack of research methodology

C. Access

Lack of data measuring access levels and affordability
Lack of official recognition of role of T/CAM providers
Need to identify safe and effective practices
Lack of cooperation between T/CAM providers and allopathic practitioners
Unsustainable use of medicinal plant resources

D. Rational Use

Lack of training for T/CAM providers
Lack of training for allopathic practitioners on T/CAM
Lack of communication between T/CAM and allopathic practitioners and between allopathic practitioners and consumers
Lack of information for the public on rational use of T/CAM

These are tasks that have been repeatedly identified by numerous groups in recent years; it would be a significant advancement if the WHO is now able to stimulate action by bringing attention, and more important, funding, to address these lacunae (WHO, 2002).

IV. A POLICY FRAMEWORK

With respect to policy action, country experience can be organized into eight broad areas of principle: (1) Equity. (2) Ethics. (3) Governance. (4) Financing. (5) Knowledge production. (6) Knowledge management and utilization. (7) Capacity development. (8) Research environment.

This framework draws on that developed by the Council on Health Research for Development (COHRED) and it served for the policy recommendations on traditional medicine made at the COHRED conference on health research priorities for the coming decade, held in Bangkok in October 2000 (Bodeker et al., 2001).

A. Equity

Research into patterns of use of modern and traditional medicine has found that the general public throughout the world use both systems according to sets of priorities that may reflect the availability of each system, its affordability, their belief in its efficacy at the symptomatic as well as etiological levels, and the cultural familiarity of the various approaches.

Research in India has found that medical pluralism was flourishing as people switched from one medical system to another depending on affordability and time (Bandyopadhyay and MacPherson, 1998). Rural women in Gujarat have been found more likely to use services that were closer to home, other things being equal. The "travel" variable (including time and travel costs) is a more important factor determining use of modern and traditional services among women in the study area than the actual direct costs of the service. In India, it has been found that the influence of family structure is significant. The presence of the mother-in-law is associated with a greater use of traditional healers (Vissandjee et al., 1997).

Inadequacies in and scarcity of modern medical services can contribute to the use of traditional health services. Less than half (44%) of Chinese immigrants studied in the United States had used Western health services in the United States within the previous 12 months; 20% reported that they had never used them. Chinese physicians stated that many Chinese patients are not satisfied with American doctors because of the inflexibility of appointments, short visit, long waiting time, distrust, and miscommunication (Ma, 1999).

With respect to the use of traditional medicine by indigenous groups, of Native American patients attending an urban Indian Health Service clinic in Wisconsin, 38% of patients see a healer, and of those who do not, 86% would consider seeing one in the future. Most patients report seeing a healer for spiritual reasons, reinforcing the point made at the beginning of this paper that traditional health systems are grounded in cultural and spiritual values that must be preserved if equity and access to high-quality traditional services is to be ensured.

Clearly, in planning the development of traditional health services, access of those who most rely on traditional medicine for their daily health needs must be ensured—namely, rural people, women-headed households, and indigenous and other ethnic communities.

India has succeeded in attracting World Bank funds to the development of traditional medical services in rural areas in a manner that will ensure that poorer sectors of society are equitably served.

Owing to the high cost and unavailability of modern medical services in rural areas of India, the Indian government has undertaken to add 10 medicines from the Ayurvedic and Unani systems into its national family welfare program. A pilot project is currently being implemented in seven Indian states for Ayurveda while Unani medicines are being introduced in four cities. The reproductive and child health project is cofunded by the World Bank and the Indian government. The medicines, which are all traditional herbal formulations, will be for anemia, edema during pregnancy, postpartum problems such as pain, uterine, and abdominal complications, lactation-related problems, nutritional deficiencies, and childhood diarrhea. Also included are massage oils for babies and mothers that are already used routinely in Indian households. Concurrent evaluation is being done to oversee acceptance levels and to ensure quality in drug administration and storage and to monitor the sustainability of the program.

Political factors are again associated with the advancement of indigenous medicine in India. After decades of underfunding, the current protradition BJP Government doubled the budget for ISM in the previous financial year (*Lancet*, April 8, 2000).

B. Ethics

1. Clinical Research

A basic starting point in clinical research into traditional and complementary medicines and therapies is that the Helsinki Declaration, which governs the use of human subjects in research, is the definitive international agreement against which clinical research standards are set. Informed consent is a key element of these standards.

While humans subjects issues remain constant, certain ethical issues also vary from the clinical evaluation of conventional drugs. For example, the ethics of providing a plant with known safety but unknown clinical effects are different in a prevention study as opposed to a treatment study. WHO guidelines for the evaluation of herbal medicines allow that in the case of traditional medicines with an established history of use, it is ethical to proceed from basic animal toxicity studies directly to Phase 3 clinical trials.

Other ethical issues include the need to protect intellectual property (IP) rights, obtaining informed consent from the community, and devising ways to share benefits and return findings to the community (Bodeker, 2003).

2. Intellectual Property

Exploitation of traditional medical knowledge for drug development without the consent of customary knowledge holders is not acceptable under international law, as set out in the International Convention on Biological Diversity (CBD). Benefit-sharing agreements should be negotiated in advance of R&D being commenced. Clinical trials on herbal medicines should be conducted in full accord with the Helsinki Agreement.

3. The Convention on Biological Diversity

The CBD is the only major international convention that assigns ownership of biodiversity to indigenous communities and individuals and asserts their right to protect this knowledge.

Article 8 (j). State Parties are required to "respect, preserve and maintain knowledge, innovations and practices of indigenous and local communities embodying traditional lifestyles relevant for the conservation and sustainable use of biological diversity and promote the wider application with the approval and involvement of the holders of such knowledge, innovations and practices and encourage the equitable sharing of the benefits arising from the utilisation of such knowledge, innovations and practices."

Article 18.4. Contracting Parties should "encourage and develop models of cooperation for the development and use of technologies, including traditional and indigenous technologies."

The CBD competes for influence with the far more powerful Trade Related Aspects of Intellectual Property Systems (TRIPS) of the World Trade Order.

TRIPS, the key international agreement promoting the harmonization of national IPR regimes, covers four types of intellectual property rights:

1. Patents
2. Geographical indications
3. Undisclosed information (trade secrets)
4. Trademarks

Despite the CBD's emphasis that any product that has been in customary use is de facto a holder of a patent for use, TRIPS makes no reference to the protection of traditional knowledge. Nor does TRIPS acknowledge or distinguish between indigenous, community-based knowledge and that of industry.

TRIPS instead makes provision "for the protection of plant varieties either by patents or by an effective sui generis system or by any combination thereof" (Art. 27(3)(b)). This, of course, applies to medicinal plants and products based on these.

4. Social and Economic Costs of Changes in IP Legislation

By requiring patents to be applied to pharmaceuticals, it is argued by many commentators that TRIPS will have the effect of pricing common drugs out of the reach of most people in poor countries. If herbal medicines are patented—either domestically or internationally—the medicines used as the first and last resort for health care by the poor will also become unaffordable. Some examples illustrate the point.

- There was a 200% increase in cost of medicines after the 1979 introduction of pharmaceutical product patents in Italy.
- Welfare loss to Argentina, Brazil, India, Mexico, Korea, and Taiwan would amount to a minimum of US$3.5 billion and a maximum of US$10.8 billion. Income gains by foreign patent owners would be between US$2.1 billion and US$14.4 billion (World Bank).
- "National health disaster" anticipated by the Indian Drug Manufacturers' Association from implementation of TRIPs in India.
  Only 30% of Indian population can afford modern medicines.
  Comparisons of prices of drugs between India and countries where patent protection exists show that drugs are up to 41 times costlier in countries with patent protection.
- Drug prices in Malaysia, where patent protection exists, are between 20% and 760% higher than in India. Profit-maximizing behavior is based on "what the market can bear" rather than on ensuring affordability of drugs to those most in need.

5. Future

1. Debate over patenting will hinge greatly on what constitutes prior informed consent. A central issues is how to determine who represents a community, what represents full consent.
2. In the case of dispute over state vs. community ownership of indigenous knowledge, there is a question as to whether states should receive royalties from knowledge that originates from communities within those states. Or whether royalties should go direct to the traditional knowledge holders.

3. Disputes over patents on herbal products—these may have an impact on local herbal use and developing country exports of herbals. The context for these kinds of disputes is the burgeoning market. The World Conservation Union estimated in 1997 that the annual global market for herbal products was in the vicinity of US$60 billion. The World Bank estimates that by 2050, the market will be valued at US$5 trillion.
4. More examples similar to the case of South African AIDS drugs—with herbals. "Patent rights vs. patients' rights."
5. Restrictions on collaborative research (e.g., India's Biodiversity Research Approval Committee now requires central government approval for all collaborative research will international partners).
6. Developing country alliances (e.g., ASEAN) working to combat prejudicial aspects of TRIPS.

C. Governance

Self-regulation by traditional health practitioners is central to the establishment and maintenance of standards of best practice. Regulation should be designed to preserve and strengthen traditional knowledge systems and practice rather than to constrict their expression and availability.

An important example is the case of New Zealand, which has allowed the registration of more than 600 Maori traditional healers who provide services within the wider health system. The government reimburses their services under health insurance schemes.

In the United Kingdom, osteopaths and chiropractors have been registered as official health professions through an Act of Parliament and the basis for maintenance of professional standards is that of self-regulation. The same principle is being applied to medical herbalists and acupuncturists, both of which professions are on track for registration in Britain.

Asia has seen the most progress in incorporating its traditional health systems into national health policy. Most of this development began 30–40 years ago and has accelerated in the past 15 or more years. In some Asian countries, e.g., China, the development has been a matter of official policy. In others, e.g., India and South Korea, change has come about as a result of a process of politicization of the traditional medicine agenda.

In China, the process of integrating traditional Chinese medicine (TCM) into the national health care system began in the late 1950s and was, in significant part, in response to national planning requirements to provide comprehensive health care services. Prior to this, TCM had been viewed of part of an imperial legacy to be replaced by a secular health care system.

The process of integration was guided by health officials trained in modern medicine, and harmonization with modern medicine was the goal of integration from the outset. This was accomplished by a science-based approach to TCM education and an emphasis on research into TCM, both supported by a substantial organizational infrastructure. Integration and development of TCM was managed via a process of centralized national planning.

More than 40 years on, the State Administration of Traditional Chinese Medicine in China now comprises eight functional departments and investment in the sector has more than quadrupled over a 15-year period (State Administration of Traditional Chinese Medicine, 1997).

However, elsewhere in the region, under Taiwan's current health care system, Chinese medicine is reported to have a subordinate role to Western medicine (Chi, 1994). This is apparent in three ways: (1) limited participation of Chinese medicine practitioners in any public health policy-making and programs; (2) small proportion of government medical resources allocated to the training, research, and practice of Chinese medicine; and (3) loose licensure system for Chinese physicians.

One commentator has outlined six recommendations for effective integration that cover many of the major salient issues:

1. Promote communication and mutual understanding among different medical systems that exist in a society.
2. Evaluate traditional medicine in its totality.
3. Integration at the theoretical level and the practical level.
4. Equitable distribution of resources between traditional and modern Western medicine.
5. An integrated training and educational program for both traditional and modern Western medicine.
6. A national drug policy that includes traditional drugs (Chi, 1994).

D. Financing

A fundamental working principle of sectoral development here is that dedicated government funding is needed to ensure that the traditional and complementary health sector develops as needed.

In the industrialized countries, where almost half of the population regularly uses complementary medicine, insurance coverage for this is still relatively new. Americans and Australians typically pay out of pocket for CM services. Americans spend more out of pocket on CM than on all U.S. hospitalizations (Eisenberg, 1998; Astin, 1998). Australians spend more on CM than on all prescription drugs (MacLennan et al., 1996). Major American medical insurers now routinely cover complementary medical services—a trend that is emerging in Britain as well.

The effect of user fees on health care utilization and health outcomes has been a subject of considerable debate in the 1990s. Much of this debate has centered on the ability and willingness of households to pay larger out-of-pocket payments for health care. Research indicates that the price elasticity among the poor is substantial, which suggests that user fee schemes would have a regressive distributional impact (Gertler and van der Gaag, 1990, cited in Hotchkiss et al., 1998).

Households may persist in paying for care, but to mobilize resources they may sacrifice other basic needs such as food and education, with serious consequences for the household and individuals within it. The opportunity costs of payment make the payment "unaffordable" because other basic needs are sacrificed.

E. Potential Conflicts Arising from Allocation of Resources to Traditional Health Care Services

Resentment can arise from underfunded sections of the modern medical sector when resources are allocated to the development of traditional medicine. A traditional birth attendant (TBA) training program in Nigeria attracted resentment from underfunded rural midwives as resources were given to birth attendants when maternity centers lacked equipment (Matthews et al., 1995).

Another potential conflict is that if traditional health care services are made available under medical insurance schemes, those who can afford to pay for insurance will be the greatest beneficiaries of traditional medicine. The poor may be relegated to purchasing unregulated drugs from unlicensed street vendors, as already happens in so many poor countries. This would stand in contrast to the customary role of traditional medicine serving as the first and last resort for available health care for the poor.

A further risk is that primary health care services in traditional medicine may remain marginal and underfunded owing to the tendency of national health budgets to favor tertiary care. In Côte d'Ivoire, the rich receive more assistance than the poor, because the poorest patients rarely use anything but primary care, whereas the Government provides generous subsidies for the tertiary level, which in practice serves the richest patients (Demery et al., 1995, cited in Brunet-Jailly, 1998). Average per capita spending on consultations differs by a ratio of 1:300 between the first and tenth deciles. The spread is extreme (1:3000) in the case of expenditures on hospitalization. It has been argued that there is injustice in the high allocation of resources to tertiary care, when household expenditures on traditional medicine and modern medicine indicate the demand and need at the primary-care level.

In Sri Lanka, Aluwihare (1997) has examined sets of figures on such indicators as infant mortality and women in the labor force. His finding is that national aggregate data do not help in the appropriate targeting of resources. Rather, the best way would be to target the parts of the country where the figures are the least satisfactory, as a dollar there would have produced a better effect than 10 dollars in an area that had better parameters. The use of data that are disaggregated by place and time is a more effective way of identifying "weak" points where specific action is needed. This would require that traditional medicine utilization studies be incorporated into national health service research as well as studies on the availability, quality, and cost of traditional health services on a region-by-region basis.

Health insurance coverage can lead to a substantial increase in the use of traditional medical services. In a Korean immigrant population in Los Angeles, 24% of the uninsured used traditional healers, compared with 59% of persons with Medicaid only and 71% of those with other types of insurance including Medicare and Medigap coverage.

In China, although traditional health services are covered by health insurance, only about 12% of the population has comprehensive medical insurance that covers the cost of hospitalisation and the proportion of uninsured people may be as high as 50% (Xhu, 1992, cited in Phillips et al., 1994; World Bank, 1997, cited in Lee, 1999). In hospital settings, insured patients are more likely to receive TCM (Phillips et al., 1997). This is due to the fact that one of the primary sources of a hospital ward's profit, under the market model of health care provision that is in place, is the 15–25% markup for prescribed medications, so the changed incentive system has become associated with increased polypharmacy (World Bank, 1992, cited in Phillips et al., 1997).

Under the market system, many TCM hospitals in China operate at a deficit, as better-equipped Western hospitals attract more patients. As TCM is largely an outpatient, low-technology specialty, most of the income of traditional hospitals comes from the sale of drugs. Even with the 25% markup allowed, it is hard to cover operational costs. Although government subsidies currently ensure survival, there is no surplus for improving services and further market reforms may threaten this subsidy system (Hesketh and Zhu, 1997).

The experience in Taiwan is that insurance coverage for traditional medicine would more than double the use of TCM. Whereas 35.4% of Taiwanese reported using TCM regularly, 86% of the public would support the coverage of Chinese medicine by the new National Health Insurance and 79% would use Chinese medicine if it does (Chi, 1994).

High profitability of traditional medicine can lead to its custodians resisting moves to provide insurance coverage for their services and products. In Korea, where the profit margin of herbal medicines is variously estimated to be 100–500% compared to their basic cost (Cho, 2000), the population utilize herbal medicines on a large scale (Han, 1997, cited in Cho, 2000). The amount of reimbursement for herbal medicine under the National Medical Insurance (NMI) scheme was approximately 50 billion Korean won in 1993. This was estimated to be only a small portion of total expenditure on herbal medicines (Moon et al., 1997, cited in Cho, 2000). The high returns on herbal medicine boosted the socioeconomic status of traditional medicine doctors to the extent that about two-thirds (64%) of them did not want herbal remedies to be included in the NMI scheme at all (Lee, 1993a, cited in Cho, 2000).

In New Zealand, which has a long tradition of universal insurance for medical and hospital services, a number of Maori organizations, as noted earlier, signed contracts with regional health authorities to provide primary health care, resulting in an increased number of Maori-controlled services throughout the country. New Zealand has allowed the registration of more than 600 Maori traditional healers and the government reimburses their services under health insurance schemes. It has been argued that the New Zealand experience showcases the importance of a funder-purchaser-provider separation and shows that this can be beneficial to indigenous health services (Scrimgeour, 1996).

In Australia, Easthope et al. (1998) showed that since the introduction of a Medicare rebate for acupuncture in 1984, use of acupuncture by medical practitioners has increased greatly. By analyzing Health Insurance Commission data on claims by all nonspecialist medical practitioners for Medicare Benefits Schedule items for an attendance where acupuncture was performed by a medical practitioner, they showed that 15.1% (about one in seven) of Australian GPs claimed for acupuncture in 1996. Claims rose from 655,000 in the financial year 1984–1985 to 960,000 in 1996–97, and Medicare reimbursements to doctors for acupuncture rose during this period from $7.7 million to $17.7 million. Acupuncture was more likely to be performed by male practitioners, by those aged 35–54 years, and by practitioners with an overseas primary medical qualification. A survey of general practices in Hobart, Tasmania, showed that although only 15% of the GPs provided acupuncture, it was available in 31% of practices.

Evaluating the health insurance records of TRM/CAM users can be an effective way of estimating cost-savings of using traditional or complementary health care for certain sectors of society. A Canadian study provides an example.

A retrospective study of Quebec health insurance enrollees compared a group of transcendental meditation (TM) practitioners with nonmeditating controls (Herron and Hillis, 2000). Earlier research had highlighted positive individual and group health effects of this practice, which derives from India's Vedic tradition. This study aimed to determine whether these health benefits translated into savings to the government in terms of possible reductions in payments to physicians for the meditating group.

The study involved a total of 2836 health insurance enrollees from Quebec. Of these, 1418 were volunteers who had been practicing the TM technique for an average of 6 years, and 1418 were controls of the same age, sex, and region who were randomly selected. Using data provided by Régie de l'Assurance-Maladie du Quebec (RAMQ), Herron and associates first established a baseline by going back 14 years and gathering information on the total amount of money paid to physicians for this group. Adjustments for inflation were made using the medical cost component of the Canadian government's Consumer Price Index (CPI). The scientists were able to determine a typical subject's rate of change in expenditure over the period using robust statistics.

Researchers found that before starting meditation, the yearly rate of increase in payments between the TM group and the control group was not significant. However, after learning meditation, the TM group's mean payments declined 1–2% each year, while the control group's mean payments increased up to 12% annually over 6 years. Thus, there was a mean annual difference between the two groups of about 13%. The research team estimated that this could translate into savings of as much as $300 million per year for the province's health insurance company, the Régie de l'Assurance-Maladie du Quebec.

An example of comparative research of a traditionally used herbal medicine and the main equivalent conventional medicine has cost-benefit implications that are important. The study, on mild to moderate depression, compared St. John's wort (*Hypericum perforatum*), with the recommended dose (150 mg) of imipramine, one of the most commonly used tricyclic antidepressants. Hippocrates, Pliny, and Galen had all described the use of *Hypericum* for the treatment of mental disorders. A randomized controlled clinical trial (RCT) was conducted involving 324 outpatients with mild to moderate depression. The study found that *Hypericum* extract is therapeutically equivalent to imipramine in treating mild to moderate depression, but that patients tolerated *Hypericum* better (Woelk, 2000). Two years of treatment with Prozac (20 mg/day) will cost US$1250 in China, about the annual income of an urban worker (Lee, 1999). A TCM equivalent of *Hypericum* would result in substantial cost savings and, if similar to *Hyper-*

icum, may be better tolerated by patients. Cost savings could be calculated on an annual, national basis, as could economic and social costs arising from reductions in side effects. Cost-benefit analysis of this type would assist countries in making informed choices about the selection of treatments to be incorporated in integrated health care services.

1. Policy Implications

1. Cost of modern medical services can be a factor in people choosing traditional medicine. Programs to develop and formalise traditional health services should not overlook this point. The risk in doing so is of depriving the poor of services that have historically been their first and last resort for health care.
2. Policy should aim to keep any user fees affordable—including those of THPs in the community.
3. Significant investment is a prerequisite for development of effective traditional health care services. Underinvestment risks perpetuating poor standards of practice and products and also contributes to maintaining old stereotypes of inferior services and knowledge in traditional medicine.

F. Knowledge Production

Comparative research should be promoted, where modern and traditional approaches to managing the same conditions are compared in terms of clinical outcomes and cost. Clinical research should follow national and international health priorities—e.g., cancer, cardiovascular disease, diabetes, TB, malaria, HIV/AIDS, etc.—and mainstream research funds should encourage a component of research into traditional means for treating specific conditions.

To ensure a rational basis for the use of plant-based medicines, priority is needed for infrastructure development in traditional medicine. This would include:

Research oriented to the safe and effective production of herbal medicines as a central feature of public health programs in nonindustrialized as well as industrialized countries

Education and training for both traditional and orthodox medical practitioners

Research policy that promotes observational and clinical studies

To justify necessary national, bilateral, and multilateral investment, a new generation of micro- and macroeconomic analyses of the traditional medicine sector is needed.

Section 4.8, "Research Environment," addresses research policy in detail.

G. Knowledge Management and Utilization

To ensure sound standards of practice based on recognized levels of training and the use of therapies that are safe and effective, information is needed on best practice across a wide range of professional and industrial issues. A coordinated development strategy with multiple national and international partners will be required to develop such an information resource to inform and support national policy development in natural health care.

Aware that other countries are also grappling with similar issues, government officials are searching for policy-related information on natural health care from the international community. To date there is no central resource on policy, trade, training, safety, evidence-based treatment modalities, sustainable use of medicinal plant biodiversity, intellectual property rights, and models of benefit sharing with customary knowledge holders. Such a resource is clearly needed.

There are many challenges. Material currently accessible online is limited in scope. Much of it consists of commercial sites containing information related to specific products being marketed. Only a small number of databases (e.g., MEDLINE, AMED, etc.) allow free access to information published in a limited number of scientific journals. Most other relevant scientific databases are accessible only on a fee-paying basis. Much of the material on policy and on trade in traditional and complementary medicine does not exist in digital form or is currently not accessible online. Each database is compiled in its own unique format and style. Data structure, indexing methods and terminology used for data retrieval, is also widely different as each database is compiled to suit specific user groups. Much of the material on Asian traditional medicine is not available in English. Identifying common strands between these data sources and devising data retrieval methodology applicable to all will be the fundamental requirement of any integrative exercise. There is also the question of financial arrangements required to ensure access and continuous input of new material from these sources.

A coordinated development strategy with multiple national and international partners will be required to develop such an information resource to inform and support national policy development in natural health care. Such a resource was called for by Commonwealth Health Ministers representing the 54 countries of the Commonwealth when, in Barbados at their 12th Commonwealth Health Ministers Meeting (Nelson, 1998) they established the Commonwealth Working Group (CWG) on Traditional and Complementary Health Systems and called for a mechanism for sharing policy experience among Commonwealth countries (Bodeker, 1999).

1. British Library

In 1985, the British Library, owing to lack of coverage on Medline, commenced work on compiling the Allied and Alternative Medicine database (AMED), which was later changed to the Allied and Complementary Medicine Database. AMED was started to assist complementary medicine practitioners and paramedical staff locate articles that were relevant to their practice. At the time that the British Library started AMED in 1985, Medline was particularly poor in the areas of complementary medicine and allied health care. AMED now covers the areas of:

Complementary medicine
Physiotherapy
Occupational therapy
Rehabilitation medicine
Podiatry
Palliative care

Since 1985 AMED has expanded its coverage and now indexes around 500 journals; the database contains nearly 120,000 references. At the same time that AMED was started, the British Library constructed a thesaurus for the database based on the Medical Subject Headings (MeSH) as used by the Medline database. The database is now available as print, through online hosts, and on CD-ROM.

While AMED covers some of the traditional medical systems, there is great need for a database that will provide accurate, relevant, and timely quality information in contrast to material of questionable quality and accuracy that is currently freely available on the Internet.

The Columbia University Project. In 1997, The Rosenthal Center for Complementary and Alternative Medicine, Columbia University, New York, brought together seven database producers, which included AMED and NAPRALERT, as partners in the production of a comprehensive web resource on complementary and alternative medicine. The purpose of this partnership was to allow cross-searching of databases in addition to some full text resources including directory information provided by the partners.

A cross-sectoral thesaurus, based on AMED, was proposed and currently funding is being sought to undertake this project. All the partners are still signed up to the project and will hope to contribute something to the success of this venture.

A freely available web-based resource on complementary and traditional medicine would make standard safety and efficacy information easily accessible and allow policy makers, consumers, and companies access to accurate evidence-based information. It would also provide rapid global updating of information on complementary and traditional medicine.

H. Capacity Development

Capacity of the traditional sector must be strengthened in the following areas: safety, efficacy, standardization, current utilization, cost-effectiveness, customer satisfaction, priority diseases (TB, malaria, AIDS, etc.), and prevention of disease.

1. Safety

A primary concern regarding traditional and complementary therapies is "Are they safe?" Recent studies in England have found that there has been adulteration with steroids of some traditional Chinese dermatological preparations. In an analysis of Chinese herbal creams prescribed for dermatological conditions, Keane et al. (1999) found that 8 of 11 creams analyzed contained steroids. Clearly, policy gaps need to be plugged and effective regulation of herbal medicines is needed, while ensuring that regulation is not simply a means of limiting public access to these preparations. Limiting access through professional controls and regulatory means can be seen as constituting monopolistic trade practice.

Safety must be the starting point for national drug development strategies for herbal medicines. While most of the published research on herbal medicine is pharmacological, WHO's *1993 Guidelines on the Evaluation of Herbal Medicines* consider that clinical evaluation is ethical where drugs have long been in traditional use. Roy Chaudhury (1992) has offered a model for the clinical evaluation of herbal medicines:

1. Toxicity testing of the plant in two species of animal for acute and subacute toxicity.
2. A modified, shorter toxicity testing if the plant has already been used in humans or is in such use now.
3. Administration of the total extract or combination of plants, if used, in exactly the same way as it is prepared and used by the population.

The differences between this approach and that of conventional drug evaluation methodology are that:

Efficacy testing is carried out on humans rather than on animals; human studies are undertaken subsequent to modified, shortened toxicology studies having shown that the substance is not toxic in animals.

The duration of the toxicity studies is reduced to 6 weeks for plants that are already in common use.
The plant or mixture of plants is administered to subjects in the same manner in which it is used in traditional medicine (Roy Chaudhury, 1992).

Research should consider best evidence for safety, including evidence for adverse effects from treatments (including magnitude, percent of people so affected, etc.), as well as from inappropriate applications of traditional therapies. Postmarket surveillance studies can provide information on adverse effects of botanical herbal preparations. Pharmacognostic and pharmacological research can provide information on the quality, efficacy, safety, or toxicity of botanical/herbal medicinal preparations.

More broadly, a basic question in addressing safety in herbal medicines is "Safe with respect to what?" Research has found that in the United States, 51% of FDA-approved drugs have serious adverse effects not detected prior to their approval. One and one-half million people are sufficiently injured by prescription drugs annually that they require hospitalization (Moore et al., 1998). Once in hospital, the problem may be compounded. The incidence of serious and fatal adverse drug reactions (ADRs) in U.S. hospitals is now ranked as between the fourth and the sixth leading cause of death in the United States, following after heart disease, cancer, pulmonary disease, and accidents (Lazarou et al., 1998).

Clearly, the safety of and risks associated with medical interventions are issues across all categories of health care.

In developing health systems for traditional medicine, safety and quality control of herbal medicines go hand in hand. A case in point is the development of new standards of safety and quality for herbal medicines produced in India. New regulations were introduced in India in July 2000 to improve the standard and quality of Indian herbal medicines. Regulations will establish standard manufacturing practices and quality control.

The new regulations outline requirements for infrastructure, manpower, quality control, and raw material authenticity and absence of contamination. Of the 9000 licensed manufacturers of traditional medicines, those who qualify can immediately seek GMP certification. The remainder have 2 years to come into compliance with the regulations and to obtain certification.

The government also set up 10 new drug-testing laboratories in 2003 for ISM and upgraded existing ones to provide high-quality evidence to licensing authorities of the safety and quality of herbal medicines. This replaces an ad hoc system of testing that was considered by the Department of ISM to be unreliable.

Randomized controlled clinical trials of selected ISM prescriptions have been initiated to document their safety and efficacy and to provide the basis for their international licensure as medicines rather than simply as food supplement (Sanjay Kumar, Reuters, July 13, 2000).

The Australian model of risk management of herbal medicines constitutes an important model of legislation and policy in this field.

The Office of Complementary Medicines of the Australian Therapeutic Goods Authority has responsibility for the regulation of drugs and other medicinal substances. The Office does not, however, regulate complementary health professionals as this is done by the various state governments of Australia.

Under the the Therapeutic Goods Act of 1989 the Therapeutic Goods Authority (TGA) established a special office for the regulation of complementary medicines, covering:

Herbal medicines
Vitamins
Minerals
Nutritional supplements
Homeopathic medicines
Aromatherapy oils

Whereas most countries regulate complementary medicines as foods, in Australia complementary medicines are regulated as medicines. The approach of the TGA in managing risks covers:

Licensing of manufactures
Premarket assessment of products
Postmarket regulatory activity.

The TGA position is that managing risk requires a balance between the premarket evaluation and postmarket vigilance. If the premarket evaluation is too little, postmarket vigilance is required. Conversely, extensive premarket evaluation means less risk to manage and less postmarket vigilance.

Accordingly, the TGA follows two paths: licensing of manufactures and premarket assessment of products.

In the case of registered products the following key steps are followed:

Quality based on good manufacturing practice
Safety through a product-by-product evaluation
Efficacy via a product-by-product evaluation

The TGA requires the following for listed medicines of lower risk:

Quality based on good manufacturing practice
Safety through a substance-by-substance evaluation
Efficacy via sponsors holding evidence to support claims and indications

Postmarket regulatory activity covers the following steps:

Postmarket review of products
Monitoring and surveillance in the marketplace
Problem reports and recalls
Laboratory testing
Adverse reaction reporting

The risk assessment framework for complementary medicines covers the following steps (F. Cumming, in Noller et al., 2001):

Characterization of substance
History and patterns of previous human use
What, if any, adverse reactions have arisen from use
Biological activity
Toxicology
Clinical trials
Conclusions and recommendations.

2. Emerging European Regulation on the Safety of Herbal Medicines

The European Community definition of a medicinal product is:

"Any substance or combination of substances presented for treating or preventing disease in human beings or animals";
"Any substance or combination of substances which may be administered to human beings or animals with a view to making a medical diagnosis or restoring, correcting or modifying physiological function in human beings or in animals is likewise considered a medicinal product"; and
Any "medicinal product" requires a product license.

Directive 65/65 requires showing through toxicology and pharmacology tests the potential toxicity of the product and any dangerous or undesirable toxic effects under proposed conditions of use. Specifically, Directive 65/65 requires:

Single-dose toxicity
Repeat-dose toxicity
Reproductive toxicity
Teratogenicity/embryo/fetal toxicity
Mutagenicity
Carcinogenicity
Pharmacokinetics
Pharmacodynamics

Local tolerance
Clinical trials:
Adverse events
Assessment of relative safety
Postmarketing experience

For products that have been in long-established use, the following is required:

Ingredients used for 10 years in Europe.
Requirements as 65/65, but:
Can replace toxicity, pharmacology, and clinical trials by reference to published reports.
Missing evidence requires additional tests.
Must show recognized efficacy and safety in normal use.

The EC's Traditional Medicines Directive makes use of the following information:

Used in Europe for 30 years (or combination Europe and another country).
Bibliographic review of safety data.
Expert report.
Additional assessment/tests may be required.
Post-marketing surveillance required.
Monographs to be developed.
Committee to provide list of acceptable ingredients.

The EC recognizes the following sources of information:

Adverse reaction reporting schemes
Poison centers
Drug information units
Postmarketing surveillance
Clinical trials
Prescription event monitoring
Existing medical and scientific literature

In Britain, where only 20% of herbal medicines are licensed, there are efforts to ensure the safety of traditional and herbal medicines via new information centers. These include:

The Chinese Herbal Database Brings Together Existing Data For:

Translation of reports of toxicity from Chinese and other literature
Production of monographs/safety reviews

Provision of information/training to medical professionals at Guy's and St Thomas' Hospitals
To be extended to other traditions of medicine
A new project at the Medical Toxicology Unit, funded by Guy's and St Thomas' Hospital Trust
Collaboration with Chinese Medicines Unit, UWS

Prescription Event Monitoring.

Pilot study to evaluate use of PEM in monitoring adverse events associated with herbal medicines
Grant application submitted
Collaboration Drug Safety Research Unit, Southampton University, National Institute of Medical Herbalists, Medical Toxicology Unit

3. Chinese Medicinal Plant Authentication Centre, Kew

Set up because of lack of quality control of Chinese medicinal herbs used in England
Identification from authenticated voucher specimens collected in China
Drug material from plants from same collection as voucher specimens
Drug fingerprints—TLC, HPLC, LC-MS, DNA
Not looking for active compounds
Independent and confidential enquiry service for practitioners, academics, suppliers, regulatory authorities

Doctors and patients need to be aware of potential for toxicity in order to identify and make reports (D. Shaw, in Noller et al, 2001).

4. Priority Diseases

There is a prevailing prejudice that traditional and complementary medicine is useful for chronic low-level conditions, whereas mainstream medicine is useful for acute and infectious disease. The development of multidrug-resistant strains of malaria and TB has challenged such views of late and there is a new search for benefits in ancient approaches.

Malaria. The two most effective drugs used in conventional medicine to treat malaria originate from plants: quinine from bark of the Peruvian cinchona tree, and artemisinin from the Chinese antipyretic *Artemisia annua* L. Other plants are likely to contain as-yet-undiscovered antimalarial substances. While much research has focused on trying to isolate and purify these from plants, there is concern that conventional isolation and extraction methods may miss synergistic mechanisms of action found in traditional antimalarials.

Currently, modern pharmaceuticals are not available in constant supply in areas most affected by malaria, particularly sub-Saharan Africa and South and Southeast Asia. With increasing drug resistance and the high cost of drugs, the use of herbal antimalarials in these regions is popular. Despite growing policy interest in traditional medicine, almost no research has been conducted on the clinical effectiveness of herbal remedies as they are used in real life.

At a December 1999 meeting in the Kilimanjaro region of Tanzania, a Research Initiative on Traditional Antimalarial Methods (RITAM) was established to develop a strategy for more effective, evidence-based use of traditional medicines for malaria. RITAM is a joint undertaking of the Global Initiative for Traditional Systems of Health (GIFTS) at Oxford University and WHO's Tropical Disease Research Programme (TDR) (Bodeker and Willcox, 2000).

RITAM members have developed four specialist groups to implement a research strategy designed to make a significant contribution to malaria control programs (Willcox et al., 2001; Willcox, Bodeker and Rasaonaive, 2004):

1. Policy, advocacy, and funding
2. Preclinical studies
3. Clinical development
4. Repellance and vector control

HIV/AIDS. In Africa and in much of Asia, the high cost and scarcity of many essential drugs as well as antiretroviral drugs has led the majority of people living with HIV/AIDS to use traditional herbal treatments for a variety of HIV-related conditions including opportunistic infections (OI). Indeed, in view of widespread use, traditional medicine is in a real sense carrying the burden of clinical care for the AIDS epidemic in Africa, a trend largely overlooked by health ministries, international agencies, and donors.

At the 1998 Bangalore meeting, Medicinal Plants for Survival, Dr. Donna Kabatesi cited clinical data on Ugandan herbal treatments effective against herpes zoster and HIV-associated chronic diarrhea and weight loss. Research being conducted by Prof. Charles Wambebe, then head of Nigeria's National Institute for Pharmaceutical Research and Development, is showing preliminary evidence that a Nigerian herbal medicine has produced steep increases in CD4 levels and improvement in HIV-related illness. Controlled clinical trials are now being conducted. The Tanga AIDS Working Group is conducting research into the efficacy of Tanzanian herbal treatments for HIV-related fungal infections.

In view of these trends, a regional Task Force on Traditional Medicine and AIDS in East and Southern Africa was inaugurated in Kampala, Uganda, on April 10, 2000. The Task Force coordinates activity related to the widespread use of traditional medicine by people living with HIV/AIDS (PLWHA) in Africa and the role of traditional healers in contributing to AIDS prevention and support.

A network of researchers and institutions is building a research program that will identify, evaluate, and develop safe and effective local treatments for HIV-related illnesses. The program uses simplified but controlled clinical protocols to conduct rapid evaluations of promising treatments. It builds databases for information sharing on successes and failures of local treatments. It is grounded in an intellectual property rights framework to protect the rights of local knowledge holders, learning lessons from a few existing programs in Africa. Recognizing the global, unsustainable pressure on wild stocks of medicinal plants, sustainable horticulture will be promoted for priority species (Bodeker et al., 2000).

In India, a conference on HIV/AIDS and Indian Systems of Medicine was hosted by the Delhi Society for the Promotion of the Rational Use of Drugs (DSPRUD) in November 2000. The Commonwealth Working Group on Traditional and Complementary Health systems and GIFTS of Health were international partners in this. This meeting brought together researchers, traditional practitioners, and policy makers to identify what work is being done in this field in India and to chart a way forward. A research agenda has been developed, a network established, and a clinical research protocol published (Chaudhury, 2001; Chaudhury and Bodeker, 2003).

I. Research Environment

Research into traditional medicine is needed at both national and international levels. If this need is to be met, dedicated funding will be required to be allocated by international funders and governments.

1. Research Priorities

To ensure a rational basis for the use of plant-based medicines, priority is needed for infrastructure development in traditional medicine. This will include:

Research oriented to the safe and effective production of herbal medicines as a central feature of public health programs in nonindustrialized as well as industrialized countries

Education and training for both traditional and orthodox medical practitioners

Research policy that promotes observational and clinical studies

2. Efficacy and Beyond: Research Methodologies for Traditional and Complementary and Medicine

Consumer satisfaction is of importance in evaluating health services. Satisfaction with care is one component of well-being, which has in turn been identified by WHO as a marker of good health. Our own research at Oxford University suggests that a search for satisfaction in the treatment of chronic disease is the primary reason why people in Britain—particularly women—seek the services of complementary health care providers. Consumer satisfaction studies merit a high place in national research into complementary and traditional health care (Ong et al., 2002).

There is an international call for evidence of what constitutes best treatments. The preferred method is through a formal approach to gathering and synthesizing research data. Evidence-based medicine (EBM) has become a worldwide movement in clinical medicine. Such high standards are now being called for by established medicine in evaluating the claims of traditional complementary health practitioners. The core of EBM is the randomized controlled clinical trial (RCT), and EBM methodology is centered around determining therapeutic effects of specific treatments via meta-analyses of clusters of RCTs.

RCTs, the unit from which the meta-analyses of EBM are built, have also been challenged as being limited in both principle and procedure (Black, 1996). RCTs are seen by some as an inadequate tool for measuring infrequent adverse outcomes such as infrequent adverse effects of drugs. They are also, owing to limitations in study size, unable to evaluate interventions designed to prevent rare events, such as accident prevention schemes. And they are unable to adequately evaluate the long-term consequences of therapies—e.g., oral contraceptives, HRT to prevent femoral fractures, and the loosening of artificial hip joints for which a 10–15-year follow-up is needed.

To address areas not readily studied using RCT methodology, and also to correctly design and interpret RCTs, observational, or cohort, studies are receiving new attention. Observational studies are based on quantitative epidemiological methods and quantitative sociological methods in which data are collected through observation. In traditional medicine, it may be assumed that a natural experiment is already taking place—practitioners are prescribing, patients are using. Observational research of existing practice allows for a first line of data to be collected without the ethical difficulties of assigning subjects to novel treatments. No one is assigned; data are gathered on what is actually happening and what the outcomes are from these interventions.

While RCTs are clearly needed, it has been suggested by Arthur Margolin of Yale University that the validity and ultimate value of RCTs of complementary therapies would be diminished if they were conducted without preliminary foundational studies. Foundational studies should investigate such issues as the reputed efficacy of the active treatment or the reputed nonefficacy of the control treatments (Margolin, 1999).

While evidence of mechanism of action is clearly not needed to promote utilization or to achieve consumer satisfaction—this is happening of its own accord—basic research into the physiological links and molecular bases of therapeutic outcomes and mechanisms of action is needed in the longer term. Where employed, basic research methodologies need to be generated to sensitively capture aspects of CM practice and theory that may appear intangible, e.g., energy (*prana, qi*) etc.

The needs of interest groups in special situations—e.g., women, children, the poor, the elderly, and those with special medical conditions—must be recognized and given priority in the development of national research agendas into CM and THC. Our own research indicates that older women with chronic conditions are the most frequent users of CM providers (Ong et al., 2002). And ethnic minority groups in Britain, for example, prefer to use their own traditional forms of medicine, such as acupuncture and traditional herbal medicine, to such Western CM systems as chiropractic and osteopathy. The specific needs, health status, and utilization patterns of special interest groups should be addressed. Also of interest are diseases for which current treatment regimens are unsatisfactory, e.g., many cancers and chronic debilitating conditions.

Prevention of disease is an area of fundamental importance in complementary health systems. Dietary and nutritional approaches to prevention provide opportunities for the study of prevention, as does the use of herbs and traditional forms of exercise (e.g., yoga) in promoting a balanced state of health. Accordingly, systematic research should be conducted into effective prevention practices.

In all therapeutic settings, Western and traditional, belief and attitude have an influence on treatment outcomes. A "placebo," or "meaning response" effect is an important component of many therapies. The extent to which therapeutic outcomes are based on expectancy is an important area of study.

WHO's Quality of Life Assessment includes spiritual dimensions in assessing an individual's quality of life. Here, "spiritual" relates to the sense of meaning regarding the self or extending beyond the self. The spiritual dimension of life and well-being is central to many traditional and complementary health systems. In Britain, 12% of those who use CM providers use the services of "spiritual healers" (Ong et al., 2002). This trend, its origin, and its outcomes are important areas of research.

A need exists for comparative evaluation of both CM and conventional medical methods for treating the same condition to identify safe and efficacious treatments that are locally available. This may also include the study of cross-cultural/cross-geographic healing practices to identify common treatments and/or to combine evidence for a specific herb or treatment regimen. Comparative studies could assess feasibility, cost-effectiveness, and environmental impact as well as specific biomedical outcomes.

Combination therapy should also be studied. For example, traditional and modern medicine are often used simultaneously in the treatment of certain chronic diseases in Asian medical systems, such as the Ayurvedic medical system of India and TCM. In addition, patients often combine modern and traditional treatments. Caution should be exercised to address cultural bias in the assumptions, methodologies, and concepts employed in comparative research.

A range of methodologies, then, can and should be employed in evaluating traditional and complementary therapies. These should be applied in a manner that is sensitive to the theoretical and clinical assumptions of the modality being evaluated to ensure that the research design adequately measures what is being studied.

A national research agenda on complementary and traditional medicine should promote research on the individual, the family and community, the wider population, and the ecosystem/environment.

Both political and scientific will are needed to support such an agenda. Legislators in industrialized countries are coming to recognize that the widespread use of complementary medicine (Eisenberg et al., 1998) is linked to votes—votes of the wealthier and more educated sectors of society. In poorer countries, the search for effective and affordable treatments for such epidemics as malaria and opportunistic infections associated with AIDS is driving renewed policy interest in traditional medicine.

In each case, substantial increases in research funding are needed. And new directions in clinical evaluation must be forged by researchers who are able to transcend limitations in research orthodoxy in the interests of providing sound information to the public on what constitutes good healthcare.

3. Policy Implications

1. Safety is the starting point in the evaluation of traditional medicines and procedures. A model for rapid toxicity testing of herbal medicines has been developed by WHO SEARO and should be examined with a view to widespread application.
2. National testing centers are needed—appropriately funded.
3. There is a concurrent need for self-regulation by THP associations, focusing on peer supervision and enforcement of standards of professional practice and conduct.

4. RCTSs are a powerful and costly tool for evaluating therapeutic efficacy. Other methods also exist for determining this. These should be used as components of a repertoire of evaluative strategies in determining what works, what works best, and what works best over time.
5. Research should be attuned to cultural concepts and issues. This is required both out of respect for the traditional medicine being studied and in view of the possibility that traditional explanatory models may provide new insights into diagnosis, disease progression, individual differences, and treatment strategies.

V. CONCLUSION

As governments grapple with the complexities of establishing regulatory and policy frameworks that will ensure safety and quality of complementary and traditional health services, it is proposed that an overarching framework for addressing policy is a beneficial means of ensuring an adequate coverage of key health policy dimensions.

In this chapter, the COHRED framework has been used, encompassing, as it does, equity, ethics, governance, financing, knowledge production, knowledge management and utilization, capacity development, and the research environment.

All of these areas require attention to ensure that public demand for access to safe and familiar complementary and traditional health services and products is met within the context of national goals for health sector development.

A vital requirement in ensuring that policies become reality is an adequate level of sectoral investment. Recent World Bank investment in the traditional health sector in China and India suggests that previous disinterest by international funders in the traditional health sector is now slowly being replaced by interest in an evidence-based approach to the development of this sector in the context of universal health care coverage and health sector reform.

This trend suggests that the way forward in policy development in this field is via a combination of concerted local consultation with all relevant interest groups, matched by an exchange of information and experience with international partners who have developed some perspectives or have experience in one or more areas of policy relevance.

To ensure that this occurs in the best interests of traditional and complementary medicine and use by a public that wants reliable access to such services, it will be essential to establish canons of best practice within the traditions, to build services around the principle of self-regulation, and for partnerships between professional bodies and regulatory agencies to be open and equitable, free of power politics associated with dominance of the sector by one or more medical interest groups.

Such a strategy has the potential to eventually lift traditional medicine and policy related to this from marginal status to a strong and internationally accepted component of comprehensive health sector development, as called for in the WHO Traditional Medicine Strategy, 2002–2005.

REFERENCES

Aluwihare APR. Ethics and practical decision-making. World Health Forum 1997; 18:120–124.

Astin JA. Why patients use alternative medicine: results of a national study. JAMA 1998; 279(19):1548–1553.

Bandyopadhyay M, MacPherson S. Women and health: tradition and culture in rural India. Brookfield, VT (USA): Ashgate Publishing, 1998.

Black N. Why we need observational studies to evaluate the effectiveness of health care. Br Med J 1996; 312:1215–1218.

Bodeker G. Traditional (i.e., indigenous) and complementary medicine in the Commonwealth: new partnerships planned with the formal health sector. J Altern Complement Med 1999; 5(1):97–101.

Bodeker G. Traditional health systems: valuing biodiversity for human health and well being. In: Posey D, et al., ed. Cultural and Spiritual Values in Biodiversity. UN Environment Programme, 2000.

Bodeker G. Planning for cost-effective traditional health services. In: Traditional Medicine: Better Science, Policy and Services for Health Development. Kobe, Japan: WHO Kobe Centre for Health Development, 2001; 337:31–70.

Bodeker G. Traditional medical knowledge, intellectual property rights and benefit sharing. Cardozo Journal of International and Comparative Law 2003; 11(2): 785–814.

Bodeker G. Lessons on integration from the developing world's experience. Br Med J 2001; 322:164–167. http://bmj.com/cgi/content/full/322/7279/164.

Bodeker G, Jenkins R, Burford G. International Conference on Health Research for Development (COHRED), Bangkok, Thailand, October 9–13, 2000: report on the Symposium on Traditional Medicine. J Alt Comp Med 2001; 7(1):101–108.

Bodeker G, Kabatesi D, Homsy J, King R. A regional task force on traditional medicine and AIDS in East and Southern Africa. Lancet 2000; 355:1284.

Bodeker G, Willcox ML. New research initiative on plant-based antimalarials. Lancet Feb 26, 2000; 355:761.

Brunet-Jailly J. AIDS and health strategy options: the case of Cote d'Ivoire. AIDS Economics Online Conference 1998. http://www.worldbank.org/aids-econ/arv/.

Chaudhury R. A clinical protocol for the study of traditional medicine and human immunodeficiency virus-related illness. J Alt Comp Med 2001; 7(5):553–566.

Chaudhury R, Bodeker G. Symposium on HIV/AIDS and Traditional Medicine of the Global Holistic Health Summit, Bangalore, Jan 14, 2003. Natl Med J India 2003; 16(2):105–106.

Chaudhury R. Herbal Medicine for Human Health. New Delhi: WHO Regional Office for SE Asia, 1992.

Chi C. Integrating traditional medicine into modern health care systems: examining the role of Chinese medicine in Taiwan. Soc Sci Med 1994; 39(3):307–321.

Cho HJ. Traditional medicine, professional monopoly and structural interests: a Korean case. Soc Sci Med 2000; 50(1):123–135.

Easthope G, Beilby JJ, Gill GF, Tranter BK. Acupuncture in Australian general practice: practitioner characteristics. Med J Aus 1998; 169:197–200.

Eisenberg DM, Davis RB, Ettner SL, Appel S, Wilkey S, Van Rompay M, Kessler RC. Trends in alternative medicine use in the United States, 1990–1997: results of a follow-up national survey. JAMA 1998; 280(18):1569–1575.

Hesketh T, Zhu WX. Health in China. Traditional Chinese medicine: one country, two systems. Br Med J 1997; 315:115–117.

Hotchkiss DR, Rous JJ, Karmacharya K, Sangraula P. Household health expenditures in Nepal: implications for health care financing reform. Health Policy Plan 1998; 13(4):371–383.

Keane FM, Munn SE, du Vivier AWP, Taylor NF, Higgins EM. Analysis of Chinese herbal creams prescribed for dermatological conditions. Br Med J 1999; 318: 563–564.

Lee S. Diagnosis postponed: shenjing shuariuo and the transformation of psychiatry in post-Mao China. Culture Med Psychiatry 1999; 23(3):349–380.

Ma GX. Between two worlds: the use of traditional and Western health services by Chinese immigrants. Jo Commun Health 1999; 24(6):421–437.

MacLennan AH, Wilson DW, Taylor AW. Prevalence and cost of alternative medicine in Australia. Lancet 1996; 347:569–572.

Margolin A. Liabilities involved in conducting randomized clinical trials of CAM therapies in the absence of preliminary, foundational studies: a case in point. J Altern Complem Med 1999; 5(1):103–104.

Matthews MK, et al. Training traditional birth attendants in Nigeria—the pictorial method. World Health Forum 1995; 16:409–414.

Moore TJ, Psaty BM, Furberg CD. Time to act on drug safety. JAMA 1998; 279(19): 1571–1573.

Nelson T. Commonwealth Health Ministers and NGO's seek health for all. Lancet 1998; 352:1766.

Ong C-K, Petersen S, Bodeker G, Stewart-Brown S. Use of complementary and alternative medical services in England: a population survey. Am J Pub Health 2002; 92(10):1653–1656.

Phillips MR, Pearson V. Future opportunities and challenges for the development of psychiatric rehabilitation in China. Br J Psychiatry 1994; 165(suppl 24):128–142.

Scrimgeour D. Funding for community control of indigenous health services. Aust NZ J Public Health 1996; 20(1):17–18.

State Administration of Traditional Chinese Medicine of the People's Republic of China. Anthology of Policies, Laws and Regulations of the People's Republic of China on Traditional Chinese Medicine. Shangdong: Shangdong University, 1997.

Vissandjee B, Barlow R, Fraser DW. Utilization of health services among rural women in Gujarat India. Public Health 1997; 111(3):135–148.

WHO Traditional Medicine Strategy 2002–2005. May 2002. http://www.who.int/medicines/organization/trm/orgtrmmain.shtml.

Willcox ML, Bodeker G, Rasoanaive P. Traditional Medicinal Plants and Malaria. London, England: CRC Press, 2004.

Willcox ML, Cosentino MJ, Pink R, Bodeker G, Wayling S. Natural products for the treatment of tropical diseases. Trends Parasitol 2001; 17(2):58–60.

Woelk H. Comparison of St John's wort and imipramine for treating depression: randomised controlled trial. Br Med J Sept 2, 2000; 321:536–539.

2

Can Traditional Medicine Coexist with Modern Medicine in the Same Health Care System?

Ping Chung Leung
Chinese University of Hong Kong
Shatin, Hong Kong, China

I. WHAT IS HEALTH?

Health is what everyone needs and everyone wants. To be able to live in well-being while being bothered by ailments and illnesses from time to time is the basic requirement for any age and race.

The biological behavior of any living organism is that the physiological activities are constantly challenged with changing needs as a result of environmental changes and aging. The biological well-being of any living organism depends on a smooth balance of physiological activities. This balance is directly challenged by specific pathological processes and indirectly affected by the environment and aging. People would love to enjoy the best constant environment. However, environmental change is something that can never be avoided. People would love to enjoy an evergreen, nonaging life. Nevertheless, the evergreen expectation has never been achieved.

Health and maintenance of health have always remained an unsettled challenge to mankind (1).

Ever since cultural activities have been recorded, endless attempts have been made to improve health. There were those efforts trying to improve the ability of the individual to resist pathological changes and to stay well. There were those efforts trying to improve the environment, as people of all regions and races realize, with more and more accumulated knowledge, that their healthy well-being very much depends on a healthy environment. The environment started with living conditions in the home, then extending outside to the community. Personal hygiene and home health must have developed together, as a consideration to keeping oneself well. Then the causes of ailment and illnesses were better known and the understanding of homeostasis revealed the existence of an internal environment that stayed in harmony with the external environment in a reasonable balance. Public health concepts and practice developed only after a reasonable understanding of both the internal and external environments.

People do want good health. They are able to understand, today, that health requires a good, balanced internal environment, as well as a good harmony between the biological self and the external environment.

The author spent some time discussing this basic concept because to understand traditional medicine, it is important to grasp this concept of balance: balance of internal biological activities (forces) and balance between the individual and his/her outside environment (2).

II. MODERN HEALTH SCIENCE

Modern science has been built on an empirical principle. There must be an objective, measurable explanation to an observation. A subjective observation must be proven with objective means, otherwise the observation was not taken as of value (3). Based on this simple concept, the successes of modern science have been remarkable.

Medical science has moved along in the same pathway and in the past 60 years we have witnessed tremendous advances. Probably all systems of healing, whether developing in the East or in the West, started in the same way, i.e., a mixture between religious idol worship (close to superstition) and reflections on observations of animal behavior. Thus religious rituals were often enriched with special inserts that were installed for the maintenance of human health. Animals possessed instincts for self-healing. Our ancesteral hunters and farmers made intelligent observations on animals around them and started applying the same "healing method." Enthusiasts would move from animal to human trials, usually self-administered trials of herbs and minerals that were believed to be "probably" doing good for a certain ailment or health problem. It was not coincidental that nearly identical legendary figures appeared historically in the history of medicine of many cultures, like Greek, Egyptian, and Chinese, in the ancient days. All of them, in their enthusiasm to know more about the property of the herbs and their effects on healing, personally consumed the herbs to experience the effects (4,5). So medical experts all started as observers of simple herbal trials. None of these experts understood the mechanism of action of the herbs even though they might be having remarkable effects on treatment. These experts would not be able to understand the mechanism of action because they had no idea about the basic structure of the organs and tissues; neither did they understand their physiological function. The modern development of medicine, following the footsteps of scientists, awaited for the knowledge of structure and function, i.e., anatomy and physiology. With the great advances during the Renaissance in human anatomy and later in human physiology, scientists became capable of exploring the abnormal processes, i.e., the pathologies. Given answers to how pathological processes happened and why they happened, healers became more capable in searching for means to counteract unwanted pathological processes.

Science development carried along a new tradition of linkage and interreliance on different specialties. Technological advances in physics and chemistry were freely applied in the medical specialty, as diagnostic means and as means to improve treatment.

The past 60 years marked the most impressive development of modern medicine. Drug therapy applied the principle of antagonism against the unwanted, supplement for the insufficient, and replacement for the deficient. The understanding of complex chemical activities enabled the development of drugs of more and more refined nature with more and more specific targets. More specific targets meant less and less adverse effects. Sophisticated diagnostic tools allowed accurate diagnosis of problems and detailed images of diseased organs. Surgical procedures therefore underwent many breakthroughs: organ transplantations, microsurgery, implant replacement, and noninvasive procedures.

When medical scientists investigated at the molecular level, more possibilities were suggested. The recent completion of human genome mapping opened up an incredible field of disease treatment in the future. The new century has been labeled the century of biological advances so that people would live to over 100 years of age, and diseases would be removed from their roots of occurrence, rather than being dealt with when discovered. Palliative means of treatment would stop being the major approach. Diseases would preferably be uprooted when the responsible genes could be specifically removed (6).

Such are the promises of modern medicine. The great strides have surpassed the imagination of most, if not all, intellectuals. The assumption could be that the ability to live to over 100 years of age might mean more satisfaction with health maintenance and more human happiness. We have to look at some of the immediate results of medical advances.

Success of modern medicine is based on deductive empirical science. The cause had to be well known in depth before the specific treatment program was developed to counteract the pathology to be corrected. When the cause of pathology was unknown, partially known, or complex, it would be most difficult to work out the effective means of cure (7).

We are all aware that there are still disease conditions where the pathology is either unknown, only partially known, or extremely complex. To cite just a few: the allergic conditions, autoimmune diseases, cancers, chronic illnesses, and viral infections. In these disease conditions, modern medicine offers control and palliative treatment, but not cure (8).

One might be surprised at the obvious deficiencies of modern medicine while the advances and future promises are so brilliant. One might be further saddened by some other outcome of the successes of modern medicine. The logic of success of modern medicine is based on identification of the specific targets that will be directly dealt with. The requirement of diagnosis and treatment implies specialization and concentration of resources in narrow areas. The result of this development is: mechanical approaches, loss of holistic care, overspecialization, decline of human care, and ever-rising costs.

While more specific problems are being solved with modern scientific concepts and technology, some essential requirements for the healing art are being lost. No wonder it is not surprising to see patients and people on the recipient end of health care getting disappointed. They do not appreciate being treated like machines and their spare parts; they are hurt by the inhuman touches; they hate being referred from one specialist to another specialist (perhaps subspecialist); more uniformly, they cannot afford the cost.

The dilemma between successful modern development on the side of the health care providers and the parallel loss of trust on the recipient side is a genuine phenomenon that might not be widely recognized by the medical world. However, objective data support the observation. These data directly affect the future of health care.

The survey done by the American Medical Association on the use of alternative medicine toward the end of the twentieth century clearly indicated that American people were shifting their expectation and trust to alternative medicine because the annual medical expenditure on complementary and alternative medicine was even greater than that spent on family medicine (9,10). The most influential research institute in the United States, the National Institutes of Health, first held a consensus conference on acupuncture in which the efficacy of acupuncture as a means of pain control was endorsed and recommended; then a special section, the National Center for Complementary Alternative Medicine (NCCAM), with a reasonable budget, was established (11,12). There was political endorsement by the White House Commission, followed by the establishment of different regional CAM centers with given specific assignments such as aging problems, women's health, or arthritis.

There is sufficient evidence to indicate that the U.S. National Institutes of Health are making a serious positive exploration of the value of CAM. Indeed, the commitment of the health providers is further exemplified by the situation in medical education. More than 90% of U.S. medical schools are now providing some form of alternative medicine within their conventional curriculum (13).

III. UNDERSTANDING CHINESE HERBAL MEDICINE

While herbal utilization as means of cure in communities in Europe and the United States might involve single herbs, Chinese herbal medicine uses a combination of different herbs. Although exceptional situations do occur when only one or two herbs are used, the majority of ancient effective formulae consist of multiple herbs.

The use of multiple herbs is based on two considerations: first, to enhance efficacy and, second, to maintain safety. Herbs of similar effects are expected to augment one another, while herbs of antagonistic effects harmonize the overall action and prevent overaction of some aggressive modalities. There is yet a more sophisticated philosophy of herbal arrangement. The components of a complex formula could be classified into four categories of function, which play four different roles: role of an emperor (君) of an adviser (臣), of a minister (佐), and of an ambassador (使). The philosophy clearly demands a balanced system that includes effectiveness, efficiency, reinforcement, moderation, and safety. By this arrangement, aggressive herbs could be used when there is the need to forcibly bring about a treatment effect; overaction is being checked with other herbs that might possess different effects; under action, on the other hand is being prevented by adding, simultaneously, supplementary varieties of herbs.

Chinese herbalists are particularly aware of the poisonous adverse effects of some herbs. They caution the use of such herbs by adding other herbs known to act as antidote. They may even try balancing off the adverse effects by using another poisonous entity that may divert the adversity of the former.

The major philosophy of treatment in Chinese herbal medicine is to maintain an overall balance. The yin-yang theory is that every human being is under three different axes of balance. Balance between heat and cold, between the "surface" and "depth," between "emptiness" and "fullness." Perhaps heat and cold could be experienced and expressed by different individuals, not "surface" and "depth," or "emptiness" and "fullness." Master healers in Chinese medicine did attempt to provide a solid description of the opposing poles of the axes of harmony. However, the definitions remained subjective and obscure to modern man. When a treatment plan has to rely on an analysis of the balance, the herbal practitioner has to develop his own system of judgment, unique to his own practice. Scientific practitioners need not be absolutely critical, because relying on diagnostic science and then giving treatment is certainly a logical means of treatment. However, short of modern diagnostic tools, one needs to initiate treatment according to logical guiding principle, which for our herbalists is the yin-yang theory. Under the yin-yang theory no one is in perfect balance. The two poles of the yin-yang axis represent the two divergent ends of a spectrum. The diseased person occupies a position somewhere along the spectrum, and the position occupied keeps changing. That is why treatment is never universal. Instead, treatment varies according to the herbal expert's judgment: whether heat or cold is dominant, whether the problem is superficial or deep, empty or solid. This changing mode of treatment aimed at the individual's specific need is contrary to the principle of generalization in modern medicine. When there is lack of generalization, research that searches for repetition of results based on generalization of symptomatology is discouraged. Indeed the herbal expert is proud of his ability to treat the same disease with different methodologies or to treat different diseases with the same means.

Actually the "disease" of the herbal expert refers more to symptoms or a syndrome than a disease entity. The healer controls symptoms with different means, but not for a specific disease. There is no knowledge about the exact pathology and sequence of events in the illness. The herbal expert can therefore, deal only with symptoms.

Symptoms reflect pathological changes. Symptoms, when controlled, reflect control of pathological adversity. This may not signify the reestablishment of balance. The reestablishment of balance depends on a holistic well-being. The balance and holistic well-being depend on the undiseased, healthy systems of function helping to cover or substitute for the deficient or pathological system. Hence herbal treatment starts by controlling the symptoms, while, either simultaneously or after the control, attempting to booster up the system or organs that are not directly under the pathological forces. In modern terminology, boostering the functional well-being of the healthy organs might refer to an effective supplement of immunological ability. The latter maneuver is achieved through herbal treatment or dietary supplement, which is always considered important in Chinese medicine (14,15).

IV. CAN THE TWO SYSTEMS OF HEALTH CARE COEXIST?

Acceptance of the value of science is universal. The reliance on science and technology as essential requirements for normal daily activities is a fact of modern life. Patients have the freedom to choose an appropriate format of treatment they prefer. Their choice is subjective and personal while at the same time they are influenced by obvious cultural, social, and economic forces. We have good evidence to confirm that today's patients have an inclination toward accepting both scientific and alternative medicine. If modern scientific practitioners take this inclination as something that arises out of superstition or cultural stubbornness or assumes that the patients are just the victims of advertising, they would not be keen to try to learn something from the alternative stream, not to speak about utilizing the alternative stream (13).

This might still be the mainline behavior among modern practitioners who, since Hippocrates, have been told not to communicate with healers of a different stream (16).

Nevertheless, with the increasing demand for alternative care among patients, there coexists an increasing curiosity among the modern practitioners who realize that, given the great advances and promises of modern medicine, there are still areas of deficiencies. This small group of modern practitioners would start exploring the pragmatic side of alternative medicine, test for its efficacy, then decide on a practical policy of application in their practice.

V. HOSPITAL SERVICE

Alternative medicine could be integrated into hospital service according to the planning of the administrator and the patients' need. Thus in China, every city, irrespective of its size, has integrated medicine or Chinese medicine hospitals, which give patient care consisting of both the modern scientific modality and traditional Chinese medicine. Even in other hospitals not labeled as such, it would be very easy to call in herbalists' support whenever required. Every hospital has its own Chinese Medicine Division ready to offer help.

China is offering a genuine integrated service whenever required. Of course this is not coincidental, but it has sociopolitical background. In the Constitution of China, it is written that both Chinese medicine and modern medicine should be developed in China. Therefore, hospitals throughout China should supply both services (17).

However, the integration is not real. In the report of a fact-finding mission taken by the University Grant Council of Hong Kong, it was stated that 50–70% of the budget of so-called Chinese medicine hospitals was spent on emergency modern medicine or diagnostics. The hidden message was that clients had a greater need of modern medicine (18).

Hospital practice by itself is modern medicine. It might not be realistic to artificially label certain hospitals "Chinese medicine hospital." It is more important to be able to supply the service to individual patients on demand. Since the hospital is basically a modern establishment created according to the concept of scientific medicine, keeping a hospital purely for the need of Chinese medicine practitioners is illogical and unnecessary. A practical means to promote integrated medicine is to accept and value Chinese medicine as a specialty that will be called on to support other treatment should the need arise. This practice therefore requires a team of herbal experts in the hospital and a specialist clinic for them. The model is being tried in some hospitals in Hong Kong. Unique individual "Chinese medicine hospitals" would be unnecessary.

VI. INTEGRATED CLINIC

An ideal arrangement might not be an integrated medicine hospital, but an integrated clinic. The integrated clinic at the University of Maryland could serve as a good example. Some other integrated clinics are being explored in the United States. The orientation would best be rehabilitation-oriented. The wide demand of chronic problems and pain related to rehabilitation would find a lot of favorable subjects who are dissatisfied with conventional medications and therapies, who would benefit from other alternatives such as massage and acupuncture (19).

Once modern practitioners become more receptive to alternative medicine and once it is proven that Chinese herbal medicine is efficacious in treating certain difficult problems, integrated clinics could be started, no longer bearing only rehabilitation orientation but catered toward evidence-based clinical trials and evidence-based clinical service. Clients do not come for general care of all disease entities, but for specific problems that modern practitioners face. Such integrated clinics deal with special problems in allergy, viral infection, degenerative diseases, metabolic disorders, chronic pain, cancers, and other pathologies. Such clinics are run for both research and service. They cannot be solely research-oriented for obvious reasons of the high demand for clinical research and the cost involved. They cannot be solely service-oriented either because efficacy tests are still much desired. The compromise needs to be careful data collection and observation for all clients irrespective of whether they belong to a research protocol or not, so that positive feedback as well as adverse effects can be recorded.

The integrated clinic would serve well as an ice-breaking medium between the uncompromising modern clinical scientists and herbal practitioners while undergraduate students in both streams should also benefit through exposures in the clinics.

VII. MEDICAL EDUCATION

We already noted that 90% of U.S. medical schools are providing various courses on alternative medicine. These are not compulsory commitments. Only some students, perhaps more mature or postgraduate students, would be interested in those courses.

Recent information from Japan indicated that starting very soon, all medical students in Japan would be required to go through 150 hr of undergraduate study in a variety of Kampo medicine (which is Chinese medicine) (20). This appears a genuinely positive commitment to herbal medicine outside China, which is providing 150–400 hr of Chinese medicine study for all modern medicine undergraduates.

Curriculum arrangements with substantial components of Chinese medicine would probably produce graduates with more dynamic caliber. However, these graduates are still rigid followers of modern science.

An advocate in Hong Kong once put forward the proposal that undergraduates could finish their modern medicine course and then spend an additional 2 years on Chinese medicine. This method of training would produce genuinely integrated medical experts who would be able to lead medicine into a new direction.

Appealing though it may appear, this view will not be supported. It might appear that cost is the major obstacle. If adopted, this medical curriculum would take 7 years to finish; i.e., 2 extra years. The extra 30% cost involved will not be bearable by any government that provides subsidy to medical education. Students might not like the idea of more prolonged study.

In fact, the major obstacle would be the concept of forcibly marrying the two different streams of medical education. When the scientific approach has long been the mainline, is it worthwhile confusing the students who enjoy the deductive theories with old concepts? They might appreciate the old concepts and adopt them selectively only later in their practice. Therefore, the important thing is to accept and establish Chinese medicine as a full specialty. Then graduates could acquire specialty knowledge after they graduate, including Chinese medicine. After all, no undergraduate should be forced to take up qualification studies in depth, on any one medical specialty.

VIII. RESEARCH

A few advocates of alternative medicine might claim that whatever modern medicine offers, the same could be achieved with alternative medicine (like herbal medicine) provided research and resources could be pumped in. Given the obvious successes of modern science, this approach of research with that amplitude of ambition is probably unnecessary.

In China, where Chinese medicine originated, political leaders called for the "modernization" of Chinese medicine, which means accepting all the concepts of traditional Chinese medicine while trying to use modern tools and concepts to explain the phenomena and to develop further. In the full enthusiasm of following this political outcry, quite a number of clinical scientists actually devoted themselves to a fervent pursuit of modernization of Chinese medicine and made themselves well known in some areas of genuine integration (21). Outside China, it would not be easy to follow this line of approach because clinical scientists, short of the sociopolitical environment, find it difficult to totally accept and adopt the traditional concepts that form the supporting pillar of their research. Neither could they make the necessary training available to themselves.

IX. THE EFFICACY-DRIVEN APPROACH

Instead of following the scientific pathway already taken by pharmaceuticals, which has had too many difficulties rather than promises, a more practical line has been endorsed. Since most, if not all, the herbs have been used for hundreds of years, there should be sufficient reliability on the safety and efficacy of the herbs. The safety and efficacy of the herbs are already well documented, but their practical utilization in specific clinical circumstances needs to be further established. The traditional use of the herbs had been focused on symptomatic control. Today, the aim of clinical management is directed toward curing a disease entity. We need to acquire an updated understanding of the effectiveness of the herbal preparations on disease entities. That is why we cannot be satisfied with records on efficacy alone but should start a series of evidence-based clinical trials to further prove the efficacy of the herbs (22).

The U.S. National Institutes of Health have openly endorsed the approach of accepting traditional methods of healing as safe measures and then putting them to proper clinical trials (12). The recognition of acupuncture as a practical, effective means of pain control started in 1997 (11). The subsequent formation of a special section devoted to research on complementary/alternative treatment followed. NCCAM was properly formed and given a substantially large budget.

X. PROBLEMS EXPECTED IN AN INTEGRATED SETTING

A. Adverse Effects of Herbal Preparations

While alternative medicine is finding more users and health food and related preparations are gaining a bigger market, adverse effects occurring after their consumption have been making headlines ever since. Thus antirheumatoid herbal preparations were found to be nephrotoxic in the Netherlands, and many mortalities have been reported in Japan, China, and Singapore after ingestion of slimming preparations. Expectedly, disasters could be related to the illegal, intentional mixing of dangerous drugs; or real, unintentional contaminations. However, the lack of full awareness of adverse effects and a deficiency of records of adverse effects with herbal consumptions are real problems experienced by those who try to selectively use herbal preparations or formulae to solve difficult problems in day-to-day practice.

Historically, great herbal masters in China in the ancient days did produce records on adverse effects and toxic problems of some herbs. As early as the Han dynasty (second century), documents were produced on herbs that need to be utilized with care or extreme care (14). This tradition was followed closely in the subsequent centuries (15).

More reports were available on methods and means by which toxicities and adverse effects could be reduced (23).

With good past experience, the prevalent belief is that Chinese medicinal herbs are safe. On the other hand, more and more reports have appeared on adverse effects and toxicities, and nonusers of herbs tend to exaggerate the reports.

When new preparations come on the market, the innovative processes of extraction and/or production might have produced or initiated new possibilities of adverse effects or toxicity. This experience is already well recorded in a number of modernized preparations, particularly those for injection (24). Among the adverse effects, allergic reactions are most common.

To date, standard instructions on clinical trials for Chinese medicine define adverse drug reaction in exactly the same way as modern scientific clinical trials, and explanations for the reactions have been identically identified (25).

Categories of adverse reactions include the following:

1. Reactions to herbs. Reactions are defined as harmful and unexpected effects when the standard dosages are used in certain drug trials. It is especially pointed out that for Chinese medicine, the harmful reactions could be due to the quality of the herb and poor choice of indication. These reactions do not include allergic responses.

2. Dosage-related adverse effects. Using an unnecessarily high dose could induce excessive effects, side effects, or even toxic effects. Secondary effects such as electrolyte imbalance might also be observed.
3. Dosage-unrelated adverse effects. These adverse effects could be the result of unfavorable preparation, contaminants in the herbs, sensitivity of the consumer, allergic reactions, or specific inductive effects of the herb.
4. Drugs interactions. Classically, records are available in old Chinese medicinal literature on combined effects of herbs, their facilitatory and antagonistic effects. Today, not only drug interactions between herbs are important, but possible interactions between herbs and commonly used pharmaceutical preparations are becoming issues of great concern since users of herbal preparations are greatly increasing.

B. Interactions Between Modern and Chinese Medicinal Drugs

The interactions between Chinese herbs and modern drugs are a common issue, yet reports on them are very rare. According to research on 1000 elderly patients admitted through the accident and emergency department, 538 of them have used over 1087 types of drugs, and 30 of them have been affected by the side effects of these drugs (26). In fact either within the hospital or outside, when patients self-prescribe, multidrug therapies are commonly practiced. Prescribed drugs, proprietary drugs, vitamins, herbal medicines, food, etc. may all interact and affect the treatment outcome.

Some drug interactions have been investigated by in vitro and in vivo experiments, but results obtained have been inconsistent. St. John's wort, an herb commonly used in Western societies, was shown to suppress monoamine oxides in vitro, but such observations were absent in in vivo studies. Hence there is insufficient evidence of the antioxidant activity of St. John's wort causing hypertensive crisis. However, recently it was reported in Switzerland that St. John's wort may interact with other drugs; e.g., the simultaneous administration of St. John's wort with digoxin, amitriptyline, or theophylline may reduce the effectiveness of the three drugs. Two patients with heart transplants were given St. John's wort when they were receiving their cyclosporin treatment. In 3 weeks' time, both had severe rejections. When the patients discontinued the herbal drug, the cyclosporin blood concentrations increased (27).

Some medications from natural products, e.g., cornu cervi pentotrichum, fructus crataegi, radix polygoni multiflori, etc., possess monoamine oxide inhibitory activity (28). If tyramine-containing food, e.g., cheese, pickled fish, chocolate, yeast, liver, beer, red wine, or yogurt, is taken when the above natural products are used, hypertension, palpitation, headache, nausea, etc. may result (29).

The Table 1 shows more examples.

C. Source of Herbs

Good clinical practice insists that the prescribed drug for the clinical trial should be thoroughly known and uniform. However, using herbal preparations for clinical trials faces the difficulties of thorough technical knowledge and uniformity.

Pharmaceutical tests demand that details be known about the chemistry, the mode of action, and metabolic pathways before clinical tests be conducted. What is the chemistry of herbs like? What are the pathways of action and metabolic degradations? Are there adverse effects in the process of metabolism? A lot of work has been done in the past 50 years on these basic questions and not much has been found out. Each and every herb contains so much complicated chemistry that many years of research might not yield much fruit. Actually at least 400 herbs are popular and have records of action and impressive efficacy. To demand thorough knowledge on just these popular herbs is just not practical, not to speak about the less commonly used additional 1000–2000 varieties (50).

Uniformity is another difficult area. Strictly speaking, since herbs are agricultural products, uniformity should start with the sites of agricultural production. The sites of production have different weather conditions, different soil contents, and different methods of plantation. At the moment, maybe more than 50% of popular Chinese herbs are produced on special farms in China. However, these farms are scattered over different provinces in China, which have widely different climatic and soil environments. Good agricultural practice demands that environmental and nurturing procedures be uniformly ensured. Procedures include soil care, watering, fertilizers, pest prevention, and harvests. When such procedures are not uniform and there are no means to ensure a common practice, good agricultural practice is not possible.

Not only is there lack of uniformity in the method of herb production, but different species of the same herb are found or planted in different regions and provinces. These different species may have different chemical contents. Herbal experts have extensive experience and knowledge about some special correlations between the effectiveness of particular herbs and their sites of production. Some commonly used herbs are even labeled jointly with the best sites of production. With the development of molecular biology, coupled with modern means of assessment for active ingredient within a chemical product,

TABLE 1 Examples of Interaction of Herbs and Medications

Herb	Drug	Interaction	Mechanism
Radix *Salviae miltiorrhizae* (Danshen)	Warfarin	Increased INR Prolonged PT/PTT (30)	Danshen decreases elimination of warfarin in rats (31)
Radix angelicae sinensis (Danggui)	Warfarin	Increased INR and widespread bruising (32)	Danggui contains coumarins
Ginseng (radix ginseng)	Alcohol	Increased alcohol clearance (33)	Ginseng decreases the activity of alcohol dehydrogenase and aldehyde dehydrogenase in mice
Garlic	Warfarin	Increased INR (34)	Postoperative bleeding (35) and spontaneous spinal epidural hemorrhage (36)
Herbal ephedra (Ma Huang)	Pargyline, isoniazid, furazolidone	Headache, nausea, vomiting, bellyache, blood pressure increase	Pargyline, isoniazid, and furazolidone interfere with the inactivation of noradrenalin and dopamine; ephedrine in herbal ephedrine can promote the release of noradrenalin and dopamine (37)
Ginkgo biloba	Aspirin	Spontaneous hyphema (38)	Ginkgolides are potent inhibitors of PAF

Cornu cervi pantotrichum (39)	Adrenomimetic	Strengthens the effect of increasing blood pressure	Natural MAOIs in Cornu cervi pantotrichum, fructus crataegi, and radix polygoni multiflori inhibit the metabolism of adrenomimetic, levodopa, and opium
Fructus crataegi (40)	Levodopa	Increased blood pressure and heart rate	
Radix polygoni multiflori	Opium	Central excitation (41)	
Bitter melon	Chlorpropamide	Decreased urea glucose (42)	Bitter melon decreases the concentration of blood glucose (43)
Liquorice	Oral contraceptives	Hypertension, edema, hypokalaemia (44)	Oral contraceptive may increase sensitivity to glycyrrhizin acid (44)
St. John's wort	Warfarin	Decreased INR	Decreases the activity of warfarin
	Cyclosporin	Decreased concentration in serum (45)	
Radix isatidis (Banlangen)	Trimethoprin (TMP)	Significantly increases anti-inflammatory effect (46)	
Liu Shen pill	Digoxin	Frequent ventricular premature beats (47)	
Tamarind	Aspirin	Increases the bioavailability of aspirin (48)	
Yohimbine	Tricyclic antidepressants	Hypertension (49)	

ACE, angiotension-converting enzyme; INR, international normalized ratio; PT, prothrombin time; PTT, partial thromboplastin time; PAF, platelet-activating factor; AUC, area under the concentration/time curve; MAOIs, monoamine oxidase inhibitors.

species-specific criteria could be identified, using the "fingerprinting" technique. Uniformity today should include screening using "fingerprinting" techniques.

When we consider the other 50% of herbs that are only available from the wilderness, i.e., around mountains, highlands, or swamps, and cannot be grown from agricultural farms, the insistence on product uniformity becomes even more difficult.

Putting together what we have discussed, to strictly insist on good clinical practice in clinical trials for herbal medicine is largely impossible. We have to accept a compromise.

Instead of following the scientific pathway already taken by pharmaceuticals, which has shown too many difficulties rather than promises, a more practical line has been endorsed. Since most, if not all, the herbs have been used for hundreds of years, there should be sufficient reliability on the safety and efficacy of the herbs. The safety and efficacy of the herbs are already well documented, but their practical utilization in specific clinical circumstances needs to be further established. The traditional use of the herbs had been focused on symptomatic control. Today, the aim of clinical management is directed toward curing a disease entity. We need to acquire an updated understanding of the effectiveness of the herbal preparations on disease entities. That is why we cannot be satisfied with records on efficacy alone but should start a series of clinical trials to further prove the efficacy of the herbs (22).

The U.S. National Institutes of Health have openly endorsed the approach of accepting traditional methods of healing as safe measures and then putting them to proper clinical trials (12). The recognition of acupuncture as a practical, effective means of pain control started in 1997 (11). The subsequent formation of a special section devoted to research on complementary/alternative treatment followed. NCCAM was properly formed and given a substantially large budget.

XI. CONCLUSION

The twenty-first century has been considered the century of biological advancement. Breakthroughs are expected on cancer treatment, viral control, and, of course, genome study. Great triumphant moments are expected in medical science, which will further endorse and glorify the success of modern science and the deductive approach. On the other hand, as we discussed earlier, scientific advances have already brought overspecialization, rigid, strict, and oversimplistic approaches that have yet failed to satisfy treatment need. The cure of many problems is still unreached. The loss of humanistic touch in the day-to-day management when target problems are emphasized much more than holistic care is going to further disappoint our patients.

Hence, as the successes and promises of medicine further demonstrate the mightiness of science, those who do not benefit might not feel that way. Scientists do feel that all problems could be solved with endless efforts of deductive wisdom. That might be true eventually as is supported by philosophers on materialism and dialectics. It might, however, take more decades. If clinical scientists, while approaching the day of mighty capability, retain their awareness of the great need for humanistic attention and holistic care, patients would enjoy more the fruits of science. Clinical scientists could therefore keep their view that eventually the scientific approach would solve all problems and there is no need to entertain alternative, unscientific medicine, without ignoring their patients' need.

Before that day though, alternative medicine, which is capable of dealing with holistic care and preventive issues, might be able to supplement deficient areas in modern medicine. We must not assume that Chinese medicine offers only practical solutions specific to problems, and that the practice could be integrated into modern medicine. In fact, the conceptual side of Chinese medicine could serve the modern scientist on numerous occasions, today and in the future. The holistic concept, the aim to maintain balance, the emphasis on the individual's responses, and the reliance on prevention could all keep the modern scientist from being overenthusiastic about deductive science, which tends to ignore the human individual. If all clinical scientists could stick to the conventional concept while engaging in the projects of their scientific frontiers, they would be able to avoid fragmented care and negligence of human need and be more sensitive to comprehensive service.

If clinical scientists fail to agree on the value of selective integration, let them be reminded that in spite of that, the long-forgotten holistic care would always help them in their treatment planning.

REFERENCES

1. Jaeschke R, Singer J. Measurement of health status. Control Clinical Trials 1989; 10:407–419.
2. Stewart AL, Greenfield, Hayo RD. Functional status and well-being of patients with chronic conditions. JAMA 1989; (262):907–913.
3. Kaptchuk TJ, Eisenberg DM. The persuasive appeal of alternative medicine. Ann Intern Med 1998; 129(12):1061–1065.
4. Bensky D, Gamble A. Chinese Herbal Medicine. Materia Medica. Seattle: Eastland Press, 1993.
5. Su WT. History of Drugs. Beijing: United Medical University Press, 1992.

6. Grlmes DA. Technology follies: the uncritical acceptance of medical innovation. JAMA 1993; (269):3030–3033.
7. Leung PC. Editorial—Seminar on evidence-based alternative medicine. Hong Kong Med J December 2001; 4:334.
8. Cohen MH. Beyond Complementary Medicine. Ann Arbor: University of Michigan Press, 2000.
9. Eisenberg DM, Kessler RC, Foster C. Unconventional medicine in the USA—prevalence, costs and patterns. N Engl J Med 328(4):246–252.
10. Eisenberg DM, Roger DB. Trends in alternative medicine use in the USA 1990–1997. JAMA 1998; 280(18):1569–1575.
11. National Institutes of Health. Acupuncture consensus statement. NIH November 3–5, 1997; 15(5):1–34.
12. National Institutes of Health. National Centre for complementary and alternative medicine. Five Year Strategic Plan 2001–2005. NIH documents.
13. Astin JA, Marie A. Review of incorporation of complementary and alternative medicine by mainstream physicians. Arch Intern Med Vol 1998; 158:2303–2309.
14. Chang CK (Han Dynasty). Discussions on Fever. Traditional Chinese Medicine Classic.
15. Li ZC (Ming Dynasty). Materia Medica. Traditional Chinese Medicine Classic.
16. Hippocrates. Hippocrates' Oath. Classic.
17. Constitution of the Peoples' Republic of China. Government Bureau, Peoples' Republic of China, 1958.
18. Medical Panel Report after a fact finding trip to Chinese Medicine Hospital in China. University Grant Council, Hong Kong. Internal publication, 1999.
19. Office of NCCAM Complementary Alternative Medicine at the NIH NCCAM clearinghouse, 2001; Vol VIII, No. 1.
20. Kampo Medicine in Japan. Proceedings of Second Congress on Integrated Medicine, Beijing September 2002.
21. Chan HK. Principle and practice of integrative medicine and Western medicine. Chinese J Integrated Traditional Western Medi 8(2):82–85.
22. Yuan R, Lin Y. Traditional Chinese medicine: an approach to scientific proof and clinical validation. Pharmacol Ther 2000; 86:191–198.
23. Suen TM (Tang Dynasty). Important Prescriptions. Traitional Chinese Medicine Classic.
24. National Bureau of Drug Supervision. Regulations on clinical trials using drugs and herbs. Bureau Publication, 1999.
25. Suen TY, Wang SF, Wang WL. Adverse Effects of Drug Treatment. Beijing: People Health Press, 1998.
26. Doucet J, Chassagne P. Drug-drug interaction related to hospital administrations in older adults: a prospective study of 1000 patients. J Am Geriatr Soc 1996; 44:944–948.
27. Ruschitzka F. Acute heart transplant rejection due to St. John's wort. Lancet 2000; 335:548–549.
28. Yang XW. Ethanol extraction of radix polygoni multiflori on the activity of monoamine oxidase in ageing mice liver and brain. China J Chinese Mater Med 1996; 21(1):48.

29. Wang JT, Yang FY. Monoamine oxidase inhibitors and their interaction. Chinese Pharma J 2000; 35(5):351–353.
30. Tam LS, Chen TYK, Leung WK, Critchley JAJH. Warfarin interactions with Chinese traditional medicines; Danshen and methyl salicylate medicated oil. Aust NZ J Med 1995; 25:257–262.
31. Chan K, Lo AC, Yeung JH, Woo KS. The effects of Danshen (*Salvia miltiorrhiza*) on warfarin pharmacodynamics and pharmacokinetics of warfarin enantiomers in rats. J Pharm Pharmacol 1995; 47:402–406.
32. Ellis GR, Stephens MR. Untitled (photograph and brief case report). Br Med J 1999; 319:650–652.
33. Lee KF, Ko JH, Park JK, Lee JS. Effects of Panax ginseng on blood alcohol clearance in man. Clin Exp Pharmacol Physiol 1987; 14:543–546.
34. De Smet PAGM, D'Arcy PF. Drug interactions with herbal and other non-toxic remedies. In: D'Arcy PF, McElnay JC, Welling PG, eds. Mechanisms of Drug Interactions. Berlin: Springer-Verlag, 1996.
35. Burnham BE. Garlic as a possible risk for postoperative bleeding. Plast Reconstruct Surg 1995; 95:213–216.
36. German K, Kuma U, Blackford HN. Garlic and the risk of TURP bleeding. Br J Urol 1995; 76:518–523.
37. Yuan Si-tong. Consideration on the problem of "ascension of the case poisoned by Chinese traditional medicines." China J Chinese Mater Med 2000; 25(10): 579–582, 588.
38. Rosenblatt M, Mindel J. Spontaneous hyphema associated with ingestion of ginkgo biloba extract. N Engl J Med 1997; 336:1108–1114.
39. Chen Xiao-guang, Jia Yue-guang, Wang Ben-xiang, et al. Inhibiting effects of extraction of cornu cervi pantotrichum on monomine oxidase of aging mice. China J Chinese Mater Med 1992; 17(2):107–114.
40. Chen Xiao-guang, Zhao Yu-zeng, Xu zhi-min, et al. Sexual hormone effects on the activity of MAO-B in liver brain of aging mice. Chinese J Gerontol 1990; 10(3):176–179.
41. Wang Jing-tian, Yang fu-yun, Zhang Yue-ying. Interactions of monoamine oxidase inhibitors. Chinese Pharm J 2000; 35(5):351–353.
42. Aslam M, Stockley IH. Interaction between curry ingredient (karela) and drug (chlorpropamide). Lancet I 1979; 607.
43. Leatherdale BA, Panesar RK, Singh G, et al. Improvement in glucose tolerance due to *Momordica charantia* (karela). Br Med J 1981; 282:1823–1824.
44. De Klerk GJ, Nieuwenhuis MG, Beutle JJ. Hypokalaemia and hypertension associated with use of liquorice flavoured chewing gum. Br Med J 1997; 314: 731–732.
45. Phytopharmaka Johanniskraut—nicht ohne Wechselwirkungen. Drugs Used in Germany 2000; 3(3):7–8.
46. Cheng Zhao-shen, Wang Qian-gen, Ling Zhi-nan, et al. Modern Prepared Traditional Chinese Medicines. Nanchang: Jiangxi Science and Technology Publishing House, 1997:17–21.
47. Zhu Jian-hua. Chinese Medicines and Western Medicines Interaction. Beijing: People's Medical Publishing House, 1991.

48. Mustapha A, Yakasai IA, Aguye IA. Effect of *Tamarindus indica* L on the bioavailability of aspirin in healthy volunteers. Eur J Drug Metab Pharmacokinet 1996; 21:223–226.
49. Lacombiez L, Bensimon G, Isnard F, et al. Effect of yohimbine on blood pressure in patients with depression and orthostatic hypertension induced by clomipramine. Clin Pharmacol Ther 1989; 45:241–248.
50. Ernst E. Harmless herbs? A review of recent literature. Am J Med 1998; 104:170–178.

3

Clinical Trials for Herbal Extracts

Bimal H. Ashar and Adrian S. Dobs
Johns Hopkins University School of Medicine
Baltimore, Maryland, U.S.A.

I. INTRODUCTION

The use of herbal medications has soared over the last decade. In 1997, an estimated 12% of the population used over-the-counter herbal products, resulting in billions of dollars in sales for the herbal industry (1). Herbal therapy has become popular for a number of reasons. First, herbs are relatively inexpensive when compared to prescription medications. They may be viewed by consumers as cost-effective alternatives to conventional therapies. Second, they are "natural" substances that are assumed to be safe. They are free from the negative stigma attached to many commonly prescribed medicines. Third, they represent a quick fix for many patients. There is the potential for disease prevention and treatment without the need for practitioner visits, prescriptions, lifestyle changes, or unpleasant procedures. Finally, herbs are easily accessible. As a result of the Dietary Supplements Health and Education Act (DSHEA) of 1994, deregulation of the herbal industry occurred. Premarket testing of products for safety or efficacy was no longer required. Supplements were suddenly assumed to be safe unless proven otherwise by the Food and Drug Administration (FDA). This has resulted in a plethora of herbal products flooding neighborhood supermarkets and drugstores.

The lack of regulation of herbal supplements poses a number of problems. At present, no standards are in place to guarantee homogeneity among different products. For example, a patient may wish to take echinacea to prevent upper respiratory infections. At the store, she will choose from a number of different echinacea products that will vary greatly in their composition. There is no assurance that the active ingredient from the plant is even present. Variation will also exist between batches from the same manufacturer due to differences in plant composition, handling, and preparation. In many instances the active ingredient(s) is unknown, thus making standardization impossible.

In general, sound scientific evidence is lacking to support the use of many of the herbs currently marketed. A number of herbal products rely on anecdotal evidence to support their use. Many of the clinical trials in the literature are of limited quality owing to small sample sizes, improper randomization, and/or the lack of adequate controls. Large-scale, randomized, controlled trials have not been undertaken by the herbal industry owing to the fact that herbs are not patentable and the potential of economic gain from positive study results is limited. A number of researchers and organizations (e.g., Cochrane Collaboration) have attempted to critically evaluate available study data through systematic reviews and meta-analyses. Many of the analyses have been equivocal. This chapter will focus on 12 popular herbal supplements used by Americans today, highlighting available clinical evidence and the potential for harm.

II. BLACK COHOSH (*CIMICIFUGA RACEMOSA*)

Black cohosh is a plant native to North America that has traditionally been used by Native Americans for a number of gynecological conditions. Its modern use has been predominantly for treatment of menopausal symptoms such as hot flashes. The active ingredients in black cohosh have yet to be identified. The estrogenic isoflavone formononetin was thought to be partially responsible for its actions; however, this isoflavone has recently been shown to be entirely absent in some black cohosh products (2). The mechanism of action of black cohosh also remains unknown. Although it was initially thought to activate estrogen receptors, recent studies regarding its estrogenic properties have been conflicting (3,4).

A recent review of alternative therapies for menopausal symptoms identified three randomized, controlled clinical trials in favor of black cohosh (5). These studies contained small sample sizes and were of short duration (6 months or less). One trial of black cohosh on hot flashes in women with breast cancer failed to reveal a positive response (6). This may represent the difficulty in treating patients with medication-induced hot flashes, rather than an overall ineffectiveness of the herbal therapy. No data currently exist to support the use of black cohosh for the prevention of osteoporosis or cardiovascular disease.

It should be noted that no published clinical trials to date have gone beyond 6 months in duration. This is important since many women may turn to using black cohosh as an alternative to long-term hormone replacement therapy. Information regarding the effects of long-term use of this herb on vaginal, endometrial, or breast tissue is not available. Short-term data on its stimulatory effect on vaginal epithelium have been conflicting (4,7).

Black cohosh has been associated with mild gastrointestinal side effects that may be self-limited (8). Overdose can lead to dizziness, tremors, headaches, nausea, and vomiting. One case report of nocturnal seizures occurring in a woman who took black cohosh, primrose oil, and chaste tree exists (9). One case of fulminant hepatic failure after 1 week of therapy with black cohosh alone has also been reported (10). No clinically significant drug interactions are known.

III. CRANBERRY (*VACCINIUM MACROCARPON*)

Folklore has for years perpetuated the use of cranberry for the treatment and prevention of urinary tract infections (UTIs). Cranberries can be consumed as fresh fruit, concentrate, sauce, and juice. Cranberry juice cocktail, which is a mixture of cranberry juice, sweetener, water, and vitamin C, has been used in a number of studies since single-strength juice is unpalatable.

Basic science research has suggested that the cranberries may inhibit the adherence of *Escherichia coli* to urinary tract epithelial cells (11). This effect may also extend to other bacteria (12). It is still unclear as to exactly what properties of cranberries account for such activity, although recent studies have suggested that proanthocyanidins (also found in blueberries) are the compounds probably responsible (13).

To date, no high-quality clinical trials have been done to suggest the efficacy of cranberry juice or extract for the *treatment* of UTIs (14). In one uncontrolled trial done in the 1960s, 73% (44 of 60) of patients had some improvement in symptoms or reduction in culture growth after 21 days of consuming 16 oz of cranberry juice. However, only four patients had completely negative cultures. Furthermore, most of the 44 patients who showed some response had a recurrence within 6 weeks of stopping therapy, suggesting that cranberry juice may be inadequate for eradication of actual infections (15).

A number of studies have suggested that cranberry juice may be effective as prophylaxis against UTIs [16–19]. One double-blind trial of 153 elderly women randomized to consuming 300 mL of cranberry juice cocktail or placebo juice showed a significant reduction in the frequency of bacteriuria with pyuria (17). The quality of this trial has been questioned owing to baseline differences between the two groups (20). Subsequent trials, however, have also suggested such a benefit (18,19). A positive effect has not been seen in children managed by intermittent bladder catheterization (21,22).

Ingestion of cranberry is generally considered quite safe. Some concern over the potential for development of nephrolithiasis exists due to increases in urinary oxalate with regular consumption (23). The clinical significance of this finding is unclear. No significant drug interactions have been documented to date.

IV. ECHINACEA (*ECHINACEA ANGUSTIFOLIA*; *ECHINACEA PALLIDA*; *ECHINACEA PURPUREA*)

Echinacea has been used as an anti-inflammatory agent and for the treatment of a number of infections caused by viruses and fungi. Traditionally, topical echinacea has been used for a number of skin conditions including boils, abscesses, skin wounds and ulcers, eczema, and psoriasis. Recently, focus has centered around its oral use for the prevention and treatment of upper respiratory infections. Although the plant genus *Echinacea* consists of a number of different species, medicinal use has predominantly centered around three of them (*E. purpurea*, *E. augustifolia*, and *E. pallida*).

No clear active ingredient within *Echinacea* plants has yet been identified. This has resulted in great variability in content of marketed products. Research has suggested that these plants may exert their activity through stimulation of cytokine production (24,25) but a clear, specific mechanism of action has yet to be defined. A number of clinical trials have been done on different preparations of echinacea for the treatment and prevention of upper respiratory infections. Some studies suggest that the duration of colds may be reduced by up to 3 days (26,27) while others have shown no significant effect (28). Conflicting results also exist for use of echinacea for the prevention of respiratory infections (28,29). A recent Cochrane review analyzed 16 randomized clinical trials of echinacea for both treatment and prevention of the common cold (30). Definitive conclusions regarding efficacy were unable to be reached owing to study limitations and variation in species of plant studied, parts of the plant used (root, leaf, flower, seed), and extraction methods. The possibility of publication bias has been raised. Echinacea has also been touted as a means for prevention of recurrent genital herpes but support for this indication is lacking at present (31).

Echinacea is thought to be quite safe for short-term use. No serious side effects have been reported although hypersensitivity reactions and anaphylaxis can occur (32). Owing to its ability to stimulate the immune system, echinacea is not recommended for patients with autoimmune disease or HIV for fear of worsening the disease. This concern remains a theoretical risk rather than an established fact. No long-term data on the safety of chronic use are available at present. No significant drug interactions have yet been identified.

V. EPHEDRA (*EPHEDRA SINICA*)

Traditional Chinese medicine has for centuries touted the use of ephedra for the treatment of asthma, congestion, and bronchitis. Also known as ma huang, it predominantly consists of two alkaloids, ephedrine and pseudoephedrine. Ephedrine is a sympathomimetic drug, structurally similar to amphetamines. Its effects on the body include central nervous system stimulation, cardiac stimulation (ionotropic and chronotropic), bronchodilation, and elevation in blood pressure. Pseudoephedrine is an isomer of ephedrine that has weaker stimulatory effects on the central nervous system and on blood pressure (33). In the United States, ephedra has become a popular ingredient in over-the-counter weight loss preparations. It is frequently combined with herbal forms of caffeine such as guarana or kola nut.

No published studies to date exist supporting the use of either ephedra or herbal caffeine *individually* for weight loss. One study of combination product Metabolife-356 (containing ma huang and guarana) has shown significant effects of a combination of these two herbs on body weight, with a loss of 4.0 kg in the treatment group vs. 0.8 kg in the placebo group ($p < 0.001$) (34). This study was limited owing to a small sample size, short-term outcomes, and a high dropout rate, primarily secondary to cardiac side effects (e.g., palpitations, hypertension, chest pain). Additionally, Metabolife-356 contans a number of other ingredients (including chromium picolinate), whose effects on weight loss are unclear. Another study by the same principal investigator looked at the effects of a combination of ma huang and kola nut on obese individuals. In this 6-month study, significant improvement in body weight and lipid profiles was seen (35). Blood pressure changes, increased heart rate, insomnia, dry mouth, and heartburn were seen more commonly in the intervention group.

While few data are published regarding the use of herbal ephedra/caffeine for weight loss, several studies exist that examine their proposed active ingredients (ephedrine/caffeine) (36–45). When used in combination and employed with intensive and monitored diet cointervention, ephedrine and caffeine induced short-term weight loss on the order of 3 kg over placebo in one study (40). It should be noted that no randomized, controlled, blinded trials have been extended beyond 24 weeks to support long-term efficacy or safety of either herbal or nonherbal forms of ephedrine/caffeine.

Reported side effects have included hypertension, nephrolithiasis, hepatitis, insomnia, arrythmias, myocardial infarction, and stroke. Cases of death and permanent disability have also been reported (46). Concomitant use of ephedra and other stimulant medications should be avoided to protect from potentiation of toxicity.

VI. FEVERFEW (*TANACETUM PARTHENIUM*)

Feverfew has been used for centuries for a variety of conditions including fever, menstrual problems, arthritis, asthma, and allergies. At present it is commonly used for the prevention of migraine headaches. Its active ingredient is thought to be the sesquiterpene lactone parthenolide; however, other parts of the plant may be partially responsible for its activity. A clear mechanism of action not yet been established but it is thought to be related to feverfew's ability to inhibit prostaglandin synthesis (47), histamine release from mast cells (48), and serotonin release from platelets (49). Additionally, it may have direct vasodilatory effects (50).

A few small clinical trials have suggested that feverfew may be effective in migraine prophylaxis (51). However, when the quality of these trials is examined, no specific conclusions regarding efficacy can be established (52). One recent, multicenter trial of 147 migraine sufferers (the largest sample size to date) failed to show improvement in migraine frequency, intensity, or duration (53). There is at present no evidence to support the use of feverfew for the treatment of acute migraine.

There are limited data regarding the long-term safety of oral feverfew. Side effects reported in short-term clinical trials were usually mild and self-limited. Hypersensitivity reactions may occur. Mouth ulceration may be seen if the feverfew plant is directly chewed. Owing to its effects on platelets, a theoretical concern about bleeding does exist although there have been no reported cases to date. For this reason, caution is advised for patients taking anticoagulants.

VII. GARLIC (*ALLIUM SATIVUM*)

Garlic is one of the most extensively studied herbal medications available. It has been thought to possess antimicrobial, anti-inflammatory, antifungal, antiprotozoal, antioxidant, antineoplastic, and antithrombotic properties that make its use as a general tonic attractive. Recent research has primarily focused on the use of garlic for the treatment of cardiovascular diseases and risk factors. Although allicin has been proposed to be the active ingredient within garlic (54,55), its poor bioavailability limits its direct effects (56). The overall effectiveness of garlic probably revolves around the synergistic effect of various organosulfur compounds produced from the metabolism of γ-glutamylcysteines found within intact garlic bulbs (56). These compounds may act to inhibit cholesterol synthesis (54,57), alter platelet function (58), and cause smooth-muscle relaxation (59).

A number of clinical trials have been performed using a variety of garlic compounds. These trials have generated conflicting results. A recent meta-analysis has suggested that garlic supplementation may decrease total cholesterol, triglycerides, and LDL levels modestly, but only in the short term (60). Analysis of studies longer than 24 weeks failed to reveal significant effects (60). High-density lipoprotein levels do not seem to be affected by garlic administration (60). When used in the short term, garlic seems to improve cholesterol levels by 4–6% (61). When compared to the 17–32% sustained decrease in cholesterol levels seen with statin drugs (62,63), the use of garlic cannot be endorsed as a viable alternative for the treatment of hypercholesterolemia. Additionally, its use for the treatment of hypertension, diabetes, or peripheral vascular disease is not supported (60,64).

Garlic toxicity is usually mild and consists of gastrointestinal upset and breath and body odor. Given its potential effects on platelet function, an increased risk of bleeding may be present. One case of a spontaneous spinal epidural hematoma has been reported with excessive garlic consumption (65). Caution should be taken with concomitant use of garlic with anticoagulants. An increase in the International Normalized Ratio of a patient taking garlic and warfarin has been reported (66). Recent concern over an interaction between garlic and protease inhibitors used for the treatment of HIV has emerged. Certain prepartations of garlic have been shown to decrease the peak levels of saquinavir by 54% (67).

VIII. GINKGO (*GINKGO BILOBA*)

Ginkgo biloba is the top-selling herb in the United States. It has been used for a variety of medical conditions including asthma, deafness, and male impotence (68). It is predominantly used currently for the treatment of dementia, memory impairment, symptomatic peripheral vascular disease, and tinnitus. It is thought to have a number of biological effects including increasing blood flow, inhibiting platelet-activating factor, altering neuronal metabolism, and working as an antioxidant (69).

Its most promising use to date seems to be for the treatment of dementia. Mild improvements in cognitive performance and social functioning in patients with Alzheimer's and multi-infarct dementia were seen in one highly publicized trial that used the ginkgo extract Egb 761 (70). A systematic review of nine randomized, double-blind, placebo-controlled trials of ginkgo for the treatment of dementia similarly showed a mild but clinically significant effect in delaying cognitive decline (71).

The evidence for the use of ginkgo biloba for impaired memory (without dementia) is also positive but limited owing to the paucity of methodologically sound studies. A systematic review of clinical trials done for this indication suggested a significant benefit over placebo. However, the authors of this review were leery of making definitive conclusions owing to the possibility of publication bias (72). There is currently no evidence that ginkgo biloba is effective for the *prevention* of dementia or for memory enhancement in adults without impairment (73).

Given its suspected ability to increase blood flow, ginkgo has used for the treatment of intermittent claudication. A meta-analysis of eight randomized, double-blind, placebo-controlled clinical trials suggested that patients taking ginkgo significantly increased their pain-free walking distance compared to those taking placebo (74). This improvement seems to be similar to that seen with pentoxifylline but less effective than seen with walking exercises (75).

Owing to its effect on blood flow and fluidity, ginkgo has also been used for the treatment of tinnitus. Current evidence does not support its use for this indication (76). Limited preliminary evidence does exist for the use of ginkgo for the prevention of acute mountain sickness (77) and sudden deafness (78).

Side effects are usually rare and usually consist of gastrointestinal complaints or headaches. Cases of spontaneous bleeding (79) and seizures (80) have been reported. Owing to the possible potentiation of anticoagulant effects, ginkgo biloba use should be avoided in patients taking warfarin.

IX. GINSENG (*PANAX SPECIES*)

Ginseng is thought of by many as a virtual panacea. Asian ginseng (*Panax ginseng*) has been used for centuries as a general tonic, stimulant, and stress reliever. In Chinese medicine, American ginseng (*Panax quinquefolius*) has been used, but is thought to possess less stimulant activity. Siberian ginseng (*Eleutherococcus senticosus*) has also gained recent popularity but belongs to a different plant species, which is often the caue of confusion. Most studies to date concentrate on the use of *Panax ginseng*. The mechanism of action for ginseng is unknown but thought to revolve around the concentration of ginsenosides that are thought to be responsible for a number of its pharmacological properities, including stimulation of the central nervous system, stimulation of the immune system, anxiolytic effects, antioxidant effects, and vasodilatory effects (81). Additionally, ginseng may accelerate hepatic lipogenesis and increase glycogen storage (82).

Numerous studies of varying quality have been published on the use of ginseng for a multitude of different indications. A systematic review of 16 double-blind, placebo-controlled clinical trials failed to provide compelling evidence for advocating ginseng use for improving physical performance, psychomotor performance, cognitive function, or immunomodulation, treating diabetes, or treating herpetic infections (83).

A recent study on American ginseng did, however, suggest a role in diabetes. In this study, diabetic and nondiabetic participants were randomized to ingesting 3 g of American ginseng or placebo before or during the administration of a 25-g oral glucose challenge. Significant reductions in capillary glucose levels were seen in both diabetic and nondiabetic subjects after ingestion of ginseng (84). The potential treatment ramifications of this finding for patients with type II diabetes has yet to be clarified.

Animal data have suggested a possible role for ginseng in cancer prevention (85). In a large prospective epidemiological study done in Korea, consumers of *Panax ginseng* had significantly lower risk of cancer compared with those not consuming ginseng (86). A dose-response relationship between ginseng and cancer was reported. Although exciting, these findings have yet to be confirmed through clinical trials.

In general, ginseng is considered safe. Reports of hypertension, insomnia, vomiting, headache, vaginal bleeding, Stevens-Johnson syndrome, and mastalgia have been cited (87). The possibility of an interaction with warfarin (reduced INR) has also been raised (88). Care should be taken in patients on anticoagulants.

X. KAVA KAVA (*PIPER METHYSTICUM*)

Kava has been used for thousands of years by inhabitants of the South Pacific. It has usually been ingested as a mildly intoxicating beverage distinct from alcohol. Current interest in kava has centered around its use as an anxiolytic agent. Its active ingredients are located in the root/rhizome of the plant and consist of compounds known as kavapyrones or kavalactones. These compounds are thought to exert anxiolytic, sedative, analgesic, and anticonvulsant effects. Kava's precise mechanism of action on the central nervous system remains unclear. It does not seem to directly bind to benzodiazepine receptors (89). It may, however, serve to indirectly enhance GABA binding in the amygdala complex (90).

A recent systematic review of seven randomized, double-blind, placebo-controlled clinical trials has suggested that kava extract is superior to placebo for the treatment of anxiety (91). Three of these trials were appropriate for meta-analysis since they used the Hamilton Rating Scale for Anxiety (HAM-A) and the same dose of kava extract. The results revealed a weighted mean difference in HAM-A score of 9.7 points (CI, 3.5–15.8) in favor of kava. One German study not included in the systematic review suggested that kava was as efficacious as the benzodiazepine oxazepam for the short-term treatment of anxiety (92).

A number of concerns have recently been raised about the safety of kava. In most studies, the number of adverse effects were similar to that of placebo (91). Undesired effects have usually consist of mild gastrointestinal upset and allergic skin reactions. Eye irritation and a yellow, scaly dry rash (kawaism) has been described with heavy, chronic use (87). Reports of extrapyramidal effects and exacerbation of Parkinson's disease do exist in the literature (93). The greatest concern regarding adverse effects has been over liver toxicity. Although rare, 25 cases of liver toxicity including hepatitis, cirrhosis, and fulminant hepatic failure have been reported in Europe (94). This has prompted the government of Switzerland to ban the sale of kava. The Food and Drug Administration is currently considering such actions in the United States.

Concomitant use of kava with other sedatives, anxiolytics, antipsychotics, or alcohol should be avoided to protect against excess sedation. No conclusive data exist to suggest that routine use of kava results in tolerance, addiction, or withdrawal. However, long-term use should probably be avoided owing to the potential for abuse.

XI. SAW PALMETTO (*SERENOA REPENS*)

Benign prostatic hyperplasia (BPH) is a common clinical condition among elderly men. Despite numerous conventional treatment options, many men choose against therapy owing to the potential for adverse effects. This has led to the popularity of saw palmetto as an agent to treat symptoms associated with an enlarged prostate. Saw palmetto seems to act by inducing contraction of prostatic epithelial tissue and by decreasing levels of tissue dihydrotestosterone, possibly through inhibition of the enzyme 5-alpha-reductase (95,96).

A recent systematic review of 21 trials that included over 3000 men with symptomatic benign prostatic hyperplasia (BPH) suggested that saw palmetto was effective in improving urological symptoms and urinary flow measures (97). The duration of the trials analyzed ranged from 4 to 48 weeks. In one head-to-head trial, saw palmetto was shown to be equivalent to finasteride (a prescribed 5-alpha-reductase inhibitor) in improving symptoms associated with BPH. Fewer sexual side effects and no change in PSA levels were seen in the group receiving the herbal treatment (98). The long-term effectiveness of saw palmetto and its ability to prevent complications from BPH such as urinary retention are not known. Additionally, there is currently no clinical evidence to support its use for the prevention of BPH or prostate cancer.

Side effects reported with the use of saw palmetto have been mild and rare. Gastrointestinal symptoms seem to be the most commonly reported complaint, occurring in less than 2% of patients (97). A case of hepatitis has been reported with the use of an herbal blend containing saw palmetto (99). A concern over bleeding and the potential for interactions with anticoagulants has also been raised owing to a single case report of intraoperative hemorrhage and animal data that suggest its role as a cyclooxygenase inhibitor (100).

XII. ST. JOHN'S WORT (*HYPERICUM PERFORATUM*)

St. John's wort has been used extensively by Americans for self-diagnosed depression and dysphoria. In Germany, it is the most widely *prescribed* antidepressant medication. It is now suggested that the active ingredient in St. John's wort that is responsible for its antidepressant effect is hyperforin and not hypericin, as previously suggested (101). Other similar compounds may also exert some effect (102). Through these active ingredients, St. John's wort is thought to selectively inhibit monamine oxidase activity as well as synaptic neurotransmitter reuptake (103). This results in elevated levels of serotonin, dopamine, and norepinephrine in specific areas of the brain.

A number of comprehensive reviews of clinical trials regarding St. John's wort have been completed. The largest meta-analysis included data from 27 trials on 2291 patients with predominantly mild-moderate depression (104). Most trials were less than 6 weeks in duration. The authors concluded that *Hypericum* preparations were significantly superior to placebo for the short-term treatment of mild to moderate depression. Effectiveness was found to be similar to tricyclic antidepressant medications (104). Additional reviews concurred with these conclusions (105,106). Head-to-head data comparing St. John's wort to selected serotonin reuptake inhibitors are limited. In one recent three-arm study, neither *Hypericum* nor sertraline showed significantly greater reduction on the Hamilton Depression Scale (HAM-D) compared with placebo (107).

In general, side effects of St. John's wort are mild and infrequent when compared to those of commonly prescribed antidepressants (108). The most commonly reported reactions include gastrointestinal irritations, allergic reactions, fatigue, dizziness, dry mouth, and headache. Reports of photosensitization and induction of mania in susceptible patients have also been documented (109,110).

Recent concerns have been raised over herb-drug interactions with use of St. John's wort. Rare cases of serotonin syndrome have been reported with the combination of St. John's wort and selective serotonin reuptake inhibitors (66). Additionally, St. John's wort has been found to induce enzymatic

TABLE 1 Potential Herb-Drug Interactions Due to St. John's Wort

Drug	Effect	Reported clinical complication
Cyclosporin	Decreased drug levels	Transplant graft rejection
Digoxin	Decreased drug levels	None to date
Indinavir	Decreased drug levels	Increase in HIV viral load
Oral contraceptives	Decreased drug effectiveness	Unplanned pregnancies
Theophylline	Decreased drug levels	None to date
Selective serotonin reuptake inhibitors (SSRIs)	Serotonin excess	Serotonin syndrome—confusion, agitation, diaphoresis, tremor, rhabdomyolysis
Warfarin	Decreased drug effectiveness	Reduced INR value

Source: Adapted from Henderson L, Yue QY, Bergquist C, Gerden B, Arlett P. St. John's wort (*Hypericum perforatum*): drug interactions and clinical outcomes. Br J Clin Pharmacol 2002; 54:349–356.

breakdown of a number of drugs through its activation of the cytochrome P450 system (111). Clinically significant interactions have been documented (Table 1).

XIII. VALERIAN (*VALERIANA OFFICINALIS*)

Insomnia is a common sleep problem throughout the world. Many available prescription medications for insomnia are associated with significant side effects including daytime somnolence and dependence. The search for a more natural and safer hypnotic has stimulated many patients to turn to herbal products such as valerian root. Although it has been used for centuries, its mechanism of action, as well as the constituents of the plant responsible for its activity, is not well defined.

As with a number of other herbs, comparison of clinical studies is difficult owing to differences in product content, preparations, and sample size. One randomized, double-blind, study of 4-week duration suggested significant improvements in sleep efficacy in patients with insomnia (112). Similar beneficial effects were found in another small study using a different compound. Sleep latency and quality were noted to be significantly improved with valerian compared to placebo (113). A more recent study suggested that valerian is equivalent to oxazepam for the treatment of insomnia (114). Definitive conclusions regarding the use of valerian for insomnia are difficult to make, however, owing to study limitations (115).

Side effects of valerian are usually mild and include headaches, nausea, nervousness, palpitations, and drowsiness. Case reports of idiosyncratic hepatotoxicity have also been reported (116). Concomitant use of valerian with alcohol or other hypnotics should be avoided to guard against excessive sedation.

XIV. CONCLUSION

In contrast to many other fields of traditional medicine (e.g., acupuncture), the use of herbal supplements fits nicely into the Western paradigm of scientific study. Public use of such supplements has uncovered the need for the design, funding, and performance of methodologically sound clinical trials. Through initiatives from the National Center for Complementary and Alternative Medicine many popular herbs are being investigated. Clinical trials examining black cohosh for the treatment of menopausal symptoms, echinacea for the prevention and treatment of the common cold, and ginkgo biloba for the prevention of dementia are a few of the studies currently underway. Hopefully, results from such trials will help guide patients and clinicians toward judicious use of herbal supplements.

REFERENCES

1. Eisenberg DM, Davis RB, Ettner SL, et al. Trends in alternative medicine use in the United States, 1990–1997. JAMA 1998; 280:1569–1575.
2. Kennelly EJ, Baggett S, Nuntanakorn P, Ososki AL, Mori SA, Duke J, Coleton M, Kronenberg F. Analysis of thirteen populations of black cohosh for formononetin. Phytomedicine 2002; 9:461–467.
3. Kruse SO, Lohning A, Pauli GF, Winterhoff H, Nahrstedt A. Fukiic and piscidic acid esters from the rhizome of *Cimicifuga racemosa* and the in vitro estrogenic activity of fukinolic acid. Planta Med 1999; 65:763–764.
4. Liske E, Hanggi W, Henneicke-von Zepelin HH, Boblitz N, Wustenberg P, Rahlfs VW. Physiological investigation of a unique extract of black cohosh (*Cimicifugae racemosae* rhizome): a 6-month clinical study demonstrates no systemic estrogenic effect. J Women's Health Gender-based Med 2002; 11:163–174.
5. Kronenberg F, Fugh-Berman A. Complementary and alternative medicine for menopausal symptoms: a review of randomized, controlled trials. Ann Intern Med 2002; 137:805–813.

6. Jacobson JS, Troxel AB, Evans J, Klaus L, Vahdat L, Kinne D, Steve Lo KM, Moore A, Rosenman PJ, Kaufman EL, Neugut AI, Grann VR. Randomized trial of black cohosh for the treatment of hot flashes among women with a history of breast cancer. J Clin Oncol 2001; 19:2739–2745.
7. Stoll W. Phytopharmacon influences atrophic vaginal epithelium—double blind study—cimicifuga vs. estrogenic substances. Therapeutikon 1987; 1:23–31.
8. Vorberg G. Therapie klimakterischer Beschwerden. Erfolgreiche hormonfreie Therapie mitt Remifemin R. Z Allgemeinmed 1984; 60:626–629.
9. Shuster J. Black cohosh root? Chasteberry tree? Seizures! Hosp Pharm 1996; 31:1553–1554.
10. Whiting PW, Clouston A, Kerlin P. Black cohosh and other herbal remedies associated with acute hepatitis. Med J Aust 2002; 177:440–443.
11. Sobota AE. Inhibition of bacterial adherence by cranberry juice: potential use for the treatment of urinary tract infections. J Urol 1984; 131:1013–1016.
12. Schmidt DR, Sobota AE. An examination of the anti-adherence activity of cranberry juice on urinary and nonurinary bacterial isolates. Microbios 1988; 55:173–181.
13. Howell AB, Vorsa N, Der Marderosian A, Foo LY. Inhibition of adherence of P-fimbriated *Escherichia coli* to uroepithelial-cell surfaces by proanthocyanidin extracts from cranberries. N Engl J Med 1998; 339:1085–1086.
14. Jepson RG, Mihaljevic L, Craig J. Cranberries for treating urinary tract infections (Cochrane Review). The Cochrane Library. Issue 4. Oxford: Update Software, 2002.
15. Papas PN, Brusch CA, Ceresia GC. Cranberry juice in the treatment of urinary tract infections. Southwest Med 1966; 47:17–20.
16. Haverkorn MJ, Mandigers J. Reduction of bacteruria and pyruia using cranberry juice [letter]. JAMA 1994; 272:590.
17. Avorn J, Monane M, Gurwitz JH, et al. Reduction of bacteriuria and pyuria after ingestion of cranberry juice. JAMA 1994; 271:751–754.
18. Kontiokari T, Sundqvist K, Nuutinen M, Pokka T, Koskela M, Uhari M. Randomised trial of cranberry-lingonberry juice and *Lactobacillus* GG drink for the prevention of urinary tract infections in women. Br Med J 2001; 322:1571–1573.
19. Stothers L. A randomized trial to evaluate effectiveness and cost effectiveness of naturopathic cranberry products as prophylaxis against urinary tract infection in women. Can J Urol 2002; 9:1558–1562.
20. Jepson RG, Mihaljevic L, Craig J. Cranberries for preventing urinary tract infections (Cochrane Review). The Cochrane Library. Issue 2. Oxford: Update Software, 2001.
21. Foda MM, Middlebrook PF, Gatfield CT, Potvin G, Wells G, Schillinger JF. Efficacy of cranberry in prevention of urinary tract infection in a susceptible pediatric population. Can J Urol 1995; 2:98–102.
22. Schlager TA, Anderson S, Trudell J, Hendley JO. Effect of cranberry juice on bacteriuria in children with neurogenic bladder receiving intermittent catheterization. J Pediatr 1999; 135:698–702.

23. Terris MK, Issa MM, Tacker JR. Dietary supplementation with cranberry concentrate tablets may increase the risk of nephrolithiasis. Urology 2001; 57:26–29.
24. Luettig B, Steinmuller C, Gifford GE, Wagner H, Lohmann-Matthes ML. Macrophage activation by the polysaccharide arabinogalactan isolated from plant cell cultures of *Echinacea purpurea*. J Natl Cancer Inst 1989; 81:669–675.
25. Burger RA, Torres AR, Warren RP, et al. Echinacea-induced cytokine production by human macrophages. Int J Immunopharmacol 1997; 19:371–379.
26. Schulten B, Bulitta M, Ballering-Bruhl B, Koster U, Schafer M. Efficacy of *Echinacea purpurea* in patients with a common cold: a placebo-controlled, randomized, double-blind clinical trial. Arzneimittelforschung 2001; 51:563–568.
27. Brinkeborn RM, Shah DV, Degenring FH. Echinaforce and other echinacea fresh plant preparations in the treatment of the common cold: a randomized, placebo controlled, double-blind clinical trial. Phytomedicine 1999; 6:1–6.
28. Grimm W, Muller HH. A randomized controlled trial of the effect of fluid extract of *Echinacea purpurea* on the incidence and severity of colds and respiratory infections. Am J Med 1999; 106:259–260.
29. Melchart D, Walther E, Linde K, Brandmaier R, Lersch C. Echinacea root extracts for the prevention of upper respiratory tract infections: a double-blind, placebo-controlled randomized trial. Arch Fam Med 1998; 7:541–545.
30. Melchart D, Linde K, Fischer P, Kaesmayr J. Echinacea for preventing and treating the common cold (Cochrane Review). The Cochrane Library. Issue 2. Oxford: Update Software, 2001.
31. Vonau B, Chard S, Mandalia S, Wilkinson D, Barton SE. Does the extract of the plant *Echinacea purpurea* influence the clinical course of recurrent genital herpes? Int J STD AIDS 2001; 12:154–158.
32. Mullins RJ. Echinacea-associated anaphylaxis. Med J Aust 1998; 168:170–171.
33. Drew CD, Knight GT, Hughes DT, Bush M. Comparison of the effects of D- (−)ephedrine and L-(+)-pseudoephedrine on the cardiovascular and respiratory systems in man. Br J Clin Pharmacol 1978; 6:221–225.
34. Boozer CN, Nasser JA, Heymsfield SB, Wang V, Chen G, Solomon JL. An herbal supplement containing mahuang-guarana for weight loss: a randomized, double-blind trial. Int J Obes Relat Metab Disord 2001; 25:316–324.
35. Boozer CN, Daly PA, Homel P, Solomon JL, Blanchard D, Nasser JA, Strauss R, Meredith T. Herbal ephedra/caffeine for weight loss: a 6-month randomized safety and efficacy trial. Int J Obes Relat Metab Disord 2002; 26: 593–604.
36. Malchow-Moller A, Larsen S, Hey H, Stokholm KH, Juhl E, Quaade F. Ephedrine as an anorectic: the story of the "Elsinore pill." Int J Obes 1981; 5:183–187.
37. Pasquali R, Baraldi G, Cesari MP, et al. A controlled trial using ephedrine in the treatment of obesity. Int J Obes 1985; 9:93–98.
38. Pasquali R, Cesari MP, Melchionda N, Stefanini C, Raitano A, Labo G. Does ephedrine promote weight loss in low-energy-adapted obese women? Int J Obes 1987; 11:163–168.

39. Krieger DR, Daly PA, Dulloo AG, Ransil BJ, Young JB, Landsberg L. Ephedrine, caffeine and aspirin promote weight loss in obese subjects. Trans Assoc Am Physicians 1990; 103:307–312.
40. Astrup A, Buemann B, Christensen NJ, et al. The effect of ephedrine/caffeine mixture on energy expenditure and body composition in obese women. Metabolism 1992; 41:686–688.
41. Astrup A, Breum L, Toubro S, Hein P, Quaade F. The effect and safety of an ephedrine/caffeine compound compared to ephedrine, caffeine and placebo in obese subjects on an energy restricted diet: a double blind trial. Int J Obes Relat Metab Disord 1992; 16:269–277.
42. Toubro S, Astrup AV, Breum L, Quaade F. Safety and efficacy of long-term treatment with ephedrine, caffeine and an ephedrine/caffeine mixture. Int J Obes Relat Metab Disord 1993; 17:S69–S72.
43. Daly PA, Krieger DR, Dulloo AG, Young JB, Landsberg L. Ephedrine, caffeine and aspirin: safety and efficacy for treatment of human obesity. Int J Obes Relat Metab Disord 1993; 17:S73–S78.
44. Breum L, Pedersen JK, Ahlstrom F, Frimodt-Moller J. Comparison of an ephedrine/caffeine combination and dexfenfluramine in the treatment of obesity-a double-blind multi-centre trial in general practice. Int J Obes Relat Metab Disord 1994; 18:99–103.
45. Molnar D, Torok K, Erhardt E, Jeges S. Safety and efficacy of treatment with an ephedrine/caffeine mixture: the first double-blind placebo-controlled pilot study in adolescents. Int J Obes Relat Metab Disord 2000; 24:1573–1578.
46. Haller CA, Benowitz NL. Adverse cardiovascular and central nervous system events associated with dietary supplements containing ephedra alkaloids. N Engl J Med 2000; 343:1833–1838.
47. Pugh WJ, Sambo K. Prostaglandin synthetase inhibitors in feverfew. J Pharm Pharmacol 1988; 40:743–745.
48. Hayes NA, Foreman JC. The activity of compounds extracted from feverfew on histamine release from rat mast cells. J Pharm Pharmacol 1987; 39:466–470.
49. Marles RJ, Kaminski J, Arnason JT, Pazos-Sanou L, Heptinstall S, Fischer NH, Crompton CW, Kindack DG, Awang DV. A bioassay for inhibition of serotonin release from bovine platelets. J Nat Prod 1992; 55:1044–1056.
50. Barsby RW, Salan U, Knight DW, Hoult JR. Feverfew extracts and parthenolide irreversibly inhibit vascular responses of the rabbit aorta. J Pharm Pharmacol 1992; 44:737–740.
51. Ernst E, Pittler MH. The efficacy and safety of feverfew (*Tanacetum parthenium* L.): an update of a systematic review. Public Health Nutr 2000; 3:509–514.
52. Pittler MH, Vogler BK, Ernst E. Feverfew for preventing migraine (Cochrane Review). The Cochrane Library. Issue 4. Oxford: Update Software, 2002.
53. Pfaffenrath V, Diener HC, Fischer M, Friede M, Henneike-von Zepelin HH. The efficacy and safety of *Tanacetum parthenium* (feverfew) in migraine prophylaxis—a double-blind, multicentre, randomized placebo-controlled dose–response study. Cephalgia 2002; 22:523–532.
54. Gebhardt R, Beck H, Wagner KG. Inhibition of cholesterol biosynthesis by

allicin and ajoene in rat hepatocytes and HepG2 cells. Biochim Biophys Acta 1994; 1213:57–62.
55. Ali M, Al-Qattan KK, Al-Enezi F, Kanafer RM, Mustafa T. Effect of allicin from garlic powder on serum lipids and blood pressure in rats fed with a high cholesterol diet. Prostaglandins Leukot Essent Fatty Acids 2000; 62:253–259.
56. Amagese H, Petesch BL, Matsuura H, Kasuga S, Itakura Y. Intake of garlic and its bioactive compounds. J Nutr 2001; 131(3s):955S–962S.
57. Yeh YY, Liu L. Cholesterol-lowering effect of garlic extracts and organosulfur compounds: human and animal studies. J Nutr 2001; 131(3s):983S–989S.
58. Steiner M, Li W. Aged garlic extract, a modulator of cardiovascular risk factors: a dose-finding study on the effects of AGE on platelet functions. J Nutr 2001; 131(3s):980S–984S.
59. Pedraza-Chaverri J, Tapia E, Medina-Campos ON, de los Angeles Granados M, Franco M. Garlic prevents hypertension induced by chronic inhibition of nitric oxide synthesis. Life Sci 1998; 62:71–77.
60. Ackermann RT, Mulrow CD, Ramirez G, Gardner CD, Morbidoni L, Lawrence VA. Garlic shows promise for improving some cardiovascular risk factors. Arch Intern Med 2001; 161:813–824.
61. Stevinson C, Pittler MH, Ernst E. Garlic for treating hypercholesterolemia: a meta-analysis of randomized clinical trials. Ann Intern Med 2000; 133:420–429.
62. Hebert PR, Gaziano JM, Chan KS, Hennekens CH. Cholesterol lowering with statin drugs, risk of stroke, and total mortality: an overview of randomized trials. JAMA 1997; 278:313–321.
63. Ross SD, Allen IE, Connelly JE, Korenblat BM, Smith ME, Bishop D, Luo D. Clinical outcomes in statin treatment trials: a meta-analysis. Arch Intern Med 1999; 159:1793–1802.
64. Jepson RG, Kleijnen J, Leng GC. Garlic for peripheral arterial occlusive disease (Cochrane Review). The Cochrane Library. Issue 4. Oxford: Update Software, 2002.
65. Rose KD, Croissant PD, Parliament CF, Levin MB. Spontaneous spinal epidural hematoma with associated platelet dysfunction from excessive garlic ingestion: a case report. Neurosurgery 1990; 26:880–882.
66. Fugh-Berman A. Herb-drug interactions. Lancet 2000; 355:134–138.
67. Piscitelli SC, Burstein AH, Welden N, Gallicano KD, Falloon J. The effect of garlic supplements on the pharmacokinetics of saquinavir. Clin Infect Dis 2002; 34:234–238.
68. Boon HS, Smith M. The Botanical Pharmacy: The Pharmacology of 47 Common Herbs. Ontario, Canada: Quarry Press, 1999.
69. Kleijnen J, Knipschild P. Ginkgo biloba. Lancet 1992; 340:1136–1139.
70. LeBars PL, Katz MM, Berman N, et al. A placebo-controlled, double-blind, randomized trial of an extract of *Ginkgo biloba* for dementia. JAMA 1997; 278:1327–1332.
71. Ernst E, Pittler MH. Ginkgo biloba for dementia: a systematic review of double-blind placebo-controlled trials. Clin Drug Invest 1999; 17:301–308.

72. Kleijnen J, Knipschild P. *Ginkgo biloba* for cerebral insufficiency. Br J Clin Pharmacol 1992; 34:352–358.
73. Solomon PR, Adams F, Silver A, Zimmer J, DeVeaux R. Ginkgo for memory enhancement: a randomized controlled trial. JAMA 2002; 288:835–840.
74. Pittler MH, Ernst E. *Ginkgo biloba* extract for the teatment of intermittent claudication: a meta-analysis of randomized trials. Am J Med 2000; 108:276–281.
75. Ernst E. The risk-benefit profile of commonly used herbal therapies: ginkgo, St. John's wort, ginseng, echinacea, saw palmetto, and kava. Ann Intern Med 2002; 136:42–53.
76. Drew S, Davies E. Effectiveness of *Ginkgo biloba* in treating tinnitus: double–blind placebo controlled trial. Br Med J 2001; 322:1–6.
77. Gertsch JH, Seto TB, Mor J, Onopa J. *Ginkgo biloba* for the prevention of severe acute mountain sickness starting one day before rapid ascent. High Alt Med Biol 2002; 3:29–37.
78. Reisser C, Weidauer H. *Ginkgo biloba* extract EGb 761 or pentoxifylline for the treatment of sudden deafness: a randomized, reference-controlled, double-blind study. Acta Otolaryngol 2001; 21:579–584.
79. Rowin J, Lewis SL. Spontaneous bilateral subdural hematomas associated with chronic *Ginkgo biloba* ingestion. Neurology 1996; 46:1775–1776.
80. Gregory PJ. Seizure associated with *Ginkgo biloba*? Ann Intern Med 2001; 134:344.
81. Blumenthal M. Herbal Medicine. Expanded Commission E Monographs. Austin, TX: American Botanical Council, 2000.
82. Yokozawa T, Seno H, Oura H. Effect of ginseng extract on lipid and sugar metabolism. I. Metabolic correlation between liver and adipose tissue. Chem Pharm Bull (Tokyo) 1975; 23:3095–3100.
83. Vogler BK, Pittler MH, Ernst E. The efficacy of ginseng: a systematic review of randomized clinical trials. Eur J Clin Pharmacol 1999; 55:567–575.
84. Vuksan V, Sievenpiper JL, Koo VYY, Fancis T, Beljan-Zdravkoic U, Xu Z, Vidgen E. American ginseng (*Panax quinquefolius* L) reduces postprandial glycemia in dondiabetic subjects and subjects with type II diabetes mellitus. Arch Intern Med 2000; 160:1009–1013.
85. Yun TK, Yun YS, Han IW. Anticarcinogenic effect of long-term oral administration of red ginseng on newborn mice exposed to various chemical carcinogens. Cancer Detect Prev 1983; 6:515–525.
86. Yun TK, Choi SY. Non-organ specific cancer prevention of ginseng: a prospective study in Korea. Int J Epidemiol 1998; 27:359–364.
87. Miller LG. Herbal medicinals: selected clinical considerations focusing on known or potential drug-herb interactions. Arch Intern Med 1998; 158:2200–2211.
88. Janetzky K, Morreale AP. Probable interaction between warfarin and ginseng. Am J Health Syst Pharm 1997; 54:692–693.
89. Davies LP, Drew CA, Duffield P, et al. Kava pyrones and resin: studies on GABAA, GABAB and benzodiazepine binding sites in rodent brain. Pharmacol Toxicol 1992; 71:120–126.

90. Jussofie A, Schmiz A, Hiemke C. Kavapyrone enriched extract from *Piper methysticum* as modulator of the GABA binding site in different regions of rat brain. Psychopharmacology 1994; 116:469–474.
91. Pittler MH, Ernst E. Kava extract for treating anxiety (Cochrane Review). The Cochrane Library. Issue 4. Oxford: Update Software, 2002.
92. Lindenberg D, Pitule-Schodel H. D,L-Kavain in comparison with oxazepam in anxiety disorders: a double-blind study of clinical effectiveness. Fortschr Med 1990; 108:49–50.
93. Meseguer E, Taboada R, Sanchez V, Mena MA, Campos V, Garcia De Yebenes J. Life-threatening parkinsonism induced by kava-kava. Mov Disord 2002; 17:195–196.
94. Food and Drug Administration letter to health care professionals, December 19, 2001. Available at http://www.cfsan.fda.gov/~dms/ds-ltr27.html. Accessed November 22, 2002.
95. Marks LS, Hess DL, Dorey FJ, Luz Macairan M, Cruz Santos PB, Tyler VE. Tissue effects of saw palmetto and finasteride: use of biopsy cores for in situ quantification of prostatic androgens. Urology 2001; 57:999–1005.
96. Marks LS, Partin AW, Epstein JI, Tyler VE, Simon I, Macairan ML, Chan TL, Dorey FJ, Garris JB, Veltri RW, Santos PB, Stonebrook KA, deKernion JB. Effects of a saw palmetto herbal blend in men with symptomatic benign prostatic hyperplasia. J Urol 2000; 163:1451–1456.
97. Wilt T, Ishani A, Mac Donald R. Serenoa repens for benign prostatic hyperplasia (Cochrane Review). The Cochrane Library. Issue 4. Oxford: Update Software, 2002.
98. Carraro JC, Raynaud JP, Koch G, Chisholm GD, Di Silverio F, Teillac P, Da Silva FC, Cauquil J, Chopin DK, Hamdy FC, Hanus M, Hauri D, Kalinteris A, Marencak J, Perier A, Perrin P. Comparison of phytotherapy (Permixon) with finasteride in the treatment of benign prostate hyperplasia: a randomized international study of 1,098 patients. Prostate 1996; 29:231–240.
99. Hamid S, Rojter S, Vierling J. Protracted cholestatic hepatitis after the use of prostata. Ann Intern Med 1997; 127:169–170.
100. Cheema P, El-Mefty O, Jazieh AR. Intraoperative haemorrhage associated with the use of extract of saw palmetto herb: a case report and review of literature. J Intern Med 2001; 250:167–169.
101. Barnes J, Anderson LA, Phillipson JD. St. John's wort (*Hypericum perforatum* L.): a review of its chemistry, pharmacology and clinical properties. J Pharm Pharmacol 2001; 53:583–600.
102. Shan MD, Hu LH, Chen ZL. Three new hyperforin analogues from *Hypericum perforatum*. J Nat Prod 2001; 64:127–130.
103. Greeson JM, Sanford B, Monti DA. St. John's wort (*Hypericum perforatum*): a review of the current pharmacological, toxicological, and clinical literature. Psychopharmacology 2001; 153:402–414.
104. Linde K, Mulrow CD. St. John's wort for depression (Cochrane Review). The Cochrane Library, Issue 4. Oxford: Update Software, 2002.
105. Stevinson C, Ernst E. Hypericum for depression: an update of the clinical evidence. Eur Neuropsychopharmacol 1999; 9:501–505.

106. Gaster B, Holroyd J. St. John's wort for depression: a systematic review. Arch Intern Med 2000; 160:152–156.
107. Hypericum Depression Trial Study Group. Effect of *Hypericum perforatum* (St. John's wort) in major depressive disorder: a randomized controlled trial. JAMA 2002; 287:1807–1814.
108. Stevinson C, Ernst E. Safety of hypericum in patients with depression. CNS Drugs 1999; 11:125–132.
109. Lane-Brown MM. Photosensitivity associated with herbal preparations of St. John's wort (*Hypericum perforatum*). Med J Aust 2000; 172:302.
110. Schulz V. Incidence and clinical relevance of the interactions and side effects of *Hypericum* preparations. Phytomedicine 200; 8:152–160.
111. Ernst E. Second thoughts about safety of St. John's wort. Lancet 1999; 354:2014–2016.
112. Vorbach EU, Gortelmeyer R, Bruning J. Efficacy and tolerability of a Baldrian preparation. Psychopharmacotherapie 1996; 3:109–115.
113. Leathwood PD, Chauffard F, Heck R. Aqueous extract of valerian root (*Valeriana officinalis* L.) improves sleep quality in man. Pharmacol Biochem Behav 1982; 17:65–71.
114. Dorn M. Efficacy and tolerability of Baldrian versus oxazepam in non-orgaic and non-psychiatric insomniacs: a randomised, doubl-blind, clinical, comparative study. Forsch Komplementarmed Klass Naturheilkd 2000; 7:79–84.
115. Stevinson C, Ernst E. Valerian for insomnia: a systematic review of randomized controlled trials. Sleep Med 2000; 1:91–99.
116. Klepser TB, Klepser ME. Unsafe and potentially safe herbal remedies. Am J Health Syst Pharm 1999; 56:125–138.

4

Herbal Medicine
Criteria for Use in Health and Disease

Eu Leong Yong and Yin Sze Loh
National University of Singapore
Singapore, Republic of Singapore

I. INTRODUCTION

Herbal, botanical, or phytomedicines are medicinal products containing active ingredients of exclusively plant origin. These medicines may be consumed as comminuted powders or as decoctions. Their production may involve concentration or purification processes resulting in extracts, tinctures, fatty or essential oils, or expressed plant juices. This review of herbal medicines excludes products that consist primarily of chemically defined constituents. The demand for herbal remedies is rising in many countries. This resurgence in the use of medicinal herbs may be due to various reasons. First, there is much disillusionment of the public with conventional medicine and its cost and inherent nonholistic approach (1–3). More important, there exists a perception among consumers that "natural" alternatives are safer than conventional medicine (2). In the United States, passage of the 1994 Dietary Supplementary Health and Education Act left the Food and Drug Administration (FDA) with limited jurisdiction over herbal products, resulting in a surge in the availability of herbal remedies to consumers. This may easily satisfy the consumers' increasing desire for convenience and personal control over their own health (2). Also, the mass media, by providing reports of the "miraculous" healing effects of herbs, are fueling this trend, increasing the awareness of the consumer of the availability of various herbal remedy options (1). Since 1990, the U.S. market for herbal supplements has grown exponentially, to more than $2 billion a year in 1997, with no signs of leveling off (2,4–6). The U.S. herbal industry, now numbering more than 1300 companies, is expected to grow at a double-digit rate annually. In 1993 it was estimated that the Australians, too, were spending almost twice as much on complementary medicines (more than $600 million per year) as on pharmaceuticals (7). This trend is seen too not only in Europe but also in Asian countries (8). Singapore's health care services are based mainly on Western medical science. However, with the development of traditional chinese medicine (TCM) particularly in China over the past two to three decades, and increasing interest in complementary medicine, Singapore's public expenditure in TCM has also risen (8). TCM practice in Singapore is confined mainly to outpatient care. More than 10% of daily outpatient attendance is estimated to be seen by TCM practitioners, the majority of whom are trained locally by TCM schools (8).

The use of herbal medicines presents unique clinical and pharmacological challenges not encountered with conventional single-compound medicines. These medicines are usually complex mixtures of many bioactive compounds and conventional "indications and uses" criteria devised for single-compound entities may not be applicable in a significant number of ways. Compared to single-agent pharmaceuticals, phytomedicines may differ in the different mechanisms of action of bioactive constituents, in their dose-response relationships, and in the synergistic/combinatorial effects of the many bioactive compounds in herbal extracts.

II. DIFFERENT MECHANISMS OF ACTION OF BIOACTIVE CONSTITUENTS

Observed effects may be the sum total of different classes of compounds having diverse mechanisms of action. The most widely used herbal medicine in Germany and Western countries is *Gingko biloba* (see Chapter 7). It is prescribed for "brain dysfunction" and to improve memory and cognition. In randomized placebo-controlled trials, the herb has been shown to improve memory impairment, cognitive performance, dementia, tinnitus, and intermittent claudication (9–11). The bioactive components of gingko are believed to include flavonoids and unique diterpenes called ginkolides. Gingkolides are potent inhibitors of the actions of platelet-activating factors, which are important for platelet activation and clotting (12). In addition, gingko extracts also exhibit antioxidation effects that are probably mediated through nitric oxide pathways (13). Thus platelet-activating and antioxidation effects could combine to reduce inflammation and increase microcirculatory blood flow and presumably improve brain function. This effect may also be augmented by the biflavone ginkgetin, which can downregulate COX-2 induction in vivo and this downregulating potential is associated with an anti-inflammatory activity (13,14). These inflammatory effects are further augmented through the activation of other pathways by the ginkolides. For example, oral administration of the ginkolide bilobalide can protect against ischemia-induced neuron death (15) by promoting expression of glial-cell-line-derived neurotrophic factor and vascular endothelial growth factor in rat astrocytes (16). Other contributing effects are membrane-stabilizing, spasmolytic, and smooth-muscle-relaxation properties exerted through alpha-adrenergic receptors and the sympathetic nervous system. Thus many pathways may converge to give the total vasodilator and microvascular effects of gingko.

Flavonoids are common compounds in plants with a role in the inhibition of interactions between plants and microbes. Soya products that contain flavonoids are thought to have potential health benefits in terms of cardiovascular health and postmenopausal symptoms and to prevent breast and prostate cancer. Genistein, one of the principal isoflavones in soy, has activity against the estrogen receptor and inhibits the tyrosine kinase receptor and DNA topoisomerase. It is also an antioxidant and affects the pathways of apoptosis (17). Ipriflavone, a synthetic isoflavone, was also shown to prevent bone loss through mechanisms that were different from the physiological estrogen (estradiol) in that it stimulated bone formation rather than suppressed bone resorption. Thus, whereas estradiol suppressed bone rate formation in ovariectomized rats, ipriflavone did not (18). Phytoestrogens also selectively activate the ER-beta more than the ER-alpha whereas the reverse is true for estradiol. Flavonoids are common in many herbal medicines including gingko and their myriad actions make analysis of outcome variables complicated.

III. SYNERGISMS AND OTHER COMBINATORIAL EFFECTS

Synergistic interactions are thought to be of importance in phytomedicines, to understand the efficacy of apparently low doses of active constituents in a herbal product. This concept, that a whole or partially purified extract of a plant offers advantages over a single isolated ingredient, also underpins the philosophy of herbal medicine. Clinical evidence to support the occurrence of synergy in phytomedicines is, however, scanty. Typically herbal medicines consist of hundreds of compounds that may vary slightly in their chemical groups but are still based on a common backbone. Thus dozens of flavanoids and flavanol glycosides have been described in epimedium including epimedokoreanoside I, icariside I, icaritin, epimedoside A, epimedins A, B, and C, anydroicaritin, tricin, korepimedoside A and B, sagittatosides A, B, and C, sagittatins A and B, diphylloside A and B, baohuosides I–VII, and baohuosu (see Chapter 10). The major components of another common herb, ligusticum, were identified to be phthalides and their hydroxylated, oxygenated derivatives, including ligustilide, butylidenephthalide, cnidilide, neocnidilide, butylphthalide, cindium lactone, sedamonic acid and sedanolide, and the dihydroxylated derivatives (senkyunolide B–L) (see Chapter on 11). The activity of the leading psychotherapeutic herb *Hypericum perfortum*, or St. John's wort, for the treatment of depression is now believed to be attributable to at least three classes of compounds: hypericins, hyperflorin, and flavonoids. Analysis of the pharmacological actions of these compounds using 42 biogenic amine receptors and transporters indicates that several pure substances in St. John's wort are potential central nervous system psychoactive agents and may contribute to the antidepressant efficacy of the plant in a complex manner (19). The biflavonoid amentoflavone significantly inhibited binding at serotonin [5-HT(1D), 5-HT(2C)], D(3)-dopamine, delta-opiate, and benzodiazepine receptors. The naphthodianthrone hypericin had significant activity at D(3)- and D(4)-dopamine receptors and beta-adrenergic receptors. Hyperflorin acted mainly on the D(1)-dopamine receptor. These data revealed unexpected interactions of pure compounds with a number of neuronal receptors, transporters, and ion channels. Similar interactions and synergistic effects have been suggested for the common psychotrophic drugs kava-kava (*Piper methysticum*) and valerian (*Valeriana officinalis*). Synergistic mechanisms have also been suggested for *Ginkgo biloba*, *Piper methysticum* (kava-kava), *Glycyrrhiza glabra*, *Cannabis sativa*, and *Salix alba* (20,21).

IV. DOSE-RESPONSE RELATIONSHIPS

Sometimes dose-dependent reversal of effects is encountered in efficacy studies, wherein higher or lower dosages can produce different effects. There are suggestions that these findings should not be interpreted to mean that phytomedicines are not efficacious. For example, extracts of goldenrod (*Solidago virgaurea*) in low doses have no diuretic effect, whereas in therapeutic doses (6–12 g dried herb per dose) diuretic effects can be demonstrated (22). Still higher doses in animals again result in antidiuretic effects. The soy phytoestrogen genistein can activate estrogen receptors (ER) at low doses but at higher doses it exhibits ER antagonistic effects. Genistein dosages that produce uterine hypertrophy in rats were 10-fold higher than that exhibiting bone protective activity (23).

V. PROBLEMS ASSOCIATED WITH THE USE OF HERBAL MEDICINES

Despite the popularity of botanical supplements, many herbal products on the market are of low quality and dubious efficacy. Scientists, clinicians, and consumers are often concerned about safety, effectiveness, and consistency of herbal preparations. Their apprehension about these qualities is due to a plurality of unknowns. These include a variety of poorly controlled factors such as raw herb quality, processing methods used to make the preparations, the complex biochemical heterogeneity of herbs, potential adulteration, unpredictable consequences when herbs are combined, unpredictable consequences when herbal remedies are combined with conventional medications, and an apparent lack of scientific validation (24–27). It is not surprising that TCM, a medical paradigm that relies mainly on anecdotal data and tradition of use, frequently cannot withstand the scrutiny of evidence-based medicine.

A. Identification, Harvesting, and Manufacturing

Herbal products can have very similar appearances, especially between subspecies or even varieties within a same family. These can be more difficult to discern if the herb is in the dried form. This poses a great problem as different species, even if they are within the same genus, can have very different chemical constituents (28,29). Misidentification of herbs leading to inappropriate usage of a herb is a cause of morbidity and mortality among consumers. An outbreak of rapidly progressive renal failure was observed in Belgium in 1992–1993 and was related to a slimming regimen involving Chinese herbs, namely *Stephania tetrandra* and *Magnolia officinalis* (30,31). Seventy-one cases were reported in 1 month in 1994, 35 of whom were on renal replacement therapy. Renal failure has been progressive in most of the cases despite withdrawal of exposure to the Chinese herbs. Renal biopsies showed an extensive interstitial fibrosis with loss of tubes, predominantly in the outer cortex. Chemical analyses of the Chinese herbs powdered extracts delivered in Belgium demonstrated a misidentification between *Stephania tetrandra* and another potentially nephrotoxic chinese herb, *Aristolochia fangchi*. Manufacturers of herbal products are not required to have good manufacturing practices (GMP) under the current regulations in the United States, Singapore, and many other countries. Often, consumers can choose from more than one manufacturing processes or formulations for a given herb. Each method may result in a different constituent in the final product, or a different percentage of the active compound (32,33). It is not surprising that inconsistencies in similar herbal remedies, or even between different batches of a specific herbal remedy, are a problem (33–36).

B. Adulteration

Herbal products are subjected to possible adulteration or contamination because regulations for herbal products are never as stringent as for conventional medicines. Adulteration may be intentional, as in the case of an herbal remedy manufactured in China and marketed in Singapore. The product, Slim 10, which is a slimming pill claimed to be totally natural, contained an adulterant, fenfluramine. It has since led to more than 10 cases of drug-induced hepatitis and thyroid disorders. One death related to acute hepatic failure has since occurred, while another consumer escaped certain mortality with a liver transplant. PC-SPES, a drug thought to be useful in prostate cancer, had to be withdrawn because of problems with contamination.

C. Lack of Scientific Evidence for Clinical Efficacy and Safety

Except for the handful of phytomedicines known in the West, the risk-benefit profile of many herbal therapies is not known. Randomized control trials are the gold standard for clinical efficacy and they have been performed only for a handful of commonly used drugs such as gingko, St. John's wort, ginseng, echinacea, saw palmetto, and kava (10). Little is known about the vast majority of the huge body of herbal extracts and formulae registered in the Chinese pharmacopoeia. The importance of well-organized, long-term clinical trials cannot be better illustrated than in the recent issue of hormone replacement therapy and its risks and benefits. Despite the long duration of clinical use of hormone replacement in postmenopausal women, it is only in recent years that certain significant risks have been well recognized and better understood.

D. Drug-herb Herb-Herb Interactions

Little more than anecdotal evidence exists regarding interactions between pharmaceutical and herbal medicines. Despite the widespread use of herbal medicines, documented herb-drug interactions are sparse. However, studies on the common herbs indicate that significant herb-drug interactions exists. Thus St. John's wort (*Hypericum perforatum*) lowers blood concentrations of cyclosporin, amitriptyline, digoxin, indinavir, warfarin, phenprocoumon, and theophylline; furthermore, it causes intermenstrual bleeding, delirium, or mild serotonin syndrome, respectively, when used concomitantly with oral contraceptives (ethinylestradiol/desogestrel), loperamide, or selective serotonin-reuptake inhibitors (sertaline, paroxetine, nefazodone). Ginkgo (*Ginkgo biloba*) interactions include bleeding when combined with warfarin, raised blood pressure when combined with a thiazide diuretic, and coma when combined with trazodone. Ginseng (*Panax ginseng*) lowers blood concentrations of alcohol and warfarin, and induces mania if used concomitantly with phenelzine (37). Garlic (*Allium sativum*) changes pharmacokinetic variables of paracetamol, decreases blood concentrations of warfarin, and produces hypoglycemia when taken with chlorpropamide. Kava (*Piper methysticum*) increases "off" periods in Parkinson patients taking levodopa and can cause a semicomatose state when given concomitantly with alprazolam. No interactions were found for echinacea (*Echinacea angustifolia*, *E. purpurea*, *E. pallida*) and saw palmetto (*Serenoa repens*). Thus, interactions between herbal medicines and synthetic drugs exist and can have serious clinical consequences (38).

E. Inadequate Regulation

Since 1994 and the passage of the Dietary Supplement Health and Education Act (DSHEA), herbal remedies in the United States are classified as dietary supplements and not as drugs or food, and are regulated far less stringently than conventional pharmaceuticals. Under the DSHEA regulations, herbal remedies are commodities sold for "stimulating, maintaining, supporting, regulating, and promoting" health rather than for treating disease. Dietary supplements may carry a statement that "describes the role of a nutrient or dietary ingredient intended to affect the structure or function in humans" or that "characterizes the documented mechanism by which a nutrient or dietary ingredient acts to maintain such structure or function." DSHEA allows general health or "structure/function" claims but does not permit therapeutic claims. Although dietary supplements are sold to affect physiological functioning, they can be removed from the market only if the FDA can prove they are not safe. For botanicals, the DSHEA regulations do not require equivalent product standardization for uniformity between production batches because herbal products, as dietary supplements, are considered more similar to foods than to drugs. The regulations also do not require the process that obtains the active component to be identified. Given the different processing methods of a particular herb, inconsistencies in chemical constituents are inevitable.

F. Insufficient Consumer Education

If a patient's perception of herbal therapies is that they are "safe and natural," like eating fruits to obtain fiber for constipation, the patient may not recognize the importance of safety issues associated with some herbal products. Use of herbal remedies can thus be less discerning and more indiscriminate as compared to use of conventional medicine. It is important for consumers to appreciate the fact that though herbal medicines have been in use for a long time, they still bring with them risks of side effects. A good example is ma huang (ephedra), commonly marketed as a natural weight loss product. Ma huang is a Chinese healing herb that has been used for thousands of years. The ephedra plant is a short, bushy shrub. Its stems contain the active constituent from which the stimulant ephedrine is now synthesized. The ephedra plant also produces ephedrine's stereoisomer, pseudoephedrine. Pseudoephedrine is the favored active ingredient in nondrowsy cold and sinus decongestants (2,39,40). Ephedrine was used traditionally to treat a variety of conditions, including asthma, hypotension, and depression. More effective medications have largely replaced it for treatment of serious disorders, but it is still available as an over-the-counter bronchodilator and an energy-enhancer. This is not to be assumed that ma huang is thus a safe herbal remedy. It can have side effects too. These include tremors, nervousness, insomnia, headache, gastrointestinal distress, high blood pressure, irregular heartbeat, hyperglycemia, and kidney stones, as reported (2,41). The *Ephedra* plant has also been linked to substance abuse. This is so because ephedrine and pseudoephedrine are used to produce the popular illicit stimulant methamphetamine (42,43).

VI. GERMAN MODEL FOR REGULATION, USE, AND SCIENTIFIC EVALUATION OF HERBAL PRODUCTS

Despite the inherent difficulties of performing clinical trials on herbal products because of their myriad constituents, different mechanisms of action of bioactive constituents, unusual dose-response relationships, and the synergistic/combinatorial effects of the many bioactive compounds, proper scientific evaluation and safe regulated use is possible. This is best exemplified by the herbal industry in Germany where herbal medicines have been regulated by imperial decree since 1901 (44). In 1976, the second medicines act was passed and sections of this act specifically addresses phytomedicines. This requires that the entire range of medicinal plants and phytomedicines be reviewed by scientific committees. In 1978, the German Minister of Health established an expert committee, Commission E, for herbal drugs and preparations. Commission E has 24 members including physicians, pharmacists, pharmacologists, toxicologists, biostatisticians, and representatives from the pharmaceutical industry. Using the grandfather principle, preparations that were already in the market were allowed to continue to be sold. The regulations were designed so that manufacturers had to provide proof of quality according to pharmaceutical standards for traditional herbal medicines. This includes statutory declarations for herbal ingredients dosage form and intended use. On the other hand, questions of safety and effectiveness were relegated to monographs published by Commission E. However, all herbal products that came into the market after 1978 had to be evaluated according to procedures for new drug approvals. Proof of quality by the manufacturer was always required, but bibliographic evidence of safety and effectiveness was acceptable for herbal drugs. By the end of 1995, 360 herbs had been evaluated by Commission E (44). Approved herbs totaling 191 include the popular herbs like gingko, St. John's wort, ginseng, soy lecithin, kava-kava, saw palmetto, echinecea, black cohosh root, primrose, and wormwood. These approved herbs have nonprescription drug status but are available only from licensed pharmacists.

For "traditionally used" herbal products that could not meet Commission E standards, a traditional medicine statute (under Commission 109a AMG76) was introduced in 1992 that permitted their registration without the need for rigorous trials and scientific study on a specific product. Provided no serious adverse effects have been associated with their use over the years and manufacturing quality is proven, the criterion for efficacy can be met by citing "that the drug has been proven useful for many years." Their medicinal claims are limited to minor conditions and preventive statements and the phrase "traditionally used in" must be on the label. They cannot be used to cure or treat a disease and such products do not qualify for reimbursement from medical health plans.

Phytotherapeutics as a subject has been legislated into medical and pharmacy school curricula since 1993 (44). It is estimated that 80% of German physicians routinely prescribe phtomedicines as part of clinical therapy. These approved phytomedicines are reimbursable by the National Health Insurance System.

VII. COMMISSION E: EVALUATION METHODS AND CRITERIA

Unlike the FDA drug reviews in which data are passively submitted for evaluation by the manufacturer, members of Commission E actively collect and review data, both published and unpublished, from various sources, including from:

Traditional sources
Experimental, pharmacological, and toxicological studies
Clinical studies
Field and epidemiological studies

Patient case records from physicians' files
Unpublished proprietary data submitted by manufacturers

Clinical data are reviewed to ensure that the herbal medicines are reasonably safe when used according to the dosage, contraindications, and other warnings provided in the monographs. With regard to efficacy, the Commission is guided by "the doctrine of reasonable certainty. The Commission will grant a positive review if the scientific data provided reasonable verification of a particular historical use." Thus some of the older herbs were given positive reviews despite the absence of a significant body of clinical studies. Since 1990, the Commission began to focus on good clinical practice studies to document the uses and have amended usage to a more restricted indication. An example is the Hawthorn (Cratageus) monograph of 1984, which initially contained indications for use in Stages I and II of the New York Heart Association (NYHA). This indication was limited in July 1994 for Stage II NYHA and only for hawthorn leaf with flower. Clinical studies using other parts of the hawthorn plant made individually from berry, leaf, or flower failed to show sufficient efficacy. These individual parts are, however, still sold as "traditionally used herbal products."

Unapproved herbs with negative evaluations are those where no plausible evidence of efficacy was available or where safety concerns outweigh the potential benefits. Even products with minor risks were eliminated if they are not balanced by an acceptable benefit. Negative monographs were also given to herbs with no traditional usage or for which there are no clinical or pharmacological studies. Herbs that pose a risk were withdrawn immediately and those unapproved drugs that do not pose a health risk can be sold in the German market only until 2004. Unapproved drugs with specified risks include angelica seed (photosensitivity caused by coumarins), ergot (wide spectrum of activity), hound's-tongue (hepatotoxic pyrrolizidine alkaloids), nutmeg (psychoactive and abortifacient effect in large doses), lemongrass (toxic alveolitis), and yohimbine (anxiety hypertension and tachycardia).

VIII. TRADITIONAL CHINESE HERBS

The pharmacopoeia of traditional Chinese herbs includes the richest and oldest sources of medicinal plants. Herbal medicines have been used for millennia in China and one of the earliest texts is the Shen Nong Ben Cao Jing published in 101 B.C. Each subsequent emperor and dynasty has continued to commission written pharmacopoeia on medicinal herbs. One of the most prominent texts, Ben Cao Gang Mu, first published in the Ming dynasty in the late 1500s, is still a reference source for current TCM practitioners. This text contains 52 volumes and includes 1160 drugs from plants and 11,096 prescription formulae. This detailed pharmacopoeia, written by Li Shih Chen, has botanical drawings of plants drawn by his son. In 1596, it was translated into Latin and later into English, French, German, Russian, and Japanese. Sadly, since then the Chinese materia medica has not been improved for hundreds of years and current TCM practices do not differ much from that of the sixteenth century. Very little modern safety and efficacy data are known for the vast majority of TCM products. What exists are in the Chinese language, and archaic nonphysiological concepts like yin, yang, coolness, dampness, "heatness," wind, and qi are used. The description of organs like lung, spleen, and kidney does not correlate with their modern anatomical meanings. These factors coupled, with the general problems in herbal medicines outlined earlier, prevent the acceptance of TCM into mainstream medical practice, despite their popularity as food supplements.

A. The Way Forward for TCM

Nevertheless it cannot be denied that this ancient Chinese materia medica harbors many potentially lifesaving bioactive compounds. The isolation of the important antimalarial drug artemesinin from the Chinese herb Qing hao su (*Artemesia annua*) is a case in point. The modernization of the TCM industry and its acceptance into mainstream medical practice will depend on how the industry addresses the problems of

- Unauthenicated botanical raw material
- Unknown mechanisms of action
- Unknown bioactive compounds
- Nonstandardization of herbal products with respect to active ingredients
- Poor manufacturing practices
- Lack of toxicology and safety data
- Lack of randomized controlled trials to demonstrate efficacy

One way forward could be the adoption of the modified German Commission E system. Here the emphasis is first on the use of authenticated raw materials, and the standardization of agricultural, processing, and storage practices. The chemical components of many herbs are increasingly being elucidated. What is important is that their mechanisms of action be clarified using modern cell and molecular biology techniques. In this regard, the advent of microarray technology and the ability to examine many protein targets and signaling systems simultaneously are ideally suited for herbal research as herbs contain multiple compounds with potentially many modes of action. The introduction of good manufacturing practices will result in herbs with standardized bioactive components. The pharmacodynamics, pharmacokinetics, safety, and efficacy of bioactive compounds can be examined scientifically in animal models. Finally, these herbal products can be tested in human studies where the outcome parameter can be refined according to the mechanisms of action defined in vitro and in animal models. The complete process will take many years and will be expensive. Here an enlightened and practical attitude on the part of legislators and regulators will help the industry move forward. Funds for research will have to be set aside from industry. Exclusive marketing rights for products that have been certified will help manufacturers recoup the costs of research and product standardization. Such a system has already been suggested by the U.S. FDA's guidance document for industry on botanical drug products (45). As in the German system, the first emphasis should be on manufacturing quality and standardization of bioactive components. Safety has to be assured in the recommended doses. Efficacy can be based partly on traditional usage, especially of herbs that are commonly consumed. In this way over the years herbal medicines will achieve the same recognition as pharmaceutical drugs. Their promise of safety and efficacy can then be fulfilled.

REFERENCES

1. Chang J. Scientific evaluation of traditional Chinese medicine under DSHEA: a conundrum. J Altern Complement Med 1999; 5(2):181–189.
2. Tinsley Joyce A. The hazards of psychotropic herbs. Minnesota Med 1999; 82(15):29–31.
3. Astin JA. Why patients use alternative medicine: results of a national study. JAMA 1998; 279:1548–1553.
4. Ronan A, deLeon D. Kava for the treatment of anxiety. Altern Med Alert 1998;1(8):85–96.
5. Plotnikoff GA. Herbalism in Minnesota: what physicians should know. Minnesota Med 1999; 82(5):12–26.
6. Eisenberg DM, Davis RB, Ettner SL, et al. Trends in alternative medicine use in the United States, 1990–1997. JAMA 1998; 280:1569–1575.
7. MacLennan A, Wilson D, Taylor A. Prevalence and cost of alternative medicine in Australia. Lancet 1996; 347:569–573.
8. Traditional Chinese Medicine—The Report by the Committee on TCM. October 1998.
9. Le Bars PL, Velasco FM, Ferguson JM, Dessain EC, Kieser M, Hoerr R. Influence of the severity of cognitive impairment on the effect of the *Ginkgo biloba* extract EGb 761 in Alzheimer's disease. Neuropsychobiology 2002; 45(1):19–26.
10. Ernst E. The risk-benefit profile of commonly used herbal therapies: ginkgo, St. John's wort, ginseng, echinacea, saw palmetto, and kava. Ann Intern Med 2002; 136(1):42–53.

11. Kennedy DO, Scholey AB, Wesnes KA. Differential, dose dependent changes in cognitive performance following acute administration of a *Ginkgo biloba/Panax ginseng* combination to healthy young volunteers. Nutr Neurosci 2001; 4(5):399–412.
12. Lenoir M, Pedruzzi E, Rais S, Drieu K, Perianin A. Sensitization of human neutrophil defense activities through activation of platelet-activating factor receptors by ginkgolide B, a bioactive component of the *Ginkgo biloba* extract EGB 761. Biochem Pharmacol 2002; 63(7):1241–1249.
13. Wong A, Dukic-Stefanovic S, Gasic-Milenkovic J, Schinzel R, Wiesinger H, Riederer P, Munch G. Anti-inflammatory antioxidants attenuate the expression of inducible nitric oxide synthase mediated by advanced glycation endproducts in murine microglia. Eur J Neurosci 2001; 14(12):1961–1967.
14. Kwak WJ, Han CK, Son KH, Chang HW, Kang SS, Park BK, Kim HP. Effects of ginkgetin from *Ginkgo biloba* leaves on Cyclooxygenases and in vivo skin inflammation. Planta Med 2002; 68(4):316–321.
15. Chandrasekaran K, Mehrabian Z, Spinnewyn B, Drieu K, Fiskum G. Neuroprotective effects of bilobalide, a component of the *Ginkgo biloba* extract (EGb 761), in gerbil global brain ischemia. Brain Res 2001; 922(2):282–292.
16. Zheng SX, Zhou LJ, Chen ZL, Yin ML, Zhu XZ. Bilobalide promotes expression of glial cell line-derived neutrophic factor and vascular endothelial growth factor in rat astrocytes. Acta Pharmacol Sin 2000; 21(2):151–155.
17. Dixon RA, Ferreira D. Genistein. Phytochemistry 2002; 60(3):205–211.
18. Arjmandi BH, Birnbaum RS, Juma S, Barengolts E, Kukreja SC. The synthetic phytoestrogen, ipriflavone, and estrogen prevent bone loss by different mechanisms. Calcif Tissue Int 2000; 66(1):61–65.
19. Butterweck V, Nahrstedt A, Evans J, Hufeisen S, Rauser L, Savage J, Popadak B, Ernsberger P, Roth BL. In vitro receptor screening of pure constituents of St. John's wort reveals novel interactions with a number of GPCRs. Psychopharmacology (Berl) 2002; 162(2):193–202.
20. Spinella M. The importance of pharmacological synergy in psychoactive herbal medicines. Altern Med Rev 2002; 7(2):130–137.
21. Williamson EM. Synergy and other interactions in phytomedicines. Phytomedicine Sep 2001; 8(5):401–409. Review.
22. Schilcher H. Quoted in German E Commission. 1998:19.
23. Ishimi Y, Miyaura C, Ohmura M, Onoe Y, Sato T, Uchiyama Y, Ito M, Wang X, Suda T, Ikegami S. Selective effects of genistein, a soybean isoflavone, on B-lymphopoiesis and bone loss caused by estrogen deficiency. Endocrinology 1999; 140(4):1893–1900.
24. Matthews H. Medicinal herbs in the United States: research needs. Environ Health Perspect 1999; 107(10).
25. Stephen MP. The Emerging Role of a Contemporary Herbal Formula in Modern Healthcare Delivery. Irvine, CA: Vita Pharmica, Hearthealth Review, 2001.
26. McIntyre M. Chinese herbs: risks, side effects, and poisoning: the case for objective reporting and analysis reveals serious misinterpretation. J Altern Complement Med 1998; 4(1):15–17.

27. Kuhn MA. Herbal remedies: drug-herb interactions. Crit Care Nurse Apr 2002; 22(2):22–28, 30, 32.
28. Chaffin J. Safety and quality concerns related to the use of herbal therapies. Minnesota Med 1999; 82(5):45–48.
29. Bakerink JA, Gospe SM, Dimand RJ, Eldridge MW. Multiple organ failure after ingestion of pennyroyal oil from herbal tea in two infants. Pediatrics 1996; 98(5):944–947.
30. Vanherweghem JL. A new form of nephropathy secondary to the absorption of Chinese herbs. Bull Mem Acad R Med Belg 1994; 149(1–2):128–135. Discussion 135–140.
31. Tanaka A, Nishida R, Yoshida T, Koshikawa M, Goto M, Kuwahara T. Outbreak of Chinese herb nephropathy in Japan: are there any differences from Belgium? Intern Med 2001; 40(4):296–300.
32. Reichling J, Saller R. Quality control in the manufacturing of modern herbal remedies. Q Rev Nat Med 1998; Spring, 21–28.
33. Wagner Hildebert. Phytomedicine research in Germany. Environ Health Perspect 1999; 107(10):779–781.
34. deWeerdt CJ. Randomized double-blind placebo-controlled trial of a fever preparation. Phytomedicine 1996; 3:225.
35. Herbal roulette. Consumer Rep 1995; 60(11):698.
36. Quality control still a problem with herbals. National Council Reliable Health Inform Newslett 1998; 21:5.
37. Coon JT, Ernst E. *Panax ginseng*: a systematic review of adverse effects and drug interactions. Drug Safety 2002; 25(5):323–344.
38. Izzo AA, Ernst E. Interactions between herbal medicines and prescribed drugs: a systematic review. Drugs 2001; 61(15):2163–2175. Review.
39. Lake CR, Quirk RS. CNS stimulants and the look-alike drugs. Psychiatr Clin North Am 1984; 7:689–701.
40. Hoffman BB, Lefkowitz J. Catecholamines and sympathomimetic drugs. In: Bilman AG, Ral TW, Nies AS, Taylor P, eds. Goodman and Gilman's the Pharmacological Basis of Therapeutics. 8th ed. New York: Pergamon Press, 1990:187–220.
41. Food and Drug Administration. Dietary supplements containing ephedrine alkaloids: proposed rule. Fed Reg 1997; 62:30677–30724.
42. Arditti J. Ma huang, from dietary supplement to abuse. Acta Clin Belg 2002; 1(suppl):34–36.
43. Tyler VE. Herbs affecting the central nervous system. Alexandria, VA: ASHS Press, 1999; 442–449.
44. Blumenthal M, Goldberg A, Gruenwald J, et al. German Commission E Monographs and American Botanical Council. Boston: Integrative Medicine Communications, 1998.
45. Guidance for Industry: Botanical Drug products (draft) US Department of Health and Human Services, Food and Drug Administration, 2000.

5

Effects of Phytochemicals in Chinese Functional Ingredients on Gut Health

Gary Williamson
Nestlé Research Center
Lausanne, Switzerland

Yongping Bao
Institute of Food Research
Norwich, England

Keli Chen
Hubei College of Chinese Traditional Medicine
Wuhan City, People's Republic of China

Peter Bucheli
Nestlé Red Centre Shanghai Ltd.
Shanghai, China

I. INTRODUCTION

China has an extensive history of understanding the links between food and well-being. The Chinese have long believed that foodstuffs and drugs come from the same source, and the importance of balanced food was discussed in *The Yellow Emperor's Classic of Internal Medicine* (West Han dynasty, 206–208 B.C.). That food could be used instead of drugs to treat diseases was discussed in a book entitled *Effective Emergency Treatments* (Tang dynasty, A.D. 618–907). For the Chinese, food was not only to be enjoyed for the taste, but also to be appreciated for its medicinal values. The most comprehensive work describing basic information about the functionality of food was carried out by Li in 1578. He devoted 27 years to study materia medica, and collected information on 1,892 different kinds of medicinal materials in a book of 25 volumes.

In Chinese medicine, foodstuffs having highly active healing effects are categorized as drugs, and those having milder effects are categorized as foods. The Chinese health authorities have listed those food materials in a special category called "Items with both food and drug properties." These would be called functional food materials in Western semantics. The Chinese health authorities have regulated the use of drugs in food since 1987, and established a list of traditional Chinese foods with medicinal effects that can be treated as food and not regulated by drug standards. This list has been updated four times to date (1988, 1991, 1998, and 2002) and consists currently of more than 87 materials, mostly of plant origin (flowers, fruits, peels, seeds, leaves, whole plant, roots). We refer to these foods as Chinese functional ingredients (CFI) because many of them are from China itself, or have been used by the Chinese in foods for a long period of time. Some of these CFI are used in China for treating digestive disorders such as diarrhea, constipation, and colitis, or to promote digestion.

In this chapter, we will discuss only the CFI that have been approved by the Chinese authorities and are food grade. We will not discuss green tea as there are already many reviews on this subject. The areas of gut health that we have considered are carcinogenesis, indigestion, constipation, vomiting, diarrhea, appetite, and promotion of digestion and bile secretion. The quality and quantity of data vary widely on each of these topics, and whereas anticarcinogenesis has been extensively studied in the scientific literature for some individual compounds, other areas of "gut comfort" have generally been studied on the unfractionated CFI itself. The information in this review is not complete and the area is changing fast, but we have tried to present an overview of CFI on gut function, and then have considered the biological activities of selected components of the CFI that may be responsible for the observed activity. Table 1 summarizes the effects of CFI on gut disorders and digestion, and some of the CFI for which scientific evidence exists for the activities are discussed below. CFI that appear in Table 1 but are not listed below are considered in China to have an effect, but we have been unable to find suitable scientific corroboration of these activities. The structures of components discussed in Section 4 are shown in Figure 1.

It should be appreciated that the dosage and frequency of CFI are part of Chinese culture and that these benefits may not directly and readily

TABLE 1 List of CFI Used in Traditional Chinese Medicine to Treat Gut Disorders and to Promote Digestion

TFI	Gut disorder
Agastache (*Agastache rugosa*)	Diarrhea
Aloe (*Aloe vera*)	Laxative
Amomum fruit (*Amomum xanthiodes*)	Diarrhea, promote digestion, excite smooth muscle
Apricot seed (*Prunus armeniaca*)	Constipation
Bamboo leaf (*Lophatherum gracile*)	Relieve vomiting
Bitter orange flower (*Citrus aurantium*)	Diarrhea, against poor appetite, bile secretion, constipation
Cassia tora seed (*Cassia tora*)	Constipation, laxative
Chinese angelica (*Angelica anomala*)	Constipation
Chinese yam (*Dioscorea opposita*)	Diarrhea, chronic enteritis
Cinnamon (*Cinnamomum cassia*)	Diarrhea, promote digestion, control smooth muscle
Clove (*Eugenia caryophyllata*)	Promote digestion, relieve vomiting, excite smooth muscle
Euryale seed (*Euryale ferox*)	Diarrhea
Fennel seed (*Foeniculum vulgare*)	Promote digestion, control smooth muscle
Ginger (*Zingiber officinale*)	Diarrhea
Hawthorn (*Crataegus cuneata*)	Diarrhea, promote digestion
Hemp seed (*Cannabis sativa*)	Constipation
Honeysuckle (*Lonicera japonica*)	Diarrhea
Job's tears (*Coix lachryma-jobi*)	Diarrhea
Kudzu root (*Pueraria lobota*)	Diarrhea, enhance appetite
Lesser galangal (*Alpinia officinarum*)	Diarrhea, promote digestion, control smooth muscle
Licorice (*Glycyrrhiza uralensis*)	Diarrhea, smooth muscle control, mucosa protection
Lotus seed (*Nelumbo nucifera*)	Diarrhea
Mandarine orange peel (*Citrus reticulata*)	Diarrhea, promote digestion
Nutmeg (*Myristica fragrans*)	Chronic diarrhea, promote digestion, control smooth muscle
Pepper (*Piper nigrum*)	Diarrhea, promote digestion
Perilla leaf (*Perilla frutescens*)	Diarrhea, excite smooth muscle
Purslane (*Portulaca oleracea*)	Diarrhea, bile secretion
Safflower (*Carthamus tinctorius*)	Enhance appetite
Smoked plum (*Prunus mume*)	Chronic diarrhea, enhance appetite, control smooth muscle, bile secretion
Star anise (*Illiicum verum*)	Bile secretion
Sword bean (*Canavalia gladiata*)	Relieve vomiting
Winter radish seed (*Raphanus sativus*)	Diarrhea, excite smooth muscle, constipation

Source: Ref. 142.

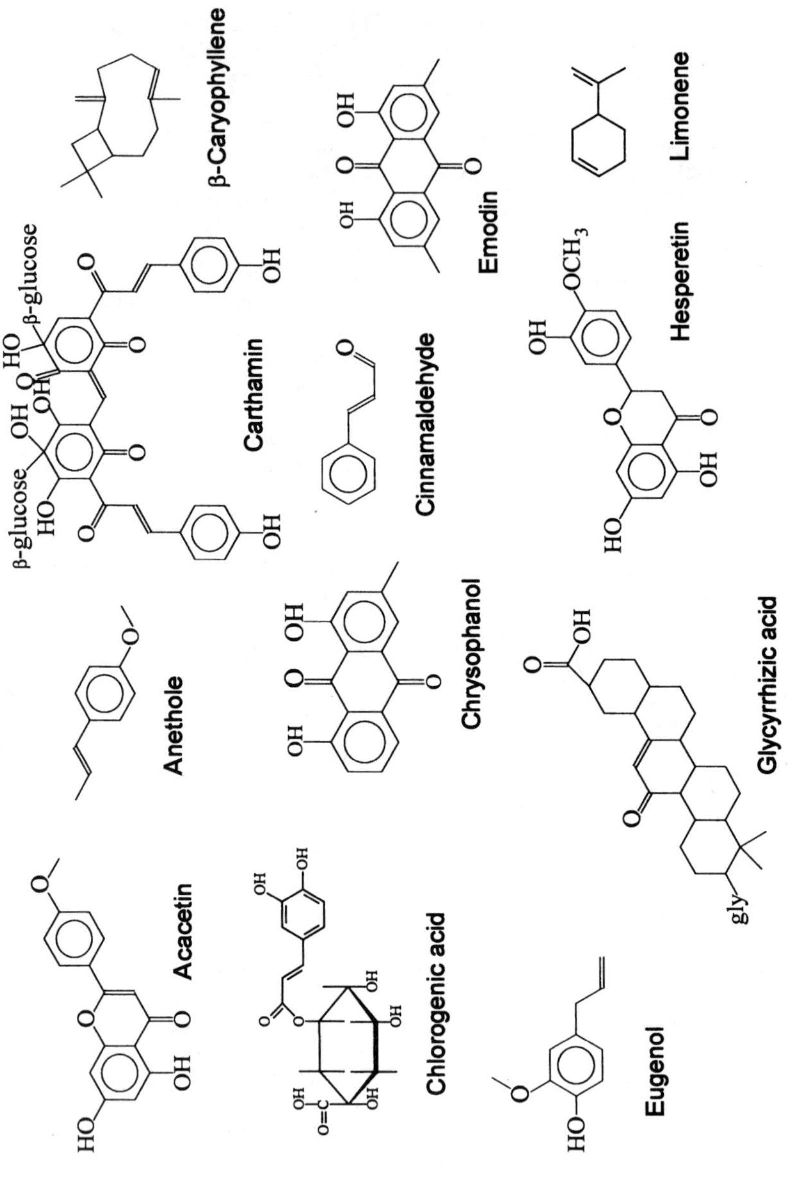

FIGURE 1 Structures of some CFI.

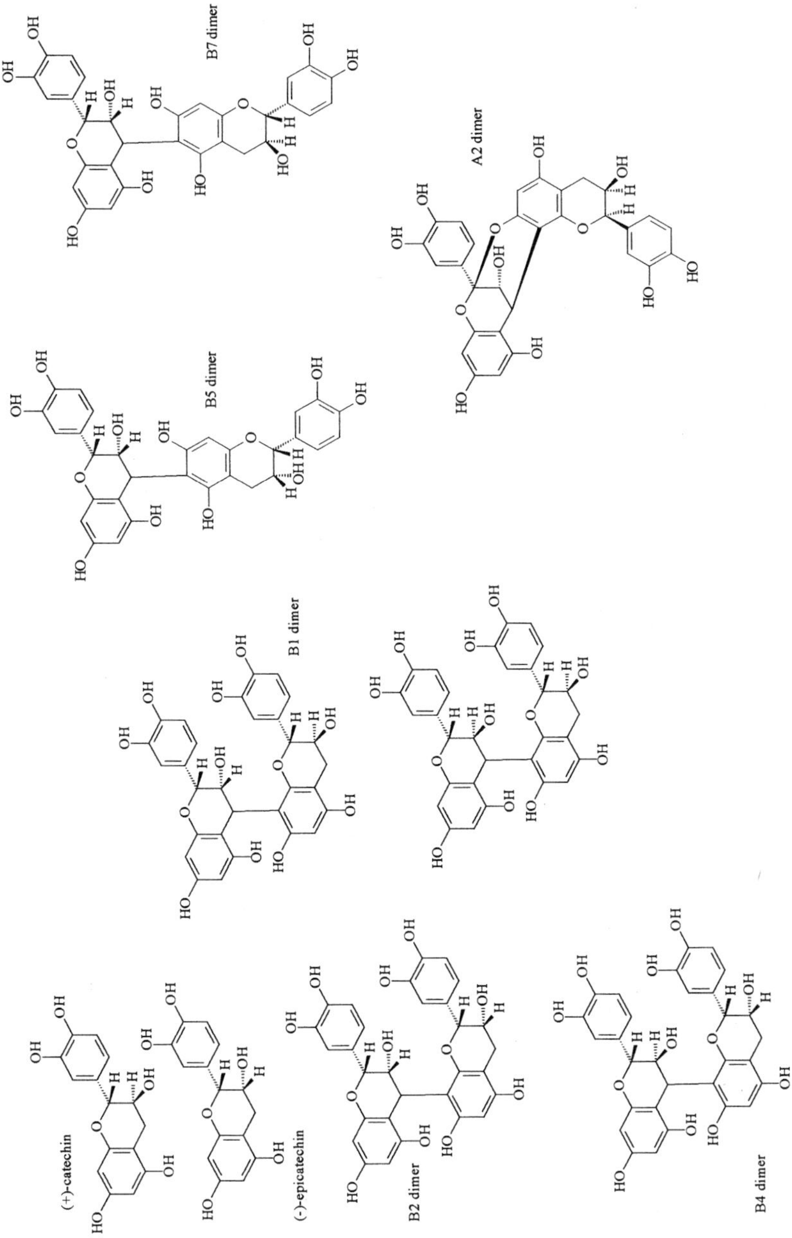

FIGURE 1 Continued.

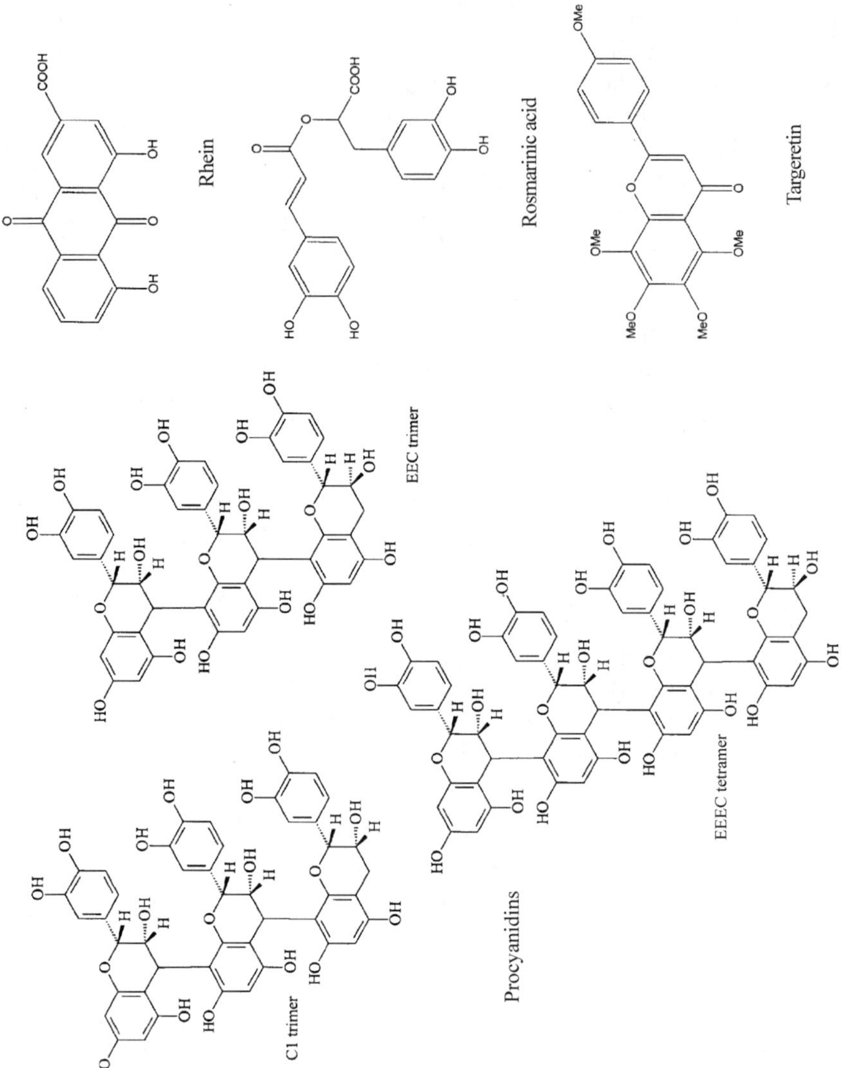

FIGURE 1 Continued.

translate into Western-style administration. This chapter makes no claims about safety of usage of any of these ingredients, since maximum doses are not always known. Furthermore, doses have been derived from traditional practices and "trial and error." There is also the possibility of contamination and variability within extracts and plant sources, and these factors need to be fully clarified before adoption into regular consumption in the West. Quality control and specification are key issues in potential systemic use of CFI to limit risk and ensure maximum benefits.

II. CHINESE FUNCTIONAL INGREDIENTS (CFI) THAT HAVE AN EFFECT ON THE GASTROINTESTINAL TRACT

A. Agastache (*Agastache rugosa*)

The aerial part of *A. rugosa* (also called Korean mint) is used in traditional medicine to treat cholera, vomiting, and miasma, and exhibits antimicrobial activity (1). Sugar, amino acid, mineral, and polyphenol composition have been described (2), and extracts contain rosmarinic acid, agastinol, and agastenol. A new diterpenoid quinone, agastaquinone, was isolated from the roots and showed nonspecific cytotoxicity against several human cancer cell lines in vitro (3). Rosmarinic acid appears to be primarily responsible for the antioxidant activity (4).

B. Aloe (*Aloe vera*)

Aloe latex or aloe juice is obtained from the yellow latex of pericyclic cells found beneath the epidermis in the leaves of *Aloe vera* and other *Aloe* species (5). It is dried to yield a solid material called "aloe" that contains anthraquinones including barbaloin, which is metabolized to the laxative aloe-emodin, iso-barbaloin, chrysophanic acid, and aloin (6,7). Because of its extremely bitter taste and its laxative effect, aloe latex or aloe juice cannot be used readily or safely in food products. The physiological effects of aloe latex and/or aloin have been widely investigated. Some of the most recent works include studies on the effect of aloe-emodin on hepatic cells (8), the protective effect of aloe extract on hepatotoxicity (9), the gastroprotective properties of aloe extract (10), the bacterial conversion of barbaloin in vivo into aloe-emodin, a genuine purgative component (11), the absorption of radio-labeled aloe-emodin (12), and many others.

C. Amomum Fruit (*Amomum xanthioides*)

Amomum Fruit is commonly decocted for use as a drink and is also called bastard "cardamon." It has an inhibitory effect on gastric acid secretion, affects gastrointestinal kinetics rather than propulsion, and is used in Chinese medicine for the treatment of gastrointestinal dyspepsia, which includes hyperchlorhydria, stomach ache, abdominal distention, anorexia, etc. (13). Oral administration of either water or methanol extracts to rabbits caused a significant decrease in gastric secretion (14). Very little information about its composition and functionality have been reported. Flavor components of the seed were determined, including α-pinene, α-phellandrene, linalool, α-terpineol, and nerolidol (15). Aqueous extracts of the related *A. villosum* were shown to have anti-gram-positive bacterium activities (16).

D. Apricot Seed (*Prunus armeniaca*)

The high amygdalin (cyanogenic glucoside, up to 8%) content of apricot seed raises safety concerns. Intensive research is being carried out on the economically important and related almond (*Prunus amygdalus*), but this is beyond the scope of this review.

E. Bamboo Leaf (*Lophatherum gracile*)

Bamboo leaf is the young stem and leaf of *L. gracile* Brongn., which have been used for bringing down fevers and diuresis. Melanosis coli has been associated with ingestion of bamboo leaf extract (17), a potential safety hazard. The histological changes in the colonic mucosa were compared with those in patients who had melanosis coli as a result of anthraquinone ingestion (aloe, etc.). Because bamboo leaf extract was not ordinarily ingested by humans, the possibility of its deposition in the intestinal mucosa has not been considered. There have been no reports on the safety of its long-term administration, and the question of safety remains open.

F. Bitter Orange (*Citrus aurantium*)

The flower of *C. aurantium daidai* is in the food-grade herb list. The dry, unripe fruits of *C. aurantium* L. and its cultivated variants are not food-grade herbs, but effective medicine, and are collected when the pericarp of the fruit is still green. The fruits are used as a digestant and expectorant and in the treatment of anal prolapse. Related citrus species are known to produce coumarins, flavanones, flavones, flavonols (which occur in the free form and/or as glycosides), and limonoids (18). The inhibitory effect of some traditional herbal medicines on the infectivity of rotavirus, which predominantly occurs in sporadic diarrhea in infants and young children, was investigated. Among the 34 kinds of herbal medicines tested, the fruit of *C. aurantium* had the most potent inhibitory activity on rotavirus infection. The active components were neohesperidin and hesperidin, 2% w/w on average (19–21). In another study,

100% of 32 patients—19 with duodenal ulcer and 19 with gastroduodenitis (including 6 with both) all of them with concomitant obstipation syndrome—were successfully treated with *Rhamus frangula*, *C. aurantium*, and *Carum carvi*. A daily defecation was attained in 91% of the patients. There was no effect on gastric mucosa or on the clinical effect of the main disease or on the percentage of the ulcer niche healing (22).

The effects of Seville orange juice on dextromethorphan pharmacokinetics were studied in 11 volunteers. Results suggest that dextromethorphan could provide some useful information on P-glycoprotein or related membrane efflux protein activity in the human gastrointestinal tract. Bioavailability of dextromethorphan increased significantly with Seville orange juice, but only returned to half the baseline value after 3 days of washout. This confirms that Seville orange juice is a long-lasting and perhaps irreversible inhibitor of gut CYP3A/Pp–glycoprotein (23). Also common in citrus are the polymethoxyflavones, tangeretin and nobiletin (24), which have some antimutagenic activity (25). Bitter orange extract plus ascorbate strongly inhibited atherosclerosis (26). We have found no recent scientific reports on *C. aurantium* flowers, except for a compositional analysis of flavonoids (27). Fruit extracts were found to be safe to use in combination with caffeine and St. John's wort for body weight loss of healthy adults (28). Use of peel is safe, although there are indications of cardiovascular toxic effects of fruit extracts in the rat (29). Bitter orange oil is widely used in perfumery and for flavoring candies, soft drinks, and baked goods (30). The polymethoxyflavonoid nobiletin specifically occurs in citrus fruits, and is a promising anti-inflammatory and anti-tumor-promoting agent.

G. *Cassia Tora* Seed (*C. tora* or *C. obtusifolia*)

An extract of *C. tora* leaves contracted smooth muscles of guinea pig ileum and rabbit jejunum in a concentration-dependent manner, and increased intestinal transit in mice dose-dependently. The studies were used to suggest that the use of *C. tora*, traditionally as a purgative and in the treatment of other ailments, is justifiable (31). Major active components are anthraquinones (chrysophanol, emodin, rhein, and others). Emodin is known for its laxative effect, and has antioxidant activity (32). A detailed composition of different varieties was recently reported (33). The related *C. obtusifolia* and its seeds, common contaminants of agricultural commodities, are toxic to cattle and poultry. Toxicity has been attributed to anthraquinones, which are major constituents of *C. obtusifolia*. Subchronic toxicity of cassia seed was investigated, and intermittent mild diarrhea was found in high-dose animals. Therefore, a dietary "no-observable-effect level" for subchronic ingestion of *C. obtusifolia* seed in rats was less than 0.15% (34).

H. Chicory

Recent research in experimental animal models revealed that inulin has possible anticarcinogenic properties since it reduced the incidence of azoxymethane (AOM)-induced aberrant cyrpt foci and tumors in the colon (35). In perfused rats, chicory extract significantly decreased cholesterol absorption by 30% in the jejunum and by 41% in the ileum, compared to the control (36,37). Recently a new type of chicory inulin with higher average chain length (DP = 25) has become commercially available. A placebo-controlled study investigated the effect of this high-performance inulin on bowel function in healthy volunteers with low stool frequency (one stool every 2–3 days). There was a significant increase in stool frequency with the high-performance inulin (38). In dogs, chicory intake resulted in increased fecal *Bifidobacterium* concentrations and some decrease in pathogenic bacteria. An increase in short-chain fatty acids was also observed, which can modulate the gut environment, facilitate absorption of nutrients, and reduce the incidence of diarrhea (39).

I. Chinese Yam (*Dioscorea opposita*)

Major constituents of chinese yam are saponins, mannan, phytic acid, and starch (40) and some varieties are rich in essential amino acids (36%) and minerals (Se, Fe, Zn, Mn) (41). The related *D. opposita*, *D. fordii*, *D. persimilis*, and *D. alata* are similar in content of polysaccharides, allatonin, and amino acids but differ in the ratio of monosaccharides. Pharmacological experiments with mice showed that they strengthen physique, help digestion, and increase immunity. It was suggested that these three kinds of Huai San Yao could be exploited as new sources of crude drugs in China (42).

J. *Chrysanthemum morifolium* Flower

The flower of *C. morifolium* Ramat is a commonly used medical herb with mild action and a popular beverage with an aromatic odor in China. It is used for treating colds and eyes with redness and pain (43). It is potentially anticarcinogenic, since the flowers contain chlorogenic acid, flavonoids, and pentacyclic triterpenes. The flavonoids from *C. morifolium* have been found to exhibit anti-HIV activity (44). Several active anti-HIV compounds, including acacetin-7-O-β-D-galactopyranoside and chrysin, have been isolated from *C. morifolium* and found to be promising compounds for the inhibition of HIV growth (45).

K. Cinnamon (*Cinnamomum cassia*)

The bark of *C. cassia* is used in traditional medicine to treat hypertension and indigestion. The growth-inhibiting activity of *C. cassia*–bark-derived materials toward five intestinal bacteria was examined (46) and the active component characterized as cinnamaldehyde. Extracts have choleretic effects in anesthetized rats, and are also analgesic (47). 2′-Hydroxycinnaldehyde was also isolated from the bark of *C. cassia*. 2′-Hydroxycinnamaldehyde inhibited the activity of farnesyl-protein transferase, an enzyme involved in the initiation of tumor formation (48).

L. Clove (*Eugenia caryophyllata*)

Bioassay-directed fractionation of clove terpenes from the plant *E. caryophyllata* has led to the isolation of the following five active known compounds: β-caryophyllene, β-caryophyllene oxide, α-humulene, α-humulene epoxide, and eugenol. These compounds showed significant activity as inducers of the detoxifying enzyme glutathione S-transferase in the mouse liver and small intestine (49). Eugenol, an active principle of clove, is an effective secretagogue in rats, causing dose-dependent augmentation of secretion. Thus, stimulation of gastric secretion at a low concentration of eugenol, i.e., 100 μg/kg body weight and below. could facilitate digestion (50). The clove ellagitannins and their related polygalloyl-glucoses inhibited maltase activity of rat intestinal α-glucosidases (51,52). Aqueous extracts of clove and cinnamon also significantly lowered the absorption of alanine from the rat intestine, and the active principle(s) in clove and cinnamon can permeate the membrane of enterocytes and inhibit the Na^+-K^+-ATPase that provides the driving force for many transport processes (53).

M. Fennel Seed (*Foeniculum vulgare*)

The fruits of *F. vulgare* Mill. are commonly employed to improve digestion in traditional systems of medicine. Rats given fennel (0.5%) and mint (1%) for 8 weeks exhibited a higher rate of secretion of bile acids and a significant enhancement of secreted intestinal enzymes, particularly lipase and amylase (54,55).

N. Ginger (*Zingiber officinale*)

Water extracts and methanol extracts of eight herbs of the Zingiberaceae were examined in intact unanesthetized rabbits for their effects on gastric secretion. Oral administration of either water or methanol extracts caused a significant decrease in gastric secretion. Since one possible cause of gastric ulcers is high acid output, water extracts of Zingiberaceae should be a rational therapy (14). Ginger extract was shown to improve gastroduodenal motility (56). Ginger contains pungent ingredients such as 6-gingerol and 6-paradol, which also have tumor antipromotion and antiproliferative effects (57).

O. Hawthorn (*Crataegus cuneata*)

The ripe fruits of hawthorn (*Crataegus* sp.) are considered to provide one of the best tonic remedies for the heart and circulatory system. In China, they are considered to act in a normalizing way upon the heart, depending on the need, stimulating or depressing its activity, but this is not scientifically validated. However, hawthorn is a rich source of the flavan-3-ol (-)-epicatechin and of proanthocyanidins (58).

P. Sea Buckthorn (*Hippophae rhamnoides*)

The fruit of *H. rhamnoides* L. is a traditional herbal medicine mainly used in Tibet and Inner Mongolia Autonomous Regions to regulate the function of stomach and intestines, and treat syndromes such as indigestion, abdominal pains, etc. (43). It has been well documented to have antioxidant, immunostimulative, regenerative, and antiulcerogenic properties (59), a protective effect against injuries in mice (60), and effects on hyperlipidemic serum cultured smooth-muscle cells in vitro (61). The alcoholic extracts of leaves and fruits of the plant at a concentration of 0.5 mg/mL were found to inhibit chromium-induced free radical production, apoptosis, and DNA fragmentation. In addition, these extracts were able to arrest the chromium-induced inhibition of lymphocyte proliferation. This suggests the alcoholic extracts have marked cytoprotective properties (62). An alcoholic extract of the berries of the plants protected against radiation-induced DNA strand breaks (63) and inhibited radiation and tertiary butyl hydroperoxide–induced DNA strand breaks at concentrations of ~0.1 mg/mL. The protection against DNA damage could mainly be attributed to direct modulation of chromatin organization (64). These studies suggest that fruit of *H. rhamnoides* can be a potential protective agent against DNA damage in chemotherapy and radiotherapy.

Q. Licorice (*Glycyrrhiza uralensis, G. glabra*)

Licorice (Gancao) is one of the most frequently used ingredients in many traditional Chinese prescriptions. It is used primarily as a demulcent, expectorant, and mild laxative. Licorice is known to exhibit many pharmacological actions, including anti-inflammatory, antiallergic, antibacterial, antiviral, antihepatotoxic, anticonvulsive, and anticancer. Licorice has been shown to possess antimutagenic activity in the Ames test using *Salmonella typhimurium* (65). Glycyrrhizic acid, an active component of licorice, was found to protect DNA damage induced by benzo[a]pyrene and ear edema induced by croton oil in mice (66,67). The extract of *G. uralensis* was also found to induce apoptosis by a p53-independent pathway in human gastric cancer cell

MGC-803; isoliquiritigenin is the main active component responsible for this action (68,69). Whe licorice was used together with other herbs such as *Chrysanthemum morifolium* and Panax notoginseng in a clinical study on 200 precancerous patients, precancerous lesions were reduced from 95.5% in the control group to 57% (70). These studies suggested that licorice possesses anti-initiating and antipromoting activities and could be a potential chemopreventive agent. The activities of licorice on cancer have been reviewed and include inhibition of cyclooxygenase and protein kinase C activities, and induction of apoptosis (71).

R. Perilla (*Perilla frutescens*)

The modulatory effect of dietary perilla oil, which is rich in the n-3 polyunsaturated fatty acid α-linolenic acid, on the development of azomethane-induced colonic aberrant crypt foci was investigated in rats. Marked increases in n-3 polyunsaturated fatty acids in membrane phospholipid fractions and decreased prostaglandin E_2 levels were observed in colonic mucosa of perilla oil–fed rats. These results suggest that perilla oil, even in small amounts, suppresses the development of aberrant crypt foci, and is therefore a possible preventive agent in the early stage of colon carcinogenesis (72). Epidemiological and experimental studies suggest that dietary fish oil and vegetable oil high in ω-3 polyunsaturated fatty acids suppress the risk of colon cancer (73). In rats the ratios of ω-2 PUFA to ω-6 PUFA in the serum and the colonic mucosa were increased parallel to the increased intake of perilla oil. The results suggested that a relatively small fraction of perilla oil, 25% of total dietary fat, may provide an appreciable beneficial effect in lowering the risk of colon cancer. Earlier results suggest that the antitumor-promoting effect of dietary perilla oil was the result of a decreased sensitivity of colonic mucosa to tumor promotors arising from the altered fatty acid composition in membrane phospholipid of colonic epithelial cells, and was not a consequence of a decrease of promotors such as bile acids (74).

S. Orange Oil (*Phyllanthus emblica*)

The fruit of *P. emblica* L. is a traditional herbal medicine mainly used in Tibet to regulate and promote the function of stomach and intestines, and treat syndromes such as indigestion, abdominal distension, etc. (43). Various parts of the medicinal plant have been used by 17 countries and nations of the world in their medical treatment. The medicinal plant is thought to have an antihepatitis, anticancer, and antitumor action and is regarded as a traditional immunomodulator and a natural adaptogen (75). The aqueous extract of the fruits can protect against nickel-induced mutagenesis and carcinogenesis (76) and *N*-nitrosodiethylamine-induced hepatocarcinogenesis in animals (77).

P. emblica, when administered orally, has been found to enhance natural killer cell activity and antibody-dependent cellular cytotoxicity on tumor-bearing animals (78).

T. Poria (*Poria cocos*)

The sclerotium of *P. cocos* has long been used as a sedative and diuretic in traditional Chinese herbal medicine. There are two reported active anticancer components in poria, triterpenes and polysacchrides. Triterpene poricoic acids G and H have antitumor-promoting activity (79). Poricoic acid B showed a strong inhibitory activity against 12-O-tetradecanoylphorbol-13-acetate-induced inflammation in mice (80). Poria extract has been shown to enhance the secretion of immune stimulators (IL-1-β, IL-6, and TNF-α) but suppressed the secretion of an immune suppressor (TGF-β), and it was suggested as an agent that can improve the immune response (81). The polysaccharides from *P. cocos* have been shown to have antitumor effects in mice (82).

III. CHINESE MEDICINE PREPARATIONS OF MIXTURES

A. Shi-Quan-Da-Bu-Tang (Ten Significant Tonic Decoction)

Food-grade herbs have been used in a famous recipe, "Shi-Quan-Da-Bu-Tang," which was formulated in the Chinese Song dynasty in A.D. 1200. It is prepared by extracting a mixture of 10 medical herbs: *Rehmannia glutinosa* (root, steamed); *Paeonia lactiflora* (root); *Ligusticum chuanxiong* (rhizome); *Angelica sinensis* (root); *Glycyrrhiza uralensis* (rhizome and root, honey-fried); *Poria cocos* (sclerotium); *Atractylodes macrocephala* (rhizome); *Panax ginseng* (root); *Astragalus membranaceus* (root, honey-fried); *Cinnamomum cassia* (bark). This potent and popular prescription has traditionally been used against anemia, anorexia, extreme exhaustion, fatigue, kidney and spleen insufficiency, and general weakness, particularly after illness. In animal studies, Shi-Quan-Da-Bu-Tang prevented body weight loss and protected against 1,2-dimethylhydrazine-induced colon cancer (83), with significant differences in mortality, fatigue, cold temperature endurance, and immune-function-related organ weight change, compared to the control animals (84). Several studies demonstrate that Shi-Quan-Da-Bu-Tang is very effective in restoring immunity in cancer patients. There is potential therapeutic activity in chemotherapy and radiotherapy because it ameliorates and/or prevents adverse toxicities (gastrointestinal disturbances such as anorexia, nausea, vomiting, hematotoxicity, immunosuppression, leukopenia, thrombocytopenia, anemia, nephropathy, etc.) of many anticancer drugs (85).

B. Jeong Dan Whan

Jeong Dan Whan is a Chinese patent medicine that is used in Korea for the treatment of acute and chronic indigestion, dyspepsia, and vomiting. This medicine consists of 14 kinds of powdered crude drugs. For the identification of the individual ingredients in such powdery mixtures, a microscopic method is often used as it requires only a small amount of material. The CFI are *Raphanus sativus*, *Brassica juncea*, *Prunus persica*, *Gardenia jasminoides*, *Alpinia oxyphylla*, and *Citrus reticulata* (86).

C. Combination of Chinese Herbs to Control Early-Weaning Diarrhea

A combination of Chinese herbs was used to control piglet early-weaning diarrhea. Chinese angelica, hawthorn fruit, licorice, and purslane were mixed with four other herbs, and decoctions (2%) made that were used to wean piglets for 4 weeks. The results showed that compared to the control, the 2% decoction reduced piglet early-weaning diarrhea by 32% (87).

D. Chungpesagan-tang

The possibility of Chungpesagan-tang, which has been recommended for stroke patients with constipation in Korean traditional clinics, as a novel antithrombotic agent was evaluated. It was found that the antithromboembolic activity of Chungpesagan-tang was activated by intestinal bacteria (88).

E. Xiao Cheng Qi Tang

Xiao cheng qi tang (minor rhubarb combination) is a Chinese herbal formula comprising *Rhei rhizoma*, *Aurantii fructus immaturus*, and *Magnoliae cortex*; it is used to treat patients with bloating, constipation, moist fever, and sinking pulse. Active components are naringin, honokiol, magnolol, sennoside B, emodin, and sennoside A (89).

IV. SELECTION OF THE ACTIVE INGREDIENTS AND THEIR MECHANISM OF ACTION

The CFI discussed above consist of a complex mixture of phytochemicals, and for most, only partial analysis has been performed. However, often (one of) the active ingredients have been identified for some of the extracts. These active ingredients are often flavonoids and hydroxycinnamates, but also terpenes, other phenolics, steroids, etc. Most flavonoids and hydroxycinnamates are found in the plant and in extracts from the plant attached to a sugar or organic acid, and consequently have a very low biological activity. For significant biological activity, the sugar or organic acid must be cleaved by glycosidases, esterases, or other hydrolytic enzymes, into the aglycone form. The site of this hydrolysis is either the small intestine (enterocyte-derived enzymes or secreted enzymes) or the colonic microflora. Fermentation of the extract also produces the same effect.

Most of the biological activities of individual compounds are associated with inhibition of carcinogenesis, since a large number of in vitro tests for anticarcinogenicity have been reported. Few assays in vitro can be used to screen for other effects on the gut, and very few clinical studies have been carried out. The activities of some examples are discussed below.

A. Acacetin

Acacetin is a flavonoid that occurs in plants as a glycoside with attached glucose, rhamnose, or glucuronic acid moieties. In the aglycone form, it is an antioxidant in vitro although this is a common property of most flavonoids. It induces UGT defense mechanisms in cells in vitro (90), inhibits cytochrome P450s CYP1A and CYP1B1 (91), induces terminal differentiation of HL-60 cells (92), inhibits topoisomerase I–catalyzed DNA ligation (93), and inhibits B(a)P-induced mutagenesis in hamster embryo-cell-mediated V79 cell mutation assay (94). All of these activities are associated with a decreased risk of carcinogenesis, incuding colon carcinogenesis.

B. Agastinol, Agastenol

These are recently reported novel lignans that inhibit etoposide-induced apoptosis of U937 cells (95). Very few data are available on effects on the gastrointestinal tract.

C. Anethole

Anethole has a broad range of biological activities related to possible action on the gastrointestinal tract. It exhibits local anesthetic activity in vivo in rats (96), is antimicrobial (97), and may possibly have antispasmodic, digestive, and secretolytic activities, although the mechanisms of these activities are not reported. At relatively high doses, anethole shows dose-related antigenotoxic effect against procarbazine and urethane in mice (98), and inhibits TNF-induced cellular responses such as NF-kB activation, TNF-induced lipid peroxidation, and reactive oxygen species, and suppresses TNF-activation of AP-1, c.jun N-terminal kinase, and MAPK-kinase (99). Possible anticarcinogenic action is suggested since rats fed anethole show induction of hepatic phase II but not phase I enzymes in the liver (100).

D. β-Caryophyllene

β-Caryophyllene shows some antibacterial activity (101), and has cytoprotective and anti-inflammataory effects in the stomach against necrotizing agents such as ethanol and acetic acid, but does not affect secretion of gastric acid and pepsin (102). Some anticarcinogenic activity is suggested since it is toxic to tumor cell lines (103), and induces small-intestinal glutathione transferase (49).

E. Chlorogenic Acid, Caffeic Acid

Chlorogenic acid is caffeic acid linked to quinic acid. Chlorogenic acid exhibits some relatively weak anticarcinogenic effects and reduces the incidence of aberrant crypt foci in rats (104). However, derivatives such as rosmarinic acid (see below) and caffeic acid phenethyl ester (from honey bee hive propiolis) have greatly enhanced biological activities.

F. Chrysophanol

Chrysophanol is antifungal (105), inhibits cytochrome P450 (106), and has potential antiallergic activity via inhibition of hyalonuridase and histamine release from mast cells (107).

G. Cinnamaldehyde, 2′-Hydroxycinnamaldehyde

Cinnamaldehyde has antimicrobial activity against some pathogens (108), inhibits rat jejunal Na^+-K^+-ATPase (53), inhibits lymphoproliferation, and induces a T-cell differentiation through the blockade of early steps in signaling pathway leading to cell growth (109).

H. Emodin

Emodin is anti-inflammatory against carageenan-induced edema in rats (110) and emodin and its metabolites have a long half-life in the plasma of rats (~50 hr) (111). Emodin exhibits a range of anticarcinogenic activities in vitro, including inhibition of formation of DNA adducts induced by 1-nitropyrene (112), modulation of cellular transformation and proliferation (113), inhibition of NF-kB activation and expression of adhesion molecules (114), inhibition of casein kinase II (114a), and induction of apoptosis (115), but emodin induces cytochromes P450 1A1 and 1B1 in human lung cell lines (116). Emodin also induced muscle contractions due to Ca^{2+} release in skeletal muscle, as a result of influx of extracellular Ca^{2+} through voltage-dependent Ca^{2+} channels of the plasma membrane (117).

I. Glycyrrhizic Acid, Glycyrrhizin

The triterpenoid glycyrrhizin is anti-inflammatory and is metabolised to the aglycone glycyrrhizic acid, which inhibits 11-β-hydroxysteroid dehydrogenase, involved in corticosteroid metabolism. The aglycone inhibited *N*-acetyltransferase activity in human colon tumor cell lines, and inhibited the formation of DNA adducts (118). Although glycyrrhizin did not directly induce apoptosis, it enhanced Fas-mediated apoptotic body formation and DNA fragmentation in T-cell lines (119). The action of licorice root, the main source of glycyrrhizin, on cancer has been reviewed (71).

J. Hesperidin, Hesperetin

Hesperetin is a flavonoid that exhibits a number of biological activities; hesperidin is the glycosylated form. Mandarin juice rich in hesperidin and β-cryptoxanthin reduced azoxymethane-induced colon carcinogenesis in rats (120); hesperidin reduced phorbol-ester induced inflammation in mouse skin (121); hesperidin was anti-inflammatory against rat colitis induced by trinitrobenzenesulfonic acid and protected against urinary bladder carcinogenesis in mice (122); and hesperidin protected against rat esophageal carcinogenesis (123). Hesperidin methylchalcone is a drug used against chronic venous insufficiency since it reduces activation of phospholipase and ameliorates the decrease in ATP in hypoxia-treated endothelial cells (124).

K. Linalool

Linalool is a monoterpene and an anticonvulsive agent (125), and is also hypnotic and hypothermic (126), via inhibition of acetylcholine release in the mouse neuromuscular junction. It is a sedative in humans (127).

L. Nobiletin

Nobiletin is a flavonoid that occurs exclusively in citrus fruits. It is antimetastatic in mice and inhibited peritoneal dissemination of gastric cancer, at least partly through inhibition of metalloproteinases (128). Nobiletin protected against the appearance of gastric hemorrhagic lesions induced by ethanol but not aspirin in the guinea pig, and alone had no effect on the potential difference. Nobiletin also relaxed the contractions induced by acetylcholine, electrical stimulation, and histamine in isolated guinea pig ileum. The anti-ulcer effects of nobiletin were ascribed to maintenance of the mucosal barrier and inhibition of gastric motor activity (129). It also suppressed azoxymethane-induced colonic aberrant crypt foci in rats (130).

M. Proanthocyanidins

Procyanidins or proanthocyanidins are oligomeric flavan-3-ol flavonoids, which occur in high amounts in some Western diets owing to their presence in cocoa/chocolate, red wine, and also in some supplements such as grape seed extract. Because they are oligomers, a number of different compounds are found naturally, consisting of either eipcatechin or catechin monomers linked in different ways with a degree of polymerization of 2–6 and more. Analytical limitations make it difficult to obtain pure oligomers above 6. Although procyanidins are only poorly bioavailable, they exert a number of effects in vivo although not specifically on the gut.

N. Rhein

Rhein is a highly biologically active anthraquinone that is a component of senna. It has a number of effects on the gastrointestinal tract, including induction of ion secretion, chemotaxis, and apoptosis in the intestinal Caco2 cell line via nitric oxide generation (131), inhibits the growth of *Helicobacter pylori* (132), modifies the peristaltic reflex of the inverted guinea pig ileum (133), inhibits glucose uptake (134), and decreases transit time in rats with a prostaglandin-dependent mechanism (135). Some anticarcinogenic activity has also been claimed, since rhein modulates topoisomerase II, and intercalates DNA (136).

O. Rosmarinic Acid

Rosmarinic acid is one of the most effective antioxidants, and it induced phase II detoxifying enzymes in rat liver but not cytochrome P450 (phase I) enzymes (137). It also inhibited cell proliferation (138), reduced lipopolysaccharide-induced liver injury in mice (138a), and may have some undefined antidepressive effects (139).

P. Tangeretin

Tangeretin is a flavonoid that affects cell-cell adhesion and downregulates the IL-2 receptor on T lymphocytes and natural killer cells (140), and may cross the blood-brain barrier in rats (141), although no specific effects on the gut have been reported.

V. SUMMARY AND POTENTIAL

Many of the effects reported have not been measured over a range of doses, there are only a few clinical studies, very little is known about the bioavailability of most of the compounds and extracts, and the reported effects in vitro may or may not be at relevant doses (i.e., similar to those found in vivo). Nevertheless, Chinese medicine clearly works in many cases, although the scientific basis of the action and the individual compounds responsible are often not known. In addition, there are a huge range of in vitro tests for anticarcinogenic activity, and it is unlikely that a single one of these tests can predict anticarcinogenicity in vivo, certainly not in humans. It is also possible that separating the active components of CFI may dilute or lose the activity, since synergy and interactions are lost. Another factor is acceptance by the Western medical community and the general public. Clearly CFI are well accepted by many Chinese, and have been used centuries. Perhaps the way forward is to consider how Western and Chinese medicines may complement each other, with conventional drugs for treatment of disease and Chinese medicines for relieving symptoms and treatment of milder complaints where Western medicine is often lacking (with the exception of painkillers).

REFERENCES

1. Song JH, Kim MJ, Kwon HD, Park IH. Antimicrobial activity and components of extracts from *Agastache rugosa* during growth period. J Food Sci Nutr 2001; 6:10–15.
2. Choi KS, Lee HY. Characteristics of useful components in the leaves of baechohyang (*Agastache rugosa, O. Kuntze*). J Korean Soc Food Sci Nutr 1999; 28:326–332.
3. Lee HK, Oh SR, Kim JI, Kim JW, Lee CO. Agastaquinone, a new cytotoxic diterpenoid quinone from *Agastache rugosa*. J Nat Products 1995; 58:1718–1721.
4. Kim JB, Kim JB, Cho KJ, Hwang YS, Park RD. Isolation, identification, and activity of rosmarinic acid, a potent antioxidant extracted from Korean *Agastache rugosa*. Hanguk Nongwhahak Hoechi 1999; 42:262–266.
5. Swanson LN. Therapeutic value of *Aloe vera*. US Pharmacist 1995; 20:26–35.
6. Leung AY. Encyclopedia of Common Natural Ingredients Used in Food, Drugs, and Cosmetics. New York: John Wiley & Sons, 1980.
7. Blumenthal M. The Complete German Commission E Monographs: Therapeutic Guide to Herbal Medicine. Austin, TX: American Botanical Council, 1998.
8. Woo SW, Nan JX, Lee SH, Park EJ, Zhao YZ, Sohn DH. Aloe emodin suppresses myofibroblastic differentiation of rat hepatic stellate cells in primary culture. Pharmacol Toxicol 2002; 90:193–198.
9. Norikura T, Kennedy DO, Nyarko AF, Kojima A, Matsui YI. Protective effect of aloe extract against the cytotoxicity of 1,4-naphthoquinone in isolated rat hepatocytes involves modulations in cellular thiol levels. Pharmacol Toxicol 2002; 90:278–284.

10. Maze G, Terpolilli RN, Lee M. *Aloe vera* extract prevents aspirin-induced acute gastric mucosal injury in rats. Med Sci Res 1997; 25:765–766.
11. Teruaki A, Che QM, Kobashi K, Hattori M, Namba T. A purgative action of barbaloin is induced by *Eubacterium* sp. strain BAR, a human intestinal anaerobe, capable of transforming barbaloin to aloe-emodin anthrone. Biol Pharm Bull 1996; 19:136–138.
12. Lang W. Pharmacokinetic-metabolic studies with ^{14}C-aloe emodin after oral administration to male and female rats. Pharmacology 1993; 47:110–119.
13. Yamazaki T, Matsushita Y, Kawashima K, Someya M, Nakajima Y, Kurashige T. Evaluation of the pharmacological activity of extracts from amomi semen on the gastrointestinal tracts. J Ethnopharmacol 2000; 71:331–335.
14. Sakai K, Miyazaki Y, Yamane T, Saitoh Y, Ikawa C, Nishihata T. Effect of extracts of Zingiberaceae herbs on gastric secretion in rabbits. Chem Pharm Bull 1989; 37:215–217.
15. Okugawa H, Moriyasu M, Saiki K, Kato A, Matsumoto K, Fujioka A, Hashimoto Y. Evaluation of crude drugs by a combination of enfleurage and chromatography. III. Flavour components in seeds of *Amomum xanthioides, Alpinia Katsumadai* and *Amomum Tsao Ko*. Shoyakugaku Zasshi 1987; 41:108–115.
16. Yu BY, Mei QC, Wang HM, Wu JJ, Xu GJ. Comparative studies on bioactivities of the resources plants of *Fructus amoni*. J Plant Res Environ 1993; 2:18–21.
17. Iseki K, Ishikawa H, Suzuki T, Murakami T, Otani T, Ishiguro S. Melanosis coli associated with ingestion of bamboo leaf extract. Gastrointest Endosc 1998; 47:305–307.
18. Benavente-Garcia O, Castillo J, del Rio Conesa AJ. Changes in neodiosmin levels during the development of *Citrus aurantium* leaves and fruits: postulation of a neodiosmin biosynthetic pathway. J Agric Food Chem 1993; 41:1916–1919.
19. Kim DH, Song MJ, Bae EA, Han MJ. Inhibitory effect of herbal medicines on rotavirus infectivity. Biol Pharm Bull (Jpn) 2000; 23:356–358.
20. Han DI, Hwang BY, Hwang SY, Park JH, Son KH, Lee SH, Chang SY, Kang SJ, Ro JS, Lee KS, Lee KS. Isolation and quantitative analysis of hesperidin from *Aurantii fructus*. Korean J Pharmacogn 2001; 32:93–97.
21. Lee, et al. Isolation and quantitative analysis of hesperidin from *Aurantii fructus*. Korean J Pharmacogn 2001; 32:93–97.
22. Matev M, Chakurski I, Stefanov G, Koichev A, Angelov I. Use of an herbal combination with laxative action on duodenal peptic ulcer and gastroduodenitis patients with a concomitant obstipation syndrome. Vutreshni bolesti (Bulgaria) 1981; 20:48–51.
23. Di Marco MP, Edvards DJ, Wainer IW, Ducharme MP. The effect of grapefruit juice and seville orange juice on the pharmakinetics of dextromethorphan: the role of gut CYP3A and P-glycoprotein. Life Sci 2002; 71:1149–1160.

24. Dugo P, Mondello L, Cogliandro E, Verzera A, Dugo G. On the genuineness of citrus essential oils. 51. Oxygen heterocyclic compounds of bitter orange oil (*Citrus aurantium* L.). J Agric Food Chem 1996; 44:544–549.
25. Miyazawa M, Okuno Y, Fukuyama M, Nakamura S, Kosaka H. Antimutagenic activity of polymethoxyflavonoids from *Citrus aurantium*. J Agric Food Chem 1999; 47:5239–5244.
26. Vinson JA, Hu SJ, Jung S, Stanski AM. A citrus extract plus ascorbic acid decreases lipids, lipid peroxides, lipoprotein oxidative susceptibility, and atherosclerosis in hypercholesterolemic hamsters. J Agric Food Chem 1998; 46: 1453–1459.
27. Carnat A, Carnat AP, Fraisse D, Lamaison JL. Note technique. Standardisation de la fleur et de la feuille d'oranger amer. Ann Pharm Fr 1999; 57:410–414.
28. Colker CM, Kalman D, Torina GC, Perlis T, Street C. Effects of *Citrus aurantium* extract, caffeine, and St. John's wort on body fat loss, lipid levels, and mood states in overweight healthy adults. Curr Ther Res 1999; 60:145–153.
29. Calapai G, Firenzuoli F, Saitta A, Squadrito F, Arlotta MR, Costantino G, Inferrera G. Antiobesity and cardiovascular toxic effects of *Citrus aurantium* extracts in the rat: a preliminary report. Fitoterapia 1999; 70:586–592.
30. Calvarano I. Contributo all'indagine analitica strumentale dell'essenza di arancio amaro. Essenz Deriv Agrum 1966; 36:5–25.
31. Chidume FC, Kwanashie HO, Adekeye JO, Wambebe C, Gamaniel KS. Antinociceptive and smooth muscle contracting activities of the methanolic extract of *Cassia tora* leaf. J Ethnopharmacol 2002; 81:205–209.
32. Yen GC, Chen HW, Duh PD. Extraction and identification of an antioxidative component from jue ming zi (*Cassia tora* L.). J Agric Food Chem 1998; 46:820–824.
33. Vadivel V, Janardhanan K. Agrobotanical traits and chemical composition of *Cassia obtusifolia* L.: a lesser-known legume of the Western Ghats region of South India. Plant Foods Hum Nutr 2002; 57:151–164.
34. Voss KA, Brennecke LH. Toxicological and hematological effects of sicklepod (*Cassia obtusifolia*) seeds in Sprague-Dawley rats: a subchronic feeding study. Official J Int Soc Toxicol 1991; 29:1329–1336.
35. Pool-Zobel B, van Loo J, Rowland I, Roberfroid MB. Experimental evidences on the potential of prebiotic fructans to reduce the risk of colon cancer. Br J Nutr 2002; 87:273–281.
36. Kim MH. The water-soluble extract of chicory reduces cholesterol uptake in gut-perfused rats. Nutr Res 2000; 20:1017–1026.
37. Kim MH, Shin HK. The water-soluble extract of chicory reduces glucose uptake from the perfused jejunum in rats. J Nutr 1996; 126:2236–2242.
38. Hond ED, Geypens B, Ghoos Y. Effect of high performance chicory inulin on constipation. Nutr Res 2000; 20:731–736.
39. Russell TJ. The effect of natural source of non-digestible oligosaccharides on the fecal microflora of the dog and effects on digestion. Friskies PetCare 1998; 19.

40. Zhang W, Jia W, Li S, Zhang J, Qu Y, Xu X. Chinese Medicated Diet. Shanghai, China: Publishing House of Shanghai College of Traditional Chinese Medicine, 1988.
41. Wang SG, Wu XZ. Analysis of nutrient components of Chinese yam in Anshun of Guizhou Province. J Mountain Agric Biol 2001; 20:191–195.
42. Hang YY, Qin HZ, Ding ZZ. A survey and quality research on the new resources of Shan Yao (*Rhizoma dioscoreae*). J Plant Resources Environ 1992; 1:10–15.
43. China Pharmacopoea (State Pharmarcopoea Committee Eds) Chemical Industry Publishing House, Beijing 2000.
44. Wang HK, Xia Y, Yang ZY, Natschke SL, Lee KH. Recent advances in the discovery and development of flavonoids and their analogues as antitumor and anti-HIV agents. Adv Exp Med Biol 1998; 439:191–225.
45. Hu CQ, Chen K. Anti-AIDS agents, Acacetin-7-O-β-D-galactopyranoside, an anti-HIV principle from *Chrysanthemum morifolium* and a structure-activity correlation with some related flavonoids. J Nat Prod 1994; 57:42–51.
46. Lee HS, Ahn YJ. Growth-inhibiting effects of *Cinnamomum cassia* bark-derived materials on human intestinal bacteria. J Agric Food Chem 1998; 46:8–12.
47. Zhu ZP, Zhang MF, Shen YQ, Chen GJ. Pharmacological study on spleen-stomach warming and analgesic action of *Cinnamomum cassia*. Presl China J Chinese Mater Med 1993; 18:553–557.
48. Kwon BM, Cho YK, Lee SH, Nam JY, Bok SH, Chun SK, Kim JA, Lee IR. 2′-Hydroxycinnamaldehyde from stem bark of *Cinnamomum cassia*. Planta Med 1996; 62:183–184.
49. Zheng GQ, Kenney PM, Lam LK. Sesquiterpenes from clove (*Eugenia caryophyllata*) as potential anticarcinogenic agents. J Nat Prod 1992; 55:999–1003.
50. Vijayalakshmi R, Quadri SSYH, Deosthale YG. Effect of eugenol on gastric function in rats. J Clin Biochem Nutr 1991; 10:161–170.
51. Toda M, Kawabata J, Kasai T. Inhibitory effects of ellagi- and gallotannins on rat intestinal α-glucosidase complexes. Biosci Biotechnol Biochem 2001; 65: 542–547.
52. Toda M, Kawabata J, Kasai T. α-Glucosidase inhibitors from clove (*Syzgium aromaticum*). Biosci Biotechnol Biochem 2000; 64:294–298.
53. Kreydiyyeh SI, Usta J, Copti R. Effect of cinnamon, clove and some of their constituents on the Na^{+}-K^{+}-ATPase activity and alanine absorption in the rat jejunum. Food Chem Toxicol 2000; 38:755–762.
54. Platel K, Srinivasan K. A study of the digestive stimulant action of select spices in experimental rats. J Food Sci Technol (Mysore) 2001; 38:358–361.
55. Platel, Srinivasan. Stimulatory influence of select spices on bile secretion in rats. Nutr Res 2000; 20:1493–1503.
56. Micklefield GH, Redeker Y, Meister V, Jung O, Greving I, May B. Effects of ginger on gastroduodenal motility. Int J Clin Pharmacol Ther 1999; 37:341–346.
57. Surh YJ. Molecular mechanisms of chemopreventive effects of selected dietary and medicinal phenolic substances. Mutat Res 1999; 428:305–327.

58. Haslam E. Natural polyphenols (vegetable tannins) as drugs: possible modes of action. J Nat Prod 1996; 59:205–215.
59. Suleyman H, Demirezer LO, Buyukokuroglu ME, Akcay MF, Gepdiremen A, Banoglu ZN, Gocer F. Antiulcerogenic effect of *Hippophae rhamnoides* L. Phytother Res 2001; 15:625–627.
60. Cheng TJ, Sai Ram M, Singh V, Ilavazhagan G, Sawhney RC. Protective action of seed oil of *Hippophae rhamnoides* L. (HR) against experimental liver injury in mice. Zhonghua Yu Fang Yi Xue Za Zhi 1992; 26:227–229.
61. Wang Y, Lu Y, Liu X, Gou Z, Hu J. The protective effect of *Hippophae rhamnoides* L. on hyperlipidemic serum cultured smooth muscle cells in vitro. Zhongguo Zhong Yao Za Zhi 1992; 17:624–626.
62. Geetha S, Sai Ram M, Singh V, Ilavazhagan G, Sawhney RC. Anti-oxidant and immunomodulatory properties of seabuckthorn (*Hippophae rhamnoides*)–an in vitro study. J Ethnopharmacol 2002; 79:373–378.
63. Goel HC, Prasad J, Singh S, Sagar RK, Kumar IP, Sinha AK. Radioprotection by a herbal preparation of *Hippophae rhamnoides*, RH-3, against whole body lethal irradiation in mice. Phytomedicine 2002; 9:15–25.
64. Kumar IP, Namita S, Goel HC. Modulation of chromatin organization by RH-3, a preparation of *Hippophae rhamnoides*, a possible role in radioprotection. Mol Cell Biochem 238:1–9.
65. Yu XY. Blockage of *Glyrrhiza uralensis* and *Chelidonium majus* in MNNG induced cancer and mutagenesis. Zhonghua Yu Fang Yi Xue Za Zhi 1992; 26: 165–167.
66. Chen XG, Han R. Effect of glycyrrhetinic acid on DNA damage and unscheduled DNA synthesis induced by benzo (a) pyrene. Yao Xue Xue Bao 1994; 29:725–729.
67. Fu N, Liu Z, Zhang R. Anti-promoting and anti-mutagenic actions of G9315. Zhongguo Yi Xue Ke Xue Yuan Xue Bao 1995; 17:349–352.
68. Ma J, Peng W, Liang D. Apoptosis of human gastric cancer cell line MGC-803 induced by *Glycyrrhiza uralensis* extract. Zhongguo Zhong Xi Yi Jie He Za Zhi 2000; 20:928–930.
69. Ma J, Fu NY, Pang DB, Wu WY, Xu AL. Apoptosis induced by isoliquiritigenin in human gastric cancer MGC-803 cells. Planta Med 2001; 67:754–757.
70. Yu XY. A prospective clinical study on reversion of 200 precancerous patients with hua-sheng-ping. Zhongguo Zhong Xi Yi Jie He Za Zhi 1993; 13:147–149.
71. Wang ZY, Nixon DW. Licorice and cancer. Nutr Cancer 2001; 39:1–11.
72. Onogi N, Okuno M, Komaki C, Moriwaki H, Kawamori T, Tanaka T, Mori H, Muto Y. Suppressing effect of perilla oil on azoxymethane-induced foci of colonic aberrant crypts in rats. Carcinogenesis 1996; 17:1291–1296.
73. Narisawa T, Fukaura Y, Yazawa K, Ishikawa C, Isoda Y, Nishizawa Y. Colon cancer prevention with a small amount of dietary perilla oil high in alpha-linolenic acid in an animal model. Cancer 1994; 73:2069–2075.
74. Narisawa T, Takahashi M, Kotanagi H, Kusaka H, Yamazaki Y, Koyama H, Fukaura Y, Nishizawa Y, Kotsugai M, Isoda Y. Inhibitory effect of dietary

perilla oil rich in the n-3 polyunsaturated fatty acid α-linolenic acid on colon carcinogenesis in rats. Jpn J Cancer Res 1991; 82:1089–1096.

75. Xia Q, Xiao P, Wan L, Kong J. Ethnopharmacology of *Phyllanthus emblica* L. Zhongguo Zhong Yao Za Zhi 1997; 22:515–518.
76. Dhir H, Agarwal K, Sharma A, Talukder G. Modifying role of *Phyllanthus emblica* and ascorbic acid against nickel clastogenicity in mice. Cancer Lett 1991; 59:9–18.
77. Jeena KJ, Joy KL, Kuttan R. Effect of *Emblica officinalis*, *Phyllanthus amarus* and *Picrorrhiza kurroa* on *N*-nitrosodiethylamine induced hepatocarcinogenesis. Cancer Lett 1999; 136:11–16.
78. Suresh K, Vasudevan DM. Augmentation of murine natural killer cell and antibody dependent cellular cytotoxicity activities by *Phyllanthus emblica*, a new immunomodulator. J Ethnopharmacol 1994; 44:55–60.
79. Ukiya M, Akihisa T, Tokuda H, Hirano M, Oshikubo M, Nobukuni Y, Kimura Y, Tai T, Kondo S, Nishino H. Inhibition of tumor-promoting effects by poricoic acids G and H and other lanostane-type triterpenes and cytotoxic activity of poricoic acids A and G from *Poria cocos*. J Nat Prod 2002; 65:462–465.
80. Kaminaga T, Yasukawa K, Kanno H, Tai T, Nunoura Y, Takido M. Inhibitory effects of lanostane-type triterpene acids, the components of *Poria cocos*, on tumor promotion by 12-O-tetradecanoylphorbol-13-acetate in two-stage carcinogenesis in mouse skin. Oncology 1996; 53:382–385.
81. Yu SJ, Tseng J. Fu-Ling, a Chinese herbal drug, modulates cytokine secretion by human peripheral blood monocytes. Int J Immunopharmacol 1996; 18:37–44.
82. Kanayama H, Togami M, Adachi N, Fukai Y, Okumoto T. Studies on the antitumor active polysaccharides from the mycelia of *Poria cocos* Wolf. III. Antitumor activity against mouse tumors. Yakugaku Zasshi 1986; 106:307–312.
83. Sakamoto S, Kudo H, Kuwa K, Suzuki S, Kato T, Kawasaki T, Nakayama T, Kasahara N, Okamoto R. Anticancer effects of a Chinese herbal medicine, juzen-taiho-to, in combination with or without 5-fluorouracil derivative on DNA-synthesizing enzymes in 1,2-dimethylhydrazine induced colonic cancer in rats. Am J Chinese Med 1991; 19:233–241.
84. Wu Y, Zhang Y, Wu JA, Lowell T, Gu M, Yuan CS. Effects of Erkang, a modified formulation of Chinese folk medicine Shi-Quan-Da-Bu-Tang, on mice. J Ethnopharmacol 1998; 61:153–159.
85. Zee-Cheng RK. Shi-quan-da-bu-tang (ten significant tonic decoction), SQT: a potent Chinese biological response modifier in cancer immunotherapy, potentiation and detoxification of anticancer drugs. Methods Find Exp Clin Pharmacol 1992; 14:725–736.
86. Park JH, Cho CH, Yun SJ. Microscopic identification of Jeong Dan Whan. Ko- rean J Pharmacognosy 2002; 33:53–56.
87. Li GP, Huang CH. Effects of Chinese medical herbs on controlling piglet early weaning diarrhoea. Chinese J Vet Sci 2002; 22:65–67.

88. Kang JK, Bae HS, Kim YS, Cho KH, Lee KS, Park EK, Kim DH. Antithrombosis of Chungpesagan-tang is activated by human intestinal bacteria. Nat Prod Sci 2001; 7:53–59.
89. Sheu SJ, Lu CF. Determination of six bioactive components of hsiao-cheng-chi-tang by capillary electrophoresis. J High Resolut Chromatogr 1995; 18:269–270.
90. Walle UK, Walle T. Induction of human UDP-glucuronosyltransferase UGT1A1 by flavonoids—structural requirements. Drug Metab Dispos 2002; 30:564–569.
91. Doostdar H, Burke MD, Mayer RT. Bioflavonoids: selective substrates and inhibitors for cytochrome P450 CYP1A and CYP1B1. Toxicology 2000; 144:31–38.
92. Kawai S, Tomono Y, Katase E, Ogawa K, Yano M. Effect of citrus flavonoids on HL-60 cell differentiation. Anticancer Res 1999; 19:1261–1269.
93. Boege F, Straub T, Kehr A, Boesenberg C, Christiansen K, Andersen A, et al. Selected novel flavones inhibit the DNA binding or the DNA religation step of eukaryotic topoisomerase I. J Biol Chem 1996; 271:2262–2270.
94. Chae YH, Ho DK, Cassady JM, Cook VM, Marcus CB, Baird WM. Effects of synthetic and naturally occurring flavonoids on metabolic activation of benzo[a]pyrene in hamster embryo cell cultures. Chem Biol Interact 1992; 82: 181–193.
95. Lee C, Kim H, Kho Y. Agastinol and agastenol, novel lignans from *Agastache rugosa* and their evaluation in an apoptosis inhibition assay. J Nat Prod 2002; 65:414–416.
96. Ghelardini C, Galeotti N, Mazzanti G. Local anaesthetic activity of monoterpenes and phenylpropanes of essential oils. Planta Med 2001; 67:564–566.
97. De M, De AK, Sen P, Banerjee AB. Antimicrobial properties of star anise (*Illicium verum* Hook f). Phytother Res 2002; 16:94–95.
98. Abraham SK. Anti-genotoxicity of trans-anethole and eugenol in mice. Food Chem Toxicol 2001; 39:493–498.
99. Chainy GB, Manna SK, Chaturvedi MM, Aggarwal BB. Anethole blocks both early and late cellular responses transduced by tumor necrosis factor: effect on NF-kappaB, AP-1, JNK, MAPKK and apoptosis. Oncogene 2000; 19:2943–2950.
100. Rompelberg CJ, Verhagen H, van Bladeren PJ. Effects of the naturally occurring alkenylbenzenes eugenol and trans- anethole on drug-metabolizing enzymes in the rat liver 76. Food Chem Toxicol 1993; 31:637–645.
101. Shafi PM, Rosamma MK, Jamil K, Reddy PS. Antibacterial activity of the essential oil from *Aristolochia indica*. Fitoterapia 2002; 73:439–441.
102. Tambe Y, Tsujiuchi H, Honda G, Ikeshiro Y, Tanaka S. Gastric cytoprotection of the non-steroidal anti-inflammatory sesquiterpene, beta-caryophyllene. Plan- ta Med 1996; 62:469–470.
103. Kubo I, Chaudhuri SK, Kubo Y, Sanchez Y, Ogura T, Saito T, et al. Cytotoxic and antioxidative sesquiterpenoids from *Heterotheca inuloides*. Planta Med 1996; 62:427–430.

104. Mori H, Kawabata K, Matsunaga K, Ushida J, Fujii K, Hara A, et al. Chemopreventive effects of coffee bean and rice constituents on colorectal carcinogenesis. Biofactors 2000; 12:101–105.
105. Agarwal SK, Singh SS, Verma S, Kumar S. Antifungal activity of anthraquinone derivatives from *Rheum emodi*. J Ethnopharmacol 2000; 72:43–46.
106. Sun MZ, Sakakibara H, Ashida H, Danno G, Kanazawa K. Cytochrome P4501A1—inhibitory action of antimutagenic anthraquinones in medicinal plants and the structure-activity relationship. Biosci Biotechnol Biochem 2000; 64:1373–1378.
107. Kim DH, Park EK, Bae EA, Han MJ. Metabolism of rhaponticin and chrysophanol 8-o-β-D-glucopyranoside from the rhizome of *Rheum undulatum* by human intestinal bacteria and their anti-allergic actions. Biol Pharm Bull 2000; 23:830–833.
108. Friedman M, Henika PR, Mandrell RE. Bactericidal activities of plant essential oils and some of their isolated constituents against *Campylobacter jejuni*, *Escherichia coli*, *Listeria monocytogenes*, and *Salmonella enterica*. J Food Protect 2002; 65:1545–1560.
109. Koh WS, Yoon SY, Kwon BM, Jeong TC, Nam KS, Han MY. Cinnamaldehyde inhibits lymphocyte proliferation and modulates T-cell differentiation. Int J Immunopharmacol 1998; 20:643–660.
110. Chang CH, Lin CC, Yang JJ, Namba T, Hattori M. Anti-inflammatory effects of emodin from ventilago leiocarpa. Am J Chinese Med 1996; 24:139–142.
111. Lang W. Pharmacokinetic-metabolic studies with 14C-aloe emodin after oral administration to male and female rats. Pharmacology 1993; 47:110–119.
112. Su HY, Cherng SH, Chen CC, Lee H. Emodin inhibits the mutagenicity and DNA adducts induced by 1- nitropyrene. Mutat Res 1995; 329:205–212.
113. Zhang L, Lau YK, Xi L, Hong RL, Kim DS, Chen CF, et al. Tyrosine kinase inhibitors, emodin and its derivative repress HER-2/neu- induced cellular transformation and metastasis-associated properties. Oncogene 1998; 16:2855–2863.
114. Kumar A, Dhawan S, Aggarwal BB. Emodin (3-methyl-1,6,8-trihydroxyanthraquinone) inhibits TNF-induced NF- kappaB activation, IkappaB degradation, and expression of cell surface adhesion proteins in human vascular endothelial cells. Oncogene 1998; 17:913–918.
114a. Yim H, Lee YH, Lee CH, Lee SK. Emodin, an anthraquinone derivative isolated from the rhizomes of *Rheum palmatum*, selectively inhibits the activity of casein kinase II as a competitive inhibitor. Planta Med 1999; 65:9–13.
115. Lee JJ, Park KH, Yu HG, Lee J, Kang SG, Yoo YD, et al. Antiproliferative effect of 2′-benzoxy-cinnamaldehyde on cultured human retinal pigment epithelial cells in vitro and safety of intravitreal 2′-benzoxy-cinnamaldehyde on rabbit eyes in vivo. Invest Ophthalmol Vis Sci 2001; 42:4351.
116. Wang HW, Chen TL, Yang PC, Ueng TH. Induction of cytochromes P450 1A1 and 1B1 by emodin in human lung adenocarcinoma cell line CL5. Drug Metab Dispos 2001; 29:1229–1235.
117. Cheng YW, Kang JJ. Emodin-induced muscle contraction of mouse

diaphragm and the involvement of Ca^{2+} influx and Ca^{2+} release from sarcoplasmic reticulum. Br J Pharmacol 1998; 123:815–820.
118. Chung DC. The genetic basis of colorectal cancer: insights into critical pathways of tumorigenesis. Gastroenterology 2000; 119:854–865.
119. Ishiwata S, Nakashita K, Ozawa Y, Niizeki M, Nozaki S, Tomioka Y, et al. Fas-mediated apoptosis is enhanced by glycyrrhizin without alteration of caspase-3-like activity. Biol Pharm Bull 1999; 22:1163–1166.
120. Tanaka T, Kohno H, Murakami M, Shimada R, Kagami S, Sumida T, et al. Suppression of azoxymethane-induced colon carcinogenesis in male F344 rats by mandarin juices rich in beta-cryptoxanthin and hesperidin. Int J Cancer 2000; 88:146–150.
121. Koyuncu H, Berkarda B, Baykut F, Soybir G, Alatli C, Gul H, et al. Preventive effect of hesperidin against inflammation in CD-1 mouse skin caused by tumor promoter. Anticancer Res 1999; 19:3237–3241.
122. Yang MZ, Tanaka T, Hirose Y, Deguchi T, Mori H, Kawada Y. Chemopreventive effects of diosmin and hesperidin on *N*-butyl-*N*-(4-hydroxybutyl)nitrosamine-induced urinary-bladder carcinogenesis in male icr mice. Int J Cancer 1997; 73:719–724.
123. Tanaka T, Makita H, Kawabata K, Mori H, Kakumoto M, Satoh K, et al. Modulation of *N*-methyl-*N*-amylnitrosamine-induced rat oesophageal tumourigenesis by dietary feeding of diosmin and hesperidin, both alone and in combination. Carcinogenesis 1997; 18:761–769.
124. Bouaziz N, Michiels C, Janssens D, Berna N, Eliaers F, Panconi E, et al. Effect of Ruscus extract and hesperidin methylchalcone on hypoxia-induced activation of endothelial cells. Int Angiol 1999; 18:306–312.
125. Brum LFS, Emanuelli T, Souza DO, Elisabetsky E. Effects of linalool on glutamate release and uptake in mouse cortical synaptosomes. Neurochem Res 2001; 26:191–194.
126. Re L, Barocci S, Sonnino S, Mencarelli A, Vivani C, Paolucci G, et al. Linalool modifies the nicotinic receptor-ion channel kinetics at the mouse neuromuscular junction. Pharmacol Res 2000; 42:177–181.
127. Sugawara Y, Hara C, Tamura K, Fujii T, Nakamura K, Masujima T, et al. Sedative effect on humans of inhalation of essential oil of linalool: sensory evaluation and physiological measurements using optically active linalools. Anal Chim Acta 1998; 365:293–299.
128. Minagawa A, Otani Y, Kubota T, Wada N, Furukawa T, Kumai K, et al. The citrus flavonoid, nobiletin, inhibits peritoneal dissemination of human gastric carcinoma in SCID mice. Jpn J Cancer Res 2001; 92:1322–1328.
129. Takase H, Yamamoto K, Hirano H, Saito Y, Yamashita A. Pharmacological profile of gastric mucosal protection by marmin and nobiletin from a traditional herbal medicine, *Aurantii fructus immaturus*. Jpn J Pharmacol 1994; 66:139–147.
130. Kohno H, Taima M, Sumida T, Azuma Y, Ogawa H, Tanaka T. Inhibitory effect of mandarin juice rich in beta-cryptoxanthin and hesperidin on 4-(methylnitrosamino)-1-(3- pyridyl)-1-butanone-induced pulmonary tumorigenesis in mice. Cancer Lett 2001; 174:141–150.

131. Raimondi F, Santoro P, Maiuri L, Londei M, Annunziata S, Ciccimarra F, et al. Reactive nitrogen species modulate the effects of rhein, an active component of senna laxatives, on human epithelium in vitro. J Pediatr Gastroenterol Nutr 2002; 34:529–534.
132. Chung JG, Tsou MF, Wang HH, Lo HH, Hsieh SE, Yen YS, et al. Rhein affects arylamine *N*-acetyltransferase activity in *Helicobacter pylori* from peptic ulcer patients. J Appl Toxicol 1998; 18:117–123.
133. Nijs G, de Witte P, Geboes K, Meulemans A, Schuurkes J, Lemli J. In vitro demonstration of a positive effect of rhein anthrone on peristaltic reflex of guinea pig ileum. Pharmacology 1993; 47:40–48.
134. Castiglione S, Fanciulli M, Bruno T, Evangelista M, Del Carlo C, Paggi MG, et al. Rhein inhibits glucose uptake in Ehrlich ascites tumor cells by alteration of membrane-associated functions. Anticancer Drugs 1993; 4:407–414.
135. Nijs G, de Witte P, Geboes K, Lemli J. Influence of rhein anthrone and rhein on small intestine transit rate in rats: evidence of prostaglandin mediation. Eur J Pharmacol 1992; 218:199–203.
136. van Gorkom BA, Timmer-Bosscha H, de Jong S, van der Kolk DM, Kleibeuker JH, de Vries EG. Cytotoxicity of rhein, the active metabolite of sennoside laxatives, is reduced by multidrug resistance-associated protein. Br J Cancer 2002; 86:1494–1500.
137. Debersac P, Vernevaut MF, Amiot MJ, Suschetet M, Siess MH. Effects of a water-soluble extract of rosemary and its purified component rosmarinic acid on xenobiotic-metabolizing enzymes in rat liver. Food Chem Toxicol 2001; 39:109–117.
138. Makino T, Ono T, Muso E, Yoshida H, Honda G, Sasayama S. Inhibitory effects of rosmarinic acid on the proliferation of cultured murine mesangial cells. Nephrol Dial Transplant 2000; 15:1140–1145.
138a. Osakabe N, Yasuda A, Natsume M, Sanbongi C, Kato Y, Osawa T, Yoshikawa T. Rosmarinic acid, a major polyphenolic component of *Perilla frutescens*, reduces lipopolysaccharide (LPS)-induced liver injury in D-galactosamine (D-GalN)-sensitized mice. Free Radic Biol Med 2002; 33:798–806.
139. Takeda H, Tsuji M, Inazu M, Egashira T, Matsumiya T. Rosmarinic acid and caffeic acid produce antidepressive-like effect in the forced swimming test in mice. Eur J Pharmacol 2002; 449:261–267.
140. Bracke ME, Boterberg T, Depypere HT, Stove C, Leclercq G, Mareel MM. The citrus methoxyflavone tangeretin affects human cell-cell interactions. Flavonoids Cell Funct 2002; 505:135–139.
141. Datla KP, Christidou M, Widmer WW, Rooprai HK, Dexter DT. Tissue distribution and neuroprotective effects of citrus flavonoid tangeretin in a rat model of Parkinson's disease. Neuroreport 2001; 12:3871–3875.
142. Liu GW, Cao LY. Chinese Herbal Medicine. Clinical Essentials of Contemporary Series of Chinese Medicine. Beijing, China: Hua Xia Publishing House, 2000.

6

Tea and Health

John H. Weisburger
American Health Foundation
Valhalla, New York, U.S.A.

I. MAIN CAUSES OF CHRONIC DISEASES

A. Reactive Oxygen Species

Living cells require oxygen to generate energy and to develop fully. However, under some circumstances cells generate from oxygen reactive oxygen species (ROS) in the form of reactive entities such as hydrogen peroxide and especially hazardous oxygen radicals (1–3).

B. Mechanisms in Cancer

Reliable and easy methods are available to determine the effect of ROS and reactive nitrogen compounds by HPLS-MS/MS analysis, especially as regards attacks on macromolecules such as DNA (4). In cancer research, we distinguish between agents that modify the DNA and generate a mutation. Such materials or synthetic chemicals are called mutagenic and genotoxic. There are chemicals or situations that enhance the development and growth of cells exposed to genotoxins. It is important to discriminate between these two classes of chemicals based on the permanence of their effect, and the doses and chronicity of exposure (5).

C. Heterocyclic Aromatic Amines

About 25 years ago, Sugimura, at the National Cancer Center, after frying or broiling of meat and fish showed that the surface of brown meat contained powerful mutagens (6). Such cooking-derived mutagens were shown to belong to a new class of carcinogens, the heterocyclic aromatic amines (HCA). When they were ingested, such chemicals also generated ROS, and damaged cells through a classic reaction of metabolically formed reactive compounds, such an acetoxy-HCA or a sulfonoxy-HCA, that modify cellular DNA in target organs. Hence, these metabolites and simultaneously formed ROS are involved in adverse effects in the development of early neoplastic cells, and also through a cellular toxic reaction, in which the cells respond by attempts to repair, leading to cell regeneration and duplication, and thus, leading to abnormal cells with an altered DNA, typical of an early cancer cell. A recent international conference updated the latest facts in the field (7).

D. Salt

Salt does not damage DNA and is not genotoxic. However, importantly, it severely impinges on the stability of cell, and cells exposed to high levels of salt undergo rapid cell duplication. Therefore, there is severe damage to the stomach with possible alteration, especially in the tissue also generating ROS and carrying a bacterium discovered in 1984, *Helicobacter pylori* (reviewed in ref. 8). Eventually, stomach cancer and possibly ulcers stem from excessive salt intake in infected cells (9). Through tradition in Japan and parts of China, people used as much as 30 g of salt per day. The Japanese have instituted a plan to progressively lower salt intake and currently, the amount consumed is about 12 g. However, only about 3 g are needed to meet physiological sodium needs.

II. TEA AS A HEALTH-PROMOTING BEVERAGE

Tea is a frequently used beverage worldwide. Tea is a hot-water extract of the leaves of the plant *Camellia sinensis*. Upon harvest, the best teas are obtained by collecting the top two leaves and the bud of the tea bush (10,11). The leaves contain the polyphenol epigallocatechin gallate and an enzyme, polyphenol oxidase. When the leaves are withered and steamed, the polyphenol oxidase is inactivated, yielding green tea upon drying. If the withering step is omitted, and the leaves are steamed, the ground product is white tea, commercially available but not used frequently. Upon more elaborate processing, crushing the leaves and incubating for about 60 min, the polyphenol oxidase converts the polyphenol to other polyphenols, such as theaflavin and thearubigin, typical of black tea (Fig. 1) (Table 1). With a lesser time of incubation, such as

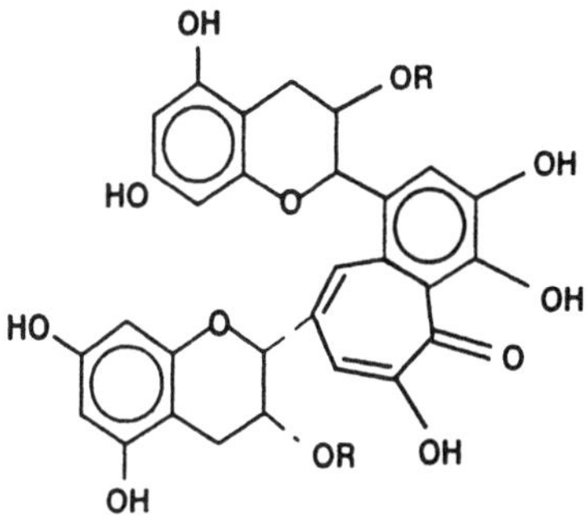

Theaflavin gallates

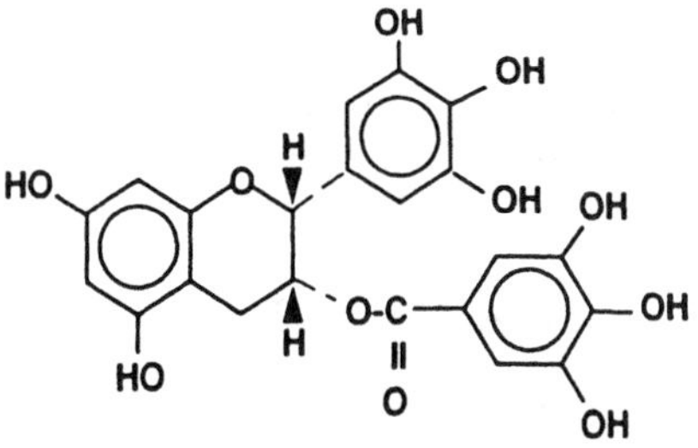

(-)-Epigallocatechin gallate

FIGURE 1 The main polyphenol in green tea is (−)-epigallocatechin gallate (EgCg) (right), which accounts usually for about 30% of the dry weight of the tea leaf. The tea leaf contains an enzyme, polyphenol oxidase, that is deactivated when the withered, macerated tea leaves are heated by steam or in a pan, yielding a product containing mainly EgCg. However, when the cut, macerated, or "rolled" leaves are transported in a moving band surrounded by warm 40°C air, the enzyme-mediated oxidation (wrongly called fermentation) occurs. One popular method of production is "crushing, tearing, curling, named CTC." Partial oxidation for about 30 min yields oolong tea. Full biochemical oxidation, which requires 90–120 min, yields black tea, containing some theaflavin (left), more complex thearubigins, and also theanine, which account, in part, for the flavor of black tea. Since the original tea leaf contains caffeine, green, oolong, and black teas contain caffeine in the amount of 40–50 mg in a 125–150-mL tea cup, made with a 2.25-g tea bag.

TABLE 1 Composition of Catechins in Polyphenols

	Percent by weight		
	Polyphenon 60	Polyphenon 100	Polyphenon B
(+)-Gallocatechin (+ GC)	—	1.4	
(−)-Epigallocatechin (EGC)	19.5	17.6	
(−)-Epicatechin (EC)	7.0	6.0	
(−)-Epigallocatechin gallate (EGCg)	29.0	54.0	
(−)-Epicatechin gallate (EGCg)	8.5	12.5	
Total catechins	64	91.5	2.8
Caffeine	12.0	0.5	0.6
Theaflavin			0.3
Thearubigins			96.3

Source: Refs. 10, 64.

about 25–35 min, an intermediate product, oolong tea, popular in southern China and in Taiwan, is obtained.

We have described the history of tea and its use worldwide, including the original discovery of tea in China some 4000 years ago, in the form of green tea, and later of black tea in northern India. Currently, green tea is used mainly in China, Japan, and North Africa (11).

A. Tea and Heart Disease Prevention

Epidemiological studies in Europe revealed that black tea drinkers had a lower incidence of heart disease (12–14). The underlying reason rests on the fact the tea polyphenols act as effective antioxidants that inhibit the oxidation of LDL cholesterol caused by reactive oxygen species, and lead to atherogenesis (15–19). In has been shown that the mechanism can be reproduced using a copper-catalyzed oxidation of LDL cholesterol, inhibited by tea polyphenols (Table 2) (20). Other investigations confirmed a lower risk of heart disease as a function of tea intake, both green and black tea (21). A

TABLE 2 Prevention of Oxidation of LDL-C by P60 and ML-1[a]

Group (n = 10)	Mean ± SE
1. Blank	0.0002 ± 0.0001
2. Control	0.3759 ± 0.0133
3. Low-dose P60A[b]	0.0154 ± 0.0026
4. High-dose P60A[c]	0.0127 ± 0.0018
5. Low-dose ML-1	0.0211 ± 0.0025
6. High-dose ML-1	0.0308 ± 0.0306

[a] MitoLife (ML) was a commercial product containing fruit juices, including green tea, the effect of which was compared to a positive control, polyphenon 60A, a polyphenol from green tea, provided by Dr. Hara, Tokyo (Table 3). Data represent absorbance at 532 nm. All groups (1, 3, 4, 5, and 6) compared to the control (LDL and cupric sulfate in buffer) were significant at $p < 0.0001$.
[b] Low-dose P60A (group 3) versus low-dose ML-1 (group 5) was significant. The low dose of P60A was 20 μM, or 1 mg, and the high dose was 40 μM, or 2 mg; with ML-1, the low dose was 1 μL, and the high dose 2 μL of a saturated solution of commercial MitoLife product.
[c] High-dose P60A (group 4) versus high-dose ML-1 (group 6) was significant at $p < 0.001$.
Source: Ref. 20.

meta-analysis of stroke and coronary heart disease "cardiovascular disease" evaluated the results of many studies and found that heart disease decreased 11% by intake of 3 cups (about 700 mL) of tea per day (22). In Japan, it was noted that the relative risk of cardiovascular disease and cancers was significantly lower with 10 cups of tea per day (23). Different approaches suggest that tea beneficially affects platelet aggregation and angiogenesis, a possible cause of heart attacks (23–29). The relevant mechanisms are complex, but may involve cell signaling that is involved in cell adhesion, migration, and clot formation in macrophages mediated by damaged LDL lipoprotein (25,26). Black and green tea were equally effective antioxidants (30). Tea had a more powerful effect, expressed as vitamin C equivalents, than the vegetables and fruits tested (31).

B. Tea and Cancer Prevention

Mutations of the cellular DNA are a key step leading to cancer (5). Mutational events can be used as markers for environmental genotoxic products that might be possible cancer risks (32). This approach is effective in research on products that might have antimutagenic and, thus, likely anticarcinogenic effects.

This method has been applied to study the effect of tea polyphenols from black tea and from green tea. It was found that both types of polyphenols decreased in a dose-related fashion the mutagenicity of different types of carcinogens (Table 3). In another series of bioassays, similar results were obtained, demonstrating the stability and reliability of these rapid tests in forecasting the chemopreventive potential of inhibitors such as tea extracts (Table 4) (33–35). Selenium potentiated the effect of green tea on the mutagenicity of 2-amino-3-methylimidazo-[4,5-f]quinoline (36). Parallel to the effects on DNA-reactive carcinogens, tea inhibited the formation of cancer of the colon and the mammary gland in rats (37–39). Even a low dose of tea was effective (Table 5) (37).

Cancer of the esophagus is decreased in animal models by tea (40), just as a lower risk is noted in parts of China of cancer of the esophagus in people who drink tea (41,42, reviewed also in Refs. 43,44). Similar results hold for oral cancer (45). There are more cigarette smokers in Japan than in the United States but the incidence of lung cancer in Japan is lower than in the United States, possibly because there are more tea drinkers in Japan, accounting for this protection. In parallel, mice and rats exposed to the tobacco-specific nitrosamines displayed a lower incidence of lung tumors when the animals were drinking tea (46). Even "spontaneous" lung tumors in mice were decreased by intake of black or green tea (47). The mechanism may depend on a reduction of oxidative stress (48). This inhibition by tea was due to lower

TABLE 3 Effect of Tea-Derived Polyphenols on Mutagenicity of Genotoxic Carcinogens

				Polyphenol, type and amount (mg)								
		S.t.[a] strain	Mutagenicity reference	60			100			B		
	μg/plate	TA	chemical	1[b]	2	3	1	2	3	1	2	3
2-Acetylaminofluorene	50	98	1196 ± 65[c]	340 ± 22[d]	113 ± 22	4.4 ± 2.5	149 ± 29	59 ± 13	7.4 ± 4.3	119 ± 17	77 ± 35	9.5 ± 5.5
2-Aminoanthracene	5	98	1865 ± 103	682 ± 123	245 ± 30	156 ± 14	620 ± 118	222 ± 48	95 ± 17	678 ± 125	245 ± 34	161 ± 17
2-Amino-3-methylimidazo-[4,5-f]-quinoline	0.0099	98	1849 ± 96	131 ± 39	0.3 ± 0.3	86 ± 86	48 ± 31	25 ± 6.2	15 ± 7.8	0 ± 0	0 ± 0	450 ± 17
2-amino-1-methyl-6-phyenlimidazo[4,5-b]-pyridine	2.3	98	1861 ± 74	277 ± 78	4.3 ± 2.6	18 ± 9	42 ± 16	17 ± 2.6	93 ± 25	482 ± 71	2.0 ± 2.0	0 ± 0
Benzidine	913	98	240 ± 24	25 ± 3.8	3 ± 2.1	6.3 ± 3.0	15 ± 3.5	4 ± 2.6	1 ± 0.3	22 ± 3.3	8 ± 2.4	2.7 ± 1.5
Aflatoxin B_1	1	98	154 ± 32	1.3 ± 1.3	4.0 ± 4.0	0 ± 0	1.3 ± 6.8	0 ± 0	8.7 ± 8.7	0 ± 0	1.3 ± 1.3	0 ± 0
Benzo[a]pyrene	5	100	341 ± 42	1.0 ± 1.0	4.0 ± 4.0	0 ± 0	0 ± 0	0 ± 0	0 ± 0	0 ± 0	0 ± 0	0 ± 0
1,2-Dibromoethane	188	100	368 ± 5.4	328 ± 5.4	320 ± 15.3	308 ± 12	293 ± 19	279 ± 9.5	227 ± 19	259 ± 8.3	250 ± 5.8	264 ± 10
2-Nitropropane	1336	100	319 ± 13	337 ± 13[e]	334 ± 9.2[e]	252 ± 26[e]	267 ± 7.0	246 ± 7.5	197 ± 2.7	247 ± 8.5	216 ± 5.1	234 ± 3.8
1-Nitropyrene	10	98	1423 ± 30	1320 ± 145[e]	1599 ± 112[e]	1814 ± 80[f]	1834 ± 105[e]	1793 ± 97[e]	1692 ± 99[e]	1837 ± 34[e]	1647 ± 117[e]	1674 ± 51[e]
2-Chloro-4-methylthio-butanoic acid[g]	16.8	1535	186 ± 21[g]	126 ± 9.8[e]	127 ± 8.7[e]	129 ± 6.7[e]	198 ± 5.5[e]	16 ± 9.6	179 ± 4.9[e]	225 ± 11[e]	183 ± 2.0[e]	209 ± 22[e]
N-Nitrosodimethylamine[h]	373	100	209 ± 11	21 ± 5.0	17 ± 11	13 ± 11	29 ± 14	16 ± 12	10 ± 2.5	68 ± 4.5	4 ± 3.5	0 ± 0
4-(*N*-Nitrosomethylamino)-1-[3-pyridyl]-1-butanone[h]	4098	100	215 ± 16	48 ± 3.5	24.0 ± 12	22 ± 4.5	25 ± 2.5	16 ± 2.5	19 ± 19	44 ± 2.0	2.5 ± 2.5	0 ± 0

[a]S.t.: *Salmonella typhimurium* strain for a given carcinogen; an S9 fraction from rat liver induced with β-naphthoflavone and phenobarbital was used in all tests, except as shown. The spontaneous revertants rate for *S. typhimurium* TA98 + S9 was 34 in DMSO (100 μL) or 32 in aqueous buffer; for TA 100 + S9 the rate was 134 in DMSO, and 124 in buffer. In all tests reported, the net values are shown, i.e., the gross data minus the appropriate background value, obtained in simultaneous determinations. Likewise, the three polyphenones (propriatory name of polyphenols) used gave background readings at the 3 dose levels used. Thus, in *S. typhimurium* TA98 + S9, polyphenon 60 gave gross readings of 30, 30, and 32 rev/plate at 1, 2, and 3 mg/plate, respectively. The corresponding values for polyphenon 100 were 45, 39, and 36 and for polyphenon B 33, 32, and 31. In *S. typhimurium* TA100 + S9, the values for 1, 3, and 3 mg polyphenon 60 were 114, 132, and 114, for polyphenon 100, 130, 114, and 108, and for polyphenon B, 124, 104, and 104. The bacterial lawn displayed no evidence of toxicity in the tests with the polyphenols alone, or in the inhibition assays involving each carcinogen and the three dose levels of the polyphenols.

[b]Polyphenols 60 and 100, from green tea, and polyphenol B, from black tea, were kind gifts from Dr. Y. Hara, Tokyo. Water solutions of the polyphenols were made by dissolving 1 g of a polyphenol in 20 mL H_2O, and using 20 μL (1 mg), 40 μL (2 mg), and 60 μL (3 mg).

[c]Revertants/plate, mean ± standard error; all tests were done in triplicate.

[d]All values were significantly different ($p \leq 0.05$) with added polyphenols, except where specifically shown.

[e]Not statistically different from mutagenicity without polyphenol.

[f]Significant ($p < 0.05$) increase over mutagenicity without polyphenol.

[g]Direct-acting mutagen; active without S9 fraction.

[h]The nitrosamines displayed no significant mutagenicity with an S9 fraction from induced rat liver; utilizing hamster liver S9 fraction at a fourfold level of protein nitrogen worked reliably in these inhibition experiments.

Source: Ref. 33.

TABLE 4 Effect of Green Tea Polyphenol P60A on the Mutagenicity of Reference Genotoxic Carcinogens[a]

Reference carcinogen	μg/plate	Mutagenicity ± SE	Carcinogen + polyphenon 60A (P60A)			
			20μL/1 mg	40 μL/2 mg	60 μL/3 mg	80 μL/4 mg
2-Acetylaminofluorene (AAF)	250	985 ± 41.0	153.5 ± 50.5[a]	17.5 ± 4.5[a]	15.5 ± 1.7[a]	10.0 ± 1.0[a]
2-Aminoanthracene (AA)	5	1936 ± 2.5	972 ± 59.5[a]	166 ± 66.0[a]	23.5 ± 6.5[a]	12.5 ± 1.5[a]
2-Amino-3-methylimidazo-[4,5-f]quinoline (IQ)	0.5	1983 ± 665	1765 ± 67.5	323 ± 43.0[a]	74.5 ± 25.5[a]	14.0 ± 8.0[a]
Aflatoxin B_1 (AFB_1)	10	1288 ± 121	73.5 ± 28.3[a]	8.0 ± 9.0[a]	7.5 ± 0.5[a]	2.0 ± 6.0[a]
Benzo[a]pyrene (BaP)	25	925 ± 88	242 ± 10.0[a]	51.5 ± 11.5[a]	5.0 ± 4.0[a]	0 ± 0.5[a]

[a] Mutagenicity in *Salmonella typhimurium* strain TA98 for AAF, AF, IQ, and AFB_1, and strain TA100 for BaP, p value of test versus revertants (rev)/plate with carcinogen $p < 0.05$ or better; dose-response trend $p < 0.04$ for AAF + P60A; trend $p < 0.008$ for AA + P60A; trend $p < 0.006$ for IQ + P60A; trend $p < 0.04$ for AFB_1 + P60A; trend $p < 0.003$ for BaP + P60A.
Source: Ref. 33.

TABLE 5 MNU-induced Colon Tumors in F344 Rats Ingesting Green Tea Extract (GTE)

Groups[a]	No. of rats examined	No. of rats with tumors	No. of tumors per rat	No. of tumors per tumor-bearing rat
Control	39	26 (67%)	1.2 ± 0.2^{b}	1.8 ± 0.2^{b}
HGTE	30	13 (43%)[c]	0.8 ± 0.2	1.8 ± 0.3
MGTE	30	12 (40%)[c]	0.5 ± 0.1^{c}	1.2 ± 0.1^{c}
LGTE	30	10 (33%)[c]	0.5 ± 0.2^{c}	1.5 ± 0.4

[a] All rats were given an intrarectal dose of 2 mg of MNU 3 times a week for 2 weeks, and received either 0% (control group), 0.05% (hGTE group), 0.01% (mGTE group), or 0.002% (1GTE group) water solution of GTE as drinking water throughout the experiment. The experiment was terminated at week 35.
[b] Mean = SEM.
[c] Significantly different from the control group: $p < 0.05$ or less.
Source: Ref. 37.

oxidation of DNA, through the tobacco-carcinogen-associated formation of ROS, yielding as marker 8-OH-dG (46). In a model of colon cancer, black tea lowered oxidative damage to the colon (49) and epigallocatechin gallate had a synergistic effect with sulindac (50). Similar interactions were observed in genetically modified mice and the heterocyclic amine 2-amino-1-methyl-6-phenylimidazo(4,5-b)pyridine (PhIP) (51). Inhibition was also demonstrated in APC (min) mice by this combination (52). Prostate cancer induction was decreased in TRAMP mice by green tea (53), and the molecular events were elucidated (54). The gene expression in human prostate LNCaP cells was altered (55).

We described above the formation of powerful mutagens during the cooking, frying, or broiling of meat, as heterocyclic aromatic amines. Epidemiological findings show that regular consumers of well-done cooked meat have a higher risk of cancer of the colon and breast (56–58). These are the target organs in rats, where cancer of the prostate and of the pancreas is also seen (59–62). The reason meats generate these kinds of compounds was discovered by a Swedish researcher, Jägerstad: namely, meats contain creatinine, which forms the 2-aminomethylimidazo part of the heterocyclic amines. Jägerstad's group developed an in vitro approach to model cooking, namely to heat glucose, creatinine, and an amino acid, such as glycine, or phenylalanine (63). We have found that addition of black tea or green tea polyphenols and caffeine to meat inhibits the mutagenicity of heterocyclic amines (64). Also, based on that experiment, we and others have shown that addition of green tea or black tea polyphenols during the frying of ground meat prevents the formation of mutagenic heterocyclic amines, which seems to be a practical way to cook "safe" hamburgers (65,66).

C. Tea Induces Detoxification Enzymes

In our laboratory, Sohn discovered that the administration of 2% solutions of black tea or green tea to rats for 6 weeks modifies the metabolic enzymes in the liver; namely, such rats display higher levels of cytochrome P450 1A1, 1A2, and 2B1, but of no other cytochromes (Table 6) (67). Note that green and black teas had similar effects. Also of great relevance, the phase II enzyme UDP-glucuronosyl transferase, which detoxifies many environmental chemicals, was significantly increased (Table 7) (68,69). On the other hand, sulfotransferase and glutathione transferases were virtually unchanged. Heterocyclic amines, described above, are subject to the biochemical activation through *N*-hydroxylation, and these *N*-hydroxy compounds are converted to the *N*-hydroxy glucuronides, a detoxified metabolite (Table 8) (69).

TABLE 6 Effects of Green or Black Tea Drinking on Phase I and II Enzymes of Male F344 Rat Liver[a]

Parameter	Predominant P450 isozymes monitored	Water	Green tea	Black tea
Phase I	1A1	4.35 ± 0.83	7.12 ± 0.31[f]	8.01 ± 0.42[f]
Ethoxyresorufin 1A2 dealkylase[b]	1A2	1.87 ± 0.39	10.10 ± 0.86[f]	11.66 ± 2.13[f]
Methoxyresorufin dealkylase[b]	2B1	2.17 ± 0.49	3.20 ± 0.15[f]	3.36 ± 0.25[f]
N-nitrosodimethylamine demethylase[c]	2E1	0.40 ± 0.06	0.49 ± 0.15	0.43 ± 0.11
Erythromycin demethylase[c]	3A4	0.49 ± 0.10	0.46 ± 0.11	0.54 ± 0.10
Phase II enzymes				
UDP-glucuronyltransferase[d]		12.00 ± 1.22	15.61 ± 1.12[f]	17.74 ± 0.84[f]
Glutathione S-transferase[e]		0.21 ± 0.02	0.23 ± 0.03	0.24 ± 0.02

[a] Data represent mean ± SD of four determinations, each derived from four different animals in each treatment group.
[b] Resorufin (pmol) produced/min/mg protein.
[c] Formaldehyde (nmol) consumed/min/mg protein.
[d] p-Nitrophenol (nmol) consumed/min/mg protein.
[e] CDNB-GSH (μmol) formed/min/mg cytosolic protein.
[f] $p < 0.01$ with respect to the control water group.
Source: Ref. 67.

TABLE 7 UDP-GT Activity in Liver Microsomes from Water- and Tea-Drinking Rats[a]

	p-NP consumed/min/mg protein	
Sample	Controls	Tea-drinking animals
1	10.8	21.8
2	11.7	16.3
3	12.1	16.9
4	9.4	16
5	11.8	13.5
6	10.5	13.3
7	10.9	19.1
Mean	11 ± 0.9	16.7 ± 3

[a] Mean ± standard deviation; $p < 0.05$ for rats on tea compared to controls.
Source: Ref. 68.

TABLE 8 Effect of Green Tea on Percent of the Total Urinary Radioactivity as Metabolites of 2-Amino-3-methylimidazo[4,5-f]quinoline (IQ) in Male and Female F344 Rats

	Percent of metabolites recovered			
	Males		Females	
Metabolites	Control	Tea	Control	Tea
1. IQ-*N*-glucuronide	6.7 ± 0.1	7.0 ± 0.2	3.2 ± 0.2	2.8 ± 0.3
2. 5-OH-IQ sulfate	13.5 ±	16.0 ± 0.3[a]	10.7 ± 0.2	14.1 ± 0.2[a]
3. *N*-OH-IQ-*N*-glucuronide	21.8 ± 0.3	24.0 ± 0.4[a]	15.4 ± 0.3	20.3 ± 0.4[a]
4. IQ sulfamate	31.0 ± 3.0	20.2 ± 0.2[a]	50.2 ± 1.1	35.3 ± 0.4[a]
5. 5-OH-IQ-glucuronide	24.0 ± 1.0	30.0 ± 3.0[a]	18.0 ± 0.2	25.1 ± 0.2[a]
6. IQ	3.0 ± 0.2	2.8 ± 0.1	2.5 ± 0.3	2.4 ± 0.4

[a] Student's *t*-test, $p < 0.05$, tea versus control. The data are the mean ± SD for the groups of 10 rats for each of the four series, in which rats were prefed 2% solutions of green tea for 6 weeks, then given a single oral dose of 40 mg/kg ^{14}C-IQ and the urines collected for 24 hr. The metabolites were separated by HPLC. The glucuronides and sulfate esters were increased, and the sulfamate was decreased in the rats on tea.
Source: Ref. 69.

Since green and black tea increased the available UDP-glucuronosyl transferase, it was observed that tea-drinking animals excrete metabolites of heterocyclic amines (69). Similar findings were made with white tea, a form of tea that is obtained by steaming of the tea leaves, without withering as is done for green tea. It is the least-processed type of tea from *Camellia sinensis*, which yielded lower levels of DNA adducts of heterocyclic amines, and fewer colonic aberrant crypts (70). Tea polyphenols also increased the liver microsomal conversion of estradiol and estrone to glucuronides (71). Earlier, we found that decaffeinated tea was less effective than regular tea in carrying out these reactions. Thus, caffeine may have a role, most likely together with the tea polyphenols as discussed in more detail below (64). Along these lines, kahweol and cafestol (found in coffee) also induced UDP-glucuronosyl transferase and GSH-transferase (72).

D. Growth Control and Apoptosis by Tea

Tea and tea polyphenols decrease the rate of growth of tumor cells through mechanisms involving alterations in gene expression (73–83). Tea even inhibited the formation of spontaneous lung tumors in A/J mice (47), which we reported in 1966 to have a stable incidence (84). Thus, the growth control effect of the polyphenols is remarkable. In addition, tea polyphenols increase the rate of apoptosis (cell death) of tumor cells and lead to their elimination (Table 9) (85–89). In cell lines derived from human head and neck squamous carcinoma it was found that EgCg decreased cyclin D1 protein, increased p21, p27 Bcl-2, and Bcl-x proteins, raised Bax protein, and activated caspase 9, suggesting an involvement of a mitochondrial pathway. Several other mechanisms are described, involving tea polyphenols and caffeine (90–102). Inhibition of angiogenesis may play a role (by blocking cell-to-cell communication) (29,103). These mechanisms may hold during tumor development by tea. Fujiki et al. (104) noted that epigallocatechin gallate affected cellular membrane tumor necrosis factor gene expression and release from cells. Also, nitric oxide (NO) synthetase gene expression and enzyme activity was inhibited, in turn affecting the associated activation and binding of nuclear factor κB to the inducible NO synthetase promoter, accounting for the inhibition of this key cellular process. Furthermore, the polyphenol epigallocatechin gallate affected the action of tumor promoters on transcription factors such as AP-1 and NF-κB, in turn controlling the activity of transforming growth factor TGF-γ. The induction of induced mammary gland cancer was inhibited by decreased promotion and progression stages with tea (38,56–58). Rectal cancer was lower in tea drinkers (105). A procedure to test the chemopreventive effect of tea with an effect on xenobiotic response elements was described (106). Reactive oxygen damage to protein was decreased

TABLE 9 Effect of PO Administration of Tea, Decaffeinated Tea, and Caffeine on Tumorigenesis, the Size of the Parametrial Fat Pads and the Thickness of the Dermal Fat Layer in SKH-1 Mice Previously Treated with UV (High-Risk Mice)

Treatment	No. of mice	No. of mice with skin nodules	No. of mice with histologically identified tumors	Total tumors (tumors per mouse)	Tumor diameter (mm/tumor)	Size of fat pads (relative units)	Thickness of dermal fat layer away from tumors (μm)	Thickness of dermal fat layer under tumors (μm)
Water	28	28	25	6.18 ± 0.71	1.90 ± 0.11	1.41 ± 0.11	162 ± 9	60 ± 4
0.6% GT	28	21	17[b]	2.00 ± 0.71[a] (68)	1.37 ± 0.18[c] (28)	0.64 ± 0.11[a] (54)	100 ± 11[a] (39)	28 ± 6[a] (53)
0.6% BT	=27	24	20	2.11 ± 0.72[a] (66)	1.23 ± 0.18[a] (35)	0.95 ± 0.11[b] (32)	88 ± 10[a] (46)	31 ± 6[a] (49)
0.6% dGT	27	22	21	4.96 ± 0.72 (20)	1.36 ± 0.13[a] (29)	1.62 ± 0.11 (0)	152 ± 10 (6)	55 ± 4 (8)
0.6% dBT	26	22	21	4.62 ± 0.74 (25)	1.38 ± 0.13[b] (28)	1.23 ± 0.12 (13)	150 ± 10 (8)	51 ± 6[a] (14)
0.044% CF	27	22	17[b]	2.41 ± 0.72[a] (61)	1.08 ± 0.17[a] (44)	0.62 ± 0.11[a] (56)	98 ± 10[a] (40)	31 ± 6[a] (49)
DGT + CF	25	21	16[b]	2.00 ± 0.75[a] (68)	1.26 ± 0.19[b] (34)	0.61 ± 0.12[a] (57)	105 ± 11[a] (35)	29 ± 6[a] (519)
DBT + CF	29	19	15[b]	1.17 ± 0.70[a] (81)	1.44 ± 0.22 (24)	0.89 ± 0.11[a] (37)	87 ± 11[a] (47)	24 ± 7[a] (61)

GT, green tea; BT, black tea; dGT, decaffeinated green tea; dBT, decaffeinated black tea; CF, caffeine.

Female SKH-1 mice were treated with UV (30 mJ/cm^2) twice a week for 22 weeks, and UV administration was stopped. These tumor-free mice had a high risk of developing skin tumors during the next several months, and they were treated for 23 weeks with 0.6% lyophilized green tea (GT, 6 mg tea solids/mL), black tea (BT, 6 mg tea solids/mL), or decaffeinated green or black tea (dGT or dBT, 6 mg tea solids/mL) as their sole source of drinking fluid. Other mice received 0.044% caffeine (CF, 0.44 mg/mL) or 0.6% lyophilized decaffeinated teas plus 0.044% caffeine. Tumors were classified by histological evaluation of skin samples from the 179 mice with skin nodules, and calculations of tumors/mouse included data from all 217 mice alive at the end of the experiment. The data for total tumors include keratoacanthomas, squamous cell carcinomas, and a small number of squamous cell papillomas.

The combined length of the two parametrial fat pads from all 217 mice alive when the experiment was terminated was measured and graded as follows: 1 (< 1 cm), 2 (1–2 cm), or 3 (>2 cm). The thickness of the dermal fat layer was measured in 5–10 representative nontumor areas of the skin (> 0.5 cm away from tumors) from 19–28 mice per group (total of 179 mice with skin nodules) using a light microscope with an ocular micrometer and 100-fold magnification. The 152 tumor-bearing mice were used for calculations of the thickness of the dermal fat layer under tumors. The values represent the mean ± SE, and the values in parentheses represent percentage decrease compared with the drinking water positive control group. Statistical evaluation of differences from the water positive control group ($^a p < 0.01$, $^b p < 0.05$, $^c p < 0.1$) was done by the Dunnett's T-test.

Source: Ref. 87.

by tea (107). A clinical trial with a polyphenol from green tea (polyphenon E) is underway (108,109).

E. Intestinal Microflora and Immune Defenses Are Improved in Tea Drinkers

Tea polyphenols affect viruses and bacteria (110). Enterobacteriaceae in the intestinal tract have mostly unpleasant properties since they generate smelly chemicals of the type of skatole and related indoles. The tea polyphenols suppress the growth of these bacteria but have no adverse effects on beneficial bacteria such as lactobacilli and biofidobacteria. Also, the consequence is a lower pH of the intestinal contents since there is increased formation of organic acids. In particular, butyric acid contributes to the chemopreventive effect. Therefore, regular tea drinkers have a healthier intestinal bacterial flora. Tea polyphenols have antiviral actions, as described in detail in the monograph of Hara (111). Studies on the human immunodeficiency virus, associated with AIDS, may provide an important application of the tea polyphenols (Z. Apostolides, personal communication and Ref. 112).

Intake of 4–5 cups of black tea for 4 weeks led to an increase of γ-δ lymphocytes and in turn of γ-interferon, reflecting a raised immune response (113).

F. Effect of Tea Polyphenols on ROS and Aging

Premature aging may also be a result of cellular ROS (114–116). The green tea polyphenol epigallocatechin gallate inhibited the markers for ROS and nitrogen species (116–118). It can be concluded that regular intake of 6 or more cups of tea per day facilitates healthy aging, which has been demonstrated on cellular systems, in animal models, and also, through studies of humans where regular tea intake is part of a health-promoting lifestyle, as in Japan and India (119). In that part of the world, one does find populations at advanced ages in good health, and a lower incidence of Alzheimer's disease in the aged (120–124).

G. Absorption and Metabolism of Tea Polyphenols

The results described above suggest that the active components in tea, namely the antioxidant polyphenols, are absorbed to generate the effects noted. This has been measured directly through a number of distinct analytical methods, such as HPLC and other chromatographic procedures, that were used to determine circulating levels in humans by several different groups. Other effects measured were the effect of intake of polyphenols from tea on biochemical parameters, such as the in vivo antioxidant effects in humans (125–127). The direct measurement of metabolites of epigallocatechin gallate utilized the tritiated chemical (128–132), through which it was discovered that there was methylation of the catecholic structure in the epigallocatechin gallate (132). Also, conjugates such as glucuronides have been found (133,134). Clearly, the effects on inhibition of carcinogenesis in various models demonstrate that the active components are absorbed and metabolized, and they are available in many tissues and organs (135).

The metabolism of dietary polyphenols, not necessarily from tea, suggests similar reacting, methylation and glucuronide formation, and opening of rings, mostly from catechol parts of the polyphenol under the influence of intestinal bacterial enzymes.

It has been suggested that the tea polyphenols might prevent the absorption of essential minerals. However, this speculation is not correct. It was found, for example, that iron is fully available (136).

H. Role of Caffeine

We have described the slightly improved antimutagenicity of regular tea containing caffeine compared to the decaffeinated version of the same tea (64) (Table 10). The tea polyphenols are active antioxidant and antimutagenic components of green or black tea but the finding that regular tea seems more active called attention to the fact that caffeine may also play a role. Thus, independent study of caffeine has described an antimutagenic effect of caffeine against heterocyclic amines and on enzyme induction in a dose-related fashion (Table 11) (64,137–141). Also, in mice exposed to ultraviolet (UV) light, a similar finding was made, namely that decaffeinated tea was somewhat less active than regular tea and that caffeine itself displayed an inhibiting effect

TABLE 10 Inhibition by Black and Decaffeinated Black Tea of the Mutagenicity Caused by PhIP in the *Salmonella typhimurium* TA98 Assay with S9 Activation

Black tea (mg/pl)	Regular tea (rev/pl)	Decaffeinated tea (rev/pl)
1	275 ± 22	424 ± 35
0.5	609 ± 22	726 ± 76
0.25	775 ± 143	845 ± 53
0.125	697 ± 258	798 ± 59

All values are for black or decaffeinated black tea with 2.5 μg PhIP. PhIP only gave 1113 ± 12 rev/pl. With 1 mg tea, the difference between regular and decaffeinated tea was significant at 0.05, but at other concentrations, the differences were not significant. The ID_{50} for black tea was 0.57 mg, and for decaffeinated tea 0.76. Each set of data is the mean ± SD from three plates. The background of 35 ± 2.3 rev/pl was subtracted from the gross data.
Source: Ref. 64.

TABLE 11 Inhibition of the Mutagenicity of PhIP by Caffeine (C)

	μg	Revertants per plate
PhIP +C	65	850 ± 166
PhIP +C	125	639 ± 47
PhIP +C	250	651 ± 21
PhIP +C	500	473 ± 17

With 2.25 μg PhIP, there were 1570 ± 126 rev/pl with *S. typhimurium* TA98 with S9, using three plates per point. The data indicated a linear dose-response. The ID_{50} for caffeine was 126 μg. The background was 40 ± 0.8 rev/pl.
Source: Ref. 64.

(139). Tea has induced several Phase I and Phase II enzymes. In this instance as well, regular tea showed increased action compared to decaffeinated tea, and a test of caffeine could induce specific cytochromes, in particular cytochrome p450 1A2 (67,137–139). In vitro, both teas and caffeine inhibited the growth of several human cancer cell lines (140). Serum concentrations of hormones and the hormone-binding globulin in women were also altered by caffeine (141). Tumor induction by tea in rodents and humans displayed improved effects with regular tea compared to decaffeinated tea, also leading to the conclusion that caffeine affects the overall effect observed (64,137–142). For example, in a lung cancer model, caffeine was noted to have an appreciable role (143).

It can be concluded that the relatively small amounts of caffeine, about 50 mg/150 mL cup of tea, made with 2.25 g of dry tea leaves, exerts an important interactive effect with the polyphenols. This potentiated action suggest that there is a joint effect between caffeine and tea polyphenols, since there is three times as much caffeine per cup of coffee, but the various effects described have not been observed with coffee. Admittedly, there have not been the detailed research results described for the amount of caffeine in coffee or coffee itself. Recently, cafestol and kahweol, diterpenes with anticarcinogenic activity, have been noted in coffee (72,144). Nonetheless, caffeine displayed a dose-response relationship when studied by itself in the various parameters examined so far. Caffeine is a stimulant and the amount present in a few cups of tea is adequate to exert a desirable effect. Clearly, additional investigations in this interesting field on the possible interaction between caffeine and the tea polyphenols in the various physiological and biochemical parameters would be of great relevance. A monograph on caffeine has appeared. It provides information on caffeine consumption, disposition and mode of action, and on development in childhood, on human behavior on withdrawal, action on bone and calcium metabolism and effect on women in relation to reproductive hazards (144). As noted, the amount of caffeine per cup of tea is limited, in comparison to other beverages. Also, there are excellent decaffeinated teas that might be suggested as a health-promoting beverage, as discussed herein, for children under age 15.

I. Tea, Weight Control, and Thermogenesis

Black, green, and oolong teas, perhaps because of their limited caffeine content, have been found to increase thermogenesis, to inhibit lipases, and to control body weight and body fat (Table 12; see also Table 9) (87,145–151). The relevant mechanism may be an effect on fat cell synthesis and the endocrine system, modulated by leptin. Green tea and caffeine increased physical activity and lowered body fat in mice. Also, tea, especially epigallo-

TABLE 12 Effect of Oral Administration of Caffeinated Beverages on the Thickness of the Dermal Fat Layer Under Tumors of Different Sizes in SKH-1 Mice Previously Treated with UV (High-Risk Mice)

	Thickness of dermal fat layer under tumors (μm)			
Tumor diameter (mm)	Noncaffeinated plus caffeinated beverages[a]	Noncaffeinated beverages[b]	Caffeinated beverages[b]	Percent decrease
≤0.5	58 ± 3 (202)	70 ± 4 (100)	45 ± 2 (102)	36
0.5–1	49 ± 3 (204)	63 ± 3 (125)	27 ± 2 (79)	57
1–2	43 ± 3 (177)	54 ± 3 (125)	16 ± 2 (52)	70
2–3	31 ± 5 (56)	39 ± 5 (42)	4 ± 1 (14)	90
>3	24 ± 5 (50)	34 ± 6 (35)	1 ± 1 (15)	97
Mean value	47 ± 1 (689)	58 ± 2 (427)	29 ± 2 (262)	50

UV-pretreated high-risk SKH-1 mice were treated orally with noncaffeinated beverages (water, dGT, dBT) or caffeinated beverages (GT, BT, CF, dGT + CF, and dBT + CF) for 23 weeks as described in Table 1. The thickness of the dermal fat layer under tumors of different sizes was measured in all 152 tumors-bearing mice (67 mice from the noncaffeinated beverage groups and 85 mice from the caffeinated beverage groups). The values in parentheses indicate the number of tumors studied. The mean value for the thickness of the dermal fat layer under tumors ± Se is given for tumors of different sizes.

[a] There was a significant negative linear association between tumor diameter and the log thickness of the dermal fat layer under tumors ($p = 0.0001$) using the random coefficient (hierarchical linear) model.

[b] The rate of decrease in thickness of the dermal fat layer under tumors of increasing size in mice treated with caffeinated beverages was significantly greater than that for mice treated with the noncaffeinated beverages ($p = 0.0001$) using the random coefficient (hierarchical linear) model.

Source: Ref. 87 (see Table 9).

catechin gallate, but not caffeine, raised insulin activity (152,153). Conceptually, those findings may be important in light of the fact that obesity is increasing, and general adoption of a health-promoting beverage, tea, may be a relatively simple means of assisting control of body weight with an otherwise healthy nutritional tradition.

III. CONCLUSION

Green tea and black tea, beverages second only to water as regards their worldwide usage, contain interesting phytochemicals, the polyphenols. A commentary on tea and health recently appeared (154). Green and black tea

TABLE 13 Multiple Mechanisms of Action of Tea (from *Camillia sinensis*)

1. In most cases black, oolong, and green tea display similar effects. Those are beverages consumed worldwide as infusions in hot water. Iced tea is prepared by adding ice to a concentrated infusion. Effects are similar at equal concentration, using a tea bag with 2.25 g tea, in 150 mL water (1.5% solution). The active principles in tea are specific polyphenols, epigallocatechin gallate (EgCg) in green tea, and theaflavins plus thearubigins in black tea.
2. Tea acts as antioxidant, decreasing the effect of ROS on cholesterol, LDL cholesterol (heart diseases), or DNA (neoplasms).
3. Tea induces several specific cytochrome P450 enzyme complexes, and UDP-glucuronosyl transferases, the latter serving to detoxify many types of carcinogens and other toxic chemicals.
4. Tea inhibits systems associated with growth of tumor cells and facilitates apoptotic cell death of neoplasms.
5. Tea modifies intestinal bacterial flora, favoring the outgrowth of beneficial bacteria and inhibiting development of bacteria with unfavorable actions.
6. Tea decreases leptins concerned with food energy utilization and fat cell growth and thus favors body weight loss and helps avoid obesity, but a leptin-receptor-independent action may account for the effects of tea.
7. Tea decreases the effect of ROS associated with cell, tissue, and body aging and hence is a means to slow the aging process and the associated diseases.
8. A number of the favorable actions of tea are mediated by its relatively low caffeine content. Seemingly the caffeine operates together with the tea polyphenols.
9. Tea can stimulate immunity through specific mechanisms, leading to improved resistance to microbial infections and possibly inhibiting tumor development.

modify host enzyme systems serving to detoxify endogenous or exogenous chemicals. They increase the level of cellular antioxidant defenses, and thus lower the risk of diseases involving adverse oxidative reactions such as heart disease and a number of types of cancer. Green and black tea have similar protective actions in most of the tests conducted. Caffeine in tea plays a role in the effects observed, since regular tea usually is slightly better than decaffeinated tea. Yet, the purified tea polyphenols available commercially are active as such at the concentrations studied. We suggest intake of 6–10 cups/day may be a useful dietary habit to assist in lowering the risk of a number of chronic diseases, especially as part of a health-promoting nutritional tradition, low in total fat (emphasis on monounsaturated and ω-3-polyunsaturated oils) and low in salt, with adequate vegetables and fruits, bran cereal, insoluble fiber, and also sources of soluble fiber (155). Total fluid intake in adults might be about 2.5 L, of which tea can be 0.7–1.4 L. It will be important to refine the mechanistic knowledge whereby tea polyphenols operate to change host physiology and biochemistry, and prevent a number of chronic diseases affecting humans (Table 13). Tea should be the beverage of choice in hospitals, which might facilitate recovery of the patients. Prevention is the definitive "cure" of chronic diseases, including most types of cancer, for which current therapy is difficult and expensive.

ACKNOWLEDGMENTS

I am indebted to Ms. Nancy Rivera and Ms. Elizabeth Appel for efficient and effective administrative support.

NOTE ADDED IN PROOF

The Proceedings of the 3rd International Scientific Symposium on Tea and Human Health have appeared (156).

REFERENCES

1. Block G, Dietrich M, Norkus EP, Morrow JD, Hudes M, Caan B, Packer L. Factors associated with oxidative stress in human populations. Am J Epidemiol 2002; 156:274–285.
2. Kasai H. Chemistry-based studies on oxidative DNA damage: formation, repair, and mutagenesis. Free Rad Biol Med 2002; 33:450–456.
3. Halliwell B. Effect of diet on cancer development: is oxidative DNA damage a biomarker? Free Rad Biol Med 2002; 32:968–974.
4. Cadet J, Douki T, Frelon S, Sauvaigo S, Pouget J-P, Ravant J-L. Assessment of oxidative base damage to isolated and cellular DNA by HPLC-MS/MS measurement. Free Rad Biol Med 2002; 33:441–449.

5. Weisburger JH, Williams GM. The distinction between genotoxic and epigenetic carcinogens and implication for cancer risk. Toxicol Sci 2000; 57:4–5.
6. Nagao M, Sugimura T, eds. Food Borne Carcinogens: Heterocyclic Amines. Chichester: John Wiley & Sons, 2000.
7. Snyderwine E, Sinha R, Felton J, Ferguson L. Highlights of the eighth international conference on carcinogenic/mutagenic *N*-substituted aryl compounds. Mutat Res 2002; 506–507:1–8.
8. Tsugane S, Tei Y, Takahashi T, Watanabe S, Sugano K. Salty food intake and risk of *Helicobacter pylori* infection. Jpn J Cancer Res 1994; 85:474–478.
9. Naito Y, Yoshikawa T. Molecular and cellular mechanisms involved in *Helicobacter pylori*–induced inflammation and oxidative stress. Free Rad Biol Med 2002; 33:323–336.
10. Wiseman SA, Balentine DA, Frei B. Antioxidants in tea. Crit Rev Food Sci Nutr 1997; 37:705–718.
11. Weisburger JH. Tea. In: Kipple K, Ornelas KC, eds. The Cambridge World History of Food. Vol 1. Cambridge, UK: Cambridge University Press, 2000:712–720.
12. Geleijnse JM, Launer LJ, Van der Kuip DA, Hofman A, Witteman JC. Inverse association of tea and flavonoid intakes with incident myocardial infarction: the Rotterdam Study. Am J Clin Nutr 2002; 75:880–886.
13. Arts ICW, Hollman PCH, Feskens EJM, Bueno de Mesquita H, Kromhout D. Catechin intake might explain the inverse relation between tea consumption and ischemic heart disease: the Zutphen Elderly Study. Am J Clin Nutr 2001; 74:227–232.
14. Hertog MG, Sweetnam PM, Fehily AM, Elwood PC, Kromhout D. Antioxidant flavonols and ischemic heart disease in a Welsh population of men: the Caerphilly Study. Am J Clin Nutr 1997; 65:1542–1543.
15. Chisolm GM, Steinberg D. The oxidative modification hypothesis of atherogenesis: an overview. Free Rad Biol Med 2000; 28:1815–1826.
16. Ishikawa T, Suzukawa M, Ito T, Yoshida H, Ayaori M, Nishiwaki M, Yonemura A, Hara Y, Nakamura H. Effect of tea flavonoid supplementation on the susceptibility of low-density lipoprotein to oxidative modification. Am J Clin Nutr 1997; 66:261–266.
17. Tokunaga S, White IR, Frost C, Tanaka K, Kono S, Tokudome S, Akamatsu T, Moriyama T, Zakouji H. Green tea consumption and serum lipids and lipoproteins in a population of healthy workers in Japan. Ann Epidemiol 2002; 12:157–165.
18. Sesso HD, Gaziano JM, Buring JE, Hennekens CH. Coffee and tea intake and the risk of myocardial infarction. Am J Epidmiol 1999; 149:162–167.
19. Feng Q, Torii Y, Uchida K, Nakamura Y, Hara Y, Osawa Y. Black tea polyphenols, theaflavins, prevent cellular DNA damage of inhibition oxidative stress and suppressing cytochrome P450 1A1 in cell cultures. J Agric Food Chem 2002; 50:213–220.
20. Weisburger JH, Hosey JR, Larios E, Pittman B, Zang E, Hara Y, Kuts-Cheraux G. Investigation of commercial MitoLife as an antioxidant and antimutagen. Nutrition 2001; 17:322–325.

21. Vinson JA. Black and green tea and heart disease: a review. Biofactors 2000; 13:127–132.
22. Peters U, Poole C, Arab L. Does tea affect cardiovascular disease? A meta-analysis. Am J Epidemiol 2001; 154:495–503.
23. Nakachi K, Matsuyama S, Mikake S, Suganuma M, Imai K. Preventive effects of drinking green tea on cancer and cardiovascular disease: epidemiological evidence for multiple targeting prevention. Biofactors 2000; 13:49–54.
24. Hodgson JM, Puddey IB, Burke V, Beilin LJ, Mori TA, Chan SY. Acute effects of ingestion of black tea on postprandial platelet aggregation in human subjects. Br J Nutr 2002; 87:141–145.
25. Wolfram RM, Oguogho A, Efthimiou Y, Budinsky AC, Sinzinger H. Effect of black tea on (iso-)prostaglandins and platelet aggregation in healthy volunteers. Prostaglandins Leukot Essent Fatty Acids 2002; 66:529–533.
26. Duffy SJ, Vita JA, Holbrook M, Swerdloff PL, Keaney JF Jr. Effect of acute and chronic tea consumption on platelet aggregation in patients with coronary artery disease. Arterioscler Thromb Bas Biol 2002; 21:1084–1089.
27. Patel RP, Moellering D, Murphy-Ullrich J, Jo H, Beckman JS, Darley-Usmar VM. Cell signaling by reactive nitrogen and oxygen species in atherosclerosis. Free Rad Biol Med 2000; 28:1780–1794.
28. Tang FY, Meydani M. Green tea catechins and vitamin E inhibit angiogenesis of human microvascular endothelial cells through suppression of IL-8 production. Nutr Cancer 2001; 41:119–125.
29. Cao Y, Cao R, Brakenhielm E. Antiangiogenic mechanisms of diet-derived polyphenols. J Nutr Biochem 2002; 13:380–390.
30. Leung LK, Su Y, Chen R, Zhang Z, Huang Y, Chen ZY. Theaflavins in black tea and catechins in green tea are equally effective antioxidants. J Nutr 2001; 131:2248–2251.
31. du Tit R, Volsteedt Y, Apostolides Z. Comparison of the antioxidant content of fruits, vegetables and teas measured as vitamin C equivalents. Toxicology 2001; 166:63–69.
32. McCann J, Choi E, Yamasaki E, Ames BN. Detection of carcinogens as mutagens in the *Salmonella*/microsome test: assay of 300 chemicals. Proc Natl Acad Sci USA 1975; 72:5135–5139.
33. Weisburger JH, Hara Y, Dolan L, Luo F-Q, Pittman B, Zang E. Tea polyphenols as inhibitors of mutagenicity of major classes of carcinogens. Mutat Res 1996; 371:57–63.
34. Kuroda Y, Hara Y. Antimutagenic and anticarcinogenic activity of tea polyphenols. Mutat Res 1999; 436:69–97.
35. Gupta S, Saha B, Giri AK. Comparative antimutagenic and anticlastogenic effects of green tea and black tea: a review. Mutat Res 2002; 512:37–65.
36. Amantana A, Santana-Rios G, Butler JA, Xu M, Whanger PD, Dashwood RH. Antimutagenic activity of selenium-enriched green tea toward the heterocyclic amine 2-amino-3-methylimidazo[4,5-f]quinoline. Biol Trace Elem Res 2002; 86:177–191.
37. Narisawa T, Fukaura Y. A very low dose of green tea polyphenols in drinking

water prevents *N*-methyl-*N*-nitrosourea-induced colon carcinogenesis in F344 rats. Jpn J Cancer Res, 1993; 1007–1009.
38. Rogers AE, Hafer LJ, Iskander YS, Yang S. Black tea and mammary gland carcinogenesis by 7,12-dimethylbenz[a]anthracene in rats fed control or high fat diets. Carcinogenesis 1998; 19:1269–1273.
39. Weisburger JH, Rivenson A, Garr K, Aliaga C. Tea, or tea and milk, inhibit mammary gland and colon carcinogenesis. Cancer Lett 1997; 114:323–327.
40. Wang ZY, Wang LD, Lee MJ, Ho CT, Huang MT, Conney AH, Yang CS. Inhibition of *N*-nitrosomethylbenzylamine-induced esophageal tumorigenesis in rats by green and black tea. Carcinogenesis 1995; 16:1243–1248.
41. Gao YT, McLaughlin JK, Blot WJ, Ji BT, Dai Q, Fraumeni JJ. Reduced risk of esophageal cancer associated with green tea consumption. J Natl Cancer Inst 1994; 86:855–858.
42. Sun CL, Yuan JM, Lee, Yang CS, Gao YT, Ross RK, Yu MC. Urinary tea polyphenols in relation to gastric and esophageal cancers: a prospective study of men in Shanghai, China. Carcinogenesis 2002; 23:1497–1503.
43. Yang CS, Maliakal P, Meng X. Inhibition of carcinogenesis by tea. Annu Rev Pharmacol Toxicol 2002; 42:25–54.
44. Mukhtar H, Ahmad N. Tea polyphenols: prevention of cancer and optimizing health. Am J Clin Nutr 2000; 71:1698S–1702S.
45. Li N, Chen X, Liao J, Yang G, Wang S, Josephson Y, Han C, Chen J, Haun M-T, Yang CS. Inhibition of 7,12-dimethylbenz[a]anthracene (DMBA)-induced oral carcinogenesis in hamsters by tea and curcumin. Carcinogenesis 2002; 23:1307–1313.
46. Weisburger JH, Chung F-L. Mechanisms of chronic disease causation by nutritional factors and tobacco products and their prevention by tea polyphenols. Food Chem Toxicol 2002; 40:1145–1154.
47. Landau JM, Wang ZY, Yang CY, Ding W, Yang CS. Inhibition of spontaneous formation of lung tumors and rhabdomyosarcomas in A/J mice by black and green tea. Carcinogenesis 1998; 19:501–507.
48. Feng Q, Kumagai T, Torii Y, Nakamura Y, Osawa T, Uchida K. Anticarcinogenic antioxidants as inhibitors against intracellular oxidative stress. Free Radic Res 2001; 35:779–788.
49. Lodovici M, Casalini C, De Filippo C, Copeland E, Xu X, Clifford M, Dolara P. Inhibition of 1,2-dimethylhydrazine-induced oxidative DNA damage in rat colon mucosa by black tea complex polyphenols. Food Chem Toxicol 2000; 38:1085–1088.
50. Ohishi T, Kishimoto Y, Miura N, Shiota G, Kohri T, Hara Y, Hasegawa J, Isemura M. Synergistic effects of (−)-epigallocatechin gallate with sulindac against colon carcinogenesis of rats treated with azoxymethane. Cancer Lett 2002; 177:49–56.
51. Orner G, Dashwood W, Blum C, Diaz G, Li Q, Al-Fageeh M, Tebbutt N, Heath J, Ernst M, Dashwood R. Response of Apc(min) and A33 (delta N beta-cat) mutant mice to treatment with tea, sulindac, and 2-amino-1-methyl-6-phenylimidazo[4,5-b]pyridine (PhIP). Mutat Res 2002; 506–507:121–127.

52. Orner GA, Dashwood WM, Blum CA, Diaz GD, Li Q, Dashwood RH. Suppression of tumorigenesis in the Apc(min) mouse: down-regulation of beta-catenin signaling by a combination of tea plus sulindac. Carcinogenesis 2003; 24:263–267.
53. Gupta S, Hastak K, Ahmad N, Lewin JS, Mukhtar H. Inhibition of prostate carcinogenesis in TRAMP mice by oral infusion of green tea polyphenols. Proc Natl Acad Sci USA 2001; 98:10350–10355.
54. Adhami VM, Ahmad N, Mukhtar H. Molecular targets for green tea in prostate cancer prevention. J Nutr 2003; 133:2417S–2424S.
55. Wang SI, Mukhtar H. Gene expression profile in human prostate LNCaP cancer cells by (−)-epigallocatechin-3-gallate. Cancer Lett 2002; 182:43–51.
56. Felton JS, Knize MG, Salmon CP, Malfatti MA, Kulp KS. Human exposure to heterocyclic amine food mutagens/carcinogens: relevance to breast cancer. Environ Mol Mutagen 2002; 39:112–118.
57. Sinha R. An epidemiologic approach to studying heterocyclic amines. Mutat Res 2002; 506–507:197–204.
58. Snyderwine EG, Venugopal M, Yu M. Mammary gland carcinogenesis by food-derived heterocyclic amines and studies on the mechanism of carcinogenesis of 2-amino-1-methyl-6-phenylimidazo[4,5-b]pyridine (PhIP). Mutat Res 2002; 506–507:145–152.
59. Shirai T, Kato K, Futakuchi M, Takahashi S, Suzuki S, Imaida K, Asamoto. Organ differences in the enhancing potential of 2-amino-1-methyl-6-phenylimidazo[4,5-b]pyridine on carcinogenicity in the prostate, colon and pancreas. Mutat Res 2002; 506–507:129–136.
60. Anderson KE, Sinha R, Kulldorff M, Gross M, Lang NP, Barber C, Harnack L, DiMagno E, Bliss R, Kadlubar FF. Meat intake and cooking techniques: associations with pancreatic cancer. Mutat Res 2002; 506–507:225–231.
61. Tanaka T, Barnes WS, Williams GM, Weisburger JH. Multipotential carcinogenicity of the fried food mutagen 2-amino-3-methylimidazo[4,5-f]quinoline in rats. Jpn J Cancer Res (GANN) 1985; 76:570–576.
62. Ohgaki H. Carcinogenicity in animals and specific organs: rodents. In: Nagao M, Sugimura T, eds. Food-borne Carcinogens: Heterocyclic Amines. New York: Wiley, 2000:198–228.
63. Skog KI, Johansson MA, Jägerstad MI. Carcinogenic heterocyclic amines in model systems and cooked foods: a review on formation, occurrence and intake. Food Chem Toxicol 1998; 36:879–896.
64. Weisburger JH, Dolan L, Pittman B. Inhibition of PhIP mutagenicity by caffeine, lycopene, daidzein, and genistein. Mutat Res 1998; 416:125–128.
65. Weisburger JH, Veliath E, Larios E, Pittman B, Zang E, Hara Y. Tea polyphenols inhibit the formation of mutagens during the cooking of meat. Mutat Res 2002; 516:19–22.
66. Kinae N, Furugori M, Takemura H, Iwazaki M, Shimoi K, Wakabayashi K. Inhibitory effect of tea extracts on the formation of heterocyclic amines during cooking of hamburger. In: Ohigashi H, Osawa T, Terao J, Watanabe S, Yoshikawa T, eds. Food Factors for Cancer Prevention. Tokyo: Springer, 1997:142–146.

67. Sohn OS, Surace A, Fiala ES, Richie JP Jr, Colosimo S, Zang E, Weisburger JH. Effects of green and black tea on hepatic xenobiotic metabolizing systems in the male F344 rat. Xenobiotica 1994; 24:119–127.
68. Embola CW, Sohn OS, Fiala ES, Weisburger JH. Induction of UDP-glucuronosyltransferase 1 (UDP-GT1) gene complex by green tea in male F344 rats. Food Chem Toxicol 2002; 40:841–844.
69. Embola CW, Weisburger JH, Weisburger MC. Urinary excretion of *N*-OH-2-amino-3-methylimidazo[4,5-f] quinoline-*N*-glucuronide in F344 rats is enhanced by green tea. Carcinogenesis 2001; 22:1095–1098.
70. Santana-Rios G, Orner GA, Xu M, Izquierdo-Pulido M, Dashwood RH. Inhibition by white tea of 2-amino-1-methyl-6-phenylimidazo[4,5-b]pyridine-induced colonic aberrant crypts in the F344 rat. Nutr Cancer 2001; 41:98–103.
71. Zhu BT, Taneja N, Loder DP, Balentine DA, Conney AH. Effects of tea polyphenols and flavonoids on liver microsomal glucuronidation of estradiol and estrone. J Steroid Biochem Mol Biol 1998; 64:207–215.
72. Huber WW, Prustomersky S, Delbanco E, Uhl M, Scharf G, Turesky RJ, Their R, Schulte-Hermann R. Enhancement of the chemoprotective enzymes glucuronosyl transferase and glutathione transferase in specific organs of the rat by the coffee components kahweol and cafestol. Arch Toxicol 2002; 76:209–217.
73. Mori H, Yamada Y, Hirose Y, Kuno T, Katayama M, Sakata K, Yoshida K, Sugie S, Hara A, Yoshimi N. Chemoprevention of large bowel carcinogenesis; the role of control of cell proliferation and significance of β-catenin-accumulated crypts as a new biomarker. Eur J Cancer Prev 2002; 11(suppl 2):S71–S75.
74. Agarwal R. Cell signaling and regulators of cell cycle as molecular targets for prostate cancer prevention by dietary agents. Biochem Pharmacol 2000; 60: 1051–1059.
75. Gupta S, Ahmad N, Nieminen AL, Mukhtar H. Growth inhibition, cell-cycle dysregulation, and induction of apoptosis by green tea constituent (−)-epigallocatechin-3-gallate in androgen-sensitive and androgen-insensitive human prostate carcinoma cells. Toxicol Appl Pharmacol 2000; 164:82–90.
76. Chung JY, Huang C, Meng X, Dong Z, Yang CS. Inhibition of activator protein 1 activity and cell growth by purified green tea and black tea polyphenols in H-ras-transformed cells: structure-activity relationship and mechanisms involved. Cancer Res 1999; 59:4610–4617.
77. Lin JK. Cancer chemoprevention by tea polyphenols through modulating signal transduction pathways. Arch Pharm Res 2002; 25:561–571.
78. von Pressentin MDM, Chen M, Guttenplan JB. Mutagenesis induced by 4-(methylnitrosamino)-1-(3-pyridyl)-1-butanone and *N*-nitrosonornicotine in *lacZ* upper aerodigestive tissue and liver and inhibition by green tea. Carcinogenesis 2002; 22:203–206.
79. Takada M, Nakamura Y, Koizumi T, Toyama H, Kamigaki T, Suzuki Y, Takeyama Y, Kuroda Y. Suppression of human pancreatic carcinoma cell growth and invasion by epigallocatechin-3-gallate. Pancreas 2002; 25:45–48.
80. Lin JK, Liang YC, Lin-Shiau SY. Cancer Chemoprevention by tea polyphenols

through mitotic signal transduction blockade. Biochem Pharmacol 1999; 58:911–915.
81. Liang YC, Lin-Shiau SY, Chen CF, Lin JK. Suppression of extracellular signals and cell proliferation through EGF receptor binding by (−)-epigallocatechin gallate in human A431 epidermoid carcinoma cells. J Cell Biochem 1997; 67:55–65.
82. Okabe S, Suganuma M, Hayashi M, Sueoka E, Komori A, Fujiki H. Mechanisms of growth inhibition of human lung cancer cell line, PC-9, by tea polyphenols. Jpn J Cancer Res 1997; 88:639–643.
83. Murase T, Nagasawa A, Suzuki J, Hase T, Tokimitsu I. Beneficial effects of tea catechins on diet-induced obesity: stimulation of lipid catabolism in the liver. Int J Obes Relat Metab Disord 2002; 26:1459–1464.
84. Shimkin MB, Weisburger JH, Weisburger EK, Gubareff N, Suntzeff V. Bioassay of 29 alkylating chemicals by the pulmonary-tumor response in strain A mice. J Natl Cancer Inst 1966; 36:124–142.
85. Lu J, Ho CT, Ghai G, Chen KY. Differential effects of theaflavin monogallates on cell growth, apoptosis, an Cox-2 gene expression in cancerous versus normal cells. Cancer Res 2000; 60:6465–6471.
86. Hayashi R, Luk H, Horio DT, Dashwood RH. Inhibition of apoptosis in colon tumors induced in the rat by 2-amino-3-methylimidazo(4,5-f)quinoline. Cancer Res 1996; 56:4307–4310.
87. Conney AH, Lu Y-P, Lou Y-R, Huang M-T. Inhibitory effects of tea and caffeine on UV-induced carcinogenesis: relationship to enhanced apoptosis and decreased tissue fat. Eur J Cancer Prev 2002; 11(suppl 2):S28–S36.
88. Zhang G, Miura Y, Yagasaki K. Induction of apoptosis and cell cycle arrest in cancer cells by in vivo metabolites of teas. Nutr Cancer 2000; 38:265–273.
89. Lambert JD, Yang CS. Mechanisms of cancer prevention by tea constituents. J Nutr 2003; 116:1345–1350.
90. Masuda M, Suzui M, Lim JT, Weinstein IB. Epigallocatechin-3-gallate inhibits activation of HER-2/neu and downstream signaling pathways in human head and neck and breast carcinoma cells. Clin Cancer Res 2003; 15:3486–3491.
91. He Z, Ma WY, Hashimoto T, Bode AM, Yang CS, Dong Z. Induction of apoptosis by caffeine is mediated by the p53, Bax, and caspase 3 pathways. Cancer Res 2003; 63:4396–4401.
92. Hastak K, Gupta S, Ahmad N, Agarwal MK, Agarwal ML, Mukhtar H. Role of p53 and NF-kappaB in epigallocatechin-3-gallate-induced apoptosis of NKCaP cells. Oncogene 2003; 22:4851–4859.
93. Il'yasova D, Hodgson ME, Martin C, Galanko J, Sandler RS. Tea consumption, apoptosis, and colorectal adenomas. Eur J Cancer Prev 2003; 12:439–443.
94. Brusselmans K, De Schrijver E, Heyns W, Verhoeven G, Swinnen JV. Epigallocatechin-3-gallate is a potent natural inhibitor of fatty acid synthase in intact cells and selectively induces apoptosis in prostate cancer cells. Int J Cancer 2003; 106:856–862.
95. Weinreb O, Mandel S, Youdim MB. Gene and protein expression profiles of anti-

and pro-apoptotic actions of dopamine, R-apomorphine, green tea polyphenol (−)-epigallocatechine-3-gallate, and melatonin. Ann NY Acad Sci 2003; 993:351–361.

96. Chung JH, Han JH, Hwang EJ, Seo JY, Cho KH, Kim KH, Youn JI, Eu HC. Dual mechanisms of green tea extract (EGCG)-induced cell survival in human epidermal keratinocytes. FASEB J 2003; 17:1913–1915.
97. Hsu S, Lewis J, Singh B, Schoenlein P, Osaki T, Athar M , Porter AG, Schuster G. Green tea polyphenol targets the mitochondria in tumor cells inducing caspase 3–dependent apoptosis. Anticancer Res 2003; 23:1533–1539.
98. Ahn WS, Huh SW, Bae SM, Lee IP, Lee JM, Namkoong SE, Kim CK, Sin JI. A major constituent of green tea, EGCG, inhibits the growth of human cervical cancer cell line, CaSki cells, through apoptosis, G(1) arrest, and regulation of gene expression. DNA Cell Biol 2003;22217–224.
99. Park AM, Dong Z. Signal transduction pathways: targets for green and black tea polyphenols. J Biochem Mol Biol 2003; 36:66–77.
100. Gupta S, Hussain T, Mukhtar H. Molecular pathway for (−)-epigallocatechin-3-gallate-induced cell cycle arrest and apoptosis of human prostate carcinoma cells. Arch Biochem Biophys 2003; 410:177–185.
101. Lin YS, Tsai YJ, Tsay JS, Lin JK. Factors affecting the levels of tea polyphenols and caffeine in tea leaves. J Agric Food Chem 2003; 51:1864–1873.
102. Roy M, Chakrabarty S, Sinha D, Bhattacharya RK, Siddiqi M. Anticlastogenic, antigenotoxic and apoptotic activity of epigallocatechin gallate: a green tea polyphenol. Mutat Res 2003; 523-524:33–41.
103. Kondo T, Ohta T, Igura K, Hara Y, Kaji K. Tea catechins inhibit angiogenesis in vitro, measured by human endothelial cell growth, migration and tube formation, through inhibition of VEGF receptor binding. Cancer Lett 2002; 180:139–144.
104. Fujiki H, Suganuma M, Okabe S, Sueoka E, Suga K, Imai K, Nakachi K. A new concept of tumor promotion by tumor necrosis factor-alpha, and cancer preventive agents (−)—epigallocatechin gallate and green tea—a review. Cancer Detect Prev 2000; 24:91–99.
105. Il'yasova D, Arab L, Martinchik A, Sdvizhkov A, Urbanovich L, Weisgerber U. Black tea consumption and risk of rectal cancer in Moscow population. Ann Epidemiol 2003; 13:405–411.
106. Chan HY, Wang H, Tsang DSC, Chen Z-Y, Leung LK. Screening of chemopreventive tea polyphenols against PAH genotoxicity in breast cancer cells by a XRE-luciferase reporter construct. Nutr Cancer 2003; 46:93–100.
107. Misra A, Chattopadhyay R, Banerjee S, Chattopadhyay DJ, Chatterjee IB. Black tea prevents cigarette smoke-induced oxidative damage of proteins in guinea pigs. J Nutr 2003; 133:2622–2628.
108. Chow HH, Cai Y, Alberts DS, Hakim I, Dorr R, Shahi F, Crowell JA, Yang CS, Hara Y. Phase I pharmacokinetic study of tea polyphenols following single-dose administration of epigallocatechin gallate and polyphenon E. Cancer Epidemiol Biomarkers Prev 2001; 10:53–58.
109. Chow HH, Cai Y, Hakim IA, Crowell JA, Shahi F, Brooks CA, Dorr RT, Hara Y, Alberts DS. Pharmacokinetics and safety of green tea polyphenols after

multiple-dose administration of epigallocatechin gallate and polyphenon E in healthy individuals. Clin Cancer Res 2003; 9:3312–3319.

110. Hara Y. Tea as preventive/protective against human diseases. Intern J Tea Sci 2002–2003; 2:20–26.
111. Hara Y. Green Tea: Health Benefits and Applications. New York: Marcel Dekker, 2001.
112. Fassina G, Buffa A, Benelli R, Varnier OE, Noonan DM, Albini A. Polyphenolic antioxidant (–)-epigallocatechin-3-gallate from green tea as a candidate anti-HIV agent. AIDS 2002; 16:939–941.
113. Kamath AB, Wang L, Das H, Li L, Reinhold VN, Bukowski JF. Antigens in tea-beverage prime human gamma delta T cells in vitro and in vivo for memory and nonmemory antibacterial cytokine responses. Proc Natl Acad Sci USA 2003; 100:6009–6014.
114. Stadtman ER. Importance of individuality in oxidative stress and aging. Free Rad Biol Med 2002; 33:597–604.
115. Smith MA, Perry G, Pryor WA. Causes and consequences of oxidative stress in Alzheimer's diseases. Free Rad Biol Med 2002; 32:1049.
116. Ferrari CKB, Torres EAFS. Biochemical pharmacology of functional foods and prevention of chronic diseases of aging. Biomed Pharmacother 2003; 57: 251–260.
117. Sohal RS, Mockett RJ, Orr WC. Mechanisms of aging: an appraisal of the oxidative stress hypothesis. Free Rad Biol Med 2002; 33:575–586.
118. Fiala ES, Sodum RS, Bhattacharya M, Li H. (–)-Epigallocatechin gallate, a polyphenolic tea antioxidant, inhibits peroxynitrite-mediated formation of 8-oxodeoxyguanosine and 3-nitrotyrosine. Experientia 1996; 9:922–926.
119. Nakachi K, Eguchi H, Imai K. Can teatime increase one's lifetime? Ageing Res Rev 2003; 2:1–10.
120. Chen L, Yang X, Jiao H, Zhao B. Tea catechins protect against lead-induced ROS formation, mitochondria dysfunction, and calcium dysregulation in PC12 cells. Chem Res Toxicol 2003; 16:1155–1161.
121. Yamamoto T, Hsu S, Lewis J, Wataha J, Dickinson D, Singh B, Bollag WB, Lockwood P, Ueta E, Osaki T, Schuster G. Green tea polyphenol causes differential oxidative environments in tumor versus normal epithelial cells. J Pharmacol Exp Ther 2003; 307:230–236.
122. Cadenas E, Davies KJA. Mitochondrial free radical generation, oxidative stress and aging. Free Rad Biol Med 2000; 29:222–230.
123. Shadlen MF, Larson EB, Yukawa M. The epidemiology of Alzheimer's disease and vascular dementia in Japanese and African-American populations: the search for etiological clues. Neurobiol Aging 2000; 21:171–181.
124. Choi YT, Jung CH, Lee SR, Bae JH, Baek WK, Suh MH, Park J, Park CW, Suh SI. The green tea polyphenol (–)-epigallocatechin gallate attenuates beta-amyloid-induced neurotoxicity in cultured hippocampal neurons. Life Sci 2001; 70:603–614.
125. Leenen R, Roodenburg AJ, Tijburg LB, Wiseman SA. A single dose of tea with or without milk increases plasma antioxidant activity in humans. Eur J Clin Nutr 2000; 54:87–92.

126. Benzie IFF, Szeto YT, Strain JJ, Tomlinson B. Consumption of green tea causes rapid increase in plasma antioxidant power in humans. Nutr Cancer 1999; 34:83–87.
127. Rechner AR, Kuhnle G, Bremner P, Hubbard GP, Moore KP, Rice-Evans CA. The metabolic fate of dietary polyphenols in humans. Free Rad Biol Med 2002; 33:220–235.
128. Swezey RR, Aldridge DE, LeValley SE, Crowell JA, Hara Y, Green CE. Absorption, tissue distribution and elimination of 4-[^{3}H]-epigallocatechin gallate in beagle dogs. Int J Toxicol 2003; 22:187–193.
129. Kohri T, Suzuki M, Nanjo F. Identification of metabolites of (−)-epicatechin gallate and their metabolic fate in the rat. J Agric Food Chem 2003; 51:5561–5566.
130. Lee M-J, Maliakal P, Chen L, Meng X, Bondoc FY, Prabhu S, Lambert G, Mohr S, Yang CS. Pharmacokinetics of tea catechins after ingestion of green tea and (−)-epigallocatechin-3-gallate by humans: formation of different metabolite and individual variability. Cancer Epidemiol Biomarkers Prev 2002; 11:1025–1032.
131. Catterall F, King LJ, Clifford MN, Ioannides C. Bioavailability of dietary doses of ^{3}H-labelled tea antioxidants (+)-catechin and (−)-epicatechin in rat. Xenobiotica 2003; 33:743–753.
132. Hong J, Lambert JD, Lee SH, Sinko PJ, Yang CS. Involvement of multidrug resistance-associated proteins in regulating cellular levels of (−)-epigallocatechin-3-gallate and its methyl metabolites. Biochem Biophys Res Commun 2003; 310:222–227.
133. Lu H, Meng X, Li C, Sang S, Patten C, Sheng S, Hong J, Bai N, Winnik B, Ho CT, Yang CS. Glucuronides of tea catechins: enzymology of biosynthesis and biological activities. Drug Metab Dispos 2003; 31:452–461.
134. Natsume M, Osakabe N, Oyama M, Sasaki M, Baba S, Nakamura Y, Osawa T, Terao J. Structures of (−)-epicatechin glucuronide identified from plasma and urine after oral ingestion of (−)-epicatechin: differences between human and rat. Free Rad Biol Med 2003; 34:840–849.
135. Suganuma M, Okabe S, Oniyama M, Tada Y, Ito H, Fujiki H. Wide distribution of [3H](−)-epigallacatechin gallate, a cancer preventive tea polyphenol, in mouse tissue. Carcinogenesis 1998; 19:1771–1776.
136. Record IR, McInerney JK, Dreosti IE. Black tea, green tea and tea polyphenols: effects on trace element status in weanling rats. Biol Trace Element Res 1996; 53:27–43.
137. Chen L, Bondoc FY, Lee MJ, Hussan AH, Thomas PE, Yang CS. Caffeine induces cytochrome P4501A2: induction of CYP1A2 by tea in rats. Drug Metab Dispos 1996; 24:529–533.
138. Bu-Abbas A, Clifford MN, Walker R, Ioannides C. Contribution of caffeine and flavanols in the induction of hepatic Phase II activities by green tea. Food Chem Toxicol 1998; 36:617–621.
139. Huang MT, Xie JG, Wang ZY, Ho CT, Lou YR, Wang CX, Hard GC, Conney AH. Effects of tea, decaffeinated tea, and caffeine on UVB light-induced complete carcinogenesis in SKH-1 mice: demonstration of caffeine as a biologically important constituent of tea. Cancer Res 1997; 57:2623–2629.

140. Valcic S, Timmermann BN, Alberts DS, Wachter GA, Krutzsch M, Wymer J. Guillen JIM. Inhibitory effect of six green tea catechins and caffeine on the growth of four selected human tumor cell lines. Anti-Cancer Drugs 1996; 7:461–468.
141. Nagata C, Kabuto M, Shimizu H. Association of coffee, green tea, and caffeine intakes with serum concentrations of estradiol and sex hormone-binding globulin in premenopausal Japanese women. Nutr Cancer 1998; 30:21–24.
142. Slattery ML, Caan BJ, Anderson KE, Potter JD. Intake of fluids and methylxanthine-containing beverages; association with colon cancer. Int J Cancer 1999; 81:199–204.
143. Chung FL, Wang M, Rivenson A, Iatropoulos MJ, Reinhardt JC, Pittman B, Ho CT, Amin SG. Inhibition of lung carcinogenesis by black tea in Fischer rats treated with a tobacco-specific carcinogen: caffeine as an important constituent. Cancer Res 1998; 58:4069–4101.
144. Mandel GH, ed. ILSI Caffeine Monograph. Food Chem Toxicol 2002; 40:1229–1310.
145. Chantre P, Lairon D. Recent findings of green tea extract AR25 (Exolise) and its activity for the treatment of obesity. Phytomedicine 2002; 9:3–8.
146. Dulloo AG, Duret C, Rohrer D, Girardier L, Mensi N, Fathi M, Chantre P, Vandermander J. Efficacy of a green tea extract rich in catechin polyphenols and caffeine in increasing 24-h energy expenditure and fat oxidation in humans. Am J Clin Nutr 1999; 70:1040–1045.
147. Kao Y-H, Hiipakka RA, Liao S. Modulation of obesity by a green tea catechin. Am J Clin Nutr 2000; 72:1232–1233.
148. Dulloo A. Modulation of obesity by a green tea catechin. Am J Clin Nutr 2000; 72:1233–1234.
149. Sayama K, Lin S, Zheng G, Oguni I. Effects of green tea on growth, food utilization and lipid metabolism in mice. In Vivo 2000; 14:481–484.
150. Kao YH, Hiipakka RA, Liao S. Modulation of endocrine systems and food intake by green tea epigallocatechin gallate. Endocrinology 2000; 141, 980–987.
151. Michna L, Lu YP, Lou YR, Wagner GC, Conney AH. Stimulatory effect of oral administration of green tea and caffeine on locomotor activity in SKH-1 mice. Life Sci 2003; 73:1383–1392.
152. Bell SJ, Goodrick GK. A functional food product for the management of weight. Crit Rev Food Sci Nutr 2002; 42:163–178.
153. Anderson RA, Polansky MM. Tea enhances insulin activity. J Agric Food Chem 2002; 50:7182–7186.
154. McKay DL, Blumberg JB. The role of tea in human health: an update. J Am Coll Nutr 2002; 21:1–13.
155. Weisburger JH. Lifestyle, health and disease prevention: the underlying mechanisms. Eur J Cancer Prev 2002; 11(suppl 2):S1–S7.
156. Blumberg J, ed. Proceedings of the Third International Scientific Symposium on Tea and Human Health: Role of Flavonoids in the Diet. J Nutr 2003; 133:3244S–3318S.

7

Ginkgo biloba
From Traditional Medicine to Molecular Biology

Yves Christen
Ipsen
Paris, France

I. INTRODUCTION

A botanical curiosity, *Ginkgo biloba* is also extremely original in its biochemical composition. This probably explains the multiplicity of effects observed with *Ginkgo biloba* extract—EGb 761. Studied at all levels of the organization of life (molecular, cellular, tissular, the entire organism, and behavior, including in humans), EGb 761 has shown particularly interesting effects in four domains: protection of the nervous system, protection of the circulatory system, protection against various diseases of the retina, and protection against some otorhinolaryngeal (ORL) diseases. Several of these effects are explained by its antioxidant action and by its effects on gene expression. As far as physiology and therapy are concerned, one remarkable aspect of EGb 761 is that it does not have a single unidirectional effect (activator or inhibitor) but rather is regulatory, promoting the adaptation of the organism to the situation at hand. This result may be due to the fact that it is a natural extract, that is, a set of molecules made by the process of natural

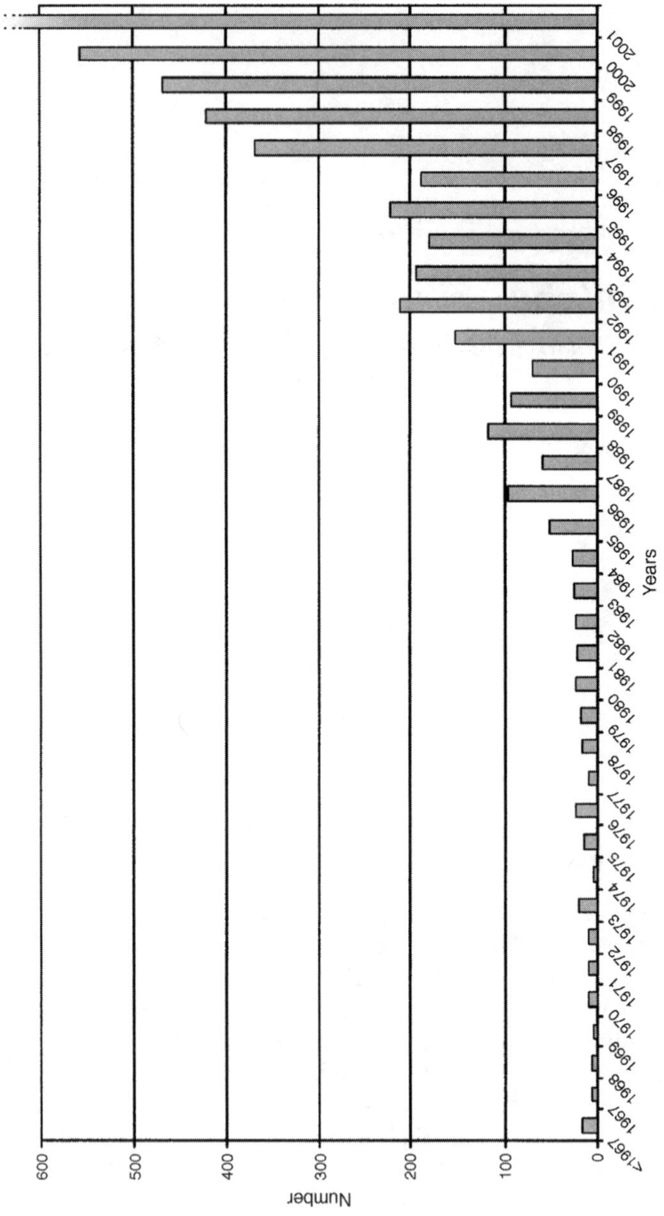

FIGURE 1 Number of publications on *Ginkgo biloba* published every year. Incomplete for the year 2001. Data from the ginkgo database. (Courtesy of F. Colmant, Medipsen, Paris.)

selection, a mechanism specialized in the making of adaptive biological systems.

Before any of its potential therapeutic uses were known, *Ginkgo biloba* was the object of study by botanists because it is an extremely original tree. For more than 30 years, an extract from the tree has also been a very popular drug, first in Europe (especially in France and Germany) and, more recently, in the United States. While several extracts of *Ginkgo biloba* exist, the reference extract, the extract that exists in standardized forms and has been the object of most of the published studies, is that known as EGb 761 (extrait de Ginkgo biloba n°761).

In recent years, the number of publications about *Ginkgo biloba* has multiplied impressively. I have described the universe of "ginkgology" elsewhere as an expanding universe (1). The concept of ginkgology is justified by the existence of a significant collection of data in very different domains but all concerning *Ginkgo biloba*: botany, evolution, ethnology and the study of traditional cultures, cultural anthropology, Asian civilizations and Far Eastern mythology, chemistry, pharmacology, medicine, etc. From this point of view, *Ginkgo biloba* is singular, perhaps unequaled in the medical world.

The increase in the number of scientific publications related to ginkgo confirms the reality of this expansion, as the analyses contained in the ginkgo database (Fig. 1) show. Although some of these studies concern nonmedical aspects of ginkgology, most examine EGb 761 and its interest to medicine. This situation is a rather paradoxical phenomenon in the history of the medical and pharmaceutical sciences: in most cases, drugs are studied primarily before their sale is approved and immediately afterward. The demands of marketing have led pharmaceutical laboratories to neglect them later, because they think they have said all that there is to be said about them and because they have found and are focusing on the next generation of drugs. Historically, the singularity of this difference is even greater than would appear from a simple reading of the statistics about the number of publications. Today, the important drugs arrive on the market with their history already established. The sponsors must argue convincingly that the research that led to their development was perfectly planned and rational and led to the specific target defined at the outset (e.g., inhibition of an enzyme or binding to a specific receptor). We might say that these drugs, conceptually, are represented in a finished universe (even though it is always possible to add new indications). EGb 761, on the other hand, exists in an open universe, into which totally new and even unforeseen data can arrive.

II. WHAT IS *GINKGO BILOBA*?

Ginkgo biloba is a tall, long-lived tree originating from China (2). Ginkgo means "silver apricot" and biloba refers to the shape of the two distinct lobes of the leaves. This species, which was classified in 1771 by Linné, is the only representative of the class of Ginkgoatae and even of its entire phylum, that of Ginkgophyta, distinct from all other trees, notably Coniferophyta and Cycadophyta. To this taxonomic singularity is added its unique status as a living fossil. Ginkgo trees already flourished 180 million years ago, when several species existed. Over the past million years, Ginkgos have progressively disappeared from most of the earth, finally surviving only in China. They have in fact nearly disappeared there, except for several rare areas, the best known of which are in Zhejiang province on the west peak of Tianmu Mountain (3). Fortunately, this disappearance in the wild has been compensated for by the cultivation of numerous specimens in China, Japan, other countries in the Far East, and even throughout the rest of the world. Many of these protected trees are very old. There are reports of more than 100 specimens in China that are more than 1000 years old (4). *Ginkgo biloba* was first introduced in Europe in 1690 by the botanist Engelbert Kaempfer, who described it as a "tree with duck feet" owing to the shape of its leaves (5). It is also an extremely hardy tree, as proved by its ability to survive the atomic bomb on Hiroshima. Today it adjusts well to pollution and is resistant to parasites; both reasons account for its success in our cities.

III. WHAT IS *GINKGO BILOBA* EXTRACT?

Ginkgo biloba extract, EGb 761, is a standardized extract of *Ginkgo biloba.* It contains 24% flavonoids and 6% terpene lactones. The flavonoids are nearly exclusively flavonol-O-glycosides (combination of the phenolic aglycones—quercetin, kaempferol, or isorhamnetin—with glucose or rhamnose or both in different positions of the flavonol moiety). The terpenoids are ginkgolides (3.1% of the extract) and bilobalide (2.9%), both found exclusively in the *Ginkgo biloba* tree. Ginkgolides are diterpenes, five of which have been identified (gingkolides A, B, C, M, and J). Bilobalide is a sesquiterpene. EGb 761 also contains proanthocyanidins (prodelphinidins) and organic acids (6). The combined activity of all the components of EGb 761 is required for its optimal therapeutic action (6). Several other extracts exist, especially in United States, where this herbal drug is not strictly regulated as in Europe. These extracts can vary in content, purity, and potency.

IV. CLINICAL INDICATIONS

The use of the ginkgo tree in traditional Chinese medicine is very ancient. The seeds have been used since at least the thirteenth century and the leaves since at least the sixteenth century. Modern Chinese pharmacopoeias mention the use of the leaves in the treatment of cardiac and pulmonary diseases but also against dysentery and filariasis (2,7). Modern Western usage of *Ginkgo biloba* extract is much more recent and results from research inspired not by traditional medicine but linked instead to the development of pharmacology. A first extract was marketed in 1965 in Germany by Dr. Willmar Schwabe Company. EGb 761 was first registered in France in 1974 and sold in 1975 by Institut Ipsen (now Ipsen Pharma) under the trademark Tanakan and in Germany as Rokan by Intersan in 1978 and as Tebonin forte by Dr. Willmar Schwabe Company in 1982. Its first therapeutic indications involved circulatory disturbances. More recently, the therapeutic effects that have been studied most are those affecting the psychobehavioral disorders associated with aging. These include cognitive disturbances, such as age-related memory disorders (grouped together today as mild cognitive impairment, MCI), or dementia, such as Alzheimer's disease. Whether these various indications (Alzheimer's disease, in particular), are included in the approved indications varies from country to country. EGb 761 is also prescribed against several diseases of the sensory organs that are often associated with aging, such as presbyacusis, tinnitus, age-related macular degeneration, glaucoma, etc.

In Europe (principally in France and Germany) these indications are officially approved, and patients are reimbursed for these health expenses. In the United States, on the other hand, *Ginkgo biloba* extract is mostly considered an herbal drug and is marketed as a health food.

In addition to the indications cited, EGb 761 has been the subject of numerous investigations that have reached definitive conclusions about its action in extremely diverse areas. Some of these indications are justified by serious studies—placebo-controlled and double-blinded—while others rest on much more fragile or uncontrolled foundations. Among the former, we note cognitive impairments associated with multiple sclerosis (8); mood disorders, particularly depression (9); sexual dysfunctions (10); and radiation-related disorders (11).

V. BIOLOGICAL PROOFS OF EFFICACY

Numerous studies have reported the principal effects of EGb 761: against neurodegenerative disorders, visual or ORL diseases, the ischemic process, and the vascular diseases associated with it (Table 1). These studies concern all levels of the organization of life: molecular, cellular, tissular, the entire organism (especially when aged or diseased), behavioral, and finally human. It is this multiplicity of findings that in its entirety constitutes the best proof of the extract therapeutic effect (12).

Many of these effects are ubiquitous. Thus, EGb 761 protects the cellular organelles, mitochondria in particular (13), the membranes, DNA, etc., and the cell as a whole against stress of diverse origins (radiation, toxic agents, etc.) and against aging. This protective effect involves diverse diseases

TABLE 1 Main Effects of *Ginkgo biloba* Extract EGb 761 and Its Clinical Applications

Therapeutic field	Molecular studies and mechanisms of action	Animal models	Clinical trial and epidemiological study
Memory impairment and MCI	Prevention: protection against oxidative stress (27); immediate effect: on gene expression (32,48)	Many experiments in rats and mice (49); protection of hippoccampus in old animals (50)	Dual coding test (51); EEG study (52) and beneficial effects on memory (53), attention and vigilance (54)
Alzheimer's disease	Protection against oxidative stress (55) and against agregation and toxicity of beta-amyloid (25,56); enhancing of alpha-secretase activity (57); induction of heme-oxygenase1 (33,58)	Beneficial effect in transgenic mice (59); enhancing of synaptic plasticity in the perforant pathway (60)	Symptomatic effect in multicenter study (61); preventive effect in epidemiological stucy (Epidos; 16)
Multiple sclerosis		Beneficial effect on experimental allergic encephalomyelitis in rat (62)	Beneficial effect on attention, memory, and functioning in patients (8)
Parkinson's disease	Protection of aged mitochondria (13); induction of Hsp70 (63)	Protection against the neurotoxic effects of MPTP (64,65)	Some positive data in uncontrolled observations
Amyotrophic lateral sclerosis	Protection against oxidative stress	Protective effect in the transgenic mice expressing the SOD1 mutation (66)	None
Stroke	Protection against oxidative stress	Protection against cerebral ischemia in gerbils and	Beneficial effect in patients with cerebrovascular

		rats; repairing of cerebral lesions	insufficiency; beneficial effect after cerebral infarct
Age-related macular degeneration	Protection against free radicals (67) and against loss of gluthatione (68)	Protection of the retina in old rats (69); protection against light-induced retinal degeneration (70)	Beneficial effect in patients (71)
Diabetic retinopathy	Protection against free radicals (27)	Protection against retinal injuries in diabetic rat (72); effect on intraocular proliferation (73)	Beneficial effect in patients (74)
Glaucoma	Protection against free radicals (75)	Effect on circulation to the optic nerve (76)	Increasing of ocular blood flow velocity in patients (77)
Vertigo		Beneficial effect on vestibular compensation in cat, rat, and guinea pig (78–80)	Beneficial effect in patients (81)
Hearing loss and sudden deafness	Improving survival of primary auditory neurons after trauma (Pujol and Puel, personal communication)	Effect on models of cochlear pathologies associated with ischemia (82)	Beneficial effect in patients (83)
Tinnitus		Attenuation of salicylate-induced tinnitus (84)	Beneficial effect in patient (85,86)
Peripheral arterial occlusive disease	Enhancing of the release of vasodilating factors such as NO/EDRF (37)	Vascular protection; vasodilator effect (37)	Several placebo-controlled multicenter studies; beneficial effect on intermittent claudication (87,88)
Trophic disorders and vasomotor changes in the extremities		Hemorheological and metabolic effects (89)	Beneficial effect on leg ulcers (90); beneficial effect in Raynaud's syndrome (91)

TABLE 1 Continued

Therapeutic field	Molecular studies and mechanisms of action	Animal models	Clinical trial and epidemiological study
Premenstrual syndrome	Vasoregulatory properties (89)		Effective against the congestive symptoms, particularly breast symptoms and neuropsychological symptoms (92)
Altitude sickness	Anti-ischemic, antihypoxic, vasoregulatory, metabolic, and antiedema properties (89)		Beneficial effect during a Himalayan expedition (93)
Protection against ionizing radiation	Protection against free radicals; inhibition of clastogenic factor (11)		Inhibition of the clastogenic factor among the Chernobyl liquidators (11)
Depression	Regulatory effect on neurotransmitters (serotonin) (44,94)	Beneficial effect on several models of stress (44,95,96)	Beneficial effect on mood among depressed patients (9)
Sexual dysfunction	Effect on phosphodiesterase (97)	Vasodilator effect (89)	Beneficial effect on sexual dysfunction (10)

of aging and not only neurodegenerative diseases. This explains the diversity of the indications for EGb 761.

To these ubiquitous effects we can add some that are much more specific, revealed by numerous studies, especially in vivo, in various pathophysiological models. For example, EGb 761 acts in vivo in models of various nervous system diseases: Alzheimer's disease (transgenic mice overexpressing a histopathological mutation of amyloid precursor protein), amyotrophic lateral sclerosis (transgenic mice expressing a harmful mutation to the superoxide dismutase gene, SOD1), Parkinson's disease (animals exposed to MPTP), stroke, head trauma, etc. EGb 761 also acts against cardiovascular disease, affecting various models of arrhythmia, myocardial ischemia and hypoxia, cerebral edema, etc. (12,14,15).

Finally, several clinical studies have confirmed its effect in the corresponding human diseases. These studies, as well as experimental research, justify expansive, large-scale prospective studies to determine whether EGb 761, which is associated with a lower prevalence of Alzheimer's disease in the Epidos epidemiological study (16), can prevent or delay the onset of this disease. The ginkgo evaluation of memory (GEM) study in United States (17) and the GuidAge study in France (18) are currently among the largest preventive studies in this field.

The clearest demonstration of the effects of EGb 761 does not concern a disease in the strict sense of the term but rather involves the duration of life. EGb 761 is the only substance that has been shown to be able to increase mean and especially maximum longevity in rats (19), which means a species of mammals. This longevity effect has also been found in the worm *Caenorhabditis elegans* (20). Although this effect does not actually involve protection against a disease, its medical importance is beyond dispute: it unambiguously demonstrates the reality of the biological action and proves how well this substance is tolerated.

VI. MECHANISMS OF ACTION

All of the various effects of EGb 761 cannot be attributed to a single mechanism of action or to a single molecule in the extract. The free-radical scavenging effect, for example, is due to flavonoids (21) but also to ginkgolides (22), the PAF-inhibiting effect (23) as well as the inhibition of peripheral benzodiazepine receptors (24) to ginkgolides, the protection against apoptosis and beta-amyloid toxicity to flavonoids (25), the increased longevity, at least in the worm *C. elegans*, to flavonoid action (20), and the upregulation of the cytochrome c oxidase gene to the biobalide (26).

Reduction to a single mechanism is certainly not necessary. Nonetheless we can explain many of EGb 761's effects by its antioxidant action and its action on gene expression, two related but distinct phenomena. Extensive experimental data have confirmed that it acts as a free-radical scavenger (21,27), including in vivo in humans (22). This finding tends to explain its protective role—of the nervous system in particular—in the harmful processes associated with aging and with traumatic, ischemic, or toxic injuries: most of the neurodegenerative disorders seems to be linked to a similar mechanism, i.e., the aggregation of toxic proteins and the effect of free radicals (28,29). More recently, effects have been observed on gene expression: EGb 761 inhibits AP-1 transcription factor (30) and increases or decreases the expression of many genes in vitro (31). Studies have also shown that EGb 761 affects in vivo gene expression in animals (32). In several cases, the gene effect involves not only mRNA expression but also production of the corresponding protein, including proteins with a clear-cut protective role, especially against neurodegenerative diseases, such as heme oxygenase 1 (33).

The free-radical-scavenging action is linked to the effect on gene expression, in that many genes, including those for transcription factors such as AP-1 and NF-kappaB, are sensitive to the free-radical concentration in cells. Nonetheless, from a biological and treatment point of view, these two mechanisms must be distinguished. Antioxidant action, in the strict sense of the term, explains the protection against degenerative mechanisms and thus the prevention or slowing down of decay. EGb 761 also exerts—for example, on attention mechanisms—effects that occur immediately or at least rapidly and cannot be explained simply by protection against cell death. Some of these effects may be due to changes in gene expression, which is a fast process. This particular mechanism can bring into play a multitude of targets within the cell, since proteins are often expressed in clusters within cells. The idea of a single target is thus illusory. The multiplicity of effects is particularly expected here because the extract contains numerous distinct molecules. The tools of molecular biology now offer new means of approaching this complexity, since DNA arrays make it possible to see, in a single experiment, an effect on several thousand genes. These are thus particularly important methods for testing the effect of such complex treatments as plant extracts, especially EGb 761 (34).

Another protective mechanism involved in many physiological and pathological situations is protection against cell death, especially apoptosis (25,35,36). Such an effect is potentially beneficial in many neurodegenerative diseases. Interestingly, EGb 761 protects cells from apoptosis in aged animals but it also exerts a cytostatic effect on tumor cells, thus showing an interesting adaptive effect (see latter on).

VII. AN ADAPTIVE EFFECT

One of the most remarkable aspects of EGb 761 is that, unlike many modern drugs, its pharmacological effects do not simply inhibit or activate a given target. On the contrary, its effect is instead regulatory, sometimes agonistic, sometimes antagonistic. Thus, at the vascular level, it does not simply exert effects on arteries, veins, and capillaries: these effects can be dilatational or constrictive, depending on the target or condition (6,37).

We know other examples of EGb 761's regulatory effects, in particular its action on apoptosis. Many experiments have shown that it protects against apoptotic phenomena, in particular in the framework of neurodegenerative processes (25), where this type of cell death plays a harmful role (38). In the presence of tumor development, however, EGb 761 acts in the opposite direction; that is, it has cytostatic properties that promote the elimination of cancers (39).

The effect of EGb 761 on the cerebral metabolism exemplifies another of these adaptive mechanisms. EGb 761 promotes oxygen and glucose consumption in the brains of animals in ischemic situations (40), but, inversely, facilitates metabolic economy in healthy subjects (41). PET imaging studies in humans have shown that the most gifted subjects tend to expend only a limited amount of brain energy for a given task compared with other individuals (42), and, inversely, that individuals with dementia use more energy than normal subjects (43). Economical energy metabolism is thus essential for optimal brain operations.

From a behavioral and neurochemical point of view, the effect of EGb 761 is similarly regulatory, promoting appropriate decision-making and neurotransmitter concentrations that help restore normality (44).

This drug thus seems to exert an adaptive effect; that is, it is sensitive to the physiological or pathological situation in which the organism finds itself (45). This may explain why it increases longevity. We note in this regard that the effects of EGb 761, which seem to differ from those of other drugs, resemble to some extent those of calorie restriction. The latter also extend life span and protect neurons against cerebral aging (46), undoubtedly by general homeostatic adaptation of the organism. By regulating energy expenditures (and modifying gene expression), calorie restriction preserves metabolic potential and limits free-radical production, itself associated with oxygen metabolism. The comparison is nonetheless incomplete, since EGb 761 intake is not accompanied by a reduction in the size of the organism, but it looks promising, especially because calorie restriction could be not very well adapted to human condition. Recent data suggest that biomarkers of calorie restriction may predict longevity in humans even in people who were not really on a diet (47). That means that it could be physiologically possible to mimic the effect of calorie restriction. EGb 761 could influence the metabolism in this way.

VIII. BOTTOM-UP VERSUS TOP-DOWN EFFECT

Modern therapeutic research is essentially based on the study of mechanisms of action: treatment targets can thus be defined and drugs developed specifically against them. The efficacy of the products thus developed should be guaranteed by the logic of this approach: they should work because they act directly on one of the steps involved in pathogenesis. This is what we might call a bottom-up strategy, which involves starting from an elementary target, located downstream, to exert a systemic effect upstream. The efficacy of this strategy requires no further proof We nonetheless note two aspects that raise questions about this type of approach. The first is that, in reality, it is impossible to define any single target in a cell that is independent from all other elementary targets. Developments in cellular and molecular biology show that cell proteins function in clusters. They have a social life: by touching one, we affect many others. Along the same line, we note that all cell signaling systems constitute cascades that involve many more or less ubiquitous enzymes. The concept of a single, well-defined target is thus less simple than we imagine, and a product "designed" to affect only one enzyme or receptor will, by a sort of domino effect, affect a multitude. To this rather theoretical comment we must add another, more bothersome in practice: the highly targeted strategies often present side effects that are the logical consequence of damage to a natural physiological system that has a rationale. In some way, disease is always a steady state or a state of compensation, in which the organism is readapting to cope with a situation—very imperfectly, of course—which is why the organism is sick. The dislocation of one of the cogs of this system is thus also a disturbance, the disruption of a compensation.

This bottom-up strategy can conceptually be opposed by another, which we can describe as top-down. Rather than aiming at a simple target, we focus on a physiological whole, hoping to modify specific molecular targets by a cascade effect. Psychotherapy is an example of this approach. It does not target a particular receptor or neuromediator (as psychoactive drugs do) but the subjects themselves. When it works, this strategy must also necessarily affect molecular targets but without focusing on them. Other examples of top-down strategies include more technologically sophisticated practices of modern science, such as transcranial magnetic stimulation or the more invasive stimulation used in the treatment of Parkinson's disease: a global target is aimed at, and the effect descends in a cascade to the molecular level.

Both strategies—bottom-up and top-down—have been used in EGb 761 studies. While many investigations have been based on a highly molecular strategy (for example, studies of the expression of some well-defined genes), others are more comprehensive (for example, its antistress effect or its effect on the duration of life, which is probably the most global parameter imaginable). The pursuit of this twofold line of research is incontestably original. The hope is that the two approaches may, as often as possible, meet at some level. This is apparently the case in neurodegenerative diseases, where we observe a comprehensive protective effect that may be explained by the data available from the study of elementary mechanisms. Other situations seem less clear; for example, some nearly immediate cognitive effects are difficult to explain by neuroprotection, as is the regulatory action of EGb 761 (that is, it works so often in the direction of adaptation to circumstances). We might simply postulate that this particularly beneficial aspect is related to the fact that EGb 761 is a natural extract, shaped by natural selection for millions of years to interact with physiological targets and to adapt to cellular complexity. There is hardly any reason for a manufactured synthetic molecule essentially designed to interact with a single target to have such a characteristics. From this point of view, it is hardly surprising that, by acting on its target, this molecule disturbs the rest of the physiological system. A natural extract (i.e., shaped by natural selection) has a greater chance of being less disruptive.

REFERENCES

1. Christen Y. The ginkgo, past, present and future. In: Van Beek TA, ed. *Ginkgo biloba*. Amsterdam: Hartwood Academic, 2000:523–532.
2. Michel PF. *Ginkgo biloba*: l'arbre qui a vaincu le temps. Paris: Editions du Félin, 1986.
3. Del Tredici P. The evolution, ecology, and cultivation of *Ginkgo biloba*. In: van Beek TA, ed. *Gingko biloba*. Amsterdam: Harwood Academic, 2000:7–23.
4. Shan-An H, Gu Y, Zi-Jie P. Resources and prospects of *Ginkgo biloba* in China. In: Hori T, Ridge RW, Tulecke W, Del Tredici P, Trémouillaux-Guiller J, Tobe H, eds. *Ginkgo biloba*—A Global Treasure: From Biology to Medicine. Tokyo: Springer, 1997:373–383.
5. Bilia AR. *Ginkgo biloba* L. Fitoterapia 2002; 73:276–279.
6. DeFeudis FV. *Ginkgo biloba* Extract (EGb 761): From Chemistry to the Clinic. Wiesbaden: Ullstein Medical, 1998.
7. Foster S, Chongxi Y. Herbal Emissaries. Rochester, VT: Healing Arts Press, 1992.
8. Kenney C, Norman M, Jacobson M, Lampinen S, Nguyen DP, Corey-Bloom J. A double-blind, placebo-controlled, modified crossover pilot study of the effects of *Ginkgo biloba* on cognitive and functional abilities in multiple sclerosis. Neurology 2002; 58(suppl 3):A458–A459.
9. Schubert H, Halama P. Primary therapy-resistant depressive instability in elderly patients with cerebral disorders: efficacy of a combination of *Ginkgo biloba* Extract (EGb 761) with antidepressants. Gritr Forsch 1993; 1:45–53.
10. Wheatley D. *Ginkgo biloba* relieves sexual dysfunction due to antidepressant drugs. Eur Neuropsychopharmacol 1999; 9(suppl 5):S253–S254.
11. Emerit I, Oganesian N, Sarkisian T, Arutyunyan R, Pogosian A, Asrian K, Levy A, Cernjavsky L. Clastogenic factors in the plasma of Chernobyl accident

recovery workers: anticlastogenic effect of *Ginkgo biloba* extract. Radiat Res 1995; 144:198–205.
12. Christen Y, Maixent JM. What is *Ginkgo biloba* extract EGb 761? An overview from molecular biology to clinical medicine. Moll Cell Biol 2002; 48:601–612.
13. Sastre J, Millan A, De la Asuncion JG, Pla R, Juan G, Pallardo FV, O'Connor E, Martin JA, Droy-Lefaix M-T, Vina J. A *Ginkgo biloba* extract (EGb 761) prevents mitochondrial aging by protecting against oxidative stress. Free Rad Biol Med 1998; 24:298–304.
14. Luo Y. Ginkgo biloba neuroprotection: therapeutic implications in Alzheimer's disease. J Alzheimer Dis 2001; 3:401–407.
15. Christen Y, ed. *Ginkgo biloba* Extract (EGb 761) as a Neuroprotective Agent: From Basic Studies to Clinical Trials. Marseille: Solal, 2001.
16. Andrieu S, Amouyal K, Reynish W, Nourhashèmi F, Vellas B, Albarède J-L, Grandjean for the Epidos Group. La consommation de vasodilatateurs et de *Ginkgo biloba* (EGB 761) dans une population de 7598 femmes âgées de plus de 75 ans. L'étude Epidos. Res Practice Alz Dis 2001; 5:58–67.
17. De Kosky ST. Antioxidants in Alzheimer's disease: intervention and prevention studies. Neurobiol Aging 2002; 23:S280.
18. Ousset PJ, Reynish E, Andrieu S, Vellas B. Etude GuidAge (Etude randomisée versus placebo de l'EGb 761 dans la prévention de la maladie d'Alzheimer sur une durée de 5 ans chez 2800 patients): rationnel. Res Practice Alz Dis 2002; 6:234–239.
19. Winter JC. The effects of an extract of *Ginkgo biloba* EGb 761, on cognitive behavior and longevity in the rat. Physiol Behav 1998; 63:425–433.
20. Wu Z, Smith JV, Paramasivam V, Butko P, Khan I, Cypser JR, Luo Y. *Ginkgo biloba* extract EGb 761 increases stress resistance and extends life span of *Caenorhabditis elegans*. Cell Mol Biol 2002; 48:725–731.
21. Packer L, Saliou C, Droy-Lefaix M-T, Christen Y. *Ginkgo biloba* extract EGb 761: antioxidant activity, and regulation of nitric oxide synthase. In: Rice-Evans CA, Packer L, eds. Flavonoids in Health and Disease. New York: Marcel Dekker, 1998:303–341.
22. Pietri S, Maurelli E, Drieu K, Culcasi M. Cardioprotective antioxidant effects of the terpenoid constituents of *Ginkgo biloba* extract (EGb 761). J Moll Cell Cardiol 1997; 29:733–742.
23. Braquet P, ed. Ginkgolides: Chemistry, Biology, Pharmacology and Clinical Perspectives. Barcelona: Prous, 1988.
24. Amri H, Ogwuegbu SO, Boujrad N, Drieu K, Papadopoulos V. In vivo regulation of the peripheral-type benzodiazepine receptor and glucocorticoid synthesis by the *Ginkgo biloba* extract EGb 761 and isolated ginkgolides. Endocrinology 1996; 137:5707–5718.
25. Bastianetto S, Ramassamy C, Doré S, Christen Y, Poirier J, Quirion R. The *Ginkgo biloba* extract (EGb 761) protects hippocampal neurons against cell death induced by β-amyloid. Eur J Neurosci 2000; 12:1882–1890.
26. Chandrasekaran K, Mehrabian Z, Spinnewyn B, Drieu K, Fiskum G. Neuroprotective effects of bilobalide, a component of the *Ginkgo biloba* extract (EGb 761), in gerbil global brain ischemia. Brain Res 2001; 922:282–292.

27. Droy-Lefaix M–T. Effect of the antioxidant action of *Ginkgo biloba* extract (EGb 761) on aging and oxidative stress. Age 1997; 20:141–149.
28. Christen Y. Des protéines et des mutations: une nouvelle vision (moléculaire) des maladies neuro-dégénératives. J Soc Biol 2002; 196:85–94.
29. Taylor JP, Hardy J, Fischbeck KH. Toxic proteins in neurodegenerative disease. Science 2002; 296:1991–1995.
30. Mizuno M, Packer L. *Ginkgo biloba* extract (EGb 761) is a suppressor of AP-1 transcription factor stimulated by PMA. Biochem Mol Biol Int 1996; 39:395–401.
31. Gohil K, Moy RK, Farzin S, Maguire JJ, Packer L. mRNA expression profile of a human cancer cell line in response to *Ginkgo biloba* extract: induction of antioxidant response and the Golgi system. Free Rad Res 2000; 33:831–849.
32. Watanabe CMH, Wolffram S, Ader P, Rimbach G, Packer L, Maguire JJ, Schultz PG, Gohil K. The in vivo neuromodulatory effects of the herbal medicine ginkgo biloba. Proc Natl Acad Sci USA 2001; 98:6577–6580.
33. Zhuang H, Pin S, Christen Y, Dore S. Neuroprotective effects of *Ginkgo biloba* is mediated by heme oxygenase. Soc Neurosci 2002; 28. In press.
34. Christen Y, Olano-Martin E, Packer L. EGb 761 in the post genomic era; new tools from molecular biology for the study of complex products such as *Ginkgo biloba* extract. Cell Mol Biol 2002; 48:593–600.
35. Smith JJ, Burdick AJ, Golik P, Khan I, Wallace D, Luo Y. Anti-apoptotic properties of *Ginkgo biloba* extract EGb 761 in differenciated cells. Cell Mol Biol 2002; 48:699–708.
36. Massieu L, Moran J, Christen Y, Effect of *Ginkgo biloba* (EGb 761) on staurosporine-induced apoptotic neuronal deathand caspase-3 activity in cortical cultures. Brain Res. In press.
37. Auguet M, Clostre F. *Ginkgo biloba* extract (EGb 761) and vasomotor adaptation. In: Papadopoulos V, Drieu K, Christen Y, eds. Advances in *Ginkgo biloba* Extract Research. Vol. 6. Adaptive Effects of *Ginkgo biloba* Extract (EGb 761). Paris: Elsevier, 1997:1–7.
38. Henderson C, Green D, Mariani J, Christen Y, eds. Neuronal Death by Accident or by Design. Heidelberg: Springer Verlag, 2001.
39. Papadopoulos V, Kapsis A, Li H, Amri H, Hardwick M, Culty M, Kasprzyk PG, Carlson M, Moreau J-P, Drieu K. Drug-induced inhibition of the peripheral-type-benzodiazepine receptor expression and cell proliferation in human breast cancer cells. Anticancer Res 2002; 20:2835–2848.
40. Karcher L, Zagermann P, Krieglstein J. Effect of an extract of *Ginkgo biloba* on rat brain energy metabolism in hypoxia. Naunyn-Schmiedeberg's Arch Pharmacol 1984; 327:31–35.
41. Lamour Y, Holloway HW, Rapoport SI, Soncrant TT. Effects of ginkgolide-B and *Ginkgo biloba* extract on local cerebral glucose utilization in the awake adult rat. Drug Dev Res 1991; 23:219–225.
42. Haier RJ. Cerebral glucose metabolism and intelligence. In: Vernon PA, ed. Biological Approaches to the Study of Human Intelligence. Norwood, NJ: Ablex Pub, 1993:317–332.
43. Bookheimer SY, Strojwas MH, Cohen MS, Saunders AM, Pericak-Vance MA,

Mazziotta JC, Small GW. Patterns of brain activation in people at risk for Alzheimer's disease. N Engl J Med 2000; 343:450–456.
44. Pardon MC, Joubert C, Perez-Diaz F, Christen Y, Launay JM, Cohen-Salmon C. In vivo regulation of cerebral monoamine oxidase activity in senescent controls and chronically stressed mice by long-term treatment with *Ginkgo biloba* extract (EGb 761). Mech Ageing Dev 2000; 113:157–168.
45. Papadopoulos V, Drieu K, Christen Y, Eds. Advances in *Ginkgo biloba* Extract Research. Vol. 6. Adaptive Effects of *Ginkgo biloba* Extract (EGb 761). Paris: Elsevier, 1997.
46. Mattson MP, Duan W, Lee J, Guo Z. Suppression of brain aging and neurodegenerative disorders by dietary restriction and environmental enrichment: molecular mechanisms. Mech Aging Dev 2001; 122:757–778.
47. Roth GS, Lane MA, Ingram DK, Mattison JA, Elahi D, Tobin JD, Muller D, Metter EJ. Biomarkers of caloric restriction may predict longevity in humans. Science 2002; 297:811.
48. Gohil K, Packer L. Global gene expression analysis identifies cell and tissue specific actions of *Ginkgo biloba* extract. EGb 761. Cell Mol Biol 2002; 48:625–632.
49. Cohen-Salmon C, Venault P, Martin B, Raffalli-Sébille MJ, Barkats M, Clostre F, Pardon MC, Christen Y, Chapouthier G. Effects of *Ginkgo biloba* extract EGb 761 on learning and memory. J Physiol (Paris) 1997; 91:291–300.
50. Barkats M, Venault P, Christen Y, Cohen-Salmon C. Effects of long term treatment with EGb 761 on age-dependent structural changes in the hippocampi of three inbred mouse strains. Life Sci 1995; 56:213–222.
51. Allain H, Raoul P, Lieury A, LeCoz F, Gandon JM, d'Arbigny P. Effect of two doses of *Ginkgo biloba* extract (EGb 761) on the dual-coding test in elderly subjects. Clin Ther 1993; 15:549–558.
52. Luthringer R, d'Arbigny P, Macher JP. *Ginkgo biloba* Extract (EGb 761), EEG and event-related potentials mapping profile. In: Christen Y, Courtois Y, Droy-Lefaix MT, eds. Advances in *Ginkgo biloba* Extract Research. Vol. 4. Effects of *Ginkgo biloba* Extract (EGb 761) on Aging and Age-Related Disorder. Paris: Elsevier, 1995:107–118.
53. Israel L, Dell'Accio E, Martin G, Hugonot R. Extrait de *Ginkgo biloba* et exercices d'entraînement de la mémoire. Evaluation comparative chez des personnes âgées ambulatoires. Psychol Méd 1987; 19:1431–1439.
54. Polich J, Gloria R. Cognitive effect of a *Ginkgo biloba*/vinpocetine compound in normal adults: systematic assessment of perception, attention and memory. Hum Psychopharmaco Clin Exp 2001; 16:409–416.
55. Ramassamy C, Averill D, Beffert U, Bastianetto S, Theroux L, Lussier-Cacan S, Cohn JS, Christen Y, Davignon J, Quirion R, Poirier J. Oxidative damage and protection by antioxidants in the frontal cortex of Alzheimer's disease is related to the apolipoprotein E genotype. Free Rad Biol Med 1999; 27:544–553.
56. Ramassamy C, Christen Y, Poirier J. *Ginkgo biloba* extract (EGb 761), β-amyloid peptide and apolipoprotein E in Alzheimer's disease. In: Christen Y, ed. Advances in *Ginkgo biloba* Extract Research. Vol. 8. *Ginkgo biloba* Extract (EGb

761) as a Neuroprotective Agent: From Basic Studies to Clinical Trials. Marseille: Solal, 2001:772–789.

57. Colciaghi F, Bellone C, Cattabeni F, Di Luca M. EGb 761 induces APPs secretion in a protein kinase C independent manner in rat hippocampal slices. In: Christen Y, ed. Advances in *Ginkgo biloba* Extract Research. Vol. 8. *Ginkgo biloba* Extract (EGb 761) as a Neuroprotective Agent: From Basic Studies to Clinical Trials. Marseille: Solal, 2001:123–137.
58. Chen JX, Zeng H, Chen X, Su CY, Lai CC. Induction of the heme oxygenase-1 by *Gingko biloba* extract but not its terpenoids partially mediated its protective effect against lysophosphatidylcholine-induced damage. Pharmacol Res 2001; 43:63–69.
59. Stackman RW, Quinn JF, Nowlin J, Eckenstein. Spatial memory deficits exhibited by a transgenic mouse model of Alzheimer's disease are blocked by *Ginkgo biloba*. Soc Neurosci 2001; 27:17191719.
60. Smriga M, Saito H, Nishiyama N. *Ginkgo biloba* facilitates synaptic plasticity in the rat perforant path: dentate gyrus projections in-vivo. Pharm Sci 1997; 3:521–523.
61. Le Bars PL, Katz MM, Berman N, Itil T, Freedman AM, Schalzberg AF. A placebo-controlled double-blind, randomized trial of an extract of *Ginkgo biloba* for dementia. JAMA 1997; 278:1327–1332.
62. Howat DW, Chand N, Moore AR, Braquet P, Willoughby DA. The effects of platelet-activating factor and its specific antagonist BN 52021 on the development of experimental allergic encephalomyelitis in rat. Int J Immunopathol Pharmacol 1988; 1:11–15.
63. Soulié C, Nicolle A, Christen Y, Ceballos-Picot I. The *Ginkgo biloba* extract EGb 761 increases viability of hNT human neurons in culture and affects the expression of genes implicated in the stress response. Cell Mol Biol 2002; 48:641–646.
64. Ramassamy C, Clostre F, Christen Y, Costentin J. In vivo *Ginkgo biloba* extract (EGb 761) protects against neurotoxic effects induced by MPTP: investigations into its mechanism(s) of action. In: Christen Y, Costentin J, Lacour M, eds. Advances in *Ginkgo biloba* Extract Research. Vol. 1. Effects of *Ginkgo biloba* Extract (EGb 761) on the Central Nervous System. Paris: Elsevier, 1992:27–36.
65. Wu WR, Zhu XZ. Involvement of monoamine oxidase inhibition in neuroprotective and neurorestorative effects of *Ginkgo biloba* extract against MPTP-induced nigrostriatal dopaminergic toxicity in C57 mice. Life Sci 1999; 65:157–164.
66. Ferrante RJ, Klein AM, Dedeoglu A, Beal MF. Therapeutic efficacy of EGb 761 (*Ginkgo biloba* extract) in a transgenic mouse model of amyotrophic lateral sclerosis. J Mol Neurosci 2001; 17:89–96.
67. Droy-Lefaix MT, Baudoin C, de Kozak Y, Doly M. Free radicals and antioxidants in pathophysiology of mammalian retina. In: Packer L, Hiramatsu M, Yoshikawa T, eds. Free Radicals in Brain Physiology and Disorders. San Diego: Academic Press, 1996:359–376.

68. Paasche G, Huster D, Reichenbach A. The glutathione content of retinal Muller (glial) cells: the effects of aging and of application of free-radical scavengers. Ophthal Res 1998; 30:351–360.
69. Droy-Lefaix M–T, Bonhomme B, Doly M. A protective effect of EGb 761 on aging rat retina. Invest Ophthalmol Vis Sci 1995; 36:S855.
70. Ranchon I, Cluzel J, Gorrand J-M, Martinez V, Doly D. Prevention of light-induced retinal neurodegeneration by *Ginkgo biloba* extract (EGb 761). In: Christen Y, ed. Advances in *Ginkgo biloba* Extract Research. Vol. 8. *Ginkgo biloba* Extract (EGb 761) as a Neuroprotective Agent: From Basic Studies to Clinical Trials. Marseille: Solal, 2001:33–52.
71. Lebuisson DA, Leroy L, Rigal G. traitement des dégénéréscences "maculaires séniles" par l'extrait de *Ginkgo biloba*: etude à double insu face au placebo. Presse Méd 1986; 15:1556–1558.
72. Besse G, Vennat JC, Betoin F, Doly M, Droy-Lefaix M-T. Extrait de *Ginkgo biloba* (EGb 761) et rétinopathie diabétique expérimentale. In: Christen Y, Doly M, Droy-Lefaix M-T, eds. Rétine, vieillissement et transplantation. Paris: Elsevier, 1994:133–138.
73. Baudouin C, Ettaiche M, Imbert F, Droy-Lefaix MT, Gastaud P, Lapalus P. Inhibition of preretinal proliferation by free radical scavengers in an experimental model of tractional retinal detachment. Exp Eye Res 1994; 59:697–706.
74. Lanthony P, Cosson JP. Evolution de la vision des couleurs dans la rétinopathie diabétique débutante traitée par extrait de *Ginkgo biloba*. J Fr Ophthalmol 1988; 11:671–674.
75. Schumer RA, Podos SM. The nerve of glaucoma! Arch Ophthalmol 1994; 112:37–44.
76. Head KA. Natural therapies for ocular disorders. Part two. Cataracts and glaucoma. Altern Med Rev 2001; 6:141–166.
77. Chung H, Harris A, Kristinsson JK, Ciulla TA, Kagemann C, Ritch R. *Ginkgo biloba* extract increases ocular blood flow velocity. J Ocular Pharmacol Ther 1999; 15:233–240.
78. Lacour M, Ez-Zaher L, Raymond J. Plasticity mechanisms in vestibular compensation in the cat are improved by an extract of *Ginkgo biloba* EGb 761. Pharmacol Biochem Behav 1991; 40:367–379.
79. Denise P, Bustany P. The effect of an extract of *Ginkgo biloba* (EGB 761) on central compensation of a total unilateral peripheral vestibular deficit in the rat. In: Lacour M, Toupet M, Denise P, Christen Y, eds. Vestibular Compensation: Fact, Theories and Clinical Perspectives. Paris: Elsevier, 1989:201–208.
80. Yabe T, Chat M, Malherbe E, Vidal PP. Effects of *Ginkgo biloba* Extract (EGb 761) on the guinea vestibular system. Pharmacol Biochem Behav 1992; 42:595–604.
81. Haguenauer JP, Cantenot F, Koskas H, Pierat H. Traitement des troubles de l'équilibre par l'extrait de *Ginkgo biloba*: etude multicetrique à double insu face au placebo. Presse Méd 1986; 15:1569–1572.
82. Cazals Y, Horner K, Didier A. Experimental models of cochlear pathologies

associated with ischemia. In: Ferradini C, Droy-Lefaix M-T, Christen Y, eds. Advances in *Ginkgo biloba* Extract Research. Vol. 2. *Ginkgo biloba* Extract (EGb 761) as a Free Radical Scavenger. Paris: Elsevier, 1993:115–122.

83. Burschka MA, Hassan HAH, Reineka T, Van Bebber L, Caird DM, Moesges R. Effect of treatment with *Ginkgo biloba* extract EGb 761 (oral) on unilateral idiopathic sudden hearing loss in a prospective randomized double-blind study of 106 outpatients. Eur Arch Oto Rhino Laryngol 2001; 258:213–219.
84. Jastreboff PJ, Zhou S, Jastreboff MM, Kwapsz U, Gryczynska U. Attenuation of salicylate-induced tinnitus by *Ginkgo biloba* extract in rats. Audiol Neurotol 1997; 2:197–212.
85. Baschek V, Steinert W. Differential diagnosis of studden deafness and therapy with high dose infusions of *Ginkgo biloba* extract. In: Claussen CF, Kirtane MV, Schlitter K, eds. Vertigo, Nausea, Tinnitus and Hypoacusia in Metabolic Disorders. Paris: Elsevier, 1998:575–582.
86. Reisser C, Weidauer H. *Ginkgo biloba* extract EGb 761 or pentoxifylline for the treatment of sudden deafness: a randomized, reference-controlled, double-blind study. Acta Oto Laryngol 2001; 121:579–584.
87. Bauer U. Six-month double-blind randomized clinical trial of *Ginkgo biloba* extract versus placebo in two parallel groups in patients suffering from peripheral arterial insufficiency. Arzneim Forsch./Drug Res 1984; 34:716–720.
88. Bulling B, Clemens N, Dankers V. Clinical uses of *Ginkgo biloba* extract in the field of peripheral arterial occlusive disease (PAOD). In: Van Beek, ed. *Ginkgo biloba*. Amsterdam: Harwood Academic, 2000:371–384.
89. Clostre F, DeFeudis FV, eds. Cardiovascular Effects of *Ginkgo biloba* Extract (EGb 761). Paris: Elsevier, 1994.
90. Maillet P, Bazex J, d'Arbigny PStudy Group Investigators. *Ginkgo biloba* extract, EGb 761 and trophic disorders of the lower limbs: contribution of EGb 761's ischemic action assiociated with local treatment. In: Clostre F, DeFeudis FV, eds. Advances in *Ginkgo biloba* Extract Research. Vol. 3. Cardiovascular Effects of *Ginkgo biloba* Extract. Paris: Elsevier, 1994:151–160.
91. Clément JL, Livecchi G, Jimenez S, Morino S, Drevard R, Eclache JP. Modifications vasomotrices des extrêmités lors de l'exposition à des conditions thermiques défavorables: méthodologie et résultat de l'étude de l'extrait de *Ginkgo biloba*. Act Angiol 1982; 7:3–8.
92. Tamborini A, Taurelle R. Intérêt de l'extrait standardisé de *Ginkgo biloba* (EGb 761) dans la prise en charge des symptômes congestifs du syndrome prémenstruel. Rev Fr Gyn Obst 1993; 88:7–9.
93. Roncin JP, Schwartz F, d'Arbigny P. EGb 761 in control of acute mountain sickness and vascular reactivity to cold exposure. Aviat Space Environ Med 1996; 67:445–452.
94. Fillion G, Fillion MP, Bolanos-Jimenez F. Serotoninergic system and Ginkgo biloba extracts. In: Papadopoulos V, Drieu K, Christen Y, eds. Advances in *Ginkgo biloba* Extract Research. Vol. 6. Adaptive Effects of *Ginkgo biloba* Extract (EGb 761). Paris: Elsevier, 1997:99–116.
95. Porsolt RD, Martin P, Lenègre A, Fromage S, Drieu K. Effects of an extract of

Ginkgo biloba (EGb 761) on "learned helplessness" and other models of stress in rodents. Pharmacol Biochem Behav 1990; 36:963–971.
96. Rapin JR, Lamproglou I, Drieu K, DeFeudis FV. Demonstration of the "anti-stress" activity of an extract of *Ginkgo biloba* (EGb 761) using a discrimination learning task. Gen Pharmacol 1994; 25:1009–1016.
97. Clostre F. *Ginkgo biloba* Extract (EGb 761): etat de connaissances à l'aube de l'an 2000. Ann Pharm Fr 1999; 57(suppl 1):1S5–1S88.

8

Ginger

Ann M. Bode and Zigang Dong
University of Minnesota
Austin, Minnesota, U.S.A.

I. INTRODUCTION

The use of "natural" or alternative medicines for treating a variety of ailments has increased significantly in the past few years. More and more older adults are using complementary and alternative medicine dietary supplements and herbal remedies without advice from a physician (1). Unfortunately much of the information regarding the effectiveness and safety of these remedies has been gleaned from anecdotal or historical accounts, which seem to be readily available from a variety of sources. For example, advice offered to pregnant women by "medical herbalists" is readily available over the Internet, and generally the advice offered is misleading and may even be dangerous (2). Plants of the ginger (*Zingiber officinale* Roscoe, Zingiberaceae) family are among the most heavily consumed dietary substances in the world (3). Although ginger has been suggested, by results of both experimental and clinical data, to be safe for therapeutic use (4), many clinicians and researchers advise caution because of the lack of a complete understanding of its mechanisms of action (5–7). The acquisition of sound scientific research data has only just become a priority for determining the mechanism of action of many dietary compounds, including ginger. A recent review emphasizes the importance of scientific appraisal to establish the safety and efficacy of potential therapeutic plant remedies (8), and the risks and benefits of herbal medicine have also been reviewed (9,10). Ginger has been purported to have a variety of powerful therapeutic effects and has been used for thousands of years for treatment of numerous ailments, including colds, nausea, arthritis, migraines, and hypertension. The medicinal, chemical, and pharmacological properties of ginger have been recently extensively reviewed (11–13). The purpose of this chapter is to critically evaluate the available scientific evidence supporting the effective and safe use of ginger and some of its various components.

II. METABOLISM OF GINGER

Although ginger is one of the most commonly consumed spices worldwide, very little is known about its metabolism or metabolites. An evaluation of the bioactivity of crude dietary compounds, including ginger, is necessary for a complete understanding of the mechanism of action and potential therapeutic effects. Although many food-derived supplements are consumed with little knowledge of their activity or safety, more attention is beginning to be given to addressing these issues.

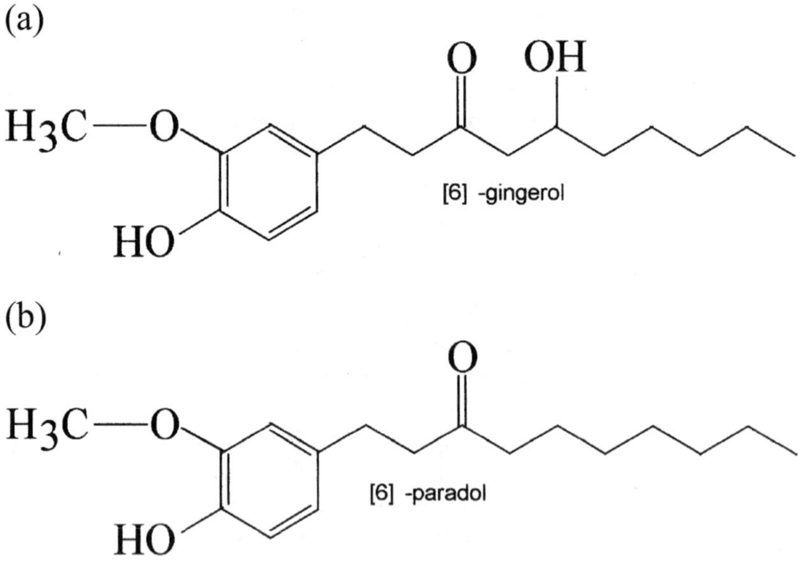

FIGURE 1 Chemical structure of (a) [6]-gingerol and (b) [6]-paradol.

The oleoresin from the root of ginger contains [6]-gingerol (1-[4′-hydroxy-3′-methoxyphenyl]-5-hydroxy-3-decanone), the major pharmacologically active component (Fig. 1a) (3), and lesser amounts of a structurally related vanilloid, [6]-paradol (1-[4′-hydroxy-3′-methyoxyphenyl]-3-decanone (Fig. 1b). An earlier study indicated that [6]-gingerol is very rapidly cleared from rat plasma following intravenous administration (3 mg/kg) (14]. In a later study, 6-gingerol was reported to be metabolized enzymatically in a stereospecific reduction to gingerdiol (15]. The careful isolation of several metabolites of [6]-gingerol after oral administration (50 mg/kg) to rats has recently been reported (16). A main metabolite, (S)-[6]-gingerol-4′-*O*-β-glucuronide, was detected in the bile and several minor metabolites were found in β-glucuronidase-treated urine, indicating that orally administered [6]-gingerol undergoes conjugation and oxidation of a phenolic side chain (16). This study may mark the beginning of the type of in vivo information that needs to be obtained, but more work is obviously needed to determine the biological activities and mechanism of action of these metabolites.

III. ANTIOXIDANT PROPERTIES OF GINGER

A common mechanism offered to explain the actions and health benefits of ginger and other herbs and spices is related to their antioxidant properties (17,18). A systematic analysis (19) of several hundred dietary plants revealed that ginger root contained a very high concentration (3.85 mmol/100 g) of total antioxidants. Only pomegranate and several types of wild berries (e.g., dog rose, blueberry, strawberry, blackberry) had a higher total antioxidant concentration (19). In addition, Zancan et al. (20) recently presented a detailed report on the development of a process to produce ginger extracts with a high content of antioxidants, suggesting that antioxidant activity is widely accepted to be important in the effectiveness of ginger.

Tumor promoters, including 12-*O*-tetradecanoylphorbol-13-acetate (TPA), are believed to act by promoting oxidative stress through the activation of the NADPH oxidase system and/or the xanthine oxidase system. Many edible Japanese plants, including mioga ginger, were reported to be very effective in suppressing TPA-induced superoxide generation from NADPH oxidase and xanthine oxidase in HL-60 cells and AS52 cells, respectively (21). Several additional studies suggest the effectiveness of ginger as an antioxidant in vitro. Ginger compounds were shown to inhibit lipid peroxidation (22,23), to inhibit superoxide production (21,24), and to decrease oxidative stress markers associated with aging (25). Recent studies suggest that ginger was effective in lowering experimentally induced lipid peroxidation and maintaining glutathione levels (26,27). Although, evidence suggests that ginger and some of its components are effective antioxidants in vitro, the physiological activity in vivo is not clear and more work using isolated, purified components of ginger is needed.

IV. ANTICARCINOGENIC EFFECTS OF GINGER

Several aspects of the chemopreventive effects of various phytochemical dietary and medicinal substances, including ginger, have been reviewed (3,28,29). Possibly because of our general failure to find a "magic cure" for cancer, the identification of plant-derived compounds or phytochemicals having the capacity to interfere with carcinogenic processes has been receiving increased interest. Many herbs and spices are known to possess an array of biochemical and pharmacological activities including antioxidant and anti-inflammatory properties that are believed to contribute to their anticarcinogenic and antimutagenic activities.

Earlier studies suggested that gingerol was an effective inhibitor of azoxymethane-induced intestinal carcinogenesis in rats (30). Several ginger components were shown to have effective antitumor-promoter activity based on their ability to inhibit TPA-induced Epstein-Barr virus early antigen (EBV-EA) in Raji cells (31,32).

The most common model used to study the effectiveness of ginger as an antitumor agent in vivo seems to be the two-stage initiation-promotion mouse skin model. In this paradigm, tumors are initiated by one application of 7, 12-dimethylbenz[a]anthracene (DMBA) followed by repeated topical applications of TPA beginning a few days later. Ginger and its constituents have been shown to inhibit tumor promotion in mouse skin (33). Another study indicated that topical application of (6)-gingerol onto the shaven backs of female ICR mice reduced the incidence of DMBA-initiated/TPA-promoted skin papilloma formation and also suppressed TPA-induced epidermal ornithine decarboxylase activity and inflammation (34). In a similar more recent study, Chung et al. (35) reported that in the DMBA/TPA skin tumor model, topical application of [6]-paradol and [6]-dehydroparadol prior to the application of TPA significantly reduced both the number of tumors per mouse and the fraction of mice with tumors (35). They suggested that the antitumor-promoting effect may be related to the ability of these compounds to suppress TPA-induced oxidative stress.

On the other hand, evidence also suggests that ginger and other related compounds may act as chemopreventive agents by inducing programmed cell death or apoptosis (36). At least two recent studies suggest that these compounds suppress proliferation of human cancer cells through the induction of apoptosis (37,38). However, very little is known regarding the molecular mechanisms by which they may exert their antitumorigenic effects. Previously, through the comparison of promotion-sensitive (P^+) and promotion-resistant (P^-) derivatives of the mouse epidermal JB6 cell lines, AP-1 was shown to have a critical role in tumor promotion (39–41). In addition, blocking the tumor-promoter-induced activation of AP-1 inhibited neoplastic transformation (40,41). Epidermal growth factor (EGF) is known to induce a relatively high level of AP-1 activity and cell transformation (39). We recently investigated the effect of two structurally related compounds of the ginger family, [6]-gingerol and [6]-paradol, on EGF-induced cell transformation and AP-1 activation (42). Our results provide the first evidence that both compounds block EGF-induced cell transformation but act by different mechanisms. [6]-Gingerol appeared to act by directly inhibiting AP-1 DNA-binding activity and transactivation, whereas [6]-paradol appeared to act by inducing apoptosis (42). Another recent study showed that [6]-paradol and other structurally related derivatives, [10]-paradol, [3]-dehydroparadol, [6]-dehydroparadol, and [10]-dehydroparadol, inhibited proliferation of KB oral squamous carcinoma cells in a time- and dose-dependent manner (43). [6]-Dehydroparadol (75 μM) was more potent than the other compounds tested and induced apoptosis through a caspase-3-dependent mechanism (43).

V. ANTI-INFLAMMATORY EFFECTS OF GINGER

Ginger and other natural compounds have been suggested to be effective against inflammation, osteoarthritis, and rheumatism (44). But because of inconsistencies in clinical studies, the effectiveness and safety of ginger for treatment of arthritis have been debated (45). Early animal studies suggested that [6]-gingerol perfused into rat hindlimb possessed thermogenic activity, characterized by increased oxygen consumption and lactate efflux (46). The thermogenesis was at least partly associated with vasoconstriction independent of adrenergic receptors or secondary catecholamine release. Large doses of ginger components also inhibited oxygen consumption, which was attributed to disruption of mitochondrial function (46). Another early study showed that ginger oil (33 mg/kg), administered orally to rats for 26 days, caused a significant repression of paw and joint swelling associated with severe chronic adjuvant arthritis (47).

In humans, one recent study showed no difference between placebo and ginger in patients with osteoarthritis of the hip or knee (48). On the other hand, patients suffering from osteoarthritis of the knee showed a consistently greater response to treatment with ginger extract compared with the control group (49). In addition, relief from pain and swelling was reported in patients suffering from rheumatoid arthritis, osteoarthritis, general muscular discomfort when they used powdered ginger as a dietary supplement for 3 months–2 years. Investigators suggested that the effectiveness of ginger may be related to its ability to inhibit prostaglandin and leukotriene biosynthesis (50). Others showed that gingerol actively inhibits arachidonate 5-lipoxygenase, an enzyme of leukotriene biosynthesis (51). [8]-Gingerol but not [6]-gingerol was shown to inhibit COX-2 expression, which is induced during inflammation to increase formation of prostaglandins (52). This suggests that the structure of ginger influences its effectiveness.

VI. GINGER AS AN ANTINAUSEA AGENT

The most common use of ginger throughout history has probably been its utilization in alleviating symptoms of nausea and vomiting. The benefits and dangers of herbal treatment in liver and gastrointestinal distress have been reviewed recently (53) and several controlled studies have shown that ginger is generally effective as an antiemetic (54). Ginger root is commonly recommended for preventing seasickness (55), but in contrast, patients receiving ginger extract for treating osteoarthritis experienced more, albeit mild, gastrointestinal adverse events than did the placebo group (49). Even though these effects of ginger have been the most well studied and reviewed extensively, the effectiveness and safety of ginger for treating nausea and vomiting is still questioned because of the often contradictory findings (5,6 and reviewed in Ref. 7). This is especially relevant for its use by pregnant women.

Nausea and vomiting during pregnancy affects the majority of pregnant women and over the years various treatments have been used to try to alleviate the condition (reviewed in Ref. 56). Unsupervised herbal or alternative therapies are often pursued and ginger is a commonly used remedy (57). Although perhaps not as potent as some treatments (58), ginger has been shown to be effective for nausea and vomiting in early pregnancy (59–61). At least one survey indicated that although overall use of dietary supplements in pregnant women appeared to be low, ginger was commonly recommended and used to prevent nausea (62). Randomized trials suggest that ginger consumption for nausea and/or vomiting in early pregnancy has very few or no adverse side effects and may be effective (60,63,64). A recent survey of a group of obstetricians and gynecologists revealed that most of them would recommend taking an antiemetic (71.3%), specifically ginger (51.8%), to patients suffering from moderate to severe nausea (65).

Animal studies indicate that oral administration of a standardized ginger extract (EV.EXT 33; 1000 mg/kg) was well tolerated by pregnant rats and had no adverse effects on the mother or development of the fetuses (66). This is somewhat in contrast to an earlier study, in which ginger tea administration to pregnant rats resulted in embryonic loss twice that of controls (5). However, surviving fetuses were significantly heavier than control. Intraperitoneal injection of ginger rhizome extract (0.5–10 g/kg) to mice was reported to have no clastogenic effects compared to ginger oil, which produced some chromosomal irregularities (67).

Ginger has been suggested to be an effective postoperative prophylactic antiemetic (68) that was not associated with an effect on gastric emptying (69). However, the effectiveness of ginger in preventing postoperative nausea and vomiting has also been debated (70). A recent study has indicated that pretreatment with ginger extracts reversed experimentally induced delay in gastric emptying in rats (71). This supports previous indications that ginger may be effective in alleviating symptoms associated with gastrointestinal illnesses, including abdominal discomfort and bloating (71). In further support of ginger increasing gastric emptying, ginger was shown to reduce food transit time in experimental rats, which was suggested to have implications for prevention of colon cancer and constipation (72). The digestive stimulatory effects of ginger and other spices have been suggested to be related to positive effects on trypsin and pancreatic lipase (73) and ginger's ability to increase gastric motility (74).

Ginger has also been recommended to combat nausea associated with chemotherapy (12,75) and 6-gingesulfonic acid, isolated from ginger root, was shown to be effective against HC1/ethanol-induced gastric lesions in rats (76). This compound showed weaker pungency and more potent antiulcer activity than 6-gingerol or 6-shogaol (77).

VII. CARDIOVASCULAR-ASSOCIATED EFFECTS OF GINGER

Caution in taking ginger and other herbal extracts has been suggested because of an apparent association with reported incidences of increased risk of bleeding following surgery (78,79) or if taken with anticoagulant drugs such as warfarin (80). However, the data are not conclusive (81). At least one study indicates that ginger has no effect on blood pressure, heart rate, or coagulation parameters and does not interact with anticoagulant drugs such as warfarin (82).

Antiplatelet therapy is an effective approach for prevention of coronary heart disease. Ginger components were suggested as a potential new class of platelet activation inhibitors without the potential side effects of aspirin, which is most commonly used in this approach. Koo et al. (83) recently compared the ability of several synthetic gingerols and analogs with aspirin in capacity to inhibit human platelet activation. The ginger compounds were less potent compared to aspirin in inhibiting arachidonic-acid-induced platelet release and aggregation and COX activity (83). However, several analogs had a significant inhibitory effect, which suggests that further development of more potent gingerol analogs has potential value as an alternative to aspirin therapy in preventing ischemic heart disease. Consumption of ginger (5 g) inhibited platelet aggregation induced in men consuming 100 g of butter daily for 7 days (84) and a later study showed that ginger enhanced fibrinolytic activity (85). Another compound isolated from ginger, (E)-8 beta, 17-epoxy-labd-12-ene-15,16-dial, has been reported to inhibit cholesterol biosynthesis (86).

At least one group found that administration or consumption of standardized ginger extract reduced aortic atherosclerotic lesion areas, plasma triglycerides and cholesterol, LDL-associated lipid peroxides, and LDL aggregation in mice (87). In rabbits fed a high-cholesterol diet, administration of ginger extract resulted in a significant antihyperlipidemic effect and a lower degree of atherosclerosis compared to the group fed cholesterol alone (88).

Ginger compounds have been shown to directly stimulate myocardial sarcoplasmic reticulum (SR) calcium uptake (89,90) but the therapeutic use of ginger in treating heart failure has not been advocated (90).

VIII. SUMMARY AND CONCLUSIONS

Ginger is recognized by the Food and Drug Administration as a food additive that is "generally recognized as safe." Ginger has been shown to possess diverse pharmacological properties but its specific biological effects are largely unknown and remain to be determined. Very few mechanistic studies exist, and as indicated in this chapter, the data regarding the effectiveness and safety of ginger administration are often contradictory. Thus as with any food or drug compound, moderate consumption is probably the best recommendation.

REFERENCES

1. Cohen RJ, Ek K, Pan CX. Complementary and alternative medicine (cam) use by older adults: a comparison of self-report and physician chart documentation. J Gerontol Biol Sci Med Sci 2002; 57:M223–M227.
2. Ernst E, Schmidt K. Health risks over the Internet: advice offered by "medical herbalists" to a pregnant woman. Wien Med Wochenschr 2002; 152:190–192.
3. Surh Y. Molecular mechanisms of chemopreventive effects of selected dietary and medicinal phenolic substances. Mutat Res 1999; 428:305–327.
4. Kaul PN, Joshi BS. Alternative medicine: herbal drugs and their critical appraisal—part ii. Prog Drug Res 2001; 57:1–75.
5. Wilkinson JM. Effect of ginger tea on the fetal development of Sprague-Dawley rats. Reprod Toxicol 2000; 14:507–512.
6. Ginger for nausea. Harvard Womens Health Watch 1999; 7:7.
7. Wilkinson JM. What do we know about herbal morning sickness treatments? A literature survey. Midwifery 2000; 16:224–228.

8. Talalay P, Talalay P. The importance of using scientific principles in the development of medicinal agents from plants. Acad Med 2001; 76:238–247.
9. Barrett B, Kiefer D, Rabago D. Assessing the risks and benefits of herbal medicine: an overview of scientific evidence. Alt Ther Health Med 1999; 5:40–49.
10. Ness J, Sherman FT, Pan CX. Alternative medicine: what the data say about common herbal therapies. Geriatrics 1999; 54:33–38, 40, 43.
11. Afzal M, Al-Hadidi D, Menon M, Pesek J, Dhami MS. Ginger: an ethnomedical, Chemical and pharmacological review. Drug Metabol Drug Interact 2001; 18:159–190.
12. Grant KL, Lutz RB. Ginger. Am J Health Syst Pharm 2000; 57:945–947.
13. Langner E, Greifenberg S, Gruenwald J. Ginger: history and use. Adv Ther 1998; 15:25–44.
14. Ding GH, Naora K, Hayashibara M, Katagiri Y, Kano Y, Iwamoto K. Pharmacokinetics of [6]-gingerol after intravenous administration in rats. Chem Pharm Bull (Tokyo) 1991; 39:1612–1614.
15. Surh YJ, Lee SS. Enzymic reduction of [6]-gingerol, a major pungent principle of ginger, in the cell-free preparation of rat liver. Life Sci 1994; 54:L321–L326.
16. Nakazawa T, Ohsawa K. Metabolism of [6]-gingerol in rats. Life Sci 2002; 70:2165–2175.
17. Aeschbach R, Loliger J, Scott BC, Murcia A, Butler J, Halliwell B, Aruoma OI. Antioxidant actions of thymol, carvacrol, 6-gingerol, zingerone and hydroxytyrosol. Food Chem Toxicol 1994; 32:31–36.
18. Ahmad N, Katiyar SK, Mukhtar H. Antioxidants in chemoprevention of skin cancer. Curr Probl Dermatol 2001; 29:128–139.
19. Halvorsen BL, Holte K, Myhrstad MC, Barikmo I, Hvattum E, Remberg SF, Wold AB, Haffner K, Baugerod H, Andersen LF, Moskaug O, Jacobs DR Jr, Blomhoff R. A systematic screening of total antioxidants in dietary plants. J Nutr 2002; 132:461–471.
20. Zancan KC, Marques MOM, Petenate AJ, Meireles MAA. Extraction of ginger (*Zingiber officinale* Roscoe) oleoresin with co2 and co-solvents: a study of the antioxidant action of the extracts. J Supercrit Fluids 2002; 000:000–000.
21. Kim HW, Murakami A, Nakamura Y, Ohigashi H. Screening of edible Japanese plants for suppressive effects on phorbol ester-induced superoxide generation in differentiated hl-60 cells and as52 cells. Cancer Lett 2002; 176:7–16.
22. Shobana S, Naidu KA. Antioxidant activity of selected indian spices. Prostagland Leukot Essent Fatty Acids 2000; 62:107–110.
23. Reddy AC, Lokesh BR. Studies on spice principles as antioxidants in the inhibition of lipid peroxidation of rat liver microsomes. Mol Cell Biochem 1992; 111:117–124.
24. Krishnakantha TP, Lokesh BR. Scavenging of superoxide anions by spice principles. Indian J Biochem Biophys 1993; 30:133–134.
25. Topic B, Tani E, Tsiakitzis K, Kourounakis PN, Dere E, Hasenohrl RU, Hacker R, Mattern CM, Huston JP. Enhanced maze performance and reduced oxidative stress by combined extracts of zingiber officinale and ginkgo biloba in the aged rat. Neurobiol Aging 2002; 23:135–143.

26. Ahmed RS, Seth V, Pasha ST, Banerjee BD. Influence of dietary ginger (*Zingiber officinales* Rosc) on oxidative stress induced by malathion in rats. Food Chem Toxicol 2000; 38:443–450.
27. Ahmed RS, Seth V, Banerjee BD. Influence of dietary ginger (*Zingiber officinales* Rosc) on antioxidant defense system in rat: comparison with ascorbic acid. Indian J Exp Biol 2000; 38:604–606.
28. Surh YJ, Lee E, Lee JM. Chemoprotective properties of some pungent ingredients present in red pepper and ginger. Mutat Res 1998; 402:259–267.
29. Surh YJ. Anti-tumor promoting potential of selected spice ingredients with antioxidative and anti-inflammatory activities: a short review. Food Chem Toxicol 2002; 40:1091–1097.
30. Yoshimi N, Wang A, Morishita Y, Tanaka T, Sugie S, Kawai K, Yamahara J, Mori H. Modifying effects of fungal and herb metabolites on azoxymethane-induced intestinal carcinogenesis in rats. Jpn J Cancer Res 1992; 83:1273–1278.
31. Vimala S, Norhanom AW, Yadav M. Anti-tumour promoter activity in Malaysian ginger rhizobia used in traditional medicine. Br J Cancer 1999; 80:110–116.
32. Kapadia GJ, Azuine MA, Tokuda H, Hang E, Mukainaka T, Nishino H, Sridhar R. Inhibitory effect of herbal remedies on 12-o-tetradecanoylphorbol-13- acetate-promoted Epstein-Barr virus early antigen activation. Pharmacol Res 2002; 45:213–220.
33. Katiyar SK, Agarwal R, Mukhtar H. Inhibition of tumor promotion in sencar mouse skin by ethanol extract of zingiber officinale rhizome. Cancer Res 1996; 56:1023–1030.
34. Park KK, Chun KS, Lee JM, Lee SS, Surh YJ. Inhibitory effects of [6]-gingerol, a major pungent principle of ginger, on phorbol ester-induced inflammation, epidermal ornithine decarboxylase activity and skin tumor promotion in icr mice. Cancer Lett 1998; 129:139–144.
35. Chung WY, Jung YJ, Surh YJ, Lee SS, Park KK. Antioxidative and antitumor promoting effects of [6]-paradol and its homologs. Mutat Res 2001; 496:199–206.
36. Thatte U, Bagadey S, Dahanukar S. Modulation of programmed cell death by medicinal plants. Cell Mol Biol (Noisy-le-grand) 2000; 46:199–214.
37. Lee E, Park KK, Lee JM, Chun KS, Kang JY, Lee SS, Surh YJ. Suppression of mouse skin tumor promotion and induction of apoptosis in hl-60 cells by *Alpinia oxyphylla* miquel (zingiberaceae). Carcinogenesis 1998; 19:1377–1381.
38. Lee E, Surh YJ. Induction of apoptosis in hl-60 cells by pungent vanilloids, [6]-gingerol and [6]-paradol. Cancer Lett 1998; 134:163–168.
39. Huang C, Ma WY, Dong Z. Requirement for phosphatidylinositol 3-kinase in epidermal growth factor-induced ap-1 transactivation and transformation in jb6 p+ cells. Mol Cell Biol 1996; 16:6427–6435.
40. Huang C, Ma W, Bowden GT, Dong Z. Ultraviolet b-induced activated protein-1 activation does not require epidermal growth factor receptor but is blocked by a dominant negative pkclambda/iota. J Biol Chem 1996; 271:31262–31268.
41. Dong Z, Birrer MJ, Watts RG, Matrisian LM, Colburn NH. Blocking of tumor

promoter-induced ap-1 activity inhibits induced transformation in jb6 mouse epidermal cells. Proc Natl Acad Sci USA 1994; 91:609–613.
42. Bode AM, Ma WY, Surh YJ, Dong Z. Inhibition of epidermal growth factor-induced cell transformation and activator protein 1 activation by [6]-gingerol. Cancer Res 2001; 61:850–853.
43. Keum YS, Kim J, Lee KH, Park KK, Surh YJ, Lee JM, Lee SS, Yoon JH, Joo SY, Cha IH, Yook JI. Induction of apoptosis and caspase-3 activation by chemopreventive [6]-paradol and structurally related compounds in kb cells. Cancer Lett 2002; 177:41–47.
44. Reginster JY, Gillot V, Bruyere O, Henrotin Y. Evidence of nutriceutical effectiveness in the treatment of osteoarthritis. Curr Rheumatol Rep 2000; 2:472–477.
45. Marcus DM, Suarez-Almazor ME. Is there a role for ginger in the treatment of osteoarthritis? Arthritis Rheum 2001; 44:2461–2462.
46. Eldershaw TP, Colquhoun EQ, Dora KA, Peng ZC, Clark MG. Pungent principles of ginger (*Zingiber officinale*) are thermogenic in the perfused rat hindlimb. Int J Obes Relat Metab Disord 1992; 16:755–763.
47. Sharma JN, Srivastava KC, Gan EK. Suppressive effects of eugenol and ginger oil on arthritic rats. Pharmacology 1994; 49:314–318.
48. Bliddal H, Rosetzsky A, Schlichting P, Weidner MS, Andersen LA, Ibfelt HH, Christensen K, Jensen ON, Barslev J. A randomized, placebo-controlled, cross-over study of ginger extracts and ibuprofen in osteoarthritis. Osteoarthritis Cartilage 2000; 8:9–12.
49. Altman RD, Marcussen KC. Effects of a ginger extract on knee pain in patients with osteoarthritis. Arthritis Rheum 2001; 44:2531–2538.
50. Srivastava KC, Mustafa T. Ginger (*Zingiber officinale*) in rheumatism and musculoskeletal disorders. Med Hypoth 1992; 39:342–348.
51. Kiuchi F, Iwakami S, Shibuya M, Hanaoka F, Sankawa U. Inhibition of prostaglandin and leukotriene biosynthesis by gingerols and diarylheptanoids. Chem Pharm Bull (Tokyo) 1992; 40:387–391.
52. Tjendraputra E, Tran VH, Liu-Brennan D, Roufogalis BD, Duke CC. Effect of ginger constituents and synthetic analogues on cyclooxygenase- 2 enzyme in intact cells. Bioorg Chem 2001; 29:156–163.
53. Langmead L, Rampton DS. Review article: Herbal treatment in gastrointestinal and liver disease—benefits and dangers. Aliment Pharmacol Ther 2001; 15:1239–1252.
54. Ernst E, Pittler MH. Efficacy of ginger for nausea and vomiting: a systematic review of randomized clinical trials. Br J Anaesth 2000; 84:367–371.
55. Schmid R, Schick T, Steffen R, Tschopp A, Wilk T. Comparison of seven commonly used agents for prophylaxis of seasickness. J Travel Med 1994; 1:203–206.
56. Murphy PA. Alternative therapies for nausea and vomiting of pregnancy. Obstet Gynecol 1998; 91:149–155.
57. Hollyer T, Boon H, Georgousis A, Smith M, Einarson A. The use of cam by women suffering from nausea and vomiting during pregnancy. BMC Complement Altern Med 2002; 2:55.

58. Jewell D, Young G. Interventions for nausea and vomiting in early pregnancy. Cochrane Database Syst Rev 2000; 22.
59. Niebyl JR. Drug therapy during pregnancy. Curr Opin Obstet Gynecol 1992; 4:43–47.
60. Jewell D, Young G. Interventions for nausea and vomiting in early pregnancy (Cochrane Review). Cochrane Database Syst Rev 2002:1.
61. Jackson EA. Is ginger root effective for decreasing the severity of nausea and vomiting in early pregnancy? J Fam Pract 2001; 50:720.
62. Tsui B, Dennehy CE, Tsourounis C. A survey of dietary supplement use during pregnancy at an academic medical center. Am J Obstet Gynecol 2001; 185:433–437.
63. Niebyl JR, Goodwin TM. Overview of nausea and vomiting of pregnancy with an emphasis on vitamins and ginger. Am J Obstet Gynecol 2002; 185:S253–S255.
64. Vutyavanich T, Kraisarin T, Ruangsri R. Ginger for nausea and vomiting in pregnancy: randomized, double-masked, placebo-controlled trial. Obstet Gynecol 2001; 97:577–582.
65. Power ML, Holzman GB, Schulkin J. A survey on the management of nausea and vomiting in pregnancy by obstetrician/gynecologists. Prim Care Update Ob/Gyns 2001; 8:69–72.
66. Weidner MS, Sigwart K. Investigation of the teratogenic potential of a *Zingiber officinale* extract in the rat. Reprod Toxicol 2001; 15:75–80.
67. Mukhopadhyay MJ, Mukherjee A. Clastogenic effect of ginger rhizome in mice. Phytother Res 2000; 14:555–557.
68. Phillips S, Ruggier R, Hutchinson SE. *Zingiber officinale* (ginger)—an antiemetic for day case surgery. Anaesthesia 1993; 48:715–717.
69. Phillips S, Hutchinson S, Ruggier R. *Zingiber officinale* does not affect gastric emptying rate: a randomised, placebo-controlled, crossover trial. Anaesthesia 1993; 48:393–395.
70. Visalyaputra S, Petchpaisit N, Somcharoen K, Choavaratana R. The efficacy of ginger root in the prevention of postoperative nausea and vomiting after outpatient gynaecological laparoscopy. Anaesthesia 1998; 53:506–510.
71. Gupta YK, Sharma M. Reversal of pyrogallol-induced delay in gastric emptying in rats by ginger (*Zingiber officinale*). Methods Find Exp Clin Pharmacol 2001; 23:501–503.
72. Platel K, Srinivasan K. Studies on the influence of dietary spices on food transit time in experimental rats. Nutr Res 2001; 21:1309–1314.
73. Platel K, Srinivasan K. Influence of dietary spices and their active principles on pancreatic digestive enzymes in albino rats. Nahrung 2000; 44:42–46.
74. Micklefield GH, Redeker Y, Meister V, Jung O, Greving I, May B. Effects of ginger on gastroduodenal motility. Int J Clin Pharmacol Ther 1999; 37:341–346.
75. Sharma SS, Gupta YK. Reversal of cisplatin-induced delay in gastric emptying in rats by ginger (*Zingiber officinale*). J Ethnopharmacol 1998; 62:49–55.
76. Yoshikawa M, Hatakeyama S, Taniguchi K, Matuda H, Yamahara J. 6-Gingesulfonic acid, a new anti-ulcer principle, and gingerglycolipids a, b, and c,

three new monoacyldigalactosylglycerols, from zingiberis rhizoma originating in Taiwan. Chem Pharm Bull (Tokyo) 1992; 40:2239–2241.
77. Yoshikawa M, Yamaguchi S, Kunimi K, Matsuda H, Okuno Y, Yamahara J, Murakami N. Stomachic principles in ginger. III. An anti-ulcer principle, 6-gingesulfonic acid, and three monoacyldigalactosylglycerols, gingerglycolipids a, b, and c, from zingiberis rhizoma originating in Taiwan. Chem Pharm Bull (Tokyo) 1994; 42:1226–1230.
78. Chang LK, Whitaker DC. The impact of herbal medicines on dermatologic surgery. Dermatol Surg 2001; 27:759–763.
79. Pribitkin ED, Boger G. Herbal therapy: what every facial plastic surgeon must know. Arch Facial Plast Surg 2001; 3:127–132.
80. Heck AM, DeWitt BA, Lukes AL. Potential interactions between alternative therapies and warfarin. Am J Health Syst Pharm 2000; 57:1221–1227; quiz 1228–1230.
81. Vaes LP, Chyka PA. Interactions of warfarin with garlic, ginger, ginkgo, or ginseng: nature of the evidence. Ann Pharmacother 2000; 34:1478–1482.
82. Weidner MS, Sigwart K. The safety of a ginger extract in the rat. J Ethnopharmacol 2000; 73:513–520.
83. Koo KL, Ammit AJ, Tran VH, Duke CC, Roufogalis BD. Gingerols and related analogues inhibit arachidonic acid-induced human platelet serotonin release and aggregation. Thromb Res 2001; 103:387–397.
84. Verma SK, Singh J, Khamesra R, Bordia A. Effect of ginger on platelet aggregation in man. Indian J Med Res 1993; 98:240–242.
85. Verma SK, Bordia A. Ginger, fat and fibrinolysis. Indian J Med Sci 2001; 55:83–86.
86. Tanabe M, Chen YD, Saito K, Kano Y. Cholesterol biosynthesis inhibitory component from zingiber officinale roscoe. Chem Pharm Bull (Tokyo) 1993; 41:710–713.
87. Fuhrman B, Rosenblat M, Hayek T, Coleman R, Aviram M. Ginger extract consumption reduces plasma cholesterol, inhibits ldl oxidation and attenuates development of atherosclerosis in atherosclerotic, apolipoprotein e-deficient mice. J Nutr 2000; 130:1124–1131.
88. Bhandari U, Sharma JN, Zafar R. The protective action of ethanolic ginger (*Zingiber officinale*) extract in cholesterol fed rabbits. J Ethnopharmacol 1998; 61:167–171.
89. Antipenko AY, Spielman AI, Kirchberger MA. Interactions of 6-gingerol and ellagic acid with the cardiac sarcoplasmic reticulum ca2+-atpase. J Pharmacol Exp Ther 1999; 290:227–234.
90. Maier LS, Schwan C, Schillinger W, Minami K, Schutt U, Pieske B. Gingerol, isoproterenol and ouabain normalize impaired post-rest behavior but not force-frequency relation in failing human myocardium. Cardiovasc Res 2000; 45:913–924.

9

Lingzhi Polyphorous Fungus (*Ganoderma lucidum*)

Sissi Wachtel-Galor and Iris F. F. Benzie
The Hong Kong Polytechnic University
Hong Kong, China

John A. Buswell
Shanghai Academy of Agricultural Sciences
Shanghai, People's Republic of China

Brian Tomlinson
The Chinese University of Hong Kong
Shatin, Hong Kong, China

I. INTRODUCTION

Mushrooms are considered a special kind of food, items of "food delicacy" because of their characteristic texture and flavor. However, it was not until the 1900s, when antibiotics were obtained from the mold *Penicillium*, that the potential medicinal value of fungi attracted worldwide attention. The chemical, biological, and biochemical properties of mushroom fruiting bodies are numerous, and higher Basidiomycetes mushrooms have been used in folk medicine throughout the world since ancient times (1–5).

Ganoderma lucidum, an Oriental fungus, has been widely used for promoting health and longevity in China, Japan, and other Asian countries (6–11). In China, *G. lucidum* is called "Lingzhi," while in Japan the name for the *Ganoderma* family is "Reishi" or "Mannentake." In Chinese, the name Lingzhi represents a combination of spiritual potency and essence of immortality. Thus, it is regarded as the "herb of spiritual potency" (9–10,12). *G. lucidum* is a large, dark mushroom with a glossy exterior, and its texture is similar to that of wood (Fig. 1). The Latin word "lucidus" means "shiny" or "brilliant" and refers to the varnished appearance of the surface of the mushroom. Among cultivated mushrooms, *G. lucidum* is unique in that the pharmaceutical rather than the nutritional value is paramount. A variety of commercial *G. lucidum* products are available in various forms, such as powders, dietary supplements, and tea, and these are produced from different parts of the mushroom, including mycelia, fruit bodies, and spores (10,13). The "love affair" of Asian people with the Lingzhi mushroom can be traced back several thousand years. More recent reports on its usage, mostly from Asia but also from North America and Europe, give credibility to some of the ancient claims of its biomedical benefits. *G. lucidum* is reputed to extend life

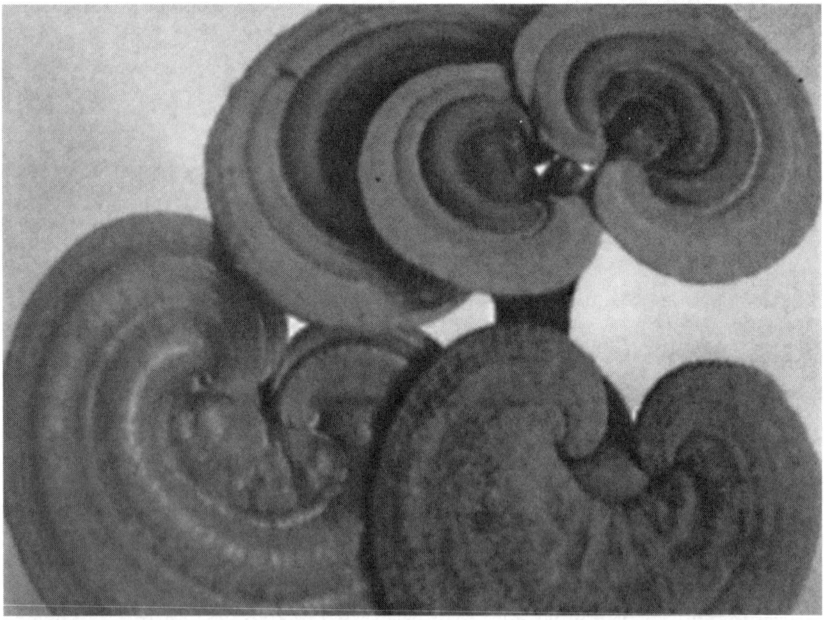

FIGURE 1 The Lingzhi mushroom (*Ganoderma lucidum*). (Courtesy of North American Reishi/Nammex.)

span and to restore youthful vigour and vitality. Specific biomedical applications and reported effects include control of hypertension, lowering of blood lipids, modulation of the immune system, and bacteriostasis (7–9,11,12). However, the beliefs regarding the health benefits of *G. lucidum* are based largely on anecdotal evidence, traditional use, and cultural mores. Most of the published reports on this mushroom are in Chinese, Korean, or Japanese and, as such, data are not readily accessible to non-Asian researchers. Furthermore, it should be noted that, in traditional Oriental medicine, the approach is holistic. Treatment is often a combination of herbs, and is aimed at the person rather than the disease. This is quite different from the reductionist perspective of Western medicine in which purified, active pharmacological agents are prescribed, each targeted toward the causes or manifestations of a specific disease. It is not easy to reconcile these very different approaches in terms of symptoms, signs, and treatment strategies. However, the desired outcome of each is the restoration and maintenance of human health, and the promotion of functional longevity. The long history and well-regarded reputation of Chinese medicines, such as *G. lucidum*, demand the respect and attention of Western scientists. The aim of this review, therefore, is to present the current evidence regarding the health effects of *G. lucidum* (Lingzhi, Reishi), and to provide an objective and scientific view of the health claims and research needs in relation to this popular Chinese herb.

II. TAXONOMY OF *G. LUCIDUM*

The family Ganodermataceae describes polypore basidiomycetous fungi having a double-walled basidiospore (14). In all, 219 species within the family have been assigned to the genus *Ganoderma* of which *G. lucidum* (W.Curt.:Fr.) P. Karsten is the species type (15). Basidiocarps of this genus have a laccate (shiny) surface that is associated with the presence of thick-walled pilocystidia embedded in an extracellular melanin matrix (15). *Ganoderma* species is found worldwide, and different characters, such as the shape and color (red, black, blue/green, white, yellow, and purple) of the fruit body (11,16,17), host specificity, and geographical origin, have been used to identify individual members of the species (18–21). The use of macroscopic characteristics has resulted in a large number of synonyms and in a confused, overlapping, and unclear taxonomy of this mushroom, and some taxonomists now consider macromorphological features to be of limited value in the identification of *Ganoderma* species owing to its high phenotypic plasticity (19,22). More reliable morphological characters for *Ganoderma* systematics are thought to include spore shape and size, context color and consistency, and the microanatomy of the pilear crust. Chlamydospore production and shape, enzymic studies, and, to a lesser extent, the range and optima of growth temperatures have also been used for differentiating morphologically similar species (15,20,23). Biochemical (triterpene constituents), genetic (mating studies), and molecular approaches (rDNA polymorphisms) have also been used in *Ganoderma* taxonomy (7,24–27). In the latter case, appropriate nucleotide sequence variation has been found in the internal transcribed spacers (ITS) of the nuclear rDNA gene (28–30).

III. HISTORY OF *G. LUCIDUM* AS A MEDICINAL MUSHROOM

The first book wholly devoted to the description of herbs and their medicinal value is called *Shen Nong Ben Cao Jing*, written in the Eastern Han dynasty of China (A.D. 25–220). This book is also known as *Classic of the Materia Medica* or *Shen-nong's Herbal Classic* and describes botanical, zoological, and mineral substances. It was composed in the second century under the pseudonym of Shen-nong, the Holy Farmer (31). The book, which has been continually updated and extended, describes the beneficial effects of several mushrooms and there is reference to the medicinal mushroom *G. lucidum* (4,11,31). In the book *Shen Nong Ben Cao Jing* ("Supplement to Classic of Materia Medica," A.D. 502–536) and in the *Ben Cao Gang Mu* by Li Shin-Zhen, which is considered to be the first pharmacopoeia in China (A.D. 1590, Ming dynasty), the mushroom was attributed with certain medicinal effects, including tonifying effects, enhancing vital energy and strengthening cardiac function, increasing memory, and having antiaging effects (17,32). However, its reputation as a panacea may have been earned more by virtue of its irregular distribution, rarity, and usage by the rich and privileged members of Chinese society than by its actual effects. According to the *Pharmacopoeia of the People's Republic of China* (33), *G. lucidum* acts to replenish Qi and ease the mind, to relieve cough and asthma, and it is recommended for dizziness, insomnia, palpitation, and shortness of breath.

IV. CULTIVATION OF *G. LUCIDUM* AND GLOBAL USAGE

Different members of the *Ganoderma* genus need different conditions for growth and cultivation (34). Moreover, different types are favored in different geographical regions. For example, in South China, black *G. lucidum* is popular, white red *G. lucidum* is preferred in Japan. Owing to its irregular distribution in the wild and to an increasing demand for *G. lucidum* as a medicinal "herb," attempts were made to cultivate the mushroom. *G. lucidum* thrives under hot and humid conditions, and many wild varieties are found in the subtropical regions of the Orient. Artificial cultivation of *G. lucidum* has been achieved using substrates such as grain, sawdust, or wood logs (10,34). Riu et al. (35) showed that the mushroom could be cultivated successfully on cork residues. Since the early 1970s, cultivation of *G. lucidum* has become a major source of the mushroom; consumption is now estimated at several thousand tons worldwide, and the market is growing rapidly. In 1995, the total estimated annual market value given by different commercial sources was US$1628 million (10).

It takes several months to culture the fruiting body of *G. lucidum* and there is a growing interest in developing fermenter-based processes for producing fungal mycelia and desirable cellular products. Such processes allow for more careful control of different growth parameters such as temperature, pH, and humidity, and should thereby facilitate improved quality control. The different growing conditions, such as the medium used, have also been reported to strongly influence mycelial growth and the production of biopolymers (e.g., polysaccharides) that are extruded from the cell (10,34,36–43). For example, Yang and Liau (38) and Yang et al. (41) reported that polysaccharide production by fermenter-grown mycelia of *G. lucidum* was optimum at 30–35°C and pH 4–4.5, and addition of supplements such as fatty acids was found to accelerate mycelial growth and the production of bioactive components.

V. DOSAGE

Even though traditional Chinese medicines (TCM) are used for their putative medicinal value, TCM is considered as a nutriceutical, and is categorized as a nutritional or dietary supplement in the United States, as defined by the Dietary Supplement Health and Education Act (DSHEA) (44). Nonetheless, a central question for any therapy is the dose that produces a desired therapeutic action without harmful side effects. *Ganoderma* as a medicinal fungus has been recommended and consumed as a tonic and panacea for over 2000 years. Although no significant toxicity has been reported, there are no standard formulations or agreed guidelines pertaining to its dosage and formulation (e.g., syrup, tablet, capsule, tea, and even aqueous extract for injection). Various species and strains of *Ganoderma* are used in the preparations, and different parts of the mushroom, i.e., the fruit body, mycelium, and/or spores, are used in treatments (13,45).

According to Teow (13,46), the effective dosage required to afford a cure or to alleviate certain symptoms ranged between 1.5 and 9 g/day of a dried commercial extract of *G. lucidum* fruit body. Chang (45) suggested a *Ganoderma* dried fruiting body (DFB) dose of 0.5–1 g/day for health maintenance,

2–5 g DFB for chronic health conditions, and up to 15 g DFB for serious illness. However, doses of up to 30 g have been used. In the *American Herbal Pharmacopoeia's* monograph (11), the recommended *G. lucidum* dosage of 6–12 g daily was adopted from the *Pharmacopoeia of the People's Republic of China* (33).

Generally, the therapeutic dose of any drug or herb is selected on the basis of toxic dose (TD), lethal dose (LD), and effective dose (ED). The LD in animals of *G. lucidum* is very high, and ranges (depending on extraction, route of administration, and duration) from 5 g/kg given to mice for 1 month to 38 g/kg given to rodents in a single intraperitoneal dose (12,45,47,48). No side effects in humans taking *G. lucidum* have been reported in the literature. However, clinicians have reported occasional mild digestive upset and skin rashes in sensitive individuals (11,12). Since the TD and LD values are high relative to human dosages of other materials, they do not pose significant limitations for the clinical usage of *G. lucidum*. Of more importance is the provision of sound scientific data confirming the putative health benefits of *G. lucidum*, and the determination and validation of the ED. However, it must be noted that data are lacking regarding possible toxic interactions with other medications, effects in pregnancy, and possible contraindications of *G. lucidum* treatment under particular conditions.

VI. MAJOR BIOACTIVE COMPONENTS OF *G. LUCIDUM*

Most mushrooms are composed of around 90% water by weight. The remaining 10% consists of 10–40% protein, 2–8% fat, 3–28% carbohydrate, 3–32% fiber, 8–10% ash, and some vitamins, with potassium, calcium, phosphorus, magnesium, iron, zinc, and copper accounting for most of the mineral content (3). In addition to these nutrients, the mushroom contains a wide variety of bioactive molecules, such as terpenoids, steroids, phenols, nucleotides and their derivatives, glycoproteins, and polysaccharides. Mushroom proteins contain all the essential amino acids and are especially rich in lysine and leucine. The low total fat content, and the high proportion of polyunsaturated fatty acids relative to total fatty acids, is considered a significant contributor to the health value of mushroom (1,3).

In a study of the nonvolatile components of *G. lucidum*, it was found that the mushroom contains 1.8% ash, 26–28% carbohydrate, 3–5% crude fat, 59% crude fiber, and 7–8% crude protein (49). One of the characteristics of the fruit body of *G. lucidum* is its bitterness, which varies in degree depending on the strain, method of cultivation, age, and other factors, The components that confer this bitterness (triterpenes) can serve as a marker for pharmacological evaluation (7,16). Polysaccharides and triterpenes are the two major physiologically active constituents of *G. lucidum*.

A. Polysaccharides

Plant polysaccharides are reported to confer anti-inflammatory, hypoglycemic, antiulcer, and anticancer effects (7,16,50). Fungi are remarkable for the variety of high-molecular-weight polysaccharide structures that they produce, and bioactive polyglycans are found in all parts of the mushroom. Polysaccharides from the *G. lucidum* mushroom have been extracted from the fruit body, mycelia, and spores, and exopolysaccharides are produced by mycelia cultured in fermenters. Analysis of the polysaccharides from *G. lucidum* indicates that glucose is the major sugar (50–55). However, *G. lucidum* polysaccharides are heteropolymers and also contain xylose, mannose, galactose, and fucose in different confirmations, including 1–3, 1–4, 1–6-linked β, and α-D (or L)-polysaccharides (16,39,51–59). Mannitol has also been found as a free sugar (49). In addition to its high concentration of high-molecular-weight polysaccharides, the mushroom consists of a matrix of the polysaccharide chitin, which is largely indigestible by the human body and is partly responsible for the physical hardness of the mushroom (11).

Polysaccharides are normally obtained by extraction with hot water followed by precipitation with ethanol or methanol, but can also be extracted with water and alkali. Various polysaccharides, including extracellular polysaccharides, can be extracted from the fruit body, spores, and mycelia (49,51–53,56,57,60). Further purification steps result in purified polysaccharides such as the glucose polymer GL-1 (98% glucose) (52). Polysaccharides isolated from *Ganoderma* species include the Ganoderans A, B, and C, which differ in their sugar and peptide composition and molecular weight (57,61). Several other polysaccharides have been isolated over the years, and some have been reported to possess significant antitumorigenic and immunostimulating effects (51–54,58,62). Branching conformation and solubility characteristics are said to affect the antitumorigenic properties of these polysaccharides (54,58,62).

B. Triterpenes

Terpenes are a class of naturally occurring compounds whose carbon skeletons are composed of isoprene C5 units. Examples of terpenes are menthol and vitamin A. Many are alkenes, but some contain other functional groups, and many are cyclical. These compounds are widely distributed throughout the plant world and are found in prokaryotes as well as eukaryotes (63,64). Terpenes have also been found to possess other properties such as anti-inflammatory, antitumorigenic, and hypolipidemic activity (65–68). For example, terpenes in *Ginko biloba* and rosemary (*Rosemarinus officinalis*) and ginseng (*Panax ginseng*) are reported to contribute to the health-promoting effects of these herbs (69–71).

Triterpenes are a subclass of terpenes and have a basic skeleton of C30. A variety of triterpenes from different plants are reviewed in Refs. 65 and 66. Many different plant species synthesize triterpenes as part as their normal program of growth and development. Some plants contain large quantities of triterpenes in their latex and resins and these are believed to contribute to disease resistance. Even though hundreds of triterpenes have been isolated from various plants, and terpenes as a class have been shown to have many potentially beneficial effects, the application of triterpenes as successful therapeutic agents is limited thus far. In general, very little is known about the enzymes and biochemical pathways involved in their biosynthesis. The genetic machinery required for the elaboration of this family of plant secondary metabolites is as yet largely uncharacterized, despite the considerable commercial interest in this important group of natural products (66,71).

In *G. lucidum*, the chemical structure of the triterpenes is based on lanostane, which is a metabolite of lanosterol (72), the biosynthesis of which is based on cyclization of squalene (71,73). Extraction of triterpenes is usually by means of methanol, ethanol, acetone, chloroform, ether, or a mixture of these solvents. The extracts can be further purified by various separation methods including normal and reverse-phase HPLC (6,7,25,27,65). The first triterpenes isolated from *G. lucidum* were the ganoderic acids A and B, which were identified in 1982 by Kubota et al. (74). Since then, more than 100 triterpenes with known chemical composition and molecular configuration have been reported to occur in *G. lucidum*. Among them, more than 50 were found to be new and unique to this fungus. The vast majority are ganoderic and lucidenic acids, but other triterpenes, such as ganoderals, ganoderiols, and ganodermic acids, have also been identified (6,27,75–90).

G. lucidum is clearly rich in triterpenes, and it is this class of compounds that gives the herb its bitter taste and, it is believed, various health benefits such as lipid-lowering and antioxidant effects. However, the triterpene content is different in the different parts and growing stages of the mushroom. The profile of the different triterpenes in *G. lucidum* can be used to distinguish this medicinal fungus from other taxonomically related species, and can serve as supporting evidence for classification. The triterpene content can also be used as a measure of quality of different *Ganoderma* samples (6,7,25,27). (See Fig. 2.)

C. Minerals, Metals, and Microbial Content

Elemental analysis of log-cultivated fruit bodies of *G. lucidum* revealed phosphorus, silica, sulfur, potassium, calcium, and magnesium to be the main mineral components. Iron, sodium, zinc, copper, manganese, and strontium were also detected in lower amounts, as were the heavy metals lead, cadmium,

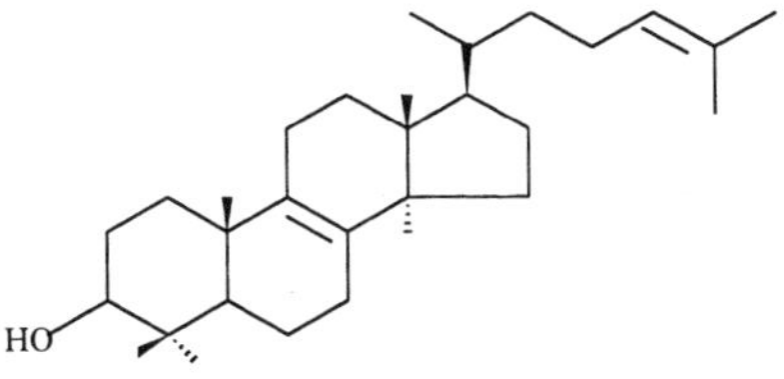

Lanosterol

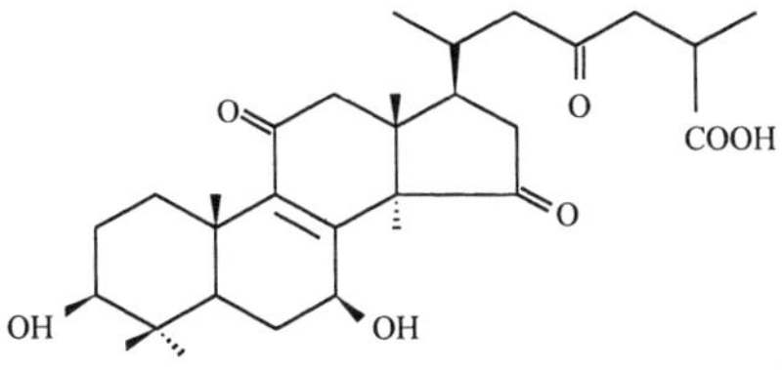

Ganoderic acid B

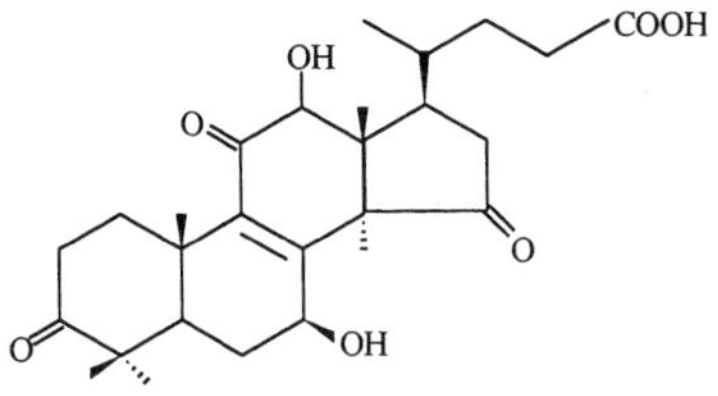

Lucidenic acid B

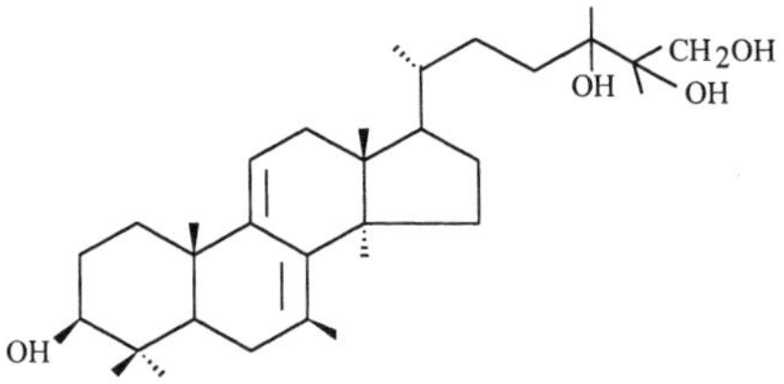

Ganoderiol A

FIGURE 2 Chemical structure of lanosterol and three of the many triterpenes isolated from *Ganoderma lucidum*. (Modified from Refs. 72,74,75,81.)

and mercury (91). Freeze-dried fruit bodies of unidentified *Ganoderma* spp collected from the wild were reported to have a mineral content of 10.2% with potassium, calcium, and magnesium the major components (48). Significantly, no cadmium, mercury, or selenium was detected in these samples. There are several reports of heavy metal accumulation in mushroom fruit bodies (92–96). However, the evidence for greater accumulation in mushrooms collected in urban areas compared with domains considered to be "pollution-free" is conflicting (94,97).

Regardless of the site of cultivation, there is a risk of contamination by heavy metals (e.g., Hg, Cd) from the environment, and of contamination by toxins from spoilage microbes and by pathogenic microbes (48,98). Natural products are not necessarily safe, and while the toxic dose of *G. lucidum* appears to be very high, the issue of contamination by heavy metals and microbial toxins must not be neglected (99). Food toxicology is a growing discipline, and this reflects a growing awareness of this possibility. Commercial preparations, therefore, must be tested, and a certificate of analysis containing information on heavy-metal and microbial content in relation to specified limits is needed.

Particular attention has been given to the germanium content of *Ganoderma* spp. Germanium was fifth highest in terms of concentration (489 μg/g) among minerals detected in *Ganoderma* fruit bodies collected from nature (48). This mineral is also present in the order of parts per billion in many plant-based foods including ginseng, aloes, and garlic (100). Germanium is not an essential element but, at low doses, has been ascribed immunopotentiating, antitumor, antioxidant, and antimutagenic activities (32,101–103). However, although the germanium content of *G. lucidum* has often been used to promote *G. lucidum*–based products, there is no firm evidence linking this element with specific health benefits associated with the mushroom.

D. Other Components of *G. lucidum*

G. lucidum contains some other compounds that may contribute to its medicinal effect, such as proteins and lectins. The protein content of dried *G. lucidum* was found to be around 7–8% (49), which is lower than that of many other mushrooms (1). Bioactive proteins are reported to contribute to the medicinal properties of *G. lucidum*. For example, a protein purified from the mycelium (LZ-8) was found to have immunosuppressive effects (104–106). The content of carbohydrate and crude fiber of the dried mushroom was examined and found to be 26–28% and 59%, respectively, showing *G. lucidum* is a good source of fiber (49). Lectins were also isolated from the fruit body and mycelium of the mushroom. "Lectins" (from the latin word "legere," to pick up, choose) are nonenzymatic proteins or glycoproteins that bind carbohydrate. Many species of animals, plants, and microorganisms produce lectins and these exhibit a wide range of functions. In animals, for example, lectins are involved in variety of cellular processes and the immune system (16,107,108). Other compounds that have been isolated from *G. lucidum* include enzymes such a metalloprotease that delays clotting time, ergosterol (provitamin D_2), nucleosides, and nucleotides such as adenosine and guanosine (13,16,32,49,85,109,110).

VII. THERAPEUTIC APPLICATIONS OF *G. LUCIDUM*

The combination of benefit without toxicity represents the desired end product in the development of effective therapeutic intervention. *G. lucidum* has been used for hundreds of years as a health promotor and treatment strategy, but it is only in recent years that objective and scientific studies of *G. lucidum* have been performed. There are now many published studies based on animal and cell culture models and on in vitro assessment of the health effects of *G. lucidum*, and there are some reports of human trials. However, there is no cohesive body of research in the Western scientific literature, and the objective evaluation of this traditional therapy in terms of human health remains to be clearly established. In the following section, studies of possible beneficial properties of *G. lucidum*, in relation to viral and bacterial infection, cancer, inflammation, immune status, cardiovascular disease, inflammatory disorders, allergy, antioxidants, and liver injury, are presented and discussed.

A. Viral Infection

The goal of research in antiviral chemotherapy is the discovery of agents that are specific for the inhibition of viral multiplication without affecting normal cells. Undesired side effects and the appearance of resistant strains make the development of new antiviral agents an urgent requirement (111). *G. lucidum* has reported potential as an antiviral agent. Isolation of various water- and methanol-soluble, high-molecular-weight, protein-bound polysaccharides (PBP) from the carpophores of *G. lucidum* showed inhibitory effects on herpes simplex virus type 1 (HSV-1), type 2 (HSV-2), and vesicular stomatitis virus New Jersey strain (VSV) in a tissue culture system. With the plaque reduction method, a significant inhibitory effect was seen at doses that showed no cytotoxicity (60,112–114). In addition, there was a marked syngergistic effect when PBP from *G. lucidum* was used in tissue culture in conjunction with the antiherpetic agents acyclovir or vidarabine and with interferon alpha (113,114). This might imply that combination therapy may be much more safe and cost-effective, as lower amounts of these cytotoxic antiviral drugs could be used, with a concomitant decrease in the risk of side effects. However, this needs further investigation by clinical trials.

Mizushina et al. (86) reported that triterpenes from the fruiting body inhibited human immunodeficiency virus type 1 (HIV-1) reverse transcriptase in vitro as measured by enzyme activity, with a 50% inhibitory concentration (IC_{50}) of <70 μM. Triterpenes from *G. lucidum* have also been reported to have an inhibitory effect against HIV-1 protease activity. Different tripterpenes demonstrated different levels of inhibition, and IC50 values ranged from 20 μM to >1000 μM (84,115). No synergistic effects with standard antiviral drugs were investigated in these studies. Furthermore, not all of the examined triterpenes showed any anti-HIV activity (115).

Few human trials have been reported in the English language scientific literature on the effect of *G. lucidum* in patients. In an open, uncontrolled clinical study of four elderly patients, a dried hot-water extract of *G. lucidum* (taken orally, and equivalent to 36 or 72 g dried mushroom per day) was used as the sole treatment for postherpetic (varicella zoster virus) neuralgia. Treatment was reported to dramatically decrease the pain and promote healing of lesions, and no toxicity was reported, even at the very high doses used (116).

A randomized, placebo-controlled trial examined the effect of mixture of *G. lucidum* with 34 other Chinese herbs on HIV-1-infected individuals (n = 68) with CD4 cell count $< 0.5 \times 10^9$/L. No improvement in clinical manifestation, plasma viral load, CD4 cell count, or quality of life was seen (117). In another small, uncontrolled clinical trial (46), four patients with hepatitis B were given 6 g/day of *G. lucidum* commercial extract for 3 months, after which the patients were HbsAg-negative and their liver enzymes (AST, ALT, ALP) had returned to normal. This is the usual course of recovery following acute hepatitis B, however, and whether *G. lucidum* contributed to the recovery was not demonstrated.

B. Bacterial Infection

In the last decade, the acceptance of traditional medicine as an alternative form of health care and the development of microbial resistance to antibiotics have led researchers to investigate the antimicrobial activity of medicinal plants and fungi (4,5,118–120), and in vitro and in vivo animal studies of *G. lucidum* have been performed. Mice injected with *G. lucidum* extract (2 mg/mouse) 1 day prior to injection with *Escherichia coli* showed markedly improved survival rates (>80% compared to 33% in controls). It is not clear if this was a direct antibacterial effect or mediated by immune modulation (121). In an in vitro study, the direct antimicrobial effect of a *G. lucidum* water extract was examined against 15 species of bacteria alone and in combination with four kinds of antibiotics (119). The results showed that *G. lucidum* had antimicrobial activity against *E. coli*, with a minimum inhibitory concentration (MIC) of 1.75 mg/mL. *G. lucidum* was also effective against *Micrococcus luteus*, *Staphylococcus aureus*, *Bacillus cereus*, *Proteus vulgaris*, and *Salmonella typhi*, with MICs in the range of 0.75–2.7 mg/mL. *G. lucidum* was less effective against other species tested, with MIC values > 5 mg/mL reported. These MICs are high compared to those of antibiotics, which are generally in the μg/mL range. Low MICs for antibiotic drugs are important to avoid their cytotoxic side effects. However, *G. lucidum* has no known toxicity, and the problem of a relatively high MIC is how and if it can be achieved in vivo. The antimicrobial combinations of *G. lucidum* with four commonly used antibiotics (119) resulted in an additive or synergistic effect in most, but not all, instances, with apparent antagonism against cefazolin and ampicillin effects on *P. vulgaris*. To date, the antimicrobial components of the crude extracts tested have not been identified, although antimicrobial polysaccharides have been identified in other fungi (4,5), and plant terpenes have been reported to have antimicrobial activity (120). In addition, the bioavailability of putative antimicrobial components of *G. lucidum* has not been established. Nonetheless, *G. lucidum* offers a potentially effective antimicrobial therapy, and may help decrease the MICs of expensive and potentially cytotoxic drugs; this deserves further study.

C. Cancer

Cancer is the leading cause of death in Hong Kong, and the second largest cause of death in the world (122,123). Despite comprehensive advances in early diagnosis of and chemotherapy for cancer, many malignancies remain difficult or impossible to cure. In searching for new cancer chemopreventive or chemotherapeutic agents over the last several years, hundreds of plant extracts, including those from mushroom, have been evaluated (2,4,5,70,124).

A number of bioactive molecules, including antitumor substances, have been identified in numerous mushroom species, including the *Ganoderma* species (2–5,125). Polysaccharides have been established to be the most potent mushroom-derived compounds with antitumor activity. It is generally accepted that some β-D-glucans, especially β-(1→3)-D-glucans obtained from fungi, including those from the *Ganoderma* family, show antitumor activity (3–5,16). This attracted attention toward the polysaccharide components of the fruiting body of *G. lucidum* and their effect on cancer.

Several studies using rats and mice have examined the possible antitumorigenic effects of *G. lucidum* (see Table 1). In 1981 Miyazaki and Nishijima (52) separated from the fruit body a polysaccharide (GL-1) that strongly inhibited (by 95–98%) the growth of transplanted sarcoma 180 tumor cells in mice when the GL-1 was injected intraperitoneally (i.p.) for 10 days. A complex of polysaccharides and protein from the mushroom was also found to show significant antitumor activity in a similar study by Kim et al. (51), with an inhibition ratio of 88% reported, and there was complete regression of tumor in a third of the test animals. In a study by Hyun et al. (53), which followed a similar protocol but used various extracted polysaccharides, inhibition ratios of 52–81% were found. The most potent fraction, labeled GL, was composed of 75% glucose, some galactose, mannose, and fucose, and 8% protein. This group also found increased superoxide production by macrophages in *G. lucidum*–treated animals, and increased antibody production, assessed by the hemolytic plaque-forming test. The authors suggested that the effect of the *G. lucidum* polysaccharides was mediated via increased cellular and humoral immunity (53).

A more recent study by Ohno et al. (121), but again using mice transplanted with sarcoma 180 cells, tested a hot-water extract (2 mg/mouse)

TABLE 1 Effect of *G. lucidum* on Tumor Growth in Animal (Mice and Rats) Studies by Year

Type of tumor	Type and amount of *G. lucidum* compound/ extract tested	Duration[a] of treatment	Route	Results	Ref.
Sarcoma 180 cells (implant)	Polysaccharide-rich extract; 50 mg/kg	10 consecutive days (+5 to +15)	i.p[b]	88% inhibition ratio[c]; tumor completely regressed in 5 of 15 animals	Kim et al. (1980)
Sarcoma 180 cells (implant)	Isolated polysaccharide (GL-1); 20 mg/kg	10 consecutive days (+1 to +11)	i.p[b]	95.6–98.5% inhibition ratio[c]; tumor completely regressed in 14/22 animals	Miyazaki and Nishijima (1981)
Sarcoma 180 cells (implant)	Isolated polysaccharides (GL, GH, CR, IN, or IA); 20 mg/kg	10 consecutive days (+3 to +13)	i.p[b]	All fraction effective; 52–81% inhibition ratios[c]; tumor completely regressed in 2/7 animals treated with GL and IN; 1/7 with GH	Hyun et al. (1990)
Lewis lung carcinoma cells (implant)	Hot-water extract; 10, 20, or 40 mg/mouse	5 times, every other day (+1,3,5,7,9)	i.p[b]	Survival time prolonged by 55% at 40 mg,	Furusawa et al. (1992)

				72% at 20 mg, and 95% at 10 mg doses (n = 6–20 per dose); possible synergistic effect with cytotoxic drugs seen; authors suggested main activity was in the ethanol-precipitable fraction	
Sarcoma 180 cells (implant)	Hot-water extract or 75% ethanol extract; 2 mg/mouse	3 times (+7,9,11 days i.p.) or 5 weeks orally (daily starting at +1)	i.p[b] or peroral	74% inhibition ratio[c] with i.p treatment; tumor completely regressed in 3/10 animals; 45–63% inhibition ratio[c] with oral treatment; however, data for water and ethanol extracts confused	Ohno et al. (1998)

TABLE 1 Continued

Type of tumor	Type and amount of *G. lucidum* compound/extract tested	Duration[a] of treatment	Route	Results	Ref.
Lung adenoma (induced)	High- and low-molecular-weight extract, individually and in combination; 2 or 10 mg/mL	6 weeks daily (starting at 0)	In drinking water	Significant inhibition of tumor incidence; authors claimed activity resides in high molecular weight rich extract	Yun (1999)
Sarcoma 180 cells (implant)	Polysaccharide (GL-B); 50, 100, or 200 mg/kg	10 consecutive days (0 to +10)	Intragastric	% inhibition ratio[c] (n = 10/experiment) 28% (20 mg/kg), 56% (100 mg/kg), 67% (200 mg/kg)	Zhang and Lin (1999)
Colon cancer (induced)	Hot-water extract of cultured mycelium and medium; 1.25%, 2%, or 5%	5 weeks daily (starting at −7)	In food	Decrease in the total number of aberrant crypts and cyst formation	Lu et al. (2001)

[a](+) or (−) signs refer to the days before (−) or after (+) tumor was implanted/induced.
[b]i.p = Intraperitoneal injection.
[c]% inhibition ratio presented was as calculated in original papers as: [(Cw − Tw)/Cw]*100, where, Cw = average tumor weight in control (untreated) group and Tw = average tumor weight in treatment group.

given i.p. for 3 days or orally daily for 5 weeks. The i.p. administration of the hot-water extract, which was reported to activate macrophages, resulted in 74% inhibition of average tumor growth, with 3 of 10 animals showing complete regression. Oral administration also showed a significant effect with an average of 45–63% inhibition. The results of this study are supported by those of Zhang and Lin (126) in which a polysaccharide isolated from *G. lucidum* and administered by intragastric tube to mice inhibited the growth of implanted sarcoma 180 cells. Ethanol-soluble fractions were tested in some of these studies and were shown to have lower percent of inhibition rate compared with the ethanol-insoluble, polysaccharide-rich fractions, although the presented data are confusing in parts (121,127). Interestingly, a pure β-(1→3) glucan (from a different source) tested in parallel with the *G. lucidum* extracts resulted in 90% inhibition of tumor growth (121). This supports the suggestion that it is the polysaccharides fraction(s) of *G. lucidum* that are the antitumorigenic components of the mushroom.

In addition to testing potential antitumorigenic effects of *G. lucidum* against sarcoma 180 tumor cells, extracts have been tested against other types of cancer cells. An aqueous extract (i.p. at 10, 20, and 40 mg/mouse) of the fruit body significantly increased the life span of mice implanted with Lewis lung carcinoma cells. However, no dose-response effect was seen (127). An additive effect was seen when *G. lucidum* was given in combination with cytotoxic antineoplastic drugs, and there was a suggestion of a possibly synergistic effect with cisplatin. The active principles in the *G. lucidum* extract were suggested to be polysaccharides, which could be concentrated from the aqueous extract by ethanol precipitation (127). In addition to the extracts from the fruiting body, these from the mycelia of *G. lucidum* have also been reported to have antitumorigenic effects. Yun (70) reported that 9 weeks of oral administration of mycelium extract significantly inhibited lung adenoma formation in mice. The activity was concentrated in the high-molecular-weight (polysaccharide) fraction. In another study (128), the hot-water extract of the mycelium/growth medium complex was given to rats. The extract was found to decrease development of abberant crypt foci (ACF), which are precancerous lesions in the colon, when given orally 1 week prior to the administration of carcinogenic agent. No toxicity effect or side effects were seen in the rats when the extract was administered for 3 months. This extract was also found to inhibit the growth of several human colon carcinoma cell lines in vitro as examined by colony formation in soft agar (128). The protective effect of *G. lucidum* seen in this study may indicate protection against colon cancer. However, it is not clear if these animal findings can be extrapolated to humans.

Whether the antitumor effect is a direct one or is mediated via effects on the immune system is an important question. Wang et al. (129) found that a polysaccharide-enriched fraction from *G. lucidum* activated cultured macrophages and T lymphocytes in vitro, increasing the levels of interleukin (IL)-1β, tumor necrosis factor (TNF)-α, and IL-6 in the culture medium. Cytokine levels in cultured cells treated with *G. lucidum* polysaccharides were 5–29-fold higher than in controls. The proliferation of leukemic cells (HL-60 and U937) in tissue culture was not affected by the polysaccharide alone, nor was the growth affected by the addition of peripheral mononuclear cells (MNCs) in culture medium. However, addition of *G. lucidum*–activated MNCs inhibited growth of leukemic cells, markedly induced leukemic cell apoptosis, and induced differentation of leukemic cells (129). The results of this study are supported by those of Zhang and Lin (126). In this study, adding the polysaccharide fraction directly to sarcoma 180 and HL-60 cell cultures in vitro did not inhibit their proliferation, nor was tumor cell apoptosis induced. However, when the extract was first added to the culture medium of macrophages and T lymphocytes, and then to the HL-60 cell cultures, cell proliferation was inhibited and apoptosis was induced. The polysaccharide significantly increased TNF-α and interferon (IFN)-γ production by macrophages and T lymphocytes in a dose-dependent and time-dependent manner, peaking at around 24 hr, with evidence of decreased cytokine production after 48 hr (126). These results strongly suggest that antitumorigenic activity is mediated by cytokines released from immune cells in response to the *G. lucidum* polysaccharides.

A similar study showed that human MNCs incubated in vitro with *G. lucidum* polysaccharide extract had antiproliferative effects and induced differentiation in U937 leukemic cells. These effects were not seen with the extract or MNC by themselves (130). In this study, the effect of *G. lucidum* polysaccharide extract on the release of cytokines from immune cells was also demonstrated and showed marked production of IL-1β and TNF-α, with a small amount of IFN-γ. Synthesis of IL-6 and nitric oxide was also found to increase in macrophage culture treated with *G. lucidum* extract, and a dose-dependent response was seen (121). A polysaccharide (GL-B) from the mushroom reportedly promoted the production of IL-2 and increased the number of cells in a mixed murine lymphocyte culture system (131), and in the study by Jia et al. (132), a hot-water extract of *G. lucidum* was reported to promote the production of a nonspecific "tumor necrosis factor" by mouse macrophages in vitro and in vivo. However, these two studies are poorly described and nonstandard methodologies were used.

It was shown that the molecular weight, water solubility, conformation, and chemical modification of the polysaccharidel all significantly affect their antitumor activities (62). For example, sulfated derivatives of polysaccharides extracted from the fruit body of *G. lucidum* showed higher antitumor activity against Ehrlich ascites carcinoma than the originals (62). In addition, polysaccharides from *G. lucidum* were reported to induce glutathione-S-transferase activity in tissue culture system (50). The glutathione-S-transferase family of "Phase II enzymes" plays an important role in the detoxification and metabolism of many xenobiotic and endobiotic compounds, and their increased activity is likely to decrease the body's mutagen load, thereby decreasing cancer risk.

Lanostanoids isolated from the mushroom may also contribute to its reputed anticancer effects. A crude chloroform extract and two isolated lanostanoids from the fruit body were found to induce NAD(P)H:quinone oxidoreductase enzyme (QR), a Phase II drug-metabolizing enzyme, in cultured hepatoma cells, as an approach to detect potential cancer chemopreventive activity (87). The crude extract and both lanostanoids increased enzyme activity in murine hepatoma cells by 1.7–2-fold at concentrations of 3–20 μg/mL (87). With another approach, this time focusing on direct DNA effects, the protection of *G. lucidum* against a mutagen (ethyl methanesulfonate) in mice was examined (48). This group used the comet assay, which is a useful method of assessing DNA damage and DNA strand breaks in individual cells such as lymphocytes (133). No evidence was found for genotoxic chromosomal breakage effect by *G. lucidum*; however, no protection was seen (48).

The cytotoxicity of several isolated triterpenes was studied against mouse sarcoma (Meth A) and carcinoma (LLC) tumor cell lines. Of 20 triterpenes tested, two showed potent cytotoxic effects, with the others showing weak to no effect compared with the positive control (88). Ethanolic extracts of broken spores were found to inhibit the growth of cervical cancer (HeLa) cells in tissue culture, but extracts of unbroken spores had no effect. An ethanol/ethyl acetate extract of broken spores was shown to arrest cells in G1 phase of the cell cycle, and there was evidence that this effect was mediated by a dose-dependent decrease in intracellular calcium level (134). A possibly additional anticancer effect of *G. lucidum* may be through effects on DNA duplication. Three terpenes from *G. lucidum* were reported to inhibit DNA polymerase from two animal species, and two cerebrosides isolated from the mushroom were found to be eukaryotic (but not prokaryotic) DNA polymerase inhibitors (86,135). Another compound, ergosterol peroxide, separated from the fruit body was found to have synergistic effect with linoleic acid on inhibition of rat DNA polymerase β, but was not effective against calf polymerase α. The compound showed no inhibitory effect by itself (109).

In two small and uncontrolled clinical trials, a commercial extract of *G. lucidum* was given to patients with Stage III nasopharyngeal carcinoma (NPC) ($n = 5$) and acute myelobastic leukemia ($n = 4$) (46). Patients received 9 g/day of the extract before, during, and after radiotherapy and/or chemotherapy. In both groups significant improvement was reported in terms of tumor size in NPC and white blood cell count in leukemia patients. However, whether *G. lucidum* contributed to this was not established owing to the poor study design.

D. Immune Status

Agents that enhance the functioning of the immune system could be expected to enhance health in terms of improved resistance to infection and removal of malignant or premalignant cells. These agents would be particularly useful in very young children and in the elderly, where immune status is often poor. Conversely, agents that suppress the immune system are sometimes necessary, and the development of immunosuppressive agents with high efficacy and minimal toxicity has been the focus of novel drug research. There is a need for such agents owing to advances in transplantation technology and for the treatment of autoimmune diseases. Traditional chinese Medicines (TCM) have been used for centuries in China to treat various immune-mediated disorders (136), and *G. lucidum* specifically has a reputation for immunomodulatory effects.

An α-1,2 polysaccharide (58% glucose) from *G. lucidum* was reported to increase the proliferation of Con A–stimulated mouse spleen cells as shown by MTT test in vitro, and to increase expression of cytokines IL-I and IL-2 and IFN-γ (55). This activity was abolished after treatment with α-1,2 fucosidase (glytolic cleavage). It seems, therefore, that the main active compound is a polysaccharide or glycoprotein fraction containing essential fucose residues with α-1,2-linkages. Polysaccharides from the mushroom increased lymphocyte proliferation in spleen cells from normal and aged mice in vivo and promoted the response to sheep red blood cells (SRBC), an indirect test of antibody production (53,137). In a similar study, a polysaccharide (1-3-α-D native and degraded) isolated from the mushroom spores showed some immunostimulating activity as assessed by increased lymphocyte proliferation and production of antibodies against SRBC, after being injected into mice (54,58). Immunostimulating results were also seen in in vitro tests of proliferation of T and B lymphocytes as measured by the MTT method. Bao et al. (59) showed similar results in a mouse model, with an isolated polysaccharide (PL-1) from the mushroom's fruit body. However, in the in vitro studies, not all tested polysaccharides showed induction of proliferation of T and B cells. ith Different derivatives of the native polysaccharides were tested in those studies with different degree of affect (54,58). Although up to now there is no accepted mechanism or agreement on the parameters that influence the glucans activities, it seems that the introduction of ionic or nonionic groups can significantly affect the physiochemical properties and immunomodulating activities of the parent glucan.

Effects of *G. lucidum* extracts on T-cell subsets in spleen, thymus, and splenocytes of γ-irradiated mice were investigated by Chen et al. (138). Mice were treated with whole-body exposure to 4 Gy γ-irradiation. A crude, water-soluble extract was given for 35 consecutive days, 7 days before and 28 days after radiation. In the study, the *G. lucidum* extract increased the thymus recovery from radiation and promoted splenocyte proliferation. In addition, results suggested that *G. lucidum* enhanced recovery of CD8+ cells in irradiated mice, and that *G. lucidum* treatment may have resulted in a slight increase in CD4+ cells in control mice (no irradiation) (138).

These animal studies indicate a possible immunopotentiating effect of *G. lucidum*. However, immunosuppressive effects of the mushroom have also been reported. A protein purified from the mycelium (LZ-8) was found to have immunosuppressive effects on human mononuclear cells. The protein Ling Zhi-8 (LZ-8) with MW 13–17 kDa was identified by Kino et al. in 1989 (104). The LZ-8 molecule consists of a homodimer of two polypeptides of 110 amino acids, which bear primary and secondary structural similarities with the immunoglobulin heavy chain. This led to the hypothesis that LZ-8 might be an ancestral protein of the immunoglobulins (106).

The administration of LZ-8 in an allografted mouse skin model resulted in an increased graft survival time, and in a rat model LZ-8 was effective in delaying the rejection process of allografted pancreatic islets (106). LZ-8 was also found to prevent systemic anaphylaxis and death (from 4/10 death in control mice to 0/10 in treated mice) when administered by intraperitoneal injection several times before shock was induced by bovine serum albumin (BSA), but had no effect if given at the same time as shock was induced (104). The authors suggested that the effect of LZ-8 was mediated by inhibition of antibody production. This was supported by the results of a later study by this group (105) in which a decrease in antibody production after immunization of mice by hepatitis B surface antigen was seen. However, this group also reported that LZ-8 showed in vitro mitogenic effects on mice spleen cells (104,105). A later study by this group suggested that LZ-8 exerts its antibody-inhibiting effect through modulation of adhesion molecules on immunocompetent cells, perhaps restoring cellular interaction that has become defective as a result of (or resulting in) autoimmune disease (139).

In a study that examined the effect of *G. lucidum* on normal human peripheral mononuclear cells, cells were incubated with methanolic extracts of *G. lucidum* in the presence of the potent immunosuppressive agent cyclosporin A, or in the presence of immunostimulatory agents (140). Results showed no convincing antagonistic effect against immunostimulatory agents except at very high concentrations (100 mg/L), which may themselves have been cytotoxic. Most of the organic extracts of *G. lucidum* appeared to increase immunosuppression in cyclosporin-treated cells at concentrations of 10 mg/L

G. lucidum. It must be noted that this study was not adequately controlled, as no cells were treated with *G. lucidum* extracts in the absence of immunostimulatory or immunoinhibitory agents. Therefore, it is not possible to say whether the effects of *G. lucidum* on cyclosporin-treated cells were additive or synergistic (140).

E. Cardiovascular Disease

Cardiovascular disease (CVD) is the leading cause of death worldwide (123), and anything that can delay or help prevent CVD will make a significant impact in both economic- and health-related terms. Established risk factors for CVD include hypertension, hypercholesterolaemia, diabetes mellitus, smoking, and increased thrombotic index, and there is an ever-increasing list of new CVD risk factors and predictors, such as homocysteine, C-reactive protein, and oxidative stress. Modulating risk factors is the key to primary prevention of CVD (141).

Morigiwa et al. (79) reported that isolated triterpenes from the fruit body of *G. lucidum* inhibited angiotensin-converting enzyme (ACE), suggesting a potential role for *G. lucidum* in the modulation of blood pressure. Three days of oral administration of mycelium extract to hypertensive rats had no hypotensive effect, but the authors reported that administration of the mycelium culture media (water and bran base) produced a decrease in blood pressure lasting up to 25 hr (142), implying production and release of hyptensive agents from the mycelium. However, this study was poorly designed and described, and apparently uncontrolled. In a study with normotensive animals (143), an ethanol-precipitable fraction of a water extract of mycelium and medium was given by intravenous injection. Blood pressure reportedly decreased in anesethetized, but not in conscious, rabbits, but did decrease in conscious rats. Heart rates did not change, but the authors reported a decreased activity in exposed renal nerves. However, this study was also uncontrolled, and results are difficult to interpret.

In a 6-month human supplementation study in Japan (144), 53 patients (40 hypertensive and 13 normotensive or mildly hypertensive control subjects) took 1.5 g (as capsules) per day of *G. lucidum* extract. After 10 days significant decreases were reported in the systolic and diastolic pressures of the hypertensive subjects, and these remained decreased until the end of the trial. The authors concluded that oral intake of *G. lucidum* resulted in lowered blood pressure in essential hypertension. The lack of significant effect in control subjects could imply an indirect effect of *G. lucidum* on blood pressure; however, it must be noted that there was no placebo-controlled group in this study. It is of interest that 6 months of supplementation with *G. lucidum* was not associated with any evidence of renal or hepatic toxicity, as no deleterious changes were seen in plasma biomarkers of kidney or liver function. Furthermore, there was a small (around 7%) but significant decrease in total cholesterol concentration (144). A cholesterol-lowering effect was also seen in a study using an in vitro rat liver homogenate model (145). One triterpene (the oxygenated lanosterol, Compound VI) from *G. lucidum* was reported to show a marked inhibitory effect on cholesterol synthesis from dihydrolanosterol, with 84% inhibition at 40 μM (145). The hypocholesterolaemic effect may be mediated by effects on cholesterol biosynthesis and by possible triterpene-mediated effects on blockage of cholesterol absorption (7,11,145).

Platelet aggregation and agents that mediate proliferation of vascular smooth muscle play a role in thrombosis and vascular spasm, key players in CVD (146). Several compounds from the *G. lucidum* mushroom have been reported to have antagonistic effects on platelet aggregation. Adenosine suppresses platelet aggregation, and a dried water extract of *G. lucidum* was reported to have an adenosine concentration of >40 mg/100 g (147). Administration of the adenosine derivative, 5-deoxy-5-methylsulfinyladenosine, isolated from *G. lucidum*, showed inhibitory effects on induction of platelet aggregation in rabbit plasma, but the effect was not as strong as that of adenosine (148).

Su et al. (149–151) showed that the triterpene ganodermic acid S (GAS), isolated from the mushroom's mycelia, inhibited platelet response to collagen, and GAS showed an additive inhibitory effect on collagen-induced platelet aggregation in the presence of prostaglandin E1. Collagen-induced aggregation is mediated by thromboxane A_2(TXA_2)-dependent signaling pathways. TXA_2 is a potent inducer of platelet activation, and agents, such as GAS, that inhibit the action of TXA_2, directly or indirectly, may have important therapeutic applications in lowering CVD risk (152).

G. lucidum has also been reported to have other antithrombotic effects. Choi and Sa (110) reported that a metalloprotease (likely a zinc metalloprotease) isolated from the mycelium of *G. lucidum* increased the thrombin-induced clotting time of human plasma in vitro, by competitive inhibition of the interaction between thrombin and fibrinogen, as well as having a fibrinolytic effect.

Diabetes mellitus is a risk factor considered equivalent to established coronary heart disease (153). Components of *G. lucidum* have been shown to have a hypoglycemic effect in animals. Ganoderans A and B, two polysaccharides isolated from fruit body water extracts and administered (dose of 100 mg/kg) by intraperitoneal injection to normal and alloxan-induced diabetic hyperglycaemic mice, significantly decreased (by up to 50%) the plasma glucose concentrations, and the hypoglycemic effect was still evident after 24 hr (61). Using a mouse model, ganoderan B was also reported to increase plasma insulin, decrease hepatic glycogen content, and modulate the activity of glucose-metabolizing enzymes in the liver (154). The same group reported that a third polysaccharide (ganoderan C) isolated from *G. lucidum* also showed significant hypoglycemic effects in mice, and that ganoderan B increased plasma insulin levels in both normal and glucose-loaded mice (57,154). In a small (n = 8) clinical trial (46) two type 1 and two type 2 diabetes mellitus patients were given 3 g/day of a commercial *G. lucidum* supplement for 2 months, while two patients in each group were given conventional therapy (insulin or oral hypoglycemic agent). After 2 months of treatment, all patients were reported to exhibit improvement in their blood glucose levels. However, the poor design, the lack of detail, and the small number of subjects mean that this study and its results have little in the way of scientific credibility, and further study is needed on potential hypoglycemic effects of *G. lucidum* in humans.

CVD can be regarded as an inflammatory disorder. Inflammation-induced increases in acute-phase proteins, such as fibrinogen, are associated with increased CVD risk, and even small increases in highly sensitive C-reactive protein (hsCRP) are regarded as predictive of CVD (155). Anti-inflammatory agents, therefore, may be useful in lowering CVD risk. *G. lucidum* has been reported to have anti-inflammatory activity, and this is described in more detail in the next section. CVD is also regarded as having a strong association with oxidative stress (155). This is relevant in that *G. lucidum* has also been reported to have antioxidant properties. These will be described later.

F. Inflammatory Disorders

The development of an inflammatory response is an important defensive mechanism. The inflammatory response is characterized by the movement of fluid, plasma proteins, cytokines, and other factors to the site of injury. However, this normal protective mechanism can cause problems if it is inadequate, uncontrolled, or inappropriate. Many chronic diseases, such as rheumatoid arthritis and systemic lupus erythematosus, involve chronic inflammation, and long-term anti-inflammatory treatment is required. These treatments, which include steroids, nonsteroidal anti-inflammatory drugs, and specific inhibitors of cycloxygenase, often bring their own problems (156,157).

G. lucidum reportedly has anti-inflammatory properties, but we have been unable to find any reports of clinical trials investigating this aspect of *G. lucidum* and its potential health benefits. A family of triterpenoids from the mushroom was reported to reduce inflammation induced by carageenan and croton oil, and a therapuetic role for *G. lucidum* has been suggested in arthritis and Alzheimer's disease (32). Streeper and Satsangi (156) studied the anti-inflammatory effect of both oral and topical treatment with water and ethyl acetate extracts of *G. lucidum* in a mouse model of croton-oil-induced irritation (to the ear). It was reported that orally administered ethyl acetate and water extracts of *G. lucidum* had significant activity that extended over a longer period of time than hydrocortisone, a commonly used anti-inflammatory treatment. Topical application of the ethyl acetate extract also resulted in significant anti-inflammatory effect, comparing favorably with hydrocortisone. The water extract, on the other hand, had little or no topical effect. This group also reported that treatment with *G. lucidum* was not associated with thymic involution, a common side effect of corticosteroid treatment (156). In another animal study (158), both oral and topical adminstration of organic extracts of *G. lucidum* was reported to ameliorate chemical-induced irritation, as measured by effects on edema, weight, and volume of affected sites (ear and paw).

The anti-inflammatory components of *G. lucidum* in these organic extracts are believed to be the triterpenes (156). In the *Handbook of Enzyme Inhibitors* (159), the triterpenes, ganoderic acids R, S, and T, are referred to as having an inhibitory effect on the enzyme phospholipase A_2 (PLA_2) from pig pancreas. PLA_2 catalyzes the rate-limiting step in the release of arachidonic acid, and mediates the inflammatory response. In addition, extracellular PLA_2, such as that secreted into body fluids during inflammation, can directly attack cell membranes, inducing cell lysis and subsequent tissue damage (160).

Jain et al. (161) studied the anti-PLA_2 activity of seven triterpenes isolated from *G. lucidum*. Three triterpenes, R, S, and T, were found to be active against enzymes from pig pancreas, but only ganoderic acid T was active also against the enzyme from bee venom and a human recombinant PLA_2 from synovial fluid. No details are given of how the ganoderic acids were purified. Hot-water extracts of *G. lucidum* have also been found to induce marked inhibition of PLA_2 from pig pancreas and bee venom (162). Giner-Larza et al. (158) also studied the PLA_2 inhibitory effect of *G. lucidum*. Mice were given *G. lucidum* extract orally 90 min before being injected in the paw with snake venom PLA2 (from *N. naja* and *N. mossambica*). Edema of the affected paw was significantly decreased 60 min after treatment, when compared to controls. However, in an in vitro study using PLA2 from *N. mossambica*, no significant inhibitory effect of *G. lucidum* was seen (158). The reason for this conflict in PLA_2 inhibition by *G. lucidum* is not clear. Analytical methods for testing PLA_2 inhibition are varied and can be problematic (161). However, it is possible that the inhibitory components of *G. lucidum* are active against only certain types of PLA_2; this deserves further study.

G. Allergy

Diagnosis of allergy is often based on identification of environmental allergens by skin tests and in vitro tests of allergen-specific IgE (157). *G. lucidum* is believed to help alleviate allergies (12). Triterpenes isolated from *G. lucidum* were shown to have an inhibitory action on histamine release from rat mast cells ex vivo; however, the methods and results in this study were poorly described (77). There are no published reports of an allergic response to ingestion of *G. lucidum*, but it should be noted that some basidiomycetes may be potential aeroallergens. Sensitization to *G. lucidum* has been reported in patients with from asthma and rhinitis (163–165), as positive skin prick and intradermal skin tests to both spores and the fruit body extract were reported in some patients (>16%), as well as elevated antibodies to the fungi and proteins separated from it. Inhalation of *G. lucidum* spores may stimulate a base level of allergic responsiveness in susceptible atopic patients. *G. lucidum* may, therefore, induce respiratory and skin allergy, and this clearly must be considered in any potential topical application of *G. lucidum*.

H. Antioxidant

Observations imply that reactive oxygen species may damage DNA, proteins, and lipids in vivo, thereby promoting development of various diseases, including cancer and CVD. Reactive oxygen species (ROS) are a partially reduced form of oxygen, and include the superoxide anion, hydrogen peroxide, and the highly reactive hydroxyl radical. These, and other ROS, are produced in various ways, such as during the course of normal aerobic metabolism, from activated phagocytes, during postischemic reperfusion, and from cigarette smoke, ionizing and ultraviolet (UV) radiation, drugs, and toxins (166–168). Oxidative damage to key biological sites is, therefore, a continuous and unavoidable physiological threat. An array of physiological antioxidants exists within the body to prevent production, inactivation, and removal of ROS, thus limiting oxidative damage. These antioxidants are of both endogenous and dietary origin. Plants contain many antioxidants, and diets rich in plant-based foods are known to be associated with improved health (166–168). While the precise components and mechanism of benefit of "healthy" diets remain to be established, it is hypothesized that antioxidants play a key role.

The antioxidant properties of *G. lucidum* have been examined in different models. Using a supercoiled bacterial DNA model, hot-water extract, water-soluble polysaccharides, and an isolated amino-polysaccharide (G009) from *G. lucidum* were reported to show good radioprotective ability, and conferred DNA protection against hydroxyl radical produced by metal-catalyzed Fenton reaction, UV irradiation, and photolysis of hydrogen peroxide (169). There were two suggested mechanisms by which the polysaccharides exerted their protective effect, metal ion binding (which prevents the Fenton reaction) and hydroxyl radical scavenging (169,170). Using a human DNA model (Raji cells) the hot-water extract (but not a cold-water extract) of *G. lucidum* was also found to markedly protect DNA from damage induced by hydrogen peroxide (171). However, it must be noted that the concentration of *G. lucidum* extract used in these antioxidant studies was very high, starting from 0.5 mg/mL (169–171), and it is not currently clear whether this concentration could be achieved in vivo.

The antioxidant activity of *G. lucidum* has also been examined in other models. The terpene and polysaccharide fractions were separated from a hot-water extract, and were screened for their antioxidative effect against pyrogallol-induced erythrocyte membrane oxidation using rat red blood cells (172). All three types (the hot-water extract and the isolated terpene and polysaccharide fractions) of extracts protected, but the polysaccharide and terpene fractions were effective at 0.1 mg/mL and above, whereas the hot-water extract was effective only at >0.25 mg/mL. The effect on lipid peroxidation was also assessed by Zhu et al. (172). Rat liver mitochondria were exposed to ferrous sulfate and ascorbic acid, which produces hydroxyl radicals, and the extent of lipid peroxidation was assessed using the thiobarbituric acid reactive substances (TBARS) reaction. TBARS levels were decreased by the addition of the *G. lucidum* extracts. The terpene fraction was the most effective, and at a concentration of 0.1 mg/mL almost all lipid peroxidation was prevented (172). A similar protocol was applied by Lee et al. (170), who used rat brain homogenate to test the amino polysaccharide (G009) fraction of *G. lucidum* at concentrations of 0.25–2.0 mg/mL. This inhibited formation of TBARS in a dose-dependent manner. Whether this was related to iron binding by the polysaccharide was not tested. In a separate experiment, the G009 polysaccharide was found to have hydroxyl-radical-scavenging effect when the hydroxylated products of hydroxyl radical trapped by salicylic acid were measured (170). This group also reported superoxide scavenging effects using two different systems of superoxide generation, a xanthine-xanthine oxidase system and a HL-60 cell culture model. In the xanthine-xanthine oxidase model, G009 mitigated superoxide-related oxidation of a chromophore in a dose-related manner. In the cell culture model, oxidation was inhibited by about 60% by 2.0 mg/mL of *G. lucidum* (170). Whether this was due to scavenging or inhibition of superoxide generation by the cells was not clear.

Using the ferric-reducing (antioxidant) power (FRAP) assay (173), we have found that hot-water extracts of *G. lucidum* show some antioxidant power, but this is not particularly high. Ascorbic acid (1 g), green tea (1 g), and *G. lucidum* (1 g) are estimated to contain 11,364 μmol, 272–1144 μmol, and

360 μmol of antioxidant power, respectively (174,175 and our unpublished data). However, we have found that there is a significant increase in plasma antioxidant capacity shortly after an oral dose of *G. lucidum*, indicating that some antioxidants in *G. lucidum* are bioavailable (Fig. 3) (175). Furthermore, using flow cytometric analysis of site-specific oxidation of membrane lipids in living cells ex vivo, we have found that membrane oxidation is inhibited by preincubation of cells with hot-water extracts of *G. lucidum* (Fig. 4) (our unpublished results).

From these, and other, data it is clear that *G. lucidum* has antioxidant properties, and that both polysaccharide and triterpene constituents contribute to these. However, it is not yet known which antioxidants are absorbed, nor is it clear whether absorbed antioxidants from *G. lucidum* have any in vivo protective effects and health benefits; further study is needed in this area.

I. Liver Injury

Hot-water and water-ether extracts of the fruit body of *G. lucidum* were found to have a potent hepatoprotective effect against carbon tetrachloride (CCl_4)-induced liver injury in rats when given orally and intraperitoneally (176,177). The measured markers for liver injury included asaparate and alanine trans-

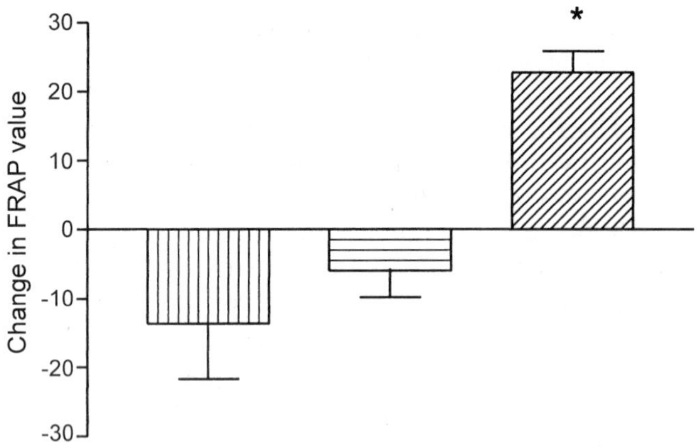

FIGURE 3 Mean + SEM change in plasma total antioxidant power (as the FRAP value) at 90 min postingestion of placebo (vertical lines), 1.1 g of *G. lucidum* extract (horizontal lines), and 3.3 g of *G. lucidum* extract (diagonal lines) in a human intervention trial ($n = 10$). A significant ($*p < 0.05$) increase in plasma FRAP was seen after the *G. lucidum* administration compared with the placebo intake, indicating an absorption of antioxidant compounds into plasma.

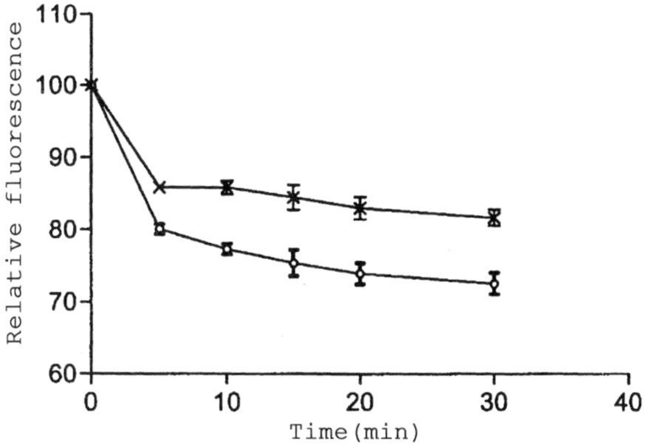

FIGURE 4 Effect of preincubation with Lingzhi (*G. lucidum*) on peroxidation within cell membranes. Each point represents the mean of three separate experiments, with 1 SD error bars shown (o = phosphate-buffered saline control; * = Lingzhi, 1.5% w/v). Preincubation with Lingzhi protected membranes, as seen by less quenching of membrane-bound fluorophore.

aminases (AST and ALT) and lactate dehydrogenase (LDH). One active compound of the extract was separated and identified as ganoderenic acid A. This was found to have potent inhibitory effect on β-glucuronidase, and the authors suggested that this inhibitory effect may have mediated the hepatoprotection seen when this isolated compound was given (177). Protection was also reported in a study in which a hot-water extract of *G. lucidum* was given orally to mice 30 min before administration of ethanol. The extract was found to show an inhibitory effect against malodialdehyde (MDA) formation, which is a degradation product of lipid peroxides, in mouse liver and renal homogenate, with evidence of a dose-response seen (178).

Hepatoprotection may also be mediated by radical-scavenging properties of *G. lucidum*. It has been hypothesized that CCl_4 and alcohol toxicity is associated with increased oxidative stress and free-radical-associated injury. Lin et al. (176) reported that hot-water extracts of *G. lucidum* showed significant radical-scavenging activity against both superoxide and hydroxyl radicals; however, the extracts were not further characterized. Interestingly, in a similar animal study of CCl_4-induced liver damage (142), oral administration of the medium in which *G. lucidum* mycelia were grown (but not the mycelium alone) had marked benefical effects, as assessed by lower 96 hr postinjury serum AST and ALT activities. No decrease was seen in the actual damage caused, as 24-hr transaminase activites were not different from levels in control animals, implying that the mycelium-medium may have promoted recovery in some way. The release of a hepatoprotective component from *G. lucidum* mycelium was also reported by Song et al. (179). In this study, an extracellular peptidoglycan (a polysaccharide/amino acid complex named WK-003) produced during mycelium fermentation was administered orally to rats for 4 days prior to CCl_4 intoxication. Serum ALT levels were significantly reduced (by 70%; $p < 0.01$) at 24 hr postinjury compared with untreated, intoxicated rats. The AST levels decreased by 27%; however, this was not statistically significant. These studies of a possible mycelial product with hepatoprotective activity being extruded into the culture medium are of interest because the mycelia of *G. lucidum* are much easier and less costly to cultivate than the fruit body.

Polysaccharides extracted from *G. lucidum* were found by Park et al. (180) to have antifibrotic properties and to ameliorate cirrhosis induced by biliary ligation. The polysaccharides were given orally for 28 days postligation, and this was found to lower collagen (hydroxyproline) content in rats liver and improved the liver morphology in comparison to control animals. The polysaccharide treatment also significantly decreased the ligation-induced increases in serum biochemical markers of liver damage (AST, ALT, alkaline phosphatase, and total bilirubin). These data suggest that polysaccharides from *G. lucidum* could be a promising antifibrotic therapy; however, no mechanisms of this putative hepatoprotective action were described, and further study is needed (180).

VIII. CONCLUDING REMARKS

G. lucidum is a well-regarded Asian herbal remedy with a long and impressive range of applications. Global consumption of *G. lucidum* is high, and an increasingly large series of patented and commercially available products that incorporate *G. lucidum* as an active ingredient are available as food supplements. These include extracts and isolated constituents in various formulations and these are marketed worldwide in the form of capsules, creams, hair tonics, and syrups (6,182). The various postulated health benefits of *G. lucidum* are outlined in Figure 5, and a summary of the experimental studies described in this chapter, with our comments, on the putative therapeutic effects of *G. lucidum* is presented in Table 2.

In conclusion, studies on *G. lucidum* composition, cultivation, and reputed effects are still being carried out, and several new studies have been published since this paper was drafted. However, convincing evidence of direct effects of *G. lucidum* on human health is lacking to date, even though the mushroom is widely promoted and consumed. Observational and anecdotal reports of benefits have not as yet been substantiated by well-controlled clinical trials or reliable scientific data. The *G. lucidum* preparations used have

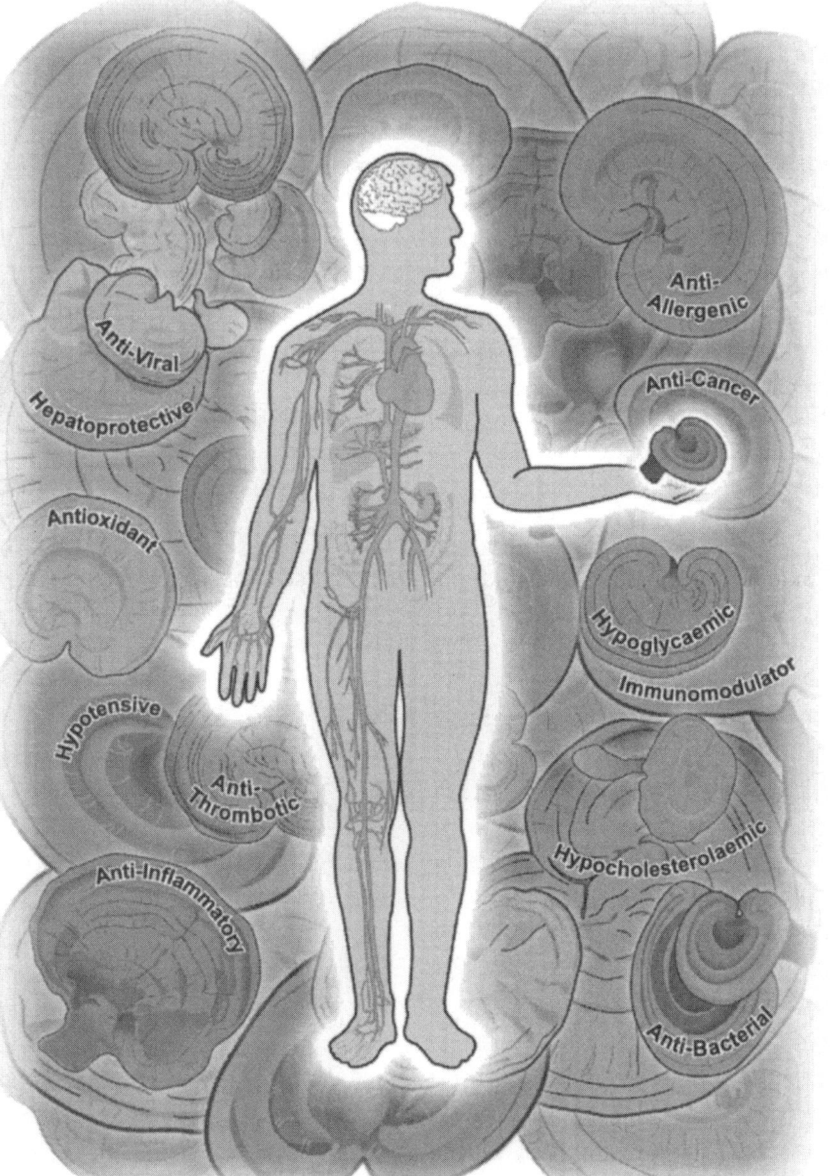

FIGURE 5 Postulated, but as yet unvalidated, health benefits of Lingzhi (*G. lucidum*).

TABLE 2 Summary of Experimental Studies[a] on the Putative Therapeutic Effects of the Lingzhi Mushroom (*Ganoderma lucidum*)

	Effect tested	Type of study	Reported effect	Comment	Ref.
Viral infection	Viral proliferation	Cell culture and in vitro	Inhibitory effect against some viruses, particularly herpes simplex; synergistic or additive effects with antiviral drugs reported. Some isolated triterpenes inhibited (HIV)-1 reverse transcriptase and protease.	*G. lucidum* may have an inhibitory effect on viral proliferation, and the possible synergistic effect with established antiviral drugs is interesting; further in vitro studies are needed.	60,84,86, 112–115
Viral infection	Recovery from or progression of viral infection	Human intervention trials	Promoted recovery from postherpetic neuralgia ($n = 4$) and reportedly also aided recovery in a small ($n = 4$) trial on hepatitis B patients. No improvement in quality of life or immune status was seen in HIV patients ($n = 68$) given a mix of Chinese herbs together with lingzhi.	Only 3 trials published to date; these were small, poorly designed, and uncontrolled studies and do not provide convincing scientific evidence for *G. lucidum* in promoting recovery from viral infection; well-planned, controlled clinical trials are needed.	46,116,117
Bacterial infection	Bacterial proliferation	In vitro and animal studies	In vitro inhibitory effect reported against some bacteria; additive or	No human trials to date; experimental evidence of possible interaction	119,121

			synergistic effect reported with antibiotic drugs, but indication of some antagonistic effect also seen.	with antibiotics is interesting, as *G. lucidum* may help lower MIC values of potentially cytotoxic drugs. However, antagonistic effects must be clarified, and testing for possible antibacterial effect against antibiotic resistant strains would be useful.	
Cancer	Tumor growth	Animal studies and human clinical trials	Administration of *G. lucidum* to animals (i.p or o.p) inhibited growth of implanted/induced tumors (see Table 1). Human studies of acute myeloblastic leukemia and advanced nasopharyngeal carcinoma reported improvement in patients treated with high-dose *G. lucidum* extract in combination with conventional therapy.	Antitumor activity appears related to polysaccharide content of mushroom. Only two human trials reported to date; there were small (n = 4 and n = 5) and uncontrolled, involved advanced illness, and *G. lucidum* was given in conjunction with standard therapy; contribution of *G. lucidum* to reported improvement in patients is not clear.	46,51–53,70, 121,126–128

TABLE 2 Continued

	Effect tested	Type of study	Reported effect	Comment	Ref.
Cancer	Growth and activation of cancer and immune cells	Cell culture and cells ex vivo and in vitro	Incubation with *G. lucidum* caused activation of cultured macrophages and T lymphocytes; increase in cytokine production; activated macrophages inhibited growth of cultured cancer cells, promoted apoptosis and differentiation; effects on cancer cells not seen with untreated macrophages or with *G. lucidum* alone; *G. lucidum* induced phase II enzymes in cultured cells; terpenes from *G. lucidum* reported to inhibit DNA polymerase in vitro.	Direct effects on cancer cells may be due to triterpene-mediated inhibition of cell division and inhibition of DNA polymerase. Indirect effects appear to be more pronounced and mediated by polysaccharide-induced effects on immune cells.	48,50,52,86–88, 109,121,126, 129—135
Immune status	Immunomodulation	Animal studies and cells ex vivo	Enhanced lymphocyte proliferation, antibody production, and recovery of the immune system in irradiated	Opposing effects—activation and suppression—seen with different constituents. Studies often poorly	53–55,58,59, 104–106, 137–140

			mice reported. An isolated protein (LZ-8) and methanolic extracts of *G. lucidum* showed immunosuppressive effects, such as delaying rejection time of allografts in mice.	described and appear uncontrolled. Further study is needed.	
CVD	Blood pressure and cholesterol synthesis	In vitro and animal studies; human intervention trial	Inhibition of cholesterol synthesis and ACE demonstrated in vitro; hypotensive effect seen in some animal studies; hypotensive and small cholesterol-lowering effect reported in human intervention trial of 40 hypertensive subjects treated with *G. lucidum* for 6 months.	Some evidence that *G. lucidum* has potential as a hypotensive and hypocholesterolemic agent; effects on blood pressure may be due to ACE inhibition; effects on cholesterol may be mediated by a combination of inhibition of cholesterol synthesis and blocking of sterol receptors in GI tract owing to structural similarity between lanosterol-derived terpenes and cholesterol. Further study needed, as only one human trial published to date.	7,11,79, 142–145

TABLE 2 Continued

	Effect tested	Type of study	Reported effect	Comment	Ref.
CVD	Platelet aggregation and blood clotting	In vitro and animal studies	Adenosine, adenosine derivative, and ganodermic acid S isolated from *G. lucidum* inhibited platelet aggregation; metalloprotease isolated from *G. lucidum* increased clotting time.	No in vivo studies published to date.	110, 147–152
CVD	Glycemic control	Animal studies and human intervention trial	Polysaccharides isolated from *G. lucidum* shown to have hypoglycemic effect in mice. In a small, poorly controlled clinical trial, *G. lucidum* supplementation was reported to improve glycemic control in type I ($n = 2$) and type II ($n = 2$) diabetes mellitus patients, compared to 4 untreated control diabetic subjects.	Positive hypoglycemic results in animal studies; however, there is a lack of data from well-designed human trials to support this claim.	46,57,61,154
Inflammation	Inflammatory response	In vitro and animal studies	Anti-inflammatory properties were shown in induced irritation	Interesting results; however, no human trials published to date,	32,156,158

			(edema) in mice after oral and topical application of organic (terpenes-containing) extracts.	and no data on mechanism of anti-inflammatory effect of triterpenes presented.	
Inflammation	PLA2 activity	In vitro	Some isolated triterpenes showed inhibitory effects against the enzyme PLA2 isolated from bee venom, hog pancreas, and snake venom. One triterpene (ganoderic acid T) reported to inhibit human recombinant PLA2.	Results indicate that different triterpenes may be active only against certain types of PLA2. Specific triterpenes should be further studied in specific models of PLA2 inhibition and the downstream antiinflammatory effects of this.	158–162
Allergy	Allergic response	In vitro and human trials	Triterpenes from *G. lucidum* reported to have inhibited histamine release in vitro. No reports of allergic response to ingestion of *G. lucidum*, but three reports of aerosensitization in atopic subjects.	No strong evidence of antiallergenic properties; further study needed. However, possible allergic reaction to *G. lucidum* should be considered, especially in patients with respiratory or allergic disorders or in association with topical application.	12,77,157, 163–165

TABLE 2 Continued

	Effect tested	Type of study	Reported effect	Comment	Ref.
Antioxidant	ROS scavenging and antioxidant bioavailability	In vitro and human intervention trial	*G. lucidum* found to possess antioxidant properties in in vitro models; reported to scavenge superoxide and hydroxyl radical, to protect DNA from ROS and decrease lipid peroxidation. In a human bioavailability study ($n = 10$), plasma antioxidant power increased after *G. lucidum* intake.	Not yet known which antioxidants from *G. lucidum* are absorbed or if the absorbed antioxidants have any in vivo protective effect. Further study needed.	169–175
Liver injury	Induced liver injury	Animal studies	*G. lucidum* reported to show antifibrotic and hepatoprotective effects after CCl4 or ethanol in animal models induced liver injury.	No histological data presented; whether the effect of *G lucidum* is truly protective, indicates faster recovery from damage, or improved clearing of plasma biomarkers of liver injury should be further investigated.	142,176–180

[a] The studies summarized in this table are those published in English in at least abstract form.

often not been well defined in terms of the source, growing conditions, means of identification of the mushroom as *G. lucidum*, contamination, heavy metal content, batch-to-batch variation, method of extraction/preparation, or dosage. Most studies have been performed on animals or in cell culture models, and experimental studies have often been small, poorly designed, and inadequately controlled. The great wealth of chemical data and anecdotal evidence on effects of *G. lucidum* needs now to be complemented by reliable experimental and clinical data from human trials to clearly establish whether the reported health-related effects are valid and significant. Quality control procedures to define and standardize *G. lucidum* preparations, in addition to well-designed animal and cell culture studies, are needed to determine mechanisms of action and to help characterize the active component(s) of this putative medicinal mushroom.

ACKNOWLEDGMENTS

The authors thank the Hong Kong Polytechnic University for funding this work.

REFERENCES

1. Chang ST, Buswell JA. Mushroom nutriceuticals. World J Micro Biotechnol 1996; 12:473–476.
2. Rajarathnam S, Shashirekha MN, Bano Z. Biodegradative and biosynthetic capacities of mushrooms: present and future strategies. Cr Rev Biotechnol 1998; 18:91–236.
3. Borchers AT, Stern JS, Hackman RM, Keen CL, Gershwin ME. Minireview: mushrooms, tumors and immunity. Proc Soc Exp Biol Med 1999; 221:281–293.
4. Wasser SP, Weis AL. Medicinal properties of substances occuring in higher basidiomycetes mushrooms: current perspectives. Int J Med Mushrooms 1999; 1:31–62.
5. Wasser SP, Weis AL. Therapeutic effects of substances occuring in higher basidiomycetes mushroom: a modern perspective. Cr Rev Immunol 1999; 19:65–96.
6. Jong SC, Birmingham JM. Medicinal benefits of the mushroom *Ganoderma*. Adv Appl Microbiol 1992; 37:101–134.
7. Shiao MS, Lee KR, Lin LJ, Wang CT. Natural products and biological activities of the Chinese medicinal fungus *Ganoderma lucidum*. Am Chem Soc Symp Series 1994; 547:342–354.
8. Chen AW, Miles PG. Biomedical research and the application of mushroom nutriceuticals from *Ganoderma lucidum*. In: Royse DJ, ed. Proceedings of the

2nd International Conference on Mushroom Biology and Mushroom Products. University Park: Penn State University, 1996:161–175.
9. Teeguarden R. The Ancient Wisdom of the Chinese Tonic Herbs. New York: Warner Books, 1998.
10. Chang ST, Buswell JA. *Ganoderma lucidum* (Curt.: Fr.) P. Karst. (Aphyllophoromycetideae)—a mushrooming medicinal mushroom. Int J Med Mushrooms 1999; 1:139–146.
11. Upton R. American Herbal Pharmacopeia and Therapeutic Compendium: Reishi Mushroom, *Ganoderma lucidum*. Standards of Analysis, Quality Control, and Therapeutics. Santa Cruz, CA, 2000.
12. Willard T. Reishi Mushroom, Herb of Spiritual Potency and Medical Wonder. Issaquah, WA: Sylvan Press, 1990.
13. Teow SS. Effective dosage of the extract of *Ganoderma lucidum* in the treatment of various ailments. In: Royse DJ, ed. Proceedings of the 2nd International Conference on Mushroom Biology and Mushroom Products. Penn State University, 1996:177–185.
14. Donk MA. A conspectus of the families of Aphyllophorales. Persoonia 1964; 3:19–24.
15. Moncalvo JM. Systematics of *Ganoderma*. In: Flood J, Bridge PD, Holderness M, eds. *Ganoderma* Diseases of Perennial Crops. Wallingford, UK: CAB International, 2000:23–45.
16. Mizuno T, Wang G, Zhang J, Kawagishi H, Nishitoba T, Reishi Li J. *Ganoderma lucidum* and *Ganoderma tsugae*: bioactive substances and medicinal effects. Food Rev Int 1995; 11:151–166.
17. Li Shizhen, Ben Cao Gang Mu, Revised ed. Beijing: Zhongguo Zhong yi yao chu ban she, 1998. Chinese.
18. Baxter AP, Eicker A. Preliminary synopsis: recorded taxa of Southern Africa Ganodermataceae. Proceedings of Contributed Symposium, 59A,B, 5th International Mycological Congress, Vancouver, Aug 14–21, 1994:3–5.
19. Zhao JD, Zhang XQ. Importance, distribution and taxonomy of Ganodermataceae in China. Proceedings of Contributed Symposium, 59A,B, 5th International Mycological Congress, Vancouver, Aug 14–21, 1994:1–2.
20. Szedlay G, Jakucs E, Boldizsar I, Boka K. Basidiocarp and mycelium morphology of *Ganoderma lucidum* Karst. strains isolated in hungary. Acta Microbiol Immunol Hung 1999; 46:41–52.
21. Woo YA, Kim HJ, Cho JH, Chung H. Discrimination of herbal medicines according to geographical origin with near infrared reflectance spectroscopy and pattern recognition techniques. J Pharm Biomed Anal 1999; 21:407–413.
22. Ryvarden L. Can we trust morphology in *Ganoderma*? In: Buchanan PK, Hseu RS, Moncalvo JM, eds. *Ganoderma*: Systematics, Phytopathology and Pharmacology. Proceedings of Contributed Symposium, 59A,B, 5th International Mycological Congress, Vancouver, Aug 14–21, 1994:19–24.
23. Gottlieb AM, Saidman BO, Wright JE. Isoenzymes of *Ganoderma* species from southern South America. Mycol Res 1998; 102:415–426.

24. Hseu RS, Wang HH, Wang HF, Moncalvo JM. Differentiation and grouping of isolates of *Ganoderma lucidum* complex by random amplified polymorphic DNA-PCR compared with grouping on the basis of internal transcribed spacer sequences. Appl Environ Microbiol 1996; 62:1354–1363.
25. Chen DH, Shiou WY, Wang KC, Huang SY, Shie YT, Tsai CM, Shie JF, Chen KD. Chemotaxonomy of triterpenoid pattern of HPLC of *Ganoderma lucidum* and *Ganoderma tsugae*. J Chinese Chem Soc 1999; 46:47–51.
26. Gottlieb AM, Ferref E, Wright JE. rDNA analyses as an aid to the taxonomy of species of *Ganoderma*. Mycol Res 2000; 104:1033–1045.
27. Su CH, Yang YZ, Ho HO, Hu CH, Sheu MT. High-performance liquid chromatographic analysis for the characterization of triterpenoids from *Ganoderma*. J Chromatogr Sci 2001; 39:93–100.
28. Moncalvo JM, Wang HF, Hseu RS. Phylogenetic relationships in *Ganoderma* inferred from the internal transcribed spacers and 25s ribosomal DNA sequences. Mycologia 1995; 87:223–238.
29. Moncalvo JM, Wang HF, Hseu RS. Gene phylogeny of the *Ganoderma lucidum* complex: comparison with traditional taxonomic characters. Mycol Res 1995; 99:1489–1499.
30. Moncalvo JM, Wang HF, Wang HH, Hseu RS. The use of rDNA nucleotide sequence data for species identification and phylogeny in the Ganodermataceae. In: Buchanan PK, Hseu RS, Moncalvo JM, eds. *Ganoderma*: Systematics, Phytopathology and Pharmacology. Proceedings of Contributed Symposia 59A,B, 5th International Mycological Congress, Vancouver, Canada, August 1994:31–44.
31. Zhu YP. Chinese Materia Medica. Singapore: Harwood Academic Publishers, 1998.
32. Patocka J. Anti-inflammatory triterpenoids from mysterious mushroom *Ganoderma lucidum* and their potential possibility in modern medicine. Acta Med (Hradec Kralove) 1999; 42:123–125.
33. Compiled by the State Pharmacopoeia Commission of P.R. China Pharmacopoeia of the People's Republic of China. English ed. Beijing, China: Chemical Industry Press, 2000.
34. Mayzumi F, Okamoto H, Mizuno T. Cultivation of Reishi. Food Rev Int 1997; 13:365–373.
35. Riu H, Roig G, Sancho J. Production of carpophores of *Lentinus edodes* and *Ganoderma lucidum* grown on cork residues. Microbiologia SEM 1997; 13:185–192.
36. Tseng TC, Shiao MS, Shieh YS, Hao YY. Studies on *Ganoderma lucidum*: liquid culture and chemical composition of mycelium. Bot Bull Acad Sin 1984; 25:149–157.
37. Cha DY, Yoo YB. Cultivation techniques of Reishi. Food Rev Int 1997; 13:373–382.
38. Yang FC, Liau CB. The influence of environmental conditions on polysaccharide formation by *Ganoderma lucidum* in submerged cultures. Process Biochem 1998; 33:547–553.

39. Lee KM, Lee SY, Lee HY. Bistage control of pH for improving exopolysaccharide production from mycelia of *Ganoderma lucidum* in an air-lift Fermentor. J Bios Bioeng 1999; 88:646–650.
40. Habijanic J, Berovic M. The relevance of solid-state substrate moisturing on *Ganoderma lucidum* biomass cultivation. Food Technol Biotechnol 2000; 38:225–228.
41. Yang F, Ke Y, Kuo S. Effect of fatty acids on the mycelial growth and polysaccharide formation by *Ganoderma lucidum* in shake flask cultures. Enzyme Microb Technol 2000; 27:295–301.
42. Fang QH, Zhong JJ. Two-stage culture process for improved production of ganoderic acid by liquid fermentation of higher fungus *Ganoderma lucidum*. Biotechnol Prog 2002; 18:51–54.
43. Kim SW, Hwang HJ, Park JP, Cho YJ, Song CH, Yun JW. Mycelial growth and exo-biopolymer production by submerged culture of various edible mushrooms under different media. Lett Appl Microbiol 2002; 34:56–60.
44. Chang J. Scientific evaluation of traditional Chinese medicine under DSHEA: a conundrum. J Altern Complem Med 1999; 5:181–189.
45. Chang R. Effective dose of *Ganoderma* in humans. Proceedings of Contributed Symposium, 59A,B, 5th International Mycological Congress, Vancouver, Aug 14–21, 1994:117–121.
46. Teow SS. The therapeutic value of *Ganoderma lucidum*. Proceedings of Contributed Symposium, 59A,B, 5th International Mycological Congress, Vancouver, Aug 14–21, 1994:105–113.
47. Kim MJ, Kim HW, Lee YS, Shim MJ. Studies on safety of *Ganoderma lucidum* [abstr]. Kor J Mycol 1986; 14:49–59.
48. Chiu SW, Wang ZM, Leung TM, Moore D. Nutritional value of *Ganoderma* extract and assessment of its genotoxicity and antigenotoxicity using comet assays of mouse lymphocytes. Food Chem Toxicol 2000; 38:173–178.
49. Mau JL, Lin HC, Chen CC. Non-volatile components of several medicinal mushrooms. Food Res Int 2001; 34:521–526.
50. Kim HS, Kacew S, Lee BM. In vitro chemopreventive effects of plant polysaccharides (aloe *Barbadensis miller*, *Lentinus endodes*, *Ganoderma lucidum* and *Coriolus versicolor*). Carcinogenesis 1999; 20:1637–1640.
51. Kim BK, Chung HS, Chung KS, Yang MS. Studies on the antineoplastic components of Korean basidiomycetes. Korean J Mycol 1980; 8:107–113.
52. Miyazaki T, Nishijima M. Studies on fungal polysaccharides. XXVII. Structural examination of water-soluble, antitumor polysaccharide of *Ganoderma lucidum*. Chem Pharm Bull 1981; 29:3611–3616.
53. Hyun JW, Choi EC, Kim BK. Studies on constituents of higher fungi of Korea (LXVII), antitumor components of the basidiocarp of *Ganoderma lucidum*. Korean J Mycol 1990; 18:58–69.
54. Bao X, Liu C, Fang J, Li X. Structural and immunological studies of a major polysaccharide from spores of *Ganoderma lucidum* (Fr.) Karst. Carbohydr Res 2001; 332:67–74.
55. Wang YY, Khoo KH, Chen ST, Lin CC, Wong CH, Lin CH. Studies on the

immuno-modulating and antitumor activities of *Ganoderma lucidum* (Reishi) polysaccharides: functional and proteomic analyses of a fucose-containing glycoprotein fraction responsible for the activities. Bioorg Med Chem 2002; 10:1057–1062.

56. Sone Y, Okuda R, Wada N, Kishida E, Misaki A. Structures and antitumor activities of the polysaccharides isolated from fruiting body and the growing culture of mycelium of *Ganoderma lucidum*. Agric Biol Chem 1985; 49:2641–2653.
57. Tomoda M, Gonda R, Kasahara Y, Hikino H. Glycan structures of ganoderans B and C, hypoglycemic glycans of *Ganoderma lucidum* fruit bodies. Phytochemistry 1986; 25:2817–2820.
58. Bao X, Duan J, Fang X, Fang J. Chemical modifications of (1→3)-α-D-glucan from spores of *Ganoderma lucidum* and investigation of their physiochemical properties and immunological activity. Carbohydr Res 2001; 336:127–140.
59. Bao X, Wang X, Dong Q, Fang J, Li X. Structural features of immunologically active polysaccharides from *Ganoderma lucidum*. Phytochemistry 2002; 59:175–181.
60. Eo SK, Kim YS, Lee CK, Han SS. Antiherpetic activities of various protein bound polysaccharides isolated from *Ganoderma lucidum*. J Ethnopharmacol 1999; 68:175–181.
61. Hikino H, Konno C, Mirin Y, Hayashi T. Isolation and hypoglycemic activity of ganoderans A and B, glycans of *Ganoderma lucidum* fruit bodies. Planta Medi 1985; 4:339–340.
62. Zhang L, Zhang M, Chen J. Solution properties of antitumor carboxymethylated derivatives of α-(1→3)-D-glucan from *Ganoderma lucidum*. Chinese J Polymer Sci 2001; 19:283–289.
63. Bettelheim FA, March J. Introduction to General, Organic and Biochemistry. Orlando, FL: Harcourt Brace College Publishers, 1995.
64. Parker SP. McGraw-Hill Dictionary of Chemistry. New York: McGraw-Hill, 1997.
65. Das MC, Mahato SB. Triterpenoids. Phytochemistry 1983; 22:1071–1095.
66. Mahato SB, Sen S. Advances in triterpenoid research, 1990–1994. Phytochemistry 1997; 44:1185–1236.
67. Safayhi H, Sailer ER. Anti-inflammatory actions of pentacyclic triterpenes. Planta Med 1997; 63:487–493.
68. Craig WJ. Health-promoting properties of common herbs. Am J Clin Nutr 1999; 70:491S–499S.
69. Mashour NK, Lin GI, Frishman WH. Herbal medicine for the treatment of cardiovascular disease: clinical considerations. Arch Intern Med 1998; 158:2225–2234.
70. Yun TK. Update from Asia—Asian studies on cancer chemoprevention. Ann NY Acad Sci 1999; 889:157–192.
71. Haralampidis K, Trojanowska M, Osbourn AE. Biosynthesis of triterpenoid saponins in plants. Adv Biochem Eng Biotechnol 2002; 75:31–49.

72. Budavari S. The Merck Index. 11th ed. Rahway, New Jersey: Merck & Co., 1989:845.
73. Abe I, Rohmer M, Prestwich GD. Enzymatic cyclization of squalene and oxidosqualene to sterols and triterpenes. Chem Rev 1993; 93:2189–2206.
74. Kubota T, Asaka Y, Miura I, Mori H. Structures of ganoderic acid A and B, two new lanostane type bitter triterpenes from *Ganoderma lucidum* (Fr.) Karst. Helv Chim Acta 1982; 65:611–619.
75. Nishitoba T, Sato H, Kasai T, Kawagishi H, Sakamura S. New bitter C27 and C30 terpenoids from fungus *Ganoderma lucidum* (Reishi). Agric Biol Chem 1984; 48:2905–2907.
76. Hirotani M, Furuya T, Shiro MA. Ganoderic acid derivative, a highly oxygenated lanostane type triterpenoid from *Ganoderma lucidum*. Phytochemistry 1985; 24:2055–2059.
77. Kohda H, Tokumoto W, Sakamoto K, Fuji M, Hirai Y, Yamasaki K, Komoda Y, Nakamura H, Ishihara S, Uchida M. The biologically active constituents of *Ganoderma lucidum* (Fr.) Karst. histamin release-inhibitory triterpenes. Chem Pharm Bull 1985; 33:1367–1374.
78. Komoda Y, Nakamura H, Ishihara S, Uchida M, Kohda H, Yamasaki K. Structures of new terpenoid constituents of *Ganoderma lucidum* (Fr.) Karst (polyporaceae). Chem Pharm Bull 1985; 33:4829–4835.
79. Morigiwa A, Kitabatake K, Fujimoto Y, Ikekawa N. Angiotensin converting enzyme-inhibitory triterpenes from *Ganoderma lucidum*. Chem Pharm Bull 1986; 34:3025–3028.
80. Nishitoba T, Sato H, Sakamura S. New terpenoids, ganolucidic acid D, ganoderic acid L, lucidone C and lucidenic acid G, from the fungus *Ganoderma lucidum*. Agric Biol Chem 1986; 50:809–811.
81. Sato H, Nishitoba T, Shirasu S, Oda K, Sakamura S. Ganoderiol A and B, new triterpenoids from the fungus *Ganoderma lucidum* (Reishi). Agric Biol Chem 1986; 50:2887–2890.
82. Lin LJ, Shiao MS. Seven new triterpenes from *Ganoderma lucidum*. J Nat Prod 1988; 51:918–924.
83. Lin LJ, Shiao MS, Yeh SF. Triterpenes from *Ganoderma lucidum*. Phytochemistry 1988; 27:2269–2271.
84. Min BS, Nakamura N, Miyashiro H, Bae K-W, Hattori M. Triterpenes from the spores of *Ganoderma lucidum* and their inhibitory activity against HIV-1 protease. Chem Pharm Bull 1998; 46:1607–1612.
85. Gonzalez AG, Leon F. Rivera A, Munoz CM, Bermejo J. Lanostanoid triterpenes from *Ganoderma lucidum*. J Nat Prod 1999; 62:1700–1701.
86. Mizushina Y, Takahashi N, Hanashima L, Koshino H, Esumi Y, Uzawa J, Sugawara F, Sakaguchi K. Lucidenic acid O and lactone, new terpene inhibitors of eukaryotic DNA polymerases from a basidiomycete, *Ganoderma Lucidum*. Bioorg Med Chem 1999; 7:2047–2052.
87. Ha TBT, Gerhauser C, Zhang WD, Ho NCL, Fouraste I. New lanostanoids from *Ganoderma Lucidum* that include NAD(P)H:quinone oxidoreductase in cultured Hepalclc7 murine hepatoma cells. Planta Med 2000; 66:681–684.

88. Min BS, Gao JJ, Nakamura N, Hattori M. Triterpenes from the spores of *Ganoderma Lucidum* and their cytotoxicity against Meth-A and LLC tumor cells. Chem Pharm Bull 2000; 48:1026–1033.
89. Wu TS, Shi LS, Kuo SC. Cytotoxicity of *Ganoderma lucidum* triterpenes. J Nat Prod 2001; 64:1121–1122.
90. Ma J, Ye Q, Hua Y, Zhang D, Cooper R, Chang MN, Chang JY, Sun HH. New lanostanoids from the mushroom *Ganoderma lucidum*. J Nat Prod 2002; 65:72–75.
91. Chen TQ, Li KB, He XJ, Zhu PG, Xu J. Micro-morphology, chemical components and identification of log-cultivated *Ganoderma Lucidum* spore. Proc '98 Nanjing Intl Symp Science and Cultivation of Mushroom, 1998: 214.
92. Byrne AR, Ravnik V. Trace element concentrations in higher fungi. Sci Tot Envir 1976; 6:65–78.
93. Stijve T, Besson R. Mercury, cadmium, lead and selenium content of mushroom species belonging to the genus *Agaricus*. Chemosphere 1976; 2:151–158.
94. Thomas K. Heavy metals in urban fungi. Mycologist 1992; 6:195–196.
95. Mejstrik V, Lepsova A. Applicability of fungi to the monitoring of environmental pollution by heavy metals. In: Markert B, ed. Plant as Biomonitors. Weinheim: VCH, 1993:365–378.
96. Vetter J. Data on arsenic and cadmium contents of some common mushrooms. Toxicon 1994; 32:11–15.
97. Michelot D, Poirier F, Melendez-Howell LM. Metal content profiles in mushrooms collected in primary forests of Latin America. Arch Environ Contam Toxicol 1999; 36:256–263.
98. Tham LX, Matsuhashi S, Kume T. Responses of *Ganoderma lucidum* to heavy metals. Mycoscience 1999; 40:209–213.
99. Ybanez N, Montoro R. Trace element food toxicology: an old and ever-growing discipline. Cr Rev Food Sci Nutr 1996; 36:299–320.
100. Mino Y, Ota N, Sakao S, Shimomura S. Determination of germanium in medicinal plants by atomic absorption spectrometry with electrothermal atomization. Chem Pharm Bull 1980; 28:2687–2691.
101. Kolesnikova OP, Tuzova MN, Kozlov VA. Screening of immunoactive properties of alkanecarbonic acid derivatives and germanium-organic compounds in vivo. Immunologiya 1997; 10:36–38.
102. Schimmer O, Eschelbach H, Breitinger DK, Gruetzner K, Wick H. Organogermanium compounds as inhibitors of the activity of direct acting mutagens in Salmonella typhimurium. Arzneim-Forsch 1997; 47:1398–1402.
103. Lee S, Park S, Oh JW, Yang CH. Natural inhibitors for protein prenyltransferase. Planta Med 1998; 64:303–308.
104. Kino K, Yamashita A, Yamaoka K, Watanabe J, Tanaka S, Shimizu K, Tsunoo H. Isolation and characterization of a new immunomodulatory protein, Ling Zhi-8 (LZ-8), from *Ganoderma lucidum*. J Biol Chem 1989; 264:472–478.
105. Kino K, Sone T, Watanabe J, Yamashita A, Tsuboi H, Miyajima H, Tsunoo H. Immunomodulator, LZ-8, prevents antibody production in mice. Int J Immunopharmac 1991; 13:1109–1115.

106. Van Der Hem L, Van Der Vliet A, Bocken CFM, Kino K, Hoitsma AJ, Tax WJM. Ling Zhi-8: studies of a new immunomodulating agent. Transplantation 1995; 60:438–443.
107. Kawagishi H, Mitsunaga SI, Yamawaki M, Ido M, Shimada A, Kinoshita T, Murata T, Usui T, Kimura A, Chiba S. A lectin from mycella of the fungus *Ganoderma lucidum*. Phytochemistry 1997; 44:7–10.
108. Wang H, Ng TB, Ooi VEC. Lectins from mushrooms. Mycol Res 1998; 102:897–906.
109. Mizushina Y, Watanabe I, Togashi H, Hanashima L, Takemura M, Ohta K, Sugawara F, Koshino H, Esumi Y, Uzawa J, Matukage A, Yoshida S, Sakaguchi K. An ergosterol peroxide, a natural product that selectively enhances the inhibitory effect of linoleic acid on DNA polymerase β. Biol Pharm Bull 1998; 21:444–448.
110. Choi HS, Sa YS. Fibrinolytic and antithrombotic protease from *Ganoderma lucidum*. Mycologia 2000; 92:545–552.
111. Flint SJ, Enquist LW, Krug RM, Racaniello VR, Skalka AM. Principles of Virology: Molecular Biology, Pathogenesis, and Control. Washington, DC: ASM Press, 2000:683–712.
112. Eo SK, Kim YS, Lee CK, Han SS. Antiviral activities of various water and methanol soluble substances isolated from *Ganoderma lucidum*. J Ethnopharmacol 1999; 68:129–136.
113. Kim YS, Eo SK, Oh KW, Lee CK, Han SS. Antiherpetic activities of acidic protein bound polysaccharide isolated from *Ganoderma lucidum* alone and in combinations with interferons. J Ethnopharmacol 2000; 72:451–458.
114. Oh KW, Lee CK, Kim YS, Eo SK, Han SS. Antiherpetic activities of acidic protein bound polysaccharide isolated from *Ganoderma lucidum* alone and in combination with acyclovir and vidarabine. J Ethnopharmacol 2000; 72:221–227.
115. El-Mekkawy S, Meselhy MR, Nakamura N, Tezuka Y, Hattori M, Kakiuchi N, Shimotohno K, Kawahata T, Otake T. Anti-HIV-1 and anti-HIV-1-protease substances from *Ganoderma lucidum*. Phytochemistry 1998; 49:1651–1657.
116. Hijikata Y, Yamada S. Effect of *Ganoderma lucidum* on postherpetic neuralgia. Am J Chinese Med 1998; 26:375–381.
117. Weber R, Christen L, Loy M, Schaller S, Christen S, Joyce CRB, Ledermann U, Ledergerber B, Cone R, Luthy R, Cohen MR. Randomized, placebo-controlled trial of Chinese herb therapy for HIV-1-infected individuals. J Acquir Immune Defic Syndr 1999; 22:56–64.
118. Robbins WJ, Kavanagh F, Hervey A. Antibiotic substances from basidiomycetes I. Pleuro. Proc Natl Acad Sci USA 1947; 33:171–176.
119. Yoon SY, Eo SK, Kim YS, Lee CK, Han SS. Antimicrobial activity of *Ganoderma lucidum* extract alone and in combination with some antibiotics. Arch Pharm Res 1994; 17:438–442.
120. Nostro A, Germano MP, D'Angelo V, Marino A, Cannatelli MA. Extraction methods and bioautography for evaluation of medicinal plant antimicrobial activity. Lett Appl Microbiol 2000; 30:379–384.

121. Ohno N, Miura NN, Sugawara N, Tokunaka K, Kirigaya N, Yadomae T. Immunomodulation by hot water and ethanol extracts of *Ganoderma lucidum*. Pharm Pharmacol Lett 1998; 4:174–177.
122. Hong Kong Department of Health Annual Report 1999/2000 at www.info.gov.hk/dh/ar9900/ar9900.htm
123. World Health Report, mortality statistics, 2001. www.who.int
124. Chihara G, Hamuro J, Maeda YY, Arai Y, Fukuoka F. Fractionation and purification of the polysaccharides with marked antitumor activity, especially lentinan, from *Lentinus edodes* (Berk.) Sing. (an edible mushroom). Cancer Res 1970; 30:2776–2781.
125. Wang G, Zhang J, Mizuno T, Zhuang C, Ito H, Mayuzumi H, Hidehumi O, Li J. Antitumor active polysaccharides from the Chinese mushroom Songshan Lingzhi, the fruiting body of *Ganoderma tsugae*. Biosci Biotechnol Biochem 1993; 57:894–900.
126. Zhang QH, Lin ZB. The antitumor activity of *Ganoderma lucidum* (Curt.:Fr.) P. Karst. (Ling Zhi) (Aphyllophoromycetideae) polysaccharides is related to tumor necrosis factor-α and interferon-γ. Int J Med Mushrooms 1999; 1:207–215.
127. Furusawa E, Chou SC, Furusawa S, Hirazumi A, Dang Y. Antitumour activity of *Ganoderma lucidum*, an edible mushroom, on intraperitoneally implanted Lewis lung carcinoma in synergenic mice. Phytother Res 1992; 6:300–304.
128. Lu H, Uesaka T, Katoh O, Kyo E, Watanabe H. Prevention of the development of preneoplastic lesions, aberrant crypt foci, by a water-soluble extract from cultured medium of *Ganoderma lucidum* (Rei-shi) mycelia in male F344 rats. Oncol Rep 2001; 8:1341–1345.
129. Wang SY, Hsu ML, Hsu HC, Tzeng CH, Lee SS, Shiao MS, Ho CK. The antitumor effect of *Ganoderma lucidum* is mediated by cytokines released from activated macrophages and T lymphocytes. Int J Cancer 1997; 70:699–705.
130. Lieu CW, Lee SS, Wang SY. The effect of *Ganoderma lucidum* on induction of differentiation in leukemic U937 cells. Anticancer Res 1992; 12:1211–1216.
131. Lei LS, Lin ZB. Effect of *Ganoderma* polysaccharides on T cell subpopulation and production of interlukin 2 in mixed lymphocyte response. Acta Pharm Sin 1992; 27:331–335.
132. Jia YF, Li H, Mori M, Zhang LX. Tumor necrosis factor production in mouse macrophages and its pharmacological modulation by *Ganoderma lucidum*. J Chinese Pharm Sci 1998; 7:29–32.
133. Szeto YT, Benzie IFF. Effects of dietary antioxidants on human DNA ex vivo. Free Rad Res 2002; 36:113–118.
134. Zhu HS, Yang XL, Wang LB, Zhao DX, Chen L. Effects of extracts from sporoderm-broken spores of *Ganoderma lucidum* on HeLa cells. Cell Biol Toxicol 2000; 16:201–206.
135. Mizushina Y, Hanashima L, Yamaguchi T, Takemura M, Sugawara F, Saneyoshi M, Matsukage A, Yoshida S, Sakaguchi K. A mushroom fruiting body-inducing substance inhibits activities of replicative DNA polymerases. Biochem Biophys Res Commun 1998; 249:17–22.

136. Ramgolam V, Ang SG, Lai YH, Loh CS, Yap HK. Traditional Chinese medicines as immunosuppressive agents. Ann Acad Med, Singapore 2000; 29:11–16.
137. Xia D, Li R, Lin Z, He Y. Effects of *Ganoderma* polysaccharides on immune function in mice. J Beij Med Univ 1989; 21:533–537.
138. Chen WC, Hau DM, Wang CC, Lin IH, Lee SS. Effects of *Ganoderma lucidum* and Krestin on subset T-cell in spleen of γ-irradiated mice. Am J Chinese Med 1995; 23:289–298.
139. Miyasaka N, Inoue H, Totsuka T, Koike R, Kino K, Tsunoo H. An Immunomodulatory protein, Ling zhi-8, facilitates cellular interaction through modulation of adhesion molecules. Biochem Biophy Res Commun 1992; 186:385–390.
140. Kim RS, Kim HW, Kim BK. Suppressive effects of *Ganoderma lucidum* on proliferation of peripheral blood mononuclear cells. Mol Cells 1997; 7:52–55.
141. Wood D, De Backer G, Fargeman O, Graham I, Mancia G, Pyorala K, together with members of the Task Force. Prevention of coronary heart disease in clinical practice. Recommendations of the second joint Task Force of European and other societies on coronary prevention. Eur Heart J 1998; 19:1434–1503.
142. Liu KC, Phounsavan SF, Huang RL, Liao C, Hsu SY, Wang KJ. Pharmacological and liver functional studies on mycelium of *Ganoderma lucidum*. Chinese Pharm J 1988; 40:21–29.
143. Lee SY, Rhee HM. Cardiovascular effects of mycelium extract of *Ganoderma lucidum*: inhibition of sympathetic outflow as a mechanism of its hypotensive action. Chem Pharm Bull 1990; 38:1359–1364.
144. Kanmatsuse K, Kajiwara N, Hayashi K, Shimogaichi S, Fukinbara I, Ishikawa H, Tamura T. Studies on *Ganoderma lucidum*: efficacy against hypertension and side effects. Yakugaku Zasshi 1985; 105:942–947. Japanese.
145. Komoda Y, Shimizu M, Sonoda Y, Sato Y. Ganoderic acid and its derivatives as cholesterol synthesis inhibitors. Chem Pharm Bull 1989; 37:531–533.
146. Dogne JM, Leval XX, Benoit P, Delarge J, Masereel B, David JL. Recent advances in antiplatelet agents. Curr Med Chem 2002; 9:577–589.
147. Shimizu A, Yano T, Saito Y, Inada Y. Isolation of an inhibitor of platelet aggregation from a fungus, *Ganoderma lucidum*. Chem Pharm Bull 1985; 33:3012–3015.
148. Kawagishi H, Fukuhara F, Sazuka M, Kawashima A, Mitsubori T, Tomita T. 5′-Deoxy-5′-methylsulphinyladenosine, a platelet aggregation inhibitor from *Ganoderma lucidum*. Phytochemistry 1993; 32:239–241.
149. Su CY, Shiao MS, Wang CT. Differential effects of ganodermic acid S on the thromboxane A2-signaling pathways in human platelets. Biochem Pharmacol 1999; 58:587–595.
150. Su CY, Shiao MS, Wang CT. Predominant inhibition of ganodermic acid S on the thromboxane A2-dependent pathway in human platelet response to collagen. Biochim Biophys Acta 1999; 1437:223–234.
151. Su CY, Shiao MS, Wang CT. Potentiation of ganodermic acid S on prostaglandin E1-induced cyclic AMP elevation in human platelets. Thromb Res 2000; 99:135–145.

152. Halushka PV. Thromboxane A2 receptors: where have you gone? Prostagland Other Lipid Media 2000; 60:175–189.
153. Expert panel on detection, evaluation, and treatment of high blood cholesterol in adults (adult treatment panel III). Executive summary of the third report of the national cholesterol education program (NCEP). JAMA 2001; 285:2486–2497.
154. Hikino H, Ishiyama M, Suzuki Y, Konno C. Mechanisms of hypoglycemic activity of ganoderan B: a glycan of *Ganoderma lucidum* fruit body. Planta Med 1989; 55:423–428.
155. Libby P, Ridker P, Maseri A. Inflammation and atherosclerosis. Circulation 2002; 105:1135–1143.
156. Streeper RT, Satsangi N. Anti-inflammatory components of mushroom extract on SUPELCOSIL ABZ + Plus HPLC columns. SUPELCO 1995; 14:1–3.
157. Stevens CD. Clinical Immunology and Serology. Philadelphia: F.A. Davis Company, 1996:166–167.
158. Giner-Larza EM, Manez S, Giner-Pons RM, Recio MC, Rios JL. On the anti-inflammatory and anti-phospholipase A2 activity of extracts from lanostane-rich species. J Ethnopharmacol 2000; 73:61–69.
159. Zollner H. Handbook of Enzyme Inhibitors. 3d ed. Weinheim, New York, Chichaster, Brisbane, Singapore, Toronto: Wiley-VCH, 1999.
160. Dan P, Dagan A, Krimsky M, Pruzanski W, Vadas P, Yedgar S. Inhibition of type I and type II phospholipase A2 by phosphatidyl-ethanolamine linked to polymeric carriers. Biochemistry 1998; 37:6199–6204.
161. Jain MK, Yu BZ, Rogers JM, Smith AE, Boger ET, Ostrander RL, Rheingold AL. Specific competitive inhibitor of secreted phospholipase A2 from berries of *Schinus terebinthifolius*. Phytochemistry 1995; 39:537–547.
162. Wachtel-Galor S, Szeto YT, Ezioni S, Buswell JA, Neeman I, Benzie IFF. Antioxidant and anti-inflammatory properties of the lingzhi mushroom. 5th Annual Nutrition Symposium, Hong Kong, Nov 10, 2001.
163. Singh AB, Gupta SK, Pereira BMJ, Prakash D. Sensitization to *Ganoderma lucidum* in patients with respiratory allergy in India. Clin Exp Allergy 1995; 25:440–447.
164. Cutten AEC, Hasnain SM, Segedin BP, Bai TR, McKay EJ. The basidiomycete *Ganoderma* and asthma: collection, quantitation and immunogenicity of the spores. NZ Med J 1988; 101:361–363.
165. Gupta SK, Pereira BMJ, Singh AB. *Ganoderma lucidum*: partial characterization of spore and whole body antigenic extracts. Invest Allergol Clin Immunol 2000; 10:83–89.
166. Thomas MJ. The role of free radicals and antioxidants: how do we know that they are working? Cr Rev Food Sci Nutr 1995; 35:21–39.
167. Strain JJ, Benzie IFF. Diet and antioxidant defence. In: Sadler M, Strain JJ, Cabellero B, eds. The Encyclopedia of Human Nutrition. London: Academic Press, 1999:95–105.
168. Young IS, Woodside JV. Antioxidants in health and disease. J Clin Pathol 2001; 54:176–186.

169. Kim KC, Kim IG. *Ganoderma lucidum* extract protects DNA from strand breakage caused by hydroxyl radical and UV irradiation. Int J Mol Med 1999; 4:273–277.
170. Lee JM, Kwon H, Jeong H, Lee JW, Lee SY, Baek SJ, Surh YJ. Inhibition of lipid peroxidation and oxidative DNA damage by *Ganoderma lucidum*. Phytother Res 2001; 15:245–249.
171. Shi Y, James AE, Benzie IFF, Buswell JA. Mushroom derived preparations in the prevention of H_2O_2-induced oxidative damage to cellular DNA. Teratog Carcinog Mutagen 2002; 22:103–111.
172. Zhu M, Chang Q, Wong LK, Chong FS, Li RC. Triterpene antioxidants from *Ganoderma lucidum*. Phytother Res 1999; 13:529–531.
173. Benzie IFF, Strain JJ. The ferric reducing ability of plasma (FRAP) as a measure of "antioxidant power": the FRAP assay. Anal Biochem 1996; 239:70–76.
174. Benzie IFF, Szeto YT. Total antioxidant capacity of teas by the ferric reducing/antioxidant power assay. J Agric Food Chem 1999; 47:633–636.
175. Wachtel-Galor S, Szeto YT, Tomlinson B, Benzie IFF. *Ganoderma lucidum* ('Lingzhi'): acute and short-term biomarker response to supplementation. Int J Food Sci Nutr 2004; 55(1):75–83.
176. Lin JM, Lin CC, Chen MF, Ujiie T, Takada A. Radical scavenger and anti-hepatotoxic activity of *Ganoderma formosanum*, *Ganoderma lucidum* and *Ganoderma neo-japonicum*. J Ethnopharmacol 1995; 47:33–41.
177. Kim DH, Shim SB, Kim NJ, Jang IS. β- Glucuronidase- inhibitory activity and hepatoprotective effect of *Ganoderma lucidum*. Biol Pharm Bull 1999; 22:162–164.
178. Shieh YH, Liu CF, Huang YK, Yang JY, Wu IL, Lin CH, Lin SC. Evaluation of the hepatic and renal protective effects of *Ganoderma lucidum* in mice. Am J Chin Med 2001; 29:501–507.
179. Song CH, Yang BK, Ra KS, Shon DH, Park EJ, Go GI, Kim YH. Hepatoprotective effect of extracellular polymer produced by submerged culture of *Ganoderma lucidum* WK-003. J Microbiol Biotechnol 1998; 8:277–279.
180. Park EJ, Ko G, Kim J, Dong HS. Antifibrotic effects of a polysaccharide extracted from *Ganoderma lucidum*, glycyrrhizin, and pentoxifylline in rats with cirrhosis induced by biliary obstruction. Biol Pharm Bull 1997; 20:417–420.
181. US Patent and Trademark Office web site: WWW.USPTO.GOV.

10

Epimedium Species

Sook Peng Yap and Eu Leong Yong
National University of Singapore
Singapore, Republic of Singapore

I. INTRODUCTION

Herba Epimedii, Berberidaceae (Chinese name "yinyanghuo," or "horny goat weed") is the dried aerial part of several species of *Epimedium*, including *E. sagittatum* (Sieb. Et Zucc), *E. koreanum* Nakai, *E. pubescens* Maxim., *E. wushanense* T.S. Ying, and *E. brevicornum* Maxim (1). Epimedium is a woody, evergreen perennial indigenous to shady mountain areas in temperate to subtropical Asia. It has broad heart-shaped leaves, and comprises over 40 species throughout the world. Most species of the genus have been used in folk medicine as yang tonic, mainly in China, Japan, and Korea. It is pungent and sweet in flavor.

A. Processing

Epimedium herb is collected in summer and fall when foliage is growing luxuriantly. The leaves are collected and removed from the thick stalks and foreign matter, then dried in the sun or in the shade.

B. Preparation and Dosage

Epimedium herb alone can be taken in the form of water-boiling extract or it can be macerated in wine for an oral infusion. It is also used together with prepared rehmania root, curculigo rhizome, dogwood fruit, and wolfberry fruit. It is often found as one of the herbs used in various proprietary products. The dosage of Epimedium herb for human consumption is in the range of 6–15 g, up to 30 g for a single use.

C. Traditional Use

Epimedium is one of the most popular and effective kidney yang tonics of Chinese herbalism. Its first recorded use dates back to the ancient text *Shen Nong Ben Cao Jing* (ca. 200 B.C.–A.D. 100). The herb is listed in the *Pharmacopoeia of the People's Republic of China* (1) as having action to "reinforce the *kidney* yang, strengthen tendons and bones, and relieve rheumatic conditions" and indicated "for impotence, seminal emission, weakness of the limbs, rheumatoid arthralgia with numbness and muscle contracture, and climacteric hypertension."

It received its colloquial name "horny goat weed" when goats grazing on the herb were observed to have excessive copulating. Oriental populations consider Epimedium an aphrodisiac and the herb is used to treat sexual dysfunction in both men and women.

In addition, herba Epimedii have been reputed to be effective in therapy for infertility, chronic nephritis, leukopenia, neurasthenia, asthenia, amnesia, or corresponding symptoms in China and Japan for over 2000 years (2,3).

D. Modern Use

In recent years, Epimedium has been extensively used for coronary diseases, hypertension, hyperlipidemia, hepatitis B, immunomodulation, as well as to alleviate menopausal discomfort (4). The herb is also thought to have anticancer and antiaging properties. It has been the subject of a number of animal and human studies to explore its medicinal values.

II. DETERMINATION OF *EPIMEDIUM* SPECIES

Classically, the species of Epimedium herb can be determined according to the spur length of its flower, and through morphological, histological, and chemotaxonomical inspection. In many cases, these methods are unreliable, as hybridization between species occurs, resulting in diversification of populations of *Epimedium* species.

A. Genetic Characterization

In plant genomes, genes for the ribosomal RNA (rDNA) are normally clustered in an array of multiple tandemly repeated copies of the cistron of 18S-ITS1-5.8S-ITS2-28S (5). The coding regions of 18S, 5.8S, and 28S rDNA sequence are highly conserved, whereas sequence homology within the ITS1 and ITS2 regions is much lower across the plant kingdom. Based on these features of the plant rDNA, molecular markers, such as random amplified polymorphic DNA (RAPD) and restriction fragment length polymorphism (RFLP), are good candidates for the identification and authentication of plant species. RAPD and PCR-RFLP have been applied to explore the DNA, generate discrete and species-specific RFLP patterns, and hence, confirm the *Epimedium* species. *E. sagittatum*, *E. koreanum*, *E. pubescens*, and *E. wushanense* were easily distinguished by a representative amplified band pattern or DNA sequences (6,7). RAPD analysis is more appropriate than RFLP analysis for the determination of species because it can be conducted by an automated procedure rapidly and no enzymatic digestion is needed; thus less plant material is required.

III. CHEMICAL CONSTITUENTS

A number of studies have been conducted to elucidate the chemical constituents and pharmacological activities of the aerial parts of Epimedium herb. Several methods such as column chromatography, liquid chromatography, pulse polarography, coulometric titration, and fluorometry have been used to study the flavonoids from *Epimedium* species (8). The main constituents in Epimedium plants are the prenylflavone glycosides. Among the important active constituents isolated from the aerial parts of these herbs are the flavonol glycosides (such as icariin and baohuoside I, Fig. 1) and flavonoids.

The glycoside icariin was first isolated from *E. macranthum* (9). The isolation of icariin from *E. brevicornum* (10–12), *E. koreanum* (11,12), *E. acuminatum* (13,14), *E. fargesii* (15), *E. wushanense* (16), *E. hunanense* (2), and *E. sagittatum* (3) was reported. The presence of icariin in *Epimedium* herb can be detected by thin-layer chromatography. However, content of other flavones might vary in different species (17).

Other compounds isolated from Epimedium herb include phenooxychromones, flavanoids, chrysoeriol, quercetin, apigenin, apigenin 7,4′-dimethyl ether, kempferol, tricin, luteolin, thalictoside, and brevicornin (8). Luteolin, a flavone, was found to have estrogenic activity with a relative potency of 58% compared to genistein (18). Apigenin and quercetin are also estrogenic. Other flavanoids and flavanol glycosides described in Epimedium include epimedokoreanoside I, icariside I, icaritin, epimedoside A, epimedins

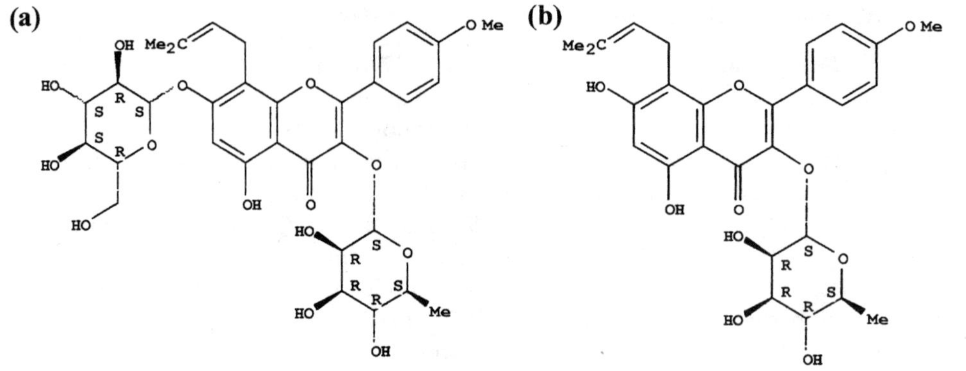

FIGURE 1 Chemical structures of bioactive compounds isolated from Epimedium: (a) icariin and (b) baohuoside I.

A, B, and C, β-anhydroicaritin, tricin, korepimedoside A and B, sagittatosides A, B, and C, sagittatins A and B, diphylloside A and B, baohuosides I–VII, and baohuosu (16,19–21). Some of these flavonol glycosides, e.g., baohuoside I (2), were reported to have immunomodulatory activity. The herb also contains ceryl alcohol linolenic acid, oleic acid, palmitic acid, sterols, benzene, tannins, fats, saponins, vitamin E, zinc, and some essential oils.

The quantitative changes of flavonoids in *E. koreanum* in different collecting periods were determined by HPLC and UV spectrophotometry. The result shows that the highest content of flavonoids is found in the flowering period (May) (22).

The seasonal fluctuation of flavonol glycosides in the leaves of *E. grandiflorum* var. thunbergianum, *E. cremeum*, and *E. sempervirens* (Berberidaceae) was also investigated (23). The total content of glycosides was greatest at flowering time, and as the leaves mature it became less fluctuating with a little decrease. The ideal period for the harvest of Epimedium leaves was 2 or 3 months after flowering.

By means of RP-HPLC, nine major flavonoids in different parts of five Epimedium plants listed in the Chinese *Pharmacopoeia* were analyzed and the total contents of nine flavonoids in the four species were found to be highest in the rhizome and roots, followed by leaves and stems (24). The composition of the main constituents and relative contents in the five species were similar in leaves and stems, but different from the rhizome and roots. These differences may affect their pharmaceutical properties.

IV. SCIENTIFIC BASIS OF THEIR BIOLOGICAL ACTIONS

Much of the work on Epimedium has focused on either the whole herb or its glycosides. Polysaccharide content of extracts may also affect its properties. It should be noted that the vast majority of these studies were performed in mainland China and they have not been replicated elsewhere.

A. Immune Effects

Epimedium has been reported to significantly enhance the phagocytic activity of macrophages (25), to stimulate the migration of T-lymphocytes from the thymus to peripheral organs, and to promote both the proliferation of bone marrow cells and the synthesis of DNA. The n-butanol fraction of *E. hunanense* and epimedin C isolated from the fraction significantly enhanced the response of spleen antibody-forming cells to nearly normal in the mice treated with the immunosuppressant hydrocortisone acetate. They also markedly enhanced lymphocyte proliferation and caused a significant recovery of interleukin-2 (IL-2) production in HCA-treated mice (2). On the other hand, a flavone analog, baohuoside I, isolated from *E. davidii* was described to significantly prolong mouse heart allograft survival (26). Assessment of the mice for appearance, behavior, biochemistry, hematology, and histology revealed no side effects even at the intraperitoneal dose of 32 mg/kg/day for 14 days. In human studies, Epimedium herbs may regulate immunodeficiency states and relieve the neuroendocrinoimmunological effect inhibited by exogenous glucocorticoid. Studies of Epimedium herbs and the effects on the immune system are summarized in Table 1.

B. Effects on the Skeletal System

The effect of Epimedium herb on osteoclastic bone resorption and osteoporosis has been studied in vitro and in vivo using ovariectomized rat models. The in vitro study (cultured osteoclasts) showed that Guizhou *Epimedium* (*E. leptorrhizum* Stearn) inhibited the osteoclastic resorption of bone. The in vivo effect of this Chinese herb was also investigated in rats with osteoporosis induced by ovariectomy and the result demonstrated that both the Epimedium and estradiol were able to increase mineral content and promote bone formation (33). Icariin-containing compounds have been isolated from aerial parts of plants of the genus *Epimedium*. The icariin-containing compositions were found to be effective in treating osteoporosis. Bone phosphorus and calcium contents, bone mineral density, and the femur strength of treated ovariectomized rats were increased significantly compared to control groups (34). Therefore, herba Epimedii may be of potential use in the treatment of

TABLE 1 Summary of Herba Epimedii and the Immunomodulating Activity

In vitro

Source	Assay	Test substance	Response	Conclusions
Li et al., 1991 (26)	Various concentrations of baohuoside I were incubated with human neutrophils, lymphocytes, K562 cells, or gibbon leukemic MLA-144 cells	Baohuoside I	Baohuoside I has significant suppressive effects on neutrophil chemotaxis, mitogen-induced lymphocyte transformation, mixed-lymphocyte culture, NK-cell cytotoxicity and IL-2 production.	Baohuoside I may have potential as an anti-inflammatory/ immunosuppressive agent.
Shan et al., 1999 (27)	Human lymphocytes were cultured with epimedium extract. Ig & IL production detected by ELISA	*E. brevicornum* crude extract	*E. brevicornum* significantly enhance IgG production by B cells and stimulate monocytes to produce IL-1.	*E. brevicornum* has immunomodulating activity on human lymphocytes in vitro.

Animal studies

Source	Test substance	Subjects	Total sample size	Response	*p*	Conclusions
Iinuma et al., 1990 (25)	*E. sagittatum* (ES)	Mice	—	ES, icariin, and epimedin C isolated from ES activated the phagocytosis of carbon by Kupffer cells in the liver.	—	ES promotes phagocytic activity of reticuloendothelial system in mice, has stimulatory effect on macrophage.

Li et al., 1994 (28)	Baohuoside I	Mice	—	Baohuoside I suppressed antibody and delayed-type hypersensitivity responses in mice in a dose-dependent fashion. In contrast, it did not significantly prolong survival of cardiac grafts or potentiate the effects of the standard antirejection drug cyclosporine.	—	The immunosuppressive properties of baohuoside I are confined to the antibody-mediated system, suggesting that it might be of value in chronic inflammatory and autoimmune diseases treatment.
Liang et al., 1997 (2)	Flavonol glycosides from *E. hunanense*, sc injection	BALB/c mice $C_{57}BL/6j$ mice $C_{57}BL/6j$ mice	21 (n = 7) 45 (n = 9) (n = 6)	n-Butanol fraction significantly improved the SAFC function in normal and HCA-suppressed BALB/c mice, significantly recovered lymphocyte proliferation and IL-2 production of HCA-suppressed $C_{57}BL/6j$ mice.	<.05	n-Butanol fraction can significantly potentiate the immune function. Epimedin C is an active compound of immuno-enhancing effects.
Chen et al., 2000 (29)	Baohuoside I	BALB/c to $C_{57}BL/10$ combination	—	Baohuoside I significantly prolonged mouse heart allograft survival. No toxic effects were observed.	=.001	Baohuoside I and its analogs useful as antirejection agents in organ transplantation.

TABLE 1 Continued

1C. Human studies						
Source	Test substance	Subjects	Total sample size	Response	*p*	Conclusions
Chen et al., 1995 (30)	*E. sagittatum* (ES)	Hemodialysis patients	—	In hemodialytic patients, levels of both sIL-2R and IL-6 could be restored to normal after treatment with ES.	<.01	ES was effective in regulating immunodeficiency states in endstage renal failure patient.
Liao et al., 1995 (31)	*E. sagittatum* (ES) decoction	Hemodialysis patients	34	IL-2 activity of peripheral blood monocytes (PBMC) stimulated by PHA increased significantly in patients treated with ES.	—	ES had therapeutic effect on sexual disorder and immunological inadequacy in chronic renal failure patients on hemodialysis.
Cai et al., 1998 (32)	*E. brevicornum* (EB) and prednisone	Patients on prednisone	65	Significant differences on ACTH, corticosterone, and lymphocyte proliferative reaction were found between treatment and control group.	<.05	EB could relieve neuroendocrino-immunological effect inhibited by exogenous glucocorticoid.

SAFC: spleen antibody-forming cells; HCA: hydrocortisone acetate.
— indicates unknown.

osteoporosis. However, the mechanisms of action for prevention of osteoporosis were not described. Table 2 summarizes the protective effects of Epimedium on bone health.

C. Endocrine Effects

It has been reported that *E. brevicornum* may reduce the cold-resistant potential of normal mice and disturb the balance of thyroid hormones in normal rats. Large doses of *E. brevicornum* may exert an unfavorable effect on normal rats, such as reducing natural weight gain and serum triiodothyronine (T3), but increasing rT3 and thyrotropin-releasing hormone levels as well as raising thyroid-stimulating hormone (40). Lower T3 and higher rT3 levels may be due to peripheral metabolism of thyroid hormones. It was concluded that large doses of this yang-restoring medicine should not be given to the organisms without symptoms of yang deficiency. Another study showed that *E. brevicornum* could raise plasma corticosterone level significantly and decreased plasma T3 level in rats, but no rise of plasma testosterone level was observed (41). In a study of 65 patients, the plasma level of adrenocorticotrophin and corticosterone decreased and lymphocyte proliferative reaction was reduced ($p < 0.05$) after treatment with *E. brevicornum* when compared with the control group (32). Epimedium herb was found to inhibit monoamine oxidase (MAO) in the hypothalamus, leading to higher levels of noradrenalin and dopamine (42). The researchers also showed that noradrenalin, adrenaline, serotonin, and dopamine levels were all elevated in animals given Epimedium. Higher levels of dopamine in particular may help to explain the apparent prosexual effect of horny goat weed. High dopamine levels encourage the release of luteinizing hormone from the pituitary gland, which in turn stimulates the testes to produce more testosterone. Stress is often accompanied by the excess release of cortical stress hormones, and Epimedium is thought to reduce the effects of corticoids on the body. Generally the herb is believed to have aphrodisiac properties.

D. Antioxidant Effects

Methanol extracts of 180 Oriental herbs were screened for their antioxidant activities by determining the peroxide values of linoleic acid during storage at 50°C (43). Among the herbal extracts tested, 44 selected herbal extracts were further studied in a methyl linoleate system for an extended storage time. Eleven herbs had particularly high antioxidant activities, where the antioxidative effects of most herbal extracts were greatly dependent on the extraction solvent used. However, *E. koreanum* Nakai extract and three other herbs appeared to show significantly strong antioxidant activities regardless of the solvents used for the extraction ($p < 0.05$). This result suggested that *E.*

TABLE 2 Summary of Herba Epimedii and Effects on Bone

In vitro

Source	Assay	Test substance	Response	Conclusions
Liu et al., 1991 (35)	Bone marrow cell cultures of "yang deficiency" animal model caused by hydroxyurea	*E. sagittatum* polysaccharides	Treatment with 100 μg of *E. sagittatum* polysaccharides increased cell multiplication and DNA synthesis rate by 72% and 68%, respectively.	*E. sagittatum* polysaccharides increased cell multiplication and DNA synthesis of bone marrow cell cultures

Animal studies

Source	Test substance	Subjects	Total sample size	Type of study	Response	p	Conclusions
Wu et al., 1996 (36)	Water extract of herba Epimedii	Rats	—	—	Herba Epimedii can prevent the side effects induced by long-term use of glucocorticoids in rats.	—	It can antagonize adrenocortical atrophy and osteoporosis.
Peng et al., 1997 (37)	*E. leptorrhizum*	Male Sprague-Dawley rats	11	—	*E. leptorrhizum* has no significant effects on endogenous cAMP in alveolar bone of orthodontic tooth.	—	cAMP was not involved to regulate the mechanism of *E. leptorrhizum* in promoting bone remodeling.

Yu et al., 1999 (33)	*E. leptorrhizum* Stearn; estradiol	Ovariectomized rats	—	—	Both Epimedium and estradiol were able to increase mineral content and promote bone formation.	—	*E. leptorrhizum* is of potential use in the treatment of osteoporosis.
Ma et al., 1999 (38)	Epimedium	Wistar ovariectomized rats	54 (n = 10)	Randomized	Trabecular volume in total bone volume (TV/TBV), and osteoid percentage increased significantly after Epimedium treatment.	$<.05$	Epimedium has some therapeutic effects on osteoporotic rat models.
Wang et al., 2000 (39)	Epimedium	Ovariectomized (OVX) rats	40 (n = 10)	Randomized	The BMD was significantly higher, but the IL-6 mRNA expression level was significantly lower in epimedium group than that in OVX group.	$<.05$ $<.01$	Epimedium can inhibit the expression of IL-6 mRNA, which may contribute to its antiresorptive effect.
Chen et al., 2000 (34)	Icariin—standardized composition	Ovariectomized Wistar rats	—	—	Bone phosphorus, calcium contents, bone mineral density, and femur strength of icariin-treated ovariectomized rats were increased significantly as compared to control.	—	Icariin-containing compositions with 20–40% icariin content by weight are still effective in treating osteoporosis.

— indicates unknown.

koreanum extract contains powerful antioxidative components. Phenolic acids and/or flavonoids might be the possible antioxidative components because methanol is a good solvent for extracting these compounds from the plant materials. Also, Epimedium compound granules, which lower blood lipid, have anti-free radicals and adjust the balance between prostacyclin I2 and thromboxane A2 in patients with kidney deficiency syndrome of ischemic cardiocerebrovascular diseases (44).

E. Anticancer Effects

Epimedium is officially listed in China as an herb that can help prevent the growth of cancer and has been listed by the Chinese Academy of Medical Sciences as one of an elite group of herbs that slow aging and promote longevity. The plant bioactive compound baohuoside I was shown to have cytotoxic and cytostatic effects on six different cancer cell lines, by means of microscopy, ^{51}Cr-release, and growth inhibition. The IC_{50} on the cells tested ranged from 2.8 to 7.5 μg/mL. At tumoricidal concentrations, inhibition of DNA and RNA synthesis, but not protein synthesis, was observed (45). Investigators at the University of Heidelberg published provocative results on herba Epimedii glycoside icariin extract. In vitro experiments showed that this herb stimulated healthy cells to produce an anticancer substance called tumor necrosis factor-α. Also, icariin purified from *E. koreanum* induced differentiation of human promyelocytic leukemic cells (HL-60) by reducing nitroblue tetrazolium and elevating the cAMP/cGMP ratio. There were many rugosities and ball-like processes on the cell surface and the mechanism might be related to elevated cAMP/cGMP ratio (46). These preliminary studies suggest that herba Epimedii may be useful against cancer.

F. Antihepatotoxic Effects

Icariin compounds display antihepatotoxic activity in cultured rat hepatocytes. Icariin was reported to significantly reduce the levels of glutamic pyruvic transaminase and sorbitol dehydrogenase release, decrease glutathione-S-transferase (GST) activity, and increase cytochrome P-450 content in CCl_4-intoxicated rat hepatocytes (47).

G. Antibacterial and Antiviral Effects

Epimedium has been shown to actively inhibit the growth of staphylococci, streptococci, and pneumococci in culture. Recent studies have shown that Epimedium has significant anti-HIV activity. Epimedium polysaccharides were found to reverse the zidovudine (AZT)-induced inhibition of DNA synthesis and reduce the toxicity of AZT (48).

H. Cardiovascular Effects

Some of the flavonol glycosides and flavonoids isolated from the genus are pharmacologically effective in dilation of the coronary artery, inhibition of platelet aggregation, and delayed formation of thrombi (8). Chen et al. (49) described the isolation of five new prenyflavones, yinyanghuo A, B, C, D, and E. Yingyanghuo A and B were shown to have significant antiplatelet activity. Flavone glycosides of *E. koreanum* (TFG) stimulated murine macrophages. The fibrinolytic activity of stimulated macrophages was approximately 2.8-fold that of the controls. In vivo experiments reported that the effect of TFG on spontaneously hypertensive and apoplexic rats was very evident. The abiotic rate of TFG-stimulated rats was 5%, while that of the control group was 90% (50). Epimedium may help to dilate the coronary vessels, increasing coronary blood flow by reducing vascular resistance (51). *E. decoctum* and its extracts give certain protection in the myocardial ischemia of rat caused by pituitrin. In rabbits, intravenously injected icariin (1 mg/kg) and water extract of *E. grandiflorum* containing icariin at a dose equivalent to 1 g plant/kg did not significantly change the heart rate and electrocardiogram. Other myocardial and circulatory indices indicated that both icariin and the extract decreased peripheral resistance, suggesting their potential use in the treatment of hypertension-complicated coronary diseases.

I. Effects on the Reproductive System

Epimedium has been reported to have proreproductive effects in the popular press. Teeguarden (52) anecdotally reported that *E. sagittatum* seemed to stimulate the sensory nerves throughout the body, particularly in the genital region. The effect of Epimedium herb on the testes, prostate gland, and levator ani muscle (which supports the body in thrusting movements) was reported to enhance male sexual function indirectly (53). *E. sagittatum* appeared to have a sexual potentiation effect and to improve the quality of life in the patients of chronic renal failure with regular hemodialysis (39). Icariin from Epimedium could inhibit contraction of arterial smooth muscle rings that restrict blood flow in the body, via a Ca^{2+} channel-blocking mechanism, further enhancing vasodilation (48). On the other hand, the chief ingredient of Epimedium herb, icariin, can promote the development of epididymes and seminal vesicle of mouse. In vitro animal studies suggest that icariin may enhance the production of testosterone (42).

J. Urinary Effects

Epimedium may improve immunological deficiencies in chronic renal failure patients on dialysis, and was reported to significantly improve blood urea nitrogen and serum creatinine levels in rats. In the gromeruli, it was reported to inhibit deposition of IgG and C3 along glomerular capillary walls in rats (54). Tan and Weng (44) reported on the efficacy of Epimedium compound pills in the treatment of "kidney-deficiency syndrome" of ischemic cardiocerebro vascular diseases. The rates of improvement were reported to be 70% in the electrocardiogram of the patients with coronary heart diseases, and 75% in the electroencephalogram of the patients with cerebral atherosclerosis.

K. Respiratory Effects

The herb acts as an antitussive and expectorant. Studies of its effectiveness in 1066 cases of chronic bronchitis demonstrated a 74.6% effectiveness rate in improving symptoms (48). It was effective in protecting guinea pigs from histamine-induced asthma.

L. Others

Methanol extracts of *E. sagittatum* were found to induce significant neurite outgrowth activity on cultured PC12H cells. Bioassay-guided fractionation yielded six prenylated flavonol glycosides, ikarisoside A, icarisid II, epimedoside A, icariin, epimedin B, and epimedokoreanoside-1, as the active ingredients (3). A recent study also demonstrated that two syringaresinol enantiomers isolated from *E. koreanum* Nakai and *Magnolia officinalis* Rehd, as well as a mixture of their glucosides, showed dose-dependent neuritogenesis in a concentration range from 0.24 to 24 μM in PC12h cells (55). *E. grandiflorum* has also been used to treat hot flashes in complex mixtures of 8 (56) or over 20 herbs (57).

V. ADVERSE EFFECTS AND TOXICITY

Epimedium is a safe and benign herb. There is no record of adverse side effects, toxicity, or contraindications to taking Epimedium by humans. In some people, ingesting it can lead to dizziness, thirst, dry mouth, vomiting, and nosebleed.

VI. SUMMARY

The use of traditional Chinese concepts like yin/yang and qi, which have no modern physiological equivalents, in chinese publications make scientific interpretation of these studies difficult. Problems are compounded by the use of terms such as "kidney" and "spleen," which often do not have the same meaning as understood in the Western medical literature. Herbs are used to treat yin/yang and qi deficiency states with no clear outcome parameters. Nevertheless these studies indicate that Epimedium herb may have biological activities that can affect cell function and therefore health status. However, the effective doses, pharmacokinetics, and cellular mechanisms have not yet been proven by science or substantiated through long-term clinical research. Owing to the limited data, no firm conclusions can be made at this time. It is critical to determine exactly which mechanisms operate in which circumstances and how these components work in view of the widespread use of this herb.

REFERENCES

1. Pharmacopoeia of the Peoples Republic of China. Vol. 1. English ed. Beijing: Chem Ind Press, 1997.
2. Liang HR, Vuorela P, Vuorela H, Hiltunen R. Isolation and immunomodulatory effect of flavonol glycosides from *Epimedium hunanense*. Planta Med 1997; 63:316–319.
3. Kuroda M, Mimaki Y, Sashida Y, Umegaki E, Yamazaki M, Chiba K, Mohri T, Kitahara M, Yasuda A, Naoi N, Xu ZW, Li MR. Flavonol glycosides from *Epimedium sagittatum* and their neurite outgrowth activity on PC12h cells. Planta Med 2000; 66(6):575–577.
4. Yang ZZ. Clinical applications of Yinyanghuo. Zhejiang J Trad Chin Med 1985; 20:478–480.
5. Hillis DM, Dixon MT. Ribosomal DNA: molecular evolution and phylogenetic inference. Q Rev Biol 1991; 66(4):410–449.
6. Nakai R, Shoyama Y, Shiraishi S. Genetic characterization of *Epimedium* species using random amplified polymorphic DNA (RAPD) and PCR-restriction fragment length polymorphism (RFLP) diagnosis. Biol Pharm Bull 1996; 19(1):67–70.
7. Wang J, Shaw PC, But PHP, Ngan FGK. Polymerase chain reaction-restriction fragment length polymorphism test for the authentication of herbal Chinese medicines. United States Patent 2001; 6,309,840.
8. Liang HR, Siren H, Jyske P, Reikkola ML. Characterization of flavonoids in extracts from four species of *Epimedium* by micellar electrokinetic capillary chromatography with diode-array detection. J Chromatogr Sci 1997; 35:117–125.
9. Akai S. Constituents of *Epimedium macranthum* Morr and Decne. I. Chemical constitution of a new glucoside of *Epimedium macranthum* Morr and Decne. I. J Pharm Soc Jpn 1935; 55:537–599.
10. Yang C, Liu HK, Wu CL. Chemical constituents of Xinyeyinyanghuo (*Epimedium brevicornum*). Chin Trad Herb Drugs 1980; 11:444.
11. Liu BQ, Ma HS, Mou P. Isolation and identification of icariin. Chin Trad Herb Drugs 1980; 11:201.
12. Liu AR, Xu LX. Analysis of active ingredients in traditional Chinese herbal drugs: assay of icariin in epimedium. Chinese J Pharm Anal 1984; 4:81–84.

13. Hu BH, Zhou LD, Liu YL. New tetrasaccharide flavonol glycoside from *Epimedium acuminatum*. J Nat Prod 1992; 55(5):672–675.
14. Dong XP, Xiao CH, Zhang R, Li W. Chemical studies of *Epimedium acuminatum* Franch. Zhongguo Zhong Yao Za Zhi 1994; 19(10):614–615.
15. Guo B, Yu J, Xiao P. Chemical constituents from the whole plant of *Epimedium fargesii* Franch. Zhongguo Zhong Yao Za Zhi 1996; 21(6):353–355.
16. Li WK, Zhang RY, Xiao PG. Flavonoids from *Epimedium wanshanense*. Phytochemistry 1996; 43(2):527–530.
17. Shi DW, Huang DJ, Bi ZQ, Wang ZW, Yang XY. Comparison of the chemical constituents and identification of the Chinese kidney-tonic yinyanghuo. Acta Acad Med Shanghai 1986; 13:13–19.
18. Rosenberg Zand RS, Jenkins DJA, Diamandis EP. Steroid hormone activity of flavonoids and related compounds. Breast Cancer Res Treat 2000; 62:35.
19. Sun PY, Chen YJ, Wen Y, Pei YP, Liu ZH, Yao XS, Takeda T, Ogihara Y. Structure determination of korepimedoside A and korepimedoside B from *Epimedium koreanum* Nakai. Yao Xue Xue Bao 1996; 31(8):602–606.
20. Li W, Guo B, Xiao P, Pan J, Lu M, Zhang R. Chemical constituents of *Epimedium wanshanense* S. Z. He et Guo. Zhongguo Zhong Yao Za Zhi 1996; 21(10): 614–616.
21. Li F, Liu YL. Studies on the isolations and structures of baohuosides-I, VI, VII and baohuosu. Yao Xue Xue Bao 1988; 23(10):739–748.
22. Chen C, Sha M, Yang S. Quantitative changes of flavonoids in *Epimedium koreanum* Nakai in different collecting periods. Zhongguo Zhong Yao Za Zhi 1996; 21(2):86–88.
23. Mizuno M, Iinuma M, Tanaka T, Iwashima S, Sakakibara N. Seasonal fluctuation of flavonol glycosides in *Epimedium* species. Yakugaku Zasshi 1989; 109(4):271–273.
24. Guo B, Xiao P. Determination of flavonoids in different parts of five epimedium plants. Zhongguo Zhong Yao Za Zhi 1996; 21(9):523–525.
25. Iinuma M, Tanaka T, Sakakibara N, Mizuno M, Matsuda H, Shiomoto H, Kubo M. Phagocytic activity of leaves of *Epimedium* species on mouse reticuloendotherial system. Yakugaku Zasshi 1990; 10(3):179–185.
26. Li SY, Teh BS, Seow WK, Liu YL, Thong YH. In vitro immunopharmacological profile of the plant flavonoid baohuoside-1. Int J Immunopharmacol 1991; 13(2-3):129–134.
27. Shan BE, Yoshida Y, Sugiura T, Yamashita U. Stimulating activity of Chinese medicinal herbs on human lymphocytes in vitro. Int J Immunopharmacol 1999; 21:149–159.
28. Li SY, Ping G, Geng L, Seow WK, Thong YH. Immunopharmacology and toxicology of the plant flavonoid baohuoside-1 in mice. Int J Immunopharmacol 1994; 16(3):227–231.
29. Chen HF, Li F, Liu LW. Flavone analogues useful as anti-rejection agents. United States Patent 2000; 6,071,883.
30. Chen X, Zhou M, Wang J. Effect of *Epimedium sagittatum* on soluble IL-2 receptor and IL-6 levels in patients undergoing hemodialysis. Zhonghua Nei Ke Za Zhi 1995; 34(2):102–104.

31. Liao HJ, Chen XM, Li WG. Effect of *Epimedium sagittatum* on quality of life and cellular immunity in patients of hemodialysis maintenance. Zhongguo Zhong Xi Yi Jie He Za Zhi 1995; 15(4):202–204.
32. Cai D, Shen S, Chen X. Clinical and experimental research of *Epimedium brevicornum* in relieving neuroendocrino-immunological effect inhibited by exogenous glucocorticoid. Zhongguo Zhong Xi Yi Jie He Za Zhi 1998; 18(1): 4–7.
33. Yu S, Chen K, Li S, Zhang K. In vitro and in vivo studies of the effect of a Chinese herb medicine on osteoclastic bone resorption. Chinese J Dent Res 1999; 2(1):7–11.
34. Chen YJ. Icariin preparations. United States Patent 2000; 6,123,944.
35. Liu F, Ding G, Li J. Effects of *Epimedium sagittatum* Maxim. polysaccharides on DNA synthesis of bone marrow cells of "yang deficiency" animal model caused by hydroxyurea. Zhongguo Zhong Yao Za Zhi 1991; 16(10):620–622.
36. Wu T, Cui L, Zhang Z, Chen Z, Li Q, Liao J, Huang L. Experimental study on antagonizing action of herba epimedii on side effects induced by glucocorticoids. Zhongguo Zhong Yao Za Zhi 1996; 21(12):748–751.
37. Peng G, Fu M, Zhang D. The experimental study about the relations between Chinese herb *Epimedium leptorrhizum* Stearn (CH-ELS) and endogenous cAMP in alveolar bone of orthodontic tooth in rats. Zhonghua Kou Qiang Yi Xue Za Zhi 1997; 32(1):40–42.
38. Ma Z, Wang R, Qiu M. Study of morphologic effects of 4 Chinese herbs by bone histomorphometry in ovariectomized rats. Zhonghua Fu Chan Ke Za Zhi 1999; 34(2):82–85.
39. Wang B, Quan J, Guo S. Effects of epimedium on the expression of interleukin-6 messenger ribonucleic acid in bone of ovariectomized rat. Zhonghua Fu Chan Ke Za Zhi 2000; 35(12):724–726.
40. Chen MD, Kuang AK, Chen JL. Influence of yang-restoring herb medicines upon metabolism of thyroid hormone in normal rats and a drug administration schedule. Zhong Xi Yi Jie He Za Zhi 1989; 9(2):93–95.
41. Kuang AK, Chen JL, Chen MD. Effects of yang-restoring herb medicines on the levels of plasma corticosterone, testosterone and triiodothyronine. Zhong Xi Yi Jie He Za Zhi 1989; 9(12):737–738.
42. Chen M, Kuang A, Chen J. Effect of monoamine neurotransmitters in the hypothalamus in a cortisol-induced rat model of yang-deficiency. Zhong Xi Yi Jie He Za Zhi 1990; 10(5):292–294.
43. Kim SY, Kim JH, Kim SK, Oh MJ, Jung MY. Antioxidant activities of selected Oriental herb extracts. J Am Oil Chem Soc 1994; 71(6):633–640.
44. Tan X, Weng W. Efficacy of epimedium compound pills in the treatment of the aged patients with kidney deficiency syndrome of ischemic cardio-cerebral vascular diseases. Hunan Yi Ke Da Xue Xue Bao 1998; 23(5):450–452.
45. Li SY, Teh BS, Seow WK, Li F, Thong YH. Effects of the plant flavonoid baohuoside-1 on cancer cells in vitro. Cancer Lett 1990; 53(2-3):175–181.
46. Zhao Y, Cui Z, Zhang L. Effects of icariin on the differentiation of HL-60 cells. Zhonghua Zhong Liu Za Zhi 1997; 19(1):53–55.
47. Lee MK, Choi YJ, Sung SH, Shin DI, Kim JW, Kim YC. Antihepatotoxic

activity of icariin, a major constituent of *Epimedium koreanum*. Planta Med 1995; 61:523–526.
48. Kee CH. The Pharmacology of Chinese Herbs. 2d ed. Boca Raton: CRC Press, 1999.
49. Chen CC, Huang YL, Sun CM, Shen CC. New prenylflavones from the leaves of *Epimedium saggitatum*. J Nat Prod 1996; 59(4):412–414.
50. Shan Y. Effect of flavone glycosides of *Epimedium koreanum* on murine fibrinolytic system and apoplectic mortality. Zhongguo Yi Xue Ke Xue Yuan Xue Bao 1992; 14(6):419–423.
51. Liu CM, Yu QH, Zhang LM. Effect of icariin on heart. Chinese Trad Herb Drugs 1982; 13:412–416.
52. Teeguarden R. Radiant Health. New York: Warner Books, 1998.
53. Bensky D, Gamble A. Chinese Herbal Medicine: Materia Medica. Seattle, WA: Eastland Press, 1993.
54. Cheng QL, Chen XM, Shi SZ. Effects of *Epimedium sagittatum* on immunopathology and extracellular matrices in rats with chronic renal insufficiency. Zhonghua Nei Ke Za Zhi 1994; 33(2):83–86.
55. Chiba K, Yamazaki M, Umegaki E, Li MR, Xu ZW, Terada S, Taka M, Naoi N, Mohri T. Neuritogenesis of herbal (+) - and (−) - syringaresinols separated by chiral HPLC in PC12h and Neuro2a cells. Biol Pharm Bull 2002; 25(6):791–793.
56. Yng W. Using complex herbal formulations to treat hot flashes. United States Patent 1999; 5.874,084.
57. Chun Z. Herbal hormone balance composition. United States Patent 2001; 6,238,707.

11

Ligusticum chuanxiong Hort.

Lis Sa Elissa Lim and Eu Leong Yong
National University of Singapore
Singapore, Republic of Singapore

I. INTRODUCTION

Ligusticum belongs to the Umbelliferae family, members of which include *L. chuanxiong* (Chuan Xiong), *L. wallichii*, *L. sinense* (Gao Ben), and *L. brachylobum*. The dried rhizome of *L. chuanxiong* is one of the most common crude drugs described in the traditional Chinese, Japanese, and Korean pharmacopoeia. In Japan, Senkyu is obtained from the dried rhizome of *L. officinale* Kitagawa (also known as *C. officinale* Makino). In China, the herb is grown in Sichuan province and the root is usually collected in the summer when the node of the plant stem becomes swollen and purplish. Once removed from the soil, it is gently baked until dry before storage.

II. PLANT/HERB RECOGNITION

The rhizome has an irregular knotty, fist-like appearance, is approximately 2–7 cm in diameter, and is yellowish in color. The external surface is rough, shrunken, and marked by parallel raised annulations. A cross-section of the root, reveals a compact, yellowish-gray matrix with scattered yellowish-brown oil cavities and a cambium in an undulated ring (Fig. 1). Chuanxiong

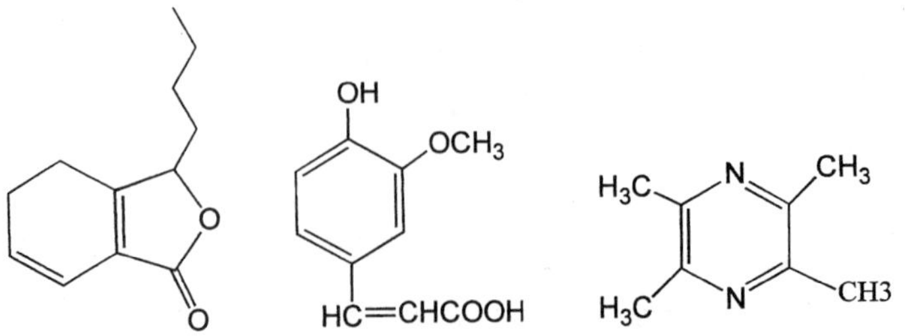

(a) (b) (c)

FIGURE 1 Structures of compounds isolated from *Ligusticum chuanxiong*: (a) senkyonolide A, (b) perulic acid, and (c) tetramethylpyrazine.

is strongly aromatic and the taste of the rhizome is slightly bitter with a sweet aftertaste. These characteristics are part of the traditional methods for identification of this herb. Other identification parameters, including the use of microscopic examination, colorimetric testing, and thin-layer chromatography, have been described in the *Pharmacopoeia of the People's Republic of China* (1).

III. USAGE

A. Traditional Usage

Ligusticum is traditionally used "to invigorate blood circulation, to promote the flow of qi, to dispel wind, and to alleviate pain." It is prescribed for headaches, abdominal pain, menstrual disorders (amenorrhea, dysmenorrhea), and for patients with pricking pain in the chest and costal regions, pain due to traumatic injury, headache, and rheumatic arthralgia (1).

B. Modern Usage

In recent years, owing to the renewed interest in herbal medicines, many inventors in the United States, Japan, and China have submitted patents based on traditional usage of *ligusticum*. Among the patents filed in the Chinese patent office are products with *L. chuanxiong* extracts that are used as detergents to prevent and treat acquired immunodeficiency syndrome (2), as a bathing lotion to promote blood circulation, and to improve skin conditions (3). In Japan, the herb has been patented for having the property to improve brain function (4). In the U.S. patent and trademark office, herbal concoctions with *L. chuanxiong* have been patented for application to the skin to help skin regeneration in patients with eczema and psoriasis (5). Tao in 2002 (6,7) submitted two patent applications for the use of *ligusticum* herbal extracts with the addition of minerals and vitamins for the treatment of brain disorders as well as to enhance brain function and for the treatment of hand and wrist discomfort.

IV. COMPOUNDS ISOLATED FROM *L. CHUANXIONG*

Isolation of the chemical constituents of *L. chuanxiong* began in the 1920s. The major components identified were ligustilide, butylidenephthalide, cnidilide, neocnidilide, butylphthalide, cindium lactone, sedamonic acid, and sedanolide (8–11). Pregnenolone, tetramethylpyrazine, coniferylferulate, senkyunolide-A, ligustilides, and their mono- and dihydroxyphthalide derivatives (senkyunolide B–L) have also been described (12–18). A significant amount of minor components, like the oxygenated phthalides (Fig. 1), have been encountered in processed material that are absent from the fresh herb. These are thought to be derivatives of the original components caused by chemical reactions during processing and storage. Thus the dihydroxyphthalides senkyunolide H and senkyunolide J are thought to be derived from the major components ligustilide and senkyunolide A. Similarly, ferulic acid is a decomposition product from coniferylferulate (19). The ligustilides and senkyunolides from *L. chuanxiong* are rather unstable and susceptible to auto-oxidation in the presence of air (14). Dimeric compounds such as levistolide A (20), wallichlide (15), and senkyunolide O and P (17) have also been described. It is anticipated that many other compounds will be described with the advent of sensitive and rapid methods for simultaneous separation and identification of compounds such as gas chromatography–mass spectrometry and high-performance liquid chromatography (HPLC)–mass spectrometry (MS).

V. ANIMAL MODELS TO INVESTIGATE/VALIDATE THE TRADITIONAL USAGE OF *L. CHUANXIONG*

A. Pharmacokinetics of *Ligusticum* Mixtures

The pharmacokinetics of most herbs and formulae used in traditional Chinese medicine (TCM) are not well understood. Mixing many different herbs together into complex formulations is a common practice in TCM. The effects of mixing different herbs together on the pharmacokinetics of individual compounds are to a large extent unknown. One of the rare efforts in this area was the attempt to investigate herb-herb interactions and the pharmacokinetics of *L. wallichii* in rat models with the use of both healthy and diseased rats (21). The results demonstrated that the pharmacokinetics of the herb in single use and in combination with other herbs displayed different properties. The investigators compared the presence in serum of two known constituents (tetramethylpyrazine and ferulic acid) of the herb after oral administration of *Ligusticum* alone and after administration of a mixture of *Ligusticum* and *Salvia miltiorrhiza*. Tetramethylpyrazine and ferulic acid were detected with HPLC, MS, and nuclear magnetic resonance (NMR). The absorption (Ka), transport (K_{21}), and distribution (Vc/F) of these two compounds were significantly lower when the second herb was present. Since *Ligusticum* and *S. miltiorrhiza* are commonly used together, the pharmacokinetics of these and other components in each herb are likely to be mutually affected when they are combined, thereby affecting their eventual toxicity and efficacy.

B. Efficacy Studies with the Crude Extract

A limited number of studies have been performed in Chinese laboratories to demonstrate the efficacy of the herb on a particular illness/treatment based on the use of the crude extracts. Most of these studies were unable to demonstrate either the specific molecular mechanism or the mode of action of the herbal extracts. The nature of the bioactive compound was also not known.

1. Muscle Function

Chuanxiong was administered to dogs to test its efficacy on muscle function, and specifically to see whether the use of a local or systemic treatment on muscle graft will increase the function of the transplanted muscle (22). The investigators subjected adult dogs to an orthotopic replantation of their bilateral rectus femoris muscles by microneurovascular anastomoses and split the subjects into a postoperative treatment group (with/without administration of chuanxiong) and a control group. They reported that therapy improved muscle function and morphology and maximal tetanic tension of the transplanted muscle. This study concluded that the combination of localized therapy and systemic injection of chuanxiong had a favorable effect on nerve regeneration as well as muscle function after a muscle transplant.

2. Effects on Central Nervous System

Chuanxiong was also reported to reduce cerebral ischemia (23) in a rabbit carotid occlusion model. Occlusion of the bilateral carotid arteries of rabbits produced bilateral partial cerebral ischemia, resulting in increased plasma and cerebrospinal fluid levels of the marker, dynorphin. *L. wallichii* Franch (*ligusticum*) pretreatment to the test group resulted in definite improvement of dynorphin levels in plasma and cerebrospinal fluid, suggesting that the severity of brain ischemic damage and neurological dysfunction in *ligusticum*-treated animals was less than that of the saline-treated group. Neither the active component nor mechanisms of action were investigated.

3. Renal Effects

L. wallichii has been reported to reduce the toxicity of cyclosporine A on renal function (24). Infusion of cyclosporine A to Sprague-Dawley rats resulted in a significant fall in glomerular filtration rate and renal plasma flow as well as an increase of plasma renin activity, angiotensin II level, and percentage of platelet aggregation. Treatment with 20% *L. wallichii* before cyclosporine A infusion significantly prevented the decline of glomerular filtration rate and renal plasma flow as well as enhancement of platelet aggregation induced by cyclosporine. These results suggested that *L. wallichii* may be beneficial for the treatment of acute nephrotoxicity induced by cyclosporine A.

4. Other Effects

Asthma and Bronchial Smooth Muscle. *L. wallichii* mixture was also reported to inhibit bronchospasm induced by histamine and acetylcholine in guinea pigs. The incubation period from antigen inhalation to asthma attack could be delayed by the *L. wallichii* mixture and the incidence of asthma and its mortality were reduced significantly in guinea pigs compared with controls (25).

Skin Permeability. Ligustici chuanxiong rhizoma (senkyu) ether extract has been reported to enhance permeability of moderately lipophilic compounds into the skin (26,27).

C. Efficacy Studies with the Use of Pure Compounds Derived from *Ligusticum*

With the characterization of components from the *L. chuanxiong*, some experiments have been performed to identify their biological function. The most well documented are tetramethylpyrazine, ferulic acid, and butylidenephthalide.

1. Cardiovascular Effects

Many investigators have focused on the cardiovascular effects of *ligusticum* since the traditional use of chuanxiong was to improve blood circulation. Tetramethylpyrazine isolated from *L. wallichii* Franch has been shown to have positive effects on portal-hypertensive rat models (28). Sprague-Dawley rats were used and portal hypertension was induced by partial ligation of the portal vein. Two weeks after the ligation, the rats were cannulated for measurement of mean arterial pressure, portal venous pressure, cardiac index, and heart rate. After the administration of tetramethylpyrazine to the rats, a dose-dependent reduction of portal venous pressure was observed and the total peripheral resistance was also significantly reduced.

Ferulic acid displayed a dose-responsive bradycardiac effect on pentobarbital-anesthetized Wistar rats, with no significant effects on blood pressure. Other effects observed from these experiments were the inhibitive effect on tachycardia and lack of activity on arterial pressure induced by phenylephrine. These results indicated that ferulinolol was a β-adrenoreceptor competitive antagonist, as it could competitively antagonize isoproterenol. Ferulinolol also demonstrated relaxant properties with isolated atria and trachea from reserpine-treated guinea pig, and at higher concentrations the compound had partial β2 agonist activity (29).

Phthalide dimers from *L. chuanxiong* (tokinolide B, levistolide A, ligustilide, and senkyunolide P) were able to relax KCl-induced contraction of rat thoracic aorta and reduced KCl-induced perfusion pressure of rat mesenteric arteries (30). Coniferylferulate reduced methoxamine-induced perfusion pressure on rat mesenteric arteries. The phthalide dimers tokinolode B and senkyunolide P and the phthalides senkyunolide, buthylphtalide, and cnidilide can decrease blood viscosity. These suggested that the herb may have important functions for activating the blood circulation and removing blood stasis. The chloroform fraction of *Cnidium* rhizome (Senkyu) exerted potent negative inotropic and chronotropic effects on isolated guinea pig atria (31). Contraction was attenuated by two major components in the chloroform fraction, ligustilide and senkyunolide, although heart rates remained unaffected by these components. Other effects of the chloroform fraction include changes in resting potential and the upstroke velocity of the action potentials.

Butylidenephthalide was reported to have a selective antianginal effect without changing blood pressure. Experiments performed to determine the mechanism of this action suggest that butylidenephthalide inhibited calcium release from calcium stores more selectively than calcium influx from extracellular space via voltage-dependent calcium channels (32). The inhibition by butylidenephthalide of calcium release from KCl-sensitive calcium stores might be similar to its inhibition of calcium release from phenylephrine-sensitive calcium stores. Senkyu phthalides have also been described as having antiarteriosclerotic properties (33). Synthetic butylidenephthalides have also been described to have inhibitory effects on mouse aorta smooth muscle cells in vitro (34).

Butylidenephthalide have been reported to strongly increase the peripheral blood flow in rats (35) and may increase the dermal absorption of radiolabeled butylidenephthalide in hairless mice (36). The results of these studies indicated that upon dermal application, the radiolabeled compound quickly permeated through the skin into the peripheral circulation. The half-life was approximately 1 hr, while the plasma concentration peaked at 2 hr postapplication. About 80% of the butylidenephthalide was excreted in the urine 24 hr postapplication, as a cystine conjugate and 5% was excreted in the feces, indicating that butylidenephthalide was not accumulated in the skin. If substantiated in humans, these studies show that butylidenephthalide may be developed into a form of treatment by skin application for an increase in blood flow.

The above studies indicate that extracts from *ligusticum* have potent biological activity and bioactive compounds contained therein may be developed into novel therapies for patients with high risk of cardiovascular diseases.

2. Antiplatelet Properties

Tetramethylpyrazine may have antiplatelet activity. The effect of this agent on platelet activation, aggregation, and thrombus formation occurring under various flow conditions was thought to be mediated by von Willebrand factor and platelet receptor proteins GP IBα and GP IIb/IIIa (37). Inhibition of platelet activation, aggregation, and thrombus formation under high sheer rates were observed. These findings suggest that tetramethylpyrazine may be effective for treating patients with thrombotic disease (38).

3. Anti-Inflammatory Properties

Tetramethylpyrazine and ferulic acid were reported to display anti-inflammatory and analgesic effects (16). When administered to guinea pigs with histamine/acetylcholine-induced bronchospasm, *Ligusticum* was found to decrease plasma levels of thromboxane B2, relax tracheal muscle, increase the forced expiratory volume, and inhibit the synthesis and release of thromboxane A2 with no adverse side effects. It has recently been reported that tetramethylpyrazine had an inhibitory effect on the elevation of aqueous flare induced by transcorneal application of prostaglandin E_2 agonists (39). Tetramethylpyrazine was able to inhibit prostaglandin E_2-induced flare. Thus tetramethylpyrazine may have applicability to treat aqueous flare; as prostaglandin E_2 is an important modulator in ocular inflammation.

4. Uterine Effects

Tetramethylpyrazine and ferulic acid have been suggested as therapeutic agents for woman with uterine hypercontractility and primary dysmenorrhea. These suggestions were based on rat uterine experiments conducted by Ozaki and Ma in 1990. In their experiments, inhibition of uterine contraction in rats was investigated by oral administration as well as intravenous administration of either tetramethylpyrazine, ferulic acid, or a combination of both agents. Their inhibitory activity was compared to that of papaverine. The results showed that tetramethylpyrazin and ferulic acid, either alone or in combination, had an inhibitory effect on spontaneous uterine contractions in estrous rats. Their therapeutic index was found to be more effective than papaverine, suggesting that these compounds may have utility as tocolytic agents (40).

5. Other Effects

CNS and Anticonvulsive Activities. Early reports suggest that 3-n-butyl phthalide may facilitate learning and memory in rats (41) and that it has a protective effect on rat brain cells (42). Recently, Chen et al. (43) investigated whether administration of tetramethylpyrazine led to any improvement in injuries related to the spinal cord. The group used rabbits and induced spinal cord ischemia via infrarenal aortic occlusion. Their results demonstrated that neurological and histopathology status of the animals in the treatment group was better than in those not treated, suggesting that tetramethylpyrazine can reduce neurological injury from the spinal cord (43).

Antibacterial/Antifungal Effects. *Ligusticum* demonstrated in vitro effects against several strains of pathogenic bacteria including *Pseudomonas aeruginosa*, *Shigella sonnei*, *Salmonella typhi*, and *Vibrio cholera* (44). The essential oil butylphthalide has been shown to inhibit dermatophytes in vitro (45).

VI. HUMAN STUDIES ON *LIGUSTICUM* HERBS

A. Cerebrovascular and Coagulation Effects

In Chinese studies, injections of *ligusticum*, ligustrazine, ligustylid, and ferulic acid were reported to have better effects on ischemic strokes than standard drugs such as papaverine, dextran, and aspirin-persantin (46). Injections of *ligusticum* extract, containing ligustrazine, ligustylid, and ferulic acid, were reported to improve brain microvascular circulation in patients with transient ischemic attacks, through inhibition of thrombus formation and platelet aggregation (47). In this study, 158 with transient ischemic attack were randomly divided into a *ligusticum* group (111 cases) and an aspirin group (47 cases). The total effective rate in the *ligusticum* group was 89.2% as compared to 61.7% in the aspirin group (47). *Ligusticum* was reported to increase cerebral blood flow, accelerate the velocity of blood flow, dilate spastic arteries, and decrease peripheral arterial resistance. The same group, in another double-blind trial, administered *L. chuanxiong* to one group (134 cases) and low-molecular-weight dextran to another group (86 cases) of 220 patients with acute cerebral infarction, to evaluate the herb's effects on neurological function and living capability (48). The total therapeutic efficacy rate in the chuanxiong group and in the dextran 40 group was reported to be 86.6% and 62.8%, respectively. It was concluded that the effect of chuanxiong in the treatment of acute cerebral infarction was significantly superior to that of low-molecular-weight dextran.

B. Anticoagulation Effects

Platelet aggregation plays a pathophysiological role in a variety of thromboembolic disorders, including myocardial infraction, atherosclerosis, and cerebrovascular diseases. Tetramethylpyrazine displayed a dose-dependent inhibition of human platelet aggregation and ATP-release reaction induced by various agonists. It was also demonstrated to have inhibitory action against monophosphate formation by collagen as well as an inhibitory effect on intracellular free calcium rise (49). The same group demonstrated that tetramethylpyrazine could significantly increase the production of nitrate and cyclic GMP in human platelet. The compound elicited a dose-dependent stimulation of endothelial type constitutive nitric oxide synthase in platelets (50). The investigators concluded that tetramethylpyrazine can provide effective prophylactic or therapeutic treatment for thromboembolic disorders. In patients with acute cerebral infarction, the levels of beta-thromboglobulin, platelet factor 4, and thromboxane B2 in plasma were significantly decreased in those treated with *ligusticum* extract, suggesting that the *ligusticum* treatment can effectively inhibit the platelet activation in vivo and correct the thromboxane A2–prostaglandin F2 imbalance in these patients (51).

VII. TOXICITY

Ligusticum is prescribed in traditional Chinese decoctions at dosages up to 9 g administered over several days. Overdose symptoms may include vomiting and dizziness (44).

VIII. CONCLUSION

Chuanxiong is a herb that has traditionally been used to promote blood circulation and treat arthralgias and menstrual disorders. Preliminary animal studies, from mainland China, indicate that administration of the crude extract may improve muscle function, reduce cerebral ischemia, and ameliorate acute nephrotoxicity induced by cyclosporine A. Tetramethylpyrazine, ferulic acid, and butylidenephthalide, pure compounds present in *ligusticum*, have been variously reported to display cardiovascular, antianginal, antiplatelet, anti-inflammatory, and tocolytic properties. Some human studies, again from mainland China, indicate that the herb may be beneficial in ischemic strokes and as anticoagulation agents. These studies, although largely uncontrolled and which have not been validated outside China, nonetheless suggest that bioactive compounds may be present in *ligusticum* that will reward scientific scrutiny.

REFERENCES

1. Chen M. The Pharmacopoeia of The People's Republic of China (English Edition 1997), Beijing, China. Chemical Industry Press.
2. Li D, Yan X, Yao G. Detergent for preventing and treating AIDS and method for preparing same. Patent No: CN116137, 1997.
3. Jiang S. Bathing lotion contg, trace elements in natural hot spring and plant extract. Patent No: CN1111990, 1995.
4. Natio T. New phthalide and brain function improver containing the same active ingredient. Patent No: JP5247022, 1993.
5. Yuen L. Herbal skin regeneration composition and method. US Patent 6,027,728, 2000.
6. Tao Y. Composition and methods for treating brain disorders and enhancing brain function. Patent Application No: US 20020009506, 2000a.
7. Tao Y. Composition and methods for treating hand and wrist discomfort. Patent No: US 20020039587, 2002b.
8. Mitsuhashi H, Nagai U. Studies on the of the constituents of umbelliferae plants. VII. Structure of ligustilide 2. Tetrahedron 1963; 19:1277–1283.
9. Mitsuhashi H, Muramatsu T. Studies on the constituents of umbelliferae plants. IX. Structure of cnilide and neocnildilide. Tetrahedron 1964; 20:1971–1982.
10. Mitsuhashi H, Nomura M. Studies on the constituents of umbelliferae plants. XII. Biogenesis of 3-butylphthalide (1). Chem Pharm Bull 1966; 14(7):777–778.
11. Bohrmann H, Stahl E, Mitsuhashi H. Studies of the constituents of umbelliferae plants. XIII. Chromatographic studies on the constituents of *Cnidium officinale* Makino. Chem Pharm Bull 1967; 15(10):1606–1608.
12. Tsuchida T, Kobayashi M, Kaneko K, Mitsuhashi H. Studies on the constituents of umbelliferase plants. XVI. Chem Pharm Bull 1987; 35:4460–4468.
13. Kobayashi M, Mitsuhashi H. Studies of three new ligustilide derivatives from *Ligusticum wallichii*. Chem Pharm Bull 1987; 35:4789–4792.
14. Kobayashi M, Fujita M, Mitsucihashi H. Studies on the constituents of umbelliferae plants. XV. Constituents of *Cindium officinale*: occurrence of coniferylferulate and hydroxphthalides. Chem Pharm Bull 1987; 35(4):1427–1433.
15. Wang P, Gao X, Wang Y, Yoshiyasu F, Iwao M, Sugawara M. Phthalides from the rhizome *Ligusticum wallichii*. Phytochemistry 1984; 23(9):2033–2038.
16. Ozaki Y. Antiinflammatory effect of tetramethylpyrazine and ferulic acid. Chem Pharm Bull 1992; 40:954–956.
17. Naito T, Katsuhara T, Niitsu K, Ikeya Y, Okada M, Mitsuhashi H. Two phthalides from *Ligusticum chuanxiong*. Phytochemistry 1992; 31:639–642.

18. Naito T, Ikeya Y, Okada M, Mistuhashi H, Maruno M. Two phthalides from *Ligusticum chuanxiong*. Phytochemistry 1996; 41(1):233–236.
19. Kobayashi M, Fujita M, Mitsuhashi H. Components of *Cnidium officinale* Makino: occurrence of pregnenolone, coniferyl ferulate, and hydroxyphthalides. Chem Pharm Bull 1984; 32(9):3770–3773.
20. Kaouadji M, Reutenauer H, Chulia AJ, Marsura A. Diligustilide, nouveau phthalide dimere: isole de *Ligusticum wallichii* Franch. Tetrahedron Lett 1983; 24(43):4677–4678.
21. Huang X, Ren P, Wen AD, Wang LL, Gao F. Pharmacokinetics of traditional Chinese syndrome and recipe: a hypothesis and its verification (I). World J Gastroenterol 2000; 6:384–391.
22. Hua J, Eritan G. Effect of postoperative treatment with a combination of chuanxiong and electret on functional recovery of muscle grafts: an experimental study in the dog. Plast Reconstr Surg 1996; 98(5):851–855.
23. Liu Z, Shi Y. Effects of *Ligusticum wallichii* on the plasma and CSF levels of dynorphin A1-13 in rabbits under acute experimental cerebral ischemia. Zhong Xi Yi Jie He Za Zhi 1990; 10:160–161.
24. Liu S. Effects of *Ligustricum Wallichii* on acute nephrotoxicity induced by cyclosporine A in rats. Zhonghua Yi Xue Za Zhi 1992; 72:345–347, 382.
25. Shao CR, Chen FM, Tang YX. Clinical and experimental study on *Ligusticum wallichii* mixture in preventing and treating bronchial asthma. Zhongguo Zhong Xi Yi Jie He Za Zhi 1994; 14(8):465–468.
26. Sekiya K, Kadota S, Katayama K, Koizumi T, Namba T. Study on baths with crude drug. III. The effect of ligustici chuanxiong rhizoma extract on the percutaneous absorption of some natural compounds. Biol Pharm Bull 1997; 20(9):983–987.
27. Namba T, Sekiya K, Kadota S, Hattori M, Katayama K, Koizumi T. Studies on the baths with crude drug: the effects of senkyu extract as skin penetration enhancer. Yakugaku Zasshi 1992; 112:638–644.
28. Chang FC, Chen KJ, Lim JG, Hong CY, Huang YT. Effects of tetramethylpyrazine on portal hypertensive rats. J Pharm Pharmacol 1998; 50(8):881–884.
29. Wu BN, Huang YC, Wu HM, Hong SJ, Chiang LC, Chen IJ. A highly selective beta adrenergic blocker with partial beta2-agonist derived from ferulic acid, an active component of *Ligusticum wallichii* Franch. J Cardiovasc Pharmacol 1998; 31(5):750–757.
30. Naito T, Kubota K, Shimoda Y, Sato T, Ikeya Y, Okada M, Maruno M. Effects of the constituents of a crude chinese drug, ligustici chuanxiong rhizoma, on vasoconstriction and blood viscosity. Nat Med 1995; 49:288–292.
31. Nakazawa K, Fujimori K, Inoue K, Sekita S, Takanaka A. Effects of extract from a herbal drug, *Cnidium rhizome* (senkyu), on contraction, heart rates and membrane potentials of isolated guinea pig atria. Yakugaku Zasshi 1989; 109:662–671.
32. Ko WC, Chang CY, Sheu JR, Tzeng SH, Chen CM. Effect of butylidenephthalide on calcium mobilization in isolated rat aorta. J Pharm Pharmacol 1998; 50:1365–1369.

33. Masayasu K. Antiarteriosclerotic. JP 1207233, 1989.
34. Mimura Y, Kobayashi S, Naitoh T, Kimura I, Kimura M. The structure-activity relationship between synthetic butylidenephthalide derivatives regarding the competence and progression of inhibition in primary cultures proliferation of mouse aorta smooth muscle cells. Biol Pharm Bull 1995; 18(9):1203–1206.
35. Yorozu H, Sato H, Komoto Y. The effects of crude extract bathing. III. The effect of phthalides from cnidii rhizoma. Jpn Assoc Phys Med Balenol Chnitol 1994; 57:123–128.
36. Sekiya K, Tezuka Y, Tanaka K, Parasain JK, Namba T, Katayama K, Koizumi T, Maeda M, Kondo T, Kadota S. Distribution, metabolism and excretion of butylidenephthalide of ligustici chuanxiong rhizoma in hairless mouse after dermal application. J Ethanopharmacol 2000; 71:401–409.
37. Liu SY, Sylvester DM. Antiplatelet activity of tetramethylpyrazine. Thromb Res 1994; 75(1):51–62.
38. Sutter MC, Wang YX. Recent cardiovascular drugs from Chinese medicinal plants. Cardiovasc Res 1993; 27(11):1891–1901.
39. Kitawawa K, Hayasaka S, Watanebe K, Nagaki Y. Aqueous flare elevation induced by transcorneal application of highly selective agonistic for prostaglandin E2 receptor subtypes in pigmented rabbits: effects of tetramethylpyrazine. Prostagland Other Lipid Metabol 2001; 65:189–198.
40. Ozaki Y, Ma JP. Inhibitory effects of tetramethylpyrazine and ferulic acid on spontaneous movement of rat uterus in situ. Chem Pharm Bull 1990; 38(6):1620–1623.
41. Yu SR, Gao NN, Li LL, Wang ZY, Chen Y, Wang WN. The protective effect of 3-butyl phthalide on rat brain cells. Yao Xue Xue Bao 1988; 23(9):656–661.
42. Yu SR, Gao NN, Li LL, Wang ZY, Chen Y, Wang WN. Facilitated performance of learning and memory in rats by 3-n-butyl phthalide. Zhongguo Yao Li Xue Bao 1988; 9(5):385–388.
43. Chen S, Xiong L, Wang Q, Sang H, Zhu Z, Dong H, Lu Z. Tetramethylpyrazine attenuates spinal cord ischemic injury due to aortic cross-clamping in rabbits. Bio Med Central Neurol 2002; 2(1):1–6.
44. Bensky D, Gamble A. Chinese Herbal Medicine: Materia Medica. Rev. ed. Seattle, WA: Eastland Press, 1993.
45. Hong YH. Oriental Materia Medica: A Concise Guide. Long Beach, CA: Oriental Healing Arts Institute, 1986.
46. Chen KJ, Chen K. Ischemic stroke treated with *Ligusticum chuanxiong*. Chinese Med J 1992; 105:870–873.
47. Chen DR. Clinical and experimental study of *Ligusticum wallichii* and aspirin in the treatment of transient ischemic attack. Zhongguo Zhong Xi Yi Jie He Za Zhi 1992b; 12:672–674.
48. Chen DR. Comparative study of chuanxiong and dextran 40 in the treatment of acute cerebral infarction. Zhongguo Zhong Xi Yi Jie He Za Zhi 1992a; 12(67):71–73.
49. Sheu JR, Kan YC, Hung WC, Ko WC, Yen MH. Mechanisms involved in the antiplatelet activity of tetramethylpyrazine in human platelets. Thromb Res 1997; 88(3):259–270.

50. Sheu JR, Kan YC, Hung WC, Lin CH, Yen MH. The anti-platelet activity of tetramethylpyrazine is mediated through activation of NO synthase. Life Sci 2000; 67:937–947.
51. Liu Z. Effects of *Ligusticum wallichii* on the plasma levels of beta-thromboglobulin, platelet factor 4, thromboxane B2 and 6-keto-PGF1 alpha in patients with acute cerebral infarction. Zhong Xi Yi Jie He Za Zhi 1991; 11: 711–713.

12

Salvia miltiorrhiza

Jin Liu
University of California
Davis, U.S.A.

Choon Nam Ong
National University of Singapore
Singapore, Republic of Singapore

I. INTRODUCTION

Salvia miltiorrhiza Bunge (SM) is a perennial herbal plant that usually grows on sunny slopes, by riversides, and on canal banks or edges of forests. It is normally 30–100 cm tall, villous, with purple flowers on the terminal or auxiliary spike (Fig. 1a). The root of SM is forked, brick-red, slender, wrinkled, with a solid and almost brittle texture (Fig. 1b). It is about 10–20 cm long and 0.3–1 cm in diameter. The part of SM used for medication is its dried root, which has a bitter and astringent taste (1).

SM, referred to as Dan Shen in traditional Chinese medicine, as an ingredient of certain medical prescriptions, has been widely used in China for the treatment of various kinds of diseases for centuries. It has been documented that the crude aqueous extract of SM has multiple pharmacological actions, for instance, promoting microcirculation, antiplatelet aggregation, and thrombosis formation, and sedative, tranquilizing, anticarbuncular, and analgesic actions (2). The decoction and injection made from SM exhibit some therapeutic effects on cardiac and cerebral ischemia as well as on liver

(a)

(b)

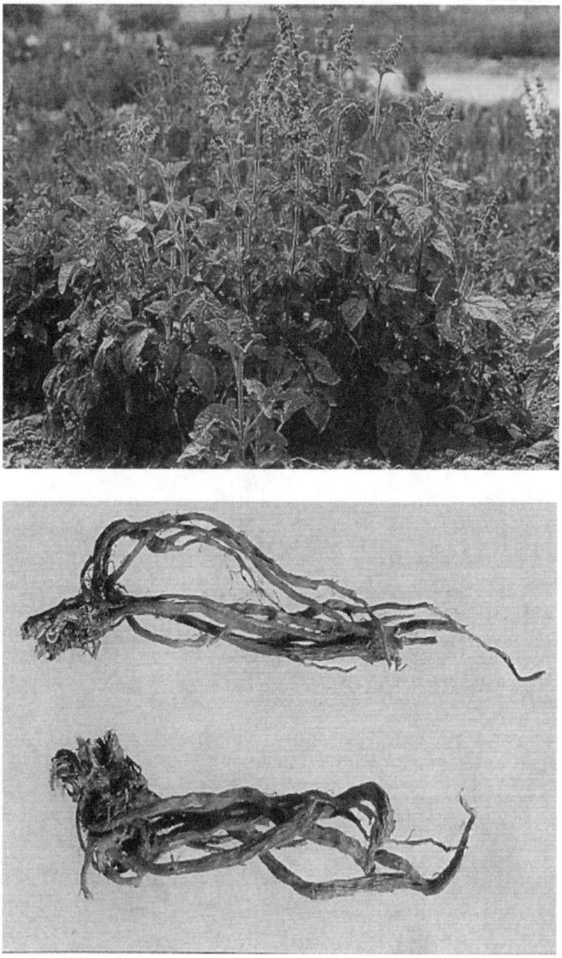

FIGURE 1 (a) Plant of *Salvia miltiorrhiza*. (b) Dried root, used for medication.

diseases, including chronic hepatitis and liver fibrosis. SM has also been used for other disorders, such as irregular menstruation, dysmenorrhea, amenorrhea, neurasthenia, irratability, and insomnia (2).

II. CHEMICAL COMPONENTS

A. Lipid-Soluble Components

In the last 50 years, many efforts have been made to study the chemical constituents of SM. Most of the studies have been focused on the lipophilic diterpenoid quinones. The major lipid-soluble components that have been identified so far include tanshinone I, dihydrotanshinone I, isotanshinone I and II, tanshinone IIA, tanshinone IIB, tanshinone V, tanshinone VI, isotanshinone, hydroxytanshinone, cryptotanshinone, isocryptotanshinone, methyltanshinonate, methylene tanshinquinone, przewaquinone A, przewaquinone B, tanshinol A, tanshinol B, tanshinol C, isotanshinone IIA, tanshiquinone A, tanshiquinone B, tanshiquinone C, miltirone, danshenxinkun B, dimethyl lithospermate, and 3,(3,4-dihydroxyphenyl)lactamide, as shown in Figure 2 (3–7).

B. Water-Soluble Components

Since the 1970s water extract of SM has been used in clinical practice in certain parts of China. Therefore, in recent years, more studies have investigated its water-soluble components. This has led to the isolation of some polyphenolic

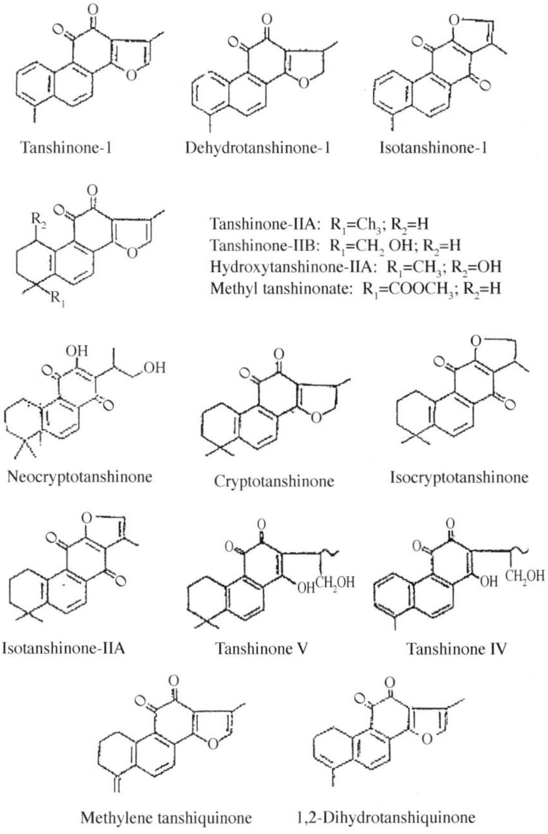

FIGURE 2 Quinones isolated from SM.

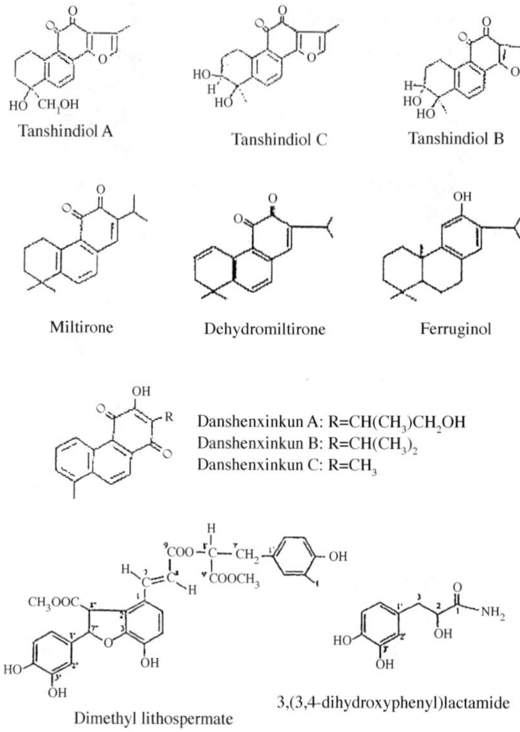

FIGURE 2 Continued.

acids from the aqueous extract of SM: salvianolic acid A, salvianolic acid B, salvianolic acid C, salvianolic acid D, salvianolic acid E, salvianolic acid F, salvianolic acid G, salvianolic acid H, salvianolic acid I, salvianolic acid J, isosalvianolic acid C, rosmarinic acid, lithospermic acid, protocatechuic aldehyde, protocatechuic acid, caffeic acid, and D(+)β3,4-dihydroxyphenol lactic acid (Danshensu, DA) (8,9).

III. BIOLOGICAL ACTIVITIES AND MECHANISMS

A. Actions on Liver Diseases

1. Liver Fibrosis

Liver fibrosis is the result of disequilibrium between synthesis and degradation of extracellular matrix (ECM) components (10). Accumulation of components of the ECM is the main pathological feature of liver fibrosis. It is often associated with hepatocellular necrosis and inflammation (11) and is a consequence of severe liver damage that occurs in many patients with chronic liver diseases, such as persistent infection with hepatitis C and B viruses, as well as alcoholic liver disease and bile duct obstruction (12). Liver stellate cells are regarded as the primary target cells for inflammatory stimuli (13). It has been shown that activation of hepatic stellate cells in injured livers leads to their proliferation and transformation into myofibroblast-like cells. The transformed cells synthesize large quantities of the major components of the ECM, including collagen types I, III, and IV, fibronectin, laminin, and proteoglycans, leading to fibrosis.

Effects of the water extract of SM on liver fibrosis have been evaluated in experimental animal models, in which liver fibrosis was induced by chronic administration of carbon tetrachloride (CCl_4) (14) or human serum albumin (15). Treatment with SM significantly reduced serum aspartate transaminase (AST), alanine transaminase (ALT), and alkaline phosphatase activities as well as total cholesterol concentration in rats of pathological control groups. The liver hydroxyproline and malondialdehyde (MDA) contents in animals treated with SM were also reduced to control levels. Moreover, the morphological characteristics of fibrotic livers were improved in rats treated with SM, as evidenced by decreased periportal and bridging necrosis, intralobular degeneration, and lobular and peripheral inflammation. These findings suggest that SM had a protective effect against liver injury and fibrosis. Effects of the water extract of SM on liver fibrosis induced by bile duct ligation and scission (BDL) were also studied and similar results were found (16). In addition, SM was able to ameliorate the portal hypertensive state (including portal venous pressure, superior mesenteric artery blood flow, cardiac index, and total peripheral resistance) in BDL rats.

As has been well studied, the accumulation of collagen type I and III is a conspicuous feature of liver fibrosis (17). There are two possible pathways by which SM reduces collagen generation. First, SM was capable of directly inhibiting gene expression of procollagen type I and III (14). Second, as the regulation of procollagen I and III synthesis is mediated primarily by transforming growth factor-β1 (TGF-β1), the decrease in TGF-β1 gene expression by SM might also contribute to the reduction of collagen synthesis (14). The cytokine TGF-β1 plays a central role in liver inflammation and fibrosis (18,19). Upon liver injury, TGF-β1 is released at the site of injury (20). It induces ECM deposition by simultaneously stimulating the synthesis of new matrix components, increasing the synthesis of the enzymes that inhibit ECM degradation, and decreasing the synthesis of matrix-degradation proteases (21,22). Hence, the inhibition of gene expression of TGF-β1 is one of the main mechanisms whereby SM exerts its antifibrotic action.

In addition to the enhanced collagen production, disruption of the normal regulation of collagenase activity may also lead to progressive liver fibrosis (23). The cytokines tissue inhibitor of metalloproteinase-1 (TIMP-1) and matrix metalloproteinase-1 (MMP-1) have been implicated in the decomposition of collagen. TIMP-1 promotes the progression of hepatic fibrosis by inhibiting the degradation of collagens (24), whereas MMP-1 belongs to a class of neutral proteases and specifically degrades the native forms of interstitial collagen type I and III (25). It was demonstrated that SM could inhibit TIMP-1 gene expression and induce MMP-1 gene expression (14). Through these effects, SM was able to promote the degradation of ECM in fibrotic rat liver, and hence prevent the deposition of type I and III collagen in the liver matrix.

Moreover, SM was reported to prevent the development of experimental liver fibrosis by inhibiting the activation and transformation of hepatic stellate cell (16,26). It was also demonstrated that salvianolic acid A, a water-soluble component of SM, significantly inhibited the proliferation and collagen production and secretion of cultured hepatic stellate cells (27). Although the mechanism of liver fibrosis is not fully understood, activated hepatic stellate cells play an important role in connective tissue synthesis and deposition during fibrogenesis. Hence, the inhibitory effects on hepatic stellate cell activation and its function of collagen synthesis are among the main mechanisms of SM action against liver fibrosis.

In addition to the antifibrotic potential, effects of SM on cell proliferation and function of cultured fibroblasts have been studied. Results from flow cytometry analysis show that SM could inhibit the proliferation of fibroblasts either by arresting cells at G0–G1 phase of the cell cycle (28) or by inducing apoptosis (29). It was also found that the production of the ECM components fibronectin, laminin, and collagen type I and III by cultured fibroblasts was significantly lower in the presence of SM (30). Furthermore, magnesium lithospermate, a component isolated from the water extract of SM, was found to posttranslationally modify enzymes proline and lysine hydroxylase in collagen biosynthesis in cultured human skin fibroblasts, thus reducing collagen secretion without affecting DNA synthesis as well as noncollagen synthesis (31).

It should be noted that oxidative stress, including reactive oxygen species (ROS) formation and lipid peroxidation (LPO), is also implicated in the pathogenesis of liver fibrosis (32,33). It has recently been reported that paracrine stimuli derived from hepatocytes undergoing oxidative stress induce hepatic stellate cell proliferation and collagen synthesis (34). Hepatic stellate cells have also been shown to be activated by free radicals generated from Fe^{2+}/ascorbate system (35) and by LPO product MDA (36) and 4-hydroxynonenal (37). Antioxidants, on the other hand, were observed to inhibit hepatic stellate cell activation induced by type I collagen (35). SM was shown to inhibit CCl_4-induced LPO in rat liver (38). In addition, it was observed that SM showed a scavenging effect on oxygen free radicals including superoxide anion and hydroxyl radical (39,40). It also increases the activity of glutathione peroxidase (GSH-Px) (41), an important enzyme in the antioxidant defense system in the liver. Based on the above evidence, it is possible that SM may exert its suppressive effects on liver fibrosis, at least in part, through its antioxidant activity.

2. Acute Liver Injury

The water extract of SM and its component lithospermate B were found to have a potent hepatoprotective activity on acute liver injuries induced by CCl_4 or D-galactosamine/lipopolysaccharide (D-GaIN/LPS) (42,43). Serum LPO, AST, ALT, and lactate dehydrogenase levels were significantly lower in SM-treated group as compared to those of the pathological control group. In addition, SM could improve histological changes of liver tissue, such as alleviate necrosis and steatosis of the liver, enhance hepatocyte regeneration, improve microcirculation, eliminate stasis of blood, and enhance albumin synthesis.

The protective effect of SM on acute liver injury is mainly due to its antioxidant activity. Free radical generation and LPO are common pathways in most of the experimental liver injuries and clinical liver diseases (44,45), especially liver injury caused by CCl_4, which is based on LPO of unsaturated fatty acids in cell membrane and intracellular organelle membrane. D-GaIN/LPS, on the other hand, is known to immunologically induce liver injury and does not involve direct oxidative tissue degradation. It is rather dependent on the release of potent mediators, such as tumor necrosis factor-α and superoxide radical from activated macrophage (43). Phenolic compounds isolated from SM could inhibit LPO of rat liver microsomes and plasma membrane induced by iron/cysteine and vitamin C/NADPH, and prevent bleb of the surface of rat hepatocytes induced by iron/cysteine (8). In addition, lithospermate B was found to have a better effect on ferrous/cysteine- and vitamin C/NADPH-induced LPO in liver mitochondria than vitamin E (46). Meanwhile, SM could enhance the enzyme activity of GSH-Px in cultured human fetal liver cells, which plays an important role in eliminating hydrogen peroxide (41). Moreover, it was observed that SM was effective in inhibiting the association of peroxidation products with DNA in liver cells and hence attenuating the decrease of cell viability (47).

3. Other Liver Diseases

In addition to experimental studies, some preliminary clinical trials have been carried out to evaluate the effect of SM in treating common liver diseases, such as chronic hepatitis (48) and portal vein hypertension (49). Although results generally support the effectiveness of SM in these cases, the mechanisms involved in its actions are far from clear.

B. Actions on Cerebral Ischemia and Reperfusion Injury

SM is commonly prescribed for ischemic cerebral vascular disease in traditional Chinese medicine. In experimental studies, SM was shown to decrease cerebral infarction and attenuate neurological deficits after ischemia and reperfusion (50–52). It was observed that SM was able to ameliorate some ultrastructural abnormalities of ischemic brain, including swollen mitochondria, partial loss of cristae, dilation of rough endoplasmic reticulum and Golgi's complex, the presence of dark neurons, swollen capillary endothelial cells and astrocytes, and active pinocytosis in the endothelial cells. SM also improved the impaired memory function after cerebral ischemia and reperfusion (53). Mechanistic studies indicate that the following properties of SM may contribute to its beneficial effects.

1. Scavenge Oxygen Free Radicals and Inhibit Lipid Peroxidation

Oxygen-derived free radicals are thought to be involved in the pathogenesis of ischemia-reperfusion injury in many organs, including brain, heart, gut, kidney, and liver (54,55). It has been demonstrated that during ischemia-reperfusion, a sequence of events leads to the formation of large quantities of superoxide radical (56). The generated superoxide radical can promote the release of iron from ferritin, probably causing the increase of free iron concentration in brain (57). Superoxide dismutase (SOD) converts the produced superoxide radical into hydrogen peroxide and molecular oxygen, whereas free iron catalyzes the conversion of superoxide radical into highly reactive hydroxyl radical that initiates free-radical chain reactions in cell membranes, causing LPO. Such peroxidation severely damages the cell membrane and causes loss of membrane fluidity and collapse of transmembrane ionic gradients. ROS have also been shown to alter endothelial and blood-brain barrier permeability and elicit brain edema and cellular injury.

Salvianolic acid A, an ingredient of SM, was able to scavenge free hydroxyl radical that generated from the ascorbic acid–ferrous system in vitro and reduce MDA content in the cortex, hippocampus, and corpus striatum of cerebral ischemia-reperfusion rats in vivo, indicating that the ameliorating effect of salvianolic acid A on learnig and memory impairment caused by cerebral ischemia-reperfusion may be related to its antioxidant activity (53). It was also found that in SM-treated rats, the cerebral SOD activity is significantly increased when compared to untreated animals (58), suggesting that SM can enhance antioxidant enzyme (SOD) and thus afford cerebroprotection against reperfusion injury.

2. Inhibit Nitric Oxide Synthase (NOS) Gene Expression and Reduce Nitric Oxide (NO) Production

Recently, the free radical NO has been identified as a messenger that carries out diverse signaling tasks in both central and peripheral nervous systems. In normal brains, NO is a nontoxic mediator of cerebral vasodilation. When present at abnormal high concentrations, NO possesses neurotoxic effects and has been implicated in the pathogenesis of cerebral injury in both permanent and transient focal ischemia (59). During ischemia, there is an increase in the extracellular concentration of excitatory amino acids (EAA) (glutamate and aspartate) (60). These EAA bind to and stimulate *N*-methyl-D-aspartate (NMDA) receptors in brain. Excessive activation of NMDA receptor allows influx of calcium into neurons, which in turn stimulates the enzyme NOS (61). NOS catalyzes the conversion of L-arginine to citrulline and NO via a calcium/calmodulin-dependent mechanism. Once formed, NO is believed to exert its cytotoxic effect by binding to the iron-sulfur centers of enzymes involved in the mitochondrial electron transport system, the citric acid cycle, and DNA synthesis. Another postulated mechanism of NO toxicity is that at high concentrations, superoxide anion and NO may react to form the peroxynitrite anion, which decomposes at acidic pH into strong oxidation (59). Thus, excessive NO generation might cause cell death in ischemia.

As NO has been proven to be involved in promoting ischemia-reperfusion cell death, any factors interfering with the production of NO may help to ameliorate ischemia-reperfusion injury. A previous investigation showed that in a four-vessel-occlusion rat model, pretreatment with SM significantly decreased cerebral NO content after 30 min of global ischemia and 15 min of reperfusion (62). This reduced NO level is attributed to the reduction of extracellular concentration of EAA by SM (63). In addition, SM can directly inhibit NOS gene expression in the cerebral cortex and caudate-putamen during ischemia (64). The inhibition of NOS gene expression as well as NO production may consitute one of the mechanisms by which SM protects against cerebral ischemia injury.

3. Inhibit Endothelin-1 (ET-1) Gene Expression

ET-1 is the most potent endogenous vasoconstrictor. Its long-lasting vasoconstriction of cerebral arteries and veins has been well documented (65). As an extracellular signaling agent in the brain, ET belongs to the class of G-protein ligands that mobilize phosphoinositide cycle and calcium influx within the cells. One consequence of phosphoinositide cycle signaling is augment of the release of EAA (66). The rise of extracellular EAA and intracellular calcium levels produced by ET may be sufficient to initiate the calcium/calmodulin-dependent NOS to generate the second-messenger NO and exert neurotoxicity in the central nervous system. Moreover, ET produced in astrocytes, which are interposed between neurons and blood vessels, can influence regional cerebral blood flow by interacting with specific receptors in the vascular smooth muscles. Furthermore, functions of the blood-brain barrier, which is composed of astrocytic processes and cerebral capillaries, may also be regulated by ET, as ET receptor is present in the capillary endothelial cells (67). Therefore, it is possible that ET plays a role in the development of neuronal cell death after cerebral ischemia and reperfusion.

ET-1 gene expression of rat brain during ischemia and reperfusion as well as the effect of SM was studied by using in situ hybridization (68). It was found that ET-1 gene expression in the cerebral cortex and caudate-putamen was markedly increased in both the 24-hr-ischemia and 24-hr-reperfusion groups. In SM-treated rats, the ET-1 gene expression of ischemia and reperfusion sides was significantly lower than that of the control, indicating that the inhibition of ET-1 gene expression may account for the protective effect of SM against cerebral ischemia and reperfusion injury.

4. Inhibit Neuron Apoptosis

Apoptosis, a form of programmed cell death, plays a critical role in the development and maintenance of many adult tissues, including those of the nervous system (69). Recent studies have provided evidence that some neuronal subpopulations may die via apoptosis after permanent or transient cerebral ischemia (70). Therefore, inhibiting apoptosis of neurons during ischemia and reperfusion may be a new approach to the treatment of ischemia cerebral vascular diseases.

The effect of SM on neuron apoptosis was studied in a left middle cerebral artery occlusion rat model (71). Results showed that 12 hr after reperfusion, a lot of apoptotic cells were found in the left ischemic cerebral cortex and caudoputamen, and the number of apoptotic cells reached the peak at 24–48 hr after reperfusion. However, in rats pretreated with SM, the number of apoptosis cells in the left cortex and caudoputamen was reduced significantly and the neuronal damage was much milder as compared to that of the saline-treated rats. Findings from this study indicate that the protection of SM against cerebral ischemia and reperfusion may be mediated, at least in part, through the reduction of apoptosis.

5. Attenuate the Dysfunction of Vasoactive Intestinal Peptide (VIP)

VIP, a basic 28-amino-acid neuropeptide, has been found in central nervous system and cerebral blood vessels. It acts as neurotransmitter and neuromodulator (72,73). Some of the VIP-containing neurons and vessels are vulnerable to ischemia, leadng to the decrease of VIP after ischemia. As has been shown, VIP is an important vasodilator. It acts directly on vascular smooth muscle to induce relaxation and increase cerebral blood flow (74). Moreover, VIP may also stimulate adenylate cyclase and increase cAMP level in the brain (75). These potent effects of VIP on cerebral vessels and cerebral oxidative metabolism suggest that VIP may be involved in the maintenance of the interrelation between local blood flow and energy generation (76). During cerebral ischemia, the low VIP level results in significantly decreased ATP production. This depletion of potential energy supply can lead to cell swelling, and hence damage cells and produce capillary compression. SM, on the other hand, has been demonstrated to increase ATP level of the brain and cAMP level in vitro and reduce neuron swelling during ischemia, thus attenuating the deleterious effects of VIP reduction after ischemia (77).

C. Actions on Cardiovascular Diseases

1. Myocardial Infarction

Tablets and injections made from pharmacologically active components isolated from SM, like DA (D(+)β3,4-dihydroxyphenol lactic acid, Danshensu) and sodium tanshinone IIA sulfonate (STS) are currently used in China for patients with various heart ailments, especially myocardial infarction. Clinical trials indicate that SM could effectively improve and protect myocardial ischemia and angina pectoris in patients with coronary heart disease, and no side effect was observed (78,79).

To explore the scientific bases for using SM to treat this disease, the protective effect of SM on myocardial infarction was studied in an experimental acute myocardial ischemia model by ligating the branch of the left coronary artery (80,81). Results showed that the degree of ST-segment elevation was decreased, and the ultimate myocardial infarction size was reduced dramatically by preadministration of SM. In addition, SM could improve ultrastructural changes of the ischemic myocardium, including severe intracellular and intercellular edema, mitochondrial enlargement, cristae ballooning and degeneration, reticulum enlargement, and cell destruction, indicating that SM is effective in protecting against infarction of the myocardium. Moreover, SM was found to accelerate the recovery of the ischemia area. The myocardial infarction caused by coronary ligation was also significantly reduced by STS (82) and DA (83). The effect of STS was comparable to that of propranolol, while DA was found to be superior to dipyridamole. In another study, SM was also found to exhibit a beneficial effect against acute myocardial ischemia and arrhythmia induced by isoproterenol or BaCl2. The death rate of the animals was significantly reduced in SM-treated animals. Moreover, SM significantly decreased premature ventricular contraction, ventricular fibrillation, bradycardia,and ECG J-point displacement (84).

Mechanistic studies from the above experiments indicate that the following properties of SM might account for its protection on ischemic myocardium: (1) inhibit the production of oxygen free radicals and LPO as well as increase antioxidant enzyme (SOD) activity, (2) block calcium influx, and (3) dilute coronary artery. Preadministration of DA was found to dilate the coronary artery and antagonize the constricting responses elicited by morphine or propranolol. It was also observed that intravenous injection of SM extract increased coronary blood flow and lowered coronary resistance in anesthetized cats. It has also been shown that STS and SM decoction could inhibit adenosine-diphosphate-induced platelet aggregation in myocardia infarction patients, possibly owing to enhanced fibrinolytic activity. Cheng et al. (84) also noted that SM promotes the regeneration of myocardial cells in the infarction region and inhibits the release of lysozymes, phagocytosis, and adhesion of meutrophils, and prevents the infiltration of white blood cells into the infarction area.

2. Myocardial Ischemia-Reperfusion Injury

The protective effect of the water extract of SM on ischemia-reperfusion injury was studied in an animal model, which was made by ligating and reopening the left ventricular branch of the coronary artery (85). SM was found to savage myocardium from reperfusion damage by inhibiting myocardial LPO and facilitating the recovery of regional myocardial blood flow. Besides the whole extract, injection of STS was also reported to reduce myocardial infarction size in rabbits with ischemia-reperfusion injury (86). This effect of STS was comparable to that of Trolox, a well-characterized antioxidant serving as a reference cytoprotector. In vitro study indicates that STS significantly prolonged the survival period of cultured human saphenous vein endothelial cells that were exposed to xanthine-oxidase-generated oxygen radicals. Endothelial cells are important in myocardial and other circulatory disorders (87). They are recognized to be the key sites of oxidant generation and attack. Thus, the cardioprotective action of STS is believed to be associated with its beneficial effect on this clinically important vascular endothelium.

In another study, when the hearts were pretreated with DA, the membrane fluidity and LPO of reperfused hearts were markedly improved (88). This protective effect of DA is mainly due to its antioxidant property. As has been established, ROS is directly involved in ischemia-reperfusion injury of the heart (89). DA was found to be more effective than sodium selenite in increasing the activity of SOD and GSH-Px, hence enhancing the antioxidant defense capability of the myocardium (90). Moreover, it was found that DA could remove superoxide radical generated from the xanthine–xanthine oxidase system and protect the mitochondrial membrane from LPO and ischemia-reperfusion injury (91).

3. Atherosclerosis

It is well known that plasma low-density lipoprotein (LDL) is the source of lipid that accumulates in atherosclerotic lesions (92). Recent studies have demonstrated that oxidized LDL plays an important role in the initiation and progression of atherosclerosis (93). Oxidized LDL in atherosclerotic lesions accelerated platelet aggregation and injured the endothelial surface or arterial wall (94). In addition, minimally modified LDL is capable of inducing gene expression in endothelial cells that may result in the acceleration of atherosclerosis (95,96). On further modification in the intima, oxidized LDL is taken up by the scavenger receptors of macrophages, gradually leading to the formation of foam cells and fibrous plaques (97). Immunochemical studies have demonstrated that oxidized LDL is present in the atherosclerotic lesions of animals and humans (92,98).

The antiatherogenic potential of SM was evaluated in rabbits fed a high-cholesterol diet (99). It was observed that SM feeding (5% water extract) reduced the plasma cholesterol level. Moreover, LDL from SM-treated group was more resistant to Cu^{2+}-induced oxidation and contained more vitamin E than did LDL from the high-cholesterol-diet group. In addition, endothelial damage, atheroscelotic area in the abdominal aorta, and cholesterol deposition in the thoracic aorta were also reduced dramatically, indicating that the severity of atheroslerosis in the SM-treated group was significantly alleviated. The reduction of atherosclerosis by SM relies not only on its cholesterol-lowering effect (SM inhibits cholesterol biosynthesis efficiently), but also on its antioxidant potential to prevent endothelial damage and to inhibit LDL oxidation modification in hypercholesterolemic animals (99). By incubating LDL from healthy persons with copper dichloride, it was found that SM had a profound anti-LPO effect (100). Moreover, salvianolic acid B, a water-soluble phenolic antioxidant isolated from SM, was found to scavenge 1,1-diphenyl-2-picrylhydrazyl radical and inhibit the oxidation of LDL more efficiently than probucol (99).

In addition to its inhibition on LDL oxidation, SM also plays a potential role in preventing the internalization of oxidized LDL. Lipid-laden foam cells, which derive predominantly from macrophage-acquired cholesterol, are the morphological hallmark of early atherosclerotic lesions (101). In most cells, the major pathway for the delivery of exogenous cholesterol is endocytosis of LDL (102). Macrophages possess LDL scavenger receptor that binds and internalizes altered forms of LDL, including copper peroxidized LDL, acetylated LDL, and MDA-modified LDL (103). In one study

(104), mouse peritoneal macrophages were incubated with peroxidized LDL (pox-LDL) and the effect of SM on the internalization of pox-LDL was observed. In the control group, LPO concentration in the medium decreased substantially after incubation of macrophage with pox-LDL. SM, on the other hand, produced a dose-dependent and much greater decrease of LPO and total cholesterol concentrations as compared to the control. Results from ultrastructural studies showed that SM induced the accumulation of lipid droplets in the cytoplasm of the macrophages, suggesting that SM could accelerate the phygocytosis and degradation of pox-LDL by macrophage, which may help to prevent and treat atherosclerosis.

In addition to oxidized LDL, the adhesion of circulating leukocytes to the vascular endothelium is also a critical early event in the development of atherosclerosis (105,106). This process depends on the interaction between cell adhesion molecules expressed on the surface of endothelial cells (EC) and their cognate ligands on leukocytes (107). Many adhesion molecules have been identified on ECs. These include vascular adhesion molecule-1 (VCAM-1), intracellular cell adhesion molecule-1 (ICAM-1), and endothelial cell selectin (E-selectin) (108). The increased expression of adhesion molecules by ECs in human atherosclerotic lesions may lead to further recruitment of leukocytes to atherosclerotic sites and play a major role in atherosclerosis (109,110).

The effects of salvianolic acid B and an ethanol extract of SM (SME) on the expression of endothelial-leukocyte adhesion molecules by tumor necrosis factor-α (TNF-α)-treated human aortic endothelial cells (HAECs) were investigated. When pretreated with salvianolic acid B and SME, the TNF-α-induced expression of VCAM-1 was notably attenuated. Dose-dependent lowering of expression of ICAM-1 was also seen with SME or Sal B. Furthermore, SME or Sal B significantly reduced the binding of the human monocytic cell line, U937, to TNF-α-stimulated HAECs (111). Based on the probable involvement of VCAM-1 and ICAM in monocyte recruitment to early atherosclerotic lesions, these findings suggest an additional mechanism by which salvianolic acid B and SME may be involved in preventing the progress of atherosclerosis.

4. Restenosis

Restenosis after successful coronary intervention remains a major limitation to the long-term outcome of this procedure (112). Intimal hyperplasia is one of the major mechanisms responsible for postangioplasty restenosis (113). The formation of intimal hyperplasia is mainly due to the phenotypic conversion and proliferation of smooth muscle cells as well as the accumulation of activated macrophages and foam cells (114,115). Activated macrophages and smooth muscle cells may express a number of cytokines, growth factors, and chemoattractant proteins, which are involved in the vessel wall remodeling, and could further exacerbate the progression of restenotic lesions (116). The monocyte chemotactic protein-1 (MCP-1) is an important mediator of monocyte recruitment into the vascular wall at sites of active inflammation or injury. It is secreted by stimulated human lymphocytes, endothelial cells, fibroblasts, monocytes, and smooth muscle cells in vitro (117–121). Increased levels of MCP-1 have been demonstrated in some animal models of postangioplasty restenosis (122,123), indicating that it may play an important role in the pathogenesis of vascular lesion formation.

To evaluate the possibility of SM on the prevention of arterial restenosis after angioplasty, the effect of SM on intimal thickening of the air-injured carotid artery of rats was studied. It was found that the maximal intimal thickness of the injured arteries was much thinner in the treatment group than that in the control group, indicating that SM could prevent experimental restenosis in rat model. Findings from in vitro study indicate that the beneficial effect of SM on restenosis might be due to its inhibition on the proliferation of smooth muscle cells (124). In another study, the effects of SM on neointimal hyperplasia and MCP-1 expression after balloon injury were evaluated. Male New Zealand white rabbits were fed a 2% cholesterol diet together with daily SM (4.8 g/kg body weight) treatment or without SM as a control for 6 weeks. The plasma cholesterol levels were lowered in the SM group. The neointimal hyperplasia in abdominal aortas was significantly inhibited in the SM group when compared with the control group. SM treatment significantly reduced MCP-1 mRNA and protein expression in balloon-injured abdominal aorta. Results from this study implied that SM might inhibit the expression of MCP-1 and thereby reduce the intimal response after balloon injury of aortas in cholesterol-fed rabbits, suggesting that SM treatment may offer some protection against postangioplasty restenosis (125).

Apoptosis has been suggested to participate in stabilizing cell number in restenosis. To determine whether SM affects vascular apoptosis, frequency of apoptotic cell death in atherosclerotic plaques and in restenotic lesions of cholesterol-fed and endothelial denudation (HC-ED) rabbits was examined. Apoptosis and associated cell types were examined in serial paraffin sections by in situ terminal deoxynucleotidyl transferase-mediated dUTP nick end labeling (TUNEL assay) and immunohistochemistry. The expression of p53, an apoptosis-related protein, was also examined. Apoptosis was mainly detected in the neointima of animals with endothelial denudation. The percentage of apoptotic cells in the SM-treated group ($68.5 \pm 5.9\%$) was significantly higher than that of the control (0%) and HC-ED ($46.1 \pm 5.4\%$) groups. The SM treatment markedly reduced the thickness of the neointima, which was mainly composed of smooth muscle cells with few macrophages.

In accordance with the apoptotic cell counts, positive immunoreactivity for p53 was observed in restenotic lesions from HC-ED and SM-treated groups but not in the control group. These results suggest that treatment with salvianolic acid B-rich fraction of SM induces apoptosis in neointima, which in turn may help prevent the neointimal thickening (126).

D. Chemopreventive Potential of SM

In recent years, the application of naturally occurring compounds, such as dietary components and herbal plants, as chemopreventive agents has attracted extensive attention. Owing to the increasing interest in this area, some preliminary studies have been carried out to explore the antitumor potential of SM.

1. In Vivo Studies

The effect of SM on aflatoxin B1 (AFB1)-induced hepatocarcinogenesis was investigated in male Fischer 344 rats. Results showed that the elevation of serum ALT and AST activities due to AFB1 dosing was almost completely abolished by the treatment of SM, indicating that SM could prevent AFB1-induced liver cell injury. It was further observed that SM substantially reduced glutathione S-transferase placenta form (GST-P) positive foci formation and GST-P mRNA expression caused by AFB1, which clearly suggests that SM is effective in preventing AFB1-induced hepatocarcinogenesis. Furthermore, the inhibition on AFB1 hepatocarcinogenesis was associated with a corresponding decrease in AFB1-DNA adducts formation as well as AFB1-induced oxidative DNA damage (8-hydroxydeoxyguanosine) in rat liver. The results also indicate that the protective effect of SM might be mediated through dual mechanisms: (1) the enhancement of AFB1 detoxification pathway, especially the induction of GST-Yc2 mRNA expression, and (2) the antioxidant property of SM (127).

Besides, the crude extract of SM was found to markedly prolong the survival period of Ehrlich ascites carcinoma-bearing mice, and STS, on the other hand, could potentiate the cytotoxic action of hydroxycamptothecine against Ehrlich ascites carcinoma (2). Yang et al. (128) reported that several tanshinones extracted from SM also exerted antitumor activities in mice. In addition, when administered orally (200 mg/kg) for 10 days, the methanol extract of SM significantly increased the life span of mice bearing sarcoma-180 cells (T/C 148%) (129). It was also found that SM injection (4.5 g/kg, ip) or low dose of cyclophosphamide (5 mg/kg) by itself had little effect on the growth of sarcoma-180 cells. However, when they were used together, the growth inhibition rate reached about 40%, which is substantially higher than that of cyclophosphamide alone (20%).

In a preliminary clinical study, 4–8 mL of SM injection with 20 mL of 10% glucose was used to treat exacerbated hepatocarcinoma patients after chemotherapy by using the technique of hepatic artery catheterization. It was found that after courses of treatment, the symptom of SM group was relieved, the tumor mass was shrunk, and the biochemical parameters were improved. The total effective rate was 65% for SM, while that of the control group was only 25% (130).

2. In Vitro Studies

Fifteen tanshinone analogs isolated from the chloroform extract of SM were examined for their cytotoxic activities against cells derived from human carcinoma of the nasopharynx (KB), cervix (Hela), colon (Colo-205), and larynx (Hep-2) by using MTT test (5). It was interesting to note that several of them were effective at concentrations below 1 μg/mL. In another in vitro study, 18 tanshinones extracted from SM were shown to exhibit profound cytotoxic activity against five cultured human cancer cell lines A549 (non-small-cell line), SK-OV-3 (ovary), SK-MEL-2 (melanoma), XF498 (central nerve system) and HCT-15 (colon) (129). The proliferation of each examined tumor cell line was significantly inhibited (IC50 value ranged from 0.2 to 8.1 μg/mL) by continuous exposure of cells to these compounds for 48 hr. It was also found that these constituents exhibited a marked, but presumably nonspecific, cytotoxicity against all examined cancer cell lines.

The cytotoxicity of tanshinones is closely related to their chemical structures. Tanshinones have a common structural feature of planar phenanthrene quinone, which resembles to a certain extent that of antitumor agents like actinomycin D, anthracyclines, and anthracenediones. These antitumor agents exert their pharmacological activity by means of DNA intercalation, which eventually causes an inhibition in DNA replication (131). It is likely that the planar phenanthrene structure of tanshinones may interact with DNA at the site of the hydrophobic core, and the hydrophilic substitution may provide additional electrophilic interactions with the phosphate backbone. Such an increase in binding affinity might explain the higher activity observed in compounds with hydrophilic substitutions. In addition to the planar phenanthrene ring, the furan ring in tanshinones plays a role in their cytotoxicity. It has been demonstrated that furan-containing compounds, e.g., nitrofurantoin and the o-quinone metabolites of etoposide (132,133), can undergo redox cycling reaction to generate superoxide anion and other free radicals. These reactive radicals are able to initiate DNA-strand scission (134). It is possible that both the furan and the o-quinone moieties of the tanshinone molecule could exert DNA-damaging action through the generation of reactive oxygen radicals at a directed site proximal to the bases. This type of antitumor mechanism is common to several naturally occurring antibiotics such as bleomycim, doxorubicin, and mitomycin C (135). This structure-activity relationship analysis indicates that the basic requirement for the cytotoxic activity of tanshinones is the presence of a furano-o-naphthoquinone in the molecule. The planar phenanthrene ring of the tanshinones may be essential for interaction with the DNA molecule whereas the furano-o-quinone moiety could be responsible for the production of oxygen free radicals in close proximity to the bases to cause DNA damage.

In addition to causing direct DNA damage, it has recently been demonstrated that tanshinone II-A was able to induce apoptosis in HL60 human premyelocytic leukemic cells and K562 human erythroleukemic cells through the activation of caspase 3, a major component in apoptotic cell death mechanism (136,137). The apoptosis-inducing property also constitutes one of the mechanisms of the cytotoxic effect of the aqueous extract of SM. It was observed that the aqueous extract of SM exerted clear cytotoxic effects and strongly inhibited the proliferation of HepG2 human hepatoma cells through the induction of apoptotic cell death (138). In the mechanistic study, a rapid decline of intracellular glutathione and protein thiol content was found in SM-treated cells. Moreover, SM treatment resulted in mitochondrial dysfunction as demonstrated by: (1) the onset of mitochondrial permeability transition; (2) the disruption of mitochondrial membrane potential; and (3) the release of cytochrome c from mitochondria into the cytosol. Subsequently, elevated level of intracellular ROS was observed prior to the onset of DNA fragmentation. However, no caspase-3 cleavage was observed throughout the whole period of SM treatment, while a caspase-3-independent poly(ADP-ribose) polymerase cleavage was noted at the late stage in SM-induced apoptosis. Taken together, results from this study suggest that SM deplete intracellular thiols, which, in turn, causes MPT and subsequent increase in ROS generation, and eventually apoptotic cell death (139).

More recently, Chen et al. (140) showed that a synthesized simplified phenolic analog of tanshinone, S-3-1, also exhibited potential activity in preventing the development of cancer. With the Ames test, S-3-1 was found to efficiently suppress the mutagenicity of benzo[α]pyrene. This result is consistent with the inhibitory effect of S-3-1 on the activation of benzo[α]pyrene by hepatic microsomal enzymes. Besides the anti-initiation effects, S-3-1 could significantly inhibit the croton-oil-induced increase of mouse skin epithermal ornithine decarboxylase activity. Moreover, S-3-1 quenched both superoxide and hydroxyl free radicals whereas it inhibited LPO in the in vitro model. These results suggest that S-3-1 might act as anti-initiation and antipromotion agents through reversing the biochemical alterations induced by carcinogen during carcinogenesis. It was also shown that S-3-1 ihibited the benzo[α]pyrene-induced transformation of V79 Chinese hamster lung fibroblasts. At 10–40 mg/kg, S-3-1 was found to inhibit the development of DMBA/croton-oil-induced skin papilloma in mice by decreasing the incidence of papilloma, prolonging the latent period of tumor occurrence, and reducing tumor number per mouse in a dose-dependent manner. Results from this study indicate that S-3-1 might be developed as a new chemopreventive drug (140).

IV. TOXICITY OF SM

So far, only a few studies have been conducted in mice or rats to evaluate the toxicity of SM. In one study, intraperitoneal injection of SM at a dose of 33.75 g/kg/day was given to mice for 14 days. No significant changes in body weight, food intake, condition of the fur, or other general appearance of the mice was observed, and also no change in blood picture, hepatic function, or liver function was found. The mice were then killed and the heart, liver, spleen, and kidney were examined pathologically. No noticeable abnormality was found except mild congestion of these organs. The LD_{50} of SM injection was found to be 61.6 ± 5.3 g/kg. In another study, two dosages of SM decoction were given to mice by intraperitoneal injection; 48-hr observation revealed no death of the animals receiving 43 k/kg of SM, whereas 2 of 10 animals given the dose of 64 g/kg died. Intragastric administration of 0.5 mL of 2% tanshinone suspension daily for 14 days in mice and 2.3 mL daily for 10 days in rats did not produce any toxic reaction, either (2).

Clinically, the following symptoms may occur in a small number of patients after administration of SM: dryness of the mouth, dizziness, lassitude, numbness and distending sensation of the hands, shortness of breath, tightness of the chest, mild irritability, precordial pain, tachycardia, nausea, vomiting, and gastrointestinal disturbance. However, these reactions usually subside or disappear spontaneously without interrupting the treatment (2). Collectively, results from experimental studies and clinical observations generally indicate that SM is a safe medicinal plant with little adverse effects.

REFERENCES

1. Institute of Chinese Materia Medica and China Academy of Traditional Chinese Medicine *Salvia miltiorrhiza* BungeMedicinal Plants in China—A Selection of 150 Commonly Used Species. Manila: World Health Organization, 1989:253.
2. Chang HM, But PP. Danshen. Pharmacology and Applications of Chinese Materia Medica. Singapore: World Scientific Publ. Co, 1986:255–268.
3. Zhang KQ, Bao Y, Wu P, Rosen RT, Ho CT. Antioxidative components of Tanshen (*Salvia miltiorrhiza* Bung). J Agric Food Chem 1990; 38:1184–1197.
4. Okamura N, Kobayashi K, Yagi A. High-performance liquid chromatography of abietane-type compounds. J Chromatogr 1991; 542:317–326.

5. Wu WL, Chang WL, Chen CF. Cytotoxic activities of tanshinones against human carcinoma cell lines. Am J Chin Med 1991; 19:207–216.
6. Kang HS, Chung HY, Jung JH, Kang SS, Choi JS. Antioxidant effect of *Salvia miltiorrhiza*. Arch Pharmacol Res 1997; 20:496–500.
7. Li HB, Che F. Preparative isolation and purification of six diterpenoids from the Chinese medicinal plant *Salvia miltiorhiza* by high-speed counter-current chromatography. J Chromatogr 2001; 925(1–2):909–914.
8. Liu GT, Zhang TM, Wang BE, Wang YW. Protective action of seven natural phenolic compounds against peroxidative damage to biomembranes. Biochem Pharmacol 1992; 43:147–152.
9. Li LN. Water soluble active components of *Salvia miltiorrhiza* and related plants. J Chin Pharmacol Sci 1997; 6:57–64.
10. Biagini G, Ballardini G. Liver fibrosis and extracellular matrix. J Hepatol 1989; 8:115–124.
11. Rojkind M, Perez-Tamayo R. Liver fibrosis. Int Rev Connect Tissue Res 1983; 10:333–393.
12. Bissell DM, Roll J. Connective tissue metabolism and hepatic fibrosis. In: Zakim D, Boyer TD, eds. Hepatology: A Textbook of Liver Disease. 2d ed. Philadelphia: WB Saunders, 1990:424–444.
13. Pinzani M. Novel insights into the biology and physiology of the Ito cell. Pharmacol Ther 1995; 66:387–412.
14. Wasser S, Ho JMS, Ang HK, Tan CEL. *Salvia miltiorrhiza* reduces experimentally-induced hepatic fibrosis in rats. J Hepatol 1998; 29:760–771.
15. Ye HJ, Wang XM, Zhang L, Zhang GR, Sun LQ, Zhang EX. Effect of Danshen injection on immunofunction of rats in experimental fibrosis. J Clin Gastroentrol 1995; 11:142–144.
16. Nan JX, Park EJ, Kang HC, Park PH, Kim JY, Sohn DH. Anti-fibrotic effects of a hot-water extract from *Salvia miltiorrhiza* roots on liver fibrosis induced by biliary obstruction in rats. J Pharm Pharmacol 2001; 53:197–204.
17. Milani S, Herbst H, Schupann D, Surrenti C, Riecken EO, Stein H. Cellular localization of type I, III and IV procollagen gene transcripts in normal and fibrotic human liver. Am J Pathol 1990; 137:59–70.
18. Czaja MJ, Weiner FR, Flanders KC, Giambrone MA, Wind R, Biempica L. In vitro and in vivo association of transforming growth factor-beta 1 with hepatic fibrosis. J Cell Biol 1989; 108:2477–2482.
19. Annoni G, Weiner FR, Zern MA. Increased transforming growth factor-beta 1 gene expression in human liver disease. J Hepatol 1992; 14:259–264.
20. Border WA, Noble NA. Transforming growth factor β in tissue fibrosis. N Engl J Med 1994; 331:1286–1292.
21. Edwards DR, Murphy G, Reynolds JJ, Whitham SE, Docherty AJP, Angel P. Transforming growth factor beta modulates the expression of collagenase and metalloproteinase inhibitor. EMBO J 1987; 6:1899–1904.
22. Weiner FR, Giambrone MA, Czaja MJ, Shah A, Annoni G, Takahashi S. Ito-cell gene expression and collagen regulation. Hepatology 1990; 11:111–117.
23. Arthur MJP. Collagenases and liver fibrosis. J Hepatol 1995; 22:43–48.

24. Iredale JP, Benyon RC, Arthur MJP, Ferris WF, Alcolado R, Winwood PJ. Tissue inhibitor of metalloproteinase-1 messenger RNA expression is enhanced relative to interstitial collagenase messenger RNA in experimental liver injury and fibrosis. Hepatology 1996; 24:176–184.
25. Birkedal-Hansen H. Proteolytic remodeling of extracellular matrix. Curr Opin Cell Biol 1995; 7:728–735.
26. Ma XH, Gong AY, Yi L, Chen XM, Zhao YC, Wang R, Han DW. Immunologic histochemistry studies on the effect of extracellular matrix of *Salvia miltiorrhiza* on experimental cirrhosis. Chin J Hepatol 1994; 2:79–89.
27. Liu CH, Liu P, Hu YY, Xu LM, Yan YZ, Wang ZN, Liu C. Effects of salvianolic acid-A on rat hepatic stellate cell proliferation and collagen production in culture. Acta Pharmacol Sin 2000; 21(8):721–726.
28. Liu J, Hua G, Wang H, Cui Y, Liu Y, Chu Y, Yang C, Chen W. Experimental study on the effect of IH764-3 on pulmonary fibrosis. Chin Med Sci J 1993; 8:9–14.
29. Ye HJ, Sun LQ, Yan XX, Song Y, He GZ. Effects of *Salvia miltiorrhiza* on proliferation and apoptosis of fibroblasts. Chin J Clin Immunol 1997; 9:25–27.
30. Wang BE, Wang HJ, Zhu JX, Liu EY. Experimental and clinical study of the therapeutic effect of composite *Salvia miltiorrhiza* on liver fibrosis. Chin J Hepatol 1993; 1:69–72.
31. Shigematsu T, Tajima S, Nishikawa T, Murad S, Pinnell SR, Nishioka I. Inhibition of collagen hydroxylation by lithospermic acid magnesium salt, a novel compound isolated from *Salvia miltiorrhiza* Radix. Biochim Biophys Acta 1994; 1200:79–83.
32. Britton RS, Bacon BR. Role of free radicals in liver diseases and hepatic fibrosis. Hepatogastroenterology 1994; 41:343–348.
33. Tsukamoto H, Rippe R, Niemela O, Lin M. Roles of oxidative stress in activation of Kupffer and Ito cells in liver fibrogenesis. J Gastroenterol Hepatol 1995; 10(suppl 1):S50–S53.
34. Baroni GS, D'Ambrosio L, Feretti G. Fibrogenic effect of oxidative stress on rat hepatic stellate cells. Hepatology 1998; 27:720–726.
35. Lee KS, Buck M, Houglum K, Chojkier M. Activation of hepatic stellate cells by TGF-β and collagen type I is mediated by oxidative stress through c-myb expression. J Clin Invest 1995; 96:2461–2468.
36. Baraona E, Liu W, Ma XL, Svegliati-Baroni G, Lieber CS. Acetaldehyde-collagen adducts in *N*-nitrosodimethylamine-induced liver cirrhosis in rats. Life Sci 1993; 52:1249–1255.
37. Parola M, Pinzani M, Casini A. Stimulation of lipid peroxidation or 4-hydroxynonenal treatment increases procollagen α (I) gene expression in human liver fat-storing cells. Biochem Biophys Res Commun 1993; 194:1044–1050.
38. Deng H, Ma X, Xu R, Chen X, Zhao Y, Yin L, Han D. Mechanisms of protective action of radix *Salviae miotiorrhizae* (RSM) against experimental hepatic injury in rats. Zhongguo Zhong Yao Za Zhi 1992; 17:233–236.
39. Lin TJ, Liu GT. Protective effect of salvianolic acid A on heart and liver

mitochondria injury induced by oxygen radicals in rats. Chin J Pharmacol Toxicol 1991; 5:276–281.
40. Zhang L, Wang XM, Zhao BL, Hou JW, Xin WJ. Scavenging effect of SM on superoxide anion radical. Acta Herbin Med Univ 1992; 26:255–259.
41. He SX, Shu CJ, Han Z, Ren YY, Li GY. Mechanistic study on the effect of *Salvia miltiorrhiza* on lipid peroxidation in cultured human fetal liver cells. J Shanxi Coll Trad Chin Med 1996; 19:29–30.
42. Hase K, Kasimu R, Basnet P, Kadota S, Namba T. Preventive effect of lithospermate B from *Salvia miltiorrhiza* on experimental hepatitis induced by carbon tetrachloride or D-galactosamine/lipopolysaccharide. Planta Med 1997; 63:22–26.
43. Qi XG. Protective mechanism of *Salvia miltiorrhiza* and *Paeonia lactiflora* on experimental liver damage. Zhong Xi Yi Jie He Za Zhi 1991; 11:102–104.
44. Sakaguchi S, Kanda N, Hsu CC, Sakaguchi O. Lipid peroxide formation and membrane damage in endotoxin-poisoned mice. Microbiol Immunol 1981; 25:229–244.
45. Suematsu T, Matsumura T, Sato N, Miyamoto T, Ooka T, Kamada T, Abe H. Lipid peroxidation in alcoholic liver disease in humans. Alcohol Clin Exp Res 1981; 5:427–430.
46. Hu YY, Liu C, Liu P. Anti-fibrotic components from Chinese herbal medicine. Zhong Cao Yao 1996; 27:183–185.
47. Cao EH, Liu XQ, Wang JJ, Xu NF. Effect of natural antioxidant tanshinone II-A on DNA damage by lipid peroxidation in liver cells. Free Rad Biol Med 1996; 20:801–806.
48. Xiong LL. Therapeutic effect of combined therapy of *Savia miltiorrhiza* and *Polyporus umbellatus* polysaccharide in the treatment of chronic hepatitis B. Zhongguo Zhong Xi Yi Jie He Za Zhi 1993; 13:533–535.
49. Li X, Yao X, Li T. Effects of radix *Salviae miltiorrhizae* on hemodynamics of portal hypertension: clinical and experimental study. Zhonghua Ne Ke Xue Za Zhi 1997; 36:450–453.
50. Leung AWN, Mo ZX, Zheng Y. Reduction of cellular damage induced by cerebral ischemia in rats. Neurochem Res 1991; 16:687–692.
51. Wu WP, Kuang PG, Zhu K. The effect of radix *Salvia miltiorrhizae* on the changes of ultrastructure in rat brain after cerebral ischemia. J Trad Chin Med 1992; 12:183–186.
52. Kuang PG, Wu WP, Zhu K. Evidence for amelioration of cellular damage in ischemic rat brain by radix *Salviae miltiorrhizae* treatment-immunocytochemistry and histopathology studies. J Trad Chin Med 1993; 13:38–41.
53. Du GH, Zhang JT. Protective effects of salvianolic acid A against impairment of memory induced by cerebral ischemia-reperfusion in mice. Chin Med J 1997; 110:65–68.
54. Cao W, Carney JM, Duchom A. Oxygen free radical involvement in ischemia and reperfusion injury to the brain. Neurosci Lett 1988; 88:233–238.
55. Hallenback JM, Dutka AT. Background review and current concepts of reperfusion injury. Arch Neurol 1990; 47:1245–1254.

56. McCord JM. Oxygen-derived free radicals in postischemic tissue injury. N Engl J Med 1985; 312:159–163.
57. Halliwell B, Gutteridge JMC. Oxygen radicals and the nervous system. Trends Neurosci 1985; 8:22–26.
58. Kuang PG, Tao Y, Tian YP. Radix *Salviae miltiorrhiza* treatment results in decreased lipid peroxidation in reperfusion injury. J Trad Chin Med 1996a; 16:138–142.
59. Nishikawa T, Kirsch JR, Kochler RC. Effect of nitric oxide synthetase inhibition on cerebral blood flow and injury volume during local ischemia in cats. Stroke 1993; 24:1717–1724.
60. Butcher SP. Correlation between amino acids release and neuropathologic outcome in rat brain following middle cerebral artery occlusion. Stroke 1990; 21:1727–1733.
61. Bredt DS, Synder SH. Isolation of nitric oxide synthetase, a calmodulin requiring enzyme. Proc Natl Acad Sci USA 1990; 87:682–685.
62. Kuang PG, Tao Y, Tian YP. Effect of radix *Salviae Miltiorrhizae* on nitric oxide cerebral ischemic-reperfusion injury. J Trad Chin Med 1996b; 16:224–227.
63. Kuang PG, Xiang J. Effect of radix *Salviae Miltiorrhizae* on EAA and IAA during cerebral ischemia in gerbils—a microdialysis study. J Trad Chin Med 1994; 14:45–50.
64. Wu WP, Kuang PG, Li ZZ. Effect of radix *Salviae Miltiorrhizae* on the gene expression of nitric oxide synthase in ischemic rat brains. J Trad Chin Med 1998a; 18:128–133.
65. Takahashi K, Ghatei MA, Jones PM. Endothelin in human brain and pituiry gland: presence of immunoreactive endothelin, endothelin messenger ribonucleic, and endothelin receptors. J Clin Endocrinol Metab 1991; 72:693–699.
66. Chuang DM, Lin WW, Lee CY. Endothelin-induced activation of phosphoinositide turnover, calcium mobilization, and transmitter release in cultured neurons and neurally related cell types. J Cardiovas Phanacol 1991; 17(suppl.7):S85–S88.
67. Yamashita K, Kataoka Y, Niwa M. Increased production of endothelins in the hippocampus of stroke-prone spontaneously hypertensive rats following transient forebrain ischemia: histochemical evidence. Cell Mol Neurobiol 1993; 13:19–23.
68. Wu WP, Kuang PG, Li ZZ. ET-1 gene expression of rat brain during ischemia and reperfusion and the protective effect of radix *Salviae Miltiorrhizae*. J Trad Chin Med 1997a; 17:59–64.
69. Raff MC. Social control on cell survival and cell death. Nature 1992; 356:397–400.
70. Li Y, Chopp M, Jiang N. Temporal profile of in situ DNA fragmentation after transient middle cerebral artery occlusion in the rats. J Cereb Blood Flow Metab 1995; 15:389.
71. Wu WP, Kuang PG, Li ZZ. Protective effect of radix *Salviae Miltiorrhizae* on apoptosis of neurons during focal cerebral ischemia and reperfusion injury. J Trad Chin Med 1997b; 17:220–225.

72. Emson PC. Vasoactive intestinal polypeptide (VIP): distribution in normal human brain and in Huntington's disease. Brain Res 1979; 173:173–178.
73. Loren I. Distribution of vasoactive intestinal polypeptide in the rat and mouse brain. Neuroscience 1979; 4:1953–1976.
74. Lee TJF. Vasoactive intestinal polypeptide-like substance. Science 1984; 224:898–901.
75. Borghi C. Vasoactive intestinal polypeptide (VIP) stimulated adenylate cyclase in selected areas of rat brain. Life Sci 1979; 14:65–70.
76. McCulloch J. Perivascular nerve fibers and the cerebral circulation. Trends Neurosci 1984; 7:133–138.
77. Kuang PG, Wu WP, Zhang FY, Liu JX, Pu CQ. The effect of radix *Salviae Miltiorrhizae* on vasoactive intestinal peptide in cerebral ischemia: an animal experiment. J Trad Chin Med 1989; 9(3):203–206.
78. Zhou S, Shao W, Duan C. Observation of preventing and treating effect of *Salvia miltiorrhiza* composita on patients with ischemic coronary heart disease undergoing non-heart surgery. Zhongguo Zhong Xi Yi Jie He Za Zhi 1999; 19(2):75–76.
79. Ji XY, Tan BK, Zhu YZ. *Salvia miltiorrhiza* and ischemic diseases. Acta Pharmacol Sin 2000; 21(12):1089–1094.
80. Zhao GC, Zhang GY, Wang XM. The effect of radix *Salvia miltiorrhiza* on lipid peroxidation in acute ischemic myocardium. Chin J Pathophysiol 1987; 3:197–200.
81. Cheng YY, Fong SM, Hon PM. Effect of *Salvia miltiorrhia* on the cardial ischemia in rats induced by ligation. Zhonguo Zhong Xi Yi Jie He Za Zhi 1992; 12(7):424–426.
82. Liu WW, Wang ED, Zhang JG. Effects of sodium tanshinone IIA sulfonate and propranolol on myocardial infarction of cats. J Hubei Med Univ 1981; 2:21–26.
83. Wang WD, Chen YH, Wang YP, Dong ZT, Yuan LX, Lu YQ, Wei PJ, Wang Y, Liu SZ. Effects of Danshensu and other water-soluble components of *Salvia miltiorrhiza* on dog ischemic myocardium and isolated pig coronary artery. Acta Shanghai Med Univ 1982; 9:14–20.
84. Cheng YY, Fong SM, Chang HM. Protective action of *Salvia miltiorrhiza* aqueous extract on chemically induced acute myocardial ischemia in rats. Zhong Xi Yi Jie He Za Zhi 1990; 10(10):609–611.
85. Han C, Wang XM, Zhang GY. The protective effect of radix *Salvia miltiorrhiza* on ischemic and post-ischemic reperfusion injury of heart. Chin J Pathophysiol 1991; 7:337–341.
86. Wu TW, Zeng LH, Fung KP, Wu J. Effect of sodium tanshinone IIA sulfonate in the rabbit myocardium and on human cardiomyocytes and vascular endothelial cells. Biochem Pharmacol 1993; 46:2327–2332.
87. Rutherford JD, Braunwald E. Chronic ischemic heart disease. In: Braunwald E, ed. Heart Disease: A Textbook of Cardiovascular Medicine. Philadelphia: WB Saunders, 1992:1292–1364.
88. Zhang L, Wang XM, Liang DQ, Zhao BL. The effect of DS-182 on

mitochondria changes induced by rat myocardial ischemia/reperfusion injury and its mechanism. Chin J Pathophysiol 1990b; 6:420–423.
89. Guarnier C. Role of oxygen in the cellular damage induced by re-oxygenation of hypoxic heart. J Mol Cell Cardiol 1980; 12:797797.
90. Tang LH, Wang XM, Liang DQ. The protection of DS-182 on reperfusion of ischemic heart. Chin J Pathophysiol 1989; 5:65–69.
91. Zhao BL, Jiang W, Zhao Y, Wu J, Xin WJ. Scavenging effects of *Salvia miltiorrhiza* on free radicals and its protection of myocardial mitochondrial membrane from ischemia-reperfusion injury. Biochem Mol Biol Intern 1996; 38:1171–1182.
92. Yla-Herttuala S, Palinski W, Butler SW, Picard S, Steinberg D, Witztum JL. Rabbit and human atherosclerotic lesions contain IgG that recognizes epitopes of oxidized LDL. Arterioscler Thromb 1994; 14:32–40.
93. Steinberg D, Parthasarathy S, Carew TE, Khoo JC, Witztum JL. Beyond cholesterol: modification of low density lipoproteins that increase its atherogenicity. N Engl J Med 1989; 320:915–924.
94. Kanazawa T, Tanaka M, Fukushi Y, Onodera K, Lee KT, Metoki H. Effects of low-density lipoprotein from normal rabbits on hypercholesterolemia and the development of atherosclerosis. Pathobiology 1991; 59(2): 85–91.
95. Cushing SD, Berliner JA, Valente AJ, Territo MC, Navab M, Parhami F. Lipoprotein induces monocyte-chemotactic protein-1 in human endothelial cells and SMC. Proc Natl Acad Sci USA 1990; 87:5134–5138.
96. Lusis AJ, Navab M. Lipoprotein oxidation and gene expression in the artery wall: new opportunities for pharmacological intervention in atherosclerosis. Biochem Pharmacol 1993; 46:2119–2126.
97. Parthasarthy S, Printz DJ, Boyd D, Joy L, Steinberg D. Macrophage oxidation of low density lipoprotein generates a modified form recognized by the scavenger receptor. Arteriosclerosis 1986; 6:505–510.
98. Palinski W, Rosenfeld ME, Yla-Herttuala S, Gurther GC, Socher SA, Butler SW, Parthasarathy S, Carew TE, Steinberg D, Wiztum JL. Low density lipoprotein undergoes oxidative modification in vivo. Proc Natl Acad Sci USA 1989; 86:1372–1376.
99. Wu YJ, Hong CY, Lin SJ, Wu P, Shiao MS. Increase of vitamin E content in LDL and reduction of atherosclerosis in cholesterol-fed rabbits by a water-soluble antioxidant-rich fraction of *Salvia miltiorrhiza*. Arterioscler Thromb Vasc Biol 1998b; 18:481–486.
100. Zhang PT, Chen ZR. Effect of *Salvia miltiorrhiza* on lipid peroxidation antioxidant enzymes activity in patients with chronic cor pulmonale. Zhongguo Zhong Xi Yi Jie He Za Zhi 1994; 14:474–477.
101. Libby P, Clinton SK. The role of macrophages in atherogenesis. Curr Opin Lipidol 1993; 4:355–363.
102. Brown MS, Goldstein JL. Lipoprotein metabolism in the macrophages: implication for cholesterol deposition in antherosclerosis. Annu Rev Biochem 1983; 52:223–361.

103. Freeman MW. Macropage scavenger receptors. Curr Opin Lipidol 1994; 5:143–148.
104. Yu SY, Kuang PG, Kanazawa T, Onodera K, Metoki H, Oike Y. The effects of radix *Salviae Miltiorrhizae* on lipid accumulation of peroxidized low density lipoprotein in mouse peritoneal macrophage-lipid analysis and morphological studies. J Trad Chin Med 1998; 18:292–299.
105. Joris I, Zand T, Nunnari JJ, Krolikowski FJ, Majno G. Studies on the pathogenesis of atherosclerosis. I Adhesion and emigration of mononuclear cells in the aorta of hypercholesterolemic rats. Am J Pathol 1983; 113:341–358.
106. Faggiotto A, Ross R, Harker L. Studies of hypercholesterolemia in the nonhuman primate. I Changes that lead to fatty streak formation. Arteriosclerosis 1984; 4:323–340.
107. Price DT, Loscalzo J. Cellular adhesion molecules and atherosclerosis. J Exp Med 1999; 107:85–97.
108. Cybulsky MI, Gimbrone MA. Endothelial expression of a mononuclear leukocyte adhesion molecule during atherosclerosis. Science 1991; 251:788–791.
109. van der Wal AC, Das PK, Tigges AJ, Becker AE. Adhesion molecules on the endothelium and mononuclear cells in human atherosclerotic lesions. Am J Pathol 1992; 141:1427–1433.
110. O'Brien KD, Allen MD, McDonald TO, Chait A, Harlan JM, Fishbein D, McCarty J, Ferguson M, Hudkins K, Benjamin CD, Lobb R, Alpers CE. Vascular cell adhesion molecule-1 is expressed in human coronary atherosclerotic plaques: implications for the mode of progression of advanced coronary atherosclerosis. J Clin Invest 1993; 92:945–951.
111. Chen YH, Lin SJ, Ku HH, Shiao MS, Lin FY, Chen JW, Chen YL. Salvianolic acid B attenuates VCAM-1 and ICAM-1 expression in TNF-α-treated human aortic endothelial cells. J Cell Biochem 2001a; 82:512–521.
112. Leimgruber PP, Roubin GS, Hollman J, Cotsonis GA, Meier B, Douglas JS, King SB Jr, Gruentzig AR. Restenosis after successful coronary angioplasty in patients with single-vessel disease. Circulation 1986; 73:710–717.
113. Post MJ, Borst C, Kuntz RE. The relative importance of arterial remodeling compared with intimal hyperplasia in lumen renarrowing after balloon angioplasty: a study in the normal rabbit and the hypercholesterolemic Yucatan micropig. Circulation 1994; 89:2816–2821.
114. Hanke H, Hassenstein S, Ulmer A, Kamenz J, Oberhoff M, Haase KK, Baumbach A. Accumulation of macrophages in the arterial vessel wall following experimental balloon angioplasty. Eur Heart J 1994; 15:691–698.
115. Chen YH, Chen YL, Lin SJ, Chou CY, Mar GY, Chang MS, Wang SP. Electron microscopic studies of phenotypic modulation of smooth muscle cells in coronary arteries of patients with unstable angina pectoris and postangioplasty restenosis. Circulation 1997; 95:1169–1175.
116. Schwartz SM, Reidy MA, O'Brien ER. Assessment of factors important in atherosclerotic occulusion and restenosis. Thromb Haemestasis 1995; 74:541–551.
117. Kaczmarek L, Calabretta B, Baserga R. Expression of cell-cycle-dependent

genes in phytohemagglutinin-stimulated human lymphocytes. Proc Natl Acad Sci USA 1985; 82:5375–5379.
118. Valente AJ, Graves DT, Vialle-Valentin CE, Delgado R, Schwartz CJ. Purification of a monocyte chemotactic factor secreted by nonhuman primate vascular cells in culture. Biochemistry 1988; 27:4162–4168.
119. Strieter RM, Wiggins R, Phan SH, Wharram BL, Showell HJ, Remick DG, Chensue SW, Kunkel SL. Monocyte chemotactic protein gene expression by cytokine-treated human fibroblasts and endothelial cells. Biochem Biophys Res Comm 1989; 162:694–700.
120. Yoshimura T, Yuhki N, Moore SK, Appella E, Lerman MI, Leonard EJ. Human monocyte chemoattractant protein-1 (MCP-1). Full-length cDNA cloning, expression in mitogen-stimulated blood mononuclear leukocytes, and sequence similarity to mouse competence gene JE. FEBS Lett 1989; 244:487–493.
121. Rollins BJ, Yoshimura T, Leonard EJ, Pober JS. Cytokine-activated human endothelial cells synthesize and secrete a monocyte chemoattractant. MCP-1/JE Am J Pathol 1990; 136:1229–1233.
122. Wysocki SJ, Zheng MH, Smith A, Lamawansa MD, Iacopetta BJ, Robertson TA, Papadimitriou JM, House AK, Norman PE. Monocyte chemoattractant protein-1 gene expression in injuried pig artery coincides with early appearance of infiltrating monocyte/macrophages. J Cell Biochem 1996; 62:303–313.
123. Merritt R, Guruge BL, Miller DD, Chaitman BR, Bora PS. Moderate alcohol feeding attenuates postinjury vascular cell proliferation in rabbit angioplasty model. J Cardiovasc Pharm 1997; 30:19–25.
124. Zhou XM, Lu ZY, Wang DW. Experimental study of *Salvia miltiorrhiza* on prevention of restenosis after angioplasty. Zhong guo Zhong Xi Yi Jie He Za Zhi 1996; 16(8):480–482.
125. Chen YL, Yang SP, Shiao MS, Chen JW, Lin SJ. *Salvia miltiorrhiza* inhibits intimal hyperplasia and monocyte chemotactic protein-1 expression after ballon injury in cholesterol-fed rabbits. J Cell Biochem 2001b; 83:484–493.
126. Hung HH, Chen YL, Lin SJ, Yang SP, Shih CC, Shiao MS, Chang CH. A salvianolic acid B-rich fraction of *Salvia miltiorrhiza* induces neointimal cell apoptosis in rabbit angioplasty model. Histol Histopathol 2001; 16(1):175–183.
127. Liu J, Yang CF, Wasser S, Shen HM, Tan CE, Ong CN. Protection of *Salvia miltiorrhiza* against aflatoxin B_1-induced hepatocarcinogenesis in Fischer 344 rats: dual mechanisms involved. Life Sci 2001a; 69(3):309–326.
128. Yang BJ, Qian MK, Qin GW, Chen ZY. Studies on the active principles of Danshen. Acta Pharmcol Sin 1981; 16:837–841.
129. Ryu SY, Lee CO, Choi SU. In vitro cytotoxicity of Tanshinone from *Salvia miltiorrhiza*. Planta Med 1997; 63:339–342.
130. Peng ZS, Rao RS, Gong ZF. Clinical effects of perfusion drugs into hepatic artery to promote blood circulation in late stage of hepatocarcinoma. Zhongguo Zhong Xi Yi Jie He Za Zhi 1993; 13:330–332.
131. Neidel S, Waring MJ. Molecular Aspects of Anti-cancer Drug Action. London: Macmillan Press, 1983.

132. Boyd MR. Biochemical mechanisms in chemical-induced lung injury: roles of metabolic activation. Crit Rev Toxicol 1980; 7:103–176.
133. Kalyanaraman B, Nemec J, Sinha BK. Characteristics of free radicals production during oxidation of etoposide (VP-16) and its catechol and quinone derivatives. Biochemistry 1989; 28:4839–4846.
134. van Maanen JMS, Lafleur MVM, Mans DRA, Akker E, Ruiter C, Kootstra PR, Pappie D, Varies J, Retil J, Pinedo HM. Effects of the orthoquinone and catechol of the antitumor drug VP-16-213 on the biological activity of single-stranded and doublestranded ox174 DNA. Biochem Pharmacol 1988; 37:3579–3589.
135. Lown JW. Molecular mechanisms of action of anti-cancer agents involving free radical intermediates. In: Pryor WA, ed. Advances in Free radical Biology and Medicine. Vol. 1. New York: Academic Press, 1985.
136. Sung HJ, Choi SM, Yoon Y, An KS. Tanshinone IIA, an ingredient of *Salvia miltiorrhiza* BUNGE , induces apoptosis in human leukemia cell lines through the activation of caspase-3. Exp Mol Med 1999; 31(4):174–178.
137. Yoon Y, Kim YO, Jeon WK, Park HJ, Sung HJ. Tanshinone IIA isolated from *Salvia miltiorrhiza* BUNGE induced apoptosis in HL60 human premyelocytic leukemia cell line. J Ethnopharmacol 1999; 68(1–3):121–127.
138. Liu J, Shen HM, Ong CN. *Salvia miltiorrhiza* inhibits cell growth and induces apoptosis in human hepatoma $HepG_2$ cells. Cancer Lett 2000b; 153(1–2):85–93.
139. Liu J, Shen HM, Ong CN. Role of intracellular thiol depletion, mitochondrial dysfunction and reactive oxygen species in *Salvia miltiorrhiza*-induced apoptosis in human hepatoma $HepG_2$ cells. Life Sci 2001b; 69(16):1833–1850.
140. Chen XG, Li Y, Yan CH, Li LN, Han R. Cancer chemopreventive activities of S-3-1, a synthetic derivative of danshinone. J Asian Nat Prod Res 2001c; 3(1):63–75.

13

Schisandrin B and Other Dibenzocyclooctadiene Lignans

Robert Kam-Ming Ko
and Duncan H. F. Mak
Hong Kong University of Science and Technology
Hong Kong, China

I. INTRODUCTION

Schisandrin B (Sch B, Fig. 1a) is the most abundant dibenzocyclooctadiene derivative (lignan) isolated from Fructus Schisandrae (FS), the fruit of *Schisandra chinensis* (Turcz.) Baillon, or Wu-Wei-Zi, meaning the fruit of five tastes in Chinese. FS is a commonly used herb in traditional Chinese medicine (TCM). The plant grows as a woody aromatic vine, with fruits occurring as bunches of berries on a short, drooping spike. The plant is native to most Eastern parts of Russia (Primorsk and Chabarowsk regions), northeastern China (Jilin, Liaoning, Heliongjiang, and Hebei provinces), North Korea, and Japan (1). In terms of pharmacological properties, TCM characterizes Wu-Wei-Zi as "warm" in nature and mainly "sour" in taste, with the regulatory/therapeutic action targeted at the "lung-kidney" as well as "liver-heart" functions. Traditionally, the herb is used as astringent and sedative, as well as in tonic formulae for invigorating the qi (vital energy) of the five viscera, namely, liver, heart, spleen, lung, and kidney, in the body (2).

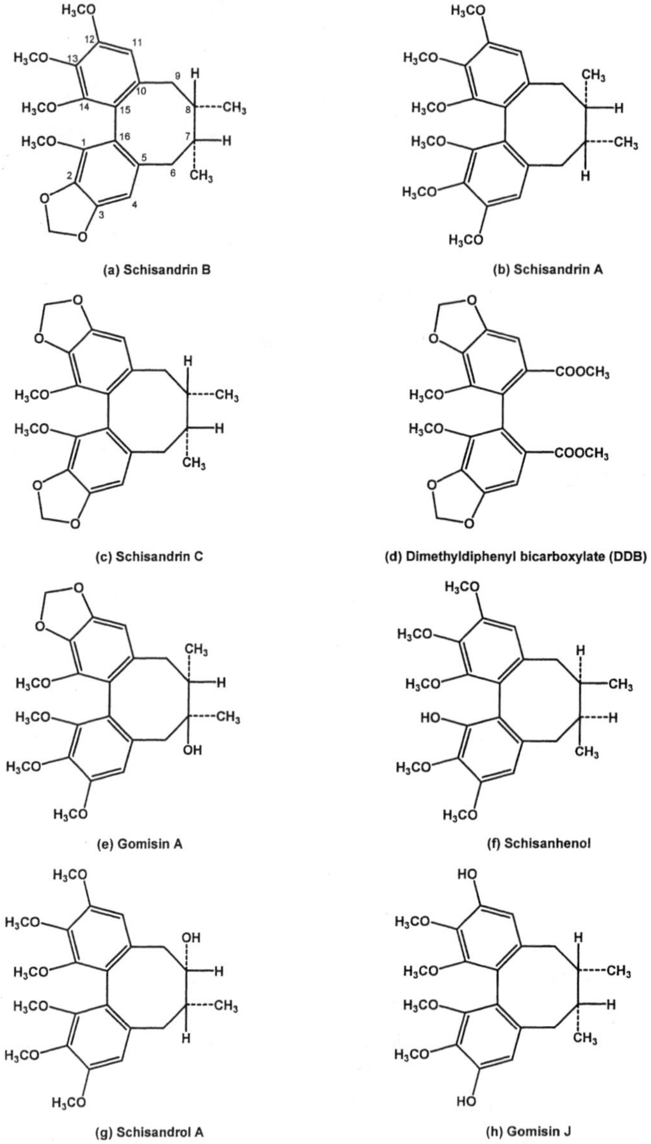

FIGURE 1 Chemical structures of schisandrin B and other dibenzocyclooctadiene lignans.

Starting from the 1950s, pharmacological studies on FS were focused mainly on examining its effect on cardiopulmonary function and the central nervous system. Since then, FS has been regarded as an adaptogen that can increase the resistance of the body against nonspecific stimuli (3). At the beginning of the 1970s, a number of clinical investigations unequivocally demonstrated the effectiveness of FS for the treatment of chronic viral and chemical hepatitis, particularly in lowering the elevated serum glutamic-pyruvate transaminase (GPT) activity (4). In an experimental model of hepatitis used as activity monitor, the activity-directed fractionation of FS extract yielded a series of lignans including Sch B (5). During the past two decades, the hepatoprotective mechanisms of Sch B and other lignans derived from Fructus Schisandrae have been extensively investigated, particularly those involving hepatic microsomal cytochrome P-450-dependent drug-metabolizing enzymes (6–8). While the tissue-protective action of Sch B was found not only limited to the liver, protection against free-radical-mediated injury was demonstrated in both heart and brain tissues in experimental animals (9,10). The apparently broad-spectrum and tissue-nonspecific protection afforded by Sch B and other lignans has attracted much interest in the area of preventive medicine. Thorough understanding of biochemical mechanism(s) of Sch B involved in tissue protection against noxious stimuli is instrumental in expediting its use in modern medicine. In the following sections, the pharmacological profile of Sch B and other structurally related lignans will be first described, followed by discussion of the biochemical mechanism(s) involved in various tissue protective actions.

II. PHARMACOLOGICAL PROFILE

A. Hepatoprotective Effects

Early pharmacological studies have demonstrated the ability of Sch B and other lignans in protecting against liver damage induced by a variety of chemicals, such as acetaminophen, carbon tetrachloride (CCl_4), thiacetamide, and immunlogical toxins, in rodents (11–18). Recent studies in our laboratory have also shown that Sch B pretreatment (0.5–4 mmol/kg/day $\times$ 3 days) protected against CCl_4 and tumor necrosis factor-α-induced hepatotoxicity in a dose-dependent manner in mice (19,20). Preliminary structure-activity relationship study, using Sch B and its lignan analogs, namely, schisandrin A (Sch A, Fig. 1b), schisandrin C (Sch C, Fig. 1c), and a synthetic intermediate of Sch C, dimethyl diphenyl bicarboxylate (DDB, Fig. 1d), indicated that the methylenedioxy group as well as the cyclooctadiene ring structure of Sch B are important structural determinants in its hepatoprotective action (21,22). Petreating mice with Sch B at a daily dose of 0.125–0.5 mmol/kg or

1 mmol/kg, respectively, for 3 days also reduced the extent of hepatic injury induced by tacrine/bis-tacrine or menadione (23,24). In addition, mice pretreated with Sch B at an oral daily dose of 1 mmol/kg for 3 days showed protective effect against galactosamine/endotoxin-induced toxicity (25). One point worth noting is that since lignans can cause irreversible inhibition on hepatic GPT (26), the inability of DDB to protect against CCl_4 hepatotoxicity, though decreasing plasma GPT activity, was evidenced by the negative histological assessment on hepatic damage (27). Paradoxically, DDB has been shown to improve liver functions of patients suffering from chronic hepatitis (28). The hepatoprotective effect of DDB may therefore be limited to certain kinds of liver injury, probably not that produced by CCl_4.

Treating rats with gomisin A [Gom A, Fig. 1e, a hydroxyl group (C_7)-containing structural analog of Sch B] at a daily dose of 30 or 100 mg/kg for 4 days could suppress the increase in serum transaminase activity and the appearance of histological changes induced in liver by CCl_4 or D-galactosamine (29). Gom A–treated rats (10–100 mg/kg/day, p.o., for 4 days) showed an accelerated proliferation of hepatocytes and recovery of liver function, as well as an increased hepatic blood flow after partial hepatectomy (30). In addition, Gom A (10 or 30 mg/kg, p.o., for 3 or 6 weeks) suppressed the fibrosis proliferation and accelerated both the liver regeneration and the recovery of liver function in CCl_4-induced chronic liver injury in rats (31).

The effect of Gom A treatment on immunologically induced liver injuries has been investigated (32–34). Gom A pretreatment (5–50 mg/kg, p.o., for 4 weeks) reduced the mortality in mice or occurrence of hepatic failure in guinea pigs subjected to immunological challenge. As for spontaneous hepatitis developed in Long Evans Cinnamon rats, Gom A treatment did not change the death rate, but the survival time was increased by 7–10 weeks when compared with that of the control (35).

B. Cardioprotective Effects

An early study in our laboratory has shown the myocardial protective effect of Shengmai San (36), a TCM formula used for the treatment of coronary heart disease (37), and the lignans derived from FS were found to contribute to the cardioprotective action (36). Pretreatment with the lignan-enriched FS extract, which has recently been shown to produce Sch B-like in vivo antioxidant activity at an equivalent potency of ~30% (w/w) (38), at an oral dose of 0.8 g/kg/day for 3 days, protected against isoproterenol-induced myocardial injury in rats and ischemia-reperfusion (IR)-induced injury in isolated perfused hearts prepared from the pretreated rats (36). The effects of Sch B treatment on myocardial IR injury in isolated rat hearts were subsequently investigated under both in vitro and ex vivo conditions (39).

In vitro administration of liposome-entrapped Sch B to the isolated-perfused hearts was found to be unable to protect against myocardial IR injury, whereas ascorbic acid and Trolox, a water-soluble analog of α-tocopherol, supplemented perfusate-produced protective effect, as evidenced by the significant decrease in the extent of lactate dehydrogenase (LDH) leakage as well as improvement in contractile force recovery. However, pretreatment with Sch B (0.6–1.2 mmol/kg/day, p.o., for 3 days) protected against IR-induced myocardial damage in a dose-dependent manner. A preliminary structure-activity relationship study indicated that both the methylenedioxy group and the cycloctadiene ring structure of Sch B are important structural determinants in mediating the protection against myocardial IR injury (40). Investigation of the possible pharmacological preconditioning effect of low doses of Sch B on the myocardium is underway in our laboratory.

C. Neuroprotective Effects

Sch B and schisanhenol (Sal, Fig. 1f, also a dibenzocyclooctadiene lignan) have been shown to protect oxidative damage induced in aging and ischemic-reperfused rat brain (41). Incubation of 8-month-old rat brain mitochondria and membrane suspension with a mixture of Fe^{2+}-cysteine resulted in the formation of malondialdehyde (MDA), an end product of lipid peroxidation, and a decrease in ATPase activity. Sch B and Sal (100 μM) completely inhibited these peroxidative damages induced by Fe^{2+}-cysteine in rat brain mitochondrial and membrane preparation [41]. Oral administration of Sch B or Sal (150 mg/kg) caused the increase in cytosolic glutathione peroxidase activity in rat brain tissue under anoxia and reoxygenation condition, with the effect of Sal being more potent (41). A recent study in our laboratory has demonstrated that Sch B pretreatment (1–2 mmol/kg, p.o., for 3 days) could reduce the mortality rate in a dose-dependent manner in mice following an intracerebroventricular injection of tert-butylhydroperoxide (42). However, DDB, when being administered at a dose of 2 mmol/kg/day, did not produce any significant effect on tert-butylhydroperoxide-induced cerebrotoxicity (43).

The ability of lignans to antagonize the effect of CNS-suppressing substances, such as barbiturates, chloral hydrate, and halothane, supports their CNS-activating activity (44). The lignan extract (1–5 mg/kg, i.p.) could inhibit the CNS suppressive effect of hexenal and chloral hydrate in rats. Moreover, the CNS-activating effect of lignans was antagonized by dopamine receptor DA_2 blocker. However, schisandrol A (Sol A, Fig. 1g, another lignan present in the extract) was found to prolong the sleeping time induced by phenobarbital and decrease the spontaneous motor activity in mice, a manifestation of CNS-depressing activity (45). Further investigation has revealed the significant elevations of dopamine and its metabolite DOPAC (in striatum) and DA (in hypothalamus) in mice after intraperitoneal administration of Sol A at a dose of 50 or 100 mg/kg (46). Furthermore, Sol A showed no affinity for dopamine D_1 and D_2 receptor, serotonin receptors, and α_1- and α_2-adrenergic receptors, nor did it affect the binding of dopamine D_1 and D_2 receptors. The inhibition exerted by schisandrol A on CNS activity may be related to the modulatory effect on dopamine metabolism in the CNS (46).

The cholinergic system is also influenced by the lignans. The lignan extract (10–30 mg/kg, p.o.) decreased the convulsant threshold and potentiated the antidiuretic action of nicotine, and potentiated the excitatory effect of carbachol on rat intestine (47,48). However, the lignans potentiated the action of reserpine only at a higher dose of 1.5 g/kg (48). In fact, the lignans affect the cholinergic system in a biphasic manner. At a lower dose of 280 mg/kg (p.o.), an indirect nicotinomimetic action was produced, whereas at a higher dose of 840 mg/kg (p.o.), a cholinolytic effect was observed (49).

A recent study has shown that pretreating mice with Sch B (0.025–0.5 mmol/kg/day, p.o., for 5 days) could enhance the passive avoidance response in mice, an indication of enhancement in cognitive function (23). This is consistent with the finding that lignan treatment (5–10 mg/day, p.o.) could improve the intellectual activity in humans (49).

D. Anticarcinogenic Effects

The effect of Gom A on hepatocarcinogenesis caused by 3′-methyl-4-dimethylaminobenzene (3′-MeDAB) in male Donryu rats has been investigated (50). Gom A treatment (30 mg/kg/day, p.o., for 5 weeks) significantly inhibited both increases in the number and size of glutathione S-transferases placental form (GST-P)-positive foci, a marker enzyme of preneoplasm, and the population of diploid nuclei, an indicator of proliferative state of hepatocytes, in the liver from rats simultaneously treated with 3′MeDAB. Gom A treatment also decreased the number of other hepatic-altered foci, such as those of the clear cell and basophilic cell type in the early stages (51). While Gom A increased GST activity in the liver by raising the level of GST-1 and 2 isozymes, it was observed that the biliary excretion of 3′MeDAB-related aminoazo dyes was increased in Gom A–treated rats, with its content in the liver being decreased in rats fed with a 3′-MeDAB-containing diet (50). Further study indicated that Gom A treatment (0.03% in the diet for 10 weeks) could reverse the 3′-MeDAB-induced increase in the ratio of diploid nuclei to tetrapoid nuclei (52). Gom A may therefore inhibit the hepatocarcingenesis induced by 3′-MeDAB by enhancing the excretion of the carcinogen from the liver as well as reversing the abnormal cytokinesis (50–53). When different types of tumor promoters such as phenobarbital (PB) and deoxycholic acid (DCA) were administered for 5 weeks after the initiation by 3′-MeDAB, preneoplastic alterations in the liver, as determined by GST-P, were markedly increased (54). Gom A (30 mg/kg/day, p.o., for 5 weeks) significantly inhibited the increases in the number and size of GST-P-positive foci, regardless of the presence of tumor promoters (54). Gom A treatment also suppressed the increase in serum bile acid concentration by DCA, but produced no effect on PB-treated animals. Since hepatocarcinogenesis has been reported to be promoted by exogenous administration of bile acids (55,56), the result suggests that the inhibitory effect of Gom A on the promotive action of DCA (but not PB) may be related to the decrease in bile acid production, presumably by improving bile acid metabolism (57).

Application (1 μg) of 1 2-O-tetradecanoylphorbol-13-acetate (TPA), a tumor promoter, to mouse ear could induce inflammation, and local administration of Gom A (0.6 mg/ear) inhibited TPA-induced inflammation (58). Furthermore, when administered at 5 μg/mouse, Gom A markedly suppressed the promotion effect of TPA (2.5 μg/mouse) on skin tumor formation in mice after initiation with 7,12-dimethylbenz[a]anthracene (50 μg/mouse) (58). The results suggest that the inhibition of tumor promotion by Gom A may be due to its anti-inflammatory activity.

E. Physical-Performance-Enhancing Effect

The effects of FS on counteracting fatigue, increasing endurance, and improving physical performance of sportsmen have long been reported (59). Until the late 1980s, no controlled studies have been documented. In a series of studies using horses, a dried ethanolic extract of FS, presumably lignan-containing, was administered orally (12 or 50 g/horse, p.o.) to thoroughbred horses 30 min prior to an 800-m race at maximum speed, and to spring horses subjected to a 12-min gallop at a speed of 400 m/min or a 5-min gallop at a speed of 700 m/min (60,61). The respiratory frequency and cardiac rate were significantly reduced in the treated horses subjected to both types of exercise, with the latter type of varied intensity, as compared to the respective control group. While plasma glucose concentration increased significantly in both types of exercise in the treated horses, the plasma lactic acid level was lower in treated horses, with the degree of decrease being more prominent in racing horses. Interestingly, horses treated with the lignan-containing FS extract were able to complete the race at an average of 1.8 sec faster, indicating an improvement in physical performance.

Poorly performing sports horses, which were found to be associated with long-lasting high serum activities of γ-glutamyltransferase (GGT), glutamate-oxaloacete transaminase (GOT), and creatine phosphokinase (CPK) (62), were orally administered with 3 g/day of the lignan-containing

FS extract (63). During the 14-day course of treatment, serum GGT and GOT activities were decreased on the seventh and fourteenth day. The decrease in serum CPK activity suggested a healing effect on muscle damage previously present in these horses (63). In this connection, a recent study in our laboratory has shown that pretreatment with a lignan-enriched FS extract, which contains biologically active lignans at ~30% (w/w) (vida infra), at a daily oral dose of 0.8 g/kg for 3 days protected against physical-exercise-induced muscle damage in rats (64).

F. Other Pharmacological Effects

Sch C and some other lignans were found to inhibit the growth of human immunodeficiency virus (HIV)-infected H9 cells at effective concentrations (EC) ranging from 0.006 to 1.2 μg/mL (65). Recently, halogenated derivatives of gomisin J (Fig. 1g) have been shown to possess anti-HIV activities by inhibiting reverse transcriptase activity as well as expressing cytoprotective action in HIV-infected H9 cells (66). In addition, the growth and clonogenicity as well as the topoisomerase II activity of hepatocarcinoma cells were inhibited by DDB (67). Sch C, with EC_{50} ranging from 0.36 to 7 μg/mL, produced cytotoxic effect on KB epidermoid carcinoma of nasopharynx, COLO-205 colon carcinoma, HEPA hepatoma, and HELA cervix tumor cells (68).

Several lignans isolated from FS were found to inhibit rat liver acetyl-CoA: cholesterol acetyltransferase activity at IC_{50} values of 25–200 mM, with gomisin N, a stereoisomer of Sch B, being most potent (69).

III. BIOCHEMICAL MECHANISMS OF ACTION

A. Detoxification/Antioxidant Actions

1. Induction of Detoxifying Enzymes

The hepatoprotection afforded by Sch B and other lignans could at least in part be attributed to the induction of hepatic cytochrome P-450-dependent (phase I) and GST (phase II) drug-metabolizing enzymes for detoxification reactions (6,7). Gom A increased the hepatic levels of microsomal cytochrome b5 and P-450, and activities of NADPH cytochrome C reductase, aminopyrine *N*-demethylase, and 7-ethoxycoumarin *O*-deethylase (11). As regards the CCl_4 hepatotoxicity, Sch B and Gom A could inhibit the CCl_4-induced lipid peroxidation as well as the binding of CCl_4 metabolites to the liver microsomal lipids (6,70,71). The ability of Sch B/Gom A to inhibit peroxidation of membrane lipids and hence maintain membrane stability of hepatocytes under oxidative stress conditions may also contribute to the hepatoprotective action against toxins that can generate reactive metabolites in the liver (72,73).

Sch B and Gom A inhibited demethylase activity induced by PB in liver microsomes in a similar manner as metyrone (70). Dual induction of Gom A and PB decreased the mutagenicity of benzo[a]pyrene (BP) by inhibiting the covalent binding of BP metabolites to DNA. Gom A also decreased the capacity of BP-induced rat microsomes to activate BP to its mutagenic metabolites (70).

2. In Vitro Antioxidant Activities

Lignans isolated from FS were found to possess antioxidant properties (74,75). Their inhibitory effect on lipid peroxidation reaction has been extensively investigated in a number of in vitro assay systems using microsomes and mitochondria prepared from brain, liver, and kidney cells/tissues as the lipid source (76–81). In all cases, the lignans, including Sch B and Gom A, were found to be more potent than α-tocopherol or its analogues, in the inhibition of lipid peroxidation. Using electron spin resonance measurement, lignans with different structures and configurations were investigated for scavenging activity on reactive oxy-radicals generated from human polymorphonuclear leukocytes stimulated by phorbol myristate acetate (82). The free-radical-scavenging activity was found to be dependent on the stereo-configurations of the lignans, in that S(-) Sch B produced a stronger effect than that of R(+) Sch B. Interestingly, the scavenging effect of S,R (±) Sch B was stronger than either that of S(-) or R(+)-Sch B (82). In this regard, a recent study in our laboratory indicated that the enantiomers of Sch B also produced differential effects on activities of hepatic glutathione antioxidant enzymes in mice (83).

3. In Vivo Antioxidant Potential

Antioxidant Actions of the Lignan-enriched FS Extract. CCl_4-induced hepatotoxicity is a commonly used model for investigating lipid peroxidation-related tissue injury (84). The involvement of free-radical-mediated reactions in the development of CCl_4-induced hepatic injury has been implicated in various in vitro and in vivo studies (85,86). The use of CCl_4 hepatotoxicity as an in vivo model for screening herbal extracts with antioxidant activities would be desirable (87). Early study examining the effect of the lignan-enriched FS extract on hepatic glutathione status in both control and CCl_4-treated rats has shown its ability to enhance hepatic glutathione status, as evidenced by increases in hepatic reduced glutathione (GSH) level and activities of hepatic glucose-6-phosphate dehydrogenase (G6PDH) and glutathione reductase (GRD), as well as a decreased susceptibility of hepatic tissue homogenates to in vitro peroxide-induced GSH depletion (88). The beneficial effect on hepatic glutathione status became more evident after CCl_4 challenge. Exposure of liver homogenates to an in vitro tert-butyl hydroperoxide challenge can be used as a means for measuring the GSH regeneration capacity (GRC) of hepatic tissues (89). Pretreatment of rats with the lignan extract caused a moderate enhancement of hepatic GRC in control rats, but the GRC-enhancing effect of the lignan pretreatment on hepatic tissues was greatly exaggerated after CCl_4 challenge (89). These results suggest that the mechanism of hepatoprotection afforded by the lignan extract may involve the facilitation of GSH regeneration via the GRD-catalyzed and NADPH-mediated reaction.

When examining the effect on rats subject to intoxication by aflatoxin B1 or cadmium chloride, which can produce hepatocellular damage through biochemical mechanisms different from that of CCl_4, the hepatoprotective action of the lignan-enriched FS extract was found to be nonhepatotoxin-specific and more effective than that of α-tocopherol (90). This supports the fundamental role of glutathione-related antioxidant and detoxification processes in the liver, which are effectively enhanced by the lignan extract treatment.

Increased physical activity is accompanied by significantly high rates of oxygen consumption and metabolism, particularly in skeletal muscle (91). Much evidence has now accumulated suggesting the involvement of reactive oxygen radicals in the development of exercise-mediated tissue injury (92). Significant elevations in plasma CPK, aspartate aminotransferases, and LDH, which are indicative of muscle damage, were observed immediately after physical activities exercise both in humans (93) and in rats (94). It has been postulated that liver may supply GSH to skeletal muscle as a protective antioxidant (95). In this regard, the protective effect of the lignan-enriched extract on physical exercise-induced muscle damage may be related to the enhancement of hepatic GSH status, thereby providing sufficient GSH for effective antioxidant protection of skeletal muscle during exercise (64).

Antioxidant Actions of Sch B. The hepatoprotection afforded by Sch B pretreatment was found to be mainly attributed to the enhancement in the functioning of the hepatic glutathione antioxidant system, possibly through stimulating the activities of glutathione related enzymes (19). A later study indicated that Sch B protected against CCl_4 toxicity by enhancing the mitochondrial glutathione redox status in mouse liver (96). However, treating mice with 1,3-bis(2-chloroethyl)-1-nitrosourea, an inhibitor of GRD, did not deplete hepatic GSH or abrogate the hepatoprotective action of Sch B in CCl_4-treated mice (96). The hepatic G6PDH-catalyzed formation of NADPH, but not GRD activity, may therefore be a limiting factor in Sch B–induced enhancement in the regeneration of GSH. A comparison between the effects of Sch B and butylated hydroxytoluene (BHT), a synthetic phenolic antioxidant, was made to identify the critical antioxidant action of Sch B involved in hepatoprotection in mice (97). The ability of Sch B, but not BHT, to sustain hepatic mitochondrial GSH level, as well as hepatic ascorbic acid and α-tocopherol levels, represents a crucial antioxidant action in protecting against CCl_4 hepatotoxicity. In further defining the antioxidant mechanism of Sch B, the effects of Sch B and α-tocopherol on ferric-chloride-induced oxidation of erythrocyte membrane lipids in vitro and CCl_4-induced lipid peroxidation in vivo were examined (98). The ability of Sch B to inhibit lipid peroxidation, while being in the absence of pro-oxidant activity as compared to α-tocopherol, would make it a more desirable antioxidant in vivo.

The antioxidant effect of Sch B can be extended to extrahepatic tissues. The myocardial protection afforded by Sch B pretreatment against myocardial IR injury was also associated with an enhancement in myocardial glutathione antioxidant status (39). In contrast, the inability of DDB to enhance myocardial glutathione antioxidant status resulted in a failure in preventing IR injury (40). Since the in vitro perfusion of isolated hearts with Sch B–containing perfusate did not protect against IR injury, the myocardial protective action of Sch B was unlikely owing to free-radical-scavenging action (39). Instead, the cardioprotection may be mainly mediated by the enhancement of myocardial glutathione antioxidant status, particularly under oxidative stress conditions. In addition, modulations in tissue level of nonenzymatic antioxidants such as ascorbic acid and α-tocopherol in response to IR challenge, which may be an effect secondary to the enhancement of myocardial glutathione status, were also observed in Sch B–pretreated hearts [99]. A recent study has shown that a single dose of Sch B treatment produced a time-dependent enhancement in myocardial mitochondrial glutathione antioxidant status (100). This effect was paralleled by the stimulation in mitochondrial ATP generation and protection against IR injury (91).

GSH plays an important role in the maintenance of cellular redox status and antioxidant defense (101). The ability of Sch B to enhance hepatic and myocardial glutathione status can offer an effective antioxidant protection by sustaining the fundamental cellular defense system against oxidative challenge. The nonenzymatic antioxidants such as GSH, ascorbic acid, and α-tocopherol work synergistically in cellular antioxidant defense (102,103), in that the enhanced cellular GSH status facilitates the regeneration of ascorbic acid and α-tocopherol from their oxidized forms (104,105). As a result, the functional integrity of the cellular antioxidant defense can be maintained even under conditions of increased oxidative stress.

Being the major site of oxygen free-radical production, mitochondrion requires strong antioxidant protection. The maintenance of mitochondrial glutathione redox status is critical for cell viability (106,107). The ability of Sch B to increase the mitochondrial GSH level therefore represents an ultimate defense against free-radical attack. In addition, liver can supply

GSH to other tissues by exporting GSH into the blood for subsequent uptake in extrahepatic tissues. The enhancement of hepatic glutathione status by Sch B may produce a generalized antioxidant effect on organs other than the liver. Sch B or the lignan extract was found to protect myocardial, brain, as well as skeletal muscle tissues against free-radical-induced damage. The generalized tissue-protective effect of Sch B may be related to its ability to produce a sustainable and GSH-mediated antioxidant effect on various tissues.

B. Enhancement/Protection of Liver Function

It has also been suggested that Gom A can enhance liver function under normal or injured conditions, in that the prevention of CCl_4-induced cholestasis can be attributed to its sustained stimulatory action on secretion of the bile-acid-independent fraction from the liver (12). Sch B and Gom A induced hypertrophy and mild hyperplasia of the liver, resulting in the increase in liver weight (108). Hepatic [^{14}C] phenylalanine incorporation, protein content, and microsomal cytochrome P-450 content were also increased (108,109). Gom A helps to regenerate the liver tissue after partial hepatectomy by enhancing ornithine decarboxylase activity, an important biochemical event in the early stages of liver regeneration in rats (110). Gom A was also found to promote hepatocyte growth after mitosis during regeneration of partially resected rat liver, and enhanced directly or indirectly the proliferative process of non-parenchymal cells, which was likely mediated by an increase expression of c-myc gene preceding DNA replication in proliferating cells (111).

Leukotrienes are potent inflammatory agents that are thought to play a role in inflammatory liver diseases (112). In immunologically induced hepatic failure, mononuclear cells are the predominant cells producing leukotrienes. The ability of Gom A to inhibit the biosynthesis of leukotrienes induced in rat peritoneal macrophages by Ca^{2+} ionophore A2318 may also be related to its antihepatotoxic effect (113). Furthermore, liver cells could be injured by antibody-dependent cell-mediated cytotoxicity (ADCC) reaction or marcophage activation. The inhibition of liver cell injury induced by ADCC or macrophage activation in vitro by Gom A may be related to the protective effect on immunologically induced liver failure (32).

Liver plays an important role in glucose synthesis by converting lactic acid or other keto-acids arising from anaerobic metabolism occurring in muscle during physical exercise back to glucose. The increase in activity of hepatic transaminase enzymes, which can deplete the level of glucose precursors by converting them into amino acids, was found to be associated with the impairment in physical performance in horses (62). An association between poor performance and high serum activities of these hepatic enzymes has been demonstrated (62). The lignans derived from FS, which can inhibit liver transaminase activities (26), can therefore sustain the blood glucose level through hepatic gluconeogenetic process during physical exercise, thereby improving the endurance and performance.

C. Heat Shock Proteins Induction

Heat shock proteins (Hsps) are a family of inducible and constitutively expressed gene products that collectively function to maintain cellular protein conformation during stress conditions. The synthesis of Hsps is induced by a variety of mild stresses, including oxidants, heat, hypoxia, and low pH, all of which can affect protein conformation (114). The synthesis of Hsps allows cells to adapt to gradual changes in their environment and to survive in otherwise lethal conditions (115). Increased production of Hsps by heat shock or other forms of stress, or gene overexpression, was found to be associated with tissue protection against noxious stimuli (116–120). The ability of Sch B to induce Hsp 70 production and protect against TNF-α–induced hepatic apoptosis in mice suggests the involvement of Hsp induction as a fundamental protective mechanism (20), in addition to the enhancement of mitochondrial glutathione antioxidant status (97), in its generalized tissue-protective action. Investigation of the correlation between induction of Hsps and enhancement of cellular/tissue antioxidant status afforded by Sch B treatment in respect to its hepato- and cardioprotective actions is currently underway in our laboratory. Preliminary results indicated that the hepatoprotective action of Sch B against CCl_4 toxicity seemed to be mediated by both enhancement of mitochondrial glutathione antioxidant status and induction of Hsp 25/70 (121).

D. Other Biochemical Actions

The effect of gomisin C (Gom C, Fig. 1h) on the respiratory burst induced by the peptide (formyl Met-Leu-Phe, FMLP) was investigated in rat neutrophils (122). Gom C was found to inhibit FMLP-induced superoxide radical formation and oxygen consumption in a concentration-dependent manner. The inhibitory action of Gom C on the respiratory burst may be mediated partly by the suppression of NADPH oxidase activity on neutrophils and partly by the decrease of cytosolic Ca^{2+} released from an agonist-sensitive intracellular store (122). This activity may contribute to the anti-inflammatory action of lignans.

The effect of lignans on the binding of platelet-activating factor on rabbit platelets was examined (123). Among the three lignans, Sch A showed the most potent antagonistic activity, and Sch C produced only marginal activity. It is therefore suggested that Sch A and Sch B may be responsible, at least in part (together with other active compounds), for the antitussive effect of FS (123).

IV. PHARMACOKINETICS AND METABOLISM

After oral administration of 15 mg Sch B to healthy male subjects, the mean value of maximum plasma concentration was found to be 96.1 ± 14.1 ng/mL (~0.25 μM) (124). The lignan molecule was metabolized by rat liver microsomes to give three main phase I metabolites. Several oxidation routes appear to be involved: (1) hydroxylation of an alkyl substitute and (2) demethylation of the -OCH3 groups on the aromatic rings (125). The metabolites were detectable in urine and bile of rats. A recent study indicated that the methoxy group of Sch B or Sch A could be demethylated by demethylase present in red blood cells and then further metabolized to produce phenolic hydroxyl group (126).

Oral administration of Gom A at a dose of 10 mg/kg resulted in a maximum serum concentration of 1446.1 ± 131.8 ng/mL in 15–30 min in rats, with over 80% of the compound being bound to serum proteins (127,128). After intravenous administration at doses of 1.6–10 mg/kg, the serum concentration of Gom A decreased biphasically, with the terminal elimination half-life being about 70 min (128). The biotransformation of Gom A to its demethylated metabolite (Met-B) was very rapid after both oral and intravenous administration, with the amount of Met-B after oral administration of Gom A at a dose of 1.6 mg/kg being relatively larger than those of other dosages. It was suggested that Gom A underwent first pass extensively, producing demethylated metabolites (127) as well as glucuronic and arylsulfate conjugates (129).

Sol A was readily absorbed after oral administration, with a half-life of 58 min in rats (130). The blood level of Sol A showed a biphasic decline after intravenous injection, with the half-life of the distribution phase and elimination phase being 1.4 and 42 min, respectively. Sol A was also detectable in urine 1 hr after oral administration. Five minutes after intravenous injection, a high level of Sol A was detected in the lungs, moderate levels in the liver, heart, brain, and kidneys, and low levels in the ileum and spleen. As regards the brain, which is the major site of action of Sol A, relatively high levels in the hypothalamus, striatum, and hippocampus and moderate levels in the cerebral cortex and cerebellum were detected. This distribution pattern may be related to the neuroleptic and anticonvulsant actions of Sol A.

V. TOXICOLOGY AND ADVERSE SIDE EFFECTS

The oral and intraperitoneal LD_{50} values of a petroleum ether extract of FS [containing 40% (w/w) lignans] were 10.5 and 4.4 g/kg, respectively (48).

Subchronic toxicity of an extract of FS (standardized to a minimum of 2% lignans) was examined in Landrace piglets at daily doses ranging from 0.07 to 0.72 g/kg for 90 days (131). Both body weight and the amount of food intake were not affected during the entire experimental period, and all blood parameters were not changed in the treated animals. No pathological changes were observed in major organs and tissues, an indication of no long-term toxicity. In another study using the same extract (0.1–0.5 g/kg/day), no fetotoxicity as well as no changes in other reproductive parameters such as implantation efficiency were observed in rats and mice.

No death was observed following a single oral dose of Sch B at 2 g/kg in rats (49). In addition, an intragastric dose of 200 mg of Sch B for 30 days caused no significant changes in body weight, blood parameters, or histological parameters of major organs in mice (49). Furthermore, Sch B, when given at 10 mg/kg daily for 4 weeks, did not affect appetite, blood parameters, liver or kidney functions, as well as liver histological parameters in dogs (49).

Gom A (0.01% or 0.03% in the diet for 40 weeks) did not cause any proliferative and neoplastic lesions in rats (50).

Information on clinical toxicity of lignans is scarce. Two cases of interaction between cyclosporin and DDB in kidney transplant patients with chronic hepatitis have been reported, in which cyclosporin was decreased to a subtherapeutic level (132).

VI. EAST-MEETS-WEST MEDICINE

According to TCM, the "five tastes" of FS bespeak much of its influence on the five visceral organs. In this regard, a renowned Chinese herbalist, Sun Simiao (A.D. 581–682), in the Tang dynasty, had noted that "taking *Schisandra* berry in May can invigorate the qi of the five viscerae." Given the indispensable role of qi in body functioning, this points to the possibility that FS can produce beneficial effect on major organs in the body. Over the past 10 years, our laboratory has attempted to define the biochemical properties of FS in regard to its purported qi invigorating action. A generalized tissue-protective action of FS or its lignan constituents has been demonstrated.

In the realm of TCM, qi, literally meaning energy, is regarded as the "root of life"; body functions are often explained in terms of qi. qi can be broadly defined as the minute substances circulating inside the body and their functional role. Alternatively, qi can be regarded as a manifestation of functional status of organs, which is in turn dependent on their neuroendocrinological regulation and energy-transforming process. Among different qi's associated with various visceral organs, the "heart-qi" and "lung-qi" are of vital importance. The normal functioning of circulatory and respiratory systems is essential to deliver oxygen and fuel molecules for maintaining cellular activities—the cellular manifestation of qi. In this connection, ischemic heart disease, the most precarious killer in industrialized countries, is a clinical manifestation of depletion of "heart-qi" and subsequently "lung-qi." Given the universal requirement of ATP—the biochemical unit of qi for energizing cellular activities, mitochondrion—the powerhouse for ATP generation in the cell—becomes the de facto cell origin of qi. However, reactive oxygen species also arise from the mitochondrial energy-transforming process. If these reactive oxidants are not removed effectively, they can cause damage in the mitochondrion as well as other cellular components.

The finding of the ability of Sch B to enhance mitochondrial glutathione antioxidant status and stimulate ATP generation not only provides a biochemical explanation for its qi-invigorating action (100), but also offers an insight into the molecular mechanism involved in generalized tissue protection. As mitochondrion is the central coordinator in regulating apoptosis (133), the Sch B–induced mitochondrial changes and the relevant signal transduction pathways leading to apoptosis will be of interest for further investigations. Given the mitochondrial decay in aging (134), the ability of Sch B to maintain mitochondrial function integrity may provide a practical approach for retarding the aging process and delaying the onset of age-related diseases such as Alzheimer's disease and Parkinson's disease.

VII. CONCLUSIONS

Over the past few decades, the pharmacological activities of Sch B and other lignans have been extensively studied. Early evidence indicated that the lignans could produce beneficial effect on liver functions, particularly in enhancing the detoxification of xenobiotics and the regeneration of liver. Later studies have also demonstrated their modulating effects on CNS activity and anticarcinogenic activity, as well as cardioprotective action. Investigations on the biochemical mechanism(s) involved in the generalized tissue protective effect afforded by Sch B and other lignans have revealed their in vitro and in vivo antioxidant activities, particularly in enhancing the mitochondrial gluthathione antioxidant status. The ability of Sch B to induce Hsps production may also represent a fundamental mechanism involved in tissue protection. Given the novel in vivo antioxidant potential, Sch B may be used for the prevention and/or treatment of free-radical-mediated tissue damage such as inflammations, radiation injury, and reperfusion injury. The beneficial effect of lignans on cardiopulmonary as well as liver function during physical exercise would make it a good candidate for sport supplement. The anticancer and anti-HIV activities of specific lignans also deserve further investigations for developing new therapeutic agents.

ACKNOWLEDGMENTS

Relevant works generated from KMK's laboratory were supported in part by a grant from Lee Kum Kee Group Ltd., Hong Kong and the Research Grants Council of Hong Kong (HKUST 6130/02M).

REFERENCES

1. Lebedev AA. Limonnik (*Schisandra chinensis*). Tashkent, Uzbek SSR: Medicina Publishing House, 1971.
2. Pharmacopoeia of the People's Republic of China. Beijing, China: The Peoples Medical Publishing House, 1988.
3. Chinese Academy of Medical Sciences Medical References 1972; 7:3.
4. Liu GT. Pharmacological actions and clinical use of fructus schizandrae. Chin Med J 1989; 102:740–749.
5. Bao TT, Tu GF, Liu GT, Sun RH, Song ZY. A comparison of the pharmacological actions of seven constituents isolated from fructus schizandrae. Yao Hsueh Hsueh Pao 1979; 14:1–7.
6. Liu KT, Cresteil T, Columelli S, Lesca P. Pharmacological properties of dibenzo[a,c]cyclooctene derivatives isolated from fructus schisandrae chinensis. II. Induction of phenobarbital-like hepatic monooxygenases. Chem Biol Interact 1982; 39:315–330.
7. Li Y, Paranawithana SR, Yoo JSH, Ning SM, Ma BL, Liu GT, Yang CS. Induction of liver microsomal cytochrome P-450 2B1 by dimethyldiphenyl bicardboxylate in rats. Acta Pharmacol Sin 1992; 13:485–490.
8. Ohtaki Y, Nomura M, Hida T, Miyamoto KI, Kanitani M, Aizawa T, Aburada M. Inhibition by gomisin A, a lignan compound, of hepatocarcinogenesis by 3′-methyl-4-diemethylaminoazobenzene in rats. Biol Pharmaceut Bull 1994; 17:808–814.
9. Lin TJ, Liu GT, Pan Y, Liu Y, Xu GZ. Protection by schisanhenol against adriamycin toxicity in rat heart mitochondria. Biochem Pharmacol 1991; 42:1805–1810.
10. Xue JY, Liu GT, Liu GT, Wei HL, Pan Y. Antioxidant activity of two dibenzocyclooctene lignans on aged and ischemic brain rats. Free Rad Biol Med 1992; 12:127–135.
11. Takeda S, Funo S, Iizyka A, Kase Y, Arai I, Ohkura Y, Sudo K, Kiuchi N, Yosida C, Maeda S. Pharmacological studies on *Schizandra* fruits. III. Effects of wuweizi C, a lignan component of *Schizandra* fruits, on experimental liver injuries in rats. Nippon Yakurigaku Zasshi 1985; 85:193–208.
12. Maeda S, Takeda S, Miyamoto Y, Aburada M, Harada M. Effects of gomisin A on liver functions in hepatotoxic chemicals–treated rats. Jpn J Pharmacol 1985; 38:347–353.
13. Takeda S, Maemura S, Sudo K, Kase Y, Arai I, Ohkura Y, Funo S, Fujii Y, Aburada M, Hosoya E. Effects of gomisin A, a lignan component of *Schizandra* fruits on experimental liver injuries and liver microsomal drug-metabolizing enzymes. Nippon Yakurigaku Zasshi 1986; 87:169–187.
14. Nagai H, Yakuo I, Aoki M, Teshima K, Ono Y, Sengoku T, Shimazawa T, Aburada M, Koda A. The effect of gomisin A on immunologic liver injury in mice. Planta Med 1989; 55:13–17.
15. Ohkura Y. Protective effects of gomisin A on the liver injury. J Osaka City Medi Cent 1991; 40:159–171.
16. Mizoguchi Y, Kawada N, Ichikawa Y, Tsutsui H. Effect of gomisin A in the prevention of acute hepatic failure induction. Planta Med 1991; 40:159–171.

17. Hikino H, Kiso Y. Natural products for liver diseases. In: Wagner H, Farnsworth N, eds. Economic and Medicinal Plant Research. New York: Academic Press Ltd, 1988:53–72.
18. Bao T, Liu G, Song Z, Xu G, Sun R. A comparison of the pharmacologic actions of 7 constituents isolated from fructus schizandrae. Chin Med J (Engl) 1980; 93:41–47.
19. Ip SP, Poon MKT, Wu SS, Che CT, Ng KH, Kong YC, Ko KM. Effect of schisandrin B on hepatic glutathione antioxidant system in mice: protection against carbon tetrachloride toxicity. Planta Med 1995; 61:398–401.
20. Ip SP, Che CT, Kong YC, Ko KM. Effects of schisandrin B pretreatment on tumor necrosis factor-α induced apoptosis and Hsp70 expression in mouse liver. Cell Stress Chaperones 2001; 6:44–48.
21. Ip SP, Ma CY, Che CT, Ko KM. Methylene group as determinant of schisandrin in enhancing hepatic mitochondrial glutathione in carbon tetrachloride–intoxicated mice. Biochem Pharmacol 1997; 54:317–319.
22. Ip SP, Yiu HY, Ko KM. Differential effect of schisandrin B and dimethyl diphenyl bicarboxylate (DDB) on hepatic mitochondrial glutathione redox status in carbon tetrachloride intoxicated mice. Mol Cell Biochem 2000; 205:111–114.
23. Pan SY, Han YF, Carlier PR, Pang YP, Mak DHF, Lam BYH, Ko KM. Schisandrin B protects against tacrine- and bis(7)-tacrine-induced hepatotoxicity and enhances cognitive function in mice. Planta Med 2002; 68:217–220.
24. Ip SP, Yiu HY, Ko KM. Schisandrin B protects against menadione-induced hepatotoxicity by enhancing DT-diapphorase activity. Mol Cell Biochem 2000; 208:151–155.
25. SP Ip. Antioxidant mechanisms of schisandrin B in protecting against carbon tetrachloride hepatotoxicity. Ph.D. thesis, Hong Kong University of Science and Technology, Hong Kong, 1998:126-130.
26. Hikino H, Kiso Y, Taguchi H, Ikeya Y. Antihepatotoxic actions of lignoids from *Schizandra chinensis* fruits. Planta Med 1984; 50:213–218.
27. Liu J, Liu Y, Klassen CD. The effect of Chinese hepatoprotective medicines on experimental liver injury in mice. J Ethnopharmacol 1994; 42:183–191.
28. Yosida T, Ueno T, Miyazaki A, Sugie H, Yosida M. Clinical effect of biphenyl dimethy dicarboxylate administration on chronic hepatitis. Jpn J Gastroenterol 1989; 86:965.
29. Takeda S, Arai I, Kase Y, Okura Y, Hasegawa M, Sekiguchi Y, Sudo K, Aburada M, Hosoya E. Pharmacological studies on antihepatotoxic action of (+)-(6S,7S,R-biar)-5,6,7,8-tetrahydro-1,2,3,12-tetramethoxy-6,7-dimethyl-10,11-methylenedioxy-6-dibenzo[a,c]cyclooctenol (TJN-101), a lignan component of *Schisandra* fruits: influences of resolvents on the efficacy of TJN-101 in experimental acute hepatic injuries. Nippon Yakurigaku Zasshi 1987; 107:517–524.
30. Takeda S, Maemura S, Sudo K, Kase Y, Ohkura Y, Funo S, Fujii T, Abarada M, Hosoya E. Effects of gomisin A, a lignan component of *Schizandra* fruits, on experimental liver injuries and liver microsomal drug-metabolizing enzymes. Nippon Yakurigaku Zasshi 1986; 87:169–187.

31. Takeda S, Kase Y, Arai I, Ohkura Y, Hasegawa M, Sekiguchi Y, Tatsugi A, Funo S, Aburada M, Hosoya E. Effects of TNJ-101, a lignan compound isolated from *Schizandra* fruits, on liver necrosis and liver regeneration after partial hepatectomy in rats with chronic liver injury induced by CCl_4. Nippon Yakurigaku Zasshi 1987; 90:51–65.
32. Ohkura Y, Mizoguchi Y, Sakagami Y, Kobayashi K, Yamamoto S, Morisawa S, Takeda S, Aburada M. Inhibitory effect of TNJ-101 ((+)-(6S,7S, R-biar)-5,6,7,8-tetrahydro-1,2,3,12-tetramethoxy-6,7-dimethyl-10,11-methylenedioxy-6-dibenzo[a,c]cyclooctenol) on immunologically induced liver injuries. Jpn J Pharmacol 1987; 44:179–185.
33. Mizoguchi Y, Shin T, Kobayashi K, Morisawa S. Effect of gomisin A in an immunologically-induced acute hepatic failure model. Planta Med 1991; 57:11–14.
34. Mizoguchi Y, Kawada N, Ichikawa S, Tsusui H. Effect of gomisin A in the prevention of acute hepatic failure induction. Planta Med 1991; 57:320–324.
35. Yokoi T, Nagayama S, Kajiwara R, Kawaguchi Y, Aizawa T, Otaki Y, Aburada M, Kamataki T. Occurrence of autoimmune antibodies to liver microsomal proteins associated with lethal hepatitis in LEC rats: effects of TJN-101 ((+)-(6S,7S,R-biar)-5,6,7,8-tetrahydro-1,2,3,12-tetramethoxy-6,7-dimethyl-10,11-methylenedioxy-6-dibenzo[a,c]cyclooctenol) on the development of hepatitis and the autoantibodies. Toxicol Lett 1995; 76:33–38.
36. Li PC, Mak DHF, Poon MKT, Ip SP, Ko KM. Myocardial protective effect of Shengmai San (SMS) and a lignan-enriched extract of fructus schisandrae, in vivo and ex vivo. Phytomedicine 1996; III:217–221.
37. Liang SM, Chen SY, Liang SQ. Shengmai San—a renowned traditional Chinese medicinal formula. In: Ko KM, ed. Traditional Herbal Medicines for Modern Times: Shengmai San. London, New York: Taylor & Francis, 2002: 1–15.
38. Chiu PY, Mak DHF, Poon MKT, Ko KM. In vivo antioxidant action of a lignan-enriched extract of *Schisandra* fruit and an anthraquinone-containing extract of *Polygonum* root in comparison to schisandrin B and emodin. Planta Med 2002; 68:951–956.
39. Yim TK, Ko KM. Schisandrin B protects against myocardial ischemia-reperfusion injury by enhancing myocardial glutathione antioxidant status. Mol Cell Biochem 1999; 196:151–156.
40. Yim TK, Ko KM. Methylenedioxy group and cyclooctadiene ring as structural determinants of schisandrin in protecting against myocardial ischemia-reperfusion injury in rats. Biochem Pharmacol 1999; 57:77–81.
41. Xue JY, Liu GT, Wei HL, Pan Y. Antioxidant activity of two dibenzocyclooctene lignans on the aged and ischemic brain in rats. Free Rad Biol Med 1992; 12:127–135.
42. BYH Lam, KM Ko, Schisandrin B protects against tert-butylhydroperoxide induced cerebral toxicity by enhancing glutathione antioxidant status in mouse brain. Mol Cell Biochem 2002; 238:181–186.
43. Lam BYH. Antioxidant effect of schisandrin B on nervous system. M.Phil.

thesis. Hong Kong University of Science and Technology, Hong Kong, 2001:75-84.
44. Niu XY, Wang WJ, Bian ZJ, Ren ZH. Effect of schisandrol on the central nervous system. Acta Pharmacol Sin, 1983; 416–421.
45. Hancke JL, Wikman G, Hernandez DE. Planta Med 1986; P85:6262. [abstract].
46. Niu XY, Bian ZJ, Ren ZH. Metabolism of schisandrol A in rats and its distribution in brain determined by TLC-UV. Acta Pharmacol Sin 1983; 18:491–495.
47. Volicer L, Jankú J, Motl O, Jircka Z. In: Chen KK, ed. Pharmacology of Oriental plants. Oxford: Pergamon Press, 1965:29–38.
48. Volicer L, Sramka M, Jankú I, Capek R, Smetana R, Ditteová V. Some pharmacological effects of *Schizandra* chinensis. Arch Int Pharmacodyn Ther 1966; 163:249–262.
49. Chang HM, But PPH. Chang HM, But PPH, eds. Pharmacology and Applications of Chinese Materia Medica. Vol. 1. Singapore: World Scientific pp. 199–209).
50. Miyamoto K, Wakusawa S, Nomura M, Sanae F, Sakai R, Sudo K, Ohtaki Y, Takeda S, Fujii Y. Effects of gomisin A on hepatocarcinogenesis by 3′-methyl-4-dimethylaminoazobenzene in rats. Jpn J Pharmacol 1991; 57:71–77.
51. Nomura M, Ohtaki Y, Hida T, Aizawa T, Wakita H, Miyamoto K. Inhibition of early 3-methyl-4-dimethylaminoazobenzene-induced hepatocarcinogenesis by gomisin A in rats. Anticancer Res 1994; 14:1967–1971.
52. Nomura M, Nakachiyama M, Hida T, Oktaki Y, Sudo K, Aizawa T, Aburada M, Miyamoto KI, Gomisin A. lignan component of *Schizandra* fruits, inhibits development of preneoplastic leasions in rat liver by 3′-methyl-4-diemethyl-aminoazobenzene. Cancer Lett 1994; 76:11–18.
53. Ohtaki Y, Nomura M, Hida T, Miyamoto K, Kanitani M, Aizawa T, Aburada M. Inhibition by gomisin A, a lignan compound, of hepatocarcinogenesis by 3′-methylaminoazobenzene in rats. Biol Pharm Bull 1994; 17:808–824.
54. Miyamoto K, Hiramatsu K, Ohtaki Y, Kanitani M, Nomura M, Aburada M. Effects of gomisin A on the promoter action and serum bile acid concentration in hepatocarcinogenesis induced by 3′-methyl-4-aminoazobenzene. Biol Pharm Bull 1995; 18:1443–1445.
55. Cameron RG, Imaida K, Tauda Ito N. Promotive effects of steroids and bile acids on hepatocarcinogenesis initiated by diethylnitrosamine. Cancer Res 1982; 42:2426–2428.
56. Porsch H, Svensson D, Blanck A. Sex-differentiated deoxycholic acid promotion of rat liver carcinogenesis is under pituitary control. Carcinogenesis 1991; 12:2035–2040.
57. Ohtaki Y, Hida T, Hiramatsu K, Kanitani M, Ohshima T, Nomura M, Wakita H, Aburada M, Miyamoto KI. Deoxycholic acid as an endogenous risk factor for hepatocarcinogenesis and effects of gomisin A, a lignan component of *Schizandra* fruits. Anticancer Res 1996; 16:751–755.
58. Yasukawa K, Ikeya Y, Mitsuhashi H, Iwasaki M, Nakagawa S, Takeuchi M, Takido M. Gomisin A inhibits tumor promotion by 12-O-tetradecanoylphor-

bol-13-acetate in two-stage carcinogenesis in mouse skin. Oncology 1992; 4: 68–71.
59. Fulder S. The drug that builds Russians. New Scientist 1980; 87(1215):576–579.
60. Ahumada F, Hermosilla J, Hola R, Peña R, Wittwer F, Hancke J, Wikman G. Studies on the effect of *Schizandra chinensis* extract on horses submitted to exercise and maximum effort. Phytother Res 1989; 3:175–179.
61. Hancke J, Burgos R, Wikman G, Ewertz E, Ahumada F. *Schizandra chinenesis*, a potential phytodrug for recovery of sport horses. Fitotherapia 1994; LXV:113–118.
62. Blood DC, Henderson JA, Radostitis OM. Medicina Veterinaria Interamericana. 6th ed. Mexico, 1986:80-85.
63. Hancke J, Burgos R, Caceres D, Brunetti F, Durigon A, Wikman G. Reduction of serum hepatic transaminases and CPK in sport horses with poor performance treated with a standardized Schizandra chinensis fruit extract. Phytomedicine 1996; 3:237–240.
64. Ko KM, Mak DHF, Li PC, Poon MKT, Ip SP. Protective effect of a lignan-enriched extract of fructus schisandrae on physical exercise induced muscle damage in rats. Phytother Res 1996; 10:450–452.
65. Chen DF, Zhang SX, Xie L, Xie JX, Chen K, Kashiwada Y, Zhou BN, Wang P, Cosentino LM, Lee KH. Anti-AIDS agent. XXVI. Structure-activity correlations of gomisin-G–related anti-HIV lignans from Kadsura interior and of related synthetic analogues. Bioorg Med Chem 1997; 5:1715–1723.
66. Fujihashi T, Hara H, Sakata T, Mori K, Higuchi H, Tanaka A, Kai H, Kaji A. Anti-human immunodeficiency virus (HIV) activities of halogenated gomisin J derivatives, new nonnucleoside inhibitors of HIV type I reverse transcriptase. Antimicrob Agents Chemother 1995; 39:2000–2007.
67. Liu Z, Chen L, Dong J, Li Y, Luo D. Anaerobic-aerobic injury in cerebrum of rabbits and the protective effect of Chinese magnoliavine (*Schisandra chinensis*) extract. Zhongcaoyao 1996; 27:355–357. [in Chinese].
68. Kuo YH, Kuo LMY, Chen CF. Four new C19 homolignans, schiarisanrins A, B and D and cytotoxic schiarisanrin C, from *Schizandra arisanensis*. J Org Chem 1997; 62:3242–3245.
69. Kwon BM, Jung HJ, Lim JH, Kim YS, Kim MK, Kim YK, Bok SH, Bae KH, Lee IR. Acetyl-CoA: cholesterol acetyltransferase inhibitory activity of lignans isolated from *Schisandra, Machilus*, and *Magnolia* species. Planta Med 1999; 65:74–76.
70. Liu KT, Lesca P. Pharmacological properties of dibenzo[a,c]cyclooctene derivatives isolated from fructus schizandrae chinensis, I. Interaction with rat liver cytochrome P-450 and inhibition of xenobiotic metabolism and mutagenicity. Chem Biol Interact 1982; 39:301–314.
71. Liu KT, Lesca P. Pharmacological properties of dibenzo[a,c]cyclooctene derivatives isolated from fructus schizandrae chinensis, III. Inhibitory effects on carbon tetrachloride-induced lipid peroxidation, metabolism and covalent binding of carbon tetrachloride to lipids. Chem Biol Interact 1982; 41:39–47.
72. Zhang TM, Wang BE, Liu GT. Effect of schisandrin B on lipoperoxidative

damage to plasma membrane of rat liver in vitro. Acta Pharmacol Sin 1992; 13:255–258.
73. Nagai H, Yakuo I, Aoki M, Teshima K, Ono Y, Sengoku T, Shimazawa T, Aburada M, Koda A. The effect of gomisin A on immunological liver injury in mice. Planta Med 1989; 55:13–17.
74. Kiso Y, Tohkin M, Hikino H, Ikeya Y, Taguchi H. Mechanism of antihepatotoxic activity of wuweizisu C and gomisin A. Planta Med 1985; 4:331–334.
75. Liu J, Xiao PG. Recent advances in the study of antioxidative effects of Chinese medicinal plants. Phytother Res 1994; 8:445–451.
76. Lu H, Liu GT. Effect of dibenzo[a,c]cyclooctene lignans isolated from fructus schisandrae on lipid peroxidation and antioxidant enzyme activity. Chem Biol Interact 1991; 78:77–84.
77. Zhang TM, Wang BE, Liu GT. Effect of schisandrin B on liperoxidative damage to plasma membrane of rat liver in vitro. Acta Pharmacol Sin 1992; 13:255–258.
78. Tongjun L, Gengtao L, Yan P. Protective effect of schisanhenol against oxygen radical induced mitochondrial toxicity on rat heart and liver. Biomed Environ Sci 1992; 5:57–64.
79. Lu H, Liu GT. Antioxidative activity of dibenzocycloctene lignans isolated from Schisandraceae. Planta Med 1992; 58:311–313.
80. Huang YS, He Y, Zhang JT. Antioxidative effect of three components isolated from fruit of schisandrae. Zhongguo Yaolixue Yu Dulixue Zazhi 1990; 4:275–277.
81. Lin TJ, Liu GT, Pan Y, Liu Y, Xu GZ. Protection by schisanhenol against adriamycin toxicity in rat heart mitochondria. Biochem Pharmacol 1991; 42:1805–1810.
82. Li XJ, Zhao BL, Liu GT, Xin WJ. Scavenging effects on active oxygen radicals by schizandrins with different structures and configurations. Free Rad Biol Med 1990; 9:99–104.
83. KM Ko, MKT Poon, SP Ip, K Wu. Protection against carbon tetrachloride liver toxicity by enantiomers of schisandrin B associated with differential changes in hepatic glutathione antioxidant system in mice. Pharmaceut Biol 2002; 40:298–301.
84. Comporti M. Lipid peroxidation and cellular damage in toxic liver injury. Lab Invest 1985; 53:599–623.
85. Fraga CG, Llesuy SF, Boveris A. Increased carbon tetrachloride–stimulated chemiluminescence in the in situ liver of barbital-treated mice. Acta Physiol Pharmacol Latinoamer 1984; 34:143–150.
86. Gee DL, Tappel AL. Production of volatile hydrocarbons by isolated hepatocytes: an in vitro model for lipid peroxidation studies. Toxicol Appl Pharmacol 1981; 60:112–120.
87. Ko KM, Yick PK, Chiu TW, Hui TY, Cheng CHK, Kong YC. Impaired hepatic antioxidant status in carbon tetrachloride intoxicated rats: an in vivo model for screening herbal extracts with antioxidant activities. Fitoterapia 1993; LXIV:539–544.

88. Ko KM, Ip SP, Poon MK, Wu SS, Che CT, Ng KH, Kong YC. Effect of a lignan-enriched fructus schisandrae extract on hepatic glutathione status in rats: protection against carbon tetrachloride toxicity. Planta Med 1995; 61:134–137.
89. Ko KM, Mak DHF, Li PC, Poon MK, Ip SP. Enhancement of hepatic glutathione regeneration capacity by a lignan-enriched extract of fructus schisandrae in rats. Jpn J Pharmacol 1995; 69:439–442.
90. Ip SP, Mak DH, Li PC, Poon MK, Ko KM. Effect of a lignan-enriched extract of *Schisandra chinensis* on aflatoxin B1 and cadmium chloride–induced hepatotoxicity in rats. Pharmacol Toxicol 1996; 78:413–416.
91. Packer L. Oxygen radicals and antioxidants in endurance exercise. In: Benzi G, Packer L, Siliprandi N, eds. Biochemical Aspects of Physical Exercise. Amsterdam: Elservier, 1988:73–92.
92. Alessio HM, Goldfarb AH. Lipid peroxidation and scavenger enzymes during exercise: adaptive response to training. J Appl Physiol 1988; 64:1333–1336.
93. Jones DA, Newham DJ, Round JM, Tolfree SE. Experimental human muscle damage: morphological changes in relation to other indices of damage. J Physiol 1986; 375:435–448.
94. Van der Meulen JH, Kuipers H, Drukker J. Relationship between exercise-induced muscle damage and enzyme release in rats. J Appl Physiol 1991; 71:999–1004.
95. Quintanilha AT. Oxidative effects of physical exercise. In: Quintanilha AT, ed. Reactive Oxygen Species in Chemistry, Biology and Medicine. New York, London: Plenum Press, 1988:187–195.
96. Ip SP, Poon MKT, Che CT, Ng KH, Kong YC, Ko KM. Schisandrin B protects against carbon tetrachloride toxicity by enhancing the mitochondrial glutathione redox status in mouse liver. Free Rad Biol Med 1996; 21:709–712.
97. Ip SP, Ko KM. The crucial antioxidant action of schisandrin B in protecting against carbon tetrachloride hepatotoxicity in mice: a comparative study with butylated hydroxytoluene. Biochem Pharmacol 1996; 52:1687–1693.
98. Mak DHF, Ip SP, Li PC, Poon MKT, Ko KM. Effects of schisandrin B and α-tocopherol on lipid peroxidation, in vitro and in vivo. Mol Cell Biochem 1996; 165:161–165.
99. Ko KM, Yiu HY. Schisandrin B modulates the ischemia-reperfusion induced changes in non-enzymatic antioxidant levels in isolated-perfused rat hearts. Mol Cell Biochem 2001; 220:141–147.
100. Chiu, PY, Ko, KM. Time-dependent enhancement in mitochondrial glutathione antioxidant and functional status by schisandrin B treatment decreases the susceptibility of rat hearts to ischemia-reperfusion injury. Proc. Second International Symposium on Antioxidants in Nutrition and Therapy: Mechanisms in Physiology-Pathology-Pharmacology, Bali, Indonesia, October 2–4, 2002.
101. Meister A, Anderson ME. Glutathione. Annu Rev Biochem 1983; 52:711–760.
102. Meister A. Glutathione-ascorbic acid antioxidant system in animals. J Biol Chem 1994; 269:9397–9400.

103. Casini AF, Maellaro E, Del Bello B, Comporti M. The role of vitamin E in the hepatotoxicity by glutathione depleting agents. Adv Exp Med Biol 1990; 264:105–110.
104. Wells WW, Xu DP, Yang YF, Rocque PA. Mammalian thioltransferase (glutaredoxin) and protein disulfide isomerase have dehydroascorbate reductase activity. J Biol Chem 1990; 265:15361–15364.
105. Chan AC, Tran K, Raynor T, Ganz PR, Chow CK. Regeneration of vitamin E in human platelets. J Biol Chem 1991; 266:17290–17295.
106. Pascoe GA, Reed DJ. Cell calcium, vitamin E, and the thiol redox system in cytotoxicity. Free Rad Biol Med 1989; 6:209–224.
107. Pascoe GA, Reed DJ. Vitamin E protection against chemical-induced cell injury. II. Evidence for a threshold effect of cellular alpha-tocopherol in prevention of adriamycin toxicity. Arch Biochem Biophys 1987; 256:159–166.
108. Liu GT, Bao TT, Wei HL, Song ZY. [Induction of hepatocyte microsomal cytochrome P-450 by schizandrin B in mice (author's transl)]. Yao Xue Xue Bao 1980; 15:206–211.
109. Liu KT, Cresteil T, Le Provost E, Lesca P. Specific evidence that schizandrins induce a phenobarbital-like cytochrome P-450 form separated from rat liver. Biochem Biophys Res Commun 1981; 103:1131–1137.
110. Kubo S, Ohkura Y, Mizoguchi Y, Matsui-Yuasa, Otani S, Morisawa S, Kinoshita H, Takeda S. Effect of gomisin A (TJN-101) on liver regeneration. Planta Med 1992; 58:489–492.
111. Hirotani Y, Kurokawa N, Takashima N, Sawada M, Iguchi K, Yanaihara N, Iwasaki M, Aburada M, Arakawa Y, Yansihara C. Effects of gomisin A on rat liver regeneration after partial hepatectomy in reference to c-myc and c-fos product levels. Biomed Res 1995; 16:43–50.
112. Keppler D, Hagmann W, Rapp S, Denslinger C, Koch HK. The relation of leukotrienes to liver injury. Hepatology 1985; 5:883–891.
113. Ohkura Y, Mizoguchi Y, Morisawa S, Takeda S, Aburada M, Hosoya E. Effect of gomisin A (TJN-101) on the arachidonic acid cascade in macrophages. Jpn J Pharmacol 1990; 52:331–336.
114. Welch WJ. Mammalian stress response: cell physiology, structure/function of stress proteins, and implications for medicine and disease. Physiol Rev 1992; 72:1063–1081.
115. Jäättela M. Heat shock proteins as cellular lifeguards. Ann Med 1999; 31:261–271.
116. Knowlton AA, Brecher P, Apstein CS. Rapid expression of heat shock protein in the rabbit after brief cardiac ischemia. J Clin Invest 1991; 87:139–147.
117. Marber MS, Latchman DS, Walker JM, Yellon DM. Cardiac stress protein elevation 24 hours after brief ischemia or heat stress is associated with resistance to myocardial infarction. Circulation 1993; 88:1264–1272.
118. Qian YZ, Bernardo NL, Nayeem MA, Chelliah J, Kukreja RC. Induction of 72-kDa heat shock protein does not produce second window of ischemic preconditioning in rat heart. Am J Physiol 1999; 276:H224–H234.

119. Ahn JH, Ko YG, Park WY, Kang YS, Chung HY, Seo JS. Suppression of ceramide-mediated apoptosis by HSP70. Mol Cells 1999; 9:200–206.
120. Nishimura H, Emoto M, Kimura K, Yoshikai Y. Hsp70 protects macrophages infected with *Salmonella choleraesuis* against TNF-alpha–induced cell death. Cell Stress Chaperones 1997; 2:50–59.
121. Tang MH, Chiu PY, Ko KM. Hepatoprotective action of schisandrin B against carbon tetrachloride toxicity was mediated by both enhancement of mitochondrial glutathione antioxidant status and induction of heat shock proteins in mice. Proc. Second International Symposium on Antioxidants in Nutrition and Therapy: Mechanisms in Physiology-Pathology-Pharmacology, Bali, Indonesia, October 2–4, 2002.
122. Wang JP, Raung SL, Hsu MF, Chen CC. Inhibition by gomisin C (a lignan from *Schizandrae chinensis*) of the respiratory burst of rat neutrophils. Br J Pharmacol 1994; 113:945–953.
123. Jung KY, Lee IS, OH SR, Kin DS, Lee HK. Lignans with platelet activating factor antagonist activity from *Schisandra chinensis* (Turcz.) Baill. Phytomedicine 1997; 4:229–231.
124. Ono H, Matsuzaki Y, Wakui Y, Takeda S, Ikeya Y, Amagaya S, Maruno M. Determination of schizandrin in human plasma by gas chromatography-mass spectrometry. J Chromatogr B Biomed Appl 1995; 674:293–297.
125. Cui YY, Wang MZ. Aspect of schizandrin metabolism in vitro and in vivo. Eur J Drug Metab Pharmacokinet 1993; 18:155–160.
126. Zheng TL, Kang JH, Chen FY, Wang PF, Chen TG, Liu QL. Difference in antioxidation for schisandrins and schisantherin between bio- and chemo-systems. Phytother Res 1997; 11:600–602.
127. Matsuzaki Y, Ischibashi E, Koguchi S, Wakui Y, Takeda S, Aburada M, Oyama T. Determination of gomisin J (TNJ-101) and its metabolites in rat serum by gas chromatography-mass spectrometry. Nippon Yakugaku Zasshi 1991; 111:617–620.
128. Matsuzaki Y, Matsuzaki T, Takeda S, Koguchi S, Ikeya Y, Mitsuhashi H, Sasaki H, Aburada M, Hosoya E, Oyama T. Studies on the metabolic fate of gomisin A (TJN-101), I. Absorption in rats. Nippon Yakugaku Zasshi 1991; 111:524–530.
129. Ikeya Y, Mitsuhashi H, Sasaki H, Matsuzaki Y, Matsuzaki T, Hosoya E. Studies on the metabolism of gomisin A (TJN-101). II. Structure determination of biliary and urinary metabolites in rat. Chem Pharm Bull (Tokyo) 1990; 38:136–141.
130. Niu XY, Bian ZJ, Ren ZH. Metabolism of schisandrol A in rats and its distribution in brain determined by TLC-UV. Acta Pharmacol Sin 1983; 491–495.
131. RA Burgos, JL Hancke. Toxicological studies on *S. chinensis*. Instituto de Farmacología Facultad de Medicina Veterinaria, Universidad Austral de Chile, Valdivia, Chile, 1992. Data on file.
132. Kim YS, Kim DH, Kim DO, Lee BK, Kim KW, Park JN, Lee JC, Choi YS,

Rim H. The effect of diphenyl-dimethyl-dicarboxylate on cyclosporine-A blood level in kidney transplants with chronic hepatitis. Korean J Intern Med 1997; 12:67–69.
133. Kroemer G, Dallaporta B, Resche-Rigon M. The mitochondrial death/life regulator in apoptosis and necrosis. Annu Rev Physiol 1998; 60:619–642.
134. Wallace DC. Mitochondrial genetics: a paradigm for aging and degenerative diseases. Science 1992; 256:628–632.

14

Spirulina
An Overview

Subramanian Sivakami
National University of Singapore
Republic of Singapore
and University of Mumbai
Mumbai, India

I. INTRODUCTION

Among the algal foods and supplements, a great deal of attention has been focused in recent times on *Spirulina* (*Arthrospira platensis*), the unicellular, filamentous, spiral-shaped, blue-green alga. Unlike some of the other medicinal plants that are used as regular dietary constituents and spices in many parts of the world, the consumption of spirulina was restricted to some communities. Traditionally, spirulina has been consumed for centuries by the people of Africa and South America where it grew naturally in lakes, being a photosynthetic organism. More recently various commercial preparations of spirulina in the form of capsules, syrup, powder, and even spirulina-incorporated noodles, cereals, and energy bars are being promoted all over the world. The most widely used species for human consumption are *Spirulina platensis* and *Spirulina maxima* though *Spirulina fusiformis* has been used for several laboratory experiments. A wide range of medicinal properties and health benefits has been attributed to spirulina. Yet systematic scientific research has been carried out only on some aspects of its nutritional and therapeutic properties. This review attempts to highlight some of the recent research in this front.

Spirulina is known to contain the highest protein content among all edible food, being in the range of 45–60% and rich in essential amino acids. This is particularly significant as it is a source of easily digestible vegetable protein. It has a high content of the pigments chlorophyll, phycocyanin, and carotenoids with phycocyanin content being as high as 14%. It is also a rich source of vitamins C, E, and B_{12}. Other phytonutrients present in spirulina are γ-linolenic acid, an essential polyunsaturated fatty acid, glycolipids, and sulfolipids.

Since spirulina grows easily in ponds and brackish waters under alkaline conditions, it is believed to grow relatively free of contamination from other algae and protozoa even in open ponds. However, for commercial production, ponds, tanks, spiral tubes, fermenters, and even large plastic bags have been employed Both open- and closed-culture systems are in use, with the cost of the latter being higher because of the need to supply lighting. Variations in different culture methods are based on differences in mixing systems, depth of the growth pond, and temperature control (1). Among different mixing systems, turbulent stirring has been shown to yield increased productivity due to better light distribution (2). More recently a continuous photobioreactor has been standardized for the cultivation of *S. platensis* with the purpose of developing it as food during space travel. Harvesting spirulina biomass is thus being studied for potential development of an auto-regenerating life support system for space travelers (3). Culturing of spirulina has also been extensively studied under laboratory conditions using varying light intensities, carbon dioxide environments, and sources of nitrogen to assess the impact of these factors on biomass, protein, carbohydrate, and phycocyanin contents (4–6). These laboratory findings when applied to large-scale cultivation can not only increase biomass productivity but also selectively increase the yield of certain phytonutrients such as pigments and polysaccharides.

An analysis of the inorganic and organic composition of various algal foods available in different parts of the world revealed no heavy metals beyond the permissible levels in spirulina and hence it was recommended as a safe food (7,8). It was also shown that *S. maxima*, when used as a food coloring and supplement for 13 weeks, did not produce any toxic effects in mice (9). Phycocyanin, the blue colorant from *S. platensis*, was also shown to be devoid of acute as well as subchronic toxicities in rats (10).

II. GENERAL HEALTH BENEFITS

The positive effects of the dietary inclusion of spirulina on general health and well-being have been shown in studies on human volunteers, fish, and birds. In

1986, it was observed by Becker et al. that spirulina can reduce the body weight of obese humans (11). Subsequently Iwata et al. in 1990 showed that it can also reduce total plasma cholesterol levels (12).

When administered in the form of syrup for 30 days, spirulina increased the mean blood hemoglobin levels by 11.65% in young anemic adult girls. However, when given as part of a wheat preparation, it brought about significantly less elevation in hemoglobin levels. This reduction in efficacy was attributed to the presence of oxalates and phytates in the grain that interfere with iron absorption (13). In another study, spirulina alone and in combination with wheat gluten resulted in higher hemoglobin content and higher iron storage (14). Supplementation of a university cafetaria diet of young healthy adults in Spain with Provital, a commercial preparation of spirulina, resulted in no significant changes in anthropometric indicators but an increase in total antioxidant capacity with increases in α-tocopherol and β-carotene levels observed only in women volunteers (15).

Partial replacement of fishmeal with spirulina showed significant increases in growth of two Indian major carps (16). Both livability and performance indices of broilers fed spirulina were shown to increase (17). Humoral and cell-mediated immune functions of chicks were also enhanced by inclusion of *S. platensis* in their diet (18). The stimulatory effects of spirulina on the immune system have prompted some workers to call it a "probiotic." Based on enhanced macrophage phagocytic functions, the group of Qureshi proposed that spirulina supplementation may improve disease resistance potential in cats (19) and chickens (20) and nitrite production in chick macrophages by increased nitric oxide synthase activity (21). A water-soluble, high-molecular-weight polysaccharide from food-grade spirulina was found to be immunostimulatory resulting in increased mRNA levels of interleukin-1β and tumor necrosis factor-α (22). A finding of great clinical significance was that an acqueous extract of *S. platensis* inhibited HIV-1 replication in human T-cell lines, peripheral blood mononuclear cells, and Langerhans cells by 50% (23). The antiviral activity was exhibited by a polysaccharide as well as a nonpolysaccharide fraction. After this, the antiviral activity of a sulfated polysaccharide, calcium spirulan, was convincingly demonstrated by studying the structural requirements for its activity (24). Two polysaccharide fractions from *S. maxima* have been also shown to possess antioxidant abilities (25).

Through assessment of a large number of enzymes such as those involved in biotransformation like cytochrome P-450 isozymes, detoxification enzymes like glutathione-S-transferase, DT-diaphorase, a battery of antioxidant enzymes like superoxide dismutase, catalase, glutathione peroxidase, glutathione reductase, and the content of glutathione itself, the chemopreventive effect of *S. platensis* was shown (26). *S. fusiformis* administration was found to depress hepatic cytochrome P-450 and induce hepatic glutathione-S-transferase with no effect on extrahepatic glutathione-S-transferase. This was interpreted by the authors to mean decreased biotransformation of xenobiotics resulting in lesser amounts of reactive electrophilic metabolites and consequent protection to the animal. A simultaneous glutathione-S-transferase induction detoxifies hydrophobic electrophiles by conjugation to glutathione (27). In addition to being chemopreventive, *S. fusiformis* has been shown to cause regression of oral leukoplakia in tobacco chewers (28).

III. ANTIOXIDANT PROPERTIES

Spirulina has a very high content of β-carotene and is believed to owe some of its potent antioxidant activity to it (29). The total carotenes in it have been shown to have a bioavailability comparable to other sources. In two very large-scale human trials with preschool children in South India, spirulina feeding led to an increase in serum retinol levels (30) and a significant decrease in "Bitot's spot," a symptom of vitamin A deficiency (31). This finding is very important in view of the prevalence of blindness and eye diseases among children of the Third World caused by vitamin A deficiency.

That a methanolic extract of *S. maxima* possesses antioxidant capacities was determined by in vitro and in vivo experiments (32). Subsequently Estrada et al. (33) fractionated a protean extract of *S. platensis* and showed that an increase in phycocyanin content was accompanied by a concomitant increase in antioxidant activities of the different fractions. Therefore, phycocyanin was identified as the component mainly responsible for antioxidant activity. However, when the antioxidant activities of phycocyanin and phycocyanobilin from *S. platensis* were systematically evaluated using a phosphatidylcholine liposome system, the results indicated that most of the antioxidant activity of phycocyanin is due to phycocyanobilin (34). This is an open-chain tetrapyrrole chromophore covalently attached to the apoprotein. Phycocyanobilin has a structure similar to the bile pigment bilirubin, also a known scavenger of reactive oxygen species (ROS). The radical scavenging activity of phycocyanobilin from *S. platensis* had been shown earlier by the same group of workers (35). Phycocyanin was also reported to protect human erythrocytes against lysis by peroxy radicals (36). It is water-extractable and both native and denatured phycocyanin possess antioxidant activities to the same extent. Spray-dried and fresh spirulina exhibit equal antioxidant abilities (34). These properties are important from the point of view of preparation of the oral food supplements in various forms.

Both the oil extract and the defatted fraction of *S. maxima* lowered total lipids and triacylglycerols in livers of rats with carbon tetrachloride (CCl_4)-induced fatty liver indicating the presence of bioactive principles in both fractions. The authors attributed the hepatoprotective effects of spirulina to its antioxidant constituents such as selenium, chlorophyll, carotene, γ-linolenic acid, and vitamins E and C (37). This observation has been confirmed by Bhat et al., who showed that C-phycocyanin significantly reduced the extent of hepatotoxicity when administered 1–3 hr before the induction of toxicity and prevented the loss of liver enzymes such as serum glutamate pyruvate transaminase (SGPT) into the serum (38). Protection was offered by phycocyanin against hepatotoxicity induced by either CCl4 or R-(+)-pulegone. The level of menthofuran, a major metabolite that appears in the urine of R-(+)-pulegone-treated rats, was significantly reduced by phycocyanin. The role of the microsomal cytochrome P-450 system in the conversion of R-(+)-pulegone to menthofuran is known. It was therefore suggested by the authors that phycocyanin interacts with cytochrome P-450 and affects the formation of 9-OH-pulegone, which acts as the precursor of menthofuran. Lowering the biotransformation of the hepatotoxins into toxic intermediates was thus proposed to be a general mechanism of protection. It was also proposed that phycocyanin scavenges haloalkane free radicals produced from CCl_4 as well as reactive metabolites formed from R-(+)-pulegone (37). These ideas are in keeping with the report of Romay et al. that phycocyanin scavenges alkoxy and hydroxy free radicals (39).

More recently, *S. maxima* has been shown to prevent fatty liver formation in male and female mice with alloxan-induced diabetes. The administration of *S. maxima* to these animals reduced the levels of thiobarbituric acid–reactive substances in serum and liver as well as triglyceride and LDL and VLDL levels (40). Spirulina has also been shown to prevent liver fibrosis (41) and arrest the progress of chronic hepatitis into hepatocirrhosis (42).

The antioxidant and anti-inflammatory properties of phycocyanin have been established using in vitro as well as in vivo assays. It was found to have the ability to inhibit glucose-oxidase-induced mouse paw inflammation, microsomal lipid peroxidation, damage to deoxyribose, and chemiluminscence response of polymorphonuclear leukocytes to strong oxidants (39). When zymosan was used to induce rheumatoid arthritis in mice, the subsequent oral administration of phycocyanin for 8 days was found to reverse the histological and ultrastructural lesions and elevated β-glucuronidase levels in the arthritic animals. This was attributed to the ROS-scavenging ability of phycocyanin. The ability of phycocyanin to inhibit arachidonic acid metabolism and cytokine production was also believed to be responsible for these antiarthritic effects (43).

Administration of C-phycocyanin extract 30 min before the induction of colitis in rats showed that it is endowed with anti-inflammatory properties. This was evident from a reduction in the level of myeloperoxidase activity as well as a reversal of histological and ultrastructural features seen in inflammatory cell infiltration in the arthritic model. Reactive oxygen species such as superoxide, H_2O_2, OH radical, and hypochlorous acid are believed to mediate human and experimental inflammatory bowel disease (IBD). Nitric oxide and peroxynitrite have also been suggested to mediate the induction of colitis (44).

Subsequently the same group of workers have shown the anti-inflammatory properties of phycocyanin in several experimental rat models such as rat paw edema induced by carrageenan, mouse ear edema induced by 12-O-tetradecanoyl phorbol 13-acetate (TPA) as well as arachidonic acid (AA) and cotton pellet granuloma (45). It was observed that the TPA-induced mouse ear edema was less effectively inhibited than that induced by AA. Since AA and its metabolites are known to take part in these models of inflammation, it was suggested that the mechanism of action of phycocyanin involves AA (45). Based on the hydroxy- and alkoxy-radical-scavenging abilities of phycocyanin in vivo and in vitro, it was proposed that this might explain the anti-inflammatory property of phycocyanin (45).

Following these observations it was shown for the first time that both phycocyanin and phycocyanobilin are able to scavenge peroxynitrite (46,47) and protect supercoiled pBR22DNA against peroxynitrite-induced strand breakage. The results also indicated that phycocyanin is more effective than phycocyanobilin. This has been attributed to the interaction of peroxynitrite with tyrosine and tryptophan residues of apophycocyanin. Similar to the peroxy-radical-mediated transformation of bilirubin to biliverdin, the chromophore of reduced phycocyanin is converted to phycocyanobilin by the peroxy radical (46,47). These findings are in line with the earlier observation by Romay and Gonzalez that phycocyanin can protect erythrocytes from lysis by peroxy radicals (36).

Because damage to DNA by reactive oxygen occurs during chronic inflammation, the anti-inflammatory activity of phycocyanin is attributable to its ability to scavenge peroxynitrite radical and other reactive oxygen species that contribute to oxidative stress, an important condition in inflammation. Since peroxynitrite can be generated in vivo by reaction between superoxide and nitric oxide, in addition to DNA strand breakage, it can cause oxidative damage to lipids, proteins, and thiols. Several anticarcinogenic agents are known to inhibit oxidative damage and in this context phycocyanin might be a potential anticarcinogenic agent. Other classes of compounds such as flavonoids and polyphenols of plant origin are also known to protect against damage mediated by peroxynitrite (47).

Using recombinant human cyclooxygenase-2, Reddy et al. showed that C-phycocyanin is a selective inhibitor of cyclooxygenase (COX-2) (48). Thus the ability of phycocyanin to protect against hepatotoxicity, inflammation, and arthritis may be due to its inhibition of COX-2 in addition to its free-radical-scavenging ability. COX-2 produces prostaglandins from AA and induction of COX-2 is believed to occur at the site of inflammation. Cyclooxygenases are also activated to produce prostaglandins as a result of free-radical-mediated processes like lipid peroxidation. In fact, cyclooxygenase-mediated inflammation is believed to be one of the responses to CCl_4-induced hepatotoxicity. The involvement of oxygen free radicals in rheumatoid arthritis and the use of inhibitors of AA metabolism in arthritis are well known. Thus COX-2 inhibition seems to explain the antiarthritic and anti-inflammatory properties of phycocyanin. These results assume a great deal of significance in view of the introduction of COX-2 inhibitors as nonsteroidal anti-inflammatory drugs (NSAID) in the market. Spirulina is rich in γ-linolenic acid (GLA), a precursor of AA, which is a proinflammatory molecule. However, recently it has been shown that dietary GLA is anti-inflammatory owing to its ability to suppress leukotriene B4 release (49). Thus the presence of GLA, in addition to phycocyanin, may contribute to the anti-inflammatory properties of spirulina. Other natural products like phytoalexin found in grapes and dietary compounds like curcumin and retinoids are known to inhibit COX-2 activity. It is interesting to note that reduced phycocyanin and phycocyanobilin, the chromphore of phycocyanin, did not possess COX-2-inhibiting ability (48). Most of the recent research described above has been carried out using purified preparations of phycocyanin from spirulina. It is clear from these experiments that the molecular basis of several of the medicinal properties of spirulina is the antioxidant potential of the biliprotein phycocyanin. Other nutritionally and clinically important constituents include carotenes and the polysaccharide spirulan. The mechanism of action of these has not been studied to the same extent as that of phycocyanin.

IV. CONCLUDING REMARKS

An important factor to be considered if spirulina is to be used as the sole food, particularly during space travel, is the bioavailability of its constituents. A report from China describes the effect of increasing concentrations of selenium on the cultivation of *S. platensis* (50). Selenium stimulated growth and biomass yield up to a point after which it was observed to be inhibitory to growth. The toxicity of higher concentrations of selenium could be overcome by addition of sulfite (50). Dietary supplementation with selenium-rich spirulina to selenium-deficient rats was found to restore the levels of enzymic and nonenzymic constituents that were altered in the deficient animals. Malondialdehyde and selenium-dependent glutathione peroxidase in plasma, erythrocytes, and homogenates of liver, kidney, and heart were restored to normal levels by selenium-enriched spirulina as well as sodium selenite (51). Subsequently, the same group of workers have shown that sodium selenite and selenomethionine were more effective than selenium-rich spirulina. This conclusion was based on the observation that selenium-rich spirulina did not restore selenium levels or glutathione peroxidase activity in most tissues to the same degree as the other forms of selenium (52). Similarly it was reported that pseudovitamin B_{12} was the predominant form in spirulina tablets and this form is known to have much less affinity to intrinsic factor (IF) and less biological activity (53). These examples indicate that all the micronutrients of spirulina may not be wholly bioavailable or biologically useful.

Blue-green algae are reported to accumulate heavy metals from contaminated pond water and consuming such food might result in metal toxicity. Interestingly, dietary *S. fusiformis* at a high dose of 800 mg/kg body weight of rats reduced lead toxicity as judged by significant enhancement in survival time, animal weight, and the weights of their testes (54). In another study, exogenous administration of spirulina at a dose of 1500 mg/kg reduced the levels of lipid peroxidation products such as malondialdehyde, conjugated diene, and hydroperoxide. Since similar effects were observed upon the adminstration of the antioxidant vitamin E or C, it was concluded that the antioxidant activity of spirulina exerted the protective effects during lead-induced toxicity (55). Thus it appears that when grown under conditions where it cannot accumulate heavy metals, spirulina can be used to reduce metal toxicity in animals. If it is to be accepted as a safe food, further controlled experiments are required to evaluate whether supplementation with large doses of the different commercial preparations of spirulina can cause or cure metal toxicity.

Though other edible algae like the green alga *Chlorella* and the blue-green alga *Aphanizomenon flos-aquae* (AFA) are known, the benefits of consuming spirulina appear to be far greater than those of others. It has been pointed out that some commercial preparations of AFA may have been contaminated with hepatotoxin and neurotoxin (56). This might prove more of a danger to health than a benefit. It is also suspected that vitamin B_{12} in spirulina preparations may have originated from bird feathers and droppings found as contamination.

These doubts and controversies notwithstanding, reports of beneficial effects of consuming spirulina are overwhelming. Since many of the nutritional deficiencies occur in the developing world, it is essential to focus on the development of palatable, inexpensive supplements. There is also a need for more stringent quality control and standardization during manufacture and marketing of the various spirulina-based products.

The rapidly growing microalgae industry in the Asia-Pacific Rim region has been reviewed succinctly giving details of all the producers in the region (57). Cultivation of spirulina is at present being done on a very large scale using different production systems in countries like China (58). It is also cultivated as a small-scale industry, which will be a source of income to small farmers and help popularize spirulina in rural communities besides reducing production costs. Being an easy-to-grow edible protein rich in antioxidant activity, spirulina has the potential to become the wonder drug and food supplement of the future.

REFERENCES

1. Borowitzka MA. Commercial production of microalgae: ponds, tanks, tubes and fermenters. J Biotechnol 1999; 70:313–321.
2. Vonshak A. *Spirulina platensis* (*Arthospira*) Physiology, Cell Biology and Biotechnology. London, UK: Taylor and Francis, 1997.
3. Morist A, Montesinos JL, Cusido JA, Godia F. Recovery and treatment of *Spirulina platensis* cells cultured in a continuous photobioreactor to be used as food. Process Biochem 2001; 37:535–547.
4. Leonardo B, Brantes M, Klaus W. High Spirulina productivity under intensive light. Arch Hydrobiol 2001; 140(suppl):151–160.
5. Tripathi U, Sarada R, Ravishankar GA. A culture method for microalgal forms using two-tier vessel providing carbon-dioxide environment: studies on growth and carotenoid production. World J Micro Biotechnol 2001; 17:325–329.
6. Vieira CJA, Leal CK, Lucielen O, Glenio M. Different nitrogen sources and growth responses of *Spirulina platensis* in microenvironments. World J Micro Biotechnol 2001; 17:439–442.
7. Yin-Mao H, Jon-Mau H, Taun-Ran Y. Inorganic elements determination for algae/spirulina food marketed in Taiwan. J Food Drug Anal 2001; 9:178–182.
8. Campanella L, Crescentini G, Avino P. Chemical composition and nutritional evaluation of some natural and commercial food products based on spirulina. Analusis 1999; 27:533–540.
9. Salaza M, Martinez E, Madrigal E, Ruiz LE, Chamorro GA. Subchronic toxicity study in mice fed *Spirulina maxima*. J Ethnopharmacol 1998; 62:235–241.
10. Naidu AK, Sarada R, Manoj G, Khan MY, Mahadeva Swamy M, Viswanatha S, Narasimha Murthy K, Ravishankar GA, Srinivas L. Toxicity assessment of phycocyanin—a blue colorant from blue green alga *Spirulina platensis*. Food Biotechnol 1999; 13:51–66.
11. Becker EW, Jakober B, Luft D. Clinical and biochemical evaluations of alga *Spirulina* with regard to its application in the treatment of obesity: a double blind crossover study. Nutr Rep Int 1986; 33:565–573.
12. Iwata K, Inayama T, Kato T. Effects of *Spirulina platensis* on plasma lipoprotein lipase activity in fructose-induced hyperlipidemic rats. J Nutr Sci 1990; 36:165–171.
13. Mani U, Sadliwala A, Iyer M, Parikh P. The effect of spirulina supplementation on blood haemoglobin levels of anaemic adult girls. J Food Sci Technol 2000; 37:642–644.
14. Kapoor R, Mehta U. Supplementary effect of spirulina on hematological status

of rats during pregnancy and lactation. Plant Foods Hum Nutr 1998; 52:315–324.

15. Garcia GI, Barrantes Perez C, Monzon Monzon Y, Romay Penabad Ch, Ledesma Rivero L. The effect of the *Spirulina* sp. microalgae "Provital" on the blood antioxidant properties and the nutritional condition of healthy young adults with a university cafeteria diet. Alimentaria 2000; 37:41–47.
16. Nandeesha MC, Gangadhara B, Manissery JK, Venkatraman LV. Growth performance of two Indian major carps, catla (*Catla catla*) and rohu (*Labeo rohita*) fed diets containing different levels of *Spirulina platensis*. Biores Technol 2001; 80:117–120.
17. Shipton TA, Britz PJ. The partial and total replacement of fishmeal with selected plant protein sources in diets for the South African abalone, *Haliotis midae* L. J Shellfish Res 2001; 20:637–645.
18. Sarma M, Sapcota D, Dutta KK, Gohain AK. Effect of dietary supplementation of herbal products on the performance of broilers. Ind J Poult Sci 2001; 36:235–236.
19. Qureshi MA, Ali RA. *Spirulina platensis* exposure enhances macrophage phagocytic function in cats. Immunopharmacol Immunotoxicol 1996; 18:457–463.
20. Qureshi MA, Garlich JD, Kidd MT. Dietary *Spirulina platensis* enhances humoral and cell-mediated immune functions in chickens. Immunopharmacol Immunotoxicol 1996; 18:465–476.
21. Al-Batshan HA, Al-Muffarerj SI, Al-Homaidan AA, Qureshi MA. Enhancement of chicken macrophage phagocytic function and nitrite production by dietary *Spirulina platensis*. Immunopharmacol Immunotoxicol 2001; 23:281–289.
22. Pugh N, Ross SA, Elsohly HN, Pasco DS. Isolation of three high molecular weight polysaccharide preparations with potent immunostimulatory activity from *Spirulina platensis*, *Aphanizomenon flos-aquae* and *Chlorella*. Planta Medica 2001; 67:737–742.
23. Ayehunie S, Belay A, Baba TW, Rupercht RM. Inhibition of HIV-1 replication by an aqueous extract of *Spirulina platensis (Arthrospira platensis)*. J AIDS Hum 1998; 18:7–12.
24. Lee JB, Srisomporn P, Hayashi K, Tanaka T, Sankawa U, Hayashi T. Effects of structural modification of calcium spirulan, a sulphated polysaccharide from *Spirulina platensis*, on antiviral activity. Chem Pharm Bull 2001; 49:108–110.
25. Zhou ZG, Liu ZL, Liu XX. Study on the isolation, purification and antioxidation properties of polysaccharides from *Spirulina maxima*. Acta Botan Sin 1997; 39:77–81.
26. Dasgupta T, Banerjee S, Yadav PK, Rao AR. Chemomodulation of carcinogen metabolizing enzymes, antioxidant profiles and skin and forestomach pailloma-genesis by *Spirulina platensis*. Mol Cell Biochem 2001; 226:27–38.
27. Mittal A, Kumar PV, Banerjee S, Rao AR, Kumar A. Modulating potential of *Spirulina fusiformis* in carcinogen metabolizing enzymes in Swiss albino mice. Phytother Res 1999; 13:111–114.
28. Mathew B, Sankaranarayanan R, Nair PP, Varghese C, Somanathan T, Amma

BP, Amma NS, Nair MK. Evaluation of chemoprevention of oral cancer with *Spirulina fusiformis*. Nutr Cancer 1995; 24:197–202.
29. Basu TK, Temple J, Ng J. Effect of dietary beta-carotene on hepatic drug metabolizing enzymes in mice. J Clin Biochem Nutr 1987; 13:95–102.
30. Annapurna VV, Bamji M. Bioavailability of spirulina carotenes in preschool children. Ind J Clin Biochem Nutr 1991; 10:145–151.
31. Seshadri CV. Large scale nutritional supplementation with *Spirulina* alga. All India coordinated Project on *Spirulina*. Shri Amm Murugappa Chettiar Res. Center, Madras, India. 1993.
32. Miranda MS, Cintra RG, Barros SB, Mancini FJ. Antioxidant activity of the microalga *Spirulina maxima*. Braz J Med Biol Res 1998; 31:1075–1079.
33. Estrada Pinero EJ, Bescos Bermejo P, del Fresno Villar. Antioxidant activity of different fractions of *Spirulina platensis* protean extract. Farmaco 2001; 56:5–7.
34. Hirata T, Tanaka M, Ooike M, Tsunomura T, Sakaguchi M. Antioxidant activities of phycocyanobilin prepared from *Spirulina platensis*. J Appl Phycol 2000; 12:435–439.
35. Hirata T, Tanaka M, Ooike M, Tsunomura T, Niizeki N, Sakaguchi M. Radical scavenging activity of phycocyanobilin prepared from the cyanobacterium, *Spirulina platensis*. Fisheries Sci 1999; 65:971–972.
36. Romay C, Gonzalez R. Phycocyanin is an antioxidant protector of human erythrocytes against lysis by peroxy radicals. J Pharm Pharmacol 2000; 52:367–368.
37. Torres-Duran PV, Miranda-Zamora R, Paredes-Carbajal MC, Mascher D, Ble-Castillo J, Diaz-Zagoya JC, Juarez-Oropeza MA. Studies on the preventive effect of *Spirulina maxima* on fatty liver development induced by carbon tetrachloride, in the rat. J Ethnopharmacol 1999; 64:141–147.
38. Bhat BV, Gaikwad NW, Madyastha KM. Hepatoprotective effect of C-phycocyanin: protection for carbon tetrachloride and R-(+)-pulegone-mediated hepatotoxicity in rats. Biochem Biophys Res Commun 1998; 249:428–431.
39. Romay C, Armesto J, Remirez D, Gonazalez R, Ledon N, Garcia I. Antioxidant and anti-inflammatory properties of C-phycocyanin from blue-green algae. Inflamm Res 1998; 47:36–41.
40. Rodriguez-Hernandez A, Ble-Castillo JL, Juarez-Oroppeza MA, Diaz Zagoya JC. *Spirulina maxima* prevents fatty liver formation in CD-1 male and female mice with experimental diabetes. Life Sci 2001; 69:1029–1037.
41. Gorban EM, Orynchak MA, Virstiuk NG, Kuprash LP, Pantele Monova TM, Sharabura LB. Clinical and experimental study of spirulina efficacy in chronic diffuse liver diseases. Okhorony Zdorov'Ia Ukrainy. 2000; 6:89–93.
42. Lu YR, Chu YJ. Effects of spirulina in prevention of liver fibrosis in rats. Zhongguo Xinyao yu Linchuang Zazhi 2001; 20:198–199.
43. Remirez D, Gonzalez A, Merino N, Gonzalez R, Ancheta O, Romay C, Rodriguez S. Effect of phycocyanin in zymosan-induced arthritis in mice-phycocyanin as an antiarrthritic compound. Drug Dev Res 1999; 48:70–75.
44. Gonzalez R, Rodriguez S, Romay C, Ancheta O, Gonzalez A, Armesto J, Remirez D, Merino N. Anti-inflammatory activity of phycocyanin extract in acetic acid–induced colitis in rats. Pharmacol Res 1999; 39:55–59.

45. Romay C, Ledon N, Gonzalez R. Further studies on anti-inflammatory activity of phycocyanin in some animal models of inflammation. Inflamm Res 1998; 47:334–338.
46. Bhat VB, Madyastha KM. C-Phycocyanin: a potent peroxy radical scavenger in vivo and in vitro. Biochem Biophys Res Commun 2000; 275:20–25.
47. Bhat VB, Madyastha KM. Scavenging of peroxynitrite by phycocyanin and phycocyanibilin from *Spirulina platensis*: protection against oxidative damage to DNA. Biochem Biophys Res Commun 2001; 285:262–266.
48. Reddy CM, Bhat VB, Kiranmai G, Reddy MN, Reddanna P, Madayastha KM. Selective inhibition of cyclooxygenase-2 by C-phycocyanin, a biliprotein from *Spirulina platensis*. Biochem Biophys Res Commun 2000; 277:599–603.
49. Kaku S, Ohkura K, Yunoki S, Nonaka M, Tachibana H, Sugano M, Yamada K. Dietary gamma-linolenic acid dose dependently modifies fatty acid composition and immune parameters in rats. Prostaglandi Leukotrienes essential fatty acids 2001; 65:205–210.
50. Zhi-yong Li, Si-yuan Guo, Lin Li. A study of the Se-rich cultivation technology of *Spirulina platensis*. Acta Hydrobiol Sin 2001; 25:386–391.
51. Cases J, Puig M, Capporiccio B, Baroux B, Baccou JC, Besancon P, Rouanet JM. Glutathione-related enzymic activities in rats receiving high cholesterol or standard diets supplemented with two forms of selenium. Food Chem 1999; 65:207–211.
52. Cases J, Vacchina V, Napolitano A, Capporiccio B, Besancon P, Lobinsky R, Rouanet JM. Selenium from selenium-rich spirulina is less bioavailable than selenium from sodium selenite and selenomethionine in selenium deficient rats. J Nutr 2001; 131:2343–2350.
53. Watanabe F, Katsura H, Takenaka S, Fujita T, Abe K, Tamura Y, Nakatsuka T, Nakano Y. Pseudovitamin B_{12} is the predominant cobamide of an algal health food, spirulina tablets. J Agr Food Chem 1999; 47:4736–4741.
54. Shastri D, Kumar M, Kumar A. Modulation of lead toxicity by *Spirulina fusiformis*. Phytother Res 1999; 13:258–260.
55. Upasani CD, Khera A, Balaraman R. Effect of lead with vitamin E, C or spirulina on malondialdehyde, conjugated dienes and hydroperoxides in rats. Ind J Exp Biol 2001; 39:70–74.
56. Carmichael WW, Drapeau C, Anderson DM. Harvesting of *Aphnizomenon flos-aquae* Ralfs ex Born. and flah. var. *flos-aquae* (*Cyanobacteria*) from Klamath Lake for human dietary use. J Appl Phycol 2000; 12:585–595.
57. Lee Yuan-Kun. Commercial production of microalgae in the Asia-Pacific Rim. J Appl Phycol 1997; 9:403–411.
58. Li Ding-Mei, Qi Yu-Zao. Spirulina industry in China: present status and future prospects. J Appl Phycol 1997; 9:25–28.

15

Averrhoa bilimbi

Peter Natesan Pushparaj,
Benny Kwong-Huat Tan,
and Chee-Hong Tan
National University of Singapore
Singapore, Republic of Singapore

I. INTRODUCTION

Averrhoa bilimbi Linn belongs to the family Oxalidaceae (Fig. 1). It is a small tree growing to 15 m tall with a trunk diameter up to 30 cm. Young parts of the tree are covered with long-persistent, yellowish to rusty, velvety hairs. Leaves are often crowded at the ends of the branches with 7–19 leaflets, each measuring up to 12 cm by 4 cm, variable in shape; lateral veins have 6–14 pairs. Flowers are borne in dense, fascicled, pendulous clusters on bare branches and on knobby protuberances along the tree trunk; the calyx is yellowish-green, petals are red to purple. Fruits are rounded to blunt, angular in cross-section, up to 10 cm by 5 cm, and fleshy and juicy but acidic when ripe. Though it is widely cultivated in the lowlands of Southeast Asia, the tree's country of origin is unknown but tropical America has been suggested. Flowering and fruiting occur intermittently throughout the year. Other names of the tree are *Averrhoa obtusangula* Stokes; Belimbing asam, Belimbing buluh, Belimbing wuluh (Malay, Javanese); Kamias, kalamias, Iba, Kolonanas (Tag); and Ta-ling-pring (Thai) (1).

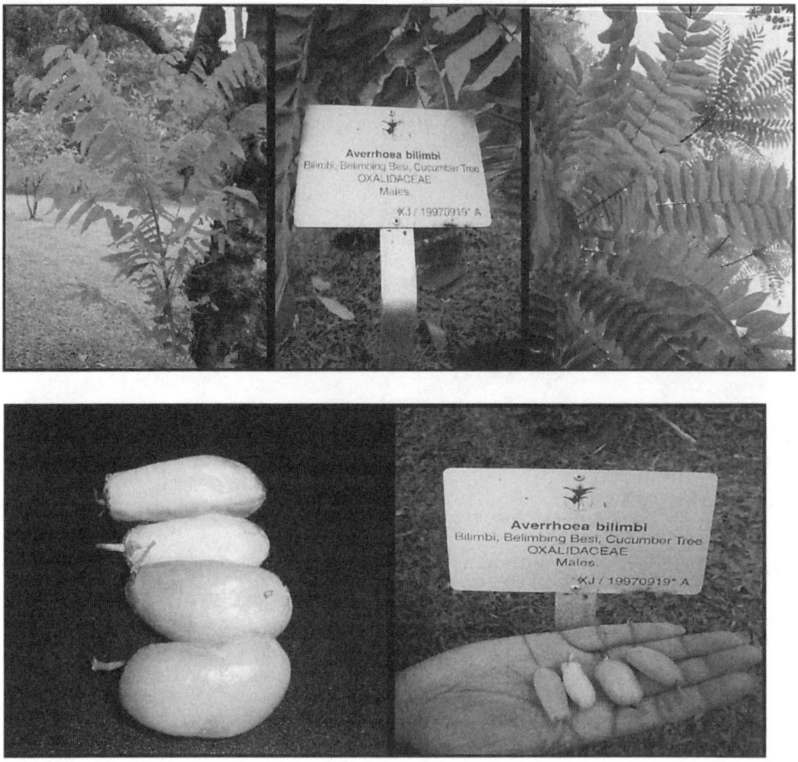

FIGURE 1 *Averrhoa bilimbi* leaves and fruits.

A. Chemical Constituents

The chemical constituents of *A. bilimbi* that have been identified include amino acids, citric acid, cyanidin-3-O-β-D-glucoside, phenolics, potassium ion, sugars, and vitamin A in fruits (2).

B. Ethnopharmacological Uses

A. bilimbi has been used as an antibacterial, antiscorbutic, astringent; postpartum protective medicine; in treatment of fever, inflammation of the rectum, and diabetes (prepared from leaves); in treatment of itches, boils, rheumatism, cough, and syphilis (paste of leaves); in treatment of scurvy, bilious colic, whooping cough, hypertension, and as a cooling drink (juice of preserved fruits); in treatment of children's cough (syrup of flowers); for stomachache (fruits), mumps, and pimples (prepared from leaves) (1).

II. HYPOGLYCEMIC ACTIVITY OF *A. BILIMBI* IN STREPTOZOTOCIN (STZ)-DIABETIC RATS

The single-high-dose-STZ-induced diabetic rat is one of the animal models of human insulin-dependent diabetes mellitus (IDDM), or type I diabetes mellitus. In this model, diabetes arises from irreversible destruction of the β-islet cells of the pancreas by streptozotocin, causing degranulation or reduction of insulin secretion. In this type I model of diabetes, the insulin is markedly depleted, but not absent (3).

The chemical structure of STZ consists of a glucose moiety (Fig. 2) with a highly reactive nitrosourea side chain that is thought to initiate its cytotoxic action. As shown in Figure 3, the glucose moiety directs this agent to the pancreatic β cells, where it binds to a membrane receptor to cause structural damage (4). The deleterious effect of STZ results from the generation of highly reactive carbonium ions (CH_3^+) that cause DNA breaks by alkylating DNA bases at various positions, resulting in activation of the nuclear enzyme poly (ADP-ribose) synthetase, thereby depleting the cellular enzyme substrate (NAD^+), leading to the cessation of NAD^+-dependent energy and protein metabolism. This in turn leads to reduced insulin secretion (5). It has been suggested that free-radical stress occurred during β-cell destruction mediated by mononuclear phagocytes and cytokines (6,7). Since free-radical scavenger was demonstrated to protect against the diabetogenic properties of STZ, it is likely the oxidative stress may play a role in determining STZ toxicity (8). However, some poly (ADP-ribose) synthetase inhibitors, such as nicotinamide and 3-aminobenzamide, could prevent the onset of diabetes (9).

A. Hypoglycemic Activity of *A. bilimbi* in STZ-Diabetic Wistar Rats

STZ-induced diabetic male Wistar rats were given five intraperitoneal (i.p.) injections of the 80% ethanolic leaf extract of *A. bilimbi* (ABe) at 300 mg/kg or the water extract of the fruits of *A. bilimbi* (ABw) at 100 mg/kg or its corresponding vehicle, daily for 7 days. Fasting blood glucose estimations and

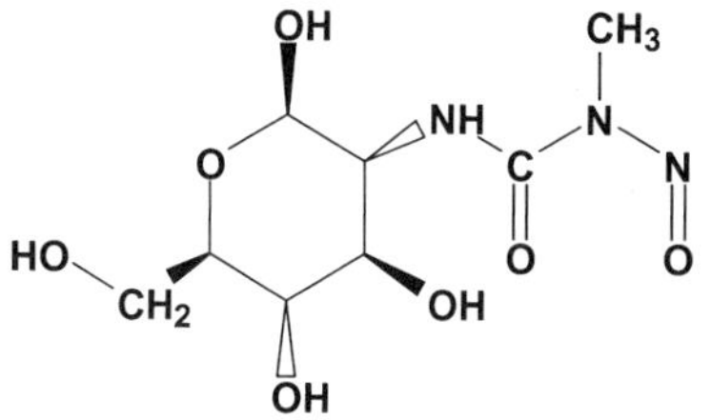

FIGURE 2 The chemical structure of streptozotocin.

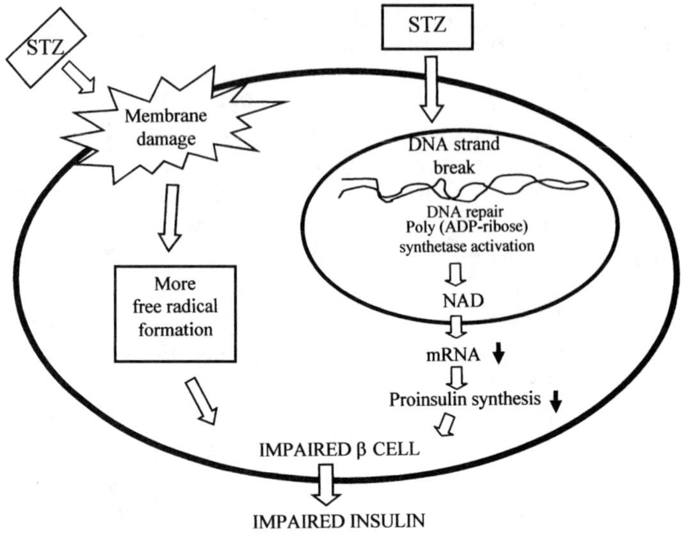

FIGURE 3 The mechanism of pancreatic β-cell destruction by streptozotocin.

food intake measurement were done on all the days of injection. The results of this preliminary study showed decreases in fasting blood glucose levels and mean daily food intake in the ABe- and ABw-treated STZ-diabetic rats (2).

B. Hypoglycemic Activity of *A. bilimbi* in STZ-diabetic Sprague-Dawley (SD) Rats

1. Effect on Oral Glucose Tolerance in Normal and Diabetic SD Rats

In the oral glucose tolerance test (OGTT) in both normal and STZ-diabetic SD rats, distilled water (control), a reference drug, metformin (500 mg/kg), or each of three different doses of ABe (125, 250, and 500 mg/kg) was orally administred to groups of four to five rats each after 16-hr fast. Thirty minutes later, glucose (3 g/kg) was orally administered to each rat with a feeding syringe (10). The blood glucose levels of the normal and diabetic rats reached a peak at 60 min after the oral administration of glucose and gradually decreased to preglucose load level. Of the three different doses, 125, 250, and 500 mg/kg, the lowest dose, i.e., 125 mg/kg, caused attenuation in the blood glucose level in both normal and diabetic rats (11). Similarly, its semipurified fractions, such as the aqueous fraction (AF) as well as the butanol fraction (BuF) at 125 mg/kg, caused attenuation in blood glucose level in STZ-diabetic rats (12). Moreover, the daily oral administration of ABe, AF, and BuF at a dose of 125 mg/kg twice a day for 14 days to STZ-diabetic SD rats caused a decrease in the blood glucose level (11,12).

2. Blood-Lipid and Cholesterol-Lowering Effect

The daily administration of ABe per orally (125 mg/kg twice a day) for 14 days to STZ-diabetic SD rats caused a reduction in the serum triglycerides and an increase in HDL cholesterol. However, ABe did not decrease the serum cholesterol and LDL cholesterol. This leads to an increase in the antiatherogenic index and HDL cholesterol:total cholesterol ratio (11). Moreover, the daily administration of ABe (125 mg/kg) and metformin (500 mg/kg) to STZ-diabetic rats twice a day for 2 weeks caused a reduction in food and water intake and an increase in body weight (11). Since ABe increased HDL cholesterol, it significantly increased the antiatherogenic index and HDL cholesterol:total cholesterol ratio. ABe thus has the potential to prevent the formation of atherosclerosis and coronary heart disease, which are the secondary diabetic complications of severe diabetes mellitus (13). In contrast, metformin failed to increase the HDL-cholesterol level and did not increase the antiatherogenic index and HDL cholesterol:total cholesterol ratio. However, it has been reported that metformin can reduce the blood lipid parameters in nondiabetic patients with coronary heart disease (14). Hence, ABe contains a hypolipidemic principle(s) that probably acts differently from metformin (11).

3. Effect of *A. bilimbi* on Liver and Kidney Thio-Barbituric-Acid-Reactive Substances (TBARS) in STZ-Diabetic SD Rats

ABe and AF treatment at a dose of 125 mg/kg in STZ-diabetic SD rats reduced the TBARS levels in the kidneys, but not in the liver. The lack of change in TBARS levels in the liver of ABe-, AF-, and BuF-treated diabetic rats could again reflect the resistance of the liver to the oxidative stress in the diabetic state. It is significant to note that neither AF nor BuF affects this capacity adversely. Since ABe and AF have the ability to reduce the formation of TBARS, they could potentially prevent platelet aggregation and thrombosis (11,12).

4. Effect of *A. bilimbi* on Insulin in STZ-Diabetic Rats

Similar to other hypoglycemic agents such as tungstate and vanadate (15–17), AF caused a time-dependent hypoglycemic effect after twice-a-day oral administration of 125 mg/kg for 7 and 14 days in STZ-diabetic SD rats. On the other hand, when the STZ-diabetic rats were treated with 125 mg of BuF/kg, the serum insulin level was higher on both day 7 and day 14. The elevation in serum insulin in the AF- and BuF-treated STZ-diabetic rats could be due to either the insulinotropic substances present in the fractions, which induce the residual functional β cells to produce insulin, or the protection of the functional β cells from further deterioration so that they remain active and produce insulin. However, except for the level in the AF-treated group on day 14, the insulin levels were well below the normal insulin level in control rats, suggesting that they may not be sufficient to lower the blood glucose to its normal level in STZ-diabetic rats (12). This indicates a possible insulin-releasing action of ABe in STZ-diabetic rats like the extracts of *Medicago sativa* (18), *Eucalyptus globulus* (19), and *Sambucus nigra* (20) which have been shown to possess insulin-releasing action both in vitro and in vivo.

5. Effect of *A. bilimbi* on Liver Glucose-6-Phosphatase Activity and Glycogen in STZ-Diabetic Rats

Glucose-6-phosphatase catalyzes the final step in glucose production by the liver and kidney. STZ has been reported to increase the expression of glucose-6-phosphatase mRNA, which contributes to the increased glucose-6-phosphatase activity in diabetes mellitus (21). Overproduction of glucose by the liver is the major cause of fasting hyperglycemia in both insulin-dependent and non-insulin-dependent diabetes mellitus. Ninety percent of partially pancreatectomized diabetic rats have a >5-fold increase in the messenger RNA and a 3–4 fold increase in the protein level of the catalytic subunit of hepatic glucose-6-phosphatase. Prolonged hyperglycemia may thus result in overproduction of glucose via increased expression of this protein (22). Normalization of the plasma glucose concentration in diabetic rats with either insulin or the glycosuric agent phlorizin normalized the hepatic glucose-6-phosphatase messenger RNA and protein within approximately 8 hr. However, phlorizin failed to decrease hepatic glucose-6-phosphatase gene expression in diabetic rats when the fall in the plasma glucose concentration was prevented by glucose infusion (22). This indicates that in vivo gene expression of glucose-6-phosphatase in the diabetic liver is regulated by glucose independently of insulin. The AF fraction, like the biguanide drug metformin, appears to control the increase in blood glucose in STZ-diabetic rats by decreasing the activity of glucose-6-phosphatase in the liver. This could be one of the mechanisms for the suppression of blood glucose concentration in the diabetic rats (12). Similarly, extracts of plants such as *Zizyphus spina-christi* reduced serum glucose level, liver phosphorylase, and glucose-6-phosphatase activities, and increased serum pyruvate level after 4 weeks of treatment. Likewise 60% ethanolic extract of *Coccinia indica* and 95% ethanolic extract of *Momordica charantia* extracts were found to lower blood glucose by depressing its synthesis, on the one hand, by depressing key gluconeogenic enzymes glucose-6-phosphatase and fructose-1, 6-bisphosphatase and, on the other, by enhancing glucose oxidation by the shunt pathway through activation of its principal enzyme, glucose -6-phosphate dehydrogenase (23). However, AF and BuF treatment in STZ-diabetic rats did not affect hepatic glycogen content (12). Similarly, vanadate compounds have been shown to inhibit hepatic glucose-6-phosphatase activity thereby reducing blood glucose levels in nonobese diabetic (NOD) mice (24).

III. FUTURE PROSPECTS

The antidiabetic studies of *A. bilimbi* in STZ-diabetic rats demonstrate that the leaves of *A. bilimbi* possess hypoglycemic, hypotriglyceridemic, anti-lipid peroxidative as well as antiatherogenic properties in STZ-diabetic rats. Hence it is believed that *A. bilimbi* leaves might have different types of active principles, each with a single or a diverse range of biological activities (11,12). However, the ethnopharmacological properties of *A. bilimbi*—such as antibacterial, antiscorbutic, astringent, postpartum protection, anti-inflammatory, as well as its use in traditional medicine for the treatment of itches, boils, rheumatism, cough, syphilis (paste of leaves); scurvy, bilious colic, whooping cough, hypertension, children's cough (syrup of flowers); stomachache (fruits), mumps, and pimples (leaf decoction)—are yet to be justified by appropriate in vivo as well as in vitro studies.

REFERENCES

1. Goh SH, Chuah CH, Mok JSL, Soepadmo E. *Malaysian Medicinal Plants for the Treatment of Cardiovascular Diseases*. Pelanduk Publications: Malaysia, 1995: 62–63.
2. Tan BKH, Fu P, Chow PW, Hsu A. Effects of *A. bilimbi* on blood sugar and food intake in streptozotocin-induced diabetic rats [abstr]. Phytomedicine 1996; 3(supp 1):271.
3. Junod A, Lambert AE, Atauffacher W, Renold AE. Diabetogenic action of streptozotocin: relationship of dose to metabolic response. J Clin Invest 1969; 48:2129–2139.
4. Johansson EB, Tjalve H. Studies on the tissue-disposition and fate of [14C] streptozotocin with special reference to the pancreatic islets. Acta Endocrinol 1978; 89:339–351.
5. Yamamoto H, Uchigata Y, Okamoto H. Streptozotocin and alloxan induce DNA strand breaks and poly (ADP-ribose) synthetase in pancreatic islets. Nature 1981; 294:284–286.
6. Pitkanen O, Martin J, Hallman M, Akerblom H. Free radical activity during development of insulin-dependent diabetes mellitus in the rat. Life Sci 1992; 50:335–339.
7. Nagy MV, Chan EK, Teruya M, Forrest LE, Likhite V, Charles MA. Macrophage-mediated islet cell cytotoxicity in BB rats. Diabetes 1989; 38(10):1329–1331.
8. Robbins MJ, Sharp RA, Slonim AE, Burr IM. Protectin against streptozotocin-induced diabetes by superoxide dismutase. Diabetologia 1980; 18:55–58.
9. Uchigata Y, Yammamoto H, Nagai H, Okamoto H. Effect of poly (ADP-ribose)

synthetase inhibitors administration to rats before and after injection of alloxan and streptozotocin on islet proinsulin synthesis. Diabetes 1983; 32:316–318.
10. Al-awadi FM, Khattar MA, Gumaa A. On the mechanism of the hypoglycaemic effect of a plant extract. Diabetologia 1985; 28:432–434.
11. Pushparaj P, Tan CH, Tan BKH. Effects of *Averrhoa bilimbi* leaf extract on blood glucose and lipids in streptozotocin-diabetic rats. J Ethnopharmacol 2000; 72:69–76.
12. Pushparaj P, Tan BKH, Tan CH. The mechanism of hypoglycemic action of the semi-purified fractions of *Averrhoa bilimbi* in streptozotocin-diabetic rats. Life Sci 2001; 70:535–547.
13. Fontbonne A, Eschwege E, Cambien F, Richard JL, Ducimetiere P, Thibult N, Warnet JM, Claude JR, Rosselin GE. Hypertriglyceridaemia as a risk factor of coronary heart disease mortality in subjects with impaired glucose tolerance or diabetes. Diabetologia 1989; 32:300–304.
14. Carlsen SM, Rossvoll O, Bjerve KS, Folling I. Metformin improves blood lipid pattern in non-diabetic patients with coronary heart disease. J Intern Med 1996; 239:227–233.
15. Weirnsperger NF. Preclinical Pharmacology of Biguanides. Germany: Springer, 1996.
16. Barbera A, Rodriquez-Gil JE, Guinovart JJ. Insulin-like actions of tungstate in diabetic rats. J Biol Chem 1994; 269:20047–20053.
17. Gil J, Miralpeix M, Carreras J, Bartrons R. Insulin-like effects of vanadate on glucokinase activity and fructose-2,6-bisphosphate levels in the liver of diabetic rats. J Biol Chem 1988; 263:1868–1871.
18. Gray AM, Flatt PR. Pancreatic and extra-pancreatic effects of the traditional anti-diabetic plant, *Medicago sativa* (Lucerne). Br J Nutr 1997; 78:325–334.
19. Gray AM, Flatt PR. Antihyperglycemic actions of *Eucalyptus globulus* (Eucalyptus) are associated with pancreatic and extrapancreatic effects in mice. J Nutr 1998; 128:2319–2323.
20. Gray AM, Abdel-Wahab YHA, Flatt PR. The traditional plant treatment, *Sambucus nigra* (elder), exhibits insulin-like and insulin-releasing actions in vitro. J Nutr 2000; 130:15–20.
21. Liu Z, Barrett EJ, Dalkin AC, Zwart AD, Chou JY. Effect of acute diabetes on rat hepatic glucose-6-phosphatase activity and its messenger RNA level. Biochem Biophys Res Commun 1994; 205:680–686.
22. Massillon D, Barzilai N, Chen W, Hu M, Rossetti L. Glucose regulates in vivo glucose-6-phosphatase gene expression in the liver of diabetic rats. J Biol Chem 1996; 271(17):9871–9874.
23. Glombitza KW, Mahran GH, Mirhom YW, Michel KG, Motawi TK. Hypoglycemic and antihyperglycemic effects of *Zizyphus spina-christi* in rats. Planta Med 1994; 60:244–247.
24. Mosseri R, Waner T, Shefi M, Shafrir E, Meyerovitch J. Gluconeogenesis in non-obese diabetic (NOD) mice: in vivo effects of vanadate treatment on hepatic glucose-6-phosphatase and phosphoenopyruvate carboxykinase. Metab Clin Exp 2000; 49:321–325.

16

Lentinus edodes
Shiitake Mushrooms

Ann-Teck Yap and Mah-Lee Ng
National University of Singapore
Singapore, Republic of Singapore

I. INTRODUCTION

For many years, mushrooms have been used as both a food and medicine in many cultures, especially in the East. The use of mushrooms to maintain health was formally recorded as early as A.D. 100 in China. Mushrooms have a long history of use in folk medicine and have been incorporated into health tonics, tinctures, teas, soups, and healthty food dishes, as well as herbal formulae (1). Within the framework of traditional medicine, mushrooms have been applied to lubricate the lungs (*Tremella fuciformis*), tone the kidneys (*Cordyceps sinesis*), reduce excessive dampness (*Grifola umbellate*), and invigorate the spleen (*Poria cocos*).

Higher Basidiomycetes mushrooms with medicinal values, such as *Ganoderma lucidum* (Curt:Fr) P. Karst. (Reishi) *Dendropolyporyus umbellatus* (Pers.:Fr) Jül., and *Tremella fuciformis* Berk. (1–6), were recorded in *Shen Norg Ben Cao Jin* (*Compendium of Materia Medica* of the godly farmer, of East Han dynasty in China, A.D. 100–200).

Large numbers of mushroom-derived compounds, both cellular components and secondary metabolites, have also stirred up much interest in the medical field. Many have been shown to affect the immune system and could be used to treat a variety of disease states (7–14). There is vast amount of literature on a large diversity of mushrooms and their medicinal properties. This chapter will concentrate on the *Lentinus edodes* and its medicinal properties.

II. *LENTINUS EDODES*

In recent years, there has been growing awareness and interest in the medicinal value of the biologically active components extracted from higher Basidiomycoto mushrooms (15–18). One such mushroom is the *Lentinus edodes*, better known as shiitake mushroom, which belongs to the family Tricholomataceae (order Agaricales and class Basidiomycetes).

The edible part of raw *L. edodes* contains about 90% water. Carbohydrates make up the major component of dried shiitake (59.2%), followed by 22.7% protein (digestibility of 80–87%), 10% fiber, 3.2% lipids (primarily linoleic acid), and 4.7% ash. *L. edodes* is currently second in terms of global production, next to *Agaricus bisporus*. For centuries, this mushroom has been consumed not only as a delicacy but also for its beneficial effects.

Shiitake mushrooms (*L. edodes*, Berk Sing, Tricholomataceae fungus) is a cultured edible fungus popular in Japan for the past three centuries. The curative powers of shiitake mushrooms are legendary. It was stated in *Ri Yong Ben Cao*, Volume 3 (1620), written by Wu-Rui of the Ming dynasty (1368–1644), that "shiitake accelerates vital energy, wards off hunger, cures colds, and defeats body fluid energy." Thus, shiitake is treated as an elixir of life, but without scientific verification (12,13). Recently, it has attracted considerable medical interest because of a multitude of medical effects, in particular for its anticancer activity and control of cholesterol level and blood pressure. In addition, it was reported to have antiviral, antibacterial, and antiparasitic activities (19).

The active substances include polysaccharides (e.g., β-glucans), nucleic acid derivatives, the hypocholesterolemic eritadenine, lipids, peptides, proteins, and glycoproteins. From the carbohydrate portion, the most important component of shiitake, several polysaccharides have been identified. They consist of water-soluble polysaccharides (1–5% of dried mushrooms), glycogen-like polysaccharides, (1→4)-, (1→6)-α-D-glucans (antitumor polysaccharides), lentinan, (1→3)-, (1→6)-β-D-glucans, (1→6)-β-D-glucan with (1→3)- and (1→4)-β-bonded heteroglucans, heterogalactan, heteromannan, and xyloglucan (8). *L. edodes* also contains vitamins (e.g., provitamin D_2, niacin, vitamin B_2 and B_1), free sugars such as trehalose, glycerol, mannitol, arabitol, glucose, mannose, and arabinose including minerals such as Cd, Zn, Cu, Fe, Mn, and Ni.

III. LENTINAN-β-D-GLUCAN

The variety of polysaccharides that have the ability to enhance the immune system are pharmacologically classified as biological response modifiers (BRM). The most active BRM has (1→3)-β-D-glucans, sometimes referred to as (1→3), (1→6)-β-D-glucans. Chihara and co-workers (7,20,21) first isolated a water-soluble antitumor polysaccharide from fruiting bodies of *L. edodes*, which was named "lentinan" after the generic name of this mushrooms. The amount of pure lentinan extracted was low. In 2001, Yap and Ng (22) designed a more efficient and simple extraction procedure that resulted in yield of more that 100-fold of pure lentinan from the same amount of mushrooms.

Lentinan is a neutral polysaccharide isolated from *L. edodes*. It is a purified β-1,3-D-glucan with β-1,6 branches in a triple helical structure. Its physical and chemical properties have been widely characterized. The molecular formula for lentinan is $(C_6H_{10}O_5)_n$, and the mean molecular mass is 500 kDa (23–25). The structure of lentinan, as shown by electrophoresis, ultracentrifugation, and other instrumental analyses, was confirmed as β-(1,3)-D-glucopyranan with a branched chain of β-(1,6)-monoglycosyl, showing a right-handed helix. The properties of lentinan are listed by Chihara and colleagues (26).

Only those that consist of a (1→3)-linked β-glucan backbone with (1→6)-linked β-D-glucopyranosyl units as branches produce strong inhibition of tumor growth (27,28). Degree of branching plays a role in producing the antitumor activity. The most active polymers [(1→3)-β-D-glucans] have degrees of branching between 0.20 and 0.33. Immunomodulating activity also depends on the distribution of the branch units along the backbone chain (29). A triple helical tertiary conformation of β-(1→3)-glucans appears to play an important role in the immunostimulating activity of medicinal mushrooms. Various degrees of antitumor activities were observed according to the structure of glucans (26,30–33).

Lentinan is insoluble in cold water, acid, and almost all of organic solvents such as alcohol, ether, chloroform, and pyridine; slightly soluble in hot water, and soluble in aqueous alkali at a raised temperature and formic acid. Infrared spectra and nuclear magnetic resonance spectra show absorptions at 890 cm^{-1} and τ 5.4, respectively, and the presence of β-glycoside linkage (21,25).

IV. OPTIMAL DOSAGE DETERMINATION

To achieve the desired highest antitumor effect, the amount of lentinan given to the experimental model should be optimized. Initially, lentinan showed little effectiveness, primarily because the dosages used were above or below what was later found to be optimal. Chihara and co-workers (7) and Aoki (34) showed that lentinan caused complete regression of sarcoma 180 transplanted into the mice at a dose of 1 mg/kg for 10 days (intraperitoneal route), while a larger dose of 80 mg/kg for 5 days yielded no antitumor activity in comparison with untreated control mice (28). Yap and Ng (22) demonstrated that 150 mg/kg lentinan is the most effective dose when administered by the oral route and achieved a tumor inhibition rate of 94.44% in murine lymphoma. Doses higher or lower than that resulted in a lower tumor inhibition rate (76–85%). These observations suggested that there might be a relationship between lentinan, types of cancer under study, route of administration, and the host's immune system, whereby a threshold of saturation for activation of lymphocytes exists. So the optimal dosage determined is a crucial consideration in treatment with lentinan.

V. THE MEDICINAL AND THERAPEUTIC VALUE OF LENTINAN

The beneficial effects of lentinan have been known for a long time and their activities have been identified. Many experiments have been conducted to demonstrate the usefulness of lentinan. Results from various experiments are promising. In Japan, lentinan is currently classified as a drug for its known effects. Lentinan has been marketed for the past 10 years in Japan for the treatment of gastric cancer, in combination with tegafur. It was safely administrated to 50,000 patients in Japan, involving a total of more than 2,000,000 doses. The usual dose in Japan is 2 mg/week (35).

A. Anticancer/Antitumor Effects

Lentinan isolated by Chihara and co-workers (7,20,26) resulted in complete regression of tumor induced from sarcoma 180 ascites cells implanted in Swiss albino mice with no cytotoxicity when given intraperitoneally. Lentinan was effective in limiting the tumor size, regardless of whether it was in an allogenic tumor-host system, syngenic tumor-host system, or autochthonous host system (31,32,36,37).

Other studies showed tumor regression in C3H/He mice when MM46 mammary carcinoma cells were subcutaneously inoculated (38). Complete regression of large Madison 109 lung carcinoma in syngeneic BALB/c mice was achieved. Evaluation of the effects of lentinan against Lewis Lung (LL) and Madison 109 (M109) lung carcinomas that were implanted in the footpads of syngeneic mice was carried out by Rose and co-workers (39). Intraperitoneal administration of lentinan was curative to mice bearing M109 lung carcinomas (50–70%) though it had no substantial effect on LL carcinomas. This contradicted the findings of Suzuki et al. (40). Their study showed inhibition of pulmonary metastasis of LL carcinoma, also in mice.

Lentinan would also be effective for patients with advanced or recurrent breast cancer (41,42). Side effects have been transitional and not serious. Use of lentinan in a combined treatment of patients with advanced or recurrent gastric or colorectal cancer has also resulted in an increased life span (26,43). In addition, lentinan was able to prevent chemical oncogenesis as shown by its suppressive effect on 3-methylcholanthrene-induced carcinogenesis (36).

For all the above studies cited so far, lentinan was administered via injections. Studies (44–48) were carried out using oral administration of powdered, dried mushroom fruiting bodies. Oral administration may be important for eliminating the side effects of $(1\rightarrow3)$-β-D-glucans, including the pain that accompanies parenteral administration. The tumor-growth-inhibitory activity increased with the concentration of the shiitake mushroom powder. When 10% L-feed (feed containing powdered shiitake fruit bodies) was used, the rate of tumor inhibition was 39.6%. Inhibition rates of 53.2% and 58.9% were achieved when 20% L-feed and 30% L-feed, respectively, were used. The degree of inhibition was proportional to the experimental diet. Administration schedule of the lentinan also influenced the rate of tumor inhibition.

In the most recent study on oral administration of lentinan conducted by Yap and Ng (22,49), male ARK mice (5–6 weeks old) were used. K36 cells (a murine lymphoma cell line) were used to induce the tumors. The mice were divided into three cohorts, namely, prefeeding for 7 days prior to inoculation of K36 cells, simultaneous feeding of the lentinan with inoculation of K36 cells, and postfeeding after 7 days of tumor induction with K36 cells. Three milligrams of lentinan were resuspended in buffer and force-fed to the mice daily.

Table 1 summarizes the data collected. It was clearly shown that lentinan feeding was very effective in preventing tumor development (between 83 and 94%). Prefeeding was the most effective regime when compared with simultaneous and postfeeding. The percentage of 83% from the postfeeding cohort indicated the regression rate of the developed tumors.

Crude mushroom homogenates also resulted in some degree of antitumor efficacy but at a much lower percentage (43–55%) The buffer-fed mice were controls (placebo). The mice with tumors are shown in Figure 1. Comparison of the sizes of the excised tumors is clearly shown.

In addition to the strong antitumor properties, the lentinan appeared to interfere with the morphogenesis of the murine lymphoma retrovirus (Fig. 2). The virus from the tumor cells of the control groups was electron-dense. However, in the lentinan-fed cohort, the virus particles from the tumor cells were empty. This indicated that the virus particles lacked the genomes and,

TABLE 1 Antitumor Properties of Lentinan

Feeding with	Average weight of tumors (g)	Tumor inhibition rate (TIR) %
Pure lentinan	0.124 (prefeed)	94.44 ($p < 0.001$)
	0.265 (S/F)	88.59 ($p < 0.001$)
	0.398 (postfeed)	83.14 ($p < 0.001$)
Crude mushroom homogenate	0.997 (prefeed)	55.20 ($p < 0.001$)
	1.272 (S/F)	45.32 ($p < 0.001$)
	1.345 (postfeed)	43.06 ($p < 0.001$)
Buffer solution	2.230 (prefeed)	0
	2.386 (S/F)	0
	2.362 (postfeed)	0

thus, were defective. This could be the reason that the induced tumors (if they occurred) were very small (Table 1) and well localized, unlike the control mice.

Past studies have shown that the efficacy of lentinan in the treatment of cancer is increased when used in conjunction with other therapies. The highest antitumor effect was achieved when bacterial lipopolysaccharide was used with lentinan (50,51). Lentinan could be used in combination with IL-2 for treating cancer (52–56). The combined administration of IL-2 and lentinan was effective against IL-2-resistant established murine tumors. Hamuro and co-workers (57) also investigated the antimetastatic effects of combined treatment with lentinan and IL-2 in spontaneous metastatic systems using murine fibrosarcoma and also showed the fruitful effects.

Marked antitumor effects were achieved when lentinan was used in conjunction with chemotherapy. The activity of pyrimidine nucleoside phosphorylase (an enzyme that converts 5′-deoxy-5-fluorouridine (5′-DFUR) to 5-fluorouracil) was induced by lentinan in tumors, but not in the spleen, thereby increasing the susceptibility of tumor cells to 5′-DFUR (58). Considerable improvement was seen in gastric and breast cancers when lentinan was used in combination with chemotherapy (59,60). Lentinan also enhanced the sensitivity of mouse colon 26 tumor to *cis*-diamminedichloro platinum (61). An in vivo study in rats with peritonitis involving the combination of lentinan with gentamicin showed a significantly better survival rate than controls (13). The tumor-regressive effect of lentinan was markedly reduced by X-irradiation of mice. 6-Benzyl thioguanosine reduced the antitumor activity of lentinan when it was injected after sarcoma 180 implantation (62). Such immunosuppressive agents should be avoided when lentinan is used to treat cancer patients.

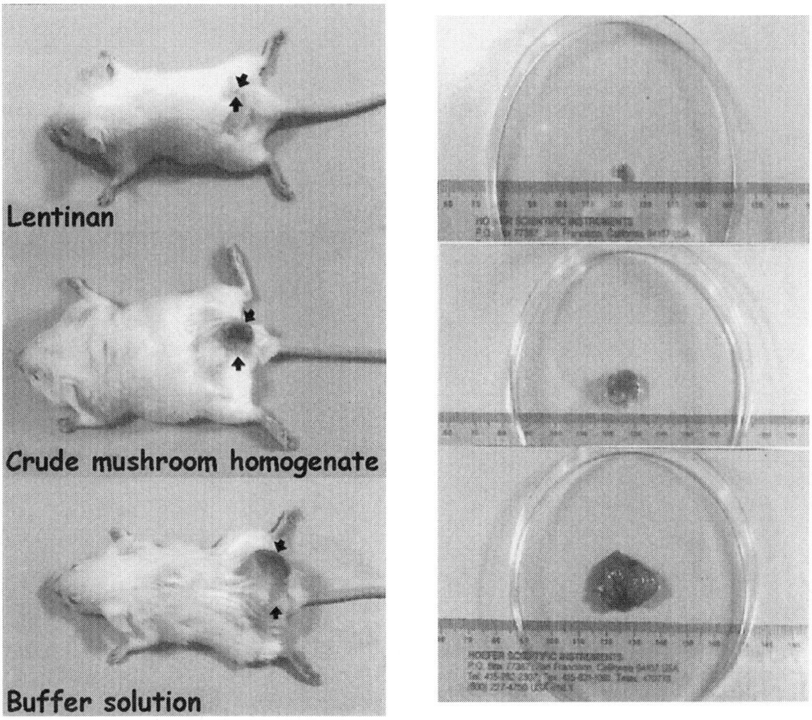

Figure 1 Comparison of tumor sizes between lentinan-, crude-mushroom-homogenate-, and buffer-fed mice. K36 cells (a murine lymphoma cell line) were used to induce the tumors. It is clearly demonstrated that the tumor excised from the buffer-fed mouse is several times larger than that from mouse fed with lentinan. Crude mushroom homogenate also offers some antitumor properties as the tumor size is smaller than that of the buffer-fed cohort. This observation is statistically significant as presented in Table 1.

The immunopotentiating ability of lentinan was postulated to play a key role in the antitumor process. Administration of lentinan to gastric cancer patients undergoing chemotherapy inhibited suppressor T-cell activity and increased the ratio of activated T cells and cytotoxic T cells in the spleen (63,64). Lentinan also increases peritoneal macrophage cytotoxicity against metastatic tumor cells in mice (65). Antimacrophage agents such as carrageenan also inhibited the effect of lentinan (26,66–68). The antitumor effect of lentinan is abolished by neonatal thymectomy and decreased by the administration of antilymphocyte serum, supporting the concept that lentinan requires immunocompetent T-cell compartments.

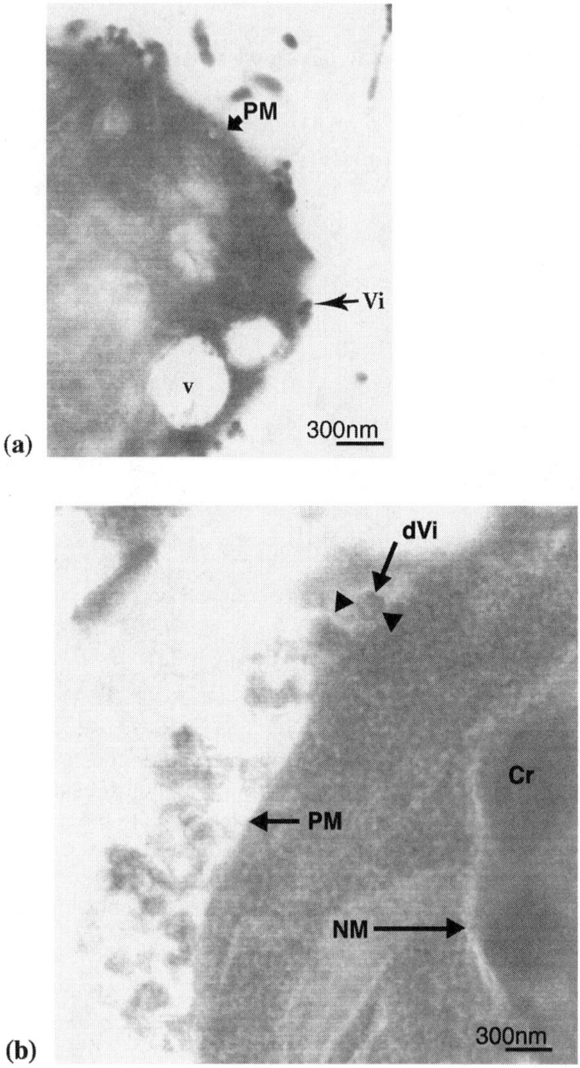

Figure 2 Electron micrograph of murine retrovirus particles budding from tumor cells. (a) In the buffer-fed regime, electron-dense infectious virus particles (Vi) are seen budding out from the plasma membrane. (b) In contrast, the virus particles budding out from the lentinan-fed cohort exhibit empty core structures. This indicates that the virus particles are defective (dVi) and lack the virus genomes.

B. Immune-Modulating Effects of Lentinan

The antitumor activity of lentinan resulted from activation of the host's immune functions rather than direct cytotoxicity to target cells (22,26,66,67, 69,70). The mechanism is postulated to involve binding of β-glucan to the surface layer of lymphocyte or specific serum protein. This activated macrophages, T cells, NK cells, and other effector cells, as well as increasing production of antibodies, interleukins, and interferons (45,71,72). Lentinan is considered to be phagocytosed by cells of macrophage lineage present in organs such as liver, spleen, and lung, and activates these cells (54,55,70,73–75). Macrophages are the first to recognize foreign bodies as nonself and give this information to lymphocytes to activate the immune system. They probably respond acutely to BRMs such as lentinan. Lentinan has been shown to facilitate the infiltration of lymphocytes and macrophages into tumor tissues (64).

Suzuki et al. (55–57) also showed that the antitumor effect was dependent on the CD-positive T lymphocytes. Lentinan stimulates the macrophages to augment their antitumor activity (76). More macrophages and T cells were found in lentinan-fed mice compared to the control group. Suzuki and co-workers (55) and Hamuro et al. (57) suggested that in addition to the augmentation of immune effector cell activity against tumors, infiltration of these cells into the tumor sites might also be involved in eradication of tumors by lentinan. Tumor-induced immunosuppression could also be overcome by lentinan treatment through enhancement of the macrophage migration inhibitory factor production (32).

The effector cells might act either selectively or nonselectively on target cells (8). Various kinds of bioactive serum factors, associated with immunity and inflammation, (such as IL-2, IL-3, vascular dilation inducer, and acute-phase protein inducer), appeared immediately after the administration of lentinan. Increments in the production of antibodies as well as interleukins (IL-1, IL-2) and interferon (IFN-γ) have also been observed (12,13,22,26,57, 63,67,70,77–86). The mechanism of lentinan-enhanced antibody-dependent, cell-mediated cytotoxicity through helper T cells (77,84) remains uncertain.

Yap and Ng further conducted a time-sequenced study on the induction of various cytokines in AKR mouse after oral feeding with lentinan. Four cytokines levels, namely IL-1α (interleukin-1 produced mainly by monocytes, promote proliferation of Th2 CD4+ T cells), IL-2 (interleukin-2 produced mainly by Th0 and Th1 CD4+ cells, as T-cell growth factor), TNF-α (produced mainly by monocytes, activates endothelial cells and other cells of immune and nonimmune systems), and IFN-γ (interferon-gamma, produced by Th1 CD4+ cells, activates NK cells, macrophages, and killer cells), rose significantly after feeding with lentinan. They peaked at different hours after feeding with lentinan but returned to baseline after 24 hr (Fig. 3a–d). The IL-1α (Fig. 3a) and IL-2 (Fig. 3b) peaked at 2 hr postfeeding with lentinan. Both the TNF-α and IFN-γ peaked at 4 hr postfeeding (Fig. 3c and 3d).

These results suggested that oral administration of lentinan may serve as a means of activating the immune system, provoking the immune responses required for disease prevention. Lentinan, once ingested, may encounter the gut-associated lymphoid tissue (GALT), which is a well-developed immune network, evolved to protect the host from infecting pathogens. Lentinan may also be absorbed into the systemic circulation, thereafter, involved in inducing immune systems against future pathogenic attack. Quantitative analysis of orally administered lentinan in murine blood carried out using limulus colorimetric test demonstrated that pure lentinan was detected in the murine blood and peaked at 0.2 mg (equivalent to the usual intravenous or intraperitoneal inoculation dosage) 30 min after feeding (Yap and Ng, unpublished data).

When fed with crude mushroom homogenates, IL-1α, IL-2, and TNF-α levels were also induced but to much lower levels when compared to lentinan-fed cohort. The IFN-γ level was not significantly induced. The lipid and protein fractions from the mushrooms did not result in noticeable induction of any of the four cytokines tested and was at the baseline like the buffer-fed cohort (control).

Many interesting biological activities of lentinan have been reported. This included an increase in the activation of nonspecific inflammatory responses such as APP (acute-phase protein) production (87), vascular dilation, and hemorrhagic necrosis of the tumors (88). Bradykinin-induced skin reaction could be used as an index of vascular reactions against lentinan and this skin reaction could be used to moniter the host sensitivity to lentinan in antitumor responses (89).

Activation and generation of helper and cytotoxic T cells (10,67,79,90–93) is an essential aspect of lentinan treatment. The augmentation of immune mediators such as IL-1 and IL-3, colony-stimulating factor(s) (94), migration inhibitory factor (32,94,95), and increasing the capacity of PBM (peripheral blood mononuclear) cells (52,53) contributed additively to the antitumor efficacy. Wang and Lin (96) postulated that the immunomodulating effect of lentinan might be relevant to change of T-cell subpopulation and increase of TNF production.

The recent study of Yap and Ng confirmed that T-lymphocytes were increased significantly (fourfold, $p < 0.001$, Student's *t*-test) after feeding with lentinan (Table 2). The CD3, CD4 (T-helper), and CD8 (T-cytotoxic) lymphocytes were isolated using T-cell-enrichment columns. All three types of CD lymphocytes were activated in comparison with the buffer-fed controls. It was noted that the placebo (controls) effects did result in some degree of

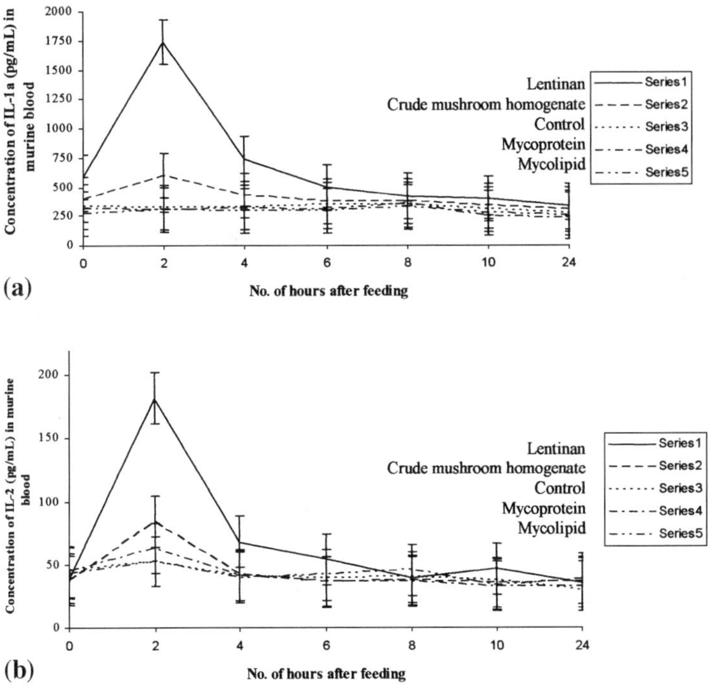

FIGURE 3 Cytokine profiles from mice fed with lentinan, crude mushroom homogenate, lipid fraction, protein fraction, and buffer (placebo). (a) IL1-α profile. There is a sharp rise 2 hr after feeding with lentinan. A small increase in level of IL1-α is seen in the mice fed with the crude mushroom homogenate. For the other three cohorts of mice, the level is at the baseline. (b) IL-2. Similar to (a), a significant rise in IL-2 level is seen in the lentinan-fed mice. This is followed in modest amount in the crude-mushroom-homogenate-fed population. Again the lipid-, protein-, and buffer-fed mice do not show any change in the level over the experimental period. (c) TNF-α. The rise in TNF-α level is seen at 4 hr after lentinan feeding. The level is also quite significant for the crude-mushroom-homogenate-fed mice. The usual low level of stimulation is seen with the other three regimes. (d) IFN-γ. The profile obtained is similar to (c) with rise at 4 hr in the lentinan-fed mice. Other than a low level of induction seen in the crude-mushroom-homogenate-fed population, the other three cohorts show minimal changes in the level of production over the 24-hr period.

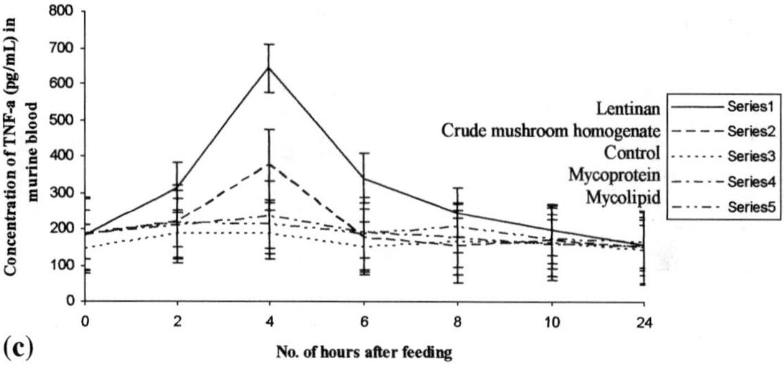

(c)

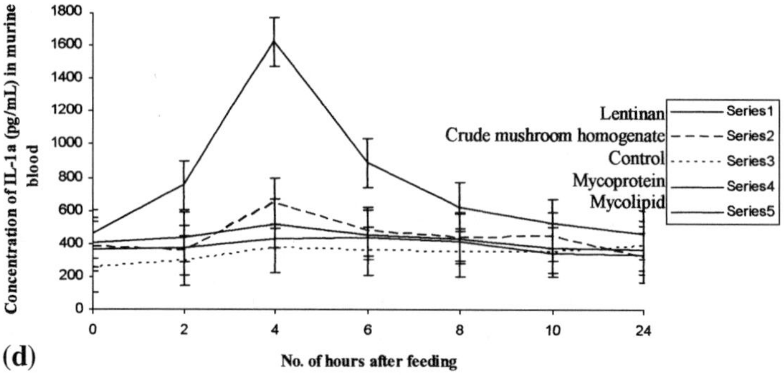

(d)

FIGURE 3 Continued.

activations of the lymphocytes. This could be due to the response of stress from force feeding of the fluid. The most activated lymphocytes were the CD4 helper lymphocytes (100%) followed by almost similar degree of activation in CD3 and CD8 lymphocytes.

Lentinan-activated lymphocytes were extracted from lentinan-fed AKR mice and reinoculated into nude (athymic) and SCID (lack immunoglobulin and lymphocytes) mice before the inoculation of human colon carcinoma cells. Six different cell lines were used representing different stages of differentiation of the carcinoma cells. Tabulated in Figure 4, the data showed that the "lentinan-activated" lymphocytes did indeed protect the immunocompromised mice effectively against human colon carcinoma development (49). These experiments showed beyond doubt that T-lymphocytes were truly activated by lentinan administration. The antitumor mechanism was a T-cell-mediated process. Figure 5 shows the proposed immunomodulating pathway after lentinan administration. Activation of

TABLE 2 Cluster of Differentiation of T-Lymphocytes

	Mice fed with	Total cell count (CD90—normal)	Cell count (CD25—activated)	Percentage of activation (%)
CD3 T-lymphocytes isolated using CD3 T-cell-enrichment column	Lentinan	13.55×10^6	9.405×10^6	69.20
	Crude mushroom homogenate	3.989×10^6	6.200×10^6	64.24
	Buffer solution	2.313×10^6	4.593×10^6	50.69
CD4 T helper lymphocytes isolated using CD4 T-cell-enrichment column	Lentinan	2.150×10^6	2.150×10^6	100.00
	Crude mushroom homogenate	1.435×10^6	0.715×10^6	49.85
	Buffer solution	0.782×10^6	0.311×10^6	40.33
CD8 T cytotoxic lymphocytes isolated using CD8 T-cell-enrichment column	Lentinan	3.393×10^6	2.263×10^6	66.80
	Crude mushroom homogenate	2.148×10^6	0.875×10^6	39.29
	Buffer solution	1.515×10^6	0.523×10^6	34.54

the immune responses against the tumor cells resulted in the process of apoptosis in these cells leading to tumor regression (49).

C. Antiviral Effects

Lentinan showed marked antiviral activity and increased host resistance against various kinds of viral infections, such as adenovirus, vesicular stomatitis virus (VSV)-encephalitis virus, Abelson virus, human immunodeficiency virus (HIV), and influenza virus.

The effect of lentinan on influenza virus infection has also been determined and reported by Irinoda et al. (97) and Maeda et al. (93). A significant level of protection in NMRI mice was noticed, even at low dosage (50 μg) of lentinan when administrated intranasally or intravenously. In 2001, Yap and Ng (22) showed that the administration of lentinan to AKR mice interfered with the maturation process of the murine leukemia retrovirus (Fig. 2).

Nude mice						
Lentinan	LoVo	SW48	SW620	SW480	SW403	SW1116
(TIR%)	85.84	87.3	88.38	88.69	89.94	91.43
SCID mice						
Lentinan (TIR%)	74.69	Test not done	70.18	Test not done	Test not done	Test not done

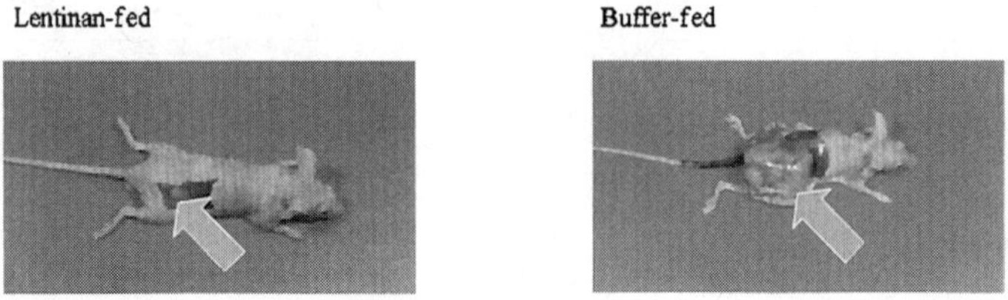

FIGURE 4 The efficacy of "lentinan-activated" lymphocytes in nude and SCID mice. Lymphocytes from AKR mice that had been fed with lentinan for 7 days were extracted and inoculated into nude or SCID mice. After inoculation of the "lentinan-activated" lymphocytes, human colon carcinoma cells were also inoculated into these mice to induce tumors. Six different human colon carcinoma cell lines were used. LoVo and SW48 represent a well-differentiated stage with signet ring formation, SW620 and SW480 are moderately differentiated, and SW403 and SW1116 are poorly differentiated with little or no signet ring formation. The tumor from the buffer-fed mouse is rather large when compared to that of the mouse that is fed with lentinan. The summary table shows that "lentinan-activated" lymphocytes do have good efficacy against tumor formation in these immunodeficient mice.

The progeny virus particles found in the induced murine lymphoma cells were defective as observed using electron microscopy.

Many AIDS patients die of opportunistic infections due to immunodysfunction, and prevention of the development of symptoms by enhancing the immune system would be useful. Effects against HIV have been found in some of the carcinostatic β-D-glucans (lentinan and others) isolated from shiitake mushrooms (98–101). A tolerance study of lentinan in HIV patients has been carried out and showed that lentinan was well tolerated and produced increases in neutrophils and natural killer (NK) cells activity (35). Lentinan also produced a trend toward improvement in CD4 cells generation and a decline in p24 antigen levels.

Tochikura et al. (101) and Iizuka (102) reported that when used in combination with azidothymidine (AZT), lentinan suppressed the surface expression of HIV on T cells more efficiently than AZT alone. It enhanced the effects against viral replication in vitro. Lentinan therefore qualified as a participant in future multidrug studies in HIV (35).

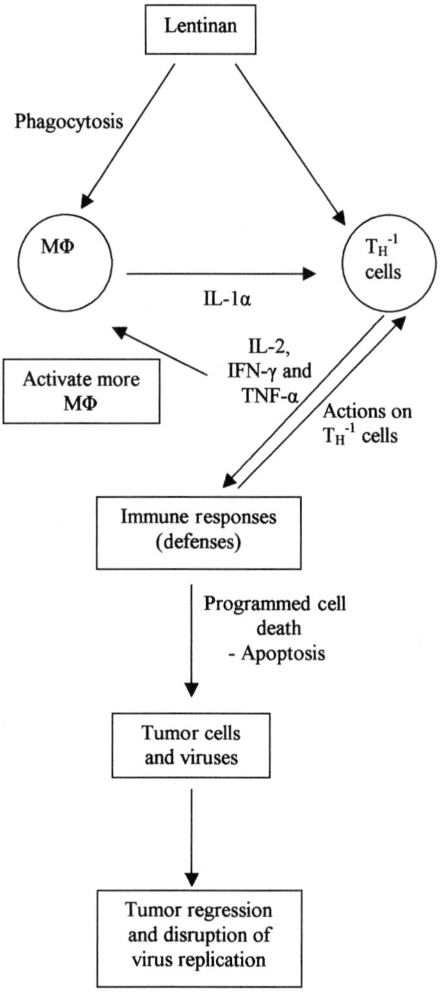

Figure 5 A proposed immunomodulation pathway of lentinan. Lentinan first comes in contact with macrophages, which in turn stimulate and activate the T cells, resulting in cytokine production. The immune response acts on the tumor cells causing apoptosis and regression of the tumor.

Lentinan has been used as an immune modulator in combination with didanosine (DDI) in a controlled study with HIV-positive patients. In vitro studies have indicated that anti-HIV effects of lentinan and DDI were additive. With promising results, it is reasonable to test the combined use of lentinan and DDI in HIV-infected individuals as well (35).

D. Antibacterial Effects

Lentinan's effectiveness against bacterial infections has been demonstrated using *Mycobacterium tuberculosis* as the test organism in IRC mice. A marked anti-infective activity was observed, and all mice completely survived when lentinan was injected intravenously once from 4 to 10 days before the infection (103). In mouse experiments, it has also been proven to be effective against relapse of tuberculosis infections (60). Peritoneal macrophages secretory activity of active oxygen was activated by lentinan and the cytokines produced enhanced the ability of polymophonuclear leukocytes to produce active oxygen with bactericidal effect (104).

E. Antiparasitic Activity of Lentinan

Lentinan was shown to be effective against parasitic infections caused by *Schistosoma mansoni*, *S. japonicum*, and *Mesocestoides corti* (93,105,106). The mechanism was concluded to be through cell-mediated immunity and was T-cell-dependent as the antiparasitic activities were not illustrated in nude mice.

VI. OTHER COMPONENTS OF LESSER INTEREST

Another active component, α-mannan peptide (KS-2), extracted from cultured mycelium of *L. edodes* was shown to be effective against sarcoma 180 and Ehrlich's carcinoma. Antitumor activity of KS-2 in mice has demonstrated a macrophage tumoricidal effect, though the actual mechanism of action of KS-2 is not clear (100).

A water-soluble, pale-brownish powder designated LEM was prepared from the culture medium of shiitake mushroom mycelia before the formation of fruit bodies. LEM is a glycoprotein containing glucose, galactose, xylose, arabinose, mannose, fructose, and various nucleic acid derivatives, vitamin B compounds, especially B_1 (thiamine), B_2 (riboflavin), and ergosterol (107). Two alcohol-insoluble fractions, LAP1 and LAP2, can be separated from LEM (108,109). LAP is a glycoprotein containing glucose, galactose, xylose, arabinose, mannose, and fructose (102). In turn, a heteroglycan fraction

(LAF1) can be prepared from LAP1 by DEAE-sepharose CL-6B column chromatography. Xylose is the major sugar in LAP or LAP1. The fraction LAF1 is composed mainly of xylose, arabinose, mannose, glucose, and galactose (111).

Both LEM and LAP components displayed strong antitumor activities (111,112). The growth of cancerous liver tumors was slowed in rats when LEM was given by injection (60). Administration of LEM (intraperitoneally) suppressed the cell proliferation of ascites hepatoma. The LEM fraction was also observed to activate the murine macrophage functions and promoted the proliferation of bone marrow cells in vitro. Cytotoxicity of NK cells was noted, and macrophages and T cells were also activated (112). LEM was found to inhibit the expression of cytopathic effects of herpes simplex virus, western equine enchepalitis virus, poliovirus, measles virus, mumps virus, and HIV (100,101,113).

The same effect was achieved when LAP was administered. The fraction LAP2 also suppressed cell proliferation of the ascites hepatoma, but the survival rate of hepatoma-bearing rats was not improved (108,109). Thus, the action of LAP1 was not cytocidal. Both LAP1 and LAF1 fractions might act as mitogens for mouse splenic macrophages and/or monocytes that are involved in cytokine induction (109,110). A protein fraction of *L. edodes* fruiting bodies known as fruiting body protein (FBP) is noted to prevent infection of plants with tobacco mosaic virus (TMV) (14).

The antiviral and immunopotentiating activities of the water-soluble, lignin-rich fraction of LEM, JLS-18, was proven. JLS-18 showed about 70 times higher antiviral activity than LEM in vitro. Release of herpes simple virus type 1 in animals is blocked by JLS-18 (9).

Studies have shown that *L. edodes* is also able to lower blood serum cholesterol (BSC) via a factor known as eritadenine (also called "lentinacin" or "lentysine"). Eritadenine was isolated from 80% ethanol extraction of *L. edodes* mushroom fruiting bodies by absorption on an Amberlite IR-120 (H^+) column, followed by elution with 4% NH_4OH (21). Addition of eritadenine (0.005%) to the diet of rats caused a 25% decrease in total cholesterol in 1 week. Eritadenine apparently reduces serum cholesterol in mice by accelerating the excretion of ingested cholesterol and its metabolic decomposition (13,114).

VII. MYCOVIRUS

Mycovirus or virus-like particles have been found in various species of fungi and most possess double-stranded RNA (ds-RNA) (115–122). These mycoviruses are heritable viruses (25) and are unusual in that they do not lyse or cause any detrimental effects in their hosts (119). The spores are an effective means for serial transmission. Three morphologically groups (25, 30, and 39 nm in diameter) have been found in partially purified preparations from both fruit bodies and mycelia of *L. edodes* (122–126).

In 1979 and 1981, Takehara and co-workers (127,128) demonstrated that viruses isolated from *L. edodes* mushrooms (including their RNA) exhibited antiviral activities in cell culture studies. It was proposed that the efficacy was from its interferon-inductive effect. Certain ds-RNA of natural and synthetic origin has been found to inhibit the growth of various transplanted tumors or leukemia in animals (58,129,130).

Suzuki and co-workers (131) reported that ds-RNA fractions extracted from *L. edodes* are highly active as an interferon inducer. They also showed the inhibitory activity was against solid tumor but not against the ascites form of the tumor, which suggested the involvement of a host-mediated immunological response to the tumor. However, Takehara and co-workers (127) demonstrated antitumor activity against Ehrlich ascites carcinoma in mice.

Owing to the lack of detailed study on the medical significance of these mycovirus, Sudhir and Ng (132) and Subha and Ng (unpublished data) carried out several experiments on this component of the *L. edodes* mushrooms. Prefeeding of AKR mice with mycovirus-extract conferred the best antitumor activity with a tumor inhibition rate (TIR) of 80.7%. Simultaneous feeding and administration of extract on induced tumors were also effective with TIR of 73.8% and 67.6%, respectively. The tumor cells used to induce the tumor were K36 murine lymphoma cells. Tumor cells in the prefeeding regime also exhibited extensive apoptotic cell death, which could be the mechanism of destroying the tumor cells (132). In addition, elevated production of T-helper lymphocytes, IFN-γ, and TNF-α was observed after oral administration of mycovirus extract.

The antiviral effect of the produced interferons appeared to interfere with the infectious retrovirus morphogenesis. The virus particles found in the mycovirus-fed tumor cells were mostly empty, i.e., without the virus genome. The defective progeny virus particles could explain the strong inhibition of tumor development in the prefed cohort.

Antiviral activity of the mycovirus was demonstrated with avian influenza virus in primary chick embryo cells. Cytopathic effects caused by the influenza virus were inhibited when the chick cells were pretreated with a suspension of the mycovirus before exposure to influenza virus (Subha and Ng, unplublished data). The mycovirus suspension was also tested against a range of bacteria (*Bacillus subtilis*, *Corynebacterium diptheriae*, *Micrococcus luteus*, *Streptococcus pyogenes*, *Staphylococcus aureus*, *Enterobacter aerogenes*, *Escherichia coli*, *Klebsiella pneumoniae*, *Salmonella typhi*, *Vibrio parachaemolyticus*, *Bacteroides fragilis*, *Clostridium perfringes*, and *Clostridium sporogenes*). The mycovirus suspension was not effective in the inhibition of any bacterial growth.

VIII. CLINICAL APPLICATION AND POSSIBLE FUTURE TRENDS

Lentinan appears to be a unique immunological adjuvant with no toxic side effects on in vivo application. It was found to have distinct antitumor and metastasis-inhibiting effect in allogenic, syngenic, and autochthonous hosts, and its mode of action has been elucidated. Several studies have been done on the antitumor activity of *L. edodes* (7,21,22,26,31–34,36,37,39,42,44–47,49,67,133–136) and it has been widely accepted that activated macrophages, cytotoxic T cells, natural killer cells, and killer T cells usually play important roles in the immunity against tumor. Lentinan has been reported to enhance the activity of these immune systems and its antitumor activity is activated through a host-mediated immune response (10,20,21,45,71,76,137–139). Hence, lentinan shows great potential as a candidate for effective therapy of cancer patients.

Several studies have shown the safety of soluble β-glucans and the absence of undesirable side effects (21,26,45,71,137). Studies involving animal models revealed that the LD_{50} is over 2500 mg/kg by intraperitoneal and 250–500 mg/kg via intravenous administration in mice and rats (26). Yap and Ng (22) and Sudhir and Ng (132) also observed no weight loss in the experimental mice experiment over a period of 1 month.

Clinical trials using lentinan in combination with chemotherapy have shown encouraging results (41,42,52,53,135,134). Taguchi (42), investigating the clinical application of lentinan, has carried out Phase I, II, and III studies of randomized control clinical trials. Results of a 4-year follow-up Phase III randomized control study of lentinan patients with advanced and recurrent stomach and colorectal cancer revealed that the combination therapy of lentinan with tegafur led to the prolongation of their life span. Increment in survival time and complete cure of micrometastases after surgical resection in cancer patients could also be achieved by using lentinan (64,140,141).

Human cancer is a disease with great diversity as compared to other infectious diseases. The tumor-host relationships may differ, depending on the stage of tumor growth, as well as the course of treatments. Hence, the use of lentinan for human cancer should be based on strict administration timing and dosage schedules in compliance with the immunological and biological changes that were observed in lentinan-treated animals. The effect of lentinan in the treatment of human cancer is increased when it is used in conjunction with other therapies, especially after surgical resection. An important field of study may be to determine the parameters for tumor-host relationships, which can then be used as indicators for the design of protocols on the use of immunopotentiators such as lentinan.

ACKNOWLEDGMENT

The authors are grateful to the National University of Singapore for the research grant (R-182-000-018-112). Thanks to Ms. R. K. Bhuvana for her kind assistance in verification of the bibliography and to Miss Patricia Netto for preparing the figures.

REFERENCES

1. Chang R. Functional properties of edible mushrooms. Nutr Rev 1996; 54(11): S91–S93.
2. Yang QY, Jong SC. Medicinal mushrooms in China. Mushroom Sci 1989; 9(1):631–643.
3. Kabi YM, Kimur S. Effect of shiitake (*Lentinus edodes*) and maitake (*Grifola frondosa*) mushrooms on blood pressure and plasma lipids of spontaneously hypertensive rats. J Nutr Sci Vitaminol 1989; 33:341–346.
4. Concise basics and current developments. In: Miles PG, Chang ST, eds. Mushroom Biology. Singapore, Hong Kong: World Scientific, 1997:1–194.
5. Wasser SP, Weis AL. In: Nevo E, ed. Medicinal Mushrooms, *Lentinus edodes* (Berk.) Sing. (Shiitake Mushroom). Haifa: Peledfus, 1997:96–127.
6. Wasser SP, Weis AL. In: Nevo E, ed. Medicinal Mushrooms, Reishi Mushroom (*Ganoderma lucidum* (Curtis:Fr.) P. Karst.). Haifa: Peledfus, 1997:39.
7. Chihara G, Maeda Y, Hamuro J, Sasaki T, Fukuoka F. Inhibition of mouse sarcoma 180 by polysaccharides from *Lentinus edodes* (Berk.) sing. Nature 1969; 222(194):687–688.
8. Jong SC, Birmingham JM, Pai SH. Immuno-modulatory substances of fungal origin. J Immunol Immunopharmacol 1991; 9(3):115–122.
9. Jong SC, Birmingham JM. Medicinal and therapeutic value of the shiitake mushroom. Adv Appl Microbiol 1993; 39:153–184.
10. Chihara G. Preclinical evaluation of lentinan in animal models. Adv Exp Med Biol 1983; 166:189–197.
11. Sakagami H, Aoki T, Simpson A, Tanuma S. Induction of immunopotentiation activity by a protein-bound polysaccharide, PSK. Anticancer Res 1991; 11(2):993–999. Review.
12. Mizuno T. Bioactive biomolecules of mushrooms: food function and medicinal effect of mushroom fungi. Food Rev Int 1995; 11(1):7–21.
13. Mizuno, Shiitake T. *Lentinus edodes*: functional properties for medicinal and food purposes. Food Rev Int 1995; 11(1):111–128.
14. Wasser SP, Weis AL. Medicinal properties of substances occurring in higher

Basidiomycetes, mushrooms: current perspectives. Int J Med Mushrooms 1999; 1:31–62. Review.

15. Ikekawa T, Nakanishi M, Uehara N, Chihara G, Fukuoka F. Antitumor action of some Basidiomycetes, especially *Phellinus linteus*. Jpn J Cancer Res (Gann) 1968; 59:155–157.
16. Kamasuka T, Momoki Y, Sakai S. Antitumor activity of polysaccharide fractions prepared from some strains of Basidiomycetes. Jpn J Cancer Res (Gann) 1968; 59(5):443–445.
17. Andreacchi AS, Wang T, Wu JH. Cardiovascular effects of the fungal extract of *Basidiomycetes* sp. YL8006. Life Sci 1997; 60(22):1987–1994.
18. Reshetnikov S, Wasser SP, Tan KK. Higher Basidiomycoto as a source of antitumour and immunostimulating polysaccharides. Intl J Med Mushrooms 2001; 3:361–394. Review.
19. Molitoris H.P. Mushrooms in medicine. Folia Microbiol 1994; 39(2):91–98.
20. Chihara G, Hamuro J, Maeda Y, Arai Y, Fukuoka F. Fractionation and purification of the polysaccharides with marked antitumour activity, especially lentinan, from *Lentinus edodes* (Berk.) Sing. (an edible mushroom). Cancer Res 1970; 30(11):2776–2781.
21. Chihara G, Hamuro J, Maeda YY, Arai Y, Fukuoka F. Antitumor polysaccharide derived chemically from natural glucan (pachyman). Nature 1970; 225:943–944.
22. Yap AT, Ng ML. An improved method for the isolation of lentinan from the edible and medicinal shiitake mushroom, *Lentinus edodes* (Berk.) Sing. (Agaricomycetideae). Int J Med Mushrooms 2001; 3:9–19.
23. Sasaki T, Takasuka N. Further study of the structure of lentinan, an antitumour polysaccharide from *Lentinus edodes*. Carbohyd Res 1976; 47(1):99–104.
24. Sasaki T, Takasuka N, Chihara G, Maeda YY. Antitumour activity of degraded products of lentinan: its correlation with molecular weight. Jpn J Cancer Res (Gann) 1976; 67(2):191–195.
25. Saito H, Ohki T, Takaoka N, Sasaki T. A ^{13}C-NMR-spectral study of a gel-forming, branched (1→3)-β-D-glucan (lentinan) from *Lentinus edodes*, and its acid degraded fractions: structure and dependence of confirmation on the molecular weight. Carbohyd Res 1977; 58:293–305.
26. Chihara G, Hamuro J, Maeda YY, Shiio T, Suga T, Takasuka N, Sasaki T. Antitumour and metastasis-inhibitory activities of lentinan as an immunomodulator: an overview. Cancer Detect Prev 1987; 1:423–443.
27. Hamuro J, Maeda YY, Fukuoka F, Chihara G. The significance of higher structure of polysaccharide lentinan and pachymaran with regard to their antitumor activity. Chem Biol Interact 1971; 3:69–71.
28. Bohn JA, BeMiller JN. (1→3)-β-D-Glucans as biological response modifiers: a review of structure-functional activity relationships. Carbohyd Polym 1995; 28:3–14.
29. Misaki A, Kishida E, Kakuta M, Tabata K. Anti-tumour fungal (1→3)-β-D-glucans: structural diversity and effects of chemical modification. In: Yalpani

M, ed. Carbohydrates and Carbohydrate Polymers. Mount Prospect, IL: ATL Press, 1993:116–129.
30. Sakai S, Takada S, Kamasuka T, Momoki Y, Sugamaya J. Antitumor action of some glucans: especially on its correlation to their chemical structure. Jpn J Cancer Res (Gann) 1968; 59:507–512.
31. Zakany J, Chihara G, Fachet J. Effect of lentinan on the production of migration inhibitory factor induced by syngeneic tumour in mice. Int J Cancer 1980; 26:783–788.
32. Zakany J, Chihara G, Fachet J. Effect of lentinan on tumour growth in murine allogeneic and syngeneic hosts. Int J Cancer 1980; 25(3):371–376.
33. Adachi K, Nanba H, Kuroda H. Potentiation of host-mediated antitumour activity in mice by β-glucan obtained from *Grifola frondosa* (Maitake). Chem Pharm Bull 1987; 35(1):262–270.
34. Aoki T. Lentinan. In: Fenichel RL, Chirigos MA, eds. Immune Modulation Agents and Their Mechanisms. New York: Marcel Dekker, 1984:63–77.
35. Gordon M, Guralnik M, Kaneko Y, Mimura T, Goodgame J, DeMarzo C, Pierce D, Baker M, Lang W. A Phase II controlled study of a combination of the immune modulator, lentinan, with didanosine (ddI) in HIV patients with CD4 cells of 200–500/mm^3. J Med 1995; 26(5–6):193–207.
36. Suga T, Shiio T, Maeda YY, Chihara G. Antitumour activity of lentinan in murine syngeneic and autochthonous hosts and its suppressive effect on 3-methylcholanthrene-induced carcinogenesis. Cancer Res 1984; 44(11):5132–5137.
37. Suzuki M, Kikuchi T, Takatsuki F, Hamuro J. The role of tumour antigen specific delayed-type hypersensitivity response in eradicating tumours by lentinan. Biotherapy 1993; 7:308–309. Japanese.
38. Masuko Y, Nakajima H, Tsusouchi J, Yamazaki M, Mizuno D, Abe S. Changes of anti-tumour immunity of hosts with murine mammary tumours regressed by lentinan: potentiation of anti-tumour delayed hypersensitivity reaction. Jpn J Cancer Res (Gann) 1987; 73(5):790–797.
39. Rose WC, Reed FC, Siminoff P, Bradner WT. Immunotherapy of Madison 109 lung carcinoma and other tumours using lentinan. Cancer Res 1984; 44:1368–1373.
40. Suzuki I, Sakurai T, Hashimoto K, Oikawa S, Masuda A, Ohsawa M, Yadomae T. Inhibition of experimental pulmonary metastasis of Lewis lung carcinoma by orally administered β-glucan in mice. Chem Pharm Bull 1991; 39(6):1606–1608.
41. Kosaka A, Wani T, Hattori Y, Yamashita A. Effect of lentinan administration of adrenalectomized rats and patients with breast cancer. Gan To Kagaku Ryoho 1982; 9(8):1474–1481.
42. Taguchi T. Effects of lentinan in advanced or recurrent cases of gastric, colorectal, and breast cancer. Gan To Kagaku Ryoho 1983; 10:387–393.
43. Nakano H, Namatame K, Nemoto H, Motohashi H, Nishiyama K, Kumada K. A multi-institutional prospective study of lentinan in advanced gastric cancer patients with unresectable and recurrent diseases: effect on prolonga-

tion of survival and improvement of quality of life. Hepato-gastroenterol 1999; 46: 2662–2668.
44. Nanba H, Mori K, Toyomasu T, Kuroda H. Antitumour action of shiitake (*Lentinus edodes*) fruit bodies orally administered to mice. Chem Pharm Bull 1987; 35(6):2453–2458.
45. Nanba H, Kuroda H. Potentiation of host mediated anti-tumour activity by orally administered mushroom (*Agaricus bisporus*) fruit bodies. Chem Pharm Bull 1988; 36(4):1437–1444.
46. Mori K, Toyomasu T, Nanba H, Kuroda H. Anti-tumour action of mushrooms by oral administration. Abstract of paper presented at Third International Mycological Congress. Tokyo, 1983.
47. Mori K, Toyomasu T, Nanba H, Kuroda H. Anti-tumour action of fruit bodies of edible mushrooms orally administered to mice. Mushroom J Tropics 1987; 7:121–126.
48. Suzuki I, Tanaka H, Kinoshita A, Oikawa S, Osawa M, Yadomae T. Effect of orally administered β-glucan on macrophage function in mice. Int J Immunopharmacol 1990; 12(6):675–684.
49. Yap AT, Ng ML. Inhibition of human colon sarcoma by lentinan from shiitake mushroom (*Lentinus edodes*). J Altern Complem Med 2002; 8(5):581–589.
50. Moriya N, Miwa H, Taketsuka S, Orita K. Antitumour effect of bacterial lipopolysaccharide (LPS) and a combination use of LPS and lentinan on C3H/He mice bearing MH-134 tumour. Gan To Kagaku Ryoho 1983; 10(7):1646–1652.
51. Moriya N, Miwa H, Orita K. Antitumour effect of bacterial lipopolysaccharide (LPS) alone and in combination with lentinan on MH-134 tumours in C3H/He mice. Acta Med Okayama 1984; 38(1):49–55.
52. Arinaga S, Karimine N, Takamuku K, Nanbara S, Nagamatsu M, Ueo H, Akiyoshi T. Enhanced production of interleukin 1 and tumor necrosis factor by peripheral monocytes after lentinan administration in patients with gastric carcinoma. Int J Immunopharmacol 1992; 14(1):43–47.
53. Arinaga S, Karimine N, Takamuku K, Nanbara S, Inoue H, Nagamatsu M, Ueo H, Akiyoshi T. Enhanced induction of lymphokine-activated killer activity after lentinan administration in patients with gastric carcinoma. Int J Immunopharmacol 1992; 14(4):535–539.
54. Suzuki M, Higuchi S, Taki Y, Taki S, Miwa K, Hamuro J. Induction of endogenous lymphokine-activated killer activity by combined administration of lentinan and interleukin 2. Int J Immunopharmacol 1990; 12:613–623.
55. Suzuki M, Iwashiro M, Takatsuki F, Kuribayashi K, Hamuro J. Reconstitution of anti-tumour effects of lentinan in nude mice: roles of delayed-type hypersensitivity reaction triggered by CD4-positive T cell clone in the infiltration of effector cells into tumour. Jpn J Cancer Res 1994; 85(4):409–417.
56. Suzuki M, Kikuchi T, Takatsuki F, Hamuro J. Curative effects of combination therapy with lentinan and interleukin-2 against established murine tumors, and the role of CD8-positive T cells. Cancer Immunol Immunother 1994; 38(1):1–8.

57. Hamuro J, Takatsuki F, Suga T, Kikuchi T, Suzuki M. Synergistic antimetastatic effects of lentinan and interleukin 2 with pre- and post-operative treatments. Jpn J Cancer Res 1994; 85(12):1288–1297.
58. Parr I, Wheeler E, Alexander P. Similarities of the anti-tumour actions of endotoxin, lipid A, and ds-RNA. Br J Cancer 1973; 27(5):370–389.
59. Maehara Y, Moriguchi S, Sakaguchu Y, Emi Y, Kohnoe S, Tsujutani S, Sugimachi K. Adjuvant chemotherapy enhances long-term survival of patients with advanced gastric cancer following curative resection. J Surg Oncol 1990; 45(3):169–172.
60. Ger E, Angelucci JA, Coleman P. Mushrooms: enjoying your medicine. Delaware Med J 1997; 69(3):149–151.
61. Murata T, Hatayama I, Kakizaki I, Satoh K, Sato K, Tsuchida S. Lentinan enhances sensitivity of mouse colon 26 tumour to cis-diamminedichloro platinum (II) and decreases glutathione transferase expression. Jpn J Cancer Res 1996; 87:1171–1178.
62. Arai Y, Tanooka H, Sekine T. Fukuoka. Effect of immuno suppressive agents on anti-tumour action of lentinan. Jpn J Cancer Res (Gann) 1971; 62(2):131–134.
63. Miyakoshi H, Aoki T, Mizukoshi M. Acting mechanisms of lentinan in human: enhancement of non-specific cell-mediated cytotoxicity as an interferon inducer. Int J Immunopharmacol 1984; 6(4):373–379.
64. Takeshita K, Watanuki S, Iida M, Saito N, Maruyama M, Sunagawa M, Habu H, Endo M. Effect of lentinan on lymphocyte subsets of peripheral blood, lymph nodes, and tumour tissues in patients with gastric cancer. Jpn J Surg 1993; 23:125–129.
65. Ladanyi A, Timar J, Lapis K. Effect of lentinan on macrophage cytotoxicity against metastatic tumor cells. Cancer Immunol Immunother 1993; 36(2):123–126.
66. Maeda YY, Chihara G. The effects of neonatal thymectomy on the antitumour activity of lentinan, carboxymethylpachymaran, and zymosan, and their effects on various immune responses. Int J Cancer 1973; 11(1):153–161.
67. Hamzsuro J, Chihara G. Lentinan, a T-cell oriented immunopotentiator; its experimental and clinical application and possible mechanism of immune modulation. In: Fenichel RL, Chirigos MA, eds. Immune Modulation Agents and Their Mechanisms. New York: Marcel Dekker, 1984:409–437.
68. Maeda YY, Hamuro J, Chihara G. The mechanisms of action of anti-tumour polysaccharides. I. The effects of antilymphocyte serum on the anti-tumour activity of lentinan. Int J Cancer 1971; 8(1):41–46.
69. Nakahara W, Fukuoka F, Maeda Y, Aoki K. The host mediated anti-tumor effect of some plant polysaccharides. Jpn J cancer Res (Gann) 1964; 55:283–288.
70. Liu M, Li J, Kong F, Lin J, Gao Y. Induction of immunomodulating cytokines by a new polysaccharide-peptide complex from culture mycelia of *Lentinus edodes*. Immunopharmacology 1998; 40(3):187–198.

71. Nanba H, Kuroda H. Antitumour mechanisms of orally administered shiitake fruit bodies. Chem Pharm Bull 1987; 35(6):2459–2464.
72. Tani M, Tanimura H, Yamaue H, Tsunoda T, Iwahashi MT, Naguchi K, Tamai M, Hotta T, Mizobata S. Augmentation of lymphokine-activated killer cell activity by lentinan. Anticancer Res 1993; 13:1773–1776.
73. O'hara Y. Fate of lentinan (antitumor polysaccharide). I. Fate of lentinan in mice, rats, and dogs. J Toxicol Sci 1980; 5(suppl):59–72.
74. Mannel DN, Mizel SB, Diamantstein T, Falk W. Induction of IL-2 responsiveness in thymocytes by synergistic action of IL-1 and IL-2. J Immunol 1985; 134(5):3108–3110.
75. Suzuki M, Takatsuki F, Maeda YY, Hamuro J, Chihara G. Antitumour and immunological activity of lentinan in comparison with lipopolysaccharide. Int J Immunopharmacol 1994; 16(5–6):463–468.
76. Mizuno M. Anti-tumor polysaccharides from mushrooms during storage. Biofactors 2000; 12:275–281.
77. Dennart G, Tucker D. Anti-tumor polysaccharide lentinan, a T-cell adjuvant. J Natl Cancer Inst 1973; 51:1727–1729.
78. Hamuro H. The role of tumour antigen specific delayed type hypersensitivity response in eradicating tumours by lentinan. Biotherapy 1993; 7:345–346. Japanese.
79. Hamuro J, Rollinghoff M, Wagner H. β(1–3)Glucan-mediated augmentation of alloreactive murine cytotoxic T lymphocytes in vivo. Cancer Res 1978; 38(9):3080–3085.
80. Moller JI. IL-2: receptors and genes. Immunol Rev 1986; 92:1–156.
81. Lowenthal JW, Cerottini JC, MacDonald HR. IL-1 dependent induction of both IL-2 secretion and IL-2 receptor expression by thymoma cells. J Immunol 1987; 137(4):1226–1231.
82. Shimizu Y, Chew J, Hirai Y, Shiokawa S, Yagi H, Katase K, Yamashiro T, Nakayama K, Teshima H, Hamada T, Fujimoto I, Yamauchi K, Hasumi K, Masubuchi K. Augmentive effect of lentinan in immune responses of pelvic lymph node lymphocytes in patients with uterine cervical cancer. Acta Obstet Gynaecol Jpn 1988; 40:1557–1558.
83. Smith KA. Interleukin-2: inception, impact and implications. Science 1988; 240:1169–1176.
84. Hanaue H, Tokuda Y, Machimura T, Kamijoh A, Kondo Y, Ogoshi K, Makuuchi H, Herlyn D, Kaneko Y, Powe J, Aoki T, Koprowski H. Monoclonal antibody-dependent murine macrophage-mediated cytotoxicity against human tumors is stimulated by lentinan. Jpn J Cancer Res (Gann) 1985; 76(1): 37–42.
85. Yamasaki K, Sone S, Yamashita T, Ogura T. Synergistic induction of lymphokine (IL-2)-activated killer activity by IL-2 and the polysaccharide lentinan, and therapy of spontaneous pulmonary metastases. Cancer Immunol Immunother 1989; 29:87–92.
86. Morinaga H, Tazawa K, Tagoh H, Muraguchi A, Fujumaki M. An in vivo study of hepatic and splenic interleukin-1β mRNA expression following

oral PSK or LEM administration. Jpn J Cancer Res 1994; 85(12):1298–1303.

87. Maeda YY, Chihara G, Ishimura K. Unique increase of serum proteins and action of antitumour polysaccharides. Nature 1974; 252(5480):250–252.
88. Maeda YY, Watanabe ST, Chihara G, Rokutanda M. T-cell mediated vascular dilatation and hemorrhage induced by antitumor polysaccharides. Int J Immunopharmacol 1984; 6(5):493–501.
89. Takatsuki F, Namiki R, Kikuchi T, Suzuki M, Hamuro J. Lentinan augments skin reaction induced by bradykinin: its correlation with vascular dilatation and hemorrhage responses and antitumour activities. Int J Immunopharmacol 1995; 17(6):465–474.
90. Dresser DW, Philips JM. The orientation of the adjuvant activities of *Salmonella typhosa* lipopolysaccharide and lentinan. Immunology 1974; 27:895–902.
91. Hosokawa M, Sawamura Y, Morikage T, Okada F, Xu ZY, Morikawa K, Itoh K, Kobayashi H. Improved therapeutic effects of interleukin 2 after the accumulation of lymphokine-activated killer cells in tumor tissue of mice previously treated with cyclophosphamide. Cancer Immunol Immunother 1988; 26(3):250–256.
92. Maeda YY, Ishimura K, Tanaka M, Sasaki T, Chihara G. In: Mizuno D, ed. Host Defence Against Cancer and Its Potentiation. Tokyo: University of Tokyo Press, 1985:1–181.
93. Maeda YY, Yonekawa H, Chihara G. Application of lentinan as cytokine inducer and host defense potentiator in immunotherapy of infectious diseases. In: Masihi KN, ed. Immunotherapy of Infections. New York: Marcel Dekker, 1984:261–280.
94. Izawa M, Ohno K, Amikura K, Hamuro J. Lentinan augments the production of IL-3 and CSF(s) by T-cells. In: Aoki T, Tsubura E, Urushizaki I, eds. Manipulation of Host Defence Mechanisms. Amsterdam: Excerpta Medica, 1984:59–69.
95. Fruehauf JP, Bonnard GD, Herberman RB. The effect of lentinan on production of interleukin-1 by human monocytes. Immunopharmacology 1982; 5:65–74.
96. Wang GL, Lin ZB. The immunomodulatory effect of lentinan. Yao Xue Xue Bao 1996; 31(2):86–90.
97. Irinoda K, Masihi KN, Chihara G, Kaneka Y, Katori T. Stimulation of microbicidal host defense mechanisms against aerosol influenza virus infection by lentinan. Int J Immunopharmacol 1992; 14(6):971–977.
98. Kaneko Y, Chihara G, Taguchi T. Activity of lentinan against cancer and AIDS. Int J Immunother 1989; 4:203–213.
99. Mizono M, Minato K, Tsuchida H. Preparation and specificity of antibodies to an anti-tumour β-glucan, lentinan. Biochem Mol Biol Int 1996; 39:679–685.
100. Suzuki H, Okubo A, Yamazaki S, Suzuki K, Mitsuya H, Toda S. Inhibition of the infectivity and cytopathic effect of human immuno-deficiency virus by

water-soluble lignin in an extract of the culture medium of *Lentinus edodes* mycelia (LEM). Biochem Biophys Res Commun 1989; 160:367–373.
101. Tochikura S, Nakashima H, Ohashi Y, Yamamoto N. Inhibition (in vitro) of replication and of the cytopathic effect of human immunodeficiency virus by an extract of the culture medium of *Lentinus edodes* mycelia. Med Microbiol Immunol 1988; 177:235–244.
102. Iizuka C. Extract of Basiomycetes especially *Lentinus edodes*, for treatment of human immunodeficiency virus (HIV). Shokin Kogyo Co., Ltd., Eur. Pat. Appl. EP 370, 673 (cl, 35.84) 30 May, JP Appl. 88/287, 316, 14 Nov 1988, approved 1990.
103. Kanai K, Kondo E, Jacques PJ, Chihara G. Immunopotentiation effect of fungal glucan as revealed by frequency limitation of post chemotherapy relapse in experimental mouse tuberculosis. Jpn J Med Sci Biol 1980; 33(6):283–293.
104. Shen SC, Nakao A, Kishimoto W, Harada A, Nonami T, Nakano M, Takagi H. The ability of polymorphonuclear leucocytes to produce active oxygen in a model of peritonitis in rats. Surg Today 1993; 24(7):603–608.
105. Byrum JE, Sher A, DiPietro J, von Lichentenberg F. Potentiation of schistosome granuloma formation by lentinan, a T-cell adjuvant. Am J Pathol 1979; 94(2):94–201.
106. White TR, Thompson RCA, Penhale WJ, Chihara G. The effect of lentinan on resistance to mice to *Mesocestoides corti*. Parasitol Res 1988; 74:563.
107. Breene WM. Nutritional and medicinal value of specialty mushrooms. J Food Prot 1990; 53(11):883–894.
108. Sugano N, Hibino Y, Choji Y, Maeda H. Anticarcinogenic actions of water-soluble and alcohol-insoluble fractions from culture medium of *Lentinus edodes* mycelia. Cancer Lett 1982; 17(12):109–114.
109. Sugano N, Choji Y, Hibino Y, Yasumura S, Maeda H. Anticarcinogenic action of an alcohol-insoluble fraction (LAP1) from culture medium of *Lentinus edodes* mycelia. Cancer Lett 1985; 27:1–6.
110. Tabata T, Watanabe W, Horita K, Kamegai J, Moriyama S, Hibino Y, Ohashi Y, Sugano N. Mitogenic activities of heteroglycan and heteroglycan-protein fractions from culture medium of *Lentinus edodes* mycelia. Immunopharmacology 1992; 24:57–64.
111. Lin Y, Huang Y. Protective action of lentinan against experimental liver injuries. J Beijing Med Univ 1987; 19:93–95.
112. Yamamoto Y, Shirono H, Kono K, Ohashi Y. Immunopotentiating activity of the water-soluble lignin rich fraction prepared from LEM—the extract of the solid culture medium of *Lentinus edodes* mycelia. Biosci Biotechnol Biochem 1997; 61(11):1909–1912.
113. Sorimachi K, Niwa A, Yamazaki S, Toda S, Yasumura Y. Antiviral activity of water-solubilized lignin derivatives in vitro. Agric Biol Chem 1990; 54:1337–1339.
114. Makita T, Hashimoto Y, Noguchi T. Mutagenic, cytogenetic and teratogenic studies on thiophanate methyl. Toxicol Appl Pharmacol 1972; 24(2):206–215.

115. Dieleman-van Zaayen A. Virus-like particles in weed mould growing on mushroom trays. Nature 1967; 216:595–596.
116. Mori K. Studies on the virus-like particles in *Lentinus edodes*. Mushroom Sci 1974; 11(1):541–566.
117. Mori K, Kuida K, Hosokawa D, Takehara M. Virus-like particles in several mushrooms. In: Mushroom Science: Proceedings of the 10th International Congress of Science and Cultivation of Edible Fungi. Bordeaux JD ed. 1978; 10(1):773–787.
118. Barton RJ, Hollings M. Purification and some properties of two viruses infecting the cultivated mushroom *Agaricus bisporus*. J Gen Virol 1979; 42:231–240.
119. Ushiyama R, Nakai Y. Intracellular virus-like particle in *Lentinus edodes*. J Gen Virol 1980; 46(2):507–509.
120. Ushiyama R, Nakai Y. Ultrastructural features of fungal virus-like particles from *Lentinus edodes*. Virology 1982; 123(1):93–101.
121. Ushiyama R, Nakai Y, Ikegami M. Evidence for double-stranded RNA from polyhedral virus-like particles in *Lentinus edodes* (Berk) Sing. Virology 1977; 77:880–883.
122. Ng ML, Goh KT, Pho LK, Tan KK. The isolation of viruses in sawdust grown *Lentinus edodes* (shiitake). In: Maher MJ, ed. Mushroom Science: Proceedings of the 13th Intrnational Congress on the Science and Cultivation of Edible Fungi 1991; 13:337–344.
123. Saksena KN, Lemke PA. Viruses in fungi. In: Fraenkel-Conrat H, Wagner RR, eds. Comprehensive Virology. New York: Plenum Press, 1978; 12:103–143.
124. Lemke PA. Viruses of eukaryotic microorganisms. Annu Rev Microbiol 1976; 30:105–145.
125. Hollings M. Mycoviruses: viruses that infect fungi. In: Smith KM, Laufer MA, eds. Advances in Virus Research. New York: Plenum Press, 1978:231–334.
126. Tavantzis SM, Romaine CP, Smith SH. Purification and partial characterization of a bacilliform virus from *Agaricus bisporus*: a single stranded RNA mycovirus. Virology 1980; 57:96–100.
127. Takehara M, Kuida K, Mori K. Anti-viral activity of virus-like particles from *Lentinus edodes*. Arch Virol 1979; 59(3):269–274.
128. Takehara M, Mori K, Kuida K, Hanawa MA. Anti-tumour effect of virus-like particles from *Lentinus edodes* (Shiitake) on Ehrlich ascites carcinoma in mice. Arch Virol 1981; 68:297–301.
129. Levy HB, Law LW, Rabson AS. Inhibition of tumour growth by polyinosinic polycytidylic acid. Proc Natl Acad Sci 1969; 62(2):357–361.
130. Gresser I. Anti-tumour effects of Interferon. Adv Cancer Res 1972; 16:97–140.
131. Suzuki F, Koide T, Tsunoda A, Ishida N. Mushroom extract as an interferon inducer. I. Biological and physiological properties of spore extracts. Proceedings of the IX International Scientific Congress on the Cultivation of Edible Fungi, Mushroom Science 1974; 9(Part I):509–539.
132. Sudhir CK, Ng ML. Antitumour activity of oral administration of mycovirus

extract from *Lentinus edodes* (Berk.) Sing. (Agaricomycetideae) on murine lymphoma. Int J Med Mushrooms 2000; 2:125–132.
133. Taguchi T. Clinical efficacy of lentinan on patients with stomach cancer: end point results of a four-year follow-up survey. Cancer Detect Prev 1987; 1(suppl):333–349.
134. Taguchi T, Furue H, Kimura T, Kondo T, Hattori T, Itoh I, Ogawa N. Results of phase III study of lentinan. Gan To Kagaku Ryoho 1985; 12(2):366–378.
135. Miyazaki K, Mizutani H, Katabuchi H, Fukuma K, Fujisaki S, Okamura H. Activated (HLA–DR+) T-lymphocyte subsets in cervical carcinoma and effects of radiotherapy and immunotherapy with sizofiran on cell-mediated immunity and survival. Gynecol Oncol 1995; 56:412–420.
136. Matsuoka H, Seo Y, Wakasugi H, Saito T, Tomoda H. Lentinan potentiates immunity and prolongs the survival time of some patients. Anticancer Res 1997; 17(4A):2751–2755.
137. Williams DL, Pretus HA, McNamee RB, Jones EL, Ensley HE, Browder IW, Di Luzio NR. Development, physicochemical characterization and glucan sulfate derived from *Saccharomyces cerevisiae*. Immunopharmacology 1991; 22:139–156.
138. Mizuno T, Saiko H, Hishitoba T, Kawagichi H. Antitumour-active substances from mushrooms. Food Rev Int 1995; 11(1):23–61.
139. Nakasaki H, Tajima T, Mitomi T, et al. Effects of oral lentinan on T-cell subsets in peripheral venous blood. Clin Ther 1989; 11(5):614–622.
140. Torisu M, Hayashi Y, Ishimitsu T, Fujimura T, Iwasaki K, Katano M, Yamamoto H, Kimura Y, Takesue M, Kondo M, Nomoto K. Significant prolongation of disease-free period gained by oral polysaccharide K (PSK) administration after curative surgical operation of colorectal cancer. Cancer Immunol Immunother 1990; 31:261–268.
141. Akiyoshi T. Enhanced induction of lymphokine-activated killer activity after lentinan administration in patients with gastric carcinoma. Int J Immunopharmacol 1992; 14:535–539.

17

Cruciferous Vegetables and Chemoprevention

The Mechanisms of Isothiocyanate-Mediated Chemoprotection in Humans

Peter Rose, Choon Nam Ong, and Matthew Whiteman

National University of Singapore
Singapore, Republic of Singapore

I. INTRODUCTION

It is well known that diet plays a fundamental role in the etiology of human cancer. Lifestyle choices such as the high consumption of alcohol, dietary fats, and smoking can all contribute to cancer risk. Extensive reviews of epidemiological evidence by Block et al. (1), among others, indicated that dietary intake of fruits and vegetables had a significant impact on several forms of cancers, the mechanisms of which have been described by Steinmetz and Potter (2–4). The general consensus is that increased consumption of fruit and vegetables was associated with a reduced risk of human cancers. Highlighted in these reviews was the strong correlation between a reduction in stomach, esophageal, lung, and colon cancer risk with high consumption of cruciferous vegetables, particularly members of the genus *Brassica* (1,5–7). The Brassicaceae comprise a large number of vegetables such as cabbage, cauliflower, brussels sprouts, broccoli, and watercress. One characteristic of cruciferous vegetables is their ability to synthesize phytochemicals known as the glucosinolates (GSLs) (Fig. 1). Upon tissue damage GSLs are hydrolyzed by endogeneous plant myrosinase or alternatively by intestinal bacteria in the gut and converted to bioactive isothiocyanates (ITCs, Fig. 1). ITCs have a wide range of biological functions including antibacterial, antifungal, and anticarcinogenic properties. Furthermore, they are involved in plant herbivore interactions; we recognize them as the characteristic spicy flavors

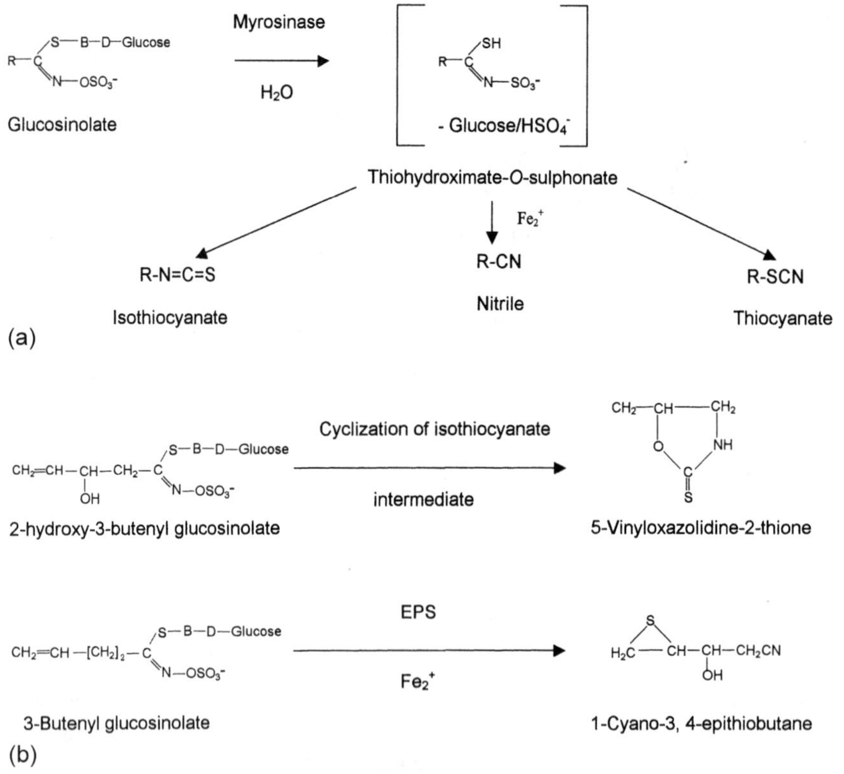

FIGURE 1 Glucosinolate-mediated hydrolysis by myrosinase. (a) Formation of isothiocyanates, nitriles, and thiocyanates from a glucosinolate precursor. (b) Hydrolysis of 4-hydroxy-3-butenyl and 3-butenyl glucosinolates to their goitrogenic products, (−) 5-vinyloxazolidine-2-thione and 1-cyano-2-hydroxy-3-butene. (Adapted from Refs. 28,33.)

associated with many of these vegetables, thus giving them their alternative name of mustard oils.

This chapter will give a brief overview of cruciferous vegetables and their potential in chemoprevention, highlighting the role of GSLs in various metabolic pathways and the formation of ITCs. The importance of these compounds on Phase I enzyme inhibition and Phase II enzyme induction, as well as apoptosis, will also be discussed. The biological significance of hydrolytic products derived from indole GSLs will not be addressed as they have been extensively reviewed (8–11). Likewise, other phytochemical constituents, such as flavonoids, isoflavones, and carotenoids, that may also contribute to the chemoprotective effects of cruciferous vegetables will not be addressed as they are beyond the scope of this chapter (12–15). Some of these compounds are covered in other chapters of this book.

II. GLUCOSINOLATES

To date, 116 GSLs have been identified in a diverse range of plant families represented in the order Capparales (16). All share a common feature of a β-D-thioglucose moiety, sulfonated oxime residue, and a variable side chain (Fig. 1; Table 1). The current chemical classification of GSLs recognizes three groups comprising aliphatic, aromatic, and indolyl GSLs based on the amino acid from which they are derived (17). The primary source of aliphatic GSLs is the amino acid methionine and to a lesser extent valine and isoleucine, while the amino acids phenylalanine, tyrosine, and tryptophan are precursors of aromatic and indolyl GSLs. The chemical diversity arises from extensive modification of the variable side chain by elongation of the primary amino acids methionine and, to a lesser extent, phenylalanine and branched-chained amino acids. After chain elongation and biosynthesis, structural modification mediated by hydroxylation, methylation, and oxidation reactions can occur leading to the formation of several structural analogs based on the initial chain-elongated molecule. The homologous series of chain-elongated GSLs can be observed for the ω-methylsulfinylalkyl (3-11 carbon), ω-methylthioalkyl (3-8 carbon), and β-phenylalkyl derivatives (Table 1).

During the early 1950s Ettlinger and Lundeen contributed much to our early knowledge of GSL chemistry with a proposed structure and the first chemical synthesis of a GSL, sinigrin (2-propenyl glucosinolate), in 1957. Further work conducted by Kjaer and additional contributions by Underhill began to expand our knowledge of GSL chemistry and biosynthesis (reviewed in Refs. 17,18). The chemical distribution of GSLs in plant taxa, particularly the agronomically important Brassicaceae, has also been the focus of much work, with detailed studies by Kjaer (18), Fenwick et al. (19), and Daxenbichler et al. (20), and reviewed by Rosa et al. (21). It was not until the

TABLE 1 Common Types of Glucosinolates and Associated Isothiocyanates Present in Cruciferous Species

Structure of R-groups	Chemical name	Carbon chain length	Trivial name	Common isothiocyanates	Common and species name
Methionine-derived aliphatic glucosinolates					
$CH_2=CH\text{-}[CH_2]_n-$	Alkenyl	*n* = 1–4	Sinigrin	Allyl	Brussels sprouts and cabbage, *Brassica oleracea*,
				3-Butenyl	Chinese mustard, *B. juncea*
$CH_2=CH\text{-}CHOH\text{-}CH_2-$	Hydroxyalkenyl	*n* = 1, 2, 3	Progoitrin	4-Hydroxyl-3-butenyl	Turnip and Swede, *B. napus*
$CH_3\text{-}S\text{-}[CH_2]_n-$	Methylthioalkyl	*n* = 2–9	Glucoerucin	4-Methylthiobutyl	Rocket, *Eruca sativa*
$CH_3\text{-}SO\text{-}[CH_2]_n-$	Methylsulfinylalkyl	*n* = 1–11	Glucoraphanin	4-Methylsulfinylbutyl	Broccoli, *B. oleracea*,
				8-Methylsulfinyloctyl	Watercress, *Rorripa nasturtium aquaticum*
				6-Methylsulphinylhexyl	Wasabi, *Wasabi japonica*
$CH_3\text{-}SO_2\text{-}[CH_2]_n-$	Methylsulfonylalkyl	*n* = 1, 2, 9	Glucoerysolin	9-Methylsulfonylnonyl	*Amaracea*
Aromatic glucosinolates			Glucotropaelin	Benzyl	Garden cress, *Lepidium sativa*, Papaya, *Carica papaya*
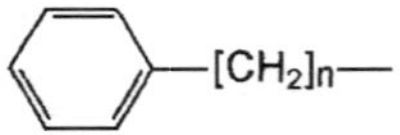	Phenylalkyl	*n* = 1–4	Gluconasturtiin	β-Phenylethyl	Watercress, *R. nasturtium aquaticum*

Source: Refs. 19, 21, 28.

latter end of the last century that any significant developments in the genetic regulation of GSL biosynthesis were made. Advances in molecular biology and comprehensive studies in *Arabidopsis thaliana* have enabled the identification of several genetic loci involved in glucosinolate biosynthesis. Contributions by Halkier and colleague have identified a role of cytochrome P450 monooxygenases (members of the CYP79 family) in the conversion of amino acids to oximes (22–26). Studies by Mithen and colleagues have characterized and cloned several genes (designated GSL-ELONG) involved in methionine chain elongation in *Arabidopsis* and *Brassica* (27–29). With additional fine mapping of the gene OHP that functions in GSL modification, its involvement in regulating the conversion of 3-methylsulphinylpropyl GSLs to 3-hydroxypropyl GSLs in *A. thaliana* has been observed (30). The data of many of these studies have a significant impact on the development of new plant breeding programs with possibilities of generating new crop varieties with increased resistance to pathogens, herbivores, and insect pests. In addition, knowledge of the genetic regulation of the GSL pathway may also contribute to the development of *Brassica* vegetables with increased anticancer properties. Such is the task of Mithen and colleagues using conventional plant-breeding methods to increase the levels of potentially anticancer GSLs in broccoli (31,32).

III. THE GLUCOSINOLATE MYROSINASE SYSTEM

Associated with the order Capparales are a group of thioglucosidases known as myrosinases [EC 3:2:2:1]. It is proposed that "myrosinase" is compartmentalized within myrosin cells and distributed throughout all parts of the plant (reviewed in Ref. 33). The separation of the myrosinase-glucosinolate system ensures that GSL degradation occurs only during tissue damage such as chewing or cutting. The catalytic degradation of GSLs initiates the cleavage of the glucose residue from the core GSL molecule, producing an unstable intermediate, the thiohydroximate-*O*-sulfonate. Further structural changes via Lossen rearrangement can lead to the formation of an ITC (Fig. 1a). However, under various physiological conditions the preferential production of ITC can be reduced in favor of other hydrolytic products such as nitriles and thiocyanates (19,33). These factors include pH, ascorbic acid concentration, Fe^{2+} ion levels, and the GSL side chain structure. For example, at low pH and high ferrous iron content the thiohydroximate-*O*-sulfonate can be converted to a nitrile by the loss of molecular sulfur. In addition to physiological parameters, interactions of proteins with myrosinase can cause the production of epithionitriles from alkenyl GSLs. For example, degradation of progoitrin (2-hydroxy-3-butenyl GSLs) in the presence of high ferrous ion concentrations and the interaction of a small labile epithiospecific protein (ESP) with myrosinase results in the formation of oxazolidine-2-thione. ESP is a small, 30–40-kDa polypeptide and was first isolated in *Crambe abyssinica* (34) and later in *Brassica napus* by Foo and Grooning (35). ESP has no direct thioglycosidase activity, but its interaction with myrosinase is required for mediating the transfer of sulfur from the S-glucose residue to the terminal alkenyl moiety (33). Recent characterization of an ESP in *A. thaliana* has also demonstrated its ability to mediate the conversion of GSLs to epithionitrile and nitriles in preference to ITCs (36).

A. Nonplant Myrosinases

Apart from the GSL-producing plant genera, myrosinase enzymes have also been characterized in insects, fungi, and bacteria (37). Endogenous myrosinase have been identified in the cabbage aphid *Brevicoryne brassicae* and the mustard aphid *Liaphis erysimi*. However, from a human nutritional perspective nonplant myrosinases present in bacteria are of greater importance. Microbial myrosinases have been isolated from *Aspergillus niger*, *Aspergillus sydowi*, and, more significantly, the gut bacteria *Enterobacter cloacae* (38,39). Indeed, the bacterial metabolism of sinigrin to its ITC and as yet other unidentified metabolites has been demonstrated by human microflora in vitro (40). Metabolism of sinigrin to its respective ITC in gnotobiotic rats inoculated with the human faecal bacteria *Bacteriodes thetaiotaomicron* has also been described. However, as yet no attempts have been made to characterize the bacterial myrosinase enzyme involved (41). The GSL myrosinase system is pivotal in the bioavailability of ITC in the human diet. Indeed, current knowledge suggests GSLs are essentially inert and it is the ITCs that are required for any biological activity in mammalian cells. Cooking methods can inactivate endogeneous myrosinase of cruciferous vegetables and this could severely hamper the bioavailability of GSL hydrolytic products.

IV. GLUCOSINOLATES AND THEIR BIOLOGICAL FUNCTION

A. Flavor Components

Glucosinolates are sulfur-containing glycosides and are some of the most abundant secondary metabolites in *Brassica* species; they function in plant insect interactions and as feeding deterrents for plant herbivores. These very same phytochemicals are also recognized by humans, particularly the ITCs, as the characteristic flavor components associated with cruciferous vegetables and salad crops. During tissue damage ITCs are often released and can be recognized by their often spicy and pungent aroma (42). In watercress, *Rorripa nasturtium aquaticum*, the primary metabolite is the volatile β-phenylethyl isothiocyanate (PEITC), which gives this plant a characteristic hot pungent flavor. In contrast, broccoli, *Brassica oleracea* L. var. *italica*, the most widely consumed *Brassica*, produces the nonvolatile, ω-methylsulphinylalkyl isothiocyanates giving broccoli its mild flavor. The bitter flavor associated with brussels sprouts, *B. oleracea* L. var. *gemmifera*, is proposed to be due to hydrolysis of 2-hydroxy-3-butenyl and 2-propenyl glucosinolates; however, interaction with other phytochemical components may also contribute.

B. Antimicrobial Properties of Dietary Isothiocyanates

The antibacterial effects of ITCs have been described on a number of occasions. The inhibitory effects of arylalkyl ITCs on the bacteria *Escherichia coli* and *Bacillus subtilis* are attributed to their reaction with cellular thiol groups disrupting cellular homeostasis. Indeed, the inhibition of polypeptide synthesis in the cell-free system of *E. coli* was attributed to the inactivation of ribosomes (43). In a study by Ono et al. identification of the active antimicrobial component in wasabi 6-methylsulfinylhexyl isothiocyanate was shown to have strong activity toward *E. coli* and *Staphylococcus aureus* (44). A comparison of the antibacterial properties of allyl isothiocyanate (AITC) with several antibacterial agents such as streptomycin, penicillin, and polymixin B has also been described. AITC induced a significant reduction in viability associated with the loss of membrane integrity in the bacteria *S. montevideo*, *E. coli*, and *Listeria monocytogenes* and was comparable to antibiotic treatments (45). More recent work conducted by Fahey and colleagues demonstrated the bacteriostatic effects of sulforaphane, a major constituent of broccoli, on the pathogenic bacterium *Helicobacter pylori*. The development of gastric and peptic ulcers induced by infection with *H. pylori* can often develop to more chronic disorders such as gastric cancer. Sulforaphane had a potent bacteriostatic effect against three reference strains and 45 clinical isolates of *H. pylori*. More promising was the fact that these properties were independent of *H. pylori* resistance to conventional antibiotics (46). Similarly, antifungal activities have been observed for AITC, 5-methylthiopentyl, 3-methylsulfinylpropyl, and PEITC against *Aspergillus niger*, *Penicillin cyclopium*, and *Rhizopus oryzae* (47). However, whether these antifungal properties have any significance to human health has yet to be properly addressed.

C. Antinutritional Effects of Glucosinolate Hydrolytic Products

It cannot be ignored that the beneficial effects of consuming cruciferous vegetables is important in the proposed prevention of chronic human disease. It must also be noted that deleterious effects can also be attributed to high exposure to ITCs and other GSL hydrolytic products. In addition to acting as feeding deterrents for herbivores, some GSL metabolites also show goitrogenic activity in mammals. For example, the use of oilseed rape meal as animal feed was severally hampered owing to high levels of 2-hydroxy-3-butenyl glucosinolate. During GSL degradation (–) 5-vinyloxazolidine-2-thione can be formed, or in the presence of ESP 1-cyano-2-hydroxy-3-butene, both compounds can have a deleterious effects in mammals (Fig. 1b). Indeed, high exposure of livestock to plants containing high levels of both these compounds can result in the development of enlarged thyroids, stunted growth, and abnormalities of the liver and kidneys (21,48,49). These abnormalities are suggested to be a result of the impairment of thyroid function by inhibition of thyroxine synthesis. Fortunately, selective breeding has reduced the levels of hydroxyalkenyl GSLs in oilseed rape and has eliminated this problem. No evidence as yet has shown that cruciferous vegetables have a goitrogenic effect in humans. Volunteers consuming 150 g of brussels sprouts showed no impairment of thyroid function as assessed by thyroid hormone levels (50).

The toxicity of ITCs in mammals has also been the subject of several investigations, albeit at levels that are generally not attainable in the human diet. The promoting effects of AITC, benzyl isothiocyanate (BITC), PEITC, and their mercapturic acid metabolites in rat urinary bladder carcinogenicity have been described. Rats pretreated with the carcinogens diethylnitrosamine and *N*-butyl-*N*-(4-hydroxybutyl)nitrosamine showed a significant increase in the incidence of urinary bladder carcinomas after feeding with either PEITC or BITC in the postinitiation phase (51,52). BITC can also induce chromosomal aberrations, sister chromatid exchange, and DNA strand breaks in cultured cells (53). The significance of these findings will be discussed later. Genotoxic effects of AITC, BITC, and PEITC have also been described using in vitro and in vivo techniques (54,55). Micronucleus induction assays in HepG2 cells and differential DNA repair assays in the bacterium *E. coli* indicate AITC to be strongly genotoxic albeit to a greater extent in bacterial systems. Similar genotoxic effects in bacteria have also been described for *Brassica* vegetable extracts. Eight different *Brassica* vegetables, including broccoli, cabbage, and brussels sprouts, were assessed on their ability to induce point mutations in the *Salmonella* strains TA98 and TA100, repairable DNA damage in *E. coli*, and clastogenic effects in mammalian cells. Induction of chromosomal aberrations and loss of cell viability were observed in mammalian cells and attributed to the GSL and ITC constituents (56). Likewise, a proposed mechanism for the genotoxic effects of AITC involving the generation of free radicals has been described. The generation of the oxidative DNA damage marker 8-oxo-7,8-dihydro-2′-deoxyguanosine in the presence of Cu^{2+} by AITC in HL-60 cells is suggested as having a possible role in carcinogenesis. However, its role in cytotoxicity and tumor promotion has not been determined (57).

Many of the toxic effects that have been described in the above studies may well be attributed to the ability of ITCs to induce apoptosis. Significant permutations in DNA damage and cellular function are often associated with the mediation of programmed cell death. Indeed, recent work has shown that DNA-damaging agents can initiate the apoptotic cascade and that this process may have a beneficial effect in removing neoplastic cells.

V. *BRASSICA* VEGETABLE CONSUMPTION AND HUMAN HEALTH: THE EPIDEMIOLOGICAL EVIDENCE

Approximately 200 studies have examined the relationship between high consumption of fruits and vegetables and their protective effect against cancer (1). Statistical analysis of 128 of 156 dietary studies revealed a reduced risk of cancers of the colon, lung, stomach, and bladder was associated with high intake of fruits and vegetables. The findings revealed that one group of the cruciferous vegetables appeared to be associated with this trend. Verhoeven et al. analyzed the data of seven cohort studies and 87 case-control studies, and found a relationship between consumption of *Brassica* vegetables and an inverse correlation with the consumption of broccoli, cabbage, and cauliflower with lung cancer risk (6,7). Implicated in the protective effects based on in vivo and in vitro data are GSLs and ultimately their hydrolytic products, the ITCs. Lin et al. observed a correlation between polymorphisms in GSTT1, broccoli consumption, and a reduction in colorectal adenomas (58). Analysis of 457 cases and 505 control subjects indicated that GSTT1-positive subjects with no broccoli intake had a higher prevalence of colorectal adenomas. In contrast, combination of both GSTM1 and GSTT1 null genotypes with high broccoli intake showed the lowest incidence of adenoma when compared to GSTM1- or GSTT1-positive subjects. Several more studies using food frequency questionnaires and/or urinary quantification of ITC metabolites have demonstrated a strong inverse correlation between *Brassica* vegetable consumption and lung cancer. Voorrips et al. analyzed 1074 cases after a 6.3-year follow-up in the Netherland Cohort Study (59). Statistically significant associations were observed in total vegetable consumption and a reduction in lung cancer. Of the several vegetable groups assessed the strongest associations were seen with the consumption of *Brassica* vegetables. In addition, London et al. demonstrated that individuals homozygous-null for GSTM1 and GSTT1 were at a lower risk of lung cancer in smokers compared to either GSTM1- or GSTT1-positive individuals (60). Both GSTM1 and GSTT1 are involved in the detoxification of both the carcinogenic polycyclic aromatic hydrocarbons (PAH) and dietary ITCs. The protective effects in null individuals were attributed to a reduction in the rate of elimination of ITCs in urine. The associated reduction of lung cancer by assessing human GST polymorphisms and ITC exposure has also been reported by Zhao et al. During evaluation of the role of genetic polymorphisms in two major GST isoenzymes, GSTM1 and GSTT1, in Chinese women a positive association between ITC exposure and a reduction in the incidence of lung cancers was observed. Data indicated that individuals null for either GSTM1 and/or GSTT1 having a high weekly intake of ITCs showed a significant inverse association to the risk of lung cancer (61). Associations have also been observed for prostate cancer risk and consumption of *Brassica* vegetables (reviewed by Kristal and Lampe). Of the 12 published studies reviewed six suggested a possible association between *Brassica* consumption and reduced risk of prostate cancer (62).

VI. CHEMOPREVENTION BY ISOTHIOCYANATE: THE IN VIVO EVIDENCE

One of the major characteristics of chemical carcinogens is their ability to act as DNA alkylating agents inducing DNA aberrations that have the potential to lead to genetic mutations. Several well-characterized carcinogens, such as benzo[a]pyrenes, nitrosamines, and aflatoxin B_1, can form DNA adducts with exposed bases in double-stranded DNA (Fig. 2). The overall consequence of this is the possible impairment of DNA replication and the induction of genetic mutation. This can be especially significant if these occur in tumor suppressor genes such as p53. A possible mechanism to prevent these deleterious effects is to use dietary agents that can alter the metabolism of carcinogens and thus reduce or prevent DNA damage. Of the many dietary compounds studied, low-dose exposure to ITCs has been proven to be highly effective in preventing DNA damage and the development of cancers in animal models (reviewed in Refs. 2,7 and summarized in Table 2). Recent experiments have focused on the inhibition of tumor formation induced by several nitrosamines and polycyclic aromatic hydrocarbons found in tobacco smoke. Of the approximately by 4000 compounds identified 43 have the potential to induce tumor formation in animal models (reviewed in Ref. 63). Two of the most effective carcinogens identified were the polycyclic aromatic hydrocarbons represented by benzo[a]pyrene and the nitrosamine 4-(methylnitrosamino)-1-(3-pyridyl)-1-butanone (NNK). Both compounds promote tumor formation in animal models. B[a]P and NNK are also suggested to be potent initiating factors in the induction of tobacco-related human cancers. Dose-dependent inhibition by arylalkyl ITCs and their *N*-acetylcysteine conjugates on NNK-induced tumor formation in rodents has been widely addressed; several of these studies are summarized in Table 2 (64–74). Common to many of these studies is a reduction in the deposition and an increase in Phase II detoxification metabolites of many of these carcinogens.

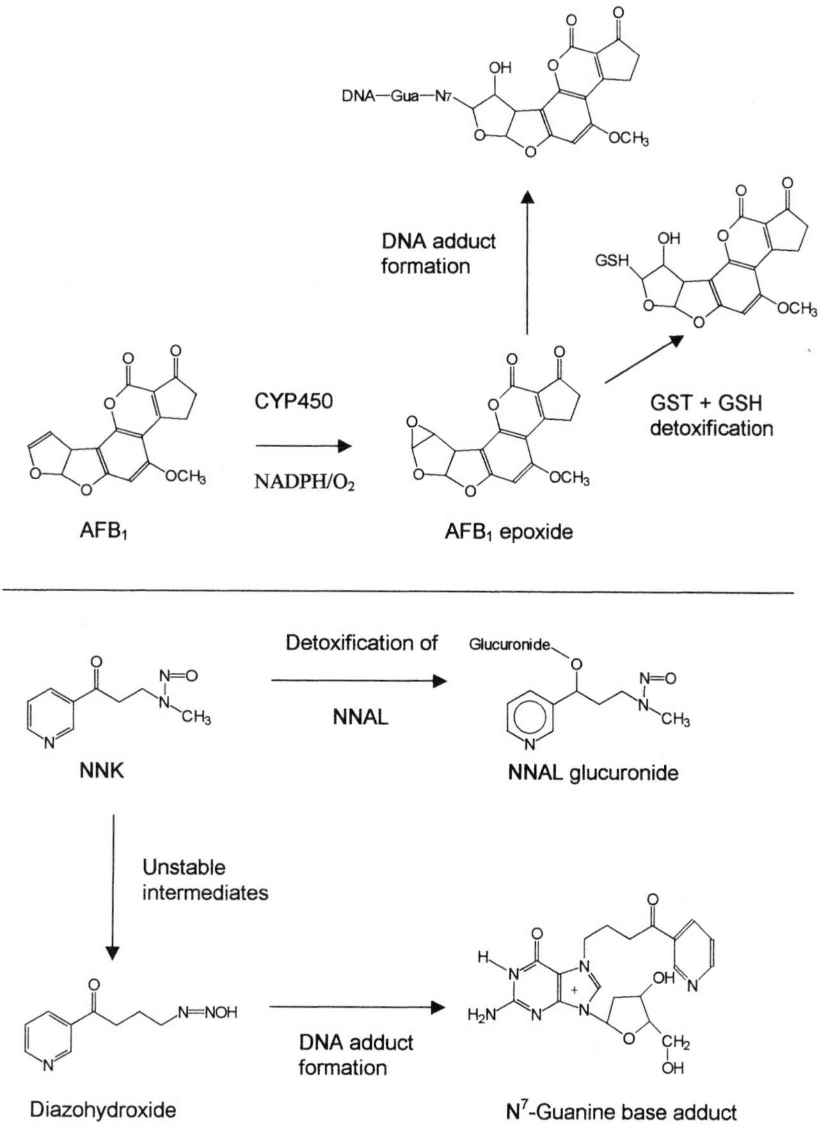

Figure 2 Metabolism, DNA adduct formation, and detoxification of the carcinogenic agents aflatoxin B1 (AFB_1) and 4-(methylnitrosamino)-1-(3 pyridyl)-1-butanone (NNK) in mammalian cells. (This figure is by no means comprehensive. See Refs. 90,95.)

TABLE 2 Summary of the In Vivo Chemopreventive Properties of Isothiocyanates in Rodents

Animal model	Tissue	Carcinogen	Isothiocyanate	Effect	Ref.
A/J mice	Pulmonary, forestomach	B[a]P	BITC	Inhibition	64
A/J mice	Lung	NNK	Aromatic ITCs	Inhibition	65
Fisher rats	Esophagus	NBMA	PEITC	Inhibition	66
ACI/N rats	Intestine	MAM	BITC	Inhibition	67
Fischer rats	Esophagus	NBMA	BITC/PBITC	No effect	68
A/J mice	Lung	NNK	PEITC	Inhibition	69
Sprague-Dawley rats	Mammary tissue	DMBA	PEITC	Inhibition	70
Fischer rats	Esophagus	NNK	PPITC	Inhibition	71
Fischer rats	Colon	AOM	Sulforaphane	Inhibition	85
Rats	Bladder	DEN and BBN	BITC/PEITC	Promotion	51
Fischer rats	Bladder and liver	DEN	PEITC	Promotion	73
A/J mice	Lung	B[a]P and NNK	BITC/PEITC	Inhibition	74
ICN mice	Stomach	B[a]P	Sulforaphane	Inhibition	46
A/J mice	Lung	B[a]P	2BITC	Inhibition	83

BITC, benzyl isothiocyanate; PEITC, phenylethyl isothiocyanate; PPITC, phenylpropyl isothiocyanate; PBITC, phenylbutyl isothiocyanate; sulforaphane, 4-methylsulfinylbutyl isothiocyanate; AOM, azoxymethane; B[a]P, benzo[a]pyrene; DEN, 1, 2-diethylnitrosamine; DMBA, 7,12-dimethylbenzanthracene; MAM, methylazomethanol acetate; NNK, 4-(methylnitroamino)-1-(3-pyridyl)-1-butanone; NBMA, *N*-nitrosobenzylmethylamine.

PEITC and BITC, both prominent isothiocyanates in watercress, garden cress, and papaya, have been the focus of much of this attention. PEITC can inhibit tumor formation induced by NNK in both rat and mouse models but it is ineffective at inhibiting tumor formation induced by B[a]P (75–79). In contrast, BITC can inhibit tumor formation induced by B[a]P while having no inhibitory effect on NNK (79–83). These contrasting differences are currently under investigation in several laboratories, and suggest that for effective chemoprevention a combination of ITCs or other phytochemicals may be necessary in preventing tumor formation. Additional research also shows both PEITC and BITC can inhibit DMBA-induced mammary tumors in rats, with PEITC being additionally effective in the inhibition of *N*-nitrosbenzylmethylamine (NBMA)-induced esophageal tumors (66,68–72). Likewise, sulforaphane, a very potent Phase II detoxfication enzyme inducer from broccoli, can inhibit DMBA-induced tumor formation in rat mammary tissues while also showing a protective effect against azoxymethane (AZO)-induced aberrant crypt foci in rats (84,85). However, it is ineffective against B[a]P-induced lung tumor formation in A/J mice (74).

Of all the in vivo studies only a few have been conducted on human subjects, many of these being coordinated by Hecht and colleagues. In humans, it is hypothesized that PEITC prevented the metabolic activation of carcinogens to more toxic forms. During the early investigation it was demonstrated that consumption of watercress in smokers significantly increased the levels of the detoxification products of the NNK metabolite NNAL and NNAL-Gluc in the urine (86). It was suggested that this effect was either due to the inhibition of NNK metabolism by CYP450 isoenzymes or due to the induction of Phase II detoxification enzymes involved in their excretion. Follow-up studies determined the latter to be the influencing factor with data suggesting that components in watercress were inducing the phase II detoxification enzyme UDP-glucuronosyltransferase (87).

Many of the in vivo traits of synthetic isothiocyanates are also observed for the respective vegetables from which they are derived. Cabbage, brussels sprouts, and broccoli have all been shown to reduce mammary tumor formation in rats exposed to DMBA (82). More recent investigations have shown that selenium-enriched broccoli is also effective at reducing intestinal tumor formation in mice exposed to dimethylhydrazine (88). Additional studies using multiple intestinal neoplasia mice as a rodent model in which the rodents are predisposed to the development of tumors in the small and large intestine show a significant reduction in the numbers of tumors when the rodents are fed selenium-enriched broccoli (89). Whether an interaction between GSL components and methylselenocysteine (the predominant seleno- compound in plants) can occur in vivo has not been determined; however, both agents do have chemopreventive properties and such effects are feasible. Nevertheless this requires further investigation.

Aflatoxin B_1 (AFB_1), a potent hepatocarcinogen, is recognized by the International Agency for Research on Cancer (IARC) as a group 1 carcinogen in humans. It is generally accepted that the formation of AFB_1-8,9-epoxide generated by the metabolism of AFB_1 by cytochrome P450 can cause the covalent binding of the epoxide to guanine bases present in DNA. More important is the finding that AFB_1 epoxide is able to induce mutations in the tumor suppressor gene p53 and K-ras oncogenes. These factors are suggested to contribute to AFB_1-induced carcinogenesis (reviewed in Ref. 90). The first study showing the modulation of AFB_1-DNA adduct formation by *Brassica* vegetables was conducted by Godlewski et al. In feeding studies GSL-containing fractions of brussels sprouts were shown to diminish the number of γ-glutamyl transpeptidase foci induced by AFB1 in hepatic tissues, a marker of hepatocarcinoma (91). Additional research indicates that the consumption of brussels sprouts had a pronounced inhibitory effect on aflatoxin B_1 DNA binding in rats. Rodents administered ^{3}H-AFB_1 either intraperitoneally or intragastrically, showed a 50–60% reduction in AFB_1 DNA binding in hepatic tissues (92). Likewise, consumption of cabbage induced an 87% reduction of AFB_1 DNA binding in weaning Fischer F344 rats (93). Associated with all three studies was a significant increase in detoxification enzyme activity in hepatic tissues. These findings could be attributed to the presence of unidentified GSL hydrolytic products in the vegetable extracts. Supporting this hypothesis is the study by Hayes et al. showing that ITCs can induce GSTA5-5, a major GST involved in the detoxification of AFB1-epoxide (94,95).

VII. THE METABOLISM OF DIETARY ISOTHIOCYANATES IN VIVO

The first step in the metabolism of dietary or synthetic ITCs involves their conjugation with the nucleophilic sulfhydryl group of glutathione in the mercapturic acid pathway (Fig. 3) (96). After GSH conjugation the resultant ITC conjugates pass through a series of catabolic steps mediated by the enzymes γ-glutamyltranspepsidase, cysteinylglycinase, aminopeptidase, and *N*-acetyltransferase to the final mercapturic acid metabolite excreted in urine, the *N*-acetylcysteine-*S* or, alternatively, *S*-*N*-(thiocarbomylisothiocyanate)-*L*-*N*-acetylcysteine conjugates. Several in vivo studies in A/J mice and rats have identified *N*-acetylcysteine conjugates of AITC, BITC, sulforaphane, and PEITC in urine, after feeding with either synthetic or plant-derived ITCs (these data are summarized in Table 3). Common to all these studies is the rapid rate at which ITCs are detoxified and excreted in the urine; typically between 30 and 80% of the total ingested ITCs is excreted within 24 hr. Disposition and pharmacokinetic studies using ^{14}C PEITC and ^{14}CPHITC in male Fischer F344 rats addressed the effects of tissue distribution on the excretion of ITCs. High localization of PEITC within the liver, lungs, and blood was observed with 88.7% of the administered dose being excreted in the urine and feces within 48 hr. In contrast, PHITC, a structural analog of PEITC (increased chain length), showed greater retention within the liver, lungs, and blood with only 7% of the dose being excreted in the urine and 47% in feces during 48 hr. The observed retention of PHITC may explain its greater efficacy at inhibiting NNK-induced lung tumor development in rodents. The data also suggest that, unlike PEITC, PHITC may also be metabolized via a different route, as large quantities are eliminated in the feces (105).

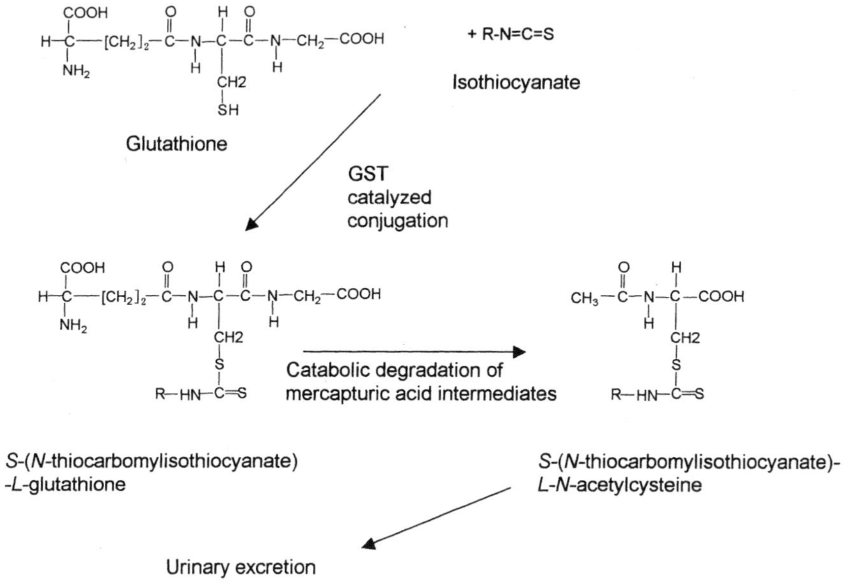

Figure 3 Detoxification of isothiocyanates occurs through the mercapturic acid pathway. The initial conjugation reaction mediated by GSTs allows for the subsequent catabolic degradation of S-(*N*-thiocarbomylisothiocyanate)-L-glutathione intermediate to its *N*-acetylcysteine derivative. NAC conjugates are routinely used for measuring isothiocyanates in urine during epidemiological and/or feeding experiments (see text).

In humans the principal urinary metabolites of ITCs are the *N*-acetylcysteine derivatives (100,102). Quantification of these has been aided by the development of the 1,2-benzenedithiol derivatization assay developed by Zhang et al. (110). Indeed, this method has often been adopted for use in feeding and epidemiological studies (60,61). In determining the role of myrosinase in the bioavailability of ITCs several studies have addressed the microbial metabolism of GSLs in humans. Getahun and Chung fed human subjects watercress with active and inactivated myrosinase and measured the urinary excretion of the *N*-acetylcysteine conjugates in urine (111). Consumption of 150 g of fresh watercress with active myrosinase resulted in the excretion of 17–77% of the administered dose of ITCs in the urine. In contrast, individuals consuming 350 g of watercress with inactivated myrosinase showed a significant reduction to only 7% of the administered dose at 24 hr. In separate experiments these investigators demonstrated the ability of human fecal samples to hydrolyze GSLs to their respective ITCs, with 18% of

TABLE 3 Summary of the Metabolic Studies Conducted Using Dietary-Derived and Synthetic Isothiocyanates In Vivo

Species investigated	Glucosinolate or isothiocyanate studied	Metabolites identified	Site of detection	Ref.
Rat, dog	BITC and its mercapturic acids	NAC conjugate	Urine Feces	97
Rat	MITC, EITC, BTITC, AITC	NAC conjugate	Urine	98
Rat	BITC, AITC, MITC, EITC, BTITC	NAC conjugate	Urine	99
Human	BITC from garden cress	NAC conjugate	Urine	100
A/J mice	PEITC	4-Hydroxy-4-carboxyl-3-phenylethylthiazolidine-2-thione and NAC conjugate	Urine and tissues	101
Human	PEITC from watercress	NAC conjugate	Urine	102
Human	AITC from brown mustard	NAC conjugate	Urine	103
Fischer F344 rats, B6C3F1 mice	AITC	Rat; NAC conjugate Mouse; -SCN ions	Urine, feces, expired air	104
Fischer F344 rats	Dose of cauliflower, sinigrin, or AITC	NAC conjugate	Urine	106
Human	PEITC from watercress	NAC conjugate	Urine	111
Fischer F344 rats	PEITC and PHITC	N/D	Urine, tissues, and expired air	105
Human	Sulforaphane from broccoli	NAC conjugates	Urine	106
Human	Broccoli sprouts containing ITCs	NAC conjugate	Urine	107
Human	Single dose of PEITC	N/D	Plasma	108
Human	Broccoli sprouts containing ITCs	N/D	Urine, plasma, serum, erythrocytes	109

AITC, allyl isothiocyanate; BITC, benzyl isothiocyanate; BTITC, butyl isothiocyanate; EITC, ethyl isothiocyanate; MITC, methyl isothiocyanate; PEITC, phenylethyl isothiocyanate; sinigrin, 2-propenyl glucosinolate.

the total GSLs being degraded with 2 hr. These data implicate colonic bacteria in the bioavailability of ITCs in the human diet. Further investigations by Shapiro et al. also demonstrated that heat inactivation can reduce the levels of ITCs metabolites in urine. In subjects consuming cooked broccoli only 10–20% of the ITCs were excreted compared to those consuming 47% in myrosinase-treated broccoli in which most of the GSLs had been converted to their respective ITCs. Furthermore, removal of colonic bacteria in subjects using antibiotic treatments almost eliminated the detection of these urinary metabolites (107). These data highlight the complex nature of the bioavailability of ITCs in the diet with a reliance on both endogeneous plant and microbial myrosinase.

VIII. THE MAMMALIAN DETOXIFICATION SYSTEM

Mammalian cells are continuously exposed to endogenous and exogenous toxins, either as by-products of metabolism or as environmental agents. These compounds are usually highly electrophilic and disrupt normal cellular function by reacting with nucleophilic centers located in and on proteins and DNA. In the extreme case, DNA adducts can be formed that result in the formation of a neoplastic cell and subsequently a cancerous cell can develop. To prevent these deleterious effects the mammalian system has developed specific pathways to stabilize and subsequently excrete xenobiotics. These pathways rely on the expression and activity of several groups of proteins known as Phase I and Phase II detoxification enzymes, such as cytochrome P450s [EC 1. 14.14.1], glutathione-*S*-transferases [EC 2.5.1.18], quinone reductase [EC 1.6.99.2], and UGT-glucoronosyltransferases [EC 2. 4.1.17]. The coordinate regulation of the latter group is generally controlled through the same transcriptional mechanism ensuring that several different Phase II detoxification enzymes may be induced by a single xenobiotic insult (112,113).

The association between Phase II detoxification enzymes and cancer risk has been the focus of much study. Deficiencies as a result of genetic polymorphisms can often lead to increased susceptibility to toxins and chemically induced carcinogenesis. These factors are emphasized in the reported increased susceptibility of smokers null for GST M1, GSTT1, and GSTP1 and additional associations with increased incidence of colon cancer, skin cancer, and ovarian cancers for individuals who are GSTM1-null (115–119). One possible means to reduce cancer risk, representing the basic principle of chemoprevention, is to modulate the activities of cellular protective enzymes using dietary supplements or dietary intervention. An increased consumption of cruciferous vegetables containing ITCs that can potentially stimulate the induction of Phase II detoxification agents may offer aid in improving human health.

Inducers of Phase II detoxification enzymes are categorized in to two main groups based on the hypothesis first highlighted by Prochaska and Talalay (114). The first group, deemed bifunctional inducers, is comprised of chemical agents, such as polycyclic aromatics and β-napthoflavone, that induce gene expression either through the antioxidant responsive element (ARE) or xenobiotic-responsive element (XRE) present within the promoter region of many of these genes. In contrast, monofunctional inducers such as ITCs induce Phase II enzymes gene expression via the ARE. Of the several groups of enzymes studied the involvement and mechanisms for CYP450s, GSTs, and NQO1 have been widely addressed and it is these enzymes that will be the focus of discussion.

IX. MODULATION OF PHASE I AND II DETOXIFICATION ENZYME ACTIVITY BY GLUCOSINOLATE HYDROLYTIC PRODUCTS

A. Phase I Enzymes

Cytochrome P450 monoxygenases constitute a superfamily of enzymes involved in oxidation and reduction reactions of both endogenous and exogenous compounds. Phase I enzymes introduce functional groups by oxidation and reduction reactions that often aid in the further metabolism of and/or excretion of chemicals. However, these fundamental processes can also lead to the generation of highly electrophilic agents that can bind to important nucleophilic sites. It is generally accepted that several CYP450 isoenzymes are involved in the bioactivation of chemical procarcinogens to more toxic forms and thus their role in human drug metabolism and cancer risk is significant. An example of this is the metabolism of the potent hepatocarcinogen aflatoxin B_1 (AFB_1) and benzo[a]pyrene (BaP), a prominent tobacco carcinogen, by CYP450 to their electrophilic epoxides. Indeed, recent evidence demonstrates the direct binding of the B[a]P epoxide to guanine bases present within both the tumor suppresser gene p53 and the oncogene K-ras (120). This finding is significant since these mutations have high prevelance in lung cancer patients. Based on current knowledge, it could be viewed that inhibition of CYP450-mediated bioactivation of procarcinogens could be a beneficial means of reducing the incidence of DNA damage associated with carcinogenesis. Intervention using dietary constituents would thus be a cheap and effective way of reducing cancers in the population. Several in vitro reports have shown synthetic BITC, PEITC, and sulforaphane are all capable of inhibiting CYP450 1A1 and 2B1 (121). In addition, Nakajima et al. demonstrated the inhibition of human CYP450 isoforms CYP450 1A2, CYP450 2A6, CYP450 2B6, CYP450 2C9, CYP450 2D6,

CYP450 2E1, and CYP450 3A4 by PEITC (122). These are important findings as CYP450 1A2 and CYP450 3A4 are involved in the bioactivation of the tobacco carcinogen NNK. Additional research shows that the inhibitory effects of BITC and butyl isothiocyanate on CYP450 2B1 and CYP450 2E1 activities are due to direct protein interaction (123). In contrast, evidence for the in vivo inhibition of CYP450s by cruciferous vegetables is conflictive. Several studies have shown whole *Brassica* vegetable extracts induce CYP450 activity in the hepatic and colonic tissues of rodents while inducing elevated levels of CYP450 1A2 in humans consuming *Brassica* vegetables (124–126). On the other hand, ingestion of watercress inhibits CYP450 2E1 in humans (127,128). These anomalies suggest that interactions with other phytochemical constituents may be involved and that these highly complex associations require further investigation.

X. PHASE II DETOXIFICATION ENZYMES

A. NQO1 Induction by Isothiocyanates

The ability of synthetic and plant-derived isothiocyanates to induce cystolic quinone reductase NQO1 [NADP(H):quinone reductase oxidoreductase], an FAD-containing flavoprotein, has been widely addressed. NQO1 exists as a homodimmer, comprised of two homo-monomeric subunits of molecular weight 32 kDa with two identical catalytic sites providing the necessary pathway to detoxify quinones to hydroquinones using NADH and NADPH as reductants (reviewed in Ref. 129). The two-electron-mediated reduction by NQO1 promotes the glucuronidation of hydroquinones that aid in their excretion (130). In addition, NQO1 also shows reductive activity toward quinone-imines and azo and nitrocompounds among others (reviewed in Ref. 131). With high localization within the liver of mammals NQO1 functions by competing with Phase I enzymes for quinone substrates. Indeed, the interaction of both NQO1 and CYP450 isoenzymes can potentially reduce the amount of free radicals produced during normal metabolic processes. BITC, PEITC, and sulforaphane, but not their respective nitriles, and several cruciferous plant extracts containing ITCs have all been demonstrated to induce NQO1 both in vitro and in vivo. Prochaska and Santamaria developed a rapid microtiter plate assay to assess the in vitro induction of NQO1 in the murine hepa1c1c7 cell line (132). Of the hundreds of compounds tested, including ITCs, diphenols, and quinones, all appear to show several common features including their ability to react with sulfhydral groups and many are substrates for GSTs (reviewed in Refs. 133,134). Indeed, the in vitro induction of NQO1 has previously been used to identify the major Phase II enzyme inducers in broccoli and watercress (135,136). Furthermore, the assay has enabled the investigation of NQO1 induction and structure function activities of a wide range of dietary constituent, including the potent ω-methylsulfinylalkyl isothiocyanates (137,138). Results from in vivo assays have also demonstrated the induction of NQO1 in several animal models. Kore et al. observed a significant increase in the NQO1 and GST activities in intestinal tissues derived from Fischer F344 rats exposed to iberin, an ITC present in broccoli (139). Likewise, Zhang et al. demonstrated the potent induction of NQO1 and GST in rodents exposed to sulforaphane (140). However, as yet no in vivo research has shown that the induction of NQO1 by dietary ITCs can alter the metabolism of, or indeed prevent, cellular damage by toxins, although current data are highly persuasive.

B. GST Induction by Isothiocyanates

The second class of detoxification enzymes, the glutathione-S-transferases (GSTs), and their functions in ITC metabolism have been of intense interest. GSTs function in detoxification of a wide range of electophilic species including aflatoxin-2,3-epoxide, tobacco carcinogens derived from benzo[a]-pyrene, and numerous pharmaceutical agents including acetaminophen. Distributed throughout the major organs and tissue such as the kidneys, lungs, intestine, skin, and the liver, GSTs catalyze the conjugation of glutathione (GSH), a tripeptide (γ-glutamyl-cysteinyl-glycine) with electophilic species, a process recognized as being the first step in the mercapturic acid pathway. Several ITCs have been demonstrated as efficient substrates for human GSTs, such as GST M1-1 and P1-1 (141,142). However, more important from a chemopreventive aspect is the ability of ITCs to induce GSTs at the transcriptional and protein level. Rodents fed ITC-enriched diets often show elevated increases in GST activity in the liver, colon, pancreas, esophagus, and stomach. Furthermore, these increases are often associated with elevated levels of the cellular antioxidant GSH and several other protective enzymes such as NQO1 and γ-glutamylcysteinesynthase (γGCS) (143,144).

XI. REGULATION OF PHASE II DETOXIFICATION ENZYMES

A. Signalling Events Associated with Phase II Enzyme Induction: The Role of Map Kinases

Chemotherapeutic drugs, natural products, and oxidative stress can modulate various extracellular signaling events and potentate stress-related gene transcription. The key components of these pathways linking extracellular events to intracellular responses are members of the mitogen-activated protein kinases (MAPK). MAPK are proline-directed serine/threonine kinases that mediate phosphorylation cascades involved in both cell survival and apoptosis. c-Jun *N*-terminal kinase (JNK), extracellular-regulated kinase (ERK), and p38 kinase are three cascades recognized in the mammalian cells. Each can function in phosphorylating transcription factors such as c-jun, ATF2, c-Myc, and Nrf2 inducing gene expression of a wide range of targets, including genes containing an ARE in their promoter regions. The importance of MAP kinases in phase II detoxification enzyme induction is exemplified by the fact that inhibitory studies using chemical agents and/or generation of dominant negative mutants significantly reduced the expression of phase II detoxification enzymes. Yu et al. demonstrated an involvement of ERK in ITC-induced NQO1 activity. In hepa1c1c7 and HepG2 cells sulforaphane stimulates ERK2 activity leading to the induction of NQO1. Blocking of the signaling cascade using specific inhibitors or a mutated ERK2 transfected into cells attenuated NQO1 activity (145). The same group also reported that p38 kinase acts as a negative regulator of ARE gene expression. Inhibition of p38 activity increased the level of ARE reporter gene activity by several enzyme inducers including sulforaphane (146). Likewise, the inhibition of ERK and p38 MAP kinases prevents the binding of the Nrf2 transcription factor to γGCS genes (147).

B. The Antioxidant Responsive Element, A Site for Nrf2 Transcription Factor Binding

As mentioned above, common to several phase II detoxification enzymes is their transcriptional regulation by a conserved element located in the promoter region designated as antioxidant responsive element (ARE). This *cis*-acting regulatory element has been identified in the 5′ flanking region of GST Ya and NQO1 genes in mammals and may also be present in other phase II enzymes. The ARE shows sequence similarity to activator protein (AP-1), and has been demonstrated to be a binding site for c-Jun, jun-B, jun-D, Fra1, and c-fos. More recent investigations have also identified a small basic leucine zipper protein (bZIP), designated Nrf-2, that can interact with the ARE, and is the prime candidate for mediating the induction of detoxification gene expression (Fig. 4). The important role of Nrf2 has been demonstrated by the work of Bloom et al. Using site-directed mutagenesis in the DNA-binding region of Nrf2, Bloom and colleagues demonstrated a decreases in Nrf2's ability to interact with the ARE (148). The overall outcome was a reduction in expression of the marker enzyme NQO1. Nrf2 can function alone or interact with c-jun, jun-B, and jun-D by formation of hetermodimers positively regulating ARE-mediated gene expression in mammalian cells (149). In contrast, interaction of Nrf2 with the small Maf proteins c-Maf, MafG,

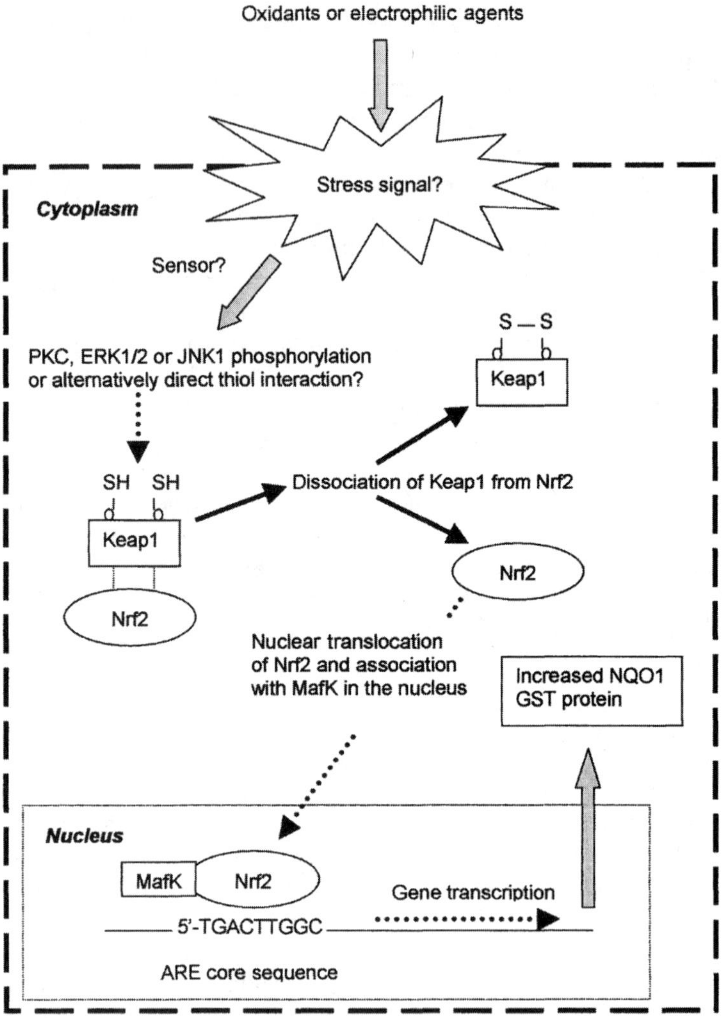

FIGURE 4 The proposed mechanism of phase II detoxification enzyme induction by oxidative stress and electrophilic agents such as isothiocyanates. PKC, protein kinase C; ERK1/2, extracellular-signaling kinases; JNK1, c-jun-n-terminal-kinase; Nrf2-, NF-E2-related factor; Keap1, Kelch-like ECH-associated protein; NQO1, quinone reductase; GST, glutathione-S-transferase. (Adapted from Refs. 148,154–156.)

and MafK in addition to c-fos negatively regulates ARE-mediated gene expression (150,151). Indeed, overexpression of MafG, MafK, and c-fos proteins in HepG2 cells suppresses the expression of ARE-related gene transcription such as the marker enzymes NQO1 and GST Ya (152).

C. Nrf2 Regulation: The Mechanism of Nrf2: Keap1 Dissociation

Nrf2 is sequested in the cytoplasm by the formation of a complex with the actin-binding protein Keap1. During insult by enzyme inducers such as ITCs, Nrf2 is released from Keap1. This allows Nrf2 to translocate to the nucleus and mediate the transcriptional activation of phase II detoxification enzymes via interaction with the ARE (153). To elucidate how Nrf2 causes enzyme induction Huang et al. focused on the mechanisms by which Keap1 dissociates from Nrf-2. Their results suggest that the involvement of protein kinase C (PKC) mediates phosphorylation of Nrf2 during oxidative stress. Once again, mutational studies were used to generate Nrf2 mutants that had an impaired ability to induce ARE-mediated transcription (154,155). Dinkova-Kostova et al. proposed an alternative mechanism by which interactions with thiol groups present in the binding domain of Keap1 are disrupted by enzyme inducers. When Keap1 was exposed to sulforaphane and bis(2-hydroxybenzylidene)acetone, the number of free thiol residues was decreased, suggesting a direct interaction with electrophiles at key sites on Keap1. The authors propose that the thiol-containing domains present on Keap1 are the sensors that allow for the dissociation of Keap1 from Nrf2, which potentiates the induction of phase II detoxification enzymes (156).

D. The In Vivo Function of Nrf2

Mice null for Nrf2(−/−) show reduced expression of several key enzymes such as GSTs, at both the mRNA and protein level, when compared to wild-type mice (Nrf2+/+). Moreover, the characteristic loss of GST expression increased the sensitivity of Nrf2 (−/−) mice to xenobiotics such as butylated hydroxyanisole and acetaminophen (157,158,160). Thimmulappa et al. using an oligonucleotide microarray approach, have identified Nrf2-regulated genes in Nrf2 (−/−) and Nrf2 (+/+) mice exposed to sulforaphane (159). Comparative analysis of treatment groups identified several genes previously showed to be induced by sulforaphane; among these were NQO1, GST, GCS, and UGT. In addition, these investigators identified several groups of genes involved in xenobiotic detoxification, antioxidant function, and biosynthetic enzymes involved in GSH and glucuronic acid pathways. Moreover, many of these enzymes were express only in the Nrf2 (+/+) mice.

XII. THE ROLE OF APOPTOSIS IN ISOTHIOCYANATE CHEMOPREVENTION

Apoptosis, also known as programmed cell death, is a means by which living organisms control abnormalities in cells that occur either by genetic or by environmental queues. Characteristic changes such as cell shrinkage, chromatin condensation, plasma membrane blebbing, DNA fragmentation, and, finally, the cell breakdown with the release of apoptotic bodies are often observed during apoptosis. The initiation of apoptosis can occur via two major pathways: through membrane-bound receptors such as the TNFα receptor, TRAIL, FADD, and the death receptors DR3, DR4, and DR5. These require interaction with extracellular ligands, which initiates an intracellular signal promoting apoptosis. Alternatively, apoptosis can be initiated via mitochondria with the release of apoptosis-inducing factors such as cytochrome c. Much cross-talk exists between both pathways and numerous components may contribute to the apoptotic cascade (reviewed in Ref. 161).

A multitude of stimuli can initiate apoptosis such as chemotherapeutic drugs, oxidative stress, ultraviolet and γ-radiation. Most induce a characteristic set of cascades that initiates proteolytic degradation of the cell (162). These biochemical and physiological events can include a decrease in cellular GSH content, generation of reactive oxygen species (ROS), cytochrome c release, and caspase activation. Furthermore, the intricate cross-talk between cellular signal transduction pathway members of the MAPkinases and the expression and/or activation of anti- and proapoptotic factors such as p53 and members of the Bcl-2 family can inhibit or potentiate the apoptotic response. In the mitochondrial pathway proapoptotic bcl-2 family proteins such as bid, bad, and bax promote mitochondrial dysfunction leading to apoptosis. These members of the proapoptotic bcl-2 proteins have the ability to either interact with components of the mitochondrial outer membrane, such as the voltage-dependent anion channel (VDAC) part of the mitochondrial permeability transition pore (MPT), or directly form channels in the outer membrane via heteroligomerization. Either one of the pathways could lead to a loss of mitochondrial membrane potential and induce the release of mitochondrial proteins that are involved in apoptotic signaling.

A. The Mechanisms of Isothiocyanate-Induced Apoptosis in Mammalian Cell

ITC-induced apoptosis has been described on only a few occasions in the literature. This pathway is summarized in Figure 5. From the available data, both extracellular signalling and the mitochondrial death pathways have been

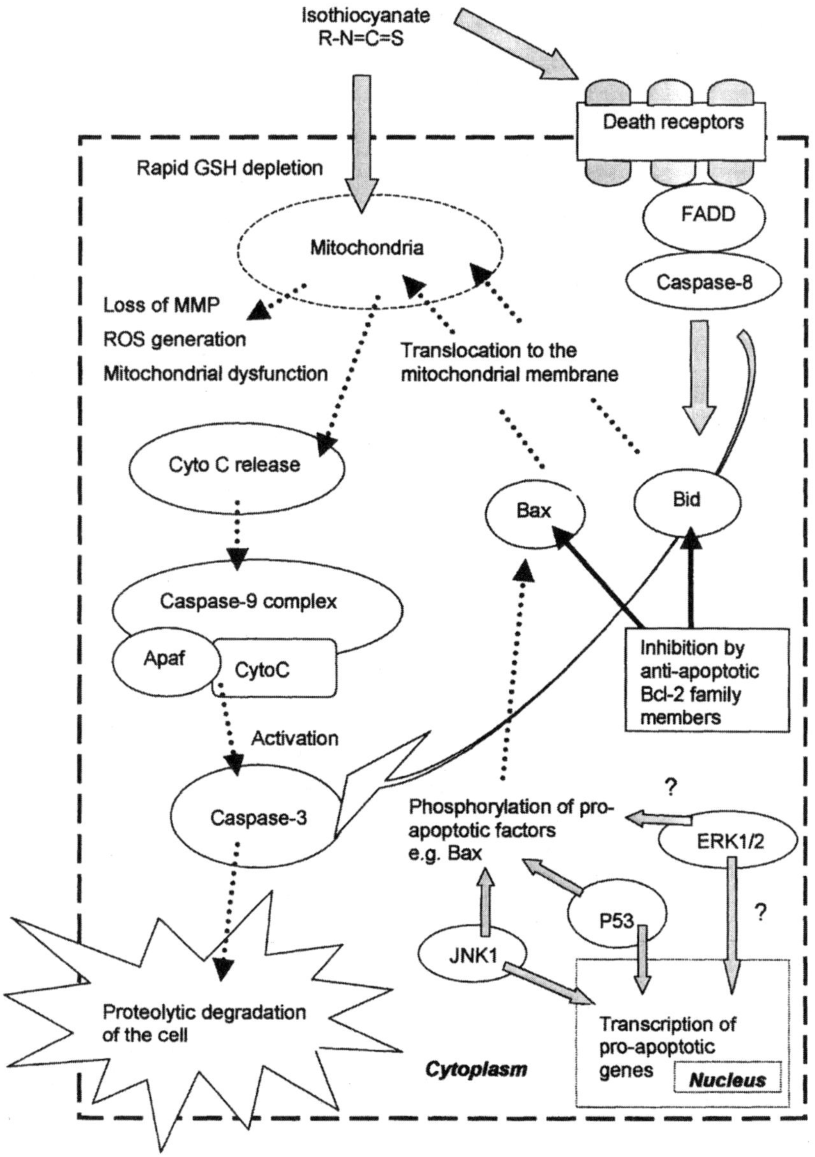

FIGURE 5 The apoptotic cascade initiated by isothiocyanates. Apaf1, apoptosis-associated factor 1; FADD, Fas-associated death domain; GSH, glutathione; MMP, mitochondrial membrane potential; ROS, reactive oxygen species. (Adapted from Refs. 166–173.)

implicated in ITC-induced apoptosis, and an overview is given below. Cancerous cells often enter cell cycle arrest when exposed to physiological concentrations of ITCs. However, at high concentrations apoptosis may occur as determined by morphological changes. For instance, AITC, BITC, and PEITC constituents of many cruciferous vegetables can inhibit cancer cell differentiation and induce selective toxicity in the human colorectal HT29 tumor cell line (163–165).

Additional data have also demonstrated G2/M-phase cell cycle arrest and apoptosis induced by sulforaphane in HT29 colon cancer cells in vitro (166). Of all the ITCs studied PEITC has received the most attention as to its role in inducing apoptosis in vitro. The time- and dose-dependent induction of apoptosis with significant increase in caspase-3-like activity has been demonstrated in HeLa cells treated with PEITC (167). This work was subsequently followed by the publications of Xu and Thornalley, who highlighted the role of caspase-8, JNK1, and Bid cleavage in human HL60 leukemia cells exposed to PEITC (168,169). The role of JNK in PEITC-induced apoptosis has also been the main focus of research for Chen and colleagues. They first demonstrated that JNK activation was important in PEITC-induced apoptosis and later showed that the transient increase in JNK activity was due to inhibition of JNK degradation by PEITC (170).

Additional studies have also suggested a role of p53 in the apoptotic cascade induced by PEITC in mouse epidemermal JB6 cells. The increased expression of p53 and the inability of PEITC to induce apoptosis in p53-deficient mouse embryonic fibroblast suggested a significant role of p53 in the induction of apoptosis (171). However, later work by Xu and Thornalley and, more recently, Xiao and Singh has shown apoptosis can occur in p53-deficient cells. Indeed, Xiao and Singh observed a role of the extracellular signaling kinases ERK 1 and 2 in PEITC-induced apoptosis in human prostate PC-3 cells (172). Inhibition of the ERK-signalling cascade prevented PEITC-induced apoptosis. In addition to extracellular signaling, the mitochondrial death pathway has been implicated in ITC-induced apoptosis. Nakamura et al. described the loss of mitochondrial membrane potential, release of cytochrome c, and activation of caspase-3 in BITC-induced apoptosis in the hepatic RL60 cell line. Associated with the loss of MMP was a dose-dependent increase in the levels of reactive oxygen species (ROS), derived from the mitochondrial electron transport chain (173). However, what role ROS has in ITC-induced apoptosis has not been determined. Investigations in our laboratory also implicate a mitochondrial death pathway in PEITC-induced apoptosis in hepatoma HepG2 cells. PEITC is observed to cause a rapid loss of cellular GSH followed by a significant decrease in mitochondrial membrane potential, cytochrome c release, and activation of caspase-3 and caspase-9 (P. Rose, unpublished observations).

B. Induction of Apoptosis by Isothiocyanates In Vivo

Although apoptosis can occur in in vitro models, it is of greater importance to know that such an event can occur in vivo. Smith et al. reported the induction of cell cycle arrest and apoptosis by AITC in colorectal crypt foci of rats treated with 1,2-dimethylhydrazine (DMH). Follow-up studies conducted using brussels sprout extracts gave similar results, confirming that isothiocyanates derived from the diet can induce apoptosis (174,175). Fisher rats F344 exposed to the carcinogen azoxymethane (AZO) develop aberrant crypt foci in colonic tissues, the formation of which is believed to be associated with the development of colon cancer. In rats fed AZO along with sulforaphane, PEITC or their respective *N*-acetylcysteine mercapturic acid metabolites show a significant reduction in the formation of aberrant crypt foci during the postinitiation phase. During the initiation phase only sulforaphane and PEITC were effective (85). More recent data have addressed the possible role of ITC-induced apoptosis in preventing lung cancer. Yang et al. demonstrated a high incidence of tumors in A/J mice exposed to a single dose of the tobacco carcinogen B[a]P. Administration of *N*-acetylcysteine conjugates of either BITC and PEITC during the postinitiation phase led to a significant reduction in tumor multiplicity. Associated with the reduction was the activation of the MAP kinases ERK1/2 and increases in activator protein 1 (AP1), phosphorylated p38 and p53, and a significant increase in the number of apoptotic cells in BITC- and PEITC-treated mice (176). Taken together these results link the apoptotic signaling pathways determined in several in vitro studies with an in vivo model.

XIII. CONCLUSIONS AND FUTURE OBJECTIVES

Our ever-expanding knowledge of how diet can influence the etiology of human disease is beginning to unravel how minor dietary components such as GSLs and their respective ITCs can prevent chronic diseases in humans. Epidemiological investigations coupled with the data from in vivo chemoprevention studies show that ITCs are effective at preventing cancers especially during the initiation phase. These chemopreventive attributes appear to be associated with the induction of phase II detoxification enzymes of which in vitro studies have determined many of the signaling mechanisms involved. Members of the MAP kinases, PKC, and the association of the transcription factor Nrf2 with ARE-mediated gene expression contribute greatly to the sequence of events leading to the induction of these protective enzymes. The role of apoptosis should also be mentioned. Under circumstances when phase II detoxification enzymes are not sufficient to prevent deleterious events caused by chemical toxins, ITCs can mediate programmed cell death. Removal of neoplastic cells by ITCs could be important in the prevention of tumor formation. Indeed, work by Yang et al. (176) suggests this to be the case.

Much work, however, still remains in accessing the biological function of chemical agents derived from cruciferous vegetables. The complexity of the glucosinolate/isothiocyanate system and disease associations still requires further research, especially in the area of bacterial metabolism, antibacterial properties, bioavailability, and interactions with other phytochemical constituents. If ITCs derived from the diet can work as effectively in humans against *H. pylori* infections, as in vitro experiments suggest, this may well be of greater importance to the prevention of cancers and possibly heart disease than previously realized. Further investigations that encompass disease states that are associated with bacterial pathogens would be advantageous, especially in a world where antibiotic-resistant bacteria are numerous. These findings pose several questions, however. Can ITCs modulate the types of bacteria in the human gut with preference to none of the harmful colonists? Or, alternatively, can ITCs alter or prevent the metabolism of toxins by colonic bacteria, reducing their potential to damage host tissues? What are the interactions of ITCs with other phytochemicals derived from cruciferous vegetables? Several classes of phytochemicals induce separate signaling events and apoptotic cascades in mammalian cells different from those of ITCs. These interactions could well potentate the chemopreventive properties of cruciferous vegetables. This would be invaluable knowledge and pertinent to future breeding programs to improve nutritional qualities of cruciferous vegetables. Currently we still rely on using the mercapturic acid as biomarkers of ITC exposure and have yet to determine other metabolites associated with the metabolism of ITCs in humans.

Are other metabolic pathways involved? What are the metabolites present within feces and do they have any biological properties? These could all have a significant effect on human health and disease incidence. Furthermore, the ability of ITCs to induce phase II enzymes is deemed a benficial property. However, what effect does this induction have on the metabolism of pharmaceutical drugs in humans? Or, more importantly, what effect does this have on chemicals that are made more toxic by metabolism by NQO1 or GSTs? Hopefully in the future many of these questions will be answered.

REFERENCES

1. Block G, Patterson B, Subar A. Fruit, vegetables, and cancer prevention: a review of the epidemiological evidence. Nutr Cancer 1992; 18(1):1–29.
2. Steinmetz KA, Potter JD. Vegetables, fruit, and cancer. II. Mechanisms. Cancer Causes Control 1991; 2(6):427–442.

3. Steinmetz KA, Potter JD. Vegetables, fruit, and cancer. I. Epidemiology. Cancer Causes Control 1991; (5):325–357.
4. Steinmetz KA, Potter JD. Vegetables, fruit, and cancer prevention: a review. J Am Diet Assoc 1996; 96(10):1027–1039.
5. Verhoeven DT, Verhagen H, Goldbohm RA, van den Brandt PA, van Poppel G. A review of mechanisms underlying anticarcinogenicity by *Brassica* vegetables. Chem Biol Interact 28 1997; 103(2):79–129.
6. Verhoeven DT, Goldbohm RA, van Poppel G, Verhagen H, van den Brandt PA. Epidemiological studies on brassica vegetables and cancer risk. Cancer Epidemiol Biomarkers Prev 1996; 5(9):733–748.
7. Van Poppel G, Verhoeven DT, Verhagen H, Goldbohm RA. *Brassica* vegetables and cancer prevention: epidemiology and mechanisms. Adv Exp Med Biol 1999; 472:159–168.
8. Preobrazhenskaya MN, Bukhman VM, Korolev AM, Efimov SA. Ascorbigen and other indole-derived compounds from *Brassica* vegetables and their analogs as anticarcinogenic and immunomodulating agents. Pharmacol Ther 1993; 60(2):301–313.
9. Broadbent TA, Broadbent HS. 1. The chemistry and pharmacology of indole-3-carbinol (indole-3-methanol) and 3-(methoxymethyl)indole. [Part II]. Curr Med Chem 1998; 5(6):469–491.
10. Broadbent TA, Broadbent HS. 1. The chemistry and pharmacology of indole-3-carbinol (indole-3-methanol) and 3-(methoxymethyl)indole. [Part I]. Curr Med Chem 1998; 5(5):337–352.
11. Brignall MS. Prevention and treatment of cancer with indole-3-carbinol. Altern Med Rev 2001; 6(6):580–589.
12. Le Marchand L. Cancer preventive effects of flavonoids: a review. Biomed Pharmacother 2002; 56(6):296–301.
13. Horvathova K, Vachalkova A, Novotny L. Flavonoids as chemoprotective agents in civilization diseases. Neoplasma 2001; 48(6):435–441.
14. Adlercreutz H. Phyto-oestrogens and cancer. Lancet Oncol 2002; 3(6):364–373.
15. Ren MQ, Kuhn G, Wegner J, Chen J. Isoflavones, substances with multi-biological and clinical properties. Eur J Nutr 2001; 40(4):135–146.
16. Fahey JW, Zalcmann AT, Talalay P. The chemical diversity and distribution of glucosinolates and isothiocyanates among plants. Phytochemistry 2001; 56(1):5–51.
17. Underhill EW, Wetter LR, Chisholm MD. Biosynthesis of glucosinolates. Biochem Soc Symp 1973; 38:303–326.
18. Kjaer A. The natural distribution of glucosinolates: a uniform class of sulphur containing glycosides. In: Bendz G, Santesson J, eds. Chemistry in Botanical Classification. London: Academic Press, 1974:229–234.
19. Fenwick GR, Heaney RK, Mullin WJ. Glucosinolates and their breakdown products in food and food plants. Crit Rev Food Sci Nutr 1983; 18(2):123–201.
20. Daxenbichler ME, Spencer GF, Carlson DG, Rose GB, Brinker AM, Powell

RG. Glucosinolate composition of seeds from 297 speices of wild plant. Phytochemistry 1991; 30(8):2623–2638.
21. Rosa E, Heaney RK, Fenwick R, Portas CAM. Glucosinolates in crop plants. Horticult Rev 1997; 19:99–215.
22. Du L, Lykkesfeldt J, Olsen CE, Halkier BA. Involvement of cytochrome P450 in oxime production in glucosinolate biosynthesis as demonstrated by an in vitro microsomal enzyme system isolated from jasmonic acid–induced seedlings of *Sinapis alba* L. Proc Natl Acad Sci USA 1995; 92(26):12505–12509.
23. Bak S, Olsen CE, Petersen BL, Moller BL, Halkier BA. Metabolic engineering of p-hydroxybenzylglucosinolate in *Arabidopsis* by expression of the cyanogenic CYP79A1 from sorghum bicolor. Plant J 1999; 20(6):663–671.
24. Hansen CH, Du L, Naur P, Olsen CE, Axelsen KB, Hick AJ, Pickett JA, Halkier BA. CYP83b1 is the oxime-metabolizing enzyme in the glucosinolate pathway in *Arabidopsis*. J Biol Chem 2001; 276(27):24790–24796.
25. Mikkelsen MD, Petersen BL, Olsen CE, Halkier BA. Biosynthesis and metabolic engineering of glucosinolates. Amino Acids 2002; 22(3):279–295.
26. Wittstock U, Halkier BA. Glucosinolate research in the *Arabidopsis* era. Trends Plant Sci 2002; 7(6):263–270.
27. de Quiros HC, Magrath R, McCallum D, Mithen R. Alpha-keto acid elongation and glucosinolate biosynthesis in *Arabidposis thaliana*. Theor Appl Genet 2000; 101(3):429–437.
28. Mithen RF, Dekker M, Verkerk R, Rabot S, Johnson IT. The nutritional significance, biosynthesis and bioavailability of glucosinolates in human foods. J Sci Food Agr 2000; 80(7):967–984.
29. Mithen R. Glucosinolates-biochemistry, genetics and biological activity. Plant Growth Regul 2001; 34(1):91–103.
30. Hall C, McCallum D, Prescott A, Mithen R. Biochemical genetics of glucosinolate modification in *Arabidopsis* and *Brassica*. Theor Appl Genet 2001; 102(2–3):369–374.
31. Faulkner K, Mithen R, Williamson G. Selective increase of the potential anticarcinogen 4-methylsulphinylbutyl glucosinolate in broccoli. Carcinogenesis 1998; 19(4):605–609.
32. Mithen R, Faulkner K, Magrath R, Rose P, Williamson G, Marquez J. Development of isothiocyanate-enriched broccoli, and its enhanced ability to induce phase 2 detoxification enzymes in mammalian cells. Theor Appl Genet 2003; 106:727–734.
33. Bones AM, Rossiter JT. The myrosinase-glucosinolate system, its organisation and biochemistry. Physiol Plant 1996; 97(1):194–208.
34. Tookey HL. *Crambe* thioglucoside glucohydrolase (EC 3.2.3.1): separation of a protein required for epithiobutane formation. Can J Biochem 1973; 51:1654–1660.
35. Foo HL, Gronning LM, Goodenough L, Bones AM, Danielsen BE, Whiting DA, Rossiter JT. Purification and characterisation of epithiospecifier protein from *Brassica napus*: enzymic intramolecular sulphur addition within alkenyl

thiohydroximates derived from alkenyl glucosinolate hydrolysis. FEBS Lett 2000; 468(2–3):243–246.

36. Lambrix V, Reichelt M, Mitchell-Olds T, Kliebenstein DJ, Gershenzon J. The *Arabidopsis* epithiospecifier protein promotes the hydrolysis of glucosinolates to nitriles and influences Trichoplusian herbivory. Plant Cell 2001; 13(12):2793–2807.
37. Rask L, Andreasson E, Ekbom B, Eriksson S, Pontoppidan B, Meijer J. Myrosinase: gene family evolution and herbivore defense in Brassicaceae. Plant Mol Biol 2000; 42(1):93–113.
38. Oginsky EL, Stein AE, Greer MA. Myrosinase activity in bacteria as demonstrated by the conversion of progoitrin to poitrin. Proc Exp Biol Med 1965; 119:360–364.
39. Tani N, Ohtsuru M, Hata T. Purification and general characteristics of bacterial myrosinase produced by *Enterobacter cloacae*. Agric Biol Chem 1974; 38:1623–1630.
40. Krul C, Humblot C, Philippe C, Vermeulen M, van Nuenen M, Havenaar R, Rabot S. Metabolism of sinigrin (2-propenyl glucosinolate) by the human colonic microflora in a dynamic in vitro large-intestinal model. Carcinogenesis 2002; 23(6):1009–1016.
41. Elfoul L, Rabot S, Khelifa N, Quinsac A, Duguay A, Rimbault A. Formation of allyl isothiocyanate from sinigrin in the digestive tract of rats monoassociated with a human colonic strain of *Bacteroides thetaiotaomicron*. FEMS Microbiol Lett 2001; 197(1):99–103.
42. Stoewsand GS. Bioactive organosulfur phytochemicals in *Brassica oleracea* vegetables: a review. Food Chem Toxicol 1995; 33(6):537–543.
43. Onderjickova O, Drobinca L, Sedlacek J, Rychlik I. The effects of thiol combining agents on polypeptide synthesis in cell free extracts from *Eshcerichia coli*. Biochem Pharmacol 1974; 23:2751–2759.
44. Ono H, Tesaki S, Tanabe S, Watanabe M. 6-Methylsulphinylhexyl isothiocyanate and its homologues as food-originated compounds with antibacterial activity against *Escherichia coli* and *Staphylococcus aureus*. Biosci Biotechnol Biochem 1998; 62:363–365.
45. Lin CM, Preston JF III, Wei CI. Antibacterial mechanism of allyl isothiocyanate. J Food Prot 2000; 63(6):727–734.
46. Fahey JW, Haristoy X, Dolan PM, Kensler TW, Scholtus I, Stephenson KK, Talalay P, Lozniewski A. Sulforaphane inhibits extracellular, intracellular, and antibiotic-resistant strains of *Helicobacter pylori* and prevents benzo[a]-pyrene-induced stomach tumors. Proc Natl Acad Sci USA 2002; 99(11): 7610–7615.
47. Drobinca L, Zemanova M, Nemec K, Antos P, Kristian A, Stullerova V, Knoppova V, Nemec JRP. Antifungal activity of isothiocyanates and related compounds. Appl Microbiol 1967; 15:701–709.
48. Nugon-Baugon L, Szylit O, Raibaud P. Production of toxic glucosinolate derivatives from rapeseed meal by intestinal microflora of rats and chicken. J Sci Food Agric 1988; 43:229–238.

49. Heaney RK, Fenwick GR. Natural toxins and protective factors in *Brassica* species, including rapeseed. Nat Toxins 1995; 3:233–237.
50. McMillan M, Spinks EA, Fenwick GR. Preliminary observations on the effect of dietary brussels sprouts on thyroid function. Hum Toxicol 1986; 5(1):15–19.
51. Hirose M, Yamaguchi T, Kimoto N, Ogawa K, Futakuchi M, Sano M, Shirai T. Strong promoting activity of phenylethyl isothiocyanate and benzyl isothiocyanate on urinary bladder carcinogenesis in F344 male rats. Int J Cancer 1998; 77(5):773–777.
52. Masutomi N, Toyoda K, Shibutani M, Niho N, Uneyama C, Takahashi N, Hirose M. Toxic effects of benzyl and allyl isothiocyanates and benzyl-isoform specific metabolites in the urinary bladder after a single intravesical application to rats. Toxicol Pathol 2001; 29(6):617–622.
53. Musk SR, Astley SB, Edwards SM, Stephenson P, Hubert RB, Johnson IT. Cytotoxic and clastogenic effects of benzyl isothiocyanate towards cultured mammalian cells. Food Chem Toxicol 1995; 33(1):31–37.
54. Kassie F, Knasmuller S. Genotoxic effects of allyl isothiocyanate (AITC) and phenethyl isothiocyanate (PEITC). Chem Biol Interact 2000; 127(2):163–180.
55. Kassie F, Pool-Zobel B, Parzefall W, Knasmuller S. Genotoxic effects of benzyl isothiocyanate, a natural chemopreventive agent. Mutagenesis 1999; 14(6):595–604.
56. Kassie F, Parzefall W, Musk S, Johnson I, Lamprecht G, Sontag G, Knasmuller S. Genotoxic effects of crude juices from *Brassica* vegetables and juices and extracts from phytopharmaceutical preparations and spices of cruciferous plants origin in bacterial and mammalian cells. Chem Biol Interact 1996; 102(1):1–16.
57. Murata M, Yamashita N, Inoue S, Kawanishi S. Mechanism of oxidative DNA damage induced by carcinogenic allyl isothiocyanate. Free Radic Biol Med 2000; 28(5):797–805.
58. Lin HJ, Zhou H, Dai A, Huang HF, Lin JH, Frankl HD, Lee ER, Haile RW. Glutathione transferase GSTT1, broccoli, and prevalence of colorectal adenomas. Pharmacogenetics 2002; 12(2):175–179.
59. Voorrips LE, Goldbohm RA, Verhoeven DT, van Poppel GA, Sturmans F, Hermus RJ, van den Brandt PA. Vegetable and fruit consumption and lung cancer risk in the Netherlands Cohort Study on diet and cancer. Cancer Causes Control 2000; 11(2):101–115.
60. London SJ, Yuan JM, Chung FL, Gao YT, Coetzee GA, Ross RK, Yu MC. Isothiocyanates, glutathione S-transferase M1 and T1 polymorphisms, and lung-cancer risk: a prospective study of men in Shanghai, China. Lancet 2000; 356(9231):724–729.
61. Zhao B, Seow A, Lee EJ, Poh WT, Teh M, Eng P, Wang YT, Tan WC, Yu MC, Lee HP. Dietary isothiocyanates, glutathione S-transferase -M1, -T1 polymorphisms and lung cancer risk among Chinese women in Singapore. Cancer Epidemiol Biomark Prev 2001; 10(10):1063–1067.
62. Kristal AR, Lampe JW. *Brassica* vegetables and prostate cancer risk: a review of the epidemiological evidence. Nutr Cancer 2002; 42(1):1–9.

63. Hecht SS. Chemoprevention by isothiocyanates. J Cell Biochem 1995; 22(suppl):195–209.
64. Wattenberg LW. Inhibitory effects of benzyl isothiocyanate administered shortly before diethylnitrosamine or benzo[a]pyrene on pulmonary and forestomach neoplasia in A/J mice. Carcinogenesis 1987; 8:1971–1973.
65. Morse MA, Eklind KI, Amin SG, Hecht SS, Chung FL. Effects of alkyl chain length on the inhibition of NNK-induced lung neoplasia in A/J mice by arylalkyl isothiocyanates. Carcinogenesis 1989; 10:1757–1759.
66. Stoner GD, Morrissey DT, Heur YH, Daniel EM, Galati AJ, Wagner SA. Inhibitory effects of phenethyl isothiocyanate on *N*-nitrosobenzylmethylamine carcinogenesis in the rat esophagus. Cancer Res 1991; 51:2063–2068.
67. Sugie S, Okamoto K, Okumura A, Tanaka T, Mori H. Inhibitory effects of benzyl thiocyanate and benzyl isothiocyanate on methylazoxymethanol acetate-induced intestinal carcinogenesis in rats. Carcinogenesis 1994; 8:1555–1560.
68. Wilkinson JT, Morse MA, Kresty LA, Stoner GD. Effect of alkyl chain length on inhibition of *N*-nitrosomethylbenzylamine-induced esophageal tumorigenesis and DNA methylation by isothiocyanates. Carcinogenesis 1995; 5:1011–1015.
69. Morse MA. Inhibition of NNK-induced lung tumorigenesis by modulators of NNK activation. Exp Lung Res 1998; 4:595–604.
70. Futakuchi M, Hirose M, Miki T, Tanaka H, Ozaki M, Shirai T. Inhibition of DMBA-initiated rat mammary tumour development by 1-*O*-hexyl-2,3,5-trimethylhydroquinone, phenylethyl isothiocyanate, and novel synthetic ascorbic acid derivatives. Eur J Cancer Prev 1998; 2:153–159.
71. Stoner GD, Adams C, Kresty LA, Amin SG, Desai D, Hecht SS, Murphy SE, Morse MA. Inhibition of *N'*-nitrosonornicotine-induced esophageal tumorigenesis by 3-phenylpropyl isothiocyanate. Carcinogenesis 1998; 12:2139–2143.
72. Hecht SS, Kenney PM, Wang M, Trushin N, Upadhyaya P. Effects of phenethyl isothiocyanate and benzyl isothiocyanate, individually and in combination, on lung tumorigenesis induced in A/J mice by benzo[a]pyrene and 4-(methylnitrosamino)-1-(3-pyridyl)-1-butanone. Cancer Lett 2000; 150:49–56.
73. Ogawa K, Hirose M, Sugiura S, Cui L, Imaida K, Ogiso T, Shirai T. Dose-dependent promotion by phenylethyl isothiocyanate, a known chemopreventer, of two-stage rat urinary bladder and liver carcinogenesis. Nutr Cancer 2001; 40:134–139.
74. Sticha KR, Kenney PM, Boysen G, Liang H, Su X, Wang M, Upadhyaya P, Hecht SS. Effects of benzyl isothiocyanate and phenethyl isothiocyanate on DNA adduct formation by a mixture of benzo[a]pyrene and 4-(methylnitrosamino)-1-(3-pyridyl)-1-butanone in A/J mouse lung. Carcinogenesis 2002; 23:1433–1439.
75. Guo Z, Smith TJ, Wang E, Eklind KI, Chung FL, Yang CS. Structure-activity relationships of arylalkyl isothiocyanates for the inhibition of 4-(methylnitrosamino)-1-(3-pyridyl)-1-butanone metabolism and the modulation of

xenobiotic-metabolizing enzymes in rats and mice. Carcinogenesis 1993; 14(6):1167–1173.
76. Jiao D, Smith TJ, Yang CS, Pittman B, Desai D, Amin S, Chung FL. Chemopreventive activity of thiol conjugates of isothiocyanates for lung tumorigenesis. Carcinogenesis 1997; 18(11):2143–2147.
77. Staretz ME, Foiles PG, Miglietta LM, Hecht SS. Evidence for an important role of DNA pyridyloxobutylation in rat lung carcinogenesis by 4-(methylnitrosamino)-1-(3-pyridyl)-1-butanone: effects of dose and phenethyl isothiocyanate. Cancer Res 1997; 57(2):259–266.
78. Matzinger SA, Crist KA, Stoner GD, Anderson MW, Pereira MA, Steele VE, Kelloff GJ, Lubet RA, You M. K-ras mutations in lung tumors from A/J and A/J × TSG-p53 F1 mice treated with 4-(methylnitrosamino)-1-(3-pyridyl)-1-butanone and phenethyl isothiocyanate. Carcinogenesis 1995; 16(10):2487–2492.
79. Lin JM, Amin S, Trushin N, Hecht SS. Effects of isothiocyanates on tumorigenesis by benzo[a]pyrene in murine tumor models. Cancer Lett 1993; 71:35–42.
80. Morse MA, Amin SG, Hecht SS, Chung FL. Effects of aromatic isothiocyanates on tumorigenicity, O6-methylguanine formation, and metabolism of the tobacco-specific nitrosamine 4-(methylnitrosamino)-1-(3-pyridyl)-1-butanone in A/J mouse lung. Cancer Res 1989; 49(11):2894–2897.
81. Wattenberg LW. Inhibition of carcinogenic effects of polycyclic hydrocarbons by benzyl isothiocyanate and related compounds. J Natl Cancer Inst 1977; 58:395–398.
82. Wattenberg LW. Inhibition of neoplasia by minor dietary constitiuents. Cancer Res 1983; 43:2448s–2453s.
83. Hecht SS, Kenney PMJ, Wang M, Upadhyaya P. Benzyl isothiocyanate: effective inhibitor of polycyclic aromatic hydrocarbon tumorigenesis in A/J mouse lung. Cancer Lett 2002; 187:87–94.
84. Zhang Y, Kensler TW, Cho GH, Posner GH, Talalay P. Anticarcinogenic activities of sulforaphane and structurally related synthetic norbornyl isothiocyanates. Proc Natl Acad Sci USA 1994; 91:3147–3150.
85. Chung FL, Conaway CC, Rao CV, Reddy BS. Chemoprevention of colonic aberrant crypt foci in Fischer rats by sulforaphane and phenylethyl isothiocyanate. Carcinogenesis 2000; 21:2287–2291.
86. Hecht SS, Chung FL, Richie JP Jr, Akerkar SA, Borukhova A, Skowronski L, Carmella SG. Effects of watercress consumption on metabolism of a tobacco-specific lung carcinogen in smokers. Cancer Epidemiol Biomark Prev 1995; 4(8):877–884.
87. Hecht SS, Carmella SG, Murphy SE. Effects of watercress consumption on urinary metabolites of nicotine in smokers. Cancer Epidemiol Biomark Prev 1999; 8(10):907–913.
88. Finley JW, Ip C, Lisk DJ, Davis GD, Hintze KJ, Whanger PD. Cancer protection properties of high selenium broccoli. J Agric Food Chem 2001; 49:2679–2683.

89. Davis CD, Zeng H, Finley JW. Selenium-enriched broccoli decreases intestinal tumorigenesis in multiple intestinal neoplasia mice. J Nutr 2002; 132:307–309.
90. Shen HM, Ong CN. Mutations of the p53 tumor suppressor gene and ras oncogenes in aflatoxin hepatocarcinogenesis. Mutat Res 1996; 366(1):23–44.
91. Godlewski CE, Boyd JN, Sherman WK, Anderson JL, Stoewsand GS. Hepatic glutathione S-transferase activity and aflatoxin B1-induced enzyme altered foci in rats fed fractions of brussels sprouts. Cancer Lett 1985; 28(2):151–157.
92. Salbe AD, Bjeldanes LF. The effects of dietary brussels sprouts and *Schizandra chinensis* on the xenobiotic-metabolizing enzymes of the rat small intestine. Food Chem Toxicol 1985; 23(1):57–65.
93. Whitty JP, Bjeldanes LF. The effects of dietary cabbage on xenobiotic-metabolizing enzymes and the binding of aflatoxin B1 to hepatic DNA in rats. Food Chem Toxicol 1987; 25(8):581–587.
94. Hayes JD, Pulford DJ, Ellis EM, McLeod R, James RF, Seidegard J, Mosialou E, Jernstrom B, Neal GE. Regulation of rat glutathione S-transferase A5 by cancer chemopreventive agents: mechanisms of inducible resistance to aflatoxin B1. Chem Biol Interact 1998; 111–112:51–67.
95. Esaki H, Kumagai S. Glutathione-S-transferase activity toward aflatoxin epoxide in livers of mastomys and other rodents. Toxicon 2002; 40(7):941–945.
96. Habig WH, Pabst MJ, Jakoby WB. Glutathione S-transferases. The first enzymatic step in mercapturic acid formation. J Biol Chem 1974; 249(22):7130–7139.
97. Brusewitz G, Cameron BD, Chasseaud LF, Gorler K, Hawkins DR, Koch H, Mennicke WH. The metabolism of benzyl isothiocyanate and its cysteine conjugate. Biochem J 1977; 162:99–107.
98. Mennicke WH, Gorler K, Krumbiegel G. Metabolism of some naturally occurring isothiocyanates in the rat. Xenobiotica 1983; 13:203–207.
99. Mennicke WH, Kral T, Krumbiegel G, Rittmann N. Determination of *N*-acetyl-S-(*N*-alkylthiocarbamoyl)-L-cysteine, a principal metabolite of alkyl isothiocyanates, in rat urine. J Chromatogr 1987; 414:19–24.
100. Mennicke WH, Gorler K, Krumbiegel G, Lorenz D, Rittmann N. Studies on the metabolism and excretion of benzyl isothiocyanate in man. Xenobiotica 1988; 18:441–447.
101. Eklind KI, Morse MA, Chung FL. Distribution and metabolism of the natural anticarcinogen phenethyl isothiocyanate in A/J mice. Carcinogenesis 1990; 11:2033–2036.
102. Chung FL, Morse MA, Eklind KI, Lewis J. Quantitation of human uptake of the anticarcinogen phenethyl isothiocyanate after a watercress meal. Cancer Epidemiol Biomark Prev 1992; 1:383–388.
103. Jiao D, Ho CT, Foiles P, Chung FL. Identification and quantification of the *N*-acetylcysteine conjugate of allyl isothiocyanate in human urine after ingestion of mustard. Cancer Epidemiol Biomark Prev 1994; 3:487–492.
104. Bollard M, Stribbling S, Mitchell S, Caldwell J. The disposition of allyl isothiocyanate in the rat and mouse. Food Chem Toxicol 1997; 35:933–943.

105. Conaway CC, Jiao D, Kohri T, Liebes L, Chung FL. Disposition and pharmacokinetics of phenethyl isothiocyanate and 6-phenylhexyl isothiocyanate in F344 rats. Drug Metab Dispos 1999; 27:13–20.
106. Conaway CC, Getahun SM, Liebes LL, Pusateri DJ, Topham DK, Botero-Omary M, Chung FL. Disposition of glucosinolates and sulforaphane in humans after ingestion of steamed and fresh broccoli. Nutr Cancer 2000; 38:168–178.
107. Shapiro TA, Fahey JW, Wade KL, Stephenson KK, Talalay P. Chemoprotective glucosinolates and isothiocyanates of broccoli sprouts: metabolism and excretion in humans. Cancer Epidemiol Biomark Prev 2001; 10:501–508.
108. Liebes L, Conaway CC, Hochster H, Mendoza S, Hecht SS, Crowell J, Chung FL. High-performance liquid chromatography–based determination of total isothiocyanate levels in human plasma: application to studies with 2-phenethyl isothiocyanate. Anal Biochem 2001; 291:279–289.
109. Ye L, Dinkova-Kostova AT, Wade KL, Zhang Y, Shapiro TA, Talalay P. Quantitative determination of dithiocarbamates in human plasma, serum, erythrocytes and urine: pharmacokinetics of broccoli sprout isothiocyanates in humans. Clin Chim Acta 2002; 316:43–53.
110. Zhang Y, Wade KL, Prestera T, Talalay P. Quantitative determination of isothiocyanates, dithiocarbamates, carbon disulfide, and related thiocarbonyl compounds by cyclocondensation with 1,2-benzenedithiol. Anal Biochem 1996; 239(2):160–167.
111. Getahun SM, Chung FL. Conversion of glucosinolates to isothiocyanates in humans after ingestion of cooked watercress. Cancer Epidemiol Biomark Prev 1998; 8(5):447–451.
112. De Long MJ, Prochaska HJ, Talalay P. Induction of NAD(P)H:quinone reductase in murine hepatoma cells by phenolic antioxidants, azo dyes, and other chemoprotectors: a model system for the study of anticarcinogens. Proc Natl Acad Sci USA 1986; 83(3):787–791.
113. Spencer SR, Xue LA, Klenz EM, Talalay P. The potency of inducers of NAD(P)H:(quinone-acceptor) oxidoreductase parallels their efficiency as substrates for glutathione transferases: structural and electronic correlations. Biochem J 1991; 273(Pt 3):711–717.
114. Prochaska HJ, Talalay P. Regulatory mechanisms of monofunctional and bifunctional anticarcinogenic enzyme inducers in murine liver. Cancer Res 1988; 48(17):4776–4782.
115. Lewis SJ, Cherry NM, Niven RM, Barber PV, Povey AC. GSTM1, GSTT1 and GSTP1 polymorphisms and lung cancer risk. Cancer Lett 2002; 180(2):165–171.
116. Sunaga N, Kohno T, Yanagitani N, Sugimura H, Kunitoh H, Tamura T, Takei Y, Tsuchiya S, Saito R, Yokota J. Contribution of the NQO1 and GSTT1 polymorphisms to lung adenocarcinoma susceptibility. Cancer Epidemiol Biomark Prev 2002; 11(8):730–738.
117. Miller DP, Liu G, De Vivo I, Lynch TJ, Wain JC, Su L, Christiani DC. Combinations of the variant genotypes of GSTP1, GSTM1, and p53 are associated with an increased lung cancer risk. Cancer Res 2002; 62(10):2819–2823.

118. Autrup H. Genetic polymorphisms in human xenobiotica metabolizing enzymes as susceptibility factors in toxic response. Mutat Res 2000; 464(1):65–76.
119. Strange RC, Jones PW, Fryer AA. Glutathione S-transferase: genetics and role in toxicology. Toxicol Lett 2000; 112–113:357–363.
120. Tretyakova N, Matter B, Jones R, Shallop A. Formation of benzo[a]pyrene diol epoxide-DNA adducts at specific guanines within K-ras and p53 gene sequences: stable isotope-labeling mass spectrometry approach. Biochemistry 2002; 41(30):9535–9544.
121. Conaway CC, Krzeminski J, Amin S, Chung FL. Decomposition rates of isothiocyanate conjugates determine their activity as inhibitors of cytochrome p450 enzymes. Chem Res Toxicol 2001; 14(9):1170–1176.
122. Nakajima M, Yoshida R, Shimada N, Yamazaki H, Yokoi T. Inhibition and inactivation of human cytochrome P450 isoforms by phenethyl isothiocyanate. Drug Metab Dispos 2001; 29(8):1110–1113.
123. Moreno RL, Kent UM, Hodge K, Hollenberg PF. Inactivation of cytochrome P450 2E1 by benzyl isothiocyanate. Chem Res Toxicol 1999; 12(7):582–587.
124. Vang O, Frandsen H, Hansen KT, Sorensen JN, Sorensen H, Andersen O. Biochemical effects of dietary intakes of different broccoli samples. I. Differential modulation of cytochrome P-450 activities in rat liver, kidney, and colon. Metabolism 2001; 50(10):1123–1129.
125. Lampe JW, King IB, Li S, Grate MT, Barale KV, Chen C, Feng Z, Potter JD. *Brassica* vegetables increase and apiaceous vegetables decrease cytochrome P450 1A2 activity in humans: changes in caffeine metabolite ratios in response to controlled vegetable diets. Carcinogenesis 2000; 21(6):1157–1162.
126. Murray S, Lake BG, Gray S, Edwards AJ, Springall C, Bowey EA, Williamson G, Boobis AR, Gooderham NJ. Effect of cruciferous vegetable consumption on heterocyclic aromatic amine metabolism in man. Carcinogenesis 2001; 22(9):1413–1420.
127. Chen L, Mohr SN, Yang CS. Decrease of plasma and urinary oxidative metabolites of acetaminophen after consumption of watercress by human volunteers. Clin Pharmacol Ther 1996; 60(6):651–660.
128. Leclercq I, Desager JP, Horsmans Y. Inhibition of chlorzoxazone metabolism, a clinical probe for CYP2E1, by a single ingestion of watercress. Clin Pharmacol Ther 1998; 64(2):144–149.
129. Faig M, Bianchet MA, Talalay P, Chen S, Winski S, Ross D, Amzel LM. Structures of recombinant human and mouse NAD(P)H:quinone oxidoreductases: species comparison and structural changes with substrate binding and release. Proc Natl Acad Sci USA 2000; 97(7):3177–3182.
130. Bianchet MA, Foster C, Faig M, Talalay P, Amzel LM. Structure and mechanism of cytosolic quinone reductases. Biochem Soc Trans 1999; 27(4):610–615.
131. Ross D, Kepa JK, Winski SL, Beall HD, Anwar A, Siegel D. NAD(P)H:quinone oxidoreductase 1 (NQO1): chemoprotection, bioactivation, gene regulation and genetic polymorphisms. Chem Biol Interact 2000; 129(1–2):77–97.
132. Prochaska HJ, Santamaria AB. Direct measurement of NAD(P)H:quinone

reductase from cells cultured in microtiter wells: a screening assay for anticarcinogenic enzyme inducers. Anal Biochem 1988; 169(2):328–336.
133. Talalay P, Zhang Y. Chemoprotection against cancer by isothiocyanates and glucosinolates. Biochem Soc Trans 1996; 24(3):806–810.
134. Fahey JW, Talalay P. Antioxidant functions of sulforaphane: a potent inducer of Phase II detoxication enzymes. Food Chem Toxicol 1999; 37(9–10): 973–979.
135. Zhang Y, Talalay P, Cho CG, Posner GH. A major inducer of anticarcinogenic protective enzymes from broccoli: isolation and elucidation of structure. Proc Natl Acad Sci USA 1992; 89(6):2399–2403.
136. Rose P, Faulkner K, Williamson G, Mithen R. 7-Methylsulfinylheptyl and 8-methylsulfinyloctyl isothiocyanates from watercress are potent inducers of phase II enzymes. Carcinogenesis 2000; 21(11):1983–1988.
137. Posner GH, Cho CG, Green JV, Zhang Y, Talalay P. Design and synthesis of bifunctional isothiocyanate analogs of sulforaphane: correlation between structure and potency as inducers of anticarcinogenic detoxication enzymes. J Med Chem 1994; 37(1):170–176.
138. Hou DX, Fukuda M, Fujii M, Fuke Y. Induction of NADPH:quinone oxidoreductase in murine hepatoma cells by methylsulfinyl isothiocyanates: methyl chain length-activity study. Int J Mol Med 2000; 6(4):441–444.
139. Kore AM, Jeffery EH, Wallig MA. Effects of 1-isothiocyanato-3-(methylsulfinyl)-propane on xenobiotic metabolizing enzymes in rats. Food Chem Toxicol 1993; 31(10):723–729.
140. Zhang Y, Kensler TW, Cho CG, Posner GH, Talalay P. Anticarcinogenic activities of sulforaphane and structurally related synthetic norbornyl isothiocyanates. Proc Natl Acad Sci USA 1994; 91(8):3147–3150.
141. Kolm RH, Danielson UH, Zhang Y, Talalay P, Mannervik B. Isothiocyanates as substrates for human glutathione transferases: structure-activity studies. Biochem J 1995; 311(Pt 2):453–459.
142. Meyer DJ, Crease DJ, Ketterer B. Forward and reverse catalysis and product sequestration by human glutathione S-transferases in the reaction of GSH with dietary aralkyl isothiocyanates. Biochem J 1995; 306(Pt 2):565–569.
143. Van Lieshout EM, Peters WH, Jansen JB. Effect of oltipraz, alpha-tocopherol, beta-carotene and phenethylisothiocyanate on rat oesophageal, gastric, colonic and hepatic glutathione, glutathione S-transferase and peroxidase. Carcinogenesis 1996; 17(7):1439–1445.
144. Wallig MA, Kingston S, Staack R, Jefferey EH. Induction of rat pancreatic glutathione S-transferase and quinone reductase activities by a mixture of glucosinolate breakdown derivatives found in brussels sprouts. Food Chem Toxicol 1998; 36(5):365–373.
145. Yu R, Lei W, Mandlekar S, Weber MJ, Der CJ, Wu J, Kong AT. Role of a mitogen-activated protein kinase pathway in the induction of phase II detoxifying enzymes by chemicals. J Biol Chem 1999; 274(39):27545–27552.
146. Yu R, Mandlekar S, Lei W, Fahl WE, Tan TH, Kong AT. p38 mitogen-activated protein kinase negatively regulates the induction of phase II drug-

metabolizing enzymes that detoxify carcinogens. J Biol Chem 2000; 275(4): 2322–2327.
147. Zipper LM, Mulcahy RT. Inhibition of ERK and p38 MAP kinases inhibits binding of Nrf2 and induction of GCS genes. Biochem Biophys Res Commun 2000; 278(2):484–492.
148. Bloom D, Dhakshinamoorthy S, Jaiswal AK. Site-directed mutagenesis of cysteine to serine in the DNA binding region of Nrf2 decreases its capacity to upregulate antioxidant response element-mediated expression and antioxidant induction of NAD(P)H:quinone oxidoreductase1 gene. Oncogene 2002; 21(14):2191–2200.
149. Venugopal R, Jaiswal AK. Nrf2 and Nrf1 in association with Jun proteins regulate antioxidant response element-mediated expression and coordinated induction of genes encoding detoxifying enzymes. Oncogene 2000; 17(24):3145–3156.
150. Dhakshinamoorthy S, Jaiswal AK. Small maf (MafG and MafK) proteins negatively regulate antioxidant response element-mediated expression and antioxidant induction of the NAD(P)H:quinone oxidoreductase1 gene. J Biol Chem 2000; 275(51):40134–40141.
151. Dhakshinamoorthy S, Jaiswal AK. c-Maf negatively regulates ARE-mediated detoxifying enzyme genes expression and anti-oxidant induction. Oncogene 2002; 21(34):5301–5312.
152. Wilkinson J IV, Radjendirane V, Pfeiffer GR, Jaiswal AK, Clapper ML. Disruption of c-Fos leads to increased expression of NAD(P)H:quinine oxidoreductase1 and glutathione S-transferase. Biochem Biophys Res Commun 1998; 253(3):855–858.
153. Zipper LM, Mulcahy RT. The Keap1 BTB/POZ dimerization function is required to sequester Nrf2 in cytoplasm. J Biol Chem 2002; 277(39):36544–36552.
154. Huang HC, Nguyen T, Pickett CB. Regulation of the antioxidant response element by protein kinase C–mediated phosphorylation of NF-E2-related factor 2. Proc Natl Acad Sci USA 2000; 97(23):12475–12480.
155. Huang HC, Nguyen T, Pickett CB. Phosphorylation of Nrf2 at Ser40 by protein kinase C regulates antioxidant response element-mediated transcription. J Biol Chem 2002; 277:42769–42774.
156. Dinkova-Kostova AT, Holtzclaw WD, Cole RN, Itoh K, Wakabayashi N, Katoh Y, Yamamoto M, Talalay P. Direct evidence that sulfhydryl groups of Keap1 are the sensors regulating induction of phase 2 enzymes that protect against carcinogens and oxidants. Proc Natl Acad Sci USA 2002; 99(18):11908–11913.
157. Chanas SA, Jiang Q, McMahon M, McWalter GK, McLellan LI, Elcombe CR, Henderson CJ, Wolf CR, Moffat GJ, Itoh K, Yamamoto M, Hayes JD. Loss of the Nrf2 transcription factor causes a marked reduction in constitutive and inducible expression of the glutathione S-transferase Gsta1, Gsta2, Gstm1, Gstm2, Gstm3 and Gstm4 genes in the livers of male and female mice. Biochem J 2002; 365(Pt 2):405–416.

158. Chan K, Han XD, Kan YW. An important function of Nrf2 in combating oxidative stress: detoxification of acetaminophen. Proc Natl Acad Sci USA 2001; 98(8):4611–4616.
159. Thimmulappa RK, Mai KH, Srisuma S, Kensler TW, Yamamoto M, Biswal S. Identification of Nrf2-regulated genes induced by the chemopreventive agent sulforaphane by oligonucleotide microarray. Cancer Res 2002; 62(18):5196–5203.
160. Ramos-Gomez M, Kwak MK, Dolan PM, Itoh K, Yamamoto M, Talalay P, Kensler TW. Sensitivity to carcinogenesis is increased and chemoprotective efficacy of enzyme inducers is lost in nrf2 transcription factor-deficient mice. Proc Natl Acad Sci USA 2001; 13;98(6):3410–3415.
161. Gupta S. Molecular steps of death receptor and mitochondrial pathways of apoptosis. Life Sci 2001; 69(25–26):2564–2957.
162. Payne CM, Bernstein C, Bernstein H. Apoptosis overview emphasizing the role of oxidative stress, DNA damage and signal-transduction pathways. Leuk Lymphoma 1995; 19(1–2):43–93.
163. Musk SR, Johnson IT. Allyl isothiocyanate is selectively toxic to transformed cells of the human colorectal tumour line HT29. Carcinogenesis 1993; 14(10):2079–2083.
164. Musk SR, Stephenson P, Smith TK, Stening P, Fyfe D, Johnson IT. Selective toxicity of compounds naturally present in food toward the transformed phenotype of human colorectal cell line HT29. Nutr Cancer 1995; 24(3):289–298.
165. Musk SR, Smith TK, Johnson IT. On the cytotoxicity and genotoxicity of allyl and phenethyl isothiocyanates and their parent glucosinolates sinigrin and gluconasturtiin. Mutat Res 1995; 348(1):19–23.
166. Gamet-Payrastre L, Li P, Lumeau S, Cassar G, Dupont MA, Chevolleau S, Gasc N, Tulliez J, Terce F. Sulforaphane, a naturally occurring isothiocyanate, induces cell cycle arrest and apoptosis in HT29 human colon cancer cells. Cancer Res 2000; 60(5):1426–1433.
167. Yu R, Mandlekar S, Harvey KJ, Ucker DS, Kong AN. Chemopreventive isothiocyanates induce apoptosis and caspase-3-like protease activity. Cancer Res 1998; 58(3):402–408.
168. Xu K, Thornalley PJ. Studies on the mechanism of the inhibition of human leukaemia cell growth by dietary isothiocyanates and their cysteine adducts in vitro. Biochem Pharmacol 2000; 60(2):221–231.
169. Xu K, Thornalley PJ. Signal transduction activated by the cancer chemopreventive isothiocyanates: cleavage of BID protein, tyrosine phosphorylation and activation of JNK. Br J Cancer 2001; 84(5):670–673.
170. Chen YR, Han J, Kori R, Kong AN, Tan TH. Phenylethyl isothiocyanate induces apoptotic signaling via suppressing phosphatase activity against c-Jun N-terminal kinase. J Biol Chem 2002; 277:39334–39342.
171. Huang C, Ma WY, Li J, Hecht SS, Dong Z. Essential role of p53 in phenethyl isothiocyanate-induced apoptosis. Cancer Res 1998; 58(18):4102–4106.
172. Xiao D, Singh SV. Phenethyl isothiocyanate-induced apoptosis in p53-deficient

PC-3 human prostate cancer cell line is mediated by extracellular signal-regulated kinases. Cancer Res 2002; 62(13):3615–3619.

173. Nakamura Y, Kawakami M, Yoshihiro A, Miyoshi N, Ohigashi H, Kawai K, Osawa T, Uchida K. Involvement of the mitochondrial death pathway in chemopreventive benzyl isothiocyanate-induced apoptosis. J Biol Chem 2002; 277(10):8492–8499.

174. Smith TK, Lund EK, Johnson IT. Inhibition of dimethylhydrazine-induced aberrant crypt foci and induction of apoptosis in rat colon following oral administration of the glucosinolate sinigrin. Carcinogenesis 1998; 19(2):267–273.

175. Johnson IT. Anticarcinogenic effects of diet-related apoptosis in the colorectal mucosa. Food Chem Toxicol 2002; 40(8):1171–1178.

176. Yang YM, Conaway CC, Chiao JW, Wang CX, Amin S, Whysner J, Dai W, Reinhardt J, Chung FL. Inhibition of benzo(a)pyrene-induced lung tumorigenesis in A/J mice by dietary *N*-acetylcysteine conjugates of benzyl and phenethyl isothiocyanates during the postinitiation phase is associated with activation of mitogen-activated protein kinases and p53 activity and induction of apoptosis. Cancer Res 2002; 62(1):2–7.

18

Pharmacological and Chemopreventive Studies of Chrysanthemum

Ranxin Shi, Choon Nam Ong, and Han-Ming Shen
National University of Singapore
Singapore, Republic of Singapore

I. INTRODUCTION

A. *Chrysanthemum morifolium* Ramat

Different from its use as an attractive flower for horticulture purposes in Europe, chrysanthemum of the Compositae family, in particular its flower, has been used as a traditional medicine in several Asian countries, such as China, Korea, and Japan, for several centuries. The flower of *Chrysanthemum morifolium* Ramat, owing to its broad pharmacological effects as well as its fragrance, is also used as a beverage—chrysanthemum tea. This chapter will focus on both the broad and specific pharmacological activities of various components of chrysanthemum, and their potential health implications.

C. morifolium Ramat is widely distributed in most habitats of China as well as Korea and Japan. In China, it is cultivated mainly in Zhejiang province along the Yangzi River. Tong Xiang City of this province, also referred to as the "City of Chrysanthemum," produces about 4000–5000 tons of chrysanthemum flower each year, which accounts for more than 90% of the total chrysanthemum production in China. Although the components of chrysanthemum may vary slightly according to the different cultivation environments, the flowers are processed using a similar method. The plants are usually grown in early spring and the flowers harvested in autumn of each year. After steam treatment, the flowers are dried under the sun and then packed into an airtight plastic bag to prevent absorption of moisture. Recently, newer technology, such as microwave sterilization and drying, has been used to enhance the production process and improve quality.

B. Applications

Chrysanthemum tea is prepared in the same way as traditional tea. The dried flowers are infused with hot water for over 10 min, and the tea is ready to serve. For clinical usage, the chrysanthemum is boiled either alone or together with various other herbs, according to the prescription to suit a specific clinical purpose.

Based on traditional usage, in addition to use as a tea, *C. morifolium* Ramat is used for the common cold, fever, migraines, conjunctivitis, eye irritation, hypertension, ulcerative colitis, vertigo, ophthalmia with swelling and pain, etc. As a mixture with other herbs, it has been claimed to be able to relieve migraines and eye irritation, improve vision, and cure keratitis. The curing rates of ulcerative colitis and hypertension are reported to be more than 90% and 80%, respectively (1,2).

Apart from the above traditional usages, there were also reports of other usage, such as antitumor activities (3,4). Chrysanthemum water extract was found to significantly inhibit growth of transplanted tumor in nude mice (Shen et al., unpublished data), suggesting that the water-soluble components of chrysanthemum may have potent chemopreventive effects. Its chemopreventive properties will be elaborated below.

Although chrysanthemum is considered to be a "mild" herb and almost with no side effect in traditional medical practice, adverse effect has been reported with its flowers, and leaves may cause skin dermatitis (5,6). In contrast, there was no report that drinking chrysanthemum tea could cause respiratory or alimentary tract irritation.

C. General Pharmacological Studies

Volatile oil and flavonoids are believed to be the main active components in *C. morifolium* Ramat. Flavonoids, in the forms of glycoside derivatives, are more polar than volatile oil and hence are readily dissolved in water. This is partly the reason that most of the studies in chrysanthemum have been focused on its flavonoids.

1. Eye Irritation

Hot-water extract of chrysanthemum has been reported to show inhibitory activity against rat lens aldose reductase. Flavones and flavone glycosides were found to be the active components responsible for this observation, among which ellagic acid showed the highest inhibitory activity. Elevated concentration of sorbitol is responsible for eye irritation (7,8). Aldose reductase, along with coenzyme nicotinamide adenine dinucleotide phosphate (NADPH), catalyzes the reduction of glucose to sorbitol.

2. Ulcerative Colitis

Chrysanthemum water extract decreases the contents of two adherent glycoproteins, CD_{44} and CD_{62p}. These two glycoproteins are responsible for the adherence and communication between cells. Their elevated levels are believed to be closely related to those in ulcerative colitis (1).

3. Hypertension

The flavonoids of chrysanthemum have been shown to increase blood circulation in experimental animals, suggesting a potential role in reducing hypertension. Several fractions from the ethanol extract also showed significant anti-myocardial ischemia and antiarrhythmia activities in rats (2).

4. Antioxidant Activities

The antioxidant properties of flavonoids extracted from chrysanthemum could have been responsible for the broad pharmacological effects of chrysanthemum. It was found that water extract showed significant antioxidant activities in the linoleic acid system in vitro. The inhibitory rate against peroxidation of linoleic acid was much higher than that of antioxidant α-tocopherol. In the liposome model system, the extract showed significant inhibitory activity against peroxidation of lecithin, suggesting that the extract may reduce lipid peroxidation and play a role in protecting against damage to the cell membrane (9).

The water extract of chrysanthemum also showed significant direct inhibitory effects on various free radicals. The extract not only showed remarkable scavenging activities on 1, 1-diphenyl-2-picrylhydrazyl (DPPH), superoxide, and hydrogen peroxide but also on hydroxyl radical, which is believed to be the free radical reacting directly and rapidly with almost every type of molecule in living cells (10). Similar to other antioxidants, chrysanthemum extract has been shown to be an electron donor with strong reducing power. The significant correlation between phenolic compounds and antioxidant activity indicates that the polyphenolic compound may contribute directly to the antioxidant activity of the extract (10,11). It was demonstrated that flavonoids, a subgroup of phenolic compounds, were responsible for the antioxidant activity of the chrysanthemum extract, which can scavenge reactive oxygen radicals, such as hydroxyl radicals and superoxide radicals. The flavonoids can also be absorbed into the cell membrane and hence protect the cells from the damage of free oxygen radicals (12). The overall observations seem to indicate that the chemical-reducing property may contribute to the free-radical-scavenging activities of chrysanthemum extract.

II. CHEMOPREVENTIVE ACTIVITIES OF CHRYSANTHEMUM

Numerous studies in the literature have reported that various components of chrysanthemum showed chemopreventive potential. These components, however, are not exclusively found in the chrysanthemum family, and based on their chemical properties, they can be classified into three major groups, namely fatty acids, triterpenoids, and flavonoids.

A. Fatty Acids

Among the saturated and unsaturated fatty acids present in the chrysanthemum flower, linoleic acid, palmitic acid, and stearic acid are believed to have significant antioxidant activities. Stearic acid and palmitic acid also showed apoptosis-inducing potential, while linoleic acid can enhance the growth of tumor cells. Stearic acid suppresses granulosa cell survival by inducing apoptosis, as evidenced by DNA ladder formation and annexin V-EGFP/propidium iodide staining of the cells (13). Palmitic acid induces apoptosis in cardiomyocytes. The apoptosis is mediated through alterations in mitochondria through cytochrome c release and caspase 3 activation (14) Palmitic acid also induces apoptosis in Chinese hamster ovary cells through generation of reactive oxygen species and a ceramide-independent pathway (15).

Although it has been reported that linoleic acid showed anticancer effect on VX-2 tumor growing in the liver of rabbits (16), another study demonstrated that linoleic acid is a tumor promoter (17). Linoleic acid has a potent growth-promoting effect on several rodent tumors, human tumor xenografts grown in immunodeficient rodents, breast cancer cells, and rat hepatoma 7288CTC (18). Linoleic acid is metabolized to the mitogen 13-hydroxyoctadecadienoic acid and thus enhances tumor growth (19). On the other hand, reduced expression of nm-23-H1, a metastasis-suppressor gene, by linoleic acid may contribute at least partly to its tumor-growth-enhancing activity (20).

B. Triterpenoids

Triterpenoids are the main components of volatile oil in chrysanthemum flower and are believed to be the main effective pharmacological components in chrysanthemum (Fig. 1). Until now, more than 50 triterpenoids have been isolated and identified, among which taraxasterol, sitosterol, and lupeol show both anti-inflammatory and antitumor activity, while lupeol shows antioxidant activity. Stigmasterol and campesterol can inhibit tumor cell growth (discussed below). Five terpenes (helianol, heliantriol C, faradiol, dammaradienol, and cycloartenol) were found to have anti-inflammatory activity while heliantriol C, faradiol, and elemene show antitumor activity.

1. Anti-Inflammatory Activity

Eleven triterpene alcohols, isolated from chrysanthemum, were tested for their inhibitory effects on TPA-induced inflammation in the ears of mice. All 11 triterpene alcohols showed remarkable inhibitory effect with a 50% inhibitory dose at 0.1–0.8 mg per ear, which was roughly at the level of indomethacin, an anti-inflammatory drug used as positive control (21). Helianol, the most predominant component in the triterpene alcohol fraction, exhibited the strongest inhibitory effect (0.1 mg per ear) among the 11 compounds tested. Since anti-inflammatory activity of the inhibitors is highly related to their anti-cancer-promoting activities, helianol is also expected to be a potent antitumor agent (22). On the other hand, cycloartenol showed anti-inflammatory properties in the mouse carrageenan peritonitis test and also show weak inhibition of phospholipase A2 activity in vitro (23).

2. Antitumor Activity

Fifteen pentacylic triterpenes isolated from chrysanthemum were screened for their anti-tumor-promoting activities. All of the compounds showed inhibi-

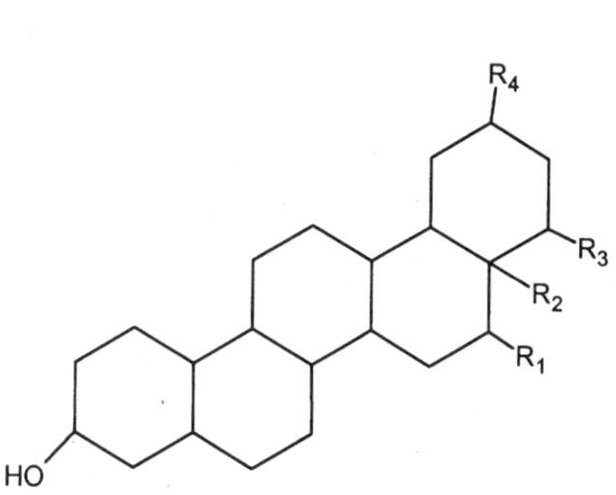

FIGURE 1 Basic structure of triterpenoids isolated from chrysanthemum.

tory effects against Epstein-Barr virus early antigen (EBV-EA) activation induced by the tumor promoter 12-*O*-tetradecanoylphorbol-13-acetate (TPA) in Raji cells (21), which have been demonstrated to closely parallel effects against tumor promotion in vivo. With 50% growth inhibitory (GI) value of less than 10 μM in sulforhodamine B protein assay, the compounds faradiol, heliantriol B_0, heliantriol, arnidiol, faradiol α-epoxide, and maniladiol showed significant inhibitory activity against almost all 60 human tumor cell lines derived from seven cancer types (lung, colon, melanoma, renal, ovarian, brain, and leukemia) (4). Arnidiol showed very significant cytotoxicity against HL-60 with a GI 50% at 0.4 μM.

β-Sitosterol, the most common plant sterol, showed cytotoxicity against cancer cell lines Colo-205, KB, HeLa, HA22T, Hep-2, GBM8401/TSGH, and H1477 (24), Vero cells (25), and colon 26-L5 carcinoma cells (26). As little as 16 μM sitosterol could induce apoptosis fourfold in LNCaP cells by increasing phosphatase 2A activity and activating the sphingomyelin cycle (27). Incorporation of sitosterol into cell membranes may alter fluidity and thus influence the activation of membrane-bound enzymes such as phosphalipase D (28).

β-Elemene has antitumor activity against HL-60 cells (29). β-Elemene exerts its cytotoxic effect on K562 leukemic cells by the induction of apoptosis, as evidence of the formation of apoptotic bodies and DNA ladder in a dose- and time-dependent manner. It has also been demonstrated that apoptosis in K562 cells induced by elemene is concomitant with decreasing expression of bcl-protein (30). Lupeol showed antitumor activity against lymphocytic leukemia P-388 cells (31). In contrast, stigmasterol inhibits growth of tumor cells Hep-2 and McCoy cells in vitro (32).

3. Antioxidant Activity

Cineol has antioxidant activity and inhibits lipoxygenase against ethanol injury in the rat (33). On the other hand, lupeol can prevent membrane peroxidation in red blood cells (34). This compound is also an effective skin chemopreventive agent that may suppress benzoyl-peroxide-induced cutaneous toxicity (35).

C. Flavonoids

Flavonoids are well-known natural antioxidant widely distributed in most edible plants. Flavonoids are believed to have putative beneficial effects due to their antioxidant activities. The evidence came from in vivo animal tests, in vitro cell culture tests, and a cohort epidemiological study. Numerous epidemiological studies show a clear correlation between fruit and vegetable consumption and lower risk of cancer of the gastrointestinal tract (36). A cohort study in Finland also supported that flavonoid intake in some circumstances may be involved in slowing the cancer process, resulting in lowered risk (37). Several studies suggested an inverse correlation with stroke and cardiovascular disease, while no relationship between flavonol intake and reduced risk of cancers was found (36).

Flavonoids are ubiquitous secondary plant metabolites with a common C6-C3-C6 structure (Fig. 2). They exist more often in the form of glycoside derivatives but less often in the aglycone form. Eleven flavonoids and flavonoid glycosides have been identified in chrysanthemum since the first report in 1974. All of them are also widely distributed in other plants, for example green tea, red wine, vegetables, and fruits. Nearly all flavonoids (luteolin, diosmetin, chrysin, apigenin, quecertin, and their glycosides) that could be isolated from chrysanthemum showed antioxidant activity and antimutagenic activity or inhibited tumor cell proliferation. Luteolin, chrysin, quecertin, and apigenin were proved to induce apoptosis and cell cycle arrest at G1 phase or G2/M or both. Flavonoids may block several points in the process of tumor promotion, including inhibiting kinases, reducing transcription factors, and regulating cell cycle (38).

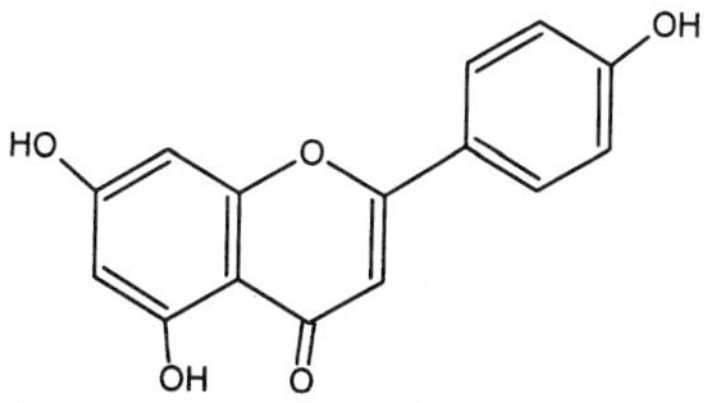

Apigenin

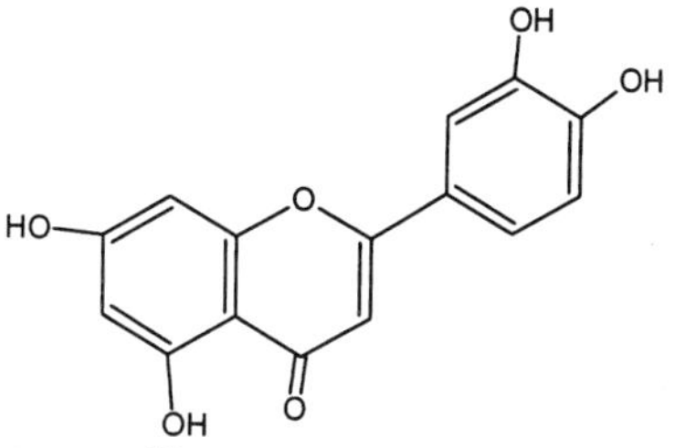

Luteolin

FIGURE 2 Structures of apigenin and luteolin, two major flavonoids in chrysanthemum. Apigenin and luteolin are two major flavonoids isolated from chrysanthemum. Both have the typical basic C6-C3-C6 structure with different hydroxyl substitution at different positions.

1. Antioxidant Activity

Reactive oxygen species (ROS), which are constantly produced mainly in mitochondria of cells, are believed to be potent harmful agents in the cells. An elevated level of ROS is damaging to the cells because ROS can readily react with many molecules, such as DNA, proteins, and phospholipids, and hence resulted in dysfunctions of these important molecules, resulting in many diseases. Therefore, it was speculated that antioxidants would be beneficial in reducing the damaging ROS. Further research on functions of ROS proved that ROS are inevitable in our cells and ROS, as second messengers, are necessary and important factors in mediating normal cell signaling. So the effects of antioxidants are probably related to their other effects, such as cytotoxicity, inducing cell cycle arrest, and inducing apoptosis.

Flavonoids have antioxidant activity in many cell-free systems. Luteolin, one of the major flavonoids of *C. morifolium* Ramat (39), inhibits lipoxygenase activity, cyclooxygenase activity, and inhibition of ascorbic-acid-stimulated malonaldehyde formation in liver lipids (40). Both luteolin and apigenin can inhibit CCl_4-induced peroxidation of rat liver microsomes (41). Further reports demonstrated that luteolin and apigenin showed remarkable antiperoxidative activity against lipid peroxidation induced in liver cell membranes by either nonenzymic or enzymic method (42). Both luteolin and apigenin also inhibit DNA damage induced by hydrogen peroxide or singlet molecular oxygen in human cells (43,44). The glycosylated form of luteolin, luteolin-7-O-glucoside, demonstrated a dose-dependent reduction of LDL oxidation with less effectiveness than luteolin. Studies of the copper-chelating properties of luteolin-7-O-glucoside and luteolin suggest that both act as hydrogen donors and metal ion chelators (45). Apigenin also inhibits xanthine oxidase and monoamine oxidase, two potent ROS-producing enzymes (46).

Oxidative stress is pivotal in many pathological processes and reduced oxidative stress is believed to prevent many diseases. Glutathione (GSH) is an important antioxidant in all cell types. Its main function is to maintain the intracellular redox balance and to eliminate xenobiotica and ROS. As well-known antioxidants, luteolin and apigenin are speculated to decrease the oxidative stress in the cells. However, the effect of luteolin and apigenin in regulating the redox balance in the cell is equivocal. In a cell-free system, apigenin can oxidize GSH to GSSH via a thiyl radical when incubated with H_2O_2 and horseradish peroxidase (HRP). Luteolin can also deplete GSH but without forming a thiyl radical or GSSG. Luteolin forms mono-GSH or bis-GSH conjugates while apigenin does not form GSH conjugates. On the contrary, quercetin increased the transcription of γ-glutamylcysteine synthetase (GCS) in COS-1 cells. The two-step synthesis of GSH is catalyzed by

GCS and glutathione synthetase. These inconsistent results suggested that the effects of flavonoids on ROS balance are far more complex than defining them as antioxidant or prooxidant agents.

2. Anti-Inflammatory Activity

Apigenin and luteolin inhibit interleukin (IL)-5, which promotes the growth and survival of eosinophils and plays an important role in eosinophilia-associated allergic inflammation (47). These two flavonoids also inhibit nitric oxide (NO) production in lipopolysaccharide (LPS)-activated RAW 264.7 cells by reducing inducible nitric oxide synthase (iNOS) expression but not inhibiting iNOS enzyme activity. NO produced by iNOS is one of the inflammatory mediators (48).

3. Antimutagenic Activity

Mutagenesis is usually the first step of several stages involved in carcinogenesis, which is a long-term, multistage process that results from accumulation of mutation and dysfunction of important molecules regulating cell proliferation. During the initiation stage, a potential carcinogen is transformed into a mutagen product by Phase I enzyme such as cytochrome P450. The mutagen product may react with cellular molecules including DNA and result in genetic mutation. The mutagen product may be detoxified by Phase II enzymes, which transform the mutagen into a form easily eliminated from the body. During the promotion stage, overgeneration of ROS resulting from overexpression of pro-oxidant enzymes will lead to accumulation of DNA mutations. Cell-proliferation-related functions are elevated to a high degree; for example, DNA synthesis is increased by overexpression or activation of DNA polymerase or topoisomerase. Cell proliferation is finally increased by changes in cell-proliferation-regulating pathways such as protein kinase C and A, mitogen-activated protein kinases (MAPK), and cyclin-dependent kinases (CDK). During the final stage, the mutations are fixed and the cells are proliferating uncontrollably (49).

Flavonoids of chrysanthemum have been demonstrated to inhibit mutagenesis and carcinogenesis by targeting various molecules at different stages. The induction of cell cycle arrest and apoptosis and interaction of several pathways will be reviewed below.

Luteolin suppresses formation of mutagenic and carcinogenic heterocyclic amines, such as 2-amino-3,8-dimethylimidazo(4,5-f) quinoxaline and 2-amino-1-methyl-6-phenylimidazo(4,5-b) pyridine (50). Luteolin also inhibits the mutagenic activity resulting from metabolic activation of benzo-pyrene and trans-7,8-dihydroxy-7,8-dihydrobenzo-pyrene by rat liver microsomes (51). Luteolin showed significant inhibitory effect on tumor expression of fibrosarcoma induced by 20-methylcholanthrene in male Swiss albino mice (52). On the other hand, apigenin is a potent inhibitor of epidermal ornithine decarboxylase inducted by TPA in a dose-dependent manner (53).

A carbonyl group at C-4 of the flavone nucleus seems to be essential for the antimutagenicity. Increasing polarity by introduction of hydroxyl groups reduced antimutagenic potency. Reducing polarity of hydroxyl flavonoids by methyl etherification, however, increased antimutagenic potency again. Of the 11 flavonoid glycosides all compounds showed antimutagenic activity except that apigenin and luteolin-7-glucoside are inactive or only weakly antimutagenic (54).

4. Estrogenic and Antiestrogenic Activity

Estrogens are involved in the proliferation and differentiation of target cells and are among the main risk factors for breast and uterine cancer (55). Antiestrogens, which inhibit estrogen action by competing for its receptors, have been used as therapy against breast cancer and have been proposed to prevent cancers.

Many flavonoids, including luteolin and apigenin, were found to have very weak estrogenic activity, 10^3–10^5-fold less than 17-β-estradial, through binding to estrogen receptor (ER) (56,57). They also show antiestrogenic activity, which is closely related to their antiproliferation activity. Luteolin, as well as other flavonoids such as daidzein, genistein, and quercetin, is able to inhibit the proliferation-stimulating activity in MCF-7 cells caused by 1 μM environmental estrogens such as diethylstilbestrol, clopmiphene, bisphenol, etc. (58,59). The suppressive effect of flavonoids suggests that these compounds have antiestrogenic and anticancer activities. Wang and Kurzer also found that 10 μM luteolin or apigenin inhibited estradiol-induced DNA synthesis (60). In an in vivo test, Holland and Roy proved that luteolin inhibited estrogen-stimulated proliferation in mammary epithelial cells of female Noble rats, which suggests it may play a protective role in estrogen-induced mammary carcinogenesis (61).

The concentration of flavonoids determines their effects on cell growth. At 0.1–10 μM, luteolin induces DNA synthesis in estrogen-depedent (MCF-7) breast cancer cells but not in estrogen-independent (MDA-MB-231) human breast cancer cells; however, at 20–90 μM, luteolin inhibits DNA synthesis in both types of cells. This suggests that additional mechanisms may be involved in the effect of high concentrations of flavonoids (60).

It is, however, important to point out that the antiestrogenicity of flavonoids does not correlate with their estrogen receptor (ER)-binding capacity, suggesting alternative signaling mechanisms may be involved in their antagonistic effects (62). Mammalian cells contain two classes of estradiol-binding sites, type I (Kd ~1.0 nM) and type II (Kd ~20 nM), designed according to their affinity (63). Luteolin competes for estradiol binding to cytosol and nuclear type II sites in rat uterine preparations but it does not interact with the rat uterine estrogen receptor (64). In an in vivo study, injection of luteolin blocked estradiol stimulation of nuclear type II sites in the immature rat uterus and this correlated with an inhibition of uterine growth. Further studies showed that luteolin could bind to nuclear type II sites irreversibly owing to covalent attachment (65). These studies suggest luteolin, through an interaction with type II sites, may be involved in cell growth regulation.

A lot of evidence demonstrated cross-talk between the estrogen pathway and the insulin-like growth factor (IGF) pathway. The IGFs can activate the ER, while the ER transcriptionally regulates genes required for IGF action. Moreover, blockade of ER function can inhibit IGF-mediated mitogenesis and interruption of IGF action can similarly inhibit estrogenic stimulation of breast cancer cells (66,67).

Apigenin, as well as chalcone and flavone, stimulates transcription factor activator protein-1 activity (AP-1). They also activate Elk-1, c-Jun, or C/EBP homologous protein (CHOP), the downstream targets of various MAPK pathways, suggesting flavonoids may affect multiple signaling pathways that converge at the level of transcriptional regulation (68).

5. Antiangiogenesis

Angiogenesis, the generation of new capillaries, occurs during many physiological processes, including development, wound healing, and formation of the corpus luteum, endometrium, and placenta (69). Angiogenesis also occurs in some pathological processes, such as solid tumor growth and metastasis, which require nutrition and oxygen owing to the fact that avascular tumors do not grow beyond a diameter of 1–2 mm (70). In response to secretion of angiogenic stimuli, such as vascular endothelial growth factor (VEGF) and matrix metalloproteases (MMP), which degrade the extracellular matrix, the endothelial cell basal membrane is degraded by the action of protease and then the endothelial cells migrate and proliferate and finally organize into capillary tubes. Several important enzymes are involved in the process. (1) VEGF is one of the most potent and specific known angiogenic factors in vivo. It increases microvascular permeability in response to hypoxia, multiple growth factors, cytokines, and estradiol (70). (2) Hyaluronic acid (HA) is one of the most abundant constituents of the extracellular matrix and acts as a barrier to neovascularization (71). Fragments of HA, as a result of catalytic activity of hyaluronidase, bind to CD44 receptor exposed on the membrane of endothelial cells and then are responsible for endothelial cell proliferation, migration, and finally angiogenesis. (3) Matrix metalloproteases (MMP) also promotes angiogenesis by degrading the extracellular matrix.

Both apigenin and luteolin inhibit the proliferation of normal and tumor cells as well as in vitro angiogenesis (72). Luteolin, on the other hand, significantly inhibits corneal neovascularization induced by basic fibroblast growth factor (bFGF), and is a potent inhibitor of corneal angiogenesis in vivo (73).

Flavonoids, including luteolin and apigenin, are competitive inhibitors of hyaluronidase (74). As inhibitor of hyaluronidase, apigenin inhibits the proliferation and the migration of endothelial cells and capillary formation in vitro. In contrast, it stimulates vascular smooth-muscle-cell proliferation. Apigenin inhibits endothelial-cell proliferation by blocking the cells in the G2/M phase. Apigenin stimulation of smooth-muscle cells is attributed to the reduced expression of two cyclin-dependent kinase inhibitors, p21 and p27, which negatively regulate the G1-phase cyclin-dependent kinase (75).

6. Antiproliferation

Many flavonoids, including luteolin and apigenin, were found to inhibit proliferation of several normal cells and cancer cells derived from nearly all tissues, such as human fibroblast HFK2, human keratinocytes HaCaT, human breast cancer MCF-7, human neuroblastoma cell SHEP and WAC2 (59,72), Raji lymphoma cell (76), pancreatic cancer cell MiaPaCa-2 (77), human leukemia HL-60 (78), hepatic stellate cells (79), human thyroid carcinoma cell lines (80), human melanoma cells OCM-1 (81), human epidermoid carcinoma A431 (82), and human prostatic tumor cells (83). Apigenin also has an antiproliferation effect in mouse erythroleukemia cells (84), B104 rat neuronal cells (85), and rat aortic vascular smooth-muscle cells (86). This exhaustive list suggests that flavonoids play an essential role in antiproliferation of numerous cancer cells.

Luteolin, as well as quercetin, kaempferol, genistein, apigenin, and myricetin, suppresses the proliferation of human prostatic tumor cells (PC-3), androgen-independent cells, indicating that flavonoids show their antiproliferation activity in an androgen-independent manner (83).

The antiproliferation effect of flavonoids may be related to their estrogenic and/or antiestrogenic activity. Luteolin exhibits cell-proliferation-inhibiting activity and is able to inhibit the proliferation-stimulating activity in MCF-7 cells caused by environmental estrogens (58,59). Both apigenin and luteolin inhibit proliferation of several human thyroid carcinoma cell lines, UCLA NPA-87-1 (with estrogen receptor ER), UCLA RO-82W-1 (with anti-estrogen-binding site AEBS), and UCLA RO-81A-1 (lacking both the AEBS and the ER), suggesting that the inhibitory activity of flavonoids may be mediated via the antiestrogen binding site (AEBS and/or type II estrogen receptor, EBS), but other mechanisms of action are involved as well (80).

Further studies showed that the inhibitory effect of apigenin on UCLA RO-81-A-1 cell proliferation is associated with an inhibition of epidermal growth factor receptor (EGFR) tyrosine autophosphorylation, phosphorylation of its downstream effector mitogen-activated protein (MAP) kinase, and phosphorylated c-Myc, a nuclear substrate for MAPK. However, protein levels of these signaling molecules were not affected (Fig. 3) (87).

The EGFR or MAPK inhibition effect of flavonoids in several other cell lines indicates that flavonoids may inhibit cell proliferation through a rather general mechanism, inhibiting activity of crucial enzymes involved in cell signaling prone to cell proliferation. The antiproliferation activity of luteolin (20 μM) in pancreatic cancer cell MiaPaCa-2 is closely related to the decreases

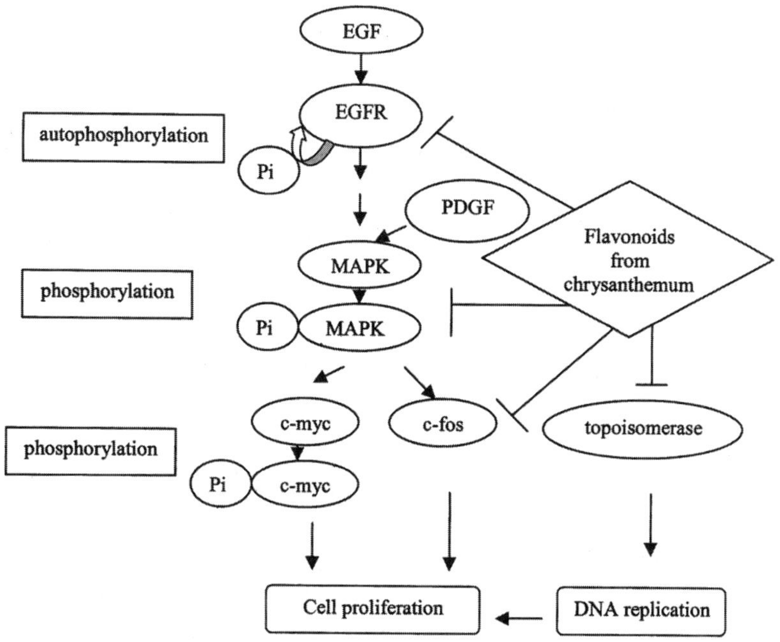

FIGURE 3 Mechanisms that could have been involved in the antiproliferation effect by flavonoids of chrysanthemum, in particular luteolin and apigenin. Growth factors, such as EGF and PDGF, promote cell proliferation through the MAP kinase pathway, in which phosphorylation and dephosphorylation of enzymes play a role in regulating activity of important molecules in cell signaling and cell proliferation. Flavonoids may inhibit cell proliferation through inhibiting EGFR autophosphorylation, phosphorylation of MAP kinase, and its nuclear substrate c-myc. As inhibitors of topoisomerase, flavonoids may show their antiproliferation activity by suppresing DNA replication.

in cellular protein phosphorylation by effectively modulating protein tyrosine kinase (PTK) activities, including that of EGFR, but not modifying the protein synthesis (88). The same group found that luteolin inhibits proliferation of human epidermoid carcinoma A431 by a similar mechanism (82). Apigenin was found to inhibit fetal bovine serum (FBS)- and platelet-derived growth factor PDGF-induced rat aortic vascular smooth muscle cell proliferation. The activity may be mediated, at least in part, by downregulation of extracellular-signal-regulated kinase ERK 1/2 and its downstream c-fos mRNA (86).

The antiproliferation effect of flavonoids is concomitant with cell cycle arrest or apoptosis in specific cell lines. For example, luteolin inhibits the proliferation of human leukemia HL-60 at 15 μM and is concomitant with apoptosis-inducing effect (78). Both apigenin and luteolin inhibit proliferation of human melanoma cells OCM-1 (89). The inhibition is mediated by arresting the cell at phase G1 or G2/M. More details about cell-cycle-arrest- or apoptosis-inducing effects of flavonoids will be elaborated below. As inhibitor of topoisomerase I and II, flavonoids may also suppress cell proliferation by inhibiting DNA synthesis (see below).

Although it seems that flavonoids inhibit proliferation of many cell lines, the antiproliferation activity is cell-type-specific as well as flavonoid-structure-specific; for example, neither apigenin nor luteolin shows significant growth-inhibitory activity in B16 melanoma 4A5 cells (81).

7. Induction of Cell Cycle Arrest

Cell cycle progression is timely regulated by cyclin-dependent kinases (CDKs) and their cyclin subunits. G1 progression and G1/S transition are regulated by CDK4-cyclin D, CDK6-cyclin D, and later CDK2-cyclin E, while CDK2 controls S-phase when associated with cyclin A and G2/M transition is regulated by CDK1 in combination with cyclins A and B (90).

Activation of CDKs is regulated by cyclin synthesis and degradation, phosphorylations and dephosphorylations on specific residues, CDK inhibitor (CKIs) synthesis, and degradation. For example, dephosphorylation of CDK1 on Thr14 and Tyr15 residues by the phosphatase CDC25C is required for the activation of CDK1. Two families of mammalian CKIs have been identified: the INK4 family, comprising p16INK4a, p15INK4b, p18INK4c, and p18INK4d, which specifically inhibit CDK4 and CDK6, and the CIP/KIP family, including p21cip1/waf1, p27kip1, and p57kip2, which have a broad range of inhibition (Fig. 4).

Recently, cell cycle checkpoints have been the targets for chemotherapeutic and chemopreventive agents. Inhibition of the cell cycle at two major checkpoints, G1 and G2/M, may be important in the antitumor activities of the flavonoids (91,92). A large number of epidemiological studies as well as

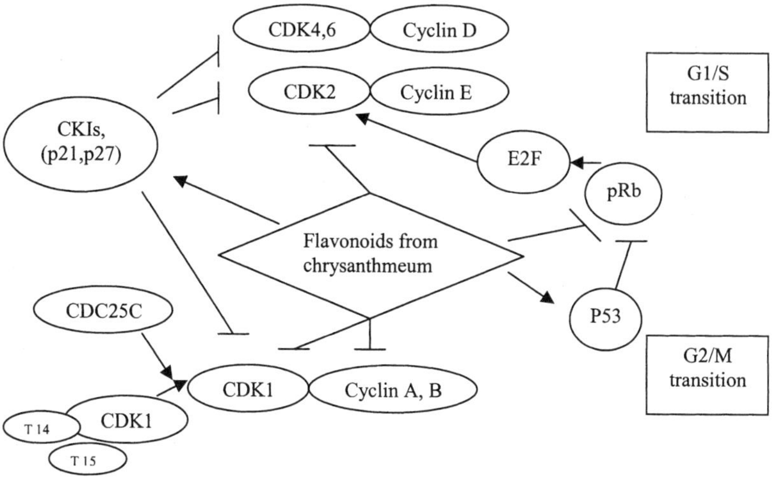

FIGURE 4 Pathways involved in the cell-cycle-arresting effect of flavonoids. Cell cycle progress is regulated directly by CDKs and cyclins, activation of which is regulated by CKIs, cdc25c, pBR, p53, etc. Flavonoids of chrysanthemum may arrest the cell cycle at G1/S transition by increasing CKIs, decreasing CDK2, or pRb activation. They also induce G2/M arrest by decreasing the protein level of CDK1 and cyclin A and B.

experiments on animal models suggest that flavonoids can prevent or inhibit cancer development. In several in vitro experiments, flavonoids have been found to inhibit the proliferation of many cancer cells by arresting cell cycle progression at either G1 or G2/M phase. The site of checkpoint arrest with a specific flavonoid can vary with cell type although apigenin and luteolin are very similar in structure.

G1 Arrest. Luteolin arrests the cell cycle at G1 phase in human gastric cancer HGC-27 cells, human melanoma cells OCM-1 (89), and human prostate cancer cells LNCaP (93). G1 cell cycle arrest induced by luteolin on OCM-1 is mediated by inhibiting the activity of CDK2 but not CDK1. Upregulation of the CDK inhibitors p27/kip1 and p21/waf1 is responsible for the inhibition of activity of CDK2 (89).

Only two cell lines, human diploid fibroblast and LNCaP, were found to be arrested at G1 phase by apigenin, while it could arrest more than 10 cell lines at G2/M phase. Apigenin induced G1 arrest on these two cell lines by inhibiting cdk2 kinase activity too (94,95). As for LNCaP cells, apigenin decreases the protein expression of cyclin D1, D2, and E and their activating partner cdk2, 4, and 6 with concomitant induction of CDK inhibitor p21/

waf1 and p27/kip1. The induction of p21/waf1 appears to be transcriptionally upregulated and is tumor-suppressor-gene-p53-dependent. In addition, apigenin inhibited the hyperphosphorylation of the pRb protein in these cells (95).

G2/M Arrest. Since the first report that apigenin inhibited the proliferation of malignant tumor cells by G2-M arrest in 1994 (85), apigenin has been found to induce G2/M arrest in 16 cell lines, including human prostate cancer cells LNCaP, human melanoma cells OCM-1, human leukemia HL-60, human colorectal cancer cells SW480, HT-29, and Caco-2, human breast cancer MCF7 and MDA-MB-468, rat hepatoma 5L and BP8, rat neuronal cells B104 (85), human prostate adenocarcinoma CA-HPV-10 (96), human endothelial cells, mouse skin cell line C50 and 308, and mouse keratinocytes (97).

G2/M arrest on most cells induced by apigenin is concomitant with change in CDK kinase activity or kinase protein level. Apigenin inhibits colon carcinoma cell SW480, HT-29, and Caco-2, mouse-skin-derived cell lines C50 and 308, and human leukemia HL-60 cell growth by inducing G2/M arrest with inhibited activity of cdc2 kinase and reduced accumulation of cyclin B1 proteins in a dose-dependent manner (97,98). Cdc2 protein level was reduced by apigenin in three colon cells while apigenin treatment did not change the steady-state level of cdc2 protein in C50, 308, and HL-60 cell lines.

Similarly, G2/M arrest in mouse keratinocytes induced by apigenin was accompanied by inhibition of both cdc2 kinase protein level and activity in a p21/waf1-independent manner (99). In contrast, apigenin arrested LNCaP prostate cancer cells at the G2/M phase by increasing p21 levels through a p53-dependent pathway (93).

Cyclin B1 and CDK1 protein levels decreased significantly in G2/M arrest on breast carcinoma cells MCF-7 and MDA-MB-468 after apigenin treatment. Apigenin reduced the protein levels of CDK4 and cyclins D1 and A, but did not affect cyclin E, CDK2, or CDK6 protein expression. Apigenin markedly reduced Rb phosphorylation in MCF-7 cells while inhibiting ERK MAP kinase phosphorylation and activation in MDA-MB-468 cells (100). On the contrary, accumulation of the hyperphosphorylated form of the retinoblastoma protein results in G2/M arrest in endothelial cell after apigenin treatment (75).

Apigenin induces G2 arrest on human melanoma cells OCM-1 by inhibiting CDK1 by 50–70% owing to the phosphorylation of the kinase on Tyr15 residue (89). Aryl hydrocarbon receptor (AHR) is believed to be a possible receptor of flavonoid in the cells. Apigenin arrests both AHR-containing rat hepatoma 5L and AHR-deficient cell line BP8 primarily in G2/M, which indicates that the cytostatic activities of apigenin do not require the AHR (101).

Only two prostate cell lines, LNCaP and PC-3, have been shown to be arrested by luteolin at the G2/M phase. Furthermore, it has been shown that luteolin can induce p21/waf1 production in a p53-independent manner (93).

8. Induction of Apoptosis

Apoptosis is a tightly regulated cell death characterized by specific morphological and biochemical changes including cell shrinkage, nuclear fragmentation, chromatin condensation, membrane blebbing, and formation of apoptotic bodies. Mitochondria are the pivotal mediator of apoptosis, which, like a big "funnel," accumulate cell death signals from both ligand-receptor interaction and stresses and then release the molecules leading to cell death such as cytochrome C, Apaf-1, procaspase-9, Smac, and apoptosis-inducing factors (AIFs). Cytochrome C with Apaf-1 and procaspase-9 trigger a caspase cascade that results in morphological and biochemical changes. The activation of mitochondria is tightly regulated by bcl-2 family proteins; for example, Bid, Bad, and Bax can induce mitochondria to release cytochrome C while Bcl-2 prevents the induction (Fig. 5). On the other hand, NF-κB is an important transcriptional factor that prevents cell death. The translocation and activation of NF-κB is regulated by the inhibitor of NF-κB (IκB).

Apoptosis is crucial for development, organ morphogenesis, tissue homeostasis, and removal of infected or damaged cells. The accumulation of damaged cells in the tissue resulting from lack of proper apoptosis is believed to lead to the generation of tumor. Many molecules involved in the apoptosis pathway, such as NF-κB, IκB, and p53, are good targets to find new chemopreventive or chemotherapic compounds. Luteolin and apigenin can induce apoptosis in both cancer cell lines and nontumor cell lines, including human epidermoid carcinoma A431, human leukemia HL-60, human prostate carcinoma LNCaP, MiaPaCa-2, normal human prostate epithelial cells, and nontumor cell line C3H10T1/2CL8 (96). Extensive research has been carried out on the apoptosis-inducing activity of apigenin and luteolin in HL-60 and LNCaP cells.

By forming a luteolin-topoII-DNA ternary complex, luteolin induces apoptosis in HL-60 cells with no increase in 8-oxodG formation but with inhibited topoisomerase II (topo II) activity and cleaved DNA (102). Apigenin can also induce HL-60 apoptosis through a rapid induction of caspase-3 activity and stimulated proteolytic cleavage of poly-(ADP-ribose) polymerase (PARP). Apigenin induced loss of mitochondrial transmembrane potential, elevation of ROS production, release of mitochondrial cytochrome c into the cytosol, and subsequent induction of procaspase-9 processing (103).

Apigenin treatment also resulted in apoptosis in human prostate carcinoma LNCaP cells as determined by DNA fragmentation, PARP cleavage, fluorescence microscopy, and flow cytometry. These effects were

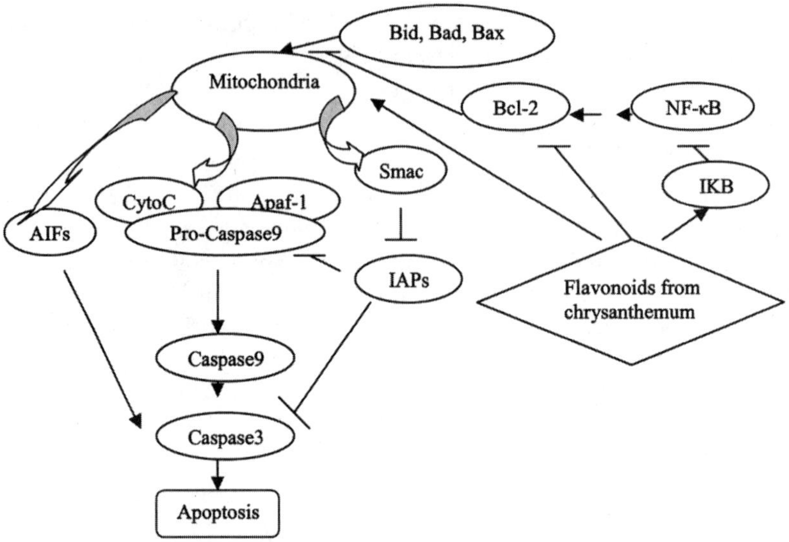

FIGURE 5 Apoptosis-inducing pathway induced by flavonoids of chrysanthemum. Cytochrome C, Apaf-1, and pro-caspase-9, released from mitochondria in response to apoptosis activators, will activate caspase-9 and then caspase-3 and finally induce apoptosis. Smac, also released from mitochondria, promotes apoptosis by inhibiting the suppressing effect of inhibitor of apoptosis proteins (IAPs). Apoptosis-inducing factors (AIFs) can induce activation of caspase-3 directly, which is believed to be the executor caspase to apoptosis. Bid, Bad, and Bax trigger the mitochondria change, which is prevented by bcl-2 protein. Flavonoids from chrysanthemum may induce apoptosis by inhibiting IκB degradation, decreasing bcl-2 protein, and triggering release of several molecules from mitochondria.

found to correlate with a shift in Bax/Bcl-2 ratio more toward apoptosis. Apigenin treatment also resulted in downmodulation of the constitutive expression of NF-kappaB/p65 (95).

The antiproliferative effect of luteolin might result from the modulation of the EGF-mediated signaling pathway. Blockade of the EGFR-signaling pathway by the protein tyrosine kinase (PTK) inhibitor luteolin significantly inhibits the growth of MiaPaCa-2 cells and induces apoptosis (88).

Treatment of WEHI 231 cells with apigenin decreased the rate of IκB turnover and nuclear levels of NF-κB (104). Apigenin blocked the LPS-induced activation of nuclear factor-κB (NF-κB) through the prevention of inhibitor κB (IκB) degradation and IκB kinase activity. This suggests that apigenin may be important in the prevention of carcinogenesis and inflammation (105).

Apigenin and luteolin also induced p53 accumulation and apoptosis in nontumor cell line C3H10T1/2CL8. The apoptosis apparently occurs in the p53-dependent G2/M phase of the cell (106).

9. Inhibition of Kinases Involved in MAPK Pathway

MAP kinase signal transduction is a typical and vital mediator of a number of cellular activities, including cell growth, proliferation, and survival. There are three major MAP kinases, extracellular signal-regulated kinases (ERKs), c-jun NH2-terminal protein kinase (JNK), and p38. Each MAP is a member of a three-protein kinase cascade including MAPKKKs, MAPKKs, and MAPK. The most extensively studied MAP kinase pathway is the Raf-MEK-ERK cascade. ERKs pathway is activated in response to the stimuli from growth factors such as insulin-like growth factor-1 (IGF-1), platelet-derived growth factor (PDGF), and epidermal growth factor (EGF) (88). Ligand-receptor interaction triggers the dimerization and activation of receptor tyrosine kinases (RTKs) due to autophosphorylation. The activated RTKs activate the Raf-MEK-ERK pathway via the protein kinase C (PKC) or phosphatidylinositol-3-kinase (PI3K) pathway (107). Once ERKs are activated, ERKs can phosphorylate and activate transcription factors, which will have an effect on the cell growth or proliferation. JNKs are activated by two MAPK kinases, MKK4 and MKK7, in response to stimuli such as inflammatory cytokines (TNF, IL-1beta), ultraviolet light, ROS, and heat shock. The activated JNKs will phosphorylate c-jun, which is an important transcription factor in effecting cell growth, inflammation, apoptosis, or differentiation. p38 is activated by MKK3 and MKK6 in response to stimuli similar to those that trigger JNKs. Chemopreventive or chemotherapeutic agents are targeted on various points along the MAPK pathway, such as inhibition of ligand-receptor interaction, inhibition of activity of receptor tyrosine kinase, PI3K, and PKC, which are also the inhibitory targets of apigenin and luteolin (108–111).

Tyrosine Protein Kinases and MAP Kinase. Apigenin and luteolin are effective inhibitors of the proliferation of certain human thyroid cancer cell lines. The dose-dependent inhibitory effect of apigenin on a human anaplastic thyroid carcinoma cell line proliferation is associated with an inhibition of both EGFR tyrosine autophosphorylation and phosphorylation of its downstream effector MAP kinase (80). Apigenin is also a proposed inhibitor of the mitogen-activated protein kinase (MAPK) pathway by inhibiting MAP kinase directly (112,113).

Luteolin inhibits the growth and reduces the cellular protein phosphorylation level by effectively inhibiting epidermal growth factor receptor (EGFR) tyrosine kinase activity of MiaPaCa-2 cancer cells. The inhibition of EGFR activity may partly contribute to the apoptosis in MianPaCa-2 cells

(77). Pretreatment of the cells with luteolin attenuates LPS-induced tyrosine phosphorylation of cellular proteins and then abolishes the decreasing effects of LPS on IκB-alpha in murine macrophages (114).

Apigenin suppresses 12-O-tetradecanoyl-phorbol-13-acetate (TPA)-mediated growth of NIH 3T3 cells by inhibiting activity of fibroblast growth factor (FGF) receptor and reducing the level of phosphorylation of cellular proteins (115). Apigenin can also reduce the level of TPA-stimulated phosphorylation of cellular proteins and inhibited TPA-induced c-jun and c-fos expression in mouse skin (111).

Protein Kinase C and Phosphoinositide 3-Kinases. Protein kinase C is a family of serine-threonine protein kinases that are involved in signal transduction pathways that regulate growth factor response, proliferation, differentiation, apoptosis, etc. The C-terminal catalytic domain contains several reactive cysteines that are targets for various chemopreventive agents. Modification of these cysteines decreases cellular PKC activity.

PKC is inhibited in a concentration-dependent manner by many flavonoids, including luteolin and apigenin (110,111). Further study showed that luteolin is a potent inhibitor of human mast cell activation through the inhibition of Ca^{2+} influx and PKC activation (116). On the other hand, apigenin inhibits PKC by competing with adenosine triphosphate (ATP). This may be an additional mechanism by which apigenin inhibits or prevents tumorigenesis.

Both luteolin and apigenin are also effective inhibitors of phosphoinositide 3-kinase PI3K, an enzyme recently shown to play an important role in signal transduction and cell transformation (109).

A. Inhibition of Other Enzymes

Topoisomerase. DNA topoisomerases are essential enzymes that catalyze the interconversion of topological isomers of DNA molecules. Acting by sequential breakage and reunion strands of DNA, two topoisomerases (topoisomerase I and topoisomerase II) are involved in many vital cellular processes, such as DNA replication, transcription, recombination, integration, and chromosomal segregation. Many anticancer agents were designed as inhibitors of these two enzymes. The DNA damage resulting from dysfunction of the vital enzymes may induce cell cycle arrest or apoptosis. Several flavonoids have been shown to exert their action by interacting with DNA topoisomerases and promoting site-specific DNA cleavage (117). Luteolin inhibits topoisomerase II activity of HL-60 cells by forming a luteolin-topo II-DNA ternary complex and then induces apoptosis in the cells (102).

By inhibiting DNA synthesis and promoting topoisomerase-II-mediated cleavage of kinetoplast DNA minicircles, luteolin inhibits the growth of

Leishmania donovani promastigotes and arrests cell cycle progression in *L. donovani* promastigotes, leading to apoptosis in vitro (118). Apigenin was found to inhibit activity of topoisomerase II and induced death of IL-2-dependent CTLL-2 cells with DNA fragmentation (119).

Other than inducing topoisomerase II–mediated apoptosis, luteolin strongly inhibits the catalytic activity of eukaryotic DNA topoisomerase I with an IC_{50} of 5 μM. Although luteolin not only intercalates directly with the enzyme but also intercalates with substrate DNA at very high concentration, the compound does not prevent the assembly of enzyme-DNA complex but stabilizes the topoisomerase-DNA covalent complex and blocks the subsequent rejoining of the DNA break (120). Apigenin inhibits topoisomerase I–catalyzed DNA relegation in a similar way as luteolin. It does not act directly on the catalytic intermediate and also does not interfere with DNA cleavage. However, formation of a ternary complex with topoisomerase I and DNA during the cleavage reaction inhibits the following DNA religation step (121).

Matrix Metalloproteinase (MMP). MMPs play a critical role in tumor cell invasion and metastasis. Luteolin suppresses the secretion of two MMPs, MMP2 and MMP9, in A431 cells (82). Apigenin also significantly reduces expression of MMP9 in SKBR-3 cells. The inhibition of expression of MMPs may be due to the inhibited MAPK activity (122).

III. PERSPECTIVES

The multifunctions of various components of chrysanthemum indicate that this plant could have potential chemoprevention properties. However, several fundamental questions still need to be answered prior to knowing the exact pharmacological effects of chrysanthemum. For example, what is the content of various active components in the *C. morifolium* Ramat? How much of the respective component is absorbed and how is it being biotransformed in the body? Obviously, more research in theses areas is needed.

A. Active Components and Intake

The beneficial effects of chrysanthemum flavonoids are highly suggested and proved in numerous experiments, which were carried out using pure flavonoids at 20–60 μM or even more than 100 μM. The actual effects, however, are related to many other factors, including content of the active components, bioavailability, and metabolism. Lack of knowledge about the contents of flavonoids in chrysanthemum makes it difficult to predict exactly how much flavonoids are effective. It has been assumed that the average intake of dietary flavonoids is about 1 g per day (123). But later investigations reduced the average intake to a few hundredths of a milligram per day, according to the flavonoid content of commonly consumed vegetables and fruits (124). For example, quercetin levels in edible vegetables are below 10 mg/kg, except for onions, kale, broccoli, and beans (up to 486 mg/kg). In most fruits, the quercetin level is about 15 mg/kg, except for apples (up to 72 mg/kg). However, green or black tea has up to 50 mg/L of three common flavonols, which is much higher than that of fruit juices (range from below 5 mg/L up to 13 mg/mL) (124). The high concentrations of catechins and especially of epigallocatechin 3-gallate (EGCG), which suppresses tumor growth and metastasis, in tea indicate the advantages of drinking several cups of tea per day. *C. morifolium* Ramat, known to contain flavonoids different from that of tea, may also have potential chemopreventive properties. However, prior to knowing the beneficial effects the content of each flavonoid and its metabolism would need to be further investigated.

In fact, there are several challenges in determining intake of flavonoids in chrysanthemum. The formation of flavonoids in chrysanthemum is influenced by numerous factors, including environmental conditions, subspecies, processing, and storage conditions. Another problem is the lack of agreement on an appropriate method to analyze the different types of flavonoids (125).

B. Bioavailability

The forms of flavonoids are as important as their content in affecting the absorption and bioactivity. It had been expected that only aglycones could be absorbed in the gastrointestinal tract, because no enzymes are secreted in the gut that could cleave the glycosidic bonds (123). However, recent studies have demonstrated that the bioavailability of specific flavonoids is much higher than previously believed. For example, quercetin glycosides were more readily absorbed than quercetin aglycone in several animal tests (126). Felgines et al. reported that naringenin glycosides, the predominant flavonone found in grapes, were efficiently absorbed after feeding to rats (127). Nevertheless, in the Caco-2 cell culture model, permeabilities of genistein aglycones were five times higher than their corresponding glycosides (128). Unfortunately, there is so far no report about the bioavailability of chrysanthemum flavonoids.

C. Equivocal Effects of Antioxidants

As mentioned earlier, the flavonoids of chrysanthemum are strong antioxidants and they may play a role in reducing the redox level in the cell. Their antioxidant effects may be also closely related to other chemopreventive properties such as anticarcinogenesis and antimutagenesis. On the other hand, recent studies revealed that flavonoids could also act as a pro-oxidant under some specific circumstances. For example, kaempferol induces significant concentration-dependent nuclear DNA degradation concurrent with lipid peroxidation. These effects were enhanced by iron(III) or copper(II) (129). Either nitric oxide or flavonoid alone does not induce strand breakage significantly in plasmid pBR322, but nitric oxide, when combined with flavonoids, significantly induces DNA single-strand breakage (130). The antioxidant and pro-oxidant behavior of flavonoids is related to their structures. In general, the more hydroxyl substitutions, the stronger the antioxidant and pro-oxidant activities. The single hydroxyl substitution at position 5 provides no activity, whereas the di-OH substitution at 3′ and 4′ is particularly important to the peroxyl-radical-absorbing activity of a flavonoid. The conjugation between rings A and B does not affect the antioxidant activity but is very important for the copper-initiated pro-oxidant action of a flavonoid. The O-methylation of the hydroxyl substitutions inactivates both the antioxidant and the pro-oxidant activities of the flavonoids (131).

The pro-oxidant properties of flavonoids are involved in their cytotoxicity on cells. For example, apigenin induces apoptosis on human prostate carcinoma LNCaP cells with increase in oxidant stress (95). Another flavonoid, baicalin, induced cytotoxicity in leukemia-derived, T-cell line, Jurkat cells as a pro-oxidant (132). These results demonstrated the pro-oxidant properties of flavonoids, which suggest their possible dual role in mutagenesis and carcinogenesis.

The actual effect of an antioxidant seems controversial. Antioxidants may show their chemopreventive properties in two ways. One is that antioxidants may protect the cells from mutation or carcinogenesis by reducing the elevated ROS because an elevated ROS level is involved in the early stage of carcinogenesis. Numerous studies supported the protective effects of antioxidants (133,134). On the other hand, there were also reports denying the protective effects of antioxidants (135). For example, antioxidant resulted in higher incidence of lung cancer and mortality in male smokers (136). In the lung cells of smokers, ROS level probably plays a role in inducing and eliminating the precancerous lung cells induced by chemical carcinogens. Antioxidant suppresses the apoptosis and potentially promotes the development of lung cancer. Thus, one must be cautious in predicting the exact effects of antioxidants under in vivo condition. Flavonoids of chrysanthemum also may show different effects in different individuals. More extensive and in-depth research is required on the relationship between the effects of chrysanthemum flavonoids in modulating oxidant level and their beneficial properties.

In summary, chrysanthemum, in particular the flower of *C. morifolium* Ramat, was found to contain several flavonoids, including apigenin and leutolin. These two compounds have been shown to have some beneficial effects, including antioxidant, antimutagenesis, anti-inflammation, antiestrogen, antiproliferation, and inhibition of several crucial enzymes involved in cell progression or tumor promotion. Pharmacological studies have also provided evidence that this plant could have some general beneficial health effect. The molecular mechanisms, however, have not been fully elucidated; more research is obviously needed to evaluate the types and content of other active compounds, as well as their pharmacological and chemopreventive properties.

REFERENCES

1. Liu Tongting, Zhao lichun, Wang Naixin, Lu Zhaotong, Sun Ziqin. Effects of Ju Hua Jian in ulcerative colitis and on the contents of CD44 and CD62p. Chin J Covalesc Med 1998; 7(6):38–39.
2. Jiang Huidi, Xia Qiang, Xu Wanhong, Cao Chunmei. Studies on cardic effects of *Chrysanthemum morifolium* Ramat and their unlying mechanism. Modern Trad Chin Med 2002; 4(2):31–34.
3. Wang HK, Xia Y, Yang ZY, Natschke SL, Lee KH. Recent advances in the discovery and development of flavonoids and their analogues as antitumor and anti-HIV agents. Adv Exp Med Biol 1998; 439:191–225.
4. Ukiya M, Akihisa T, Tokuda H, Suzuki H, Mukainaka T, Ichiishi E, Yasukawa K, Kasahara Y, Nishino H. Constituents of Compositae plants. III. Anti-tumor promoting effects and cytotoxic activity against human cancer cell lines of triterpene diols and triols from edible chrysanthemum flowers. Cancer Lett 2002; 177(1):7–12.
5. Sharma SC, Tanwar RC, Kaur S. Contact dermatitis from chrysanthemums in India. Contact Dermat 1989; 21(2):69–71.
6. Singhal V, Reddy BS. Common contact sensitizers in Delhi. J Dermatol 2000; 27(7):440–445.
7. Terashima S, Shimizu M, Horie S, Morita N. Studies on aldose reductase inhibitors from natural products. IV. Constituents and aldose reductase inhibitory effect of *Chrysanthemum morifolium*, *Bixa orellana* and *Ipomoea batatas*. Chem Pharm Bull (Tokyo) 1991; 39(12):3346–3347.
8. Matsuda H, Morikawa T, Toguchida I, Harima S, Yoshikawa M. Medicinal flowers. VI. Absolute stereostructures of two new flavanone glycosides and a phenylbutanoid glycoside from the flowers of *Chrysanthemum indicum* L.: their inhibitory activities for rat lens aldose reductase. Chem Pharm Bull (Tokyo) 2002; 50(7):972–975.
9. Duh Pin-Der, Gow-Chin Yen. Antioxidative activity of three herbal water extracts. Food Chem 1997; 60(4):639–645.
10. Duh Pin-Der, Yang-Ying Tu, Gow-Chin Yen. Antioxidant activity of water extract of Harng Jyur (*Chrysanthemum morifolium* Ramat). Lebensm-Wiss-Technol 1999; 32:269–277.

11. Zhang Erxian, Fang Li, Zhang Jie, Yu Lijun, Xiao Xiang. Research on the antioxidantive activities of chrysanthemum extract. Shi Pin Ke Xue 2000; 21(7):6–9.
12. Duthie SJ, Dobson VL. Dietary flavonoids protect human colonocyte DNA from oxidative attack in vitro. Eur J Nutr 1999; 38(1):28–34.
13. Mu YM, Yanase T, Nishi Y, Tanaka A, Saito M, Jin CH, Mukasa C, Okabe T, Nomura M, Goto K, Nawata H. Saturated FFAs, palmitic acid and stearic acid, induce apoptosis in human granulosa cells. Endocrinology 2001; 142(8):3590–3597.
14. Sparagna GC, Hickson-Bick DL, Buja LM, McMillin JB. Fatty acid-induced apoptosis in neonatal cardiomyocytes: redox signaling. Antioxid Redox Signal 2001; 3(1):71–79.
15. Listenberger LL, Ory DS, Schaffer JE. Palmitate-induced apoptosis can occur through a ceramide-independent pathway. J Biol Chem 2001; 276(18):14890–14895.
16. Hayashi Y, Fukushima S, Kishimoto S, Kawaguchi T, Numata M, Isoda Y, Hirano J, Nakano M. Anticancer effects of free polyunsaturated fatty acids in an oily lymphographic agent following intrahepatic arterial administration to a rabbit bearing VX-2 tumor. Cancer Res 1992; 52(2):400–405.
17. Zusman I, Gurevich P, Madar Z, Nyska A, Korol D, Timar B, Zuckerman A. Tumor-promoting and tumor-protective effects of high-fat diets on chemically induced mammary cancer in rats. Anticancer Res 1997; 17(1A), 349–356.
18. Sauer Leonard A, Dauchy Robert T, Blask David E. Blask Mechanism for the antitumor and anticachectic effects of n-3 fatty acids. Cancer Res 2000; 60:5289–5295.
19. Sauer LA, Dauchy RT, Blask DE. Polyunsaturated fatty acids, melatonin, and cancer prevention. Biochem Pharmacol 2001; 61(12):1455–1462.
20. Jiang WG, Hiscox S, Bryce RP, Horrobin DF, Mansel RE. The effects of n-6 polyunsaturated fatty acids on the expression of nm-23 in human cancer cells. Br J Cancer 1998; 77(5):731–738.
21. Ukiya M, Akihisa T, Yasukawa K, Kasahara Y, Kimura Y, Koike K, Nikaido T, Takido M. Constituents of compositae plants. 2. Triterpene diols, triols, and their 3-o-fatty acid esters from edible chrysanthemum flower extract and their anti-inflammatory effects. J Agric Food Chem 2001; 49(7):3187–3197.
22. Akihisa T, Yasukawa K, Oinuma H, Kasahara Y, Yamanouchi S, Takido M, Kumaki K, Tamura T. Triterpene alcohols from the flowers of compositae and their anti-inflammatory effects. Phytochemistry 1996; 43(6):1255–1260.
23. Ahumada C, Saenz T, Garcia D, De La Puerta R, Fernandez A, Martinez E. The effects of a triterpene fraction isolated from *Crataegus monogyna* Jacq. on different acute inflammation models in rats and mice: leucocyte migration and phospholipase A2 inhibition. J Pharm Pharmacol 1997; 49(3):329–331.
24. Chiang HC, Tseng TH, Wang CJ, Chen CF, Kan WS. Experimental antitumor agents from *Solanum indicum* L. Anticancer Res 1991; 11(5):1911–1917.
25. Mohanan PV, Devi KS. Cytotoxic potential of the preparations from *Solanum trilobatum* and the effect of sobatum on tumour reduction in mice. Cancer Lett 1996; 110(1–2):71–76.

26. Banskota AH, Tezuka Y, Tran KQ, Tanaka K, Saiki I, Kadota S. Methyl quadrangularates A–D and related triterpenes from *Combretum quadrangulare*. Chem Pharm Bull (Tokyo) 2000; 48(4):496–504.
27. von Holtz RL, Fink CS, Awad AB. Beta-sitosterol activates the sphingomyelin cycle and induces apoptosis in LNCaP human prostate cancer cells. Nutr Cancer 1998; 32(1):8–12.
28. Awad AB, Gan Y, Fink CS. Effect of beta-sitosterol, a plant sterol, on growth, protein phosphatase 2A, and phospholipase D in LNCaP cells. Nutr Cancer 2000; 36(1):74–78.
29. Yang H, Wang X, Yu L. The antitumor activity of elemene is associated with apoptosis. Zhonghua Zhong Liu Za Zhi 1996; 18(3):169–172.
30. Zou L, Liu W, Yu L. Beta-elemene induces apoptosis of K562 leukemia cells. Zhonghua Zhong Liu Za Zhi 2001; 23(3):196–198.
31. Miles DH, Kokpol U. Tumor inhibitors. II. Constituents and antitumor activity of *Sarracenia* flava. J Pharm Sci 1976; 65(2):284–285.
32. Gomez MA, Garcia MD, Saenz MT. Cytostatic activity of *Achillea ageratum* L. Phytother Res 2001; 15(7):633–634.
33. Santos FA, Rao VS. 1,8-Cineol, a food flavoring agent, prevents ethanol-induced gastric injury in rats. Dig Dis Sci 2001; 46(2):331–337.
34. Vidya L, Malini MM, Varalakshmi P. Effect of pentacyclic triterpenes on oxalate-induced changes in rat erythrocytes. Pharmacol Res 2000; 42(4):313–316.
35. Saleem M, Alam A, Arifin S, Shah MS, Ahmed B, Sultana S. Lupeol, a triterpene, inhibits early responses of tumor promotion induced by benzoyl peroxide in murine skin. Pharmacol Res 2001; 43(2):127–134.
36. Hollman PC, Feskens EJ, Katan MB. Tea flavonols in cardiovascular disease and cancer epidemiology. Proc Soc Exp Biol Med 1999; 220(4):198–202.
37. Knekt P, Jarvinen R, Seppanen R, Hellovaara M, Teppo L, Pukkala E, Aromaa A. Dietary flavonoids and the risk of lung cancer and other malignant neoplasms. Am J Epidemiol 1997; 146(3):223–230.
38. Birt DF, Hendrich S, Wang W. Dietary agents in cancer prevention: flavonoids and isoflavonoids. Pharmacol Ther 2001; 90(2-3):157–177.
39. Arisawa M, Ishiwari Y, Nakaoki T, Sekino S, Takakuwa T. Unutilized resources. III. Components of *Juncus* genus plants, the leaves of *Aesulus turbinate*, and the petals of *Chrysanthemum morifolium*. Shoyakugaku Zasshi 1969; 23(2):49–52.
40. Robak J, Shridi F, Wolbis M, Krolikowska M. Screening of the influence of flavonoids on lipoxygenase and cyclooxygenase activity, as well as on non-enzymic lipid oxidation. Pol J Pharmacol Pharm 1988; 40(5):451–458.
41. Cholbi MR, Paya M, Alcaraz MJ. Inhibitory effects of phenolic compounds on CC14-induced microsomal lipid peroxidation. Experientia 1991; 47(2):195–199.
42. Galvez J, de la Cruz JP, Zarzuelo A, Sanchez de la Cuesta F. Flavonoid inhibition of enzymic and nonenzymic lipid peroxidation in rat liver differs from its influence on the glutathione-related enzymes. Pharmacology 1995; 51(2): 127–133.

43. Devasagayam TP, Subramanian M, Singh BB, Ramanathan R, Das NP. Protection of plasmid pBR322 DNA by flavonoids against single-stranded breaks induced by singlet molecular oxygen. J Photochem Photobiol B 1995; 30(2-3):97–103.
44. Noroozi M, Angerson WJ, Lean ME. Effects of flavonoids and vitamin C on oxidative DNA damage to human lymphocytes. Am J Clin Nutr 1998; 67(6): 1210–1218.
45. Brown JE, Rice-Evans CA. Luteolin-rich artichoke extract protects low density lipoprotein from oxidation in vitro. Free Radic Res 1998; 29(3):247–255.
46. Lin CM, Chen CS, Chen CT, Liang YC, Lin JK. Molecular modeling of flavonoids that inhibits xanthine oxidase. Biochem Biophys Res Commun 2002; 294(1):167–172.
47. Park KY, Lee SH, Min BK, Lee KS, Choi JS, Chung SR, Min KR, Kim Y. Inhibitory effect of luteolin 4′-O-glucoside from *Kummerowia striata* and other flavonoids on interleukin-5 bioactivity. Planta Med 1999; 65(5):457–459.
48. Kim HK, Cheon BS, Kim YH, Kim SY, Kim HP. Effects of naturally occurring flavonoids on nitric oxide production in the macrophage cell line RAW 264.7 and their structure-activity relationships. Biochem Pharmacol 1999; 58(5):759–765.
49. Depeint F, Gee JM, Williamson G, Johnson IT. Evidence for consistent patterns between flavonoids structures and cellular activities. Proc Nutr Soc 2002; 61:97–103.
50. Oguri A, Suda M, Totsuka Y, Sugimura T, Wakabayashi K. Inhibitory effects of antioxidants on formation of heterocyclic amines. Mutat Res 1998; 402(1-2):237–245.
51. Huang MT, Wood AW, Newmark HL, Sayer JM, Yagi H, Jerina DM, Conney AH. Inhibition of the mutagenicity of bay-region diol-epoxides of polycyclic aromatic hydrocarbons by phenolic plant flavonoids. Carcinogenesis 1983; 4(12):1631–1637.
52. Elangovan V, Sekar N, Govindasamy S. Chemopreventive potential of dietary bioflavonoids against 20-methylcholanthrene-induced tumorigenesis. Cancer Lett 1994; 87(1):107–113.
53. Wei H, Tye L, Bresnick E, Birt DF. Inhibitory effect of apigenin, a plant flavonoid, on epidermal ornithine decarboxylase and skin tumor promotion in mice. Cancer Res 1990; 50(3):499–502.
54. Edenharder R, von Petersdorff I, Rauscher R. Antimutagenic effects of flavonoids, chalcones and structurally related compounds on the activity of 2-amino-3-methylimidazo[4,5-f]quinoline (IQ) and other heterocyclic amine mutagens from cooked food. Mutat Res 1993; 287(2):261–274.
55. Miller WR. Estrogens and the risk of breast cancer. In: Miller WR, ed. Estrogen and Breast Cancer. New York: Springer, Berlin Heidelberg, 1996:35–62.
56. Davis SR, Murkies AL, Wilcox G. Phytoestrogens in clinical practice. Integr Med 1998; 1:27–34.
57. Zand RS, Jenkins DJ, Diamandis EP. Steroid hormone activity of flavonoids and related compounds. Breast Cancer Res Treat 2000; 62(1):35–49.

58. Han DH, Tachibana H, Yamada K. Inhibition of environmental estrogen-induced proliferation of human breast carcinoma MCF-7 cells by flavonoids. In Vitro Cell Dev Biol Anim 2001; 37(5):275–282.
59. Han DH, Denison MS, Tachibana H, Yamada K. Relationship between estrogen receptor-binding and estrogenic activities of environmental estrogens and suppression by flavonoids. Biosci Biotechnol Biochem 2002; 66(7):1479–1487.
60. Wang C, Kurzer MS. Effects of phytoestrogens on DNA synthesis in MCF-7 cells in the presence of estradiol or growth factors. Nutr Cancer 1998; 31(2):90–100.
61. Holland MB, Roy D. Estrone-induced cell proliferation and differentiation in the mammary gland of the female Noble rat. Carcinogenesis 1995; 16(8):1955–1961.
62. Collins-Burow BM, Burow ME, Duong BN, McLachlan JA. Estrogenic and antiestrogenic activities of flavonoid phytochemicals through estrogen receptor binding-dependent and -independent mechanisms. Nutr Cancer 2000; 38(2):229–244.
63. Markaverich BM, Shoulars K, Brown MA. Purification and characterization of nuclear type II [(3)H] estradiol binding sites from the rat uterus: covalent labeling with [(3)H]luteolin. Steroids 2001; 66(9):707–719.
64. Markaverich BM, Roberts RR, Alejandro MA, Johnson GA, Middleditch BS, Clark JH. Bioflavonoid interaction with rat uterine type II binding sites and cell growth inhibition. J Steroid Biochem 1988; 30(1-6):71–78.
65. Markaverich BM, Gregory RR. Preliminary assessment of luteolin as an affinity ligand for type II estrogen—binding sites in rat uterine nuclear extracts. Steroids 1993; 58(6):268–274.
66. Westley BR, Clayton SJ, Daws MR, Molloy CA, May FE. Interactions between the oestrogen and insulin-like growth factor signalling pathways in the control of breast epithelial cell proliferation. Biochem Soc Symp 1998; 63:35–44.
67. Yee D, Lee AV. Crosstalk between the insulin-like growth factors and estrogens in breast cancer. J Mamm Gland Biol Neoplas 2000; 5(1):107–115.
68. Frigo DE, Duong BN, Melnik LI, Schief LS, Collins-Burow BM, Pace DK, McLachlan JA, Burow ME. Flavonoid phytochemicals regulate activator protein-1 signal transduction pathways in endometrial and kidney stable cell lines. J Nutr 2002; 132(7):1848–1853.
69. Folkman J. Angiogenesis in cancer, vascular, rheumatoid and other disease. Nature Med 1995; 1:27–31.
70. Benassayag C, Perrot-Applanat M, Ferre F. Phytoestrogens as modulators of steroid action in target cells. J Chromatogr B 2002; 777(1-2):233–248.
71. Trochon V, Mabilat-Pragnon C, Bertrand P, Legrand Y, Soria J, Soria C, Bertrand D, Lu H. Hyaluronectin blocks the stimulatory effect of hyaluronan-derived fragments on endothelial cells during angiogenesis in vitro. FEBS Lett 1997; 418(1-2):6–10.
72. Fotsis T, Pepper MS, Aktas E, Breit S, Rasku S, Adlercreutz H, Wahala K, Montesano R, Schweigerer L. Flavonoids, dietary-derived inhibitors of cell proliferation and in vitro angiogenesis. Cancer Res 1997; 57(14):2916–2921.

73. Joussen AM, Rohrschneider K, Reichling J, Kirchhof B, Kruse FE. Treatment of corneal neovascularization with dietary isoflavonoids and flavonoids. Exp Eye Res 2000; 71(5):483–487.
74. Kuppusamy UR, Khoo HE, Das NP. Structure-activity studies of flavonoids as inhibitors of hyaluronidase. Biochem Pharmacol 1990; 40(2):397–401.
75. Trochon V, Blot E, Cymbalista F, Engelmann C, Tang RP, Thomaidis A, Vasse M, Soria J, Lu H, Soria C. Apigenin inhibits endothelial-cell proliferation in G(2)/M phase whereas it stimulates smooth-muscle cells by inhibiting P21 and P27 expression. Int J Cancer 2000; 85(5):691–696.
76. Ramanathan R, Das NP, Tan CH. Effects of gamma-linolenic acid, flavonoids, and vitamins on cytotoxicity and lipid peroxidation. Free Radic Biol Med 1994; 16(1):43–48.
77. Lee LT, Huang YT, Hwang JJ, Lee PP, Ke FC, Nair MP, Kanadaswam C, Lee MT. Blockade of the epidermal growth factor receptor tyrosine kinase activity by quercetin and luteolin leads to growth inhibition and apoptosis of pancreatic tumor cells. Anticancer Res 2002a; 22(3):1615–1627.
78. Ko WG, Kang TH, Lee SJ, Kim YC, Lee BH. Effects of luteolin on the inhibition of proliferation and induction of apoptosis in human myeloid leukaemia cells. Phytother Res 2002; 16(3):295–298.
79. Zhao W, Liang C, Chen Z, Pang R, Zhao B, Chen Z. Luteolin inhibits proliferation and collagen synthesis of hepatic stellate cells. Zhonghua Gan Zang Bing Za Zhi 2002; 10(3):204–206.
80. Yin F, Giuliano AE, Van Herle AJ. a. Growth inhibitory effects of flavonoids in human thyroid cancer cell lines. Thyroid 1999a; 9(4):369–376.
81. Iwashita K, Kobori M, Yamaki K, Tsushida T. Flavonoids inhibit cell growth and induce apoptosis in B16 melanoma 4A5 cells. Biosci Biotechnol Biochem 2000; 64(9):1813–1820.
82. Huang YT, Hwang JJ, Lee PP, Ke FC, Huang JH, Huang CJ, Kandaswami C, Middleton E Jr, Lee MT. Effects of luteolin and quercetin, inhibitors of tyrosine kinase, on cell growth and metastasis-associated properties in A431 cells overexpressing epidermal growth factor receptor. Br J Pharmacol 1999; 128(5): 999–1010.
83. Knowles LM, Zigrossi DA, Tauber RA, Hightower C, Milner JA. Flavonoids suppress androgen-independent human prostate tumor proliferation. Nutr Cancer 2000; 38(1):116–122.
84. Jing Y, Waxman S. Structural requirements for differentiation-induction and growth-inhibition of mouse erythroleukemia cells by isoflavones. Anticancer Res 1995; 15(4):1147–1152.
85. Sato F, Matsukawa Y, Matsumoto K, Nishino H, Sakai T. Apigenin induces morphological differentiation and G2-M arrest in rat neuronal cells. Biochem Biophys Res Commun 1994; 204(2):578–584.
86. Kim TJ, Zhang YH, Kim Y, Lee CK, Lee MK, Hong JT, Yun YP. Effects of apigenin on the serum- and platelet derived growth factor-BB-induced proliferation of rat aortic vascular smooth muscle cells. Planta Med 2002; 68(7):605–609.

87. Yin F, Giuliano AE, Van Herle AJ. b. Signal pathways involved in apigenin inhibition of growth and induction of apoptosis of human anaplastic thyroid cancer cells (ARO). Anticancer Res 1999b; 19(5B):4297–4303.
88. Lee JT, McCubrey JA. The Raf/MEK/ERK signal transduction cascade as a target for chemotherapeutic intervention in leukemia. Leukemia 2002b; 16:486–507.
89. Casagrande F, Darbon JM. Effects of structurally related flavonoids on cell cycle progression of human melanoma cells: regulation of cyclin-dependent kinases CDK2 and CDK1. Biochem Pharmacol 2001; 61(10):1205–1215.
90. Donjerkovic D, Scott DW. Regulation of the G1 phase of the mammalian cell cycle. Cell Res 2000; 10(1):1–16.
91. Lindenmeyer F, Li H, Menashi S, Soria C, Lu H. Apigenin acts on the tumor cell invasion process and regulates protease production. Nutr Cancer 2001; 39(1):139–147.
92. Zi X, Feyes DK, Agarwal R. Anticarcinogenic effect of a flavonoid antioxidant, silymarin, in human breast cancer cells MDA-MB 468: induction of G1 arrest through an increase in Cip1/p21 concomitant with a decrease in kinase activity of cyclin-dependent kinases and associated cyclins. Clin Cancer Res 1998; 4(4): 1055–1064.
93. Kobayashi T, Nakata T, Kuzumaki T. Effect of flavonoids on cell cycle progression in prostate cancer cells. Cancer Lett 2002; 176(1):17–23.
94. Lepley DM, Pelling JC. Induction of p21/WAF1 and G1 cell-cycle arrest by the chemopreventive agent apigenin. Mol Carcinog 1997; 19(2):74–82.
95. Gupta S, Afaq F, Mukhtar H. Involvement of nuclear factor-kappa B, Bax and Bcl-2 in induction of cell cycle arrest and apoptosis by apigenin in human prostate carcinoma cells. Oncogene 2002; 21(23):3727–3738.
96. Gupta S, Afaq F, Mukhtar H. Selective growth-inhibitory, cell-cycle deregulatory and apoptotic response of apigenin in normal versus human prostate carcinoma cells. Biochem Biophys Res Commun 2001; 287(4):914–920.
97. Lepley DM, Li B, Birt DF, Pelling JC. The chemopreventive flavonoid apigenin induces G2/M arrest in keratinocytes. Carcinogenesis 1996; 17(11):2367–2375.
98. Wang W, Heideman L, Chung CS, Pelling JC, Koehler KJ, Birt DF. Cell-cycle arrest at G2/M and growth inhibition by apigenin in human colon carcinoma cell lines. Mol Carcinog 2000; 28(2):102–110.
99. McVean M, Weinberg WC, Pelling JC. A p21(waf1)-independent pathway for inhibitory phosphorylation of cyclin-dependent kinase p34(cdc2) and concomitant G(2)/M arrest by the chemopreventive flavonoid apigenin. Mol Carcinog 2002; 33(1):36–43.
100. Yin F, Giuliano AE, Law RE, Van Herle AJ. Apigenin inhibits growth and induces G2/M arrest by modulating cyclin-CDK regulators and ERK MAP kinase activation in breast carcinoma cells. Anticancer Res 2001; 21(1A):413–420.
101. Reiners JJ Jr, Clift R, Mathieu P. Suppression of cell cycle progression by flavonoids: dependence on the aryl hydrocarbon receptor. Carcinogenesis 1999; 20(8):1561–1566.

102. Yamashita N, Kawanishi S. Distinct mechanisms of DNA damage in apoptosis induced by quercetin and luteolin. Free Radic Res 2000; 33(5):623–633.
103. Wang IK, Lin-Shiau SY, Lin JK. Induction of apoptosis by apigenin and related flavonoids through cytochrome c release and activation of caspase-9 and caspase-3 in leukaemia HL-60 cells. Eur J Cancer 1999; 35(10):1517–1525.
104. Shen J, Channavajhala P, Seldin DC, Sonenshein GE. Phosphorylation by the protein kinase CK2 promotes calpain-mediated degradation of IkappaBalpha. J Immunol 2001; 167(9):4919–4925.
105. Liang YC, Huang YT, Tsai SH, Lin-Shiau SY, Chen CF, Lin JK. Suppression of inducible cyclooxygenase and inducible nitric oxide synthase by apigenin and related flavonoids in mouse macrophage. Carcinogenesis 1999; 20(10):1945–1952.
106. Plaumann B, Fritsche M, Rimpler H, Brandner G, Hess RD. Flavonoids activate wild-type p53. Oncogene 1996; 13(8):1605–1614.
107. Grammer TC, Blenis J. Evidence for MEK-independent pathways regulating the prolonged activation of the ERK-MAP kinases. Oncogene 1997; 14(14): 1635–1642.
108. Fujita-Yamaguchi Y, Kathuria S. Characterization of receptor tyrosine-specific protein kinases by the use of inhibitors: staurosporine is a 100-times more potent inhibitor of insulin receptor than IGF-I receptor. Biochem Biophys Res Commun 1988; 157(3):955–962.
109. Agullo G, Gamet-Payrastre L, Manenti S, Viala C, Remesy C, Chap H, Payrastre B. Relationship between flavonoid structure and inhibition of phosphatidylinositol 3-kinase: a comparison with tyrosine kinase and protein kinase C inhibition. Biochem Pharmacol 1997; 53(11):1649–1657.
110. Ferriola PC, Cody V, Middleton E Jr. Protein kinase C inhibition by plant flavonoids: kinetic mechanisms and structure-activity relationships. Biochem Pharmacol 1989; 38(10):1617–1624.
111. Lin JK, Chen YC, Huang YT, Lin-Shiau SY. Suppression of protein kinase C and nuclear oncogene expression as possible molecular mechanisms of cancer chemoprevention by apigenin and curcumin. J Cell Biochem 1997; 28–29(suppl)):39–48.
112. Galve-Roperh I, Haro A, Diaz-Laviada I. Induction of nerve growth factor synthesis by sphingomyelinase and ceramide in primary astrocyte cultures. Brain Res Mol Brain Res 1997; 52(1):90–97.
113. Carrillo C, Cafferata EG, Genovese J, O'Reilly M, Roberts AB, Santa-Coloma TA. TGF-beta1 up-regulates the mRNA for the Na+/Ca2+ exchanger in neonatal rat cardiac myocytes. Cell Mol Biol (Noisy-le-grand) 1998; 44(3):543–551.
114. Xagorari A, Roussos C, Papapetropoulos A. Inhibition of LPS-stimulated pathways in macrophages by the flavonoid luteolin. Br J Pharmacol 2002; 136(7):1058–1064.
115. Huang YT, Kuo ML, Liu JY, Huang SY, Lin JK. Inhibitions of protein kinase C and proto-oncogene expressions in NIH 3T3 cells by apigenin. Eur J Cancer, 1996, (1):146–151.

116. Kimata M, Shichijo M, Miura T, Serizawa I, Inagaki N, Nagai H. Effects of luteolin, quercetin and baicalein on immunoglobulin E-mediated mediator release from human cultured mast cells. Clin Exp Allergy 2000; 30(4):501–508.
117. Constantinou A, Mehta R, Runyan C, Rao K, Vaughan A, Moon R. Flavonoids as DNA topoisomerase antagonists and poisons: structure-activity relationships. J Nat Prod 1995; 58(2):217–225.
118. Mittra B, Saha A, Chowdhury AR, Pal C, Mandal S, Mukhopadhyay S, Bandyopadhyay S, Majumder HK. Luteolin, an abundant dietary component is a potent anti-leishmanial agent that acts by inducing topoisomerase II-mediated kinetoplast DNA cleavage leading to apoptosis. Mol Med 2000; 6(6):527–541.
119. Azuma Y, Onishi Y, Sato Y, Kizaki H. Effects of protein tyrosine kinase inhibitors with different modes of action on topoisomerase activity and death of IL-2-dependent CTLL-2 cells. J Biochem (Tokyo) 1995; 118(2):312–318.
120. Chowdhury AR, Sharma S, Mandal S, Goswami A, Mukhopadhyay S, Majumder HK. Luteolin, an emerging anti-cancer flavonoid, poisons eukaryotic DNA topoisomerase I. Biochem J 2002; 366(Pt 2):653–661.
121. Boege F, Straub T, Kehr A, Boesenberg C, Christiansen K, Andersen A, Jakob F, Kohrle J. Selected novel flavones inhibit the DNA binding or the DNA religation step of eukaryotic topoisomerase I. J Biol Chem 1996; 271(4):2262–2270.
122. Reddy KB, Krueger JS, Kondapaka SB, Diglio CA. Mitogen-activated protein kinase (MAPK) regulates the expression of progelatinase B (MMP-9) in breast epithelial cells. Int J Cancer 1999; 82(2):268–273.
123. Kuhnau J. The flavonoids: a class of semi-essential food components: their role in human nutrition. World Rev Nutr Diet 1976; 24:117–191.
124. Hertog MG, Hollman PC, Katan MB, Kromhout D. Intake of potentially anticarcinogenic flavonoids and their determinants in adults in the Netherlands. Nutr Cancer 1993; 20(1):21–29.
125. Ross JA, Kasum CM. Dietary flavonoids: bioavailability, metabolic effects, and safety. Annu Rev Nutr 2002; 22:19–34.
126. Hollman PC, van Trijp JMP, Buysman NCP, van der Gaag MS, Mengelers MJB. Relative bioavailibility of the antioxidant flavonoid quercetin from various foods in man. FEBS Lett 1997; 418:152–156.
127. Felgines C, Texier O, Morand C, Manach C, Scalbert A. Bioavailability of the flavanone naringenin and its glycosidese in rats. Am J Physiol Gastrointest Liver Physiol 2000; 279:G1148–G1154.
128. Liu Y, Hu M. Absorption and metabolism of flavonoids in the caco-2 cell culture model and a perused rat intestinal model. Drug Metab Dispos 2002; 30(4):370–377.
129. Sahu SC, Gray GC. Kaempferol-induced nuclear DNA damage and lipid peroxidation. Cancer Lett 1994; 85(2):159–164.
130. Ohshima H, Yoshie Y, Auriol S, Gilibert I. Antioxidant and pro-oxidant actions of flavonoids: effects on DNA damage induced by nitric oxide, peroxynitrite and nitroxyl anion. Free Radic Biol Med 1998; 25(9):1057–1065.

131. Cao G, Sofic E, Prior RL. Antioxidant and prooxidant behavior of flavonoids: structure-activity relationships. Free Radic Biol Med 1997; 22(5):749–760.
132. Ueda S, Nakamura H, Masutani H, Sasada T, Takabayashi A, Yamaoka Y, Yodoi J. Baicalin induces apoptosis via mitochondrial pathway as prooxidant. Mol Immunol 2002; 38(10):781–791.
133. Curtin JF, Donovan M, Cotter TG. Regulation and measurement of oxidative stress in apoptosis. J Immunol Methods 2002; 265(1–2):49–72.
134. Das S. Vitamin E and the genesis and prevention of cancer: a review. Acta Oncol 1994; 33:615–619.
135. Rawe PM. Beta-carotene takes a collective beating. Lancet 1996; 347:249.
136. Heinonen OP, Albanes D, Virtamo J, Taylor PR, Huttunen JK, Hartman AM, Haapakoski J, Malila N, Rautalahti M, Ripatti S, Maenpaa H, Teerenhovi L, Koss L, Virolainen M, Edwards BK. Prostate cancer and supplementation with alpha-tocopherol and beta-carotene: incidence and mortality in a controlled trial. J Natl Cancer Inst 1998; 90(6):440–446.

19

Andrographis paniculata and the Cardiovascular System

Benny Kwong-Huat Tan
National University of Singapore
Singapore, Republic of Singapore

Amy C. Y. Zhang
Epitomics, Inc.
Burlingame, California, U.S.A.

I. INTRODUCTION

Andrographis paniculata (Burm. f) Nees (Acanthaceae) is a well-known bitter medicinal herb found in the Far East (specifically in India, Southeast Asia, the northern parts of the Malayan peninsula, Java, and southern parts of China). It is also cultivated commercially. It is an erect, stiff herb, growing up to 1 m tall, with quadrangular stems that are thickened above the nodes. The leaves are opposite, lanceolate (3–12 cm by 1–3 cm) while flowers are narrow, white, tube-like, and appear as laxly branched terminal or axillary inflorescences (Fig. 1).

The herb is known by several other names—*Justicia paniculata* Burm. f.; Hempedu bumi, Sambiloto, Sambiroto (Javanese/Malay), Chuan xin lian (Chinese).

FIGURE 1 *Andrographis paniculata* (Burm. f) Nees (Acanthaceae). (Courtesy of Dr. Andrew Wee Kien Han.)

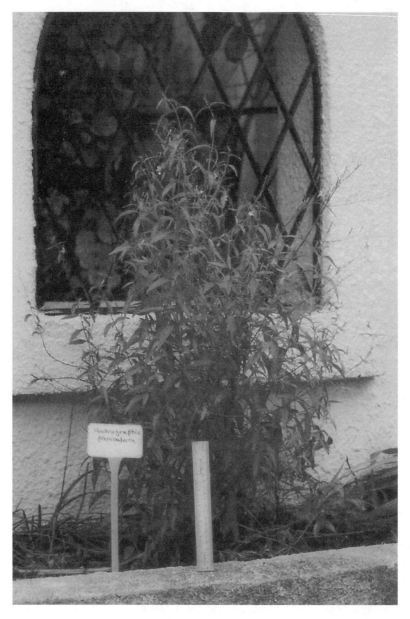

II. CHEMICAL CONSTITUENTS OF *A. PANICULATA*

The chemical constituents of *A. paniculata* are mainly diterpenoids (which all contain hydroxyl, α,β-unsaturated-γ lactone, and exomethylene groups in their chemical structures) and flavonoids. The diterpenoids include andrographolide (1), 14-deoxyandrographolide (DA), 14-deoxy-11,12-didehydroandrographolide (DDA), 14-deoxy-11-oxoandrographolide (2), neoandrographolide (3), andrographiside (di-deoxyandrographolide), deoxyandrographoside (andropanoside), andrograpanin, deoxyandrographolide 19-D-glucoside, and 14-deoxy-12-methoxy-andrographolide (4–7).

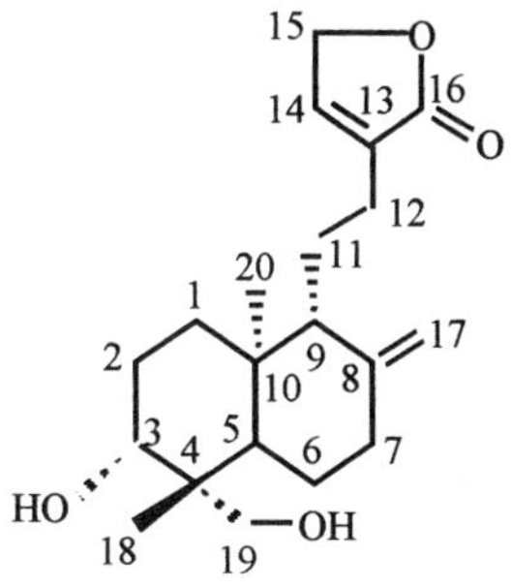

1

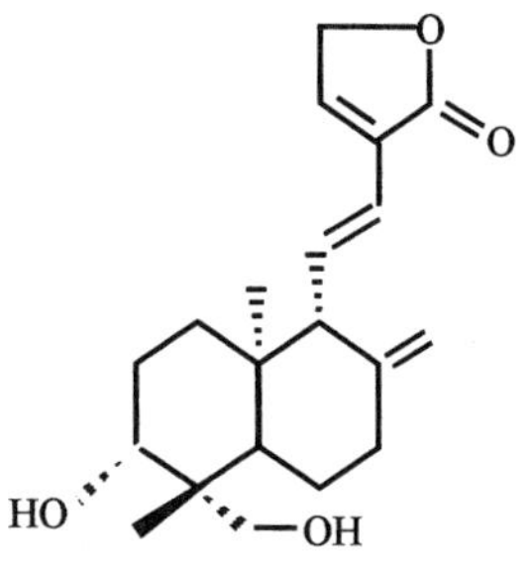

2

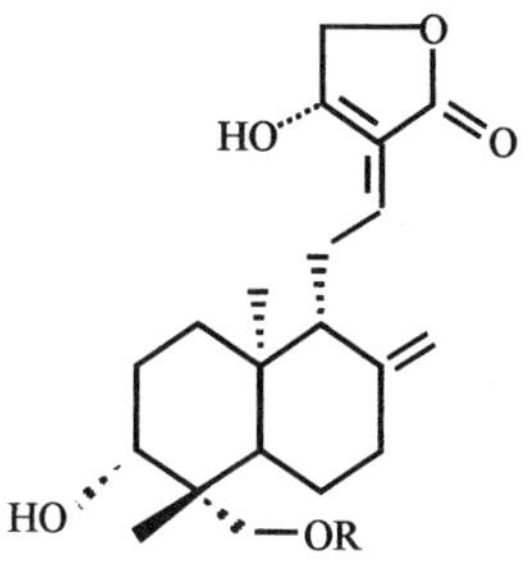

3: R=H
4: R=Glucoside

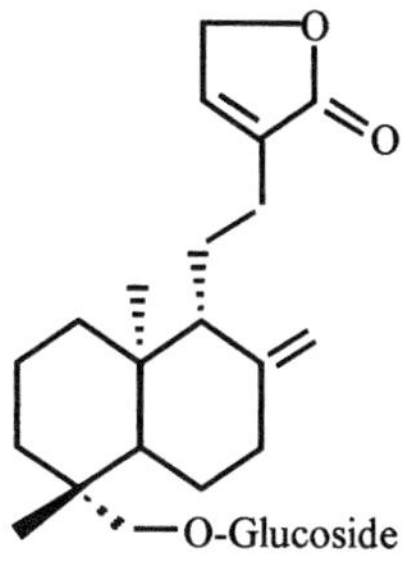

5

FIGURE 2 Chemical structures of DA (1), DDA (2), andrographolide (3) andrographiside (4), and neoandrographolide (5).

Matsuda et al. (8) reported the isolation of six new diterpenoids of the ent-labdane type, viz. 14-epi-andrographolide, isoandrographolide, 14-deoxy-12-hydroxyandrographolide, and 14-deoxy-11-hydroxyandrographolide and the diterpene glucosides 14-deoxy-11, 12-didehydrographiside, and 6′acetyl-eoandrographolide. Four new diterpene dimers, bis-andrographolides, A, B, C, and D, from the aerial parts (including seeds, stem, and leaves) of *A. paniculata* were also isolated and their structure determined by chemical and spectral analysis (8).

From the root of the plant, a new flavonone glucoside, andrographidine (A), and five new flavone glucosides, andrographidine B, C, D, E, and F, were isolated along with 5-hydroxy-7, 8, 2′-, 3′-tetramethoxyflavone, and 7, 8-dimethoxy-5-hydroxyflavone. They have uncommon O-substitution pattern including 5,7-8-,2′-,3′- and 4′O-substituents (9). Tang and Eisenbrand (10) reported that the main constituent of *A. paniculata* was andrographolide.

DA (Fig. 2,1), $C_{20}H_{30}O_4$, is a colorless plate crystal (from methanol) with hydroxyl, α,β-unsaturated-γ-lactone, and exo-methylene groups in its chemical structure. It was reported to possess antipyretic and anti-inflammatory effects (10,11).

DDA (Fig. 2,2), C20H28O4, is a colorless needle crystal (from methanol) with hydroxyl, α,β-unsaturated-γ-lactone, and exo-methylene groups present in its chemical structure (2). This is very similar to that of 14-deoxyandrographolide, with the exception of a double bond at C-11 and 12. So far, there has been no literature report on the biological activities of DDA.

III. BIOLOGICAL EFFECTS OF *A. PANICULATA*

A. paniculata has been reported to have multiple pharmacological activities, including the lowering of blood pressure. Anecdotally, it is taken as a bitter infusion from six to seven leaves for lowering very high blood pressure. A published report by Ahmad and Asmawi (12) indicated that the extract of this plant was used among Malays in Malaysia for the treatment of hypertension. Wang and Zhao (13) reported that the extract could alleviate atherosclerotic artery stenosis induced by both deendothelialization and a high-cholesterol diet. This chapter reviews the authors' investigations into the cardiovascular effects of a crude water extract of *A. paniculata*, its semipurified fractions, and some of its diterpenoid compounds.

The effects of an intraperitoneally administered aqueous extract of *A. paniculata* on systolic blood pressure (SBP), plasma and lung angiotensin-converting enzyme (ACE) activities, and also the free radical content in the kidneys of male spontaneously hypertensive rats (SHR) and normotensive Wistar-Kyoto (WKY) rats were also evaluated.

It is well known that ACE plays an important role in blood pressure regulation by (a) catalyzing the conversion of angiotensin I to angiotensin II, which has potent vasoconstrictor effects, and (b) promoting inactivation of the natriuretic vasodilator bradykinin. These actions lead to an elevation in blood pressure. Cushman and Cheung (14) reported that the lungs and kidneys had large amounts of this enzyme.

Suryaprabha et al. (15) reported that in hypertensive states, there is an increased amount of free radicals. Elevated levels of free radicals have in turn been associated with increased amounts of ACE in the kidneys (16). Free radicals, especially superoxide ions, can also inactivate the vasodilators nitric oxide (NO) and prostacyclin (PGI_2) (17). All these factors can potentially aggravate the hypertension. We decided to evaluate whether the extract of *A. paniculata* could affect these parameters and also the blood pressure of the experimental rats.

Chronic intraperitoneal infusion of three different doses of the extract (0.7, 1.4, and 2.8 mg/kg) was administered by osmotic pumps (ALZA Corp., USA) to SHR over 14 days. The extract produced significant dose-dependent reductions in the SBP of SHR compared with vehicle-treated controls. Peak reductions in SBP occurred on day 2 with all three doses (Fig. 3). The lowest of the three doses was thus chosen as the optimum hypotensive dose of the extract.

A follow-up study was done using this optimum dose in SHR and WKY rats. We showed that the extract significantly lowered SBP in both these strains of rats. Plasma but not lung ACE activity in extract-treated SHR was found to be significantly lower than that in vehicle-treated SHR. However, no significant difference was found in plasma and lung ACE activities between extract and vehicle-treated WKY rats.

Interestingly, the kidney TBARS value in vehicle-treated SHR was significantly higher than that in vehicle-treated WKY rats. This appears to be consistent with the expectation that free-radical levels are elevated in hypertension. The level of lipid peroxidation products in the kidneys [as reflected by estimation of thiobarbituric-acid-reacting substance (TBARS)] was also found to be significantly lower in extract-treated SHR but not WKY rats when compared to their corresponding vehicle-treated controls. More recently, it was reported that *A. paniculata* has antioxidant properties by production of reactive oxygen species (18) or increasing the levels of antioxidant enzymes (19). It will thus have the capacity to reduce free-radical activity. However, the extract was found to lower TBARS content in SHR but not WKY rats. This may be because there are higher levels in the SHR.

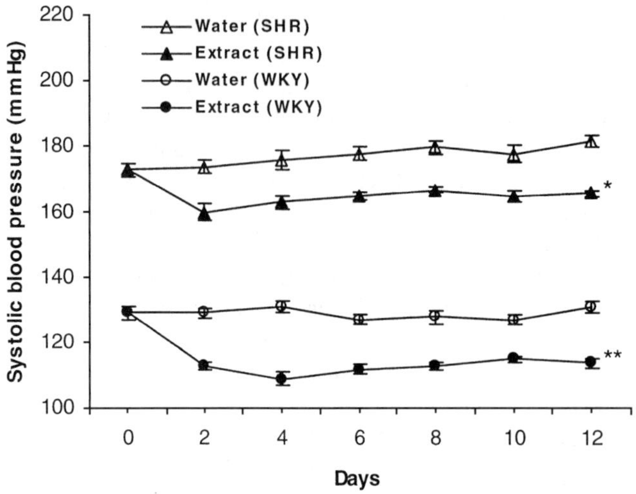

FIGURE 3 Changes in mean systolic blood pressure (SBP) of SHR and WKY rats over a 13-day intraperitoneal infusion of an aqueous extract of *A. paniculata* (0.7 g/kg) or distilled water. Values shown are the mean ± SEM. SBP of seven animals in each group (except extract-treated SHR, $n = 8$). *Significantly lower than the vehicle-treated SHR ($p = 0.0001$, two-way ANOVA). **Significantly lower than the vehicle-treated WKY ($p = 0.0001$, two-way ANOVA).

It appeared from this initial study that the hypotensive responses to *A. paniculata* were related neither to the basal level of SBP nor to the strain of rat. The finding that ACE activity was depressed in the plasma but not lungs of extract-treated SHR suggests that the extract may exert its hypotensive effect in SHR by selectively inhibiting the activity of the circulating renin-angiotensin system. However, no change in either plasma or lung ACE activities occurred in the extract-treated WKY rats, which also had a significant fall in SBP. This suggests that in the normotensive rat, *A. paniculata* extract may have a different mode of hypotensive action, such as calcium channel blockade, resulting in vascular smooth muscle relaxation, or interaction with the sympathetic nervous system and its receptors at either central or peripheral levels.

Captopril, an ACE inhibitor that is widely used in the treatment of human hypertension, has the ability to scavenge free radicals (20). This could result in the sparing of PGI_2 and NO degradation, thus indicating the possibility of a second, and possibly indirect, mode of hypotensive action. Our finding that the hypotensive effect of the *A. paniculata* extract was associated with reduced ACE activity and reduced kidney lipid peroxidation level indicates some similarity to the effects of captopril.

IV. FURTHER STUDIES WITH FRACTIONS OF *A. PANICULATA* EXTRACT AND SOME DITERPENOID DERIVATIVES

A. paniculata extract was fractionated with solvents to obtain three fractions with different polarity—FA (ethyl acetate fraction), FB (butanol fraction), and FC (aqueous fraction). These were tested in the anesthetized normotensive Sprague-Dawley (SD) rat to evaluate their effects on the mean arterial blood pressure (MAP). MAP is the average systolic pressure that drives blood through the systemic organs and is thus a critical cardiovascular parameter. We found that FA did not reduce MAP in the anesthetized SD rat, while the crude aqueous extract of *A. paniculata* (WE), FB, and FC produced a significant fall in MAP in a dose-dependent manner without significant decrease in heart rate, the ED_{50} values for WE, FB, and FC being 11.4, 5.0, and 8.6 mg/kg, respectively (Fig. 4). These findings suggested that the hypotensive substance(s) in the crude water extract was concentrated in FB.

The lack of significant change in the heart rate suggests also that the hypotensive compound(s) in the FB fraction of *A. paniculata* extract may not have a direct action on the heart.

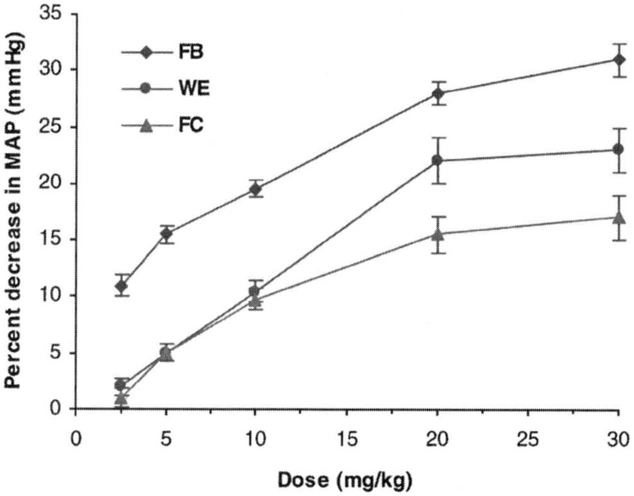

FIGURE 4 The effects of a crude water extract of *A. paniculata* (WE), its semi-purified butanol fraction (FB), and aqueous fraction (FC) on MAP of anaesthetized SD rats. Points represent the mean percent change in MAP of six animals in each group; bars indicate the SEM.

Pharmacological antagonist studies were performed using the FB fraction (5 mg/kg) to further evaluate the mechanism(s) of hypotensive action. The findings showed that the α-adrenoceptor, muscarinic cholinergic receptor, and ACE were not involved in the hypotensive action of FB. This was because this action was not affected by propranolol, atropine, and captopril, respectively (Fig. 5). Furthermore, in the presence of hexamethonium, pyrilamine, and cimetidine, the decreases in MAP induced by FB were significantly attenuated, suggesting that the hypotensive action of FB might involve the autonomic ganglion and histaminergic systems. In addition, the data also indicated that the α-adrenoceptors are involved, since phentolamine almost completely abolished the hypotensive effect.

The following diterpenoids from *A. paniculata* were tested for their effects on the MAP of anesthetized SD rats: DA, DDA, andrographolide, andrographiside, neoandrographolide. We found that andrographolide, andrographiside, and neoandrographolide were without effect on the MAP

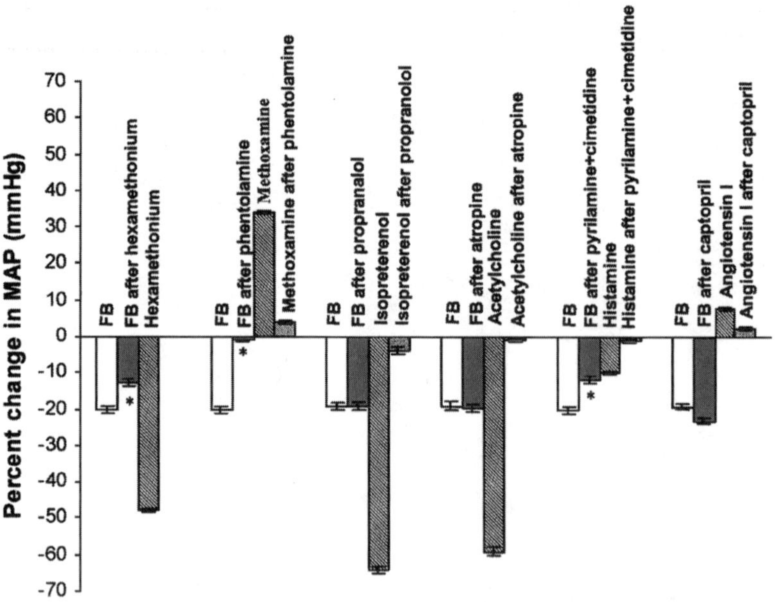

FIGURE 5 The effects of ganglionic, α- and β-adrenergic, muscarinic cholinergic, and histaminergic receptor blocking agents, and captopril on the hypotensive action of butanol fraction (FB) from crude water extract of *A. paniculata*. Columns represent the mean percent change in MAP of six animals; bars indicate the SEM. *Denotes that hypotensive responses of FB were significantly reduced from those of control.

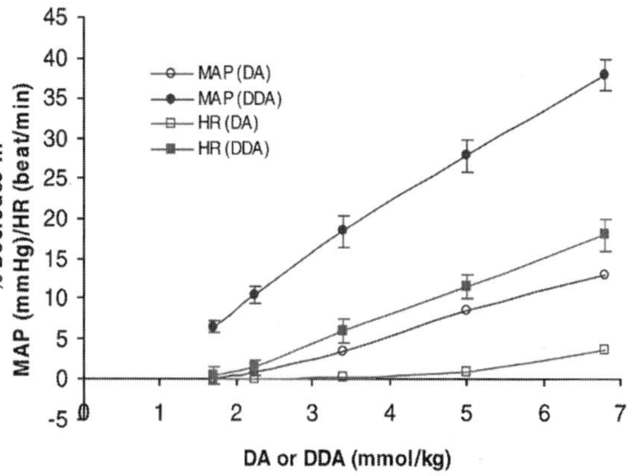

Figure 6 Effects of DA or DDA on MAP and HR of anesthetized SD rats. Each point represents the mean percentage decrease in MAP or HR of eight animals; bars indicate the SEM.

of the anesthetized rat. DDA dose-dependently decreased MAP and heart rate while DA had a weaker effect on these parameters than DDA (Fig. 6). It thus appeared that the hypotensive effect of *A. paniculata* could be contributed by at least these two diterpenoids.

V. EFFECTS OF DA AND DDA ON ISOLATED RAT THORACIC AORTA

Further studies were done with DA and DDA to investigate their effects on phenylephrine- and high-K^+-induced contractions of the rat thoracic aorta.

The results showed that both DA and DDA had a vasorelaxant property as they inhibited contractions induced by phenylephrine and high K^+ in a concentration-dependent manner in endothelium-intact aorta. They also antagonized the concentration-response curve of phenylephrine in a noncompetitive manner. The effect was attenuated in endothelium-denuded aorta without modifying the maximal response. This suggested that the vasorelaxant effect of DA and DDA was partly dependent on the endothelium.

The vascular endothelium plays an important role in controlling the vascular tone via secretion of both relaxant and contractile factors (21). The most potent known are the vasodilators NO and PGI_2 and the vasoconstrictors angiotensin II and endothelin. NO is synthesized from the amino acid L-arginine, a family of nitric oxide synthetase (NOS) isoenzymes, including endothelial NOS (eNOS), neuronal NOS (nNOS), and inducible NOS (iNOS). NO stimulates cyclic GMP production by activating soluble guanylate cyclase (21) and thus causes vasodilatation.

Like verapamil, both DA and DDA produced a much greater vasorelaxant effect in aorta precontracted by KCl than by phenylephrine. In Ca^{2+}-free medium, these diterpenoids antagonized Ca^{2+}-induced vasoconstraction in a concentration-dependent manner and almost abolished both caffeine- and norepinephrine-induced transient contractions. Their vasorelaxant effects were partly antagonized by the competitive nitric oxide (NO)-synthase inhibitor N^G-nitro-L-arginine methyl ester (L-NAME), and also by methylene blue, a soluble guanylate cyclase inhibitor, but were unaffected by both indomethacin, a cyclo-oxygenase inhibitor and glibenclamide, an ATP-sensitive K^+-channel blocker. These results suggest that the vasorelaxant activity of DA and DDA may be mediated via the activation of nitric oxide synthase and guanylate cyclase, as well as the blockade of Ca^{2+} influx through both voltage- and receptor-operated Ca^{2+} channels. Compared to DA, DDA had a stronger vasorelaxant activity.

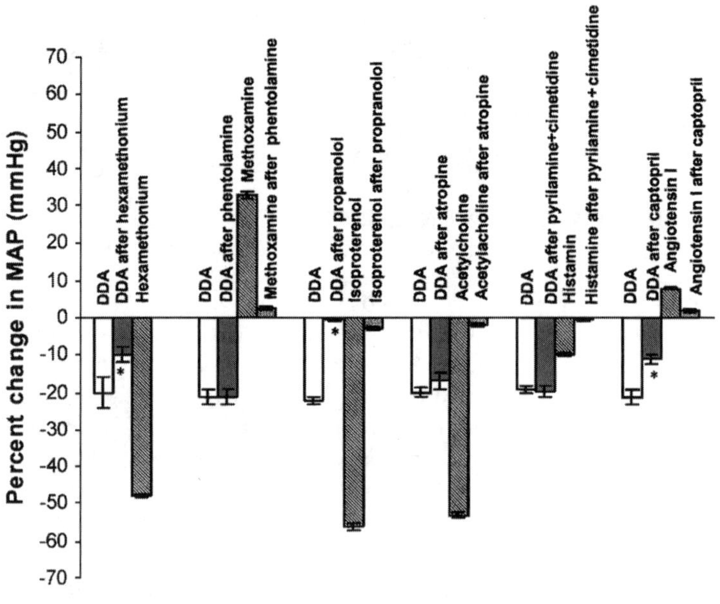

FIGURE 7 The effects of ganglionic, α- and β-adrenergic, muscarinic cholinergic and histaminergic receptor blocking agents, and captopril on the hypotensive acatin of DDA. Columns represent the mean percent change in MAP of six animals; bars indicate the SEM. *Denotes that hypotensive responses of DDA were significantly reduced from those of control ($p < 0.05$, t-test).

VI. EFFECTS OF DDA IN ANESTHETIZED SD RATS AND ISOLATED RAT RIGHT ATRIA

We found that DDA produced significant decreases in both MAP and heart rate in a dose-dependent manner (Fig. 6). The ED50 value for MAP was 3.4 mmol/kg. Pharmacological antagonist studies were subsequently done with this dose. We found that the hypotensive action of DDA was not mediated through effects on the α-adrenoceptor, muscarinic cholinergic, or histaminergic receptors, for it was not affected by phentolamine, atropine, pyrilamine, or cimetidine (Fig. 7). However, in the presence of propranolol, hexamethonium, and captopril, the hypotensive effect was negated or attenuated, suggesting the involvement of β-adrenoceptors, autonomic ganglia receptor, and ACE.

In spontaneously beating isolated rat right atria, DDA caused a negative chronotropic effect (Fig. 8), indicating that it may have direct β_1-adrenoceptor blocking action on the heart in addition to its α-adrenergic receptor inhibitory activity. The bradycardic effect of DDA may also contribute to the hypotensive action. This discordant finding, compared to

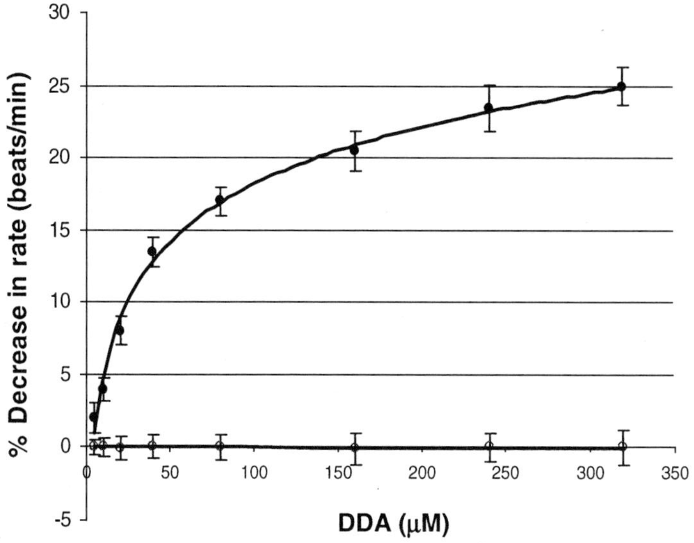

FIGURE 8 Effect of DDA (•, $n = 10$) on the beating rate of isolated right atria from normotensive rats. Vehicle-treated control group (DMSO, o, $n = 5$). Points represent the mean ± SEM of values. All points on the DDA curve were significantly different from the corresponding points on the control ($p < 0.05$, t-test).

the earlier finding of a lack of effect of FB on the heart of the anesthetized SD rat, may be explained by the fact that DDA is either absent or else present in FB in such small amounts as to have no significant effect on the heart rate.

VII. EFFECTS OF DA AND DDA ON ENDOTHELIAL CELL PRODUCTION OF NITRIC OXIDE

As our earlier studies suggested that the relaxation of the isolated rat aorta caused by DA and DDA may be mediated through the L-arginine-NO synthase pathway and NO activation of guanylate cyclase, it was decided to study the effects of DDA on NO production by human endothelial cell cultures. NO was quantified spectrometrically by the accumulation of nitrite produced by endothelial cells cultured in F12 medium for up to 48 hr. This method has been documented by previous workers (22,23).

We found that DA and DDA significantly stimulated NO production by endothelial cells in a concentration-dependent manner. This suggests another possible mechanism for their hypotensive effect.

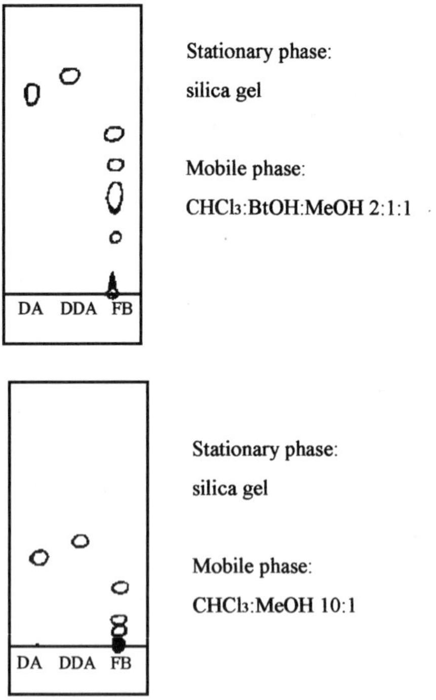

FIGURE 9 Comparison of DA, DDA, and FB by TLC.

VIII. THIN-LAYER CHROMATOGRAPHIC (TLC) ANALYSIS OF FB FOR THE PRESENCE OF DA AND DDA

As our studies thus far suggested that DA and DDA were compounds that, like FB, had significant effects on the cardiovascular parameters of experimental rats, the FB fraction was analyzed by TLC to confirm the presence of these bioactive compounds. No detectable amounts of either DA or DDA were, however, found in FB (Fig. 9). This provided the explanation for a lack of effect of FB on heart rate (unlike DDA) and suggested that the bioactivity in FB could be attributed to compounds other than DA and DDA and that furthermore there were other compound(s) in the crude water extract of *A. paniculata* that could produce a hypotensive effect.

IX. CONCLUSION

This series of studies have shown that DA and DDA, having pharmacological actions that lead to a lowering in blood pressure, could serve as potential lead molecules for the development of new antihypertensive compounds. Further purification of FB could yield new compound(s) with hypotensive properties. Last but not least, our studies indicate that the practice of drinking an infusion of leaves of this bitter herb for treating hypertension may indeed have some scientific merit.

ACKNOWLEDGMENTS

The authors acknowledge the generosity of Professor Masanori Kuroyanagi, School of Pharmaceutical Sciences, University of Shizuoka, 52-1 Yada, Shizuoka-shi 422, Japan in supplying andrographolide, DA, and DDA for our studies. We also thank the National University of Singapore for providing the research grant (RP960329) for the study and the research scholarship awarded to C.-Y. Zhang.

REFERENCES

1. Cava MP, Chan WR, Stein RP, Willis CR. Andrographolide, further transformations and stereochemical evidence: the structure of andrographolide. Tetrahedron 1965; 21:2617–2632.
2. Balmain A, Connolly JD. Minor diterpenoid constituents of *Andrographis paniculata* Nees. J Chem Soc Perk Trans 1973; 1:1247–1251.
3. Chan WR, Taylor DR, Willis CR, Bodden RL. The structure on stereochemistry of neoandrographolide, a diterpene glucoside from *Andrographis paniculata*. Tetrahedron 1971; 27:5081–5091.
4. Chen WM, Liang XT. Deoxyandrographolide-19-D-glucoside from the leaves of *Andrographis paniculata*. Planta Med 1987; 53:245–246.

5. Hu CQ, Zhao BN. Studies on the diterpenes of Chun Xin Lian (*Andrographis paniculata*). Chin Trad Herb Drugs 1981; 12:531.
6. Fujita T, Fujitani R, Takeda Y, Takaishi Y, Yamada T, Kido M, Muira I. On the diterpenoid of *Andrographis paniculata*: Xray crystallographic analysis of andrographolide and structure determination of new minor diterpenoids. Chem Pharm Bull 1984; 32:2117–2225.
7. Hu CQ, Zhao BN, Chou PN. Isolation and structure of two new diterpenoid glucosides from *Andrographis paniculata* Nee. Acta Pharmacol Sin 1982; 17: 435–440.
8. Matsuda T, Kuroyanagi M, Sugiyama S, Umehara K, Ueno A, Nishi K. Cell differentiation-inducing diterpenes from *Andrographis paniculata* Nees. Chem Pharm Bull 1994; 42:1216–1225.
9. Kuroyanagi M, Sato M, Ueno A, Nishi K. Flavonoids from *Andrographis paniculata*. Chem Pharm Bull 1987; 35:4429–4435.
10. Tang W, Eisenbrand G. Chinese Drugs of Plant Origin: Chemistry, Pharmacology, Use in Traditional and Modern Medicine. Berlin: Springer-Verlag, 1992: 97–103.
11. Deng WL, Nie RJ, Liu JY. Comparison of pharmacological effect of four andrographolides. Chin Pharm Bull 1982; 17:195–198.
12. Ahmad M, Asmawi MZ. Some pharmacological effects of aqueous extract of *Andrographis paniculata* Nees. In: Gan EK, ed. The International Conference on the Use of Traditional Medicine and other Natural Products in Health Care. School of Pharmaceutical Sciences, University of Science, Malaysia, June 8–11, 1993. [abstr]
13. Wang DW, Zhao HY. Promotion of atherosclerotic stenosis and restenosis after angioplasty with *Andrographis paniculata* Nees and fish oil: experimental studies of effects and mechanism. Chin Med J (Eng). 1994; 107:464–470.
14. Cushman DW, Cheung HS. Studies in vitro of angiotensin converting enzyme of lung and other tissues. In: Genest J, Koiw E, eds. Hypertension. Berlin: Springer, 1972:532–541.
15. Suryaprabha P, Das UN, Koratkar R, Sangeetha SP, Ramesh G. Free radical generation, lipid peroxidation and essential fatty acids in uncontrolled essential hypertension. Prostag Leuko Essent Fatty Acids 1990; 41:27–33.
16. Ikemoto F, Song GB, Tominaga M, Yamamoto K. Oxidation-induced increase in activity of angiotensin converting enzyme in the rat kidney. Biochem Biophys Res Commun 1988; 153:1017–1031.
17. Gryglewski RJ, Palmer RMG, Moncada S. Superoxide anion is involved in the breakdown of endothelium-derived vascular relaxing factor. Nature 1986; 320:454–456.
18. Shen YC, Chen CF, Chiou WF. Suppression of rat neutrophil reactive oxygen species production and adhesion by the diterpenoid alctone andrographolide. Planta Med 2000; 6694:314–317.
19. Zhang XF, Tan BKH. Antihyperglycaemic and anti-oxidant properties of *Andrographis paniculata* in normal and diabetic rats. Clin Exp Pharmacol Physiol 2000; 27(5–6):358–363.

20. Bagchi D, Prasad R, Das DK. Direct scavenging effects of free radicals by captopril, an angiotensin converting enzyme inhibitor. Biochem Biophys Res Commun 1989; 158:52–57.
21. McQuillan LP, Leung GK, Marsden PA, Kostyk SK, Keurembanas S. Hypoxia inhibits expression of eNOS via transcriptional and post-transcriptional mechanisms. Am J Physiol 1994; 267:H1921–H1297.
22. Feder LS, Laskin DL. Regulation of hepatic endothelial cell and macrophage proliferation and nitric oxide production by GM-CSF, M-CSF and IL-1β following acute endotoxaemia. J Leucocyte Biol 1994; 55:507–513.
23. Li JM, Fenton RA, Cutler BS, Dobson JG, Jr. Adenosine enhances nitric oxide production by vascular endothelial cells. Am J Physiol 1995; 269(Cell Physiol 38):C519–C523.

20

Rosemary

Elizabeth Offord
Nestlé Research Center
Lausanne, Switzerland

I. ROSEMARY EXTRACTS: PREPARATION AND COMPOSITION

A. Preparation

The leaves of the plant *Rosmarinus officinalis* L. are best known as a spice and flavoring agent but they are also reported as a herbal remedy with antioxidant, anti-inflammatory, anticarcinogenic, antidiuretic, and hepatotoxic protective properties (1–3). Crude and refined extracts of *R. officinalis* L. are commercially available in the form of powders and liquids at different concentrations of the active components (e.g., Robertet S.A., Grasse, France; LycoRed Natural Products Industries, Beer Sheva, Israel; Kalsec Inc., Michigan, USA).

To overcome the problem of odor, color, and taste associated with rosemary components, refined rosemary extracts are prepared. Manufacturing procedures generally involve two steps. In the first step, the essential oils of rosemary are removed by steam distillation or selective solvent extraction. The residue (dried leaves) is extracted with different solvents, such as hexane, methanol, ethanol, and acetone (4–8), or, alternatively, by supercritical fluid processing with carbon dioxide (9). The final preparation is almost without odor and color and has a high antioxidant capacity, similar to the synthetic antioxidants butylated hydroxyanisole (BHA) and butylated hydroxytoluene (BHT).

B. Composition

The composition of rosemary extracts varies according to their extraction procedure. A large number of antioxidant components have been identified (5,6,10–14). The most potent antioxidant components are the diterpenes carnosol and carnosic acid, which account for 90% of the antioxidant potential in certain extracts (15). Interestingly, in the plant, carnosic acid is localized to subcellular compartments and its function is to protect chloroplasts against oxidative stress (16). Other phenolics and minor constituents such as rosmanol, isorosmanol, rosmaridiphenol, and rosmariquinone also have antioxidant activity (11–14). Some components of rosemary extracts that do not have strong antioxidant activity but may be involved in the

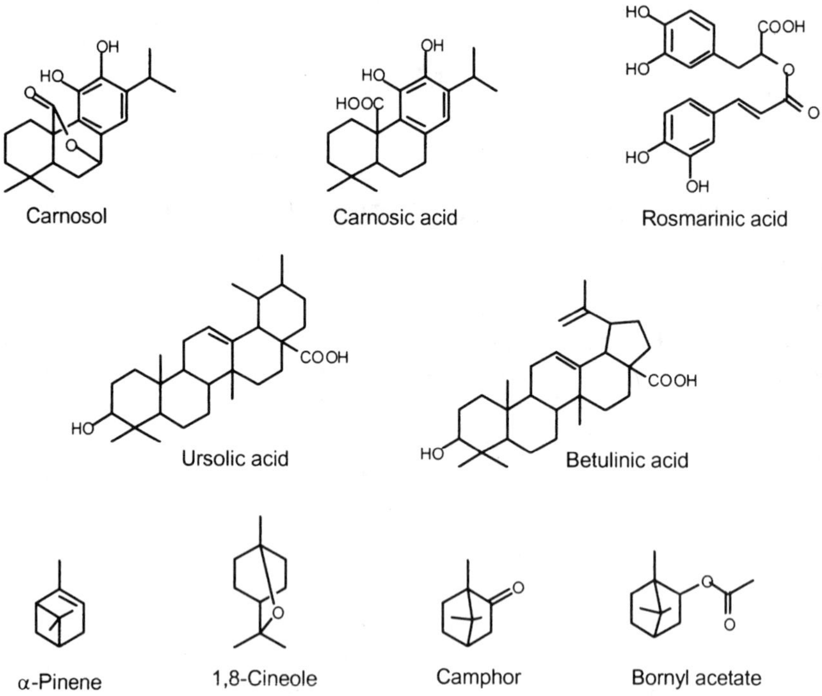

FIGURE 1 Structures of some typical components of rosemary extracts or essential oils.

anticarcinogenic activity include the triterpenic acids ursolic acid, oleanolic acid, and betulinic acid (17–19).

Analysis of a commercially available water-soluble extract (Robertet S.A., France) showed a high content of rosmarinic acid (1.2%), flavones (glycoside and glucuronide of 6-hydroxyluteolin and aglyones derived from apigenin and chrysin, around 3%), and some monoterpenes (verbenone, α-terpineol, 1,8-cineole, camphor, and limonene) (20). A dichloromethane extract contained mainly flavonoids and phenolic diterpenes (21). Two flavones were identified as cirsimaritin and genkwanin. Phenolic diterpenes were carnosic acid and its derivatives, carnosol, rosmanol, epirosmanol methyl ether, and traces of epirosmanol. The triterpene ursolic acid was not detected. Glucuronides of the flavonoid luteolin, together with hesperedin, were isolated from 50% aqueous methanol extract of rosemary leaves (22).

The essential oil of rosemary is obtained primarily from the apical part of the plant and the leaves (23). Around 50 constituents have been identified but the essential oil is principally rich in monoterpenes and sesquiterpene hydrocarbons, which vary according to the geographic origin (24). Spanish oils were found to be rich in α-pinene, 1,8-cineole, and camphor while the French oils possessed α-pinene, 1,8 cineole, and bornyl acetate and Moroccan oils were typically rich in 1,8-cineole. Some minor constituents include β-pinene, β-caryophylene, camphene, limonene, myrcene, camphor, borneol, α-terpineol, and terpinen-4-ol (21,24)(Fig. 1).

II. CHEMICAL AND BIOLOGICAL ACTIVITIES

A. Antioxidant Properties in Food and Biological Systems

During storage of prepared or dehydrated food, lipid autoxidative degradation products such as hydroperoxides, malondialdehydes, aldehydes, ketones, and hydroxy fatty acids may occur if the food is not properly protected by antioxidants. These products not only result in unpleasant flavors but may also be a health risk (25). Lipid oxidation is an autocatalyzed radical chain reaction induced by free radicals (26). Polyphenolic antioxidants possess a relatively reactive phenolic hydrogen atom, which functions as a donor, allowing formation of the antioxidant phenoxyl radical. Various extracts have been shown to act as effective antioxidants in food systems such as stabilization of animal fats and vegetable oils as well as wheat, rice, oat or potato flakes, frozen ground pork patties, and dehydrated chicken meat (27–32). Extracts of rosemary containing the polyphenolic antioxidants, or preparations of the essential oil, show potent antimicrobial properties, inhibiting the growth and survival of food-borne microorganisms (33–35). Rosemary extracts also show antiviral activity in vitro (36).

The high antioxidant capacity of rosemary components suggests a beneficial effect not only in combatting degeneration of foods through oxidation or microbial contamination but also to health in scavenging free radicals that are implicated in human disease. Rosemary extracts carnosol and carnosic acid inhibit lipid peroxidation and deoxyribose damage and scavenge hydrogen peroxide, hypochlorous acid, peroxynitrite, peroxyl, and hydroxyl radicals in lipid and nonlipid systems (15,37,38). Rosemary extract and antioxidant components inhibit oxidation of low-density lipoprotein (LDL) and show a synergistic effect with lycopene from oleoresin (39,40).

B. Chemoprotective Properties of Rosemary

Carcinogenesis is a multistage process consisting of initiation, promotion, and progression. Protection against both the initiation and tumor promotion stages of carcinogenesis is one of the important findings obtained with phenolic antioxidants such as teas and rosemary (1,2).

1. Animal Studies

Topical application of a methanol extract of rosemary, carnosol, or ursolic acid to mouse skin inhibited the covalent binding of benzo(a)pyrene [B(a)P] to epidermal DNA and inhibited tumor initiation by B(a)P and 7,12-dimethylbenz(a)anthracene (DMBA) (19). Dietary intake of 0.5–1% crude rosemary extract by rats for 2–3 weeks before administration of DMBA reduced mammary gland tumor incidence and inhibited in vivo binding of DMBA metabolites to mammary epithelial cell DNA (41–43).

Many chemoprotective agents act through induction of Phase II detoxifying enzymes such as glutathione S-transferase (GST), NAD(P)H:quinone reductase (QR), or UDP-glucuronosyltransferase (UGT) (44,45). In rats fed rosemary as 0.25–1.0% of their diet, the activities of liver GST and QR enzymes were induced 3–4-fold (46). Similarly, rats fed various (water or dichloromethane) extracts of rosemary at 0.5% of their diet for 2 weeks resulted in stimulation of GST, QR, and UGT enzyme activities (20,21). Surprisingly, in contrast to the results reported with ethanolic extracts in human cells (described below), the water extract of rosemary also induced the Phase I, cytochrome P450 (CYP450) enzymes. This difference in effect on CYP450 enzymes may be due to the composition of the water (rich in rosmarinic acid) and ethanolic (rich in carnosol and carnosic acid) extracts. Alternatively, it may be due to a species difference between rat and human CYP450 metabolism or to the generation of secondary metabolites in vivo with different effects from the intact molecules administered in in vitro studies.

Topical application of a methanol extract of rosemary, carnosol, or ursolic acid to mouse skin resulted in strong inhibitory effects on 12-O-tetradecanoylphorbol-13-acetate (TPA)-induced inflammation, omithine decarboxylase (ODC) activity, and tumor promotion, as well as on arachidonic-acid-induced inflammation (19). Anti-tumor-promoting activity in mouse skin has also been reported for betulinic acid and oleanolic acid (17,18).

2. Cellular Mechanisms

The antimutagenic (47) and antigenotoxic effects of rosemary components may be partly mediated by their antioxidant properties in scavenging free radicals involved in DNA oxidation. Indeed, carnosic acid, carnosol, rosmarinic acid, and ursolic acid effectively inhibited DNA strand breakage induced by the Fenton reaction, suggesting effective scavenging of the hydroxyl radical (48), and an ethanolic extract of rosemary showed antigenotoxic effects against DNA damage induced by H_2O_2 in CaCo-2 colon cancer cells and in hamster lung cells V79 (49).

Modulation of metabolic enzymes involved in activation and detoxification of carcinogens is an important mechanism in chemoprotection. An ethanolic extract of rosemary extract, carnosol and carnosic acid, inhibited DNA adduct formation by the lung carcinogen B(a)P in human bronchial (BEAS-2B) cells through inhibition of the activity of the CYP450 enzyme CYP1A1, involved in the activation of B(a)P to its DNA-binding epoxide, benzo(a)pyrene-(+)-anti-7,8-dihydrodiol-9,10-epoxide (anti-BPDE) (50). Furthermore, carnosol (3 μM) induced expression of the Phase II enzyme glutathione S-transferase π (GST π) involved in the detoxification of the proximate carcinogenic metabolite of B(a)P. Therefore, in human bronchial cells rosemary extract acts by a dual mechanism involving inhibition of Phase I–activating enzymes and induction of Phase II–detoxifyig enzymes. Similarly, in human liver cells expressing CYP1A2 or CYP3A4, rosemary extract inhibited the formation of DNA adducts by the epoxide of the mycotoxin aflatoxin B_1 (AFB_1) through inhibiting the enzyme activity of CYP1A2 and CYP3A4 (51). In the human liver, it is not clear how aflatoxin epoxide (AFBO) is detoxified, as none of the GSTs have a strong affinity for AFBO; therefore, inhibition of CYP450 metabolism may be the dominant mechanism of protection against AFB_1-induced genotoxicity.

The enzyme NADPH:quinone reductase (QR) is important for detoxification of highly reactive quinone intermediates and has been associated with anticarcinogenic activity (45). Many chemoprotective agents induce QR by a transcriptional activation mechanism acting through upstream promoter sequences (52). Indeed, carnosol induced QR mRNA levels in human bronchial cells (50). Quinone reductase activity has been conveniently studied in the mouse hepatoma cell line Hepa 1c1c7 (53). Rosemary components effectively induce QR in these cells (54). In our studies, we found that QR activity was induced twofold by 1.0 μM carnosol compared to 0.2 μM sulforaphane, a component of broccoli known to be a potent inducer of QR.

Cellular mechanisms relevant to tumor promotion are affected by rosemary components. Growth inhibitory and differentiation effects of carnosic acid (2.5–10 μM) were shown in human leukemic cells (55). Carnosic acid inhibited cell proliferation through interference with cell cycle progression without induction of apoptotic or necrotic cell death. Low concentrations of carnosic acid significantly potentiated the action of the differentiation agents all-*trans* retinoic acid and 1,25-dihydroxyvitamin D_3. In contrast, in another study with carnosol and leukemic cell lines, carnosol induced apoptotic cell death and downregulated Bcl-2 (56).

Nitric oxide (NO) is a small, short-lived molecule that is synthesized from L-arginine by NO synthase (NOS) and released from cells in response to a number of homeostatic and pathological stimuli (57). NO is involved in diverse physiological and pathological processes such as vasodilation, neurotransmission, inflammation and the immune response, platelet inhibition, cellular signalling, and free radical (peroxynitrite)-induced cytotoxicity and can be regulated by dietary factors (58,59). The inducible form of NOS (iNOS) is upregulated under inflammatory conditions and in response to cytokines, resulting in a relatively high and sustained level of NO production. Overproduction of NO may lead to production of damaging reactive nitrogen species such as nitrate, nitrite, peroxynitrite, and 3-nitrotyrosine with cytotoxic and genotoxic consequences (60,61). Carnosol has been shown to inhibit lipopolysaccharide and interferon-gamma induced NO production in activated mouse macrophages in a concentration-related manner (2–10 μM) (48,62). The mechanism involves inhibition of iNOS mRNA and protein expression by blocking activation of the transcription factor NF-κB through interference with the signal-induced phosphorylation of its inhibitor, IκB (48). The NF-κB family of transcription factors regulates the expression of many genes involved in immune and inflammatory responses. Therefore, inhibition of NF-κB activation provides a possible mechanism for the anti-inflammatory and anti-tumor-promoting action of carnosol.

The lipoxygenase pathways of arachidonic acid metabolism produce reactive oxygen species, which may play a role in inflammation and tumor promotion. Rosemary extracts carnosol and ursolic acid inhibited soybean 15-lipoxygenase activity (31). Since soybean lipoxygenase bears many similarities to the mammalian lipoxygenase enzyme (63), these results further suggest that rosemary components have the potential to inhibit lipoxygenase enzymes, which is another potential mechanism for the anti-tumor-promoting activity of rosemary components.

III. OTHER HEALTH BENEFITS ASSOCIATED WITH ROSEMARY

A. Diruetic Effects

Herbal remedies are widely used in the pharmacopoeia. Among them, rosemary extracts are recommended for urinary ailments. An experimental study in rats demonstrated a diuretic effect after 5–6 days of oral administration of an aqueous extracts of *R. officinalis* L. by measuring changes in urinary volume and electrolyte excretion (64).

B. Hepatoprotective Effects

An essential oil and ethanolic extract from *R. officinalis* L. showed hepatoprotective effects in rats treated with carbon tetrachloride (65). *R. tomentosus* is a vegetal species closely related to the culinary rosemary *R. officinalis*. A dried ethanol extract of the aerial parts of *R. tomentosus* and its major fraction separated by column chromatography showed antihepatotoxic activity in rats with acute liver damage but the active compounds were not identified (66).

C. Cosmetic Benefits

Dietary antioxidants such as vitamin C, vitamin E, and β-carotene show a potential to combat the oxidative processes involved in skin ageing (67). An alcoholic extract of rosemary leaves, Rosm1, with strong antioxidant properties was shown to inhibit oxidative alterations to skin surface lipids (68) and to attenuate oxidative-stress-induced modifications in heat shock protein expression and modification in cellular thiol and carbonyl content in human skin fibroblasts (69). Carnosic acid (1–3 μM), like vitamin E, showed photoprotective effects against ultraviolet A (UVA) radiation in human skin fibroblasts by suppressing the UVA-induced rise in metalloproteinase-1 mRNA expression (70). Taken together, these results suggest a potentially interesting application of rosemary extract, or its components, in cosmetic dermatology.

IV. POTENTIAL ADVERSE EFFECTS

Very few studies have addressed the question of adverse effects of consuming high quantities of spice extracts or polyphenolic antioxidants. Since one of the postulated mechanisms of antioxidant action is chelation of pro-oxidant metals such as iron, a recent human study examined the effect of polyphenolic-rich green tea and rosemary extracts on the absorption of nonheme iron (71). It was found that green tea and rosemary extracts added to foods decreased absorption of nonheme iron by around 20%, indicating that indeed iron was chelated by the extracts. Therefore, caution is required in dealing with iron-deficient populations.

A study was carried out investigating the embryotoxic effects of rosemary extract in pregnant rats (72). Twenty-six milligrams of a 30% (w/v) *R. officinalis* aqueous extract was administered by gavage during two different periods of Wistar rat pregnancy. No effects of rosemary extract were observed on postimplantation loss or fetus anomalies but a slight, though not significant, increase in preimplantation loss was observed. The authors conclude that this finding might explain the use of the plant aqueous extract as an abortive in Brazilian folk medicine, but further studies using higher doses would be required to demonstrate a significant effect.

V. CLINICAL EFFICACY TRIALS

Until now, no human efficacy trials have been performed with rosemary extracts and no detailed pharmacokinetic data exist. Therefore, there is a clear need to perform clinical studies addressing the uptake and metabolism of rosemary components and their efficacy on biomarkers of human health. Studies in animals suggest a problem of bioavailability of individual components of rosemary extracts when given orally. For example, although dietary administration of rosemary extract enhanced the activity of Phase II enzymes in the rat, carnosol exhibited this effect only when given intraperitoneally (36,43). Similarly, an aqueous extract of rosemary, but neither carnosic acid nor rosmarinic acid, stimulated Phase II enzymes in the rat possibly owing to a problem of absorption of the individual components (20). Rosemary extract provides a natural mixture of bioactive components that may turn out to be more effective than single components, especially when delivered in foods. Therefore, it will be important to investigate the bioavailability of single rosemary components compared to whole extracts or even the leaves themselves and to determine the active dose for health benefits.

VI. CONCLUSIONS AND FUTURE PERSPECTIVES

Rosemary extracts and their polyphenolic components may have an application in the food industry that exceeds that of traditional flavoring and stabilizing agents. Their potential impact on human health is now a challenging concept for the development of natural, healthy foods. Although spices have been used in cooking and flavoring for centuries, they have not been consumed in the higher quantities used in the experimental studies summarized here. Therefore, before any health claims can be made, it is necessary to carry out safety and efficacy trials and to determine the active dose. Efficacy, safety, and regulatory issues are linked to composition of the complex plant extracts and their pleiotrophic effects. Clearly, the success of human efficacy trials will depend on the availability of a valid biomarker approach as indicator of improved health or reduced disease status. In conclusion, although rosemary has many interesting flavoring, food-stabilizing, and therapeutic properties, no health claims can be made until efficacy has been demonstrated in clinical trials.

REFERENCES

1. Ho C-T, Ferraro T, Chen Q, Rosen RT, Huang M-T. Phytochemicals in teas and rosemary and their cancer-preventive properties. In: Ho C-T, Toshihiko O, Huang M-T, Rosen RT, eds. Food Phytochemicals for Cancer Prevention II. Washington, DC: ACS Symposium Series 547. 1994:2–19.
2. Offord EA, Guillot F, Aeschbach R, Löliger J, Pfeifer AMA. Antioxidant and biological properties of rosemary components: Implications for food and health. In: Shahidi F, ed. Natural Antioxidants: Chemistry, Health Effects, and Applications. Champaign, IL: AOCS Press, 1997:88–96.
3. Wargovich MJ, Woods C, Hollis DM, Zander ME. Herbals, cancer prevention and health. J Nutr 2001; 131:3034S–3036S.
4. Bracco U, Löliger J, Viret J-L. Production and use of natural antioxidants. J Am Oil Chem Soc 1981; 58:686–690.
5. Wu JW, Lee MH, Ho CT, Chang SS. Elucidation of the chemical structures of natural antioxidants isolated from rosemary. J Am Oil Chem Soc 1982; 59:339–345.
6. Chang SS, Biserka O-M, Hsieh OAL, Huang C-L. Natural antioxidants from rosemary and sage. J Food Sci 1977; 42:1102–1106.
7. Löliger J, Wille HJ. Natural antioxidants. Oils Fats Int 1993; 9:18–22.
8. Ho CT, Wang M, Wei G, Huang T, Huang M. Chemistry and antioxidative factors in rosemary and sage. Biofactors 2000; 13:161–166.
9. Lopez-Sebastian S, Ramoz E, Ibanez E, Bueno J, Ballester L, Tabera J, Reglero G. Dearomatization of antioxidant rosemary extracts by treatment with supercritical carbon dioxide. J Agric Food Chem 1998; 46:13–19.
10. Inatani R, Nakatani N, Fuwa H, Seto H. Structure of a new antioxidative phenolic diterpene isolated from rosemary (*Rosmarinus officinalis* L.). Agric Biol Chem 1982; 46:1661–1666.
11. Inatani R, Nakatani N, Fuwa H. Antioxidative effect of the constituents of rosemary (*Rosmarinus officinalis* L.) and their derivatives. Agric Biol Chem 1983; 47:521–528.
12. Nakatani N, Inatani R. Two antioxidative diterpenes from rosemary (*Rosmarinus officinalis* L) and a revised structure for rosmanol. Agric Biol Chem 1984; 48:2081–2085.
13. Houlihan CM, Ho C-T, Chang SS. Elucidation of the chemical structure of a novel antioxidant, rosmaridiphenol, isolated from rosemary. J Am Oil Chem Soc 1984; 61:1036–1039.

14. Houlihan CM, Ho C-T, Chang SS. The structure of rosmariquinone—a new antioxidant isolated from *Rosmarinus officinalis* L. J Am Oil Chem Soc 1985; 62:96–99.
15. Aruoma OI, Halliwell B, Aeschbach R, Löliger J. Antioxidant and pro-oxidant properties of active rosemary constituents: carnosol and carnosic acid. Xenobiotica 1992; 22:257–268.
16. Munne-Bosch S, Alegre L. Subcellular compartmentation of the diterpene carnosic acid and its derivatives in the leaves of rosemary. Plant Physiol 2001; 125:1094–1102.
17. Tokuda H, Ohigashi H, Koshimizu K, Ito Y. Inhibitory effects of ursolic acid and oleanic acid on skin tumor promotion by 12-O-tetradecanoylphorbol-13-acetate. Cancer Lett 1986; 33:279–285.
18. Yasukawa K, Takido M, Matsumoto T, Takeuchi M, Nakagawa S. Sterol and triterpene derivatives from plants inhibit the effects of a tumor promoter, and sitosterol and betulinic acid inhibit tumor formation in mouse skin two-stage carcinogenesis. Oncology 1991; 48:72–76.
19. Huang M-T, Ho C-T, Wang ZY, Ferraro T, Lou Y-R, Stauber K, Ma W, Gerogiadis C, Laskin JD, Conney AH. Inhibition of skin tumorigenesis by rosemary and its constituents camosol and ursolic acid. Cancer Res 1994; 54:701–708.
20. Debersac P, Vernevaut M-F, Amiot M-J, Suschetet M, Siess M-H. Effects of a water-soluble extract of rosemary and its purified component rosmarinic acid on xenobiotic metabolizing enzymes in rat liver. Food Chem Toxicol 2001; 39:109–117.
21. Debersac P, Heydel J-M, Amiot M-J, Goudonnet H, Artur Y, Suschetet M, Siess M-H. Induction of cytochrome P450 and/or detoxification enzymes by various extracts of rosemary: description of specific patterns. Food Chem Toxicol 2001; 39:907–918.
22. Okamura N, Haraguchi H, Hashimoto K, Yagi A. Flavonoids in *Rosmarinus officinalis* leaves. Phytochemistry 1994; 37:1463–1466.
23. Flamini G, Cioni P, Morelli I, Macchia M, Ceccarini L. Main agronomic-productive characteristics of two ecotypes of *Rosmarinus officinalis* L. and chemical composition of their essential oils. J Agric Food Chem 2002; 50:3512–3517.
24. Chalchat JC, Garry R-P, Michet A, Benjilali B, Chabart JL. Essential oils of rosemary (*Rosmarinus officinalis* L): the chemical composition of oils of various origins (Morocco, Spain, France). J Essent Oil Res 1993; 5:613–618.
25. Addis PB, Warner GJ. The potential health aspects of lipid oxidation products in foods. In: Aruoma O, Halliwell B, eds. Free Radicals and Food Additives. London: Taylor & Francis, 1991:77–119.
26. Kappus H. Lipid peroxidation: Mechanism and biological relevance. In: Aruoma OI, Halliwell B, eds. Free Radicals and Food Additives. London: Taylor & Francis, 1991:59–75.
27. Löliger J. The use of antioxidants in foods. In: Aruoma OI, Halliwell B, eds. Free Radicals and Food Additives. London: Taylor & Francis, 1991:121–150.
28. Frankel EN, Huang S-W, Prior E, Aeschbach R. Evaluation of antioxidant

activity of rosemary extracts, carnosol and carnosic acid in bulk vegetable oils and fish oil and their emulsions. J Agric Food Chem 1996; 72:201–208.
29. Frankel EN, Huang S-W, Aeschbach R, Prior E. Antioxidant activity of a rosemary extract and its constituents, carnosic acid, carnosol, and rosmarinic acid, in bulk oil and oil-in-water emulsion. J Agric Food Chem 1996; 44:131–135.
30. Huang SW, Frankel EN, Schwarz K, Aeschbach R, German JB. Antioxidant activity of carnosic acid and methyl carnosate in bulk oils and oil-in-water emulsions. J Agric Food Chem 1996; 44:2951–2956.
31. Chen Q, Huang S, Ho C-T. Effects of rosemary extracts and major constituents on lipid oxidation and soybean lipoxygenase activity. J Am Oil Chem Soc 1992; 69:999–1002.
32. Nissen L, Mansson L, Bertelsen G, Huynh-Ba T, Skibsted L. Protection of dehydrated chicken meat by natural antioxidants as evaluated by electron spin resonance spectrometry. J Agric Food Chem 2000; 48:5548–5556.
33. Collin MA, Charles HP. Antimicrobial activity of carnosol and ursolic acid. Food Microbiol 1987; 4:311–315.
34. Del Campo J, Amiot MJ, Nguyen-The C. Antimicrobial effect of rosemary extracts. J Food Prot 2000; 63:1359–1368.
35. Elgayyar M, Draughon FA, Golden DA, Mount JR. Antimicrobial activity of essential oils from plants against selected pathogenic and saprophytic micro-organisms. J Food Prot 2001; 64:1019–1024.
36. Aruoma OI, Spencer JP, Rossi R, Aeschbach R, Khan A, Mahmood N, Munoz A, Murcia A, Butler J, Halliwell B. An evaluation of the antioxidant and antiviral action of extracts of rosemary and Provencal herbs. Food Chem Toxic 1996; 34:449–456.
37. Martinez-Tome M, Jimenez A, Ruggieri S, Frega N, Strabbioli R, Murcia M. Antioxidant properties of Mediterranean spices compared with common food additives. J Food Prot 2001; 64:1412–1419.
38. Choi HR, Choi JS, Han YN, Bae SJ, Chung HY. Peroxynitrite scavenging activity of herb extracts. Phytother Res 2002; 16:364–367.
39. Pearson DA, Frankel EN, Aeschbach R, German JB. Inhibition of endothelial cell–mediated oxidation of low-density lipoprotein by rosemary and plant phenolics. J Agric Food Chem 1997; 45:578–582.
40. Fuhrman B, Volkova N, Rosenblat M, Aviram M. Lycopene synergistically inhibits LDL oxidation in combination with vitamin E, glabridin, rosmarinic acid, carnosic acid or garlic. Antioxid Redox Signal 2000; 2:491–506.
41. Singletary KW, Nelshoppen JM. Inhibition of 7,12-dimethylbenz(a)anthracene (DMBA)-induced mammary tumorigenesis and of in vivo formation of mammary DMBA-DNA adducts by rosemary extract. Cancer Lett 1991; 60:169–175.
42. Singletary KW, MacDonald C, Wallig M. Inhibition by rosemary and carnosol of 7,12-dimethylbenz(a)anthracene(DMBA)-induced rat mammary tumorigenesis and in vivo DMBA-DNA adduct formation. Cancer Lett 1996; 104:43–48.
43. Amagase H, Sakamoto K, Segal ER, Milner JA. Dietary rosemary suppresses 7,12-dimethylbenz(a)anthracene binding to rat mammary cell DNA. J Nutr 1996; 126:1475–1480.

44. Hayes JD, Pulford DJ. The glutathione S-transferase supergene family—regulation of GST and the contribution of the isoenzymes to cancer chemoprotection and drug resistance. Crit Rev Biochem Mol Biol 1995; 30:445–600.
45. Kensler TW, Davidson NE, Groopman JD, Roebuck BD, Prochaska HJ, Talalay PT. Chemoprotection by inducers of electrophile detoxication enzymes. In: Bronzetti G, ed. Antimutagenesis and Anticarcinogenesis Mechanisms III. New York: Plenum Press, 1993:127–136.
46. Singletary KW. Rosemary extract and carnosol stimulate rat liver glutathione S-transferase and quinone reductase activities. Cancer Lett 1996; 100:139–144.
47. Minnuni M, Wolleb U, Mueller O, Pfeifer A, Aeschbacher HU. Natural antioxidants as inhibitors of oxygen species induced mutagenicity. Mutat Res 1992; 269:193–200.
48. Lo AH, Liang YC, Lin-Shiau SY, Ho CT, Lin JK. Carnosol, an antioxidant in rosemary, suppresses inducible nitric oxide synthase through down-regulating nuclear factor-kappa B in mouse macrophages. Carcinogenesis 2002; 23:983–991.
49. Slamenova D, Kuboskova K, Horvathova E, Robichova S. Rosemary-stimulated reduction of DNA strand breaks and FPG-sensitive sites in mammalian cells treated with H_2O_2 or visible light-excited methylene blue. Cancer Lett 2002; 177:145–153.
50. Offord EA, Macé K, Ruffieux C, Malnoë A, Pfeifer AMA. Rosemary components inhibit benzo(a)pyrene-induced genotoxicity in human bronchial cells. Carcinogenesis 1995; 16:2057–2062.
51. Offord EA, Macé K, Avanti O, Pfeifer A. Mechanisms involved in the chemoprotective effects of rosemary extract studied in human liver and bronchial cells. Cancer Lett 1997; 114:1–7.
52. Prestera T, Talalay P. Electrophile and antioxidant regulation of enzymes that detoxify carcinogens. Proc Natl Acad Sci USA 1995; 92:8965–8969.
53. Prochaska HJ, Santamaria AB, Talalay P. Rapid detection of inducers of enzymes that protect against carcinogens. Proc Natl Acad Sci USA 1992; 89: 2394–2398.
54. Tawfiq N, Wanigatunga S, Heaney RK, Musk SRR, Williamson G, Fenwick GR. Induction of the anti-carcinogenic enzyme quinone reductase by food extracts using murine hepatoma cells. Eur J Cancer Prev 1994; 3:285–292.
55. Steiner M, Priel I, Giat J, Levy J, Sharoni Y, Danilenko M. Carnosic acid inhibits proliferation and augments differentiation of human leukemic cells induced by 1,25-dihydroxyvitamin D_3 and retinoic acid. Nutr Cancer 2001; 41:135–144.
56. Dorrie J, Sapala K, Zunino SJ. Carnosol-induced apoptosis and downregulation of Bcl-2 in B-lineage leukemia cells. Cancer Lett 2001; 170:33–39.
57. Moncada S, Palmer RM, Higgs EA. Nitric oxide: physiology, pathophysiology and pharmacology. Pharmacol Rev 1991; 43:109–142.
58. Wu G, Meininger CJ. Regulation of nitric oxide synthesis by dietary factors. Annu Rev Nutr 2002; 22:61–86.
59. Fredstrom S. Nitric oxide, oxidative stress, and dietary antioxidants. Nutrition 2002; 18:537–539.

60. Liu RH, Hotchkiss JH. Potential genotoxicity of chronically elevated nitric oxide: a review. Mutat Res 1995; 339:73–89.
61. Drew B, Leewenburgh C. Aging and the role of reactive nitrogen species. Ann NY Acad Sci 2002; 959:66–81.
62. Chan MM, Ho CT, Huang HI. Effects of three phytochemicals from tea, rosemary and turmeric on inflammation-induced nitrite production. Cancer Lett 1995; 96:23–29.
63. Percival MD. Human 5-lipoxygenase contains an essential iron. J Biol Chem 1991; 266:10058–10061.
64. Haloui M, Louedec L, Michel JB, Lyoussi B. Experimental diuretic effects of *Rosmarinus officinalis* and *Centaurium erythraea*. J Ethnopharmacol 2000; 71:465–472.
65. Fahim FA, Esmat AY, Fadel HM, Hassan KF. Allied studies on the effect of *Rosmarinus officinalis* L. on experimental hepatotoxicity and mutagenesis. Int J Food Sci Nutr 1999; 50:413–427.
66. Galisteo M, Suarez A, del Pilar Montilla M, del Pilar Utrilla M, Jiminez J, Gil A, Faus MJ, Navarro M. Antihepatotoxic activity of *Rosmarinus tomentosus* in a model of acute hepatic damage induced by thioacetamide. Phytother Res 2000; 14:522–526.
67. Fuchs J. Potential and limitations of the natural antioxidants RRR-alpha-tocopherol, L-ascorbic acid and β-carotene in cutaneous photoprotection. Free Rad Biol Med 1998; 25:848–873.
68. Calabrese V, Scapagnini G, Catalano C, Dinotta F, Ceraci D, Morganti P. Biochemical studies of a natural antioxidant isolated from rosemary and its application in cosmetic dermatology. Int J Tissue React 2000; 22:5–13.
69. Calabrese V, Scapagnini G, Catalano C, Bates TE, Dinotta F, Micali G, Giuffrida Stella AM. Induction of heat shock protein synthesis in human skin fibroblasts in response to oxidative stress: regulation by a natural antioxidant from rosemary extracts. Int J Tissue React 2001; 23:51–58.
70. Offord EA, Gautier J-C, Avanti O, Scaletta C, Runge F, Krämer K, Applegate LA. Photoprotective potential of lycopene, β-carotene, vitamin E, vitamin C and carnosic acid in UVA-irradiated human skin fibroblasts. Free Rad Biol Med 2002; 32:1293–1303.
71. Samman S, Sandstrom B, Toft MB, Bukhave K, Jensen M, Sorensen SS, Hansen M. Green tea or rosemary extract added to foods reduces nonheme-iron absorption. Am J Clin Nutr 2001; 73:607–612.
72. Lemonica IP, Damasceno DC, di-Stasi LC. Study of the embryotoxic effects of an extract of rosemary (*Rosmarinus officinalis* L). Braz J Med Biol Res 1996; 29:223–227.

21

Crataegus (Hawthorn)

Walter K. K. Ho, Zhen Yu Chen, and Yu Huang
Chinese University of Hong Kong
Shatin, Hong Kong, China

I. INTRODUCTION

Hawthorn refers to the plant *Crataegus* and is widely distributed throughout the northern temperate regions of the world with approximately 280 species primarily in East Asia, Europe, and North America. Hawthorn fruit tastes sour and sweet and is traditionally used as herbal medicine in China to cure scurvy, constipation, digestive ailment, dyspnea, and kidney stones. In the last several decades, hawthorn fruits have been primarily used in China and Europe for treatment of various cardiovascular disorders (1–4). Consumption of hawthorn fruit has been shown to have long-term medicinal benefits to the cardiovascular system (5,6). The hawthorn fruit has positive effect in treatment of the early stages of congestive heart failure (7,8) and angina pectoris (9). To explore the biochemical mechanisms by which hawthorn fruit possesses such beneficial effects, this chapter focuses mainly on the three major biological properties of hawthorn fruits, viz., hypolipidemic, antioxidant, and blood-vessel-relaxing activity. As many species of the hawthorn plant are distributed throughout the world, the research data we present in this chapter were from the species *Crataegus pinnatifida* Bge. Var. major N.

E.Br. This species is grown mostly in northeastern China and is used frequently in traditional Chinese medicine.

II. HYPOCHOLESTEROLEMIC ACTIVITY

Hawthorn fruit has hypolipidemic activity. Chen et al. (10) demonstrated that serum total cholesterol, triglyceride, and apo-B decreased by 15%, 10%, and 8%, respectively, with HDL cholesterol being unchanged, in 30 hyperlipidemic humans who consumed hawthorn fruit drinks. In a recent unpublished study, we have also evaluated the clinical efficacy of hawthorn in lowering blood cholesterol using a randomized, double-blinded, placebo-controlled, crossover design. Seventy-three mildly hypercholesterolemic patients were asked to take a 250-mL hawthorn or placebo drink three times a day for 4 weeks. At the end of this period, a washout of 4 weeks was implemented before the crossover. Blood samples were taken at baseline and week 4, 9, and 12 for total cholesterol, LDL cholesterol, HDL cholesterol, and triglyceride for analysis. Toxicity was monitored by blood chemistry. The results of this study are shown in Table 1 and Table 2. The hawthorn group had a 7.8% reduction in total blood cholesterol and a 12.4% reduction in LDL cholesterol versus a 0.8% and 4.8% reduction, respectively, in the placebo group in the first phase of the trial. After the crossover, the hawthorn group still had a significant reduction in both total cholesterol (6.7% vs. 3.4%) and LDL cholesterol (13.8% vs. 5.0%) compared with the placebo group. Neither blood triglyceride nor HDL-cholesterol was significantly changed after the intake of hawthorn juice. Analysis of the blood chemistry results indicated

TABLE 1 Serum Total Cholesterol Level (mg/dL) After Intake of Hawthorn Juice or Placebo for 4 Weeks

Group	Baseline	Week 4	Difference	Significance
Group A: hawthorn	268 ± 57	247 ± 55	-21 ± 33	$p < 0.05$
Group C: placebo	254 ± 40	252 ± 47	-2 ± 35	ns
	Week 9	Week 12	Difference	Significance
Group A: placebo	235 ± 39	227 ± 41	-8 ± 29	ns
Group C: hawthorn	239 ± 38	223 ± 33	-16 ± 29	$p < 0.05$

Subjects were given 250 mL hawthorn or placebo drink three times per day for 4 weeks. Starting at the fifth week treatment was stopped until week 9. Then the two groups of subjects were crossed over for treatment for an additional period of 4 weeks. Blood samples were analyzed at baseline, week 4, week 9, and week 12. The hawthorn drink given contained 8% water-soluble material from the fruit. The placebo drink contained artificial coloring and flavor and had the same caloric content as the hawthorn drink.

TABLE 2 Serum LDL Cholesterol (mg/dL) After Intake of Hawthorn Juice or Placebo for 4 Weeks

Group	Baseline	Week 4	Difference	Significance
Group A: hawthorn	186 ± 59	163 ± 54	−23 ± 32	$p < 0.05$
Group C: placebo	168 ± 38	160 ± 38	−8 ± 34	ns
	Week 9	Week 12	Difference	Significance
Group A: placebo	161 ± 39	153 ± 42	−8 ± 24	ns
Group C: hawthorn	159 ± 31	137 ± 24	−22 ± 26	$p < 0.05$

See footnote to Table 1 for experimental details.

that no significant changes in blood cell counts, liver and kidney function as well as other indexes were observed after consumption of hawthorn. Out of the 73 subjects studied, only 7 patients dropped out, 3 of them attributed to intolerance to the acidity of the juice (pH 3.5) while the remaining had problems unrelated to the trial.

In rats, the hypocholesterolemic potency of hawthorn fruit drink was even more pronounced. One of our previous studies (11) examined the hypolipidemic activity of hawthorn fruit in three groups of New Zealand white rabbits fed with one of three diets, a control diet without addition of cholesterol (NC), a 1.0% high-cholesterol diet (HC), and a HC diet supplemented with 2.0% hawthorn fruit powder (HC-H). The results showed that inclusion of 2% dry hawthorn fruit powder led to 23% lower serum total cholesterol and 22% lower serum triglyceride in rabbits (Table 3). In addition, hawthorn fruit supplementation led to 51% less cholesterol accumulation in the aorta of rabbits (Table 3). In hamsters, significant reduction in the serum total cholesterol by 10% and triglyceride by 13% was also observed after they were fed a diet supplemented with 0.5% hawthorn fruit ethanolic extract (Table 4) (12). However, supplementation of hawthorn fruit ethanolic extract had no effect on the serum HDL-cholesterol level (Table 4). All these observations confirm that hawthorn fruit modulates blood lipids favorably.

The mechanism by which dietary hawthorn fruit decreases serum cholesterol may involve multifaceted interactions of cholesterol metabolism. The decrease in cholesterol biosynthesis would lead directly to a lower blood cholesterol level. Rajendran et al. (13) followed cholesterol synthesis by measuring the incorporation of [^{14}C]-acetate into the liver cholesterol in rats fed a diet supplemented with hawthorn ethanolic extract. It was found that supplementation of hawthorn ethanolic extract led to 33% lower cholesterol biosynthesis in rats. However, we found that inclusion of hawthorn fruit in the diet had no effect on the 3-hydroxy-3-methyl glutaryl coenzyme A (HMG-

TABLE 3 Serum and Aortic Lipids, and Fecal Neutral and Acidic Sterols of New Zealand White Rabbits Fed a Reference Diet (NC), a High-Cholesterol Diet (HC), or a High-Cholesterol Diet Supplemented with 2.0% Dry Hawthorn Fruit Powder (HC-H) for 4 Weeks

	NC	HC	HC-H
Serum			
Total cholesterol (mmol/L)	0.5 ± 0.2^{c}	24.7 ± 2.8^{a}	18.9 ± 4.7^{b}
HDL cholesterol (mmol/L)	0.3 ± 0.1^{a}	0.2 ± 0.1^{b}	0.3 ± 0.1^{a}
Triglycerides (mmol/L)	0.6 ± 0.1^{c}	2.2 ± 0.5^{a}	1.7 ± 0.3^{b}
Aorta			
Total cholesterol (μmol/g)	1.5 ± 0.7^{c}	28.3 ± 14.3^{a}	13.9 ± 8.1^{b}
Triglycerides (μmol/g)	31.8 ± 2.8^{b}	52.0 ± 24.2^{a}	49.6 ± 24.8^{a}
Liver total cholesterol (μmol/g)	3.0 ± 0.4^{c}	95.0 ± 24.2^{a}	58.0 ± 14.4^{b}
Heart total cholesterol (μmol/g)	2.8 ± 0.3^{c}	7.4 ± 2.4^{a}	5.5 ± 0.9^{b}
Kidney total cholesterol (μmol/g)	6.9 ± 0.6^{c}	17.7 ± 1.8^{a}	14.2 ± 2.6^{b}
Fecal total neutral sterols (mg/g)	51.1 ± 10.1^{c}	134.1 ± 19.6^{b}	264.4 ± 36.1^{a}
Fecal total acidic sterols (mg/g)	13.2 ± 2.1^{c}	18.1 ± 2.4^{b}	35.5 ± 4.8^{a}

Values are means ± SD.
[a,b,c] Means at a row with different letters differ significantly, $p < 0.05$.

TABLE 4 Serum Lipids, Fecal Neutral and Acidic Sterols, Liver 3-Hydroxy-3-Methyl Glutaryl Coenzyme A (HMG-CoA) Reductase, Liver Cholesterol-7α-Hydroxylase (CH), and Intestinal Acyl CoA:Cholesterol Acyltransferase (ACAT), in Hamsters Fed the Control High-Cholesterol Diet or the Same High-Cholesterol Diet Supplemented with 0.5% Hawthorn Fruit Ethanolic Extract

	Control	Hawthorn
Serum total cholesterol (mmol/L)	4.6 ± 0.5	4.1 ± 0.5^{a}
Serum HDL cholesterol (mmol/L)	2.3 ± 0.3	2.4 ± 0.3
Serum triglycerides (mmol/L)	3.3 ± 0.7	2.9 ± 0.4^{a}
Fecal total neutral sterols (mg/g)	8.6 ± 1.4	11.8 ± 2.0^{a}
Fecal total acidic sterols (mg/g)	3.3 ± 0.9	4.8 ± 1.0^{a}
HMG-CoA reductase (pm/min/mg protein)	6.6 ± 2.50	6.4 ± 2.5
CH (pm/min/mg protein)	53.0 ± 29.2	148.9 ± 57.2^{a}
ACAT (nm/min/mg protein)	1.0 ± 0.3	0.8 ± 0.2^{a}

Values are means ± SD.
[a] Means at a row differ significantly, $p < 0.05$.

CoA) reductase activity in hamsters and rabbits (11,12), suggesting that the cholesterol-lowering effect of hawthorn fruit is not mediated by a downregulation of HMG-CoA reductase.

The inhibition of cholesterol absorption in the intestine could also be responsible for the hypocholesterolemic activity of hawthorn fruits. As shown in Tables 3 and 4, supplementation of hawthorn fruit in the form of either crude water-soluble extract powder or ethanolic extract significantly increased cholesterol excretion in the rabbit and hamster. The effect of hawthorn fruit supplementation on intestinal acyl CoA:cholesterol acyltransferase (ACAT) activity was studied because intestinal ACAT may play a key role in the absorption of cholesterol by esterification of cholesterol prior to absorption (14). The results in hamsters demonstrated that supplementation of hawthorn fruit ethanolic extract was associated with a lower intestinal ACAT activity (12), suggesting that inhibition of cholesterol absorption of dietary cholesterol is at least partly mediated by downregulation of intestinal ACAT activity.

Bile acids are the major metabolites of cholesterol. Greater excretion of bile acids could also lead to a lower level of serum cholesterol. We found that the fecal excretion of both primary (cholic and chenodeoxycholic) and secondary (lithocholic and deoxycholic) bile acids was greater in hamsters and rabbits (11,12) fed diets supplemented with hawthorn fruit (Tables 3 and 4). The liver cholesterol 7α-hydroxylase (CH) is a regulatory enzyme in the metabolic pathway from cholesterol to bile acids. Hawthorn fruit supplementation in the diet significantly increased the liver CH activity compared with the control group (Table 4), suggesting that the increased excretion of bile acids is partly mediated by upregulation of this enzyme.

Blood total and LDL-cholesterol level is maintained in a steady balance in which the rate of entry of cholesterol into the blood is equal to the removal of cholesterol from the blood. A reduced serum cholesterol level indicates a shift in this steady state, resulting from either a decrease in the rate of entry or an increase in the rate of removal by peripheral tissues. The rate by which LDL cholesterol is taken up by peripheral tissues is mediated by LDL receptors. Upregulation of LDL receptors is probably an alternative mechanism responsible for the hypocholesterolemic activity of hawthorn fruits. We have investigated the effect of hawthorn extract on LDL receptor level in HepG2 cells and found that hawthorn fruit extract could prevent the downregulation of LDL receptors by LDL in a dose-dependent manner (Fig. 1) (15). A similar effect was observed in a study by Rajendran et al. (13), who showed that supplementation of 0.5 mL ethanolic extract per 100 g body weight per day for 6 weeks was associated with a 25% increase in hepatic LDL-receptor activity, resulting in greater influx of plasma cholesterol into the liver. It is concluded that hawthorn fruit lowers serum cholesterol by a

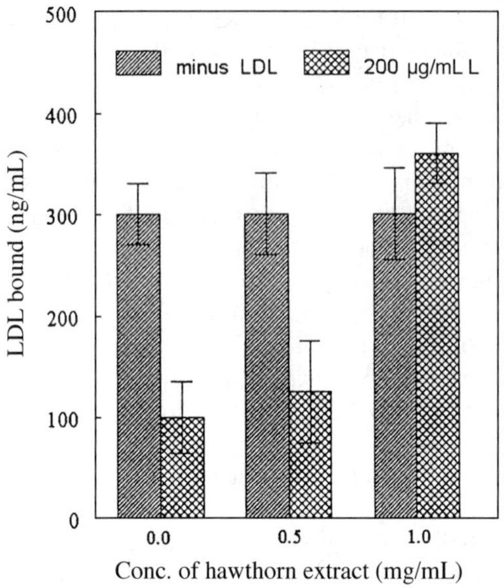

FIGURE 1 Inhibition of LDL-receptor downregulation by hawthorn water-soluble extract. HepG2 cells were incubated in the presence and absence of hawthorn with and without 500 μg LDL/mL. In the absence of hawthorn, LDL receptor was downregulated by LDL to maximum level. The presence of 0.5 and 1.0 mg/mL of hawthorn extract prevented this downregulation in a proportional manner.

combination of mechanisms involving increasing LDL receptor activity and reducing cholesterol absorption and bile acid reabsorption.

III. ANTIOXIDANT ACTIVITY

Pharmacological studies of hawthorn fruits focus on its cardiovascular protective, hypotensive, and cholesterol-lowerig activity (1,4–7,9). However, mechanisms of these beneficial effects are still being investigated. Dietary antioxidants may reduce the initiation and propagation of free radicals in vivo, and therefore minimize the free-radical-induced damage to the heart tissue and cardiovascular vessels. In recent years, it has been generally accepted that oxidation of human LDL is one of the risk factors in the development of cardiovascular disease (16–19). In vitro and in vivo experiments support the view that hawthorn fruit has strong antioxidant activity (20–22).

Hawthorn fruit is a rich source of phenolic antioxidants (22). To quantify these phenolic antioxidants present in hawthorn fruits, a HPLC method was developed in our laboratory. As shown in Figure 2, at least eight flavonoids were identified in hawthorn fruit. The structures of these compounds are shown in Figure 3. The HPLC analysis found that epicatechin was most abundant (1.78 g/kg dry fruit) followed by chlorogenic acid (0.65 g/kg), hyperoside (0.25 g/kg), isoquercitrin (0.13 g/kg), protocatechuic acid (0.03 g/kg), rutin (0.03 g/kg), and quercetin (0.01 g/kg). The eight flavonoids purified from hawthorn fruit demonstrated varying antioxidant activity (Fig. 4). When incubated with LDL, ursolic acid showed no antioxidant activity while

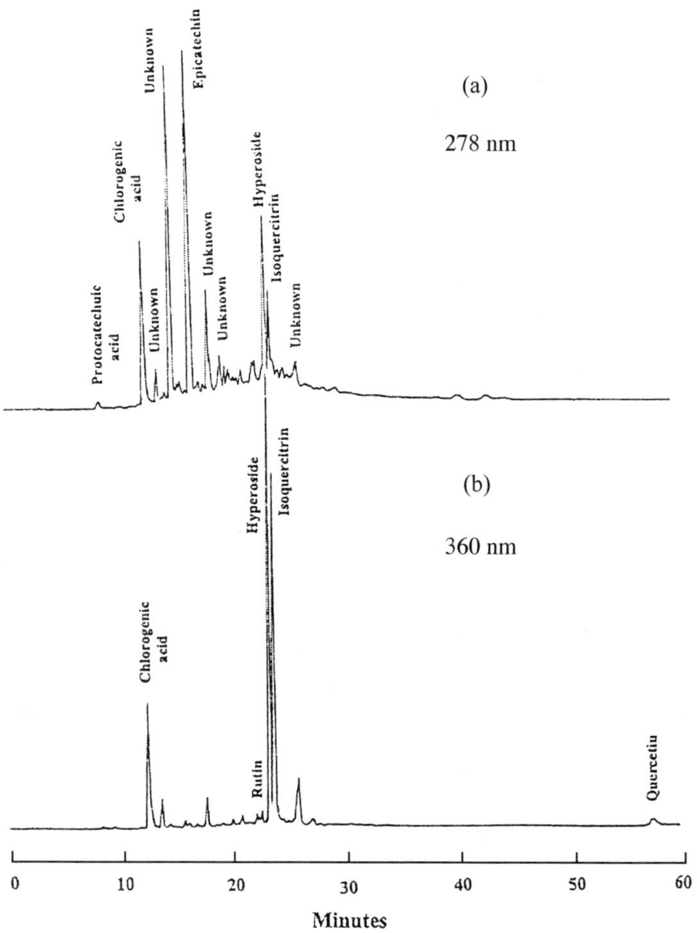

FIGURE 2 High-performance liquid chromatographic profile of hawthorn fruit phenolics. See Ref. 22 for the conditions.

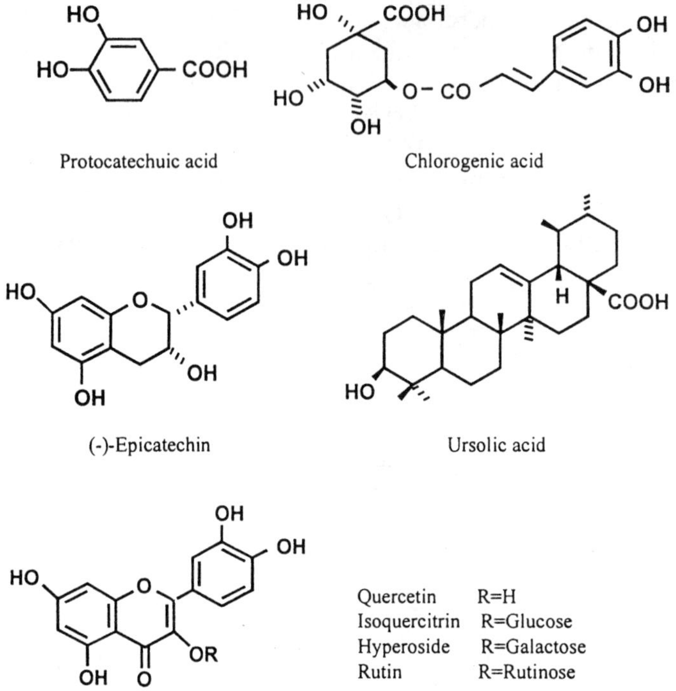

FIGURE 3 Chemical structures of chlorogenic acid, epicatechin, hyperoside, isoquercitrin, protocatechuic acid, quercetin, rutin, and usolic acid.

hyperoside was most protective to human LDL followed by quercetin and isoquercitrin (Fig. 4). Under the same experimental conditions, the antioxidant activity of epicatechin, chlorogenic acid, and rutin was similar but it was weaker than that of hyperoside, quercetin, and isoquercitrin (Fig. 4).

α-Tocopherol is the major antioxidant in human LDL. The flavonoids purified from hawthorn fruit were also effective in protecting α-tocopherol from free-radical-induced degradation in human LDL (22). Supplementation of hawthorn fruit in the diet (2%) significantly increased serum α-tocopherol in rats (Fig. 5). At the end of 3 weeks, serum α-tocopherol in the hawthorn-fruit-supplemented group was increased by 18% as compared with that of the control rats. At the end of 6 weeks, serum α-tocopherol in the hawthorn-fruit-supplemented group was increased by 20% as compared with that of the control rats (Fig. 5). Epidemiological studies showed that flavonoid consumption was negatively associated with coronary heart disease mortality (23). If the consumption of hawthorn fruit is associated with a significantly

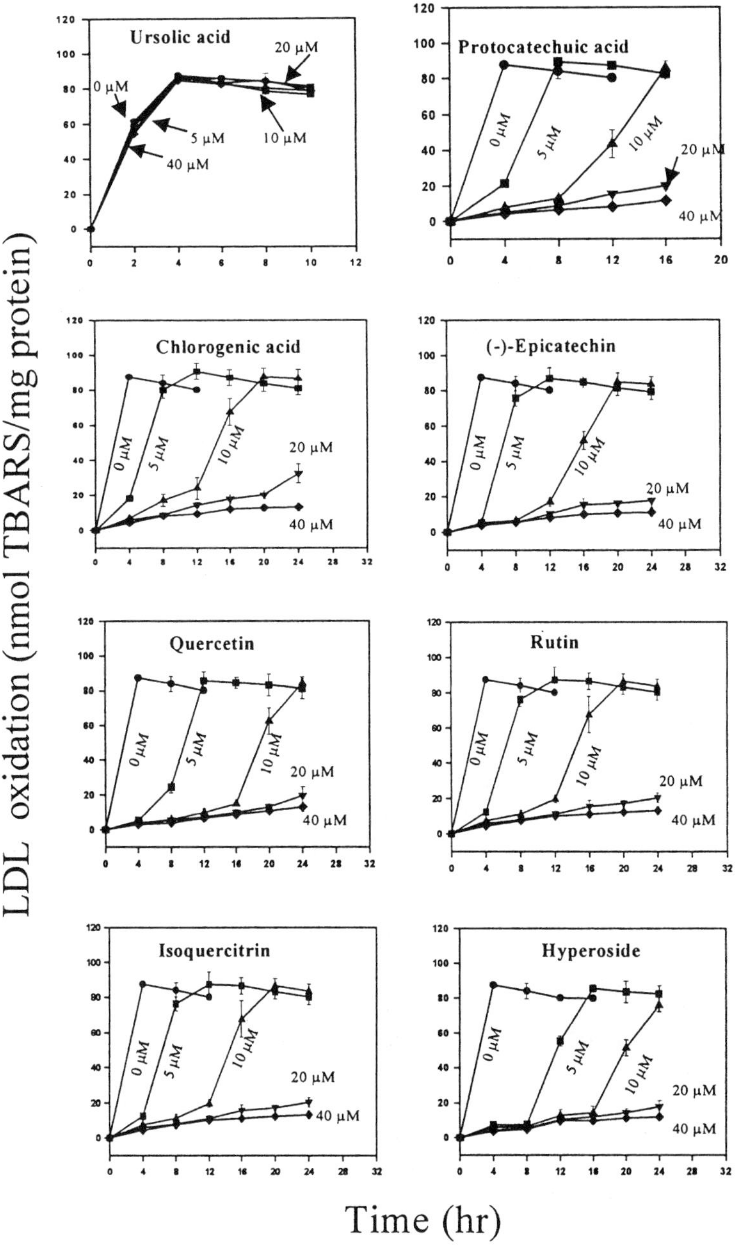

FIGURE 4 Effect of hawthorn fruit phenolics on production of thiobarbituric acid-reactive substances (TBARS) in Cu^{2+}-mediated oxidation of human LDL.

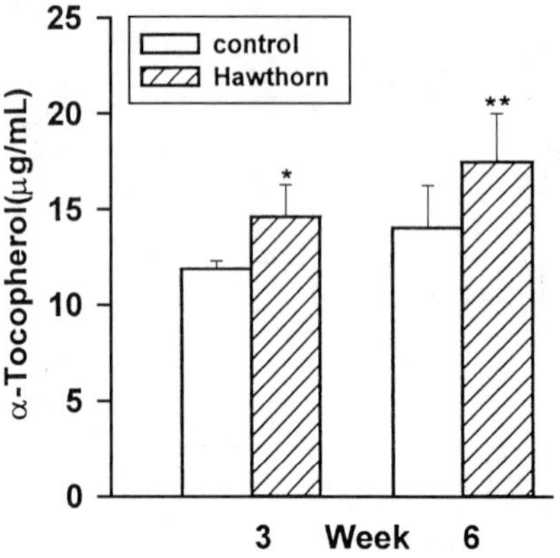

FIGURE 5 Effect of hawthorn fruit powder supplementation (2%) in diet on serum α-tocopherol in rats. Means at a given time point differ significantly. $*p < 0.05$; $**p < 0.01$. See Ref. 22 for the experimental conditions.

lower risk of cardiovascular disease in humans, part of the mechanism may also involve the protective role of these antioxidants to α-tocopherol and human LDL from oxidation.

To correlate the pharmacological action of the hawthorn flavonoids with their apparent health benefits, we also studied the absorption kinetics and excretion of four major hawthorn flavonoids, viz., epicatechin, chlorogenic acid, hyperoside, and isoquercitrin, after oral administration to rats. As chlorogenic acid and hyperoside could not be detected in the plasma, urine, or feces after oral administration, their pharmacokinetics could not be assessed. For isoquercitrin, the systemic absorption rate was very rapid and maximum level was observed in the blood after 10 min. In contrast, epicatechin was absorbed much slower reaching a T_{max} at 66 min. The absolute bioavailability of the two compounds was 61% and 34%, respectively. Based on this limited study, different flavonoids from hawthorn may have very different oral absorption and clearance characteristics. More detailed studies are needed to delineate the pharmacological benefits of these compounds as some of them might have limited bioavailability. Isoquercitrin and hyperoside are structurally very similar except one is a glucoside and the other is a galactoside. Yet, one of them is absorbed into the bloodstream quickly while the other is not. Hence, it is likely that some flavonoids may be preferentially uptaken in the gastrointestinal tract and this information would be essential to determine the health benefits of dietary supplements even though they may contain high amounts of flavonoids.

IV. CARDIOVASCULAR EFFECTS

Many species of hawthorns in the genus *Crataegus* have been widely used as folk medicines in China for centuries. Hawthorn berry is probably the best-known cardiotonic. It reduces peripheral flow resistance and lowers blood pressure; it dilates coronary vasculature, improves blood flow to the heart, and is used to treat angina pectoris.

A. Human Studies

Hawthorn extract is well noted in Europe as an antihypertensive remedy, particularly useful in the treatment of mild forms of heart failure and angina pectoris, which are usually related to impaired coronary blood supply (24). Hawthorn reduces the incidence of anginal attacks and lessens patients' complaints of chest pain. In patients with decreased coronary perfusion due to coronary sclerosis, hawthorn lowers oxygen utilization during exercise. This effect may explain a significant decrease of the ischemic reaction in 40 of 52 patients after intravenous administration of hawthorn extract for over 13 days (25).

More recently, the efficacy and tolerance of a standardized hawthorn extract WS 1442 have been tested in a multicenter utilization observational study. Treatment with WS 1442 in patients with cardiac insufficiency stage NYHA II improves cardiac performance (improved ejection fraction), lowers blood pressure, and reduces the number of patients showing ST depression, arrhythmias, and ventricular extrasystoles during exercise (26). This and other randomized, placebo-controlled, doubled-blind studies suggest that hawthorn medication is a clinically effective and well-tolerated therapeutic alternative for patients with congestive heart failure corresponding to NYHA class I (4,27–30).

B. Animal Studies

Studies with isolated perfused rat heart indicate a cardioprotective effect of hawthorn extracts on the ischemic-reperfused heart and this effect is not accompanied by the increase in coronary flow (31). This protection may be coupled to the antioxidative properties of hawthorn extract, which inhibits formation of free radicals (32,33) and subsequent injury to the heart. A significant reduction in the time spent on ventricular fibrillation was observed by infusion of an extract from flowering tops of *Crataegus meyei* A. Pojark. In anesthetized rats, a bolus injection of the extract lowered blood pressure (34). These effects indicate that the extract of *C. meyei* may have a hypotensive and an antiarrthymic action on ischemic myocardium.

Cardioprotective effects of WS 1442 may be partly attributable to the strong free-radical-scavenging activity of some bioactive constituents such as flavonoids and oligomeric procyanidins. Oral administration of WS 1442 at a dose of 100 mg/kg/day to rats shows a significant protection against ischemia-reperfusion–induced pathologies (35).

C. In Vitro Studies

Even though both human and animal studies show the hypotensive effect of hawthorn extract, the underlying cellular mechanisms are completely unclear. It is possible that hawthorn extract may target both endothelium and vascular smooth muscle cells to cause vasodilation. We have recently demonstrated that hawthorn extract produces dose-dependent relaxation mainly in an endothelium-dependent manner in isolated rat mesenteric arteries. Figure 6

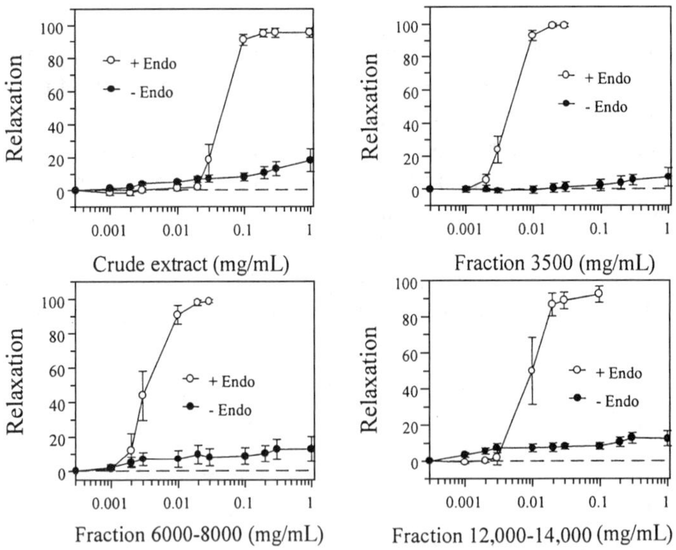

FIGURE 6 The cumulative dose-response curves for the relaxant response to an extract from a hawthorn drink following dialysis in both endothelium-intact (○) and -denuded (●) rings prepared from rat mesenteric arteries. The rings were preconstricted by 50 nM U46619. Data are means ± SEM of six experiments. The molecular weight cutoffs of the dialysis membranes to remove small molecules are as indicated. The active material appears to be retained between 3500 and 8000 molecular weight cutoff.

shows that in U46619-preconstracted rat mesenteric artery rings, hawthorn extract from a fruit drink (the same one we used to perform the clinical trial in Section II) induces primarily endothelium-dependent relaxation after removal of small molecules via dialysis with membranes of molecular weight cutoff at 3500, 6000–8000, and 12,000–14,000 kDa.

Removal of the functional endothelium abolishes the relaxant effect of hawthorn extract. The hawthorn-extract-induced relaxation can be readily washed out and is highly repeatable. The relaxant effect of hawthorn extract is concentration-dependently attenuated by pretreatment of rat mesenteric arteries with an inhibitor of nitric oxide synthase, N^G-nitro-L-arginine methyl ester, or an inhibitor of gunaylate cyclase, methylene blue, while L-arginine, the nitric oxide precursor, partly antagonizes the effect of N^G-nitro-L-arginine methyl ester (36). In addition to nitric oxide, the endothelium also releases prostacyclin or endothelium-derived hyperpolarizing factor in response to various stimuli. However, indomethacin (an inhibitor of cyclooxygenase that catalyzes biosynthesis of prostacyclin), glibenclamide (a blocker of vascular ATP-sensitive potassium channels), or iberiotoxin (a blocker of calcium-activated potassium channel) did not influence the vasorelaxant response to hawthorn extract, suggesting that the relaxing prostanoids or calcium-activated or ATP-sensitive potassium channels are not involved. Hawthorn extract produces significantly less relaxant effect in endothelium-intact artery rings preconstricted by 60 mM extracellular potassium. In endothelium-denuded rings contracted by elevated potassium, hawthorn extract was still able to induce relaxation albeit to much lesser degree. Raising extracellular potassium would bring the membrane potential nearer to the new equilibrium potential for potassium efflux; thus the effect of potassium channel activation on transmembrane calcium movement should be minimized. Reduced effect on high potassium-induced contraction indicates that hawthorn extract may also stimulate release of some unknown endothelium-derived factors that could hyperpolarize the cell membrane of the underlying vascular smooth muscle via opening of potassium channels. The endothelial nitric-oxide-mediated relaxation is supported by the ability of hawthorn extract to raise the tissue content of cyclic GMP in endothelium-intact rat aortas. This effect can be abolished by endothelium denuation or by inhibitors of nitric-oxide-mediated relaxation, such as N^G-nitro-L-arginine (personal communication).

Endothelial nitric oxide seems to play a differential role in hawthorn-extract-induced relaxation in the rat arteries prepared from different vascular beds. For example, hawthorn extract only produces endothelium-independent relaxation in isolated rat cerebral, carotid, and coronary arteries (37) since neither endothelial removal nor nitric oxide synthase inhibitors had an effect. It is currently unknown what has caused this discrepancy in the vascular response to hawthorn extract in different arteries. It is suggested that some bioactive components in hawthorn extract may have a direct muscle relaxant action, e.g., possible inhibition of calcium influx in arterial smooth muscle cells (38).

One recent study described that procyanidins in hawthorn extract (*Crataegus oxyacantha*, L.) may be responsible for the endothelium/nitric-oxide-dependent relaxation in rat aortas, probably through activation of tetraethylammonium-sensitive potassium channels (38). However, our results indicate other unknown ingredients may be involved since procyanidins were undetectable in the dialyzed hawthorn extract sample on HPLC. Monoacetyl-vitexinrhamnoside, a flavonoid with phosphodiesterase-inhibitory property contained in another *Crataegus* species (hawthorn, Rosaceas), was also found to induced relaxation in rabbit isolated femoral arteries and this relaxation was inhibited by N^G-nitro-L-arginine (39). In Langendorff- rabbit hearts, monoacetyl-vitexinrhamnoside enhanced heart rate, cardiac contractility, and coronary flow (39), suggesting that this flavonoid has an anti-ischemic effect probably through improvement of myocardial perfusion.

In addition to antioxidant and hypocholesterolemic activity of hawthorn extract, the vasorelaxant effect on various blood vessels suggests the potential preventive action of this plant against cerebral or coronary circulation-associated disease such as cerebral vasospasm and coronary artery disease. The endothelium/nitric-oxide-dependent action indicates that hawthorn fruit extract may have a wide spectrum of benefits in the cardiovascular system.

ACKNOWLEDGMENTS

The research mentioned in this report was supported by grants from the Hong Kong Jockey Club and the Innovation Technology Commission of Hong Kong (AF/247/97). We wish to thank Dr. Q. Chang, Dr. Z. S. Zhang, Dr. A. James, Professor M. Chow, Professor B. Tomlinson, and Professor Min Zhu for their help in carrying out some of the studies.

REFERENCES

1. Ammon HPT, Händel M. *Crataegus*, toxicology and pharmacology. I. Toxicity. Planta Med 1981; 43:105–120.
2. Huang KC. The Pharmacology of Chinese Herbs. Boca Raton, FL: CRC Press, 1999:117–127.
3. Weiss RF, Fintelman V. Herbal Medicine. New York: Georg Thieme Verlag, 2000:140–148.

4. Rigelsky JM, Sweet BV. Hawthorn: pharmacology and therapeutic uses. Am J Health Syst Pharma 2002; 59:417–422.
5. Ammon HPT, Händel M. *Crataegus*, toxicology and pharmacology. II. Pharmacodynamics. Planta Med 1981; 43:209–239.
6. Ammon HPT, Händel M. *Crataegus*, toxicology and pharmacology. III. Pharmacodynamics and pharmacokinetics. Planta Med 1981; 43:313–322.
7. Weihmayr T, Emst E. Therapeutic effectiveness of *Crataegus*. Forsch Med 1996; 114:27–29.
8. Schussler M, Holzl J, Fricke U. Myocardial effects of flavonoids from *Crataegus* species. Arzneim-Forsch Drug Res 1995; 45:842–845.
9. Hanack T, Bruckel MH. The treatment of mild stable forms of angina pectoris using *Crategutt novo*. Therapiewoche 1983; 33:4331–4333.
10. Chen JD, Wu YZ, Tao ZL, Chen ZM, Liu XP. Hawthorn (Shan Zha) drink and its lowering effect on blood lipid levels in humans and rats. World Rev Nutr Diet 1995; 77:147–154.
11. Zhang Z, Ho WKK, Huang Y, James AE, Lam LW, Chen ZY. Hawthorn fruit is hypolipidemic in rabbits fed a high cholesterol diet. J Nutr 2002; 132:5–10.
12. Zhang Z, Ho WKK, Huang Y, Chen ZY. Hypocholesterolemic activity of hawthorn fruit is mediated by regulation of cholesterol-7α-hydroxylase and acyl CoA:cholesterol acyltransferase. Food Res Int 2002; 35:885–891.
13. Rajendran S, Deepalakshmi PD, Parasakthy K, Devarj H, Niranjali Devaraji S. Effect of tincture of *Crataegus* on the LDL-receptor activity of hepatic plasma membrane of rats fed an atherogenic diet. Atherosclerosis 1996; 123: 235–241.
14. Wrenn SM, Parks JS Jr, Immermann FW, Rudel LL. ACAT inhibitors CL283,546 and CL283,796 reduce LDL cholesterol without affecting cholesterol absorption in African green monkeys. J Lipid Res 1995; 36:1199–1210.
15. Ho WKK, Chang HM, Lee CM. Method and compositions for lowering blood lipids. US Patent Number 5665359, September 9, 1997.
16. Steinberg D, Parthasarathy S, Carew TW, Knoo JC, Witztum JL. Beyond cholesterol: modification of low-density lipoprotein that increases its atherogenicity. N Engl J Med 1989; 320:915–924.
17. Witztum JL, Steinberg D. Role of oxidized low-density lipoprotein in atherosclerosis. J Clin Invest 1991; 88:1785–1792.
18. Jessup W, Dean RT, de Whalley CV, Rankin SM, Leak DS. The role of oxidative modification and antioxidants in LDL metabolism and atherosclerosis. Adv Exp Med Biol 1990; 264:139–142.
19. Knipping G, Rothneder M, Striegl G, Esterbauder H. Antioxidants and resistance against oxidation of porcine LDL subfractions. J Lipid Res 1990; 31:1965–1972.
20. Bahorun T, Gressier B, Trotin F, Brunet C, Dine T, Luyckx M, Vasseur J, Cazin M, Cazin JC, Pinas M. Oxygen species scavenging activity of phenolic extracts from hawthorn fresh organs and pharmaceutical preparations. Arzneimitteforschung 1996; 46:1086–1089.
21. Stroka Z, Cisowski W, Seredynska M, Luczkiewicz M. Phenolic extracts from

meadowsweet and hawthorn flowers have antioxidative properties. Z Naturforsch 2001; 56:739–744.
22. Zhang Z, Chang Q, Zhu M, Huang Y, Ho WKK, Chen ZY. Characterization of antioxidants present in hawthorn fruits. J Nutr Biochem 2000; 12:144–152.
23. Hertog MGL, Feskens EJM, Hollman PCH, Katan MB, Kromhout D. Dietary antioxidant flavonoids and risk of coronary heart disease: the Zutphen Elderly Study. Lancet 1993; 342:1007–1011.
24. Weiss RF, Fintelmann V. Herbal Medicine. New York: Georg Thieme Verlag, 2000.
25. Kandziora J. Crataegutt-wirkung bei koronarendurchblu-tungsstoerungen. Muench Med Wochenschr 1969; 6:295–298.
26. Tauchert M, Gildor A, Lipinski J. High-dose *Crataegus* extract WS 1442 in the treatment of NYHA stage II heart failure. Herz 1999; 24:465–474.
27. Leuchtgens H. *Crataegus* special extract WS 1442 in NYHA II heart failure: a placebo controlled randomized double-blind study. Fortschr Med 1993; 111: 352–354.
28. Weikl A, Assmus KD, Neukum-Schmidt A, Schmitz J, Zapfe G, Noh HS, Siegrist J, *Crataegus* special extract WS 1442: assessment of objective effectiveness in patients with heart failure (NYHA II). Fortschr Med 1996; 114:291–296.
29. Rietbrock N, Hamel M, Hempel B, Mitrovic V, Schmidt T, Wolf GK. Actions of standardized extracts of *Crataegus* berries on exercise tolerance and quality of life in patients with congestive heart failure. Arzneimittelforschung 2001; 51:793–798.
30. Walker AF, Marakis G, Morris AP, Robinson PA. Promising hypotensive effect of hawthorn extract: a randomized double-blind pilot study of mild, essential hypertension. Phytother Res 2002; 16:48–54.
31. Nasa Y, Hashizume H, Hoque AN, Abiko Y. Protective effect of *Crataegus* extract on the cardiac mechanical dysfunction in isolated perfused working rat heart. Arzneimittelforschung 1993; 43:945–949.
32. Bahorun T, Trotin F, Pommery J, Vasseur J, Pinkas M. Antioxidant activities of *Crataegus monogyna* extracts. Planta Med 1994; 60:323–328.
33. Bahorun T, Gressier B, Trotin F, Brunet C, Dine T, Luyckx M, Vasseur J, Cazin M, Cazin JC, Pinkas M. Oxygen species scavenging activity of phenolic extracts from hawthorn fresh plant organs and pharmaceutical preparations. Arzneimittelforschung 1996; 46:1086–1089.
34. Garjani A, Nazemiyeh H, Maleki N, Valizadeh H. Effects of extracts from flowering tops of *Crataegus meyeri* A. Pojark. on ischaemic arrhythmias in anaesthetized rats. Phytother Res 2000; 14:428–431.
35. Chatterjee SS, Koch E, Jaggy H, Krzeminski T. In vitro and in vivo studies on the cardioprotective action of oligomeric procyanidins in a *Crataegus* extract of leaves and blooms. Arzneimittelforschung 1997; 47:815–821.
36. Chen ZY, Zhang ZS, Kwan KY, Zhu M, Ho WKK, Huang Y. Endothelium-dependent relaxation induced by hawthorn extract in rat mesenteric artery. Life Sci 1998; 63:1983–1991.
37. Chan HY, Chen ZY, Yao XQ, Lau CW, Zhang ZS, Ho WKK, Huang Y.

Differential role of endothelium in hawthorn fruit extract–induced relaxation of rat cerebral, coronary, carotid arteries and aorta. Orient Pharm Exp Med 2002. In press.

38. Kim SH, Kang KW, Kim KW, Kim ND. Procyanidins in crataegus extract evoke endothelium-dependent vasorelaxation in rat aorta. Life Sci 2000; 67:121–131.
39. Schüssler M, Holzl J, Rump AF, Fricke U. Functional and antiischaemic effects of monoacetyl-vitexinrhamnoside in different in vitro models. Gen Pharmacol 1995; 26:1565–1570.

22

Resveratrol
The Promise Therein

Shazib Pervaiz

National University of Singapore
Singapore, Republic of Singapore

I. INTRODUCTION

The use of herbal ingredients and plant extracts for their pharmacological properties dates back to the earliest human endeavors in medicinal chemistry. Indeed, a number of pharmacological agents in use today are a direct outcome of these remarkable observations. With the rapid advances made over the last two decades in biomedical research, there has been an unprecedented interest in unraveling the magical properties ofsome of the commonly used natural products. Thanks to modern technology, chemists and biologists today are extremely well equipped in the art of identifying and screening the biological activities of plant and herbal ingredients. As a result, many of these natural products are under scrutiny for their clinical potential, in terms of both disease prevention and treatment.

Among the long list of compounds being tested for their beneficial effects on human health is a family of polymers given the name viniferin. Compounds belonging to this category elicit strong antifungal properties and are therefore included under the broad class of plant antibiotics known as phytoalexins (Soleas et al., 1997). One remarkable compound in this list is resveratrol (RSV), a major active ingredient of stilbene phytoalexins, first isolated from the roots of the oriental medicinal plant *Polygonum capsidatum* (Ko-jo-kon in Japanese) (Nonomura et al., 1963). That this compound was an active ingredient of a wondrous folk plant known for its remedial effects against a long list of human afflictions (Kubo et al., 1981; Nonomura et al., 1963), and the observation that it was synthesized by leaf tissue in response to fungal infection of grapevines (*Vitis vinifera*) (Langcake and Pryce, 1976) provided the impetus for the tremendous increase in activity surrounding RSV in the field of biomedical research. Consequently, over the past several years a substantial amount of work has focused on studying the biological activity of this phytoalexin and its derivatives. These studies have demonstrated the tremendous potential of RSV as a preventive and therapeutic compound in biological systems, such as cardiovascular and immune systems.

The relatively high concentration of RSV in wine (Siemann and Creasy, 1992) and its documented cardioprotective effect (Sato et al., 2002) form the basis for the so-called "French paradox" (Kopp, 1998). However, since the reported cancer chemopreventive activity in animal models of carcinogenesis (Jang et al., 1997), the interest has shifted mostly to the mechanism of the anticancer activity of RSV and its potential as a chemotherapeutic agent. As a result, the positive or negative effects of RSV on some important physiological pathways have been proposed as possible mechanisms for its observed cancer chemopreventive activity. These include: suppression of cellular proliferation via inhibition of key steps in the signal transduction pathways (Haworth and Avkiran, 2001; Mgbonyebi et al., 1998; Pozo-Guisado et al., 2002; Tou and Urbizo, 2001) and cyclin-dependent kinases (cdks) (Ragione et al., 1998); promotion of cellular differentiation (Mizutani et al., 1998); scavenging/suppression of intracellular reactive oxygen species (ROS) (Manna et al., 2000); induction of apoptotic cell death through activation of mitochondria-dependent or -independent pathways (Clement et al., 1998a; Hsieh and Wu, 1999; Huang et al., 1999); anti-inflammatory activity via downregulation of proinflammatory cytokines (Rotondo et al., 1998; Wadsworth and Koop, 1999); and inhibition of androgen receptor function and estrogenic activity (Lu and Serrero, 1999; Mitchell et al., 1999). This review is intended to provide the reader with an appreciation of the diverse biological effects of this remarkable compound that holds great promise for the future. Starting with a brief overview of the sources and chemistry, the chapter presents an overview and appraisal of the potential chemopreventive and chemotherapeutic properties of RSV.

II. OCCURRENCE, SYNTHESIS, AND CHEMISTRY

Nonflavonoid classes of phenolic compounds, such as RSV, are synthesized by a variety of plants in response to injury or fungal infection (Langcake and

Pryce, 1976). Although RSV does not enjoy a wide distribution in the plant kingdom, its occurrence has been documented in trees, including eucalyptus, spruce, and the tropical deciduous tree *Bauhinia racemosa*, in a few flowering plants such as *Veratrum grandiflorum* and *Veratrum formosanum* (two species of lilly), in *Pterolobium hexapetallum* (nonedible legume), in peanuts and groundnuts, and in grapevines (Soleas et al., 1997). One of the richest sources of RSV is the weed *Polygonum capsidatum*, root extracts of which have been used extensively in Oriental fold medicine (Kubo et al., 1981; Nonomura et al., 1963). Since the first reported detection of trans-RSV in grapvines (*Vitis vinifera*) in 1976 (Langcake and Pryce, 1976) and later in wine in 1992 (Siemann and Creasy, 1992), most interest has centered on RSV in grapevine. This was mainly due to the fact that compounds found in grapevines were implicated in epidemiological data demonstrating an inverse correlation between red wine consumption and incidence of cardiovascular disease—the "French paradox" (Kopp, 1998). The pioneering work of Langcake and associates also indicated that phytoalexins like RSV were not present in healthy vine leaves or berries, but were quite abundant in mature vine wood.

Exposure to ultraviolet (UV) rays stimulates the synthesis of RSV as well as other viniferins (Langcake and Pryce, 1977b), and the formation of viniferins from RSV involves oxidative dimerization that could be reproduced in vitro by exposure of the parent compound to horseradish peroxidase–hydrogen peroxide system in vitro (Langcake and Pryce, 1977a). The synthetic potential is highest just before the grapes reach maturity, and is low in buds, flowers, and mature fruits, and resistant species produced significantly higher amounts than susceptible ones (Jeandet et al., 2002). Higher amounts are also observed in healthy areas around necrotic lesions following fungal infection of grape berry skins, and this seems to be an inherent protective mechanism to limit the spread. Studies conducted in the wine-producing French area of Burgundy demonstrated that RSV production enables the vines to withstand *Botrytis* attack, and that the stimulus for RSV synthesis in healthy berries away from the site of infection must involve a chemical signal generated by the pathogen or the host for regulating the activity of stilbene synthase, the terminal enzyme in the biosynthesis of RSV (Jeandet et al., 1995a). In a typical cycle, fungal infection triggers RSV synthesis, which leads to its accumulation around the infected area; however, 48–72 hr later the pathogen upregulates the activity of the enzyme stilbene oxidase, which leads to oxidative degradation of RSV (Hoos and Blaich, 1988). Thus a tricky hide-and-seek battle goes on with the ultimate winner determined by the environment, the virulence of the pathogen, the stage in development of the plant, and the bolus of infection.

The determination of RSV content has not been restricted to plant components including leaves, skins, and petals, but also involves wines and grape juices. Initial attempts failed owing to the absence of good methodology to recover RSV and prevent its oxidative degradation; however, more recent application of HPLC and GC-MS to the detection of RSV in wines has shown that both *cis* and *trans* isomers are present in wines with the latter found in significantly higher concentration (Lamuela-Raventos et al., 1995; Soleas et al., 2001b). Generally, white wines contain 1–5% of the RSV content of most red wines. The highest concentration of *trans*-RSV has been reported in wines prepared from Pinot noir grapes (averaging 5.13 mg/L) (Lamuela-Raventos et al., 1995).

Chemically, RSV is comprised of two phenols linked by a styrene double bond to generate 3,4′,5 trihydroxysulbene (Fig. 1), a structure related to the synthetic estrogen diethylstilbestrol.

The precursor for RSV synthesis is the amino acid phenylalanine, which is deaminated by phenylalanine ammonia lyase to cinnamic acid. Hydroxylation of cinnamic acid by cinnamate-4-hydroxylase generates p-coumaric acid, which in turn is converted by a specific CoA ligase to p-coumaroyl CoA. Condensation of p-coumaroyl CoA with three molecules of melanoyl CoA by stilbene synthase (or resveratrol synthase) results in the formation of RSV (Jeandet et al., 1995c). Stilbene synthase is normally not active or expressed in nonstressed seedlings; however, within 6 hr of exposure to UV radiation or fungal infection the enzyme activity is upregulated and peaks by 30 hr. Soluble β-glucans present in bacterial cell walls are potent inducers of stilbene

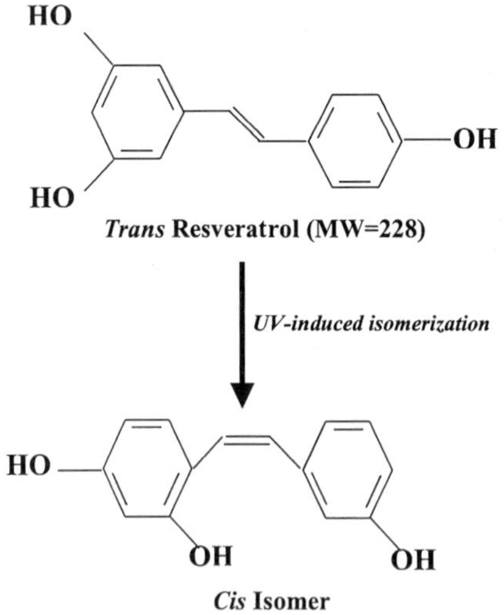

FIGURE 1 Structure of resveratrol (3,4′,5 trihydroxystilbene).

synthase, and reports also suggest that the presence of Ca^{2+} seems critical for the enzyme activity (Ebel, 1986). RSV exists as *cis* and *trans* isomeric forms with *trans*-to-*cis* isomerization facilitated by UV exposure. *Trans*-RSV (MW = 228) is commercially available and is relatively stable if protected from high pH and light (Soleas et al., 1997). The difference in absorption maxima (307 nm for the *trans* and 288 nm for the *cis* isomer) allows for their separation and detection by HPLC using a C18 reverse-phase column (Jeandet et al., 1995b). More recently gas chromatography (GC) has been used to measure concentrations of *cis* and *trans* isomers in plasma and cells (Soleas et al., 2001b). Oxidative modification (dimerization) of RSV gives rise to another class of compounds called viniferins. The potential of grapevines to synthesize RSV and viniferins has been shown to provide resistance against a variety of plant diseases. To that end, gene transfer of full-length stilbene synthase into plants lacking this activity resulted in rapid induction of the enzyme and accumulation of RSV upon UV irradiation, and conferred resistance to microbial infection (Hain et al., 1990, 1993).

III. FROM THE GRAPEVINE TO MAMMALIAN BIOLOGY

As mentioned earlier, the diverse beneficial effects of extracts prepared from the plant *P. capsidatum* against a host of human afflictions had been documented decades before the actual identification of RSV as a potent ingredient of this Oriental folk medicine. Since this reported observation in the mid-seventies, a lot of work went into the actual synthesis in plants and the factors that promoted expression of RSV-producing enzymes. This led to its classification as a phytoalexin that is rapidly synthesized in response to fungal infection or UV irradiation and, when genetically expressed in plants that lacked RSV synthase activity, provided resistance from fungal infection. Subsequent identification of RSV as a major phenolic constituent of wines and its association with decreased cardiovascular disease risk in moderate wine consumers have resulted in a tremendous increase in interest in elucidating the effects of this polyphenolic compound and its derivatives on human health and disease. Consequently, the diverse biological activities and potential beneficial effects of RSV have been studied in the past 5 years. In the following sections, I will provide an overview of the many biochemical properties and biological effects of RSV that could have potential clinical implications.

A. Antioxidant Activity of RSV—Potential Cardioprotective Effect

Normal cellular metabolism generates reactive oxygen intermediates (ROI), such as superoxide (O_2^-), hydrogen peroxide (H_2O_2), and hydroxyl radical

($OH^{\cdot}$). Excessive accumulation of ROI is kept in check by the cellular antioxidant defense mechanism comprised of a number of intracellular enzymes, such as glutathione (GSH), superoxide dismutase (SOD), and catalase (Halliwell and Gutteridge, 1999). A defect in the cells' inherent ability to counteract the production of ROI results in their abnormal accumulation, a state commonly referred to as "oxidative stress." Exposure of cellular macromolecules (lipids, proteins, and nuclei acids) to ROI results in their oxidative modifications with deleterious potential (Packer, 1992). A classic example of this is the oxidative modification of low-density lipoproteins (LDL) (Esterbauer et al., 1992), the so-called "bad" cholesterol implicated in atherosclerosis and increased incidence of coronary artery disease. Generated by lipolytic remodeling of VLDL, normal circulating LDL is endocytosed via the specific LDL receptor. While the endocytosis of normal LDL is tightly regulated, oxidized LDL is taken up by a nonregulated scavenger receptor system resulting in an abnormal accumulation of LDL in monocytic subendothelial cells (foam cells) (Steinberg et al., 1989). Oxidized lipoproteins provide a permissive environment for atheroma formation and platelet aggregation, thereby fueling the process of atherosclerosis (Steinberg et al., 1989).

Phenolic compounds present in red wine elicit antioxidant activity and prevent LDL oxidation (Whitehead et al., 1995). In line with this, epidemiological studies have linked moderate intake of wine with an appreciable decrease in the risk of coronary artery disease, particularly in regions of France where the diet is high in fat (Fuhrman et al., 1995). Studies have demonstrated that RSV is a potent inhibitor of the oxidation of polyunsaturated fatty acids (PUFA) found in LDL, which plays a major role in atherosclerosis (Miller and Rice-Evans, 1995). Other reports indicate that RSV is more potent than flavonoids in preventing copper-catalyzed oxidation, and as LDL has high affinity for copper, this copper-chelating activity impedes oxidative modification of LDL (Frankel et al., 1993). Further evidence of the protective effect of RSV on lipid accumulation was reported in human hepatocarcinoma cells HepG2, which elicit most of the normal liver parenchymal functions (Goldberg et al., 1995; Soleas et al., 1997). Addition of RSV to the culture medium resulted in a dose-dependent decrease in the intracellular concentration of Apo B, and a significant reduction in the rate of secretion of cholesterol esters and triglycerides. The latter is an indication of fewer VLDL and therefore lower LDL production. Although these observations provide evidence for antilipogenic and atherosclerosis-inhibitory effect of RSV, in vivo data fall short of corroborating these findings; studies using hyperlipidemic rabbits fed on RSV showed no decreases in serum cholesterol levels or in atherosclerotic lesions (Wilson et al., 1996).

Through its inhibitory effect on membrane lipid peroxidation, RSV has also been shown to reduce the toxic effects of ROI in living cells. For example, rat adrenal pheochromocytoma cells (PC12) exposed to ethanol-induced oxidative death were remarkably protected in the presence of RSV (Sun et al., 1997). In similar experiments this death inhibitory activity was attributed to the ability of RSV to block internalization of oxidized lipoproteins. In addition, oxidized lipoprotein-induced cell death was inhibited in neuronal cells in the presence of RSV, indicating neuroprotective activity (Draczynska-Lusiak et al., 1998). The antioxidant activity of RSV has also been shown to inhibit proliferation of hepatic stellate cells (Kawada et al., 1998), a major factor in the development of liver fibrosis, thereby suggesting a hepatoprotective effect. The antioxidant activity of RSV has been further corroborated by studies demonstrating its inhibitory effect on intracellular ROI production induced by the tumor promoter phorbol ester (Martinez and Moreno, 2000), thereby preventing the development of a pro-oxidant milieu that favors carcinogenesis (Cerutti, 1985). However, more recent data and our unpublished results provide an interesting insight into the effect of this compound on intracellular redox state. These data seem to support both an anti- and pro-oxidant activity of RSV, depending on the concentration of RSV and the cell type. For example, in human leukemia cells RSV induces an increase in intracellular ROI, whereas in prostate cancer cells a dose-dependent decrease in intracellular ROI, in particular O_2^-, is observed (Li and Pervaiz, unpublished results).

In addition to the anti-oxidant property of RSV, two other biological effects of RSV support its cardioprotective ability. First, wine phenolics such as RSV have been shown to modulate the production of nitric oxide (NO) from vascular endothelium, a nitrogen species involved in inflammatory responses (Hattori et al., 2002; Hung et al., 2000). Increased levels of NO can cause vascular damage thereby contributing to the development of atheromatous plaques. Second, RSV has been shown to inhibit platelet aggregation, another major contributor in the process of atherosclerosis (Olas et al., 2001; Orsini et al., 1997). Platelets stick to the endothelial surface of blood vessels, can activate the process of thrombus formation, and their aggregation could set into motion the process of vascular occlusion. Platelets have also been linked to the synthesis of eicosanoids from arachidonic acid that contributes to platelet adhesion (Fremont, 2000). A dose-dependent decrease in platelet aggregation has been demonstrated with RSV, further lending support to its preventive activity against coronary artery disease. This has been linked to the ability of RSV to inhibit eicosanoid synthesis (Soleas et al., 1997) (discussed in more detail in a later section).

The observations presented in the preceding section are further supported by human in vivo studies demonstrating increased antioxidant activity in blood of moderate red wine consumers (Whitehead et al., 1995); however, much more research needs to be done to establish that the reported beneficial effects on human cardiovascular, neurological, and hepatic systems are indeed a function of RSV.

B. Anticyclooxygenase, Antilipoxygenase Activities, and Regulation of Cytokine Secretion: Immunomodulatory Effect

Among the various beneficial effects of the extract prepared from the roots of *P. capsidatum* (the plant from which RSV was first isolated) were its magical effects on allergic and inflammatory diseases. Invariably, these pathological states are a direct or indirect outcome of a hyperactive immune system as a result of an increase in activity of leukocytes that churn out excess of biological response modifiers. The two enzyme systems involved in the synthesis of proinflammatory mediators such as 5-HETE (5-hydroxy-6,8,11,14-eicosatetraenoic acid), thromboxane A2, prostaglandins (PG), and HTT (12-hydroxy-5,8,10-heptadecatrienoic acid) are the cycloxygenase (COX) and the lipoxygenase pathways (Cuendet and Pezzuto, 2000). COX-1 (also referred to as PGH synthase) is constitutively expressed, whereas an inducible COX-2 is also expressed constitutively in certain regions of the brain, kidneys, and cancerous tissues. COX-2 activity, usually undetected in normal tissues, generates proinflammatory substances by the oxygenation of arachidonic acid to PGs (PGD2 and PGE2) (Cuendet and Pezzuto, 2000). In addition, COX-2 can catalyze the formation of chemotactic substances such as HHT and thromboxone A2 from PGH2 via the thromboxone synthetase (Gierse et al., 1995). This chemotactic activity can in turn lead to platelet aggregation. The leukocyte lipoxygenase is known to catalyze the initial reaction that leads to the formation of 5-HETE, a stable derivative of the peroxy form 5-HPETE (Kimura et al., 1995). These substances have high chemotactic activity and are potent inducers of histamine release from basophil.

The PGs have been implicated in promoting cell proliferation, suppressing immune surveillance, and stimulating tumorigenesis (Gusman et al., 2001). Owing to these deleterious effects of PGs and other inflammatory substances generated by COX and lipoxygenase pathways, identification of molecules with the potential to inhibit these pathways has been a major focus of biomedical research. In this regard, the effects of stilbenes, in particular RSV, on COX and leukocyte lipoxygenase pathways have produced interesting results. RSV was found to inhibit the 5-lipoxegenase product 5-HETE and the COX products HHT and thromboxane B2 (Kimura et al., 1985). Based on these results, the researchers further established that this inhibitory activity was directly responsible for the antiplatelet aggregation induced by RSV.

The COX and lipoxygenase inhibitory activities of RSV have also been reported to account for its protective effect against oxidative-stress-induced death of human erythroleukemia K562 cells (MacCarrone et al., 1999). The mechanism of this death-inhibitory activity of RSV involved inhibition of H_2O_2-induced increases in PGE2 (product of COX activity) and leukotriene B4 (product of lipoxygenase activity) concentrations. This inhibitory effect on COX and lipoxygenase activities has been proposed as a possible mechanism for the antitumor activity of RSV; however, our studies (in HL60 leukemia and T47D breast carcinoma cells) and recent data from other groups provide evidence that the antitumor activity may, in part, be due to its ability to trigger apoptotic death in tumor cells (Ahmad et al., 2001; Clement et al., 1998a; Ding and Adrian, 2002; Ferry-Dumazet et al., 2002; Huang et al., 1999; Morris et al., 2002). Nevetheless, given the role that inflammatory mediators play in the induction and promotion of carcinogenesis, it is plausible that both these observed activities may play a role in cancer chemoprevention.

The anti-inflammatory activity of RSV has also been demonstrated in a rat model of carrageenan-induced paw edema (Gentilli et al., 2001). RSV inhibited both acute and chronic phases of this inflammatory process, with an activity greater than that of indomethacin or phenylbutazone. This effect was also attributed to the impairment of PG synthesis via selective inhibition of COX-1. Similarly, preincubation with RSV decreased arachidonic acid release and COX-2 induction in mouse peritoneal macrophages stimulated with tumor promoter PMA, ROI, or lipopolysaccharides (LPS) (Tsai et al., 1999). Gene transfer experiments using a reporter construct containing *COX-2-luciferase* confirmed that RSV-mediated decrease in COX-2 activity was indeed due to its inhibitory effect on protein kinase C (PKC)-driven activation of *COX-2* transcription (Subbaramaiah et al., 1998). A more detailed account of the effect of RSV on gene transcription and transcriptional factors will be presented in a later section.

The effect of RSV on macrophages and polymorphonuclear cells (PMN) has also been evaluated. These cells are the major players in the body's response to immunogenic challenges, and biological response modifier secreted from these cells can contribute to the development of disease states such as allergy and inflammation (Harlan, 1987). One classic model of macrophage activation is the bacterial LPS. Under normal physiological settings this activation leads to a moderate increase in iNOS activity resulting in NO production that has bactericidal effects. However, abnormally high concentrations of NO and its derivatives peroxynitrite and nitrogen dioxide give rise to inflammation and have been shown to contribute to the process of carcinogenesis (Halliwell, 1994). In this regard, exposure of RAW 264.7 macrophage cells to LPS resulted in the induction of iNOS and the resultant release of nitrite into the culture medium (Tsai et al., 1999; Wadsworth and

Koop, 1999). Preincubation of cells with RSV resulted in a dose-dependent inhibition of *iNOS* induction, and decreases in the steady-state levels of iNOS mRNA and protein. In contrast, RSV has also been shown to activate NO production through the induction of NOS activity in cultured bovine pulmonary artery endothelial cells (Hsieh et al., 1999b). In this model the vasodilatory activity of NO has been proposed as a possible mechanism for the prevention of initiation of atherosclerosis.

The effect of RSV on PMN-induced proinflammatory signals has also been investigated. In these series of experiments, PMN were stimulated by exposure to formyl methionyl leucyl phenylalanine (fMLP), the complement fragment C5a, the Ca^{2+} ionophore A23187, or a monoclonal antibody to the β2-integrin Mac-1, and the effects on ROI production, neutrophil degranulation, and the cell surface expression of Mac-1 were assessed (Rotondo et al., 1998). Enhanced ROI generation by PMN can result in membrane lipid peroxidation, endothelial damage, and increase in vascular permeability. Degranulation of neutrophils can result in the release of enzymes such as elastase and β-glucoronidase, which have also been linked to endothelial damage and subendothelial smooth muscle proliferation (Harlan, 1987; Totani et al., 1994). A third major contributor to endothelial injury is the increase in the cell surface expression of adhesion molecules of the β-2 integrin family such as CD11a/CD18 (LFA1), CD11b/CD18 (Mac-1), and CD11c/CD18 (p150/95) (Arnaout, 1990). RSV remarkably inhibited ROI production, release of elastase and β-glucoronidase from neutrophil granules, and the cell surface expression of the β2 integrin MAC-1, upon PMN stimulation. These results strongly indicate that RSV elicits inhibitory effect at all physiological phases of the inflammatory response, i.e., from the initial recruitment of PMNs to their activation and the subsequent release of inflammatory mediators. As the inflammatory response is a critical common denominator in the development of many systemic disorders, such as atherosclerosis and carcinogenesis, the strong anti-inflammatory activity of RSV could have tremendous clinical implications.

C. RSV and Transcription Factors: Regulation of Gene Expression

Thus far we have discussed the biological effects of RSV on a variety of critical biochemical pathways involved in normal cellular physiology. This includes a direct or indirect effect on gene expression, a process controlled by a class of proteins called transcription factors. Transcription factors bind to upstream DNA sequences to activate the transcription of DNA to mRNA. The upstream signals to trigger nuclear localization (for those transcription factors that are normally extranuclear) and DNA binding of these transcription factors vary depending on the stimulus, the cell type, and the intended response. One of the most striking biological activities of polyphenolics such as RSV is their remarkable anti-inflammatory potential (as described in the preceding section). Owing to this association, there has been a lot of interest in investigating the effect(s) of RSV and its derivatives on transcription factors that regulate the expression of inflammatory mediators, such as tumor necrosis alpha (TNF-α), interleukin 1(IL-1), IL-6, and iNOS (Manna et al., 2000; Wadsworth and Koop, 1999). These include C/EBP, *fos/jun*, AP-1, and the Rel family of transcription factors, in particular NF-κB.

The proinflammatory, carcinogenic, and growth-modulating effects of many compounds are mediated by NF-κB (Miagkov et al., 1998; Suganuma et al., 1999), and therefore, considering the anti-inflammatory and growth-inhibitory properties of RSV, a significant amount of work is underway to elucidate the effect of RSV on NF-κB activity. NF-κB is comprised of two proteins of 50 kD and 65 kD and in its unstimulated form resides in the cytosol in a complex with an inhibitory subunit IκB. Activation-induced phosphorylation of IκB results in its degradation, thus allowing NF-κB to enter the nucleus and activate gene transcription (Pahl, 1999). The effect of RSV on the activation of NF-κB induced by a variety of inflammatory agents was investigated in myeloid (U937), lymphoid (Jurkat), and epithelial (HeLa) cell lines. Results indicated that the presence of RSV prevented the activation of NF-κB triggered by exposure of these cell types to TNF, PMA, H_2O_2, LPS, okadaic acid, and ceramide (Manna et al., 2000).

Inhibition of TNF-induced activation by RSV was not only shown by electrophoretic gel moblity shift assays (EMSA), but also confirmed by specific antibodies against the p50 and p65 subunits (of NF-κB) and by the ability of the cold NF-κB to completely inhibit the shift in gel mobility. The mechanism of RSV-induced inhibition of NF-κB activity is distinctly different from that reported with chemical modifiers of NF-κB subunits that prevent its DNA-binding activity, such as herbimycin A and caffeic acid phenylethyl ester; RSV does not affect DNA-binding activity of NF-κB or other transcription factors such as SP-1 or Oct-1. However, the report provides evidence to support inhibition of TNF-induced phosphorylation and nuclear localization of the p65 subunit by RSV. Alternatively, RSV has also been shown to inhibit the phosphorylation (inactivation) and degradation of IκBα (Holmes-McNary and Baldwin, 2000), which sequesters NF-κB in the cytoplasm, although results to the contrary have also been reported (Ashikawa et al., 2002).

The ability of RSV to inhibit NF-κB activation triggered by a diverse class of stimuli that engage different intracellular signaling complexes suggests that RSV interferes with the activation of this critical transcription factor at a step common to many stimuli and signal transduction pathways. In this regard, an attractive candidate could be the intracellular level of ROI, as ROI are induced by most of the stimuli mentioned in the particular study. Considering that NF-κB is a pleiotropic transcription factor involved in diverse pathways ranging from endotoxin-induced inflammation to cell proliferation and oncogenesis to signals that turn on the cells' suicide program, molecules such as RSV that interfer with the activation of NF-κB are of particular interest to biologists and clinicians. However, it must be pointed out that there is some controversy regarding the inhibitory activity of RSV on NF-κB. For example, in a macrophage model of LPS-induced inflammatory response RSV had no effect on NF-κB activation (Wadsworth and Koop, 1999), and the authors contended that RSV had a more selective action on genes activated by LPS independent of NF-κB.

NF-κB is not the only transcription factor affected by RSV. Most agents that activate NF-κB also activate another transcription factor, AP-1 (activator protein 1) (Karin et al., 1997). RSV has been shown to inhibit TNF-induced activation of AP-1 (Manna et al., 2000). The activation of AP-1 is mediated by JNK (c-Jun N-terminal protein kinase) and the upstream kinase MEK (mitogen-activated protein kinase kinase, or MAPKK) (Karin and Delhase, 1998). TNF-induced activities of JNK and MEK were inhibited by RSV, thus providing a possible mechanism for AP-1 inhibition (Manna et al., 2000). Interestingly, among the proteins induced upon activation of NF-κB and AP-1 are iNOS and COX-2 (Hwang et al., 1997; von Knethen et al., 1999), two enzymes inhibited by RSV. Thus it is possible that RSV inhibits iNOS and COX-2 via its inhibitory effect on these transcription factors. It is also plausible that the expression of other genes regulated by NF-κB or AP-1, such as matrix metalloproteinase 9 (MMP-9), and cell surface adhesion molecules ICAM-1 and VCAM-1 (Collins et al., 1995; Sato and Seiki, 1993), which have been implicated in carcinogenesis, may also be muted upon exposure to RSV. Consistent with this, a recent report has demonstrated that RSV suppresses carcinogenesis in rats via downregulation of MMP9 (Banerjee et al., 2002).

The expression/function of the androgen receptor (AR), a transcription factor belonging to the nuclear steroid hormone receptor family, is also inhibited by RSV in prostate cancer cells (Mitchell et al., 1999). This transcription factor is an essential mediator of androgen action, controls the transcription of androgen-inducible genes such as PSA (prostate-specific antigen), and is implicated in the development of prostate cancer (Culig et al., 2002). Exposure of LNCaP (prostate cancer cell line) cells to RSV resulted in inhibition of growth of this androgen-responsive cell line via pathways that involved a decrease in the expression and function of the AR; the transcriptional activity of PSA was dramatically reduced upon RSV treatment of the prostate cancer cell line (Hsieh and Wu, 1999, 2000). In addition, RSV has been shown to possess both estrogen agonist and antagonist activities (Basly et al., 2000; Lu and Serrero, 1999). Estrogens act via binding to the estrogen receptor (ER), another member of the nuclear receptor superfamily. This ligand-receptor binding brings about transcriptional activation of estrogen-responsive target genes (Gusman et al., 2001). In studies using human breast carcinoma cells (MCF-7), exposure to RSV resulted in activation of transcription of genes (transfected in MCF-7 cells) responsive to estrogen (Gehm et al., 1997). This activity was dependent upon the presence of the estrogen response element (ERE) sequence and the type of ER; higher transcriptional activity with ERβ than ERα. However, the reported superagonist activity of RSV in the presence of estradiol was contradicted by reports demonstrating antiestrogenic activity of RSV; RSV suppressed estradiol-induced progesterone receptor expression (Lu and Serrero, 1999).

In another breast cancer cell line, T47D (estrogen dependent), low concentrations of RSV (10 μM) resulted in an increase in cell proliferation and growth (Gehm et al., 1997), whereas at relatively higher concentrations the cells underwent apoptotic death (Clement et al., 1998a). These opposing actions of RSV have given rise to some controversy with respect to the use of RSV or similar compounds as therapeutic agents against ER+ breast cancer cells. The estrogenic activity of RSV has also been demonstrated in ER+ pituitary cells, which undergo a significant increase in prolactin secretion (Stahl et al., 1998), and in MC3T3-E1 osteoblastic cells, which respond to RSV by increasing alkaline phosphatase and hydroxylase activity (Mizutani et al., 1998), indicating estrogenic and bone loss preventive effect. Despite this in vitro evidence suggesting strong estrogenic activity of RSV, in vivo studies (so far) using rat models have failed to corroborate the in vitro data (Ashby et al., 1999; Freyberger et al., 2001; Turner et al., 1999).

In the first reported cancer chemopreventive activity in vivo, RSV was shown to inhibit tumor formation induced by the aryl hydrocarbon DMBA (7,12-dimethylbenzanthracene) (Jang et al., 1997). The genotoxicity of aryl hydrocarbons is a function of their metabolic activation via binding to the aryl hydrocarbon receptor (AHR), a cytosolic protein that translocates to the nucleus upon ligand binding (Hayashi et al., 1994). Once in the nucleus, AHR forms a heterodimer with the aryl hydrocarbon nuclear translocator, thus forming a transcription factor that initiates the transcription of a number of genes (Rowlands and Gustafsson, 1997). The best-characterized response to AHR activation is the increase in transcription of the *CYP1A1* gene, which encodes for the cytochrome P450 (CYP450) isozyme CYP1A1 (Ciolino et al., 1998). CYP450 isozymes belong to a family of constitutive and inducible heme-containing enzymes involved in the metabolism of a wide variety of substances, including carcinogens such as aromatic hydrocarbons and heterocyclic amines (Murray, 2000; Nelson et al., 1996). The metabolized active forms of carcinogens can subsequently interact with human DNA and cause mutations.

Considering their carcinogenic potential, approaches aimed at directly inhibiting enzyme activity or upstream inhibition of the transcription of *CYP450* genes have been proposed as probable strategies for cancer prevention (Murray, 2000). The effect of RSV on AHR function and *CYP1A1* transcription has been the focus of intense investigations. These studies provide ample evidence that RSV inhibits AH-induced *CYP1A1* expression at the mRNA and protein levels (Casper et al., 1999; Ciolino et al., 1998; Ciolino and Yeh, 1999). In experiments done with DMBA, RSV inhibited the binding of the nuclear AHR to the xenobiotic-response element of the *CYP1A1* promoter without directly binding to the AHR (Chang et al., 2001). Similar effects of RSV on other CYP450 isozymes, such as CYP1A2 and CYP3A4, have also been documented (Bhat and Pezzuto, 2002; Chan and Delucchi, 2000). Considering that CYP450s are overexpressed in a variety of human tumors, the strong inhibitory effect of RSV and similar compounds could have tremendous implications for the prevention and treatment of cancer.

Any discussion on transcription factors will not be complete without the mention of the tumor suppressor p53. p53 serves as the guardian of the genome by regulating the cell cycle (prevents progression through S phase) and activating the transcription of DNA repair enzymes such as GADD45, thereby preventing damaged DNA from being replicated (Steele et al., 1998). In addition, p53 can activate the transcription of genes involved in the apoptotic pathway, thus ensuring deletion of damaged or unwanted cells (Flatt et al., 2000). Loss-of-function mutations of p53 are associated with an increased incidence of tumor formation (Hussain et al., 2000). The effect of RSV on intracellular p53 level and its transcriptional activity has been studied in cancerous and noncancerous cell lines. In one such study involving cultured bovine pulmonary artery endothelial cells, RSV was shown to induce accumulation of p53 with the resultant increase in transcription of the cyclin-dependent kinase (cdk) inhibitor $p21^{Wafl/Cipl}$ and cell cycle arrest (Hsieh et al., 1999b). This prevents proliferation of endothelial cells, a factor that may explain the cardioprotective effect of red wine polyphenols. In a different model using mouse JB6 epidermal cell line, RSV was shown to increase the transactivation of p53 activity by specifically activating phosphorylation at serine 15, mutation of which abrogates the apoptotic activity of p53 (She et al., 2001). This was linked to an upstream activation of the MAP kinases, in particular ERKs (extracellular signal-regulated protein kinase) and p38 kinase. Similarly, gene knockout of p53 (p53−/−) in mouse fibroblasts resulted in complete resistance to RSV-induced death, further supporting the involvement of p53 in the biological activity of RSV (Huang et al., 1999).

D. Regulation of Cell Proliferation and Apoptosis: Cancer Chemopreventive Activity

Since its reported cancer chemopreventive activity in a mouse model of carcinogenesis, there has been a flurry of papers reporting the effects of RSV on critical events that regulate cellular proliferation and growth. In this regard, biochemical pathways involved in differentiation, transformation, cell cycle regulation, and cell death induction have all been demonstrated as potential targets of RSV (Bhat and Pezzuto, 2002; Gusman et al., 2001; Joe et al., 2002; Soleas et al., 2001a). In the preceding sections describing the diverse signaling networks impacted by RSV, I touched on some of the intricate pathways operational in carcinogenic transformation of cells. These include intracellular generation of ROI, activation of protein kinases, induction of enzymes that generate proinflammatory mediators such as COX and lipoxygenase, activation of transcription factors such as NF-κB, AP-1, CYP1A1, AHR, and p53, growth stimulation of estrogen-responsive cells, etc. As remarkable as it seems, the regulatory/inhibitory effect of RSV on these signal transduction pathways has generated tremendous interest in its clinical chemopreventive and chemotherapeutic potential.

Depending on its concentration, RSV can both stimulate (as shown with ER+ breast cancer and pituitary cells (Mizutani et al., 1998) and inhibit cell proliferation (Clement et al., 1998a; Joe et al., 2002; Pervaiz, 2001). Generally, at the concentrations used in vitro the effect is predominantly antiproliferative, as demonstrated in a variety of cancer cell lines (Bhat and Pezzuto, 2002). The mechanism(s) for this growth inhibitory activity of RSV could be due to its ability to block ribonucleotide reductase, a complex enzyme that catalyzes the reduction of ribonucleotides into the corresponding deoxyribonucleotides (Fontecave et al., 1998). Inhibitors of ribonucleotide reductases, such as gemcitabine (2'-difluoro-2'-deoxycytidine), have been in clinical use owing to their inhibitory effect on DNA synthesis (Grunewald et al., 1992). A second probable mechanism for the observed antiproliferative activity of RSV could be its ability to inhibit DNA polymerase (Tsan et al., 2002) or ornithine decarboxylase (Schneider et al., 2000), a key enzyme involved in polyamine synthesis that is increased in cancer growth. The antioxidant activity of RSV could be yet another mechanism for growth inhibition, as a slight prooxidant intracellular milieu, an invariable finding in cancer cells (Cerutti, 1985), is a strong stimulus for proliferation. However, recent findings and our unpublished data (Li Ying and S. Pervaiz) provide evidence to suggest that RSV can both inhibit and stimulate intracellular ROI production, depending on the cell type. These data may help to explain the conflicting data demonstrating pro- and antiproliferative effects of RSV on mammalian cells.

Acquisition of the cancer phenotype is a process that involves dysregulated growth, an outcome of enhanced proliferation and resistance to apoptotic triggers. Regulation of growth and proliferation in untransformed cells is maintained by tight control of the cell cycle by the cell cycle checkpoint proteins, in particular p53, Rb, p27, and the cdk-inhibitor $p21^{Wafl/Cipl}$. Any alteration in the normal functioning of these proteins allows for the cells to undergo unabated cycling resulting in accumulation of DNA mutations, a prerequisite for carcinogenesis. A number of studies have now established that RSV inhibits cellular proliferation by inducing cell cycle arrest in the G1/S phase (Bhat and Pezzuto, 2002). In CEM-C7H2 acute leukemia cells and MCF-7 breast cancer cells exposure to RSV resulted in accumulation of cells in the S phase (Bernhard et al., 2000; Joe et al., 2002). Exposure to RSV also resulted in a transient increase in the expression of G1/S regulators, such as cyclin D1, cdk4, and cyclin E, in MCF-7 cells (Pozo-Guisado et al., 2002); cyclins D1 and E are responsible for S-phase entry. These cells ultimately undergo apoptotic death, unlike the breast cancer cell line MDA-MB-231 where cell cycle activation or upregulation of p21, p53, or p27 did not occur and the mode of inhibition of cell proliferation was attributed to nonapototic death of the cells (Pozo-Guisado et al., 2002). Interestingly, the compound was extremely effective against a highly invasive breast carcinoma cell line, MDA-MB-435 (Hsieh et al., 1999a). Similarly, RSV treatment has been shown to induce cell cycle arrest in human promyelocytic leukemia HL60 cells at the S/G2 phase transition and a subsequent increase in the number of cells in the G1/S phase, brought about by an increase in cyclins A and E and inactivation of cdc2 (Ragione et al., 1998).

In another study using A431 epidermoid cancer cells, RSV decreased the levels of cyclins D1, D2, E, and cdk2 and cdk4/6 (Ahmad et al., 2001). RSV has also been shown to induce changes in the cell cycle in prostate cancer LNCaP cells with a significant decrease in the levels of prostate-specific antigen (PSA) (Hsieh and Wu, 1999). Suppression of cell cycle progression through the S and G2 phase and a concomitant increase in the expression of p53 and $p21^{Wafl/Cipl}$ has also been demonstrated in pulmonary epithelial cells upon exposure to RSV (Hsieh et al., 1999b). In contrast, RSV has been shown to stimulate proliferation and differentiation of MC3T3-E1 osteoblast cells as shown by an increase in DNA synthesis, alkaline phosphatase, and hydroxylase activity–estrogenic effect (Mizutani et al., 1998). Collectively, the effect of RSV on growth and cell cycle control proteins seems to vary between cell types.

Although, some of the in vitro biological effects of RSV have not been corroborated in vivo, there is evidence to support the antiproliferative and growth-inhibitory activity in animal models of carcinogenesis. For instance, RSV-treated mice developed fewer tumors in response to DMBA and PMA (Jang et al., 1997). Similar effects were observed in a rat tumor model (Carbo et al., 1999). Our group was the first to investigate the mechanism of the reported cancer-chemopreventive activity of RSV. Using HL60 human leukemia and T47D breast carcinoma cells, we showed that the decrease in incidence of tumors in RSV-treated mice could be due to targeted killing of the tumor cells by RSV. Both cell lines exhibited classic hallmarks of apoptotic death (Clement et al., 1998a; Pervaiz, 2001). Apoptosis is a programmed series of events triggered in response to death receptor ligation, such as CD95/Apo1/Fas or TNF-r, or exposure to genotoxic agents such as anticancer drugs, or exposure to UV irradiation (Hengartner, 2000). The commitment and execution phases of this death pathway depend on an intricate cross-talk between the caspase family of intracellular cystine proteases and amplification factors derived from the mitochondria (Pervaiz et al., 1999b; Thornberry, 1998). In a classic death receptor model (CD95 ligation) early recruitment and activation of the initiator caspase-8 results in direct activation of downstream caspases leading to the executioner caspase-3 activation and cellular disassembly or can engage the mitochondrial death pathway to trigger the release of apoptogenic factors such as Cyt.C, apoptosis-inducing factor (AIF), and Smac/Diablo. Cyt.C can complex with cytosolic Apaf-1 (apoptosis-protease-activating factor-1) and procaspase 9 in the presence of dATP to form the apoptosome (Scaffidi et al., 1998). Once assembled, this complex then activates caspase 9, which then engages caspase 3, resulting in DNA fragmentation and death.

Caspase-8-dependent recruitment of the mitochondria is facilitated by the proapoptotic Bcl-2 family proteins Bax and Bid (Korsmeyer, 1999), which can translocate to the mitochondria and trigger mitochondrial permeability transition by changing the conformation of the mitochondrial inner membrane pore (PT pore) (Green and Kroemer, 1998). Owing to the critical role that mitochondria play in the execution of the apoptotic signal and the fact that the death inhibitory protein Bcl-2 was first isolated as a mitochondrial protein, they have become attractive candidates for the design of targeted therapies. Our initial findings showed that exposure of HL60 cells to RSV resulted in changes in the mitochondrial transmembrane potential and release of Cyt.C, suggesting a mitochondrial-specific activity of RSV (Clement et al., 1998a; Pervaiz, 2001). Since these observations, a number of other reports have corroborated the mitochondrial-dependent apoptotic activity of RSV against a variety of tumor cell lines (Dorrie et al., 2001; Mahyar-Roemer et al., 2001; Roman et al., 2002; Tinhofer et al., 2001).

There are also reports indicating upregulation of the proapoptotic protein Bax and downregulation of Bcl-2 upon exposure to RSV (Tessitore et al., 2000). However, a recent report (Mahyar-Roemer et al., 2002) and our data (K. Ahmad and S. Pervaiz; unpublished results) seem to suggest that RSV-mediated apoptosis is independent of Bax as gene knockout of Bax (Bax−/−) did not alter tumor cell sensitivity to RSV. In addition, we showed that pretreatment of cells with relatively low doses of RSV can sensitize the cells to drug-induced apoptosis (Pervaiz, 2001), thereby suggesting a potential synergistic activity that could be of clinical relevance. However, our more recent findings indicate that RSV can facilitate or inhibit the death signal and that this effect is dependent on whether RSV elicits a pro- or antioxidant effect in the cell type. For example, exposure of HL60 and LNCaP cells to similar concentrations of RSV resulted in a distinctly different effect on the cellular redox state; RSV increase intracellular O_2^- in HL60 cells whereas a dose-dependent drop is observed in LNCaP cells (Li and Pervaiz; unpublished results).

The involvement of p53 and p21 (as discussed in the preceding section) has also been reported in the apoptotic response elicited by RSV. As p53 controls the transcription of a number of essential mediators of apoptosis, such as CD95/Apo1/Fas, Bax, p21, etc., the p53 dependence of RSV-induced apoptosis is of particular importance. In our earlier report we showed that RSV-induced apoptosis in HL60 and T47D cells was mediated by upregulation of CD95-CD95L interaction, thereby resulting in death of CD95-expressing cells (Clement et al., 1998a). A number of other apoptosis-inducing agents have been shown to sensitize tumor cells by enhancing the interaction between the CD95 receptor and its ligand (Micheau et al., 1997). However, CD95-independent death signaling has also been demonstrated in other cell lines (Bernhard et al., 2000; Tsan et al., 2000). In a recent report, suppression of DMBA-induced mammary carcinogenesis by RSV in rats was linked to the inhibition of COX-2 and MMP9 expression and blocking of NF-κB activation (Banerjee et al., 2002).

In contrast to its apoptosis-inducing activity, RSV has also been shown to inhibit apoptosis in some systems. In this regard, an earlier report indicated that RSV interfered with H_2O_2-induced apoptotic signal (MacCarrone et al., 1999). We have previously shown that H_2O_2 triggers apoptosis by decreasing intracellular O_2^- and cytosolic pH (Clement et al., 1998b), thus creating a permissive intracellular milieu for death execution (Pervaiz and Clement, 2002). A slight increase in intracellular O_2^- can inhibit receptor or drug-induced apoptosis via direct or indirect effect on spase activation pathways (Clement and Stamenkovic, 1996; Pervaiz et al., 1999a). Our recent data (K. Ahmad and S. Pervaiz; unpublished results) indicate that the inhibitory effect of RSV on H_2O_2-induced apoptosis is mediated by its prooxidant activity in HL60 cells (increase in intracellular O_2^-), which prevents H_2O_2-mediated drop in intracellular O_2^- and cytosolic pH, thus creating a nonconducive environment for apoptotic execution.

IV. CONCLUDING REMARKS

The body of evidence presented in this chapter speaks volumes for the clinical potential of wine polyphenolics such as RSV and related compounds. The relatively simple chemical structure enables RSV to interact with receptors and enzymes, giving rise to biological effects such as suppression of growth, induction of differentiation, inhibition of ROS production, cell cycle regulation, inhibition of lipid peroxidation, downregulation of proinflammatory mediators, regulation of gene expression by impacting transcription factor activity, and upregulation of death-inducing factors. These in vitro effects have been corroborated in some studies demonstrating the beneficial effects on the cardiovascular, neurological, and hepatic systems; however, the most exciting in vivo data relate to its cancer chemopreventive and chemotherapeutic activity. Because of the diverse biological activity, RSV and related compounds have joined with many other promising agents being investigated for their disease-preventive and therapeutic potential. Being a natural constituent of wine, fruits, and nuts, and owing to the fact that it has no untoward effects on normal cells or tissues, RSV is under preclinical scrutiny. The outcome of these studies will provide the definite answer to the real clinical potential of this remarkable compound.

ACKNOWLEDGMENTS

I would like to extend my sincere apologies to those whose invaluable contributions could have been inadvertently overlooked. I wish to acknowledge the National Medical Research Council and the Biomedical Research Council of Singapore and the Academic Research Fund, National University of Singapore, for the funding support.

REFERENCES

Ahmad N, Adhami VM, Afaq F, Feyes DK, Mukhtar H. Resveratrol causes WAF-1/p21-mediated G(1)-phase arrest of cell cycle and induction of apoptosis in human epidermoid carcinoma A431 cells. Clin Cancer Res 2001; 7:1466–1473.

Arnaout MA. Structure and function of the leukocyte adhesion molecules CD11/CD18. Blood 1990; 75:1037–1050.

Ashby J, Tinwell H, Pennie W, Brooks AN, Lefevre PA, Beresford N, Sumpter JP. Partial ad weak oestrogenicity of the red wine constituent resveratrol: consideration of its superagonist activity in MCF-7 cells and its suggested cardiovascular protective effects. J Appl Toxicol 1999; 19:39–45.

Ashikawa K, Majumdar S, Banerjee S, Bharti AC, Shishodia S, Aggarwal BB. Piceatannol inhibits TNF-induced NF-kappaB activation and NF-kappaB-

mediated gene expression through suppression of IkappaBalpha kinase and p65 phosphorylation. J Immunol 2002; 169:6490–6497.
Banerjee S, Bueso-Ramos C, Aggarwal BB. Suppression of 7,12-dimethylbenz(a)anthracene-induced mammary carcinogenesis in rats by resveratrol: role of nuclear factor-kappaB, cyclooxygenase 2, and matrix metalloprotease 9. Cancer Res 2002; 62:4945–4954.
Basly JP, Marre-Fournier F, Le Bail JC, Habrioux G, Chulia AJ. Estrogenic/antiestrogenic and scavenging properties of (E)- and (Z)- resveratrol. Life Sci 2000; 66:769–777.
Bernhard D, Tinhofer I, Tonko M, Hubl H, Ausserlechner MJ, Greil R, Kofler R, Csordas A. Resveratrol causes arrest in the S-phase prior to Fas-independent apoptosis in CEM-C7H2 acute leukemia cells. Cell Death Differ 2000; 7:834–842.
Bhat KP, Pezzuto JM. Cancer chemopreventive activity of resveratrol. Ann NY Acad Sci 2002; 957:210–229.
Carbo N, Costelli P, Baccino FM, Lopez-Soriano FJ, Argiles JM. Resveratrol, a natural product present in wine, decreases tumour growth in a rat tumour model. Biochem Biophys Res Commun 1999; 254:739–743.
Casper RF, Quesne M, Rogers IM, Shirota T, Jolivet A, Milgrom E, Savouret JF. Resveratrol has antagonist activity on the aryl hydrocarbon receptor: implications for prevention of dioxin toxicity. Mol Pharmacol 1999; 56:784–790.
Cerutti PA. Prooxidant states and tumor promotion. Science 1985; 227:375–381.
Chan WK, Delucchi AB. Resveratrol, a red wine constituent, is a mechanism-based inactivator of cytochrome P450 3A4. Life Sci 2000; 67:3103–3112.
Chang TK, Chen J. Differential inhibition and inactivation of human CYP1 enzymes by trans- resveratrol: evidence for mechanism-based inactivation of CYP1A2. J Pharmacol Exp Ther 2001; 299:874–882.
Ciolino HP, Daschner PJ, Yeh GC. Resveratrol inhibits transcription of CYP1A1 in vitro by preventing activation of the aryl hydrocarbon receptor. Cancer Res 1998; 58:5707–5712.
Ciolino HP, Yeh GC. Inhibition of aryl hydrocarbon-induced cytochrome P-450 1A1 enzyme activity and CYP1A1 expression by resveratrol. Mol Pharmacol 1999; 56:760–767.
Clement MV, Hirpara JL, Chawdhury SH, Pervaiz S. Chemopreventive agent resveratrol, a natural product derived from grapes, triggers CD95 signaling-dependent apoptosis in human tumor cells. Blood 1998a; 92:996–1002.
Clement MV, Ponton A, Pervaiz S. Apoptosis induced by hydrogen peroxide is mediated by decreased superoxide anion concentration and reduction of intracellular milieu. FEBS Lett 1998b; 440:13–18.
Clement MV, Stamenkovic I. Superoxide anion is a natural inhibitor of FAS-mediated cell death. EMBO J 1996; 15:216–225.
Collins T, Read MA, Neish AS, Whitley MZ, Thanos D, Maniatis T. Transcriptional regulation of endothelial cell adhesion molecules: NF-kappa B and cytokine-inducible enhancers. FASEB J 1995; 9:899–909.

Cuendet M, Pezzuto JM. The role of cyclooxygenase and lipoxygenase in cancer chemoprevention. Drug Metabol Drug Interact 2000; 17:109–157.

Culig Z, Klocker H, Bartsch G, Hobisch A. Androgen receptors in prostate cancer. Endocr Relat Cancer 2002; 9:155–170.

Ding XZ, Adrian TE. Resveratrol inhibits proliferation and induces apoptosis in human pancreatic cancer cells. Pancreas 2002; 25:e71–e76.

Dorrie J, Gerauer H, Wachter Y, Zunino SJ. Resveratrol induces extensive apoptosis by depolarizing mitochondrial membranes and activating caspase-9 in acute lymphoblastic leukemia cells. Cancer Res 2001; 61:4731–4739.

Draczynska-Lusiak B, Doung A, Sun AY. Oxidized lipoproteins may play a role in neuronal cell death in Alzheimer disease. Mol Chem Neuropathol 1998; 33:139–148.

Ebel J. Phytoalexin synthesis: the biochemical analysis of the induction process. Annu Rev Phytopathol 1986; 24:235–264.

Esterbauer H, Gebicki J, Puhl H, Jurgens G. The role of lipid peroxidation and antioxidants in oxidative modification of LDL. Free Rad Biol Med 1992; 13:341–390.

Ferry-Dumazet H, Garnier O, Mamani-Matsuda M, Vercauteren J, Belloc F, Billiard C, Dupouy M, Thiolat D, Kolb JP, Marit G, et al. Resveratrol inhibits the growth and induces the apoptosis of both normal and leukemic hematopoietic cells. Carcinogenesis 2002; 23:1327–1333.

Flatt PM, Polyak K, Tang LJ, Scatena CD, Westfall MD, Rubinstein LA, Yu J, Kinzler KW, Vogelstein B, Hill DE, Pietenpol JA. p53-Dependent expression of PIG3 during proliferation, genotoxic stress, and reversible growth arrest. Cancer Lett 2000; 156:63–72.

Fontecave M, Lepoivre M, Elleingand E, Gerez C, Guittet O. Resveratrol, a remarkable inhibitor of ribonucleotide reductase. FEBS Lett 1998; 421:277–279.

Frankel EN, Waterhouse AL, Kinsella JE. Inhibition of human LDL oxidation by resveratrol. Lancet 1993; 341:1103–1104.

Fremont L. Biological effects of resveratrol. Life Sci 2000; 66:663–673.

Freyberger A, Hartmann E, Hildebrand H, Krotlinger F. Differential response of immature rat uterine tissue to ethinylestradiol and the red wine constituent resveratrol. Arch Toxicol 2001; 74:709–715.

Fuhrman B, Lavy A, Aviram M. Consumption of red wine with meals reduces the susceptibility of human plasma and low-density lipoprotein to lipid peroxidation. Am J Clin Nutr 1995; 61:549–554.

Gehm BD, McAndrews JM, Chien PY, Jameson JL. Resveratrol, a polyphenolic compound found in grapes and wine, is an agonist for the estrogen receptor. Proc Natl Acad Sci U S A 1997; 94:14138–14143.

Gentilli M, Mazoit JX, Bouaziz H, Fletcher D, Casper RF, Benhamou D, Savouret JF. Resveratrol decreases hyperalgesia induced by carrageenan in the rat hind paw. Life Sci 2001; 68:1317–1321.

Gierse JK, Hauser SD, Creely DP, Koboldt C, Rangwala SH, Isakson PC, Seibert K. Expression and selective inhibition of the constitutive and inducible forms of human cyclo-oxygenase. Biochem J 1995; 305:479–484.

Goldberg DM, Hahn SE, Parkes JG. Beyond alcohol: beverage consumption and cardiovascular mortality. Clin Chim Acta 1995; 237:155–187.

Green D, Kroemer G. The central executioners of apoptosis: caspases or mitochondria? Trends Cell Biol 1998; 8:267–271.

Grunewald R, Kantarjian H, Du M, Faucher K, Tarassoff P, Plunkett W. Gemcitabine in leukemia: a phase I clinical, plasma, and cellular pharmacology study. J Clin Oncol 1992; 10:406–413.

Gusman J, Malonne H, Atassi G. A reappraisal of the potential chemopreventive and chemotherapeutic properties of resveratrol. Carcinogenesis 2001; 22:1111–1117.

Hain R, Bieseler B, Kindl H, Schroder G, Stocker R. Expression of a stilbene synthase gene in *Nicotiana tabacum* results in synthesis of the phytoalexin resveratrol. Plant Mol Biol 1990; 15:325–335.

Hain R, Reif HJ, Krause E, Langebartels R, Kindl H, Vornam B, Wiese W, Schmelzer E, Schreier PH, Stocker RH, et al. Disease resistance results from foreign phytoalexin expression in a novel plant. Nature 1993; 361:153–156.

Halliwell B. Free radicals, antioxidants, and human disease: curiosity, cause, or consequence? Lancet 1994; 344:721–724.

Halliwell B, Gutteridge JMC. Free Radicals in Biology and Medicine. 2d ed. Oxford, England: Clarendon Press, 1999.

Harlan JM. Neutrophil-mediated vascular injury. Acta Med Scand Suppl 1987; 715(suppl):123–129.

Hattori R, Otani H, Maulik N, Das DK. Pharmacological preconditioning with resveratrol: role of nitric oxide. Am J Physiol Heart Circ Physiol 2002; 282:H1988–H1995.

Haworth RS, Avkiran M. Inhibition of protein kinase D by resveratrol. Biochem Pharmacol 2001; 62:1647–1651.

Hayashi S, Watanabe J, Nakachi K, Eguchi H, Gotoh O, Kawajiri K. Interindividual difference in expression of human Ah receptor and related P450 genes. Carcinogenesis 1994; 15:801–806.

Hengartner MO. The biochemistry of apoptosis. Nature 2000; 407:770–776.

Holmes-McNary M, Baldwin AS. Chemopreventive properties of *trans*-resveratrol are associated with inhibition of activation of the IkappaB kinase. Cancer Res 2000; 60:3477–3483.

Hoos G, Blaich R. Metabolism of stilbene phytoalexin in grapevines: oxidation of resveratrol in single cell culture. Vitis 1988; 27:1–12.

Hsieh TC, Burfeind P, Laud K, Backer JM, Traganos F, Darzynkiewicz Z, Wu JM. Cell cycle effects and control of gene expression by resveratrol in human breast carcinoma cell lines with different metastatic potentials. Int J Oncol 1999a; 15:245–252.

Hsieh TC, Juan G, Darzynkiewicz Z, Wu JM. Resveratrol increases nitric oxide synthase, induces accumulation of p53 and p21 (WAF1/CIP1), and suppresses cultured bovine pulmonary artery endothelial cell proliferation by perturbing progression through S and G2. Cancer Res 1999b; 59:2596–2601.

Hsieh TC, Wu JM. Differential effects on growth, cell cycle arrest, and induction of apoptosis by resveratrol in human prostate cancer cell lines. Exp Cell Res 1999; 249:109–115.

Hsieh TC, Wu JM. Grape-derived chemopreventive agent resveratrol decreases prostate- specific antigen (PSA) expression in LNCaP cells by an androgen receptor (AR)-independent mechanism. Anticancer Res 2000; 20:225–228.

Huang C, Ma WY, Goranson A, Dong Z. Resveratrol suppresses cell transformation and induces apoptosis through a p53-dependent pathway. Carcinogenesis 1999; 20:237–242.

Hung LM, Chen JK, Huang SS, Lee RS, Su MJ. Cardioprotective effect of resveratrol, a natural antioxidant derived from grapes. Cardiovasc Res 2000; 47:549–555.

Hussain SP, Hollstein MH, Harris CC. p53 tumor suppressor gene: at the crossroads of molecular carcinogenesis, molecular epidemiology, and human risk assessment. Ann NY Acad Sci 2000; 919:79–85.

Hwang D, Jang BC, Yu G, Boudreau M. Expression of mitogen-inducible cyclooxygenase induced by lipopolysaccharide: mediation through both mitogen-activated protein kinase and NF-kappaB signaling pathways in macrophages. Biochem Pharmacol 1997; 54:87–96.

Jang M, Cai L, Udeani GO, Slowing KV, Thomas CF, Beecher CW, Fong HH, Farnsworth NR, Kinghorn AD, Mehta RG, et al. Cancer chemopreventive activity of resveratrol, a natural product derived from grapes. Science 1997; 275:218–220.

Jeandet P, Bessis R, Sbaghi M, Meunier P. Production of the phytoalexin resveratrol by grape berries as a response to Botrytis attack under natural conditions. J Phytopathol 1995a; 143:135–139.

Jeandet P, Bessis R, Sbaghi M, Meunier P, Trollat P. Resveratrol content of wines of different ages: relationship with fungal disease pressure in the vineyard. Am J Enol Vitic 1995b; 46:1–4.

Jeandet P, Douillet-Breuil AC, Bessis R, Debord S, Sbaghi M, Adrian M. Phytoalexins from the Vitaceae: biosynthesis, phytoalexin gene expression in transgenic plants, antifungal activity, and metabolism. J Agric Food Chem 2002; 50:2731–2741.

Jeandet P, Sbaghi M, Bessis R, Meunier P. The potential relationship of stilbene (resveratrol) synthesis to anthocyanin content in grape berry skin. Vitis 1995c; 34:91–94.

Joe AK, Liu H, Suzui M, Vural ME, Xiao D, Weinstein IB. Resveratrol induces growth inhibition, S-phase arrest, apoptosis, and changes in biomarker expression in several human cancer cell lines. Clin Cancer Res 2002; 8:893–903.

Karin M, Delhase M. JNK or IKK, AP-1 or NF-kappaB, which are the targets for MEK kinase 1 action? Proc Natl Acad Sci USA 1998; 95:9067–9069.

Karin M, Liu Z, Zandi E. AP-1 function and regulation. Curr Opin Cell Biol 1997; 9:240–246.

Kawada N, Seki S, Inoue M, Kuroki T. Effect of antioxidants, resveratrol, quercetin, and *N*-acetylcysteine, on the functions of cultured rat hepatic stellate cells and Kupffer cells. Hepatology 1998; 27:1265–1274.

Kimura Y, Okuda H, Arichi S. Effects of stilbenes on arachidonate metabolism in leukocytes. Biochim Biophys Acta 1985; 834:275–278.

Kimura Y, Okuda H, Kubo M. Effects of stilbenes isolated from medicinal plants on arachidonate metabolism and degranulation in human polymorphonuclear leukocytes. J Ethnopharmacol 1995; 45:131–139.

Kopp P. Resveratrol, a phytoestrogen found in red wine: a possible explanation for the conundrum of the 'French paradox'? Eur J Endocrinol 1998; 138:619–620.

Korsmeyer SJ. BCL-2 gene family and the regulation of programmed cell death. Cancer Res 1999; 59:1693s–1700s.

Kubo M, Kimurta Y, Shin H, Haneda T, Tani T, Namba K. Studies on the anti-fungal substances of crude drug. II. On the roots of *Polygonum capsidatum* Sieb et Zucc. (Polygonaceae). Shoyakugaku Zasshi 1981; 35:58–61.

Lamuela-Raventos RM, Romero-Perez AI, Waterhouse AL, de la Torre-Boronat MC. Direct HPLC analysis of *cis* and *trans*-resveratrol and piecid isomers in Spanish red *Vitis vinifera* wines. J Agric Food Chem 1995; 43:281–283.

Langcake P, Pryce RJ. The production of resveratrol by *Vitis vinifera* and other members of the vitaceae as a response to infection or injury. Physiol Plant Pathol 1976; 9:77–86.

Langcake P, Pryce RJ. Oxidative dimerization of 4-hydroxystilbenes in vitro: production of a grapevine phytoalexin mimic. J Chem Soc Commun 1977a; 1412:208–210.

Langcake P, Pryce RJ. The production of resveratrol and the viniferins by grapevines in response to ultraviolet irradiation. Phytochemistry 1977b; 16: 1193–1196.

Lu R, Serrero G. Resveratrol, a natural product derived from grape, exhibits antiestrogenic activity and inhibits the growth of human breast cancer cells. J Cell Physiol 1999; 179:297–304.

MacCarrone M, Lorenzon T, Guerrieri P, Agro AF. Resveratrol prevents apoptosis in K562 cells by inhibiting lipoxygenase and cyclooxygenase activity. Eur J Biochem 1999; 265:27–34.

Mahyar-Roemer M, Katsen A, Mestres P, Roemer K. Resveratrol induces colon tumor cell apoptosis independently of p53 and precede by epithelial differentiation, mitochondrial proliferation and membrane potential collapse. Int J Cancer 2001; 94:615–622.

Mahyar-Roemer M, Kohler H, Roemer K. Role of Bax in resveratrol-induced apoptosis of colorectal carcinoma cells. BMC Cancer 2002; 2:2727.

Manna SK, Mukhopadhyay A, Aggarwal BB. Resveratrol suppresses TNF-induced activation of nuclear transcription factors NF-kappa B., activator protein-1, and apoptosis: potential role of reactive oxygen intermediates and lipid peroxidation. J Immunol 2000; 164:6509–6519.

Martinez J, Moreno JJ. Effect of resveratrol, a natural polyphenolic compound, on reactive oxygen species and prostaglandin production. Biochem Pharmacol 2000; 59:865–870.

Mgbonyebi OP, Russo J, Russo IH. Antiproliferative effect of synthetic resveratrol on human breast epithelial cells. Int J Oncol 1998; 12:865–869.

Miagkov AV, Kovalenko DV, Brown CE, Didsbury JR, Cogswell JP, Stimpson SA, Baldwin AS, Makarov SS. NF-kappaB activation provides the potential link between inflammation and hyperplasia in the arthritic joint. Proc Natl Acad Sci USA 1998; 95:13859–13864.

Micheau O, Solary E, Hamman A, Martin F, Dimanche-Boitrel MT. Sensitization of cancer cells treated with cytotoxi drugs to fas-mediated cytotoxicity. J Natl Cancer Inst 1997; 89:783–789.

Miller NJ, Rice-Evans CA. Antioxidant activity of resveratrol in red wine. Clin Chem 1995; 41:1789.

Mitchell SH, Zhu W, Young CY. Resveratrol inhibits the expression and function of the androgen receptor in LNCaP prostate cancer cells. Cancer Res 1999; 59:5892–5895.

Mizutani K, Ikeda K, Kawai Y, Yamori Y. Resveratrol stimulates the proliferation and differentiation of osteoblastic MC3T3-E1 cells. Biochem Biophys Res Commun 1998; 253:859–863.

Morris GZ, Williams RL, Elliott MS, Beebe SJ. Resveratrol induces apoptosis in LNCaP cells and requires hydroxyl groups to decrease viability in LNCaP and DU 145 cells. Prostate 2002; 52:319–329.

Murray GI. The role of cytochrome P450 in tumour development and progression and its potential in therapy. J Pathol 2000; 192:419–426.

Nelson DR, Koymans L, Kamataki T, Stegeman JJ, Feyereisen R, Waxman DJ, Waterman MR, Gotoh O, Coon MJ, Estabrook RW, et al. P450 superfamily: update on new sequences, gene mapping, accession numbers and nomenclature. Pharmacogenetics 1996; 6:1–42.

Nonomura S, Kanagawa H, Makimoto A. Chemical constituents of polygonaceous plants. I. Studies on the components of Ko-jo-kon. (*Polygonum capsidatum*-SIEB et ZUCC). Yakugaku Zasshi 1963; 83:988–990.

Olas B, Wachowicz B, Szewczuk J, Saluk-Juszczak J, Kaca W. The effect of resveratrol on the platelet secretory process induced by endotoxin and thrombin. Microbios 2001; 105:7–13.

Orsini F, Pelizzoni F, Verotta L, Aburjai T, Rogers CB. Isolation, synthesis, and antiplatelet aggregation activity of resveratrol 3-*O*-beta-D-glucopyranoside and related compounds. J Nat Prod 1997; 60:1082–1087.

Packer L. Interactions among anti-oxidants in health and diseases: vitamin E and its redox cycle. Proc Soc Exp Biol Med 1992; 200:271–276.

Pahl HL. Activators and target genes of Rel/NF-kappaB transcription factors. Oncogene 1999; 18:6853–6866.

Pervaiz S. Resveratrol—from the bottle to the bedside? Leuk Lymphoma 2001; 40:491–498.

Pervaiz S, Clement MV. A permissive apoptotic environment: function of a decrease in intracellular superoxide anion and cytosolic acidification. Biochem Biophys Res Commun 2002; 290:1145–1150.

Pervaiz S, Ramalingam JK, Hirpara JL. Superoxide anion inhibits drug-induced tumor cell death. FEBS Lett 1999a; 459:343–348.

Pervaiz S, Seyed MA, Hirpara JL, Clement MV, Loh KW. Purified photoproducts of merocyanine 540 trigger cytochrome C release and caspase 8-dependent apoptosis in human leukemia and melanoma cells. Blood 1999b; 93:4096–4108.

Pozo-Guisado E, Alvarez-Barrientos A, Mulero-Navarro S, Santiago-Josefat B, Fernandez-Salguero PM. The antiproliferative activity of resveratrol results in apoptosis in MCF-7 but not in MDA-MB-231 human breast cancer cells: cell-specific alteration of the cell cycle. Biochem Pharmacol 2002; 64:1375–1386.

Ragione FD, Cucciolla V, Borriello A, Pietra VD, Racioppi L, Soldati G, Manna C, Galletti P, Zappia V. Resveratrol arrests the cell division cycle at S/G2 phase transition. Biochem Biophys Res Commun 1998; 250:53–58.

Roman V, Billard C, Kern C, Ferry-Dumazet H, Izard JC, Mohammad R, Mossalayi DM, Kolb JP. Analysis of resveratrol-induced apoptosis in human B-cell chronic leukaemia. Br J Haematol 2002; 117:842–851.

Rotondo S, Rajtar G, Manarini S, Celardo A, Rotillo D, de Gaetano G, Evangelista V, Cerletti C. Effect of trans-resveratrol, a natural polyphenolic compound, on human polymorphonuclear leukocyte function. Br J Pharmacol 1998; 123:1691–1699.

Rowlands JC, Gustafsson JA. Aryl hydrocarbon receptor-mediated signal transduction. Crit Rev Toxicol 1997; 27:109–134.

Sato H, Seiki M. Regulatory mechanism of 92 kDa type IV collagenase gene expression which is associated with invasiveness of tumor cells. Oncogene 1993; 8:395–405.

Sato M, Maulik N, Das DK. Cardioprotection with alcohol: role of both alcohol and polyphenolic antioxidants. Ann NY Acad Sci 2002; 957:122–135.

Scaffidi C, Fulda S, Srinivasan A, Friesen C, Li F, Tomaselli KJ, Debatin KM, Krammer PH, Peter ME. Two CD95 (APO-1/Fas) signaling pathways. EMBO J 1998; 17:1675–1687.

Schneider Y, Vincent F, Duranton B, Badolo L, Gosse F, Bergmann C, Seiler N, Raul F. Anti-proliferative effect of resveratrol, a natural component of grapes and wine, on human colonic cancer cells. Cancer Lett 2000; 158:85–91.

She QB, Bode AM, Ma WY, Chen NY, Dong Z. Resveratrol-induced activation of p53 and apoptosis is mediated by extracellular-signal-regulated protein kinases and p38 kinase. Cancer Res 2001; 61:1604–1610.

Siemann EH, Creasy LL. Concentration of the phytoalexin resveratrol in wine. An J Eno Vitic 1992; 43:49–52.

Soleas GJ, Diamandis EP, Goldberg DM. Resveratrol: a molecule whose time has come? And gone? Clin Biochem 1997; 30:91–113.

Soleas GJ, Diamandis EP, Goldberg DM. The world of resveratrol. Adv Exp Med Biol 2001a; 492:159–182.

Soleas GJ, Yan J, Goldberg DM. Measurement of *trans*-resveratrol, (+)-catechin, and quercetin in rat and human blood and urine by gas chromatography with mass selective detection. Meth Enzymol 2001b; 335:130–145.

Stahl S, Chun TY, Gray WG. Phytoestrogens act as estrogen agonists in an estrogen-responsive pituitary cell line. Toxicol Appl Pharmacol 1998; 152:41–48.

Steele RJ, Thompson AM, Hall PA, Lane DP. The p53 tumour suppressor gene. Br J Surg 1998; 85:1460–1467.

Steinberg D, Parsatharathy S, Carew TE, Khoo JC. Beyond cholesterol: modifications of low-density lipoprotein that increases its atherogenicity. N Engl J Med 1989; 320:915–924.

Subbaramaiah K, Chung WJ, Michaluart P, Telang N, Tanabe T, Inoue H, Jang M, Pezzuto JM, Dannenberg AJ. Resveratrol inhibits cyclooxygenase-2 transcription and activity in phorbol ester-treated human mammary epithelial cells. J Biol Chem 1998; 273:21875–21882.

Suganuma M, Okabe S, Marino MW, Sakai A, Sueoka E, Fujiki H. Essential role of tumor necrosis factor alpha (TNF-alpha) in tumor promotion as revealed by TNF-alpha-deficient mice. Cancer Res 1999; 59:4516–4518.

Sun AY, Chen YM, James-Kracke M, Wixom P, Cheng Y. Ethanol-induced cell death by lipid peroxidation in PC12 cells. Neurochem Res 1997; 22:1187–1192.

Tessitore L, Davit A, Sarotto I, Caderni G. Resveratrol depresses the growth of colorectal aberrant crypt foci by affecting bax and p21(CIP) expression. Carcinogenesis 2000; 21:1619–1622.

Thornberry NA. Caspases: key mediators of apoptosis. Chem Biol 1998; 5:97–103.

Tinhofer I, Bernhard D, Senfter M, Anether G, Loeffler M, Kroemer G, Kofler R, Csordas A, Greil R. Resveratrol, a tumor-suppressive compound from grapes, induces apoptosis via a novel mitochondrial pathway controlled by Bcl-2. FASEB J 2001; 15:1613–1615.

Totani L, Piccoli A, Pellegrini G, Di Santo A, Lorenzet R. Polymorphonuclear leukocytes enhance release of growth factors by cultured endothelial cells. Arterioscler Thromb 1994; 14:125–132.

Tou J, Urbizo C. Resveratrol inhibits the formation of phosphatidic acid and diglyceride in chemotactic peptide- or phorbol ester-stimulated human neutrophils. Cell Signal 2001; 13:191–197.

Tsai SH, Lin-Shiau SY, Lin JK. Suppression of nitric oxide synthase and the down-regulation of the activation of NFkappaB in macrophages by resveratrol. Br J Pharmacol 1999; 126:673–680.

Tsan MF, White JE, Maheshwari JG, Bremner TA, Sacco J. Resveratrol induces Fas signalling-independent apoptosis in THP-1 human monocytic leukaemia cells. Br J Haematol 2000; 109:405–412.

Tsan MF, White JE, Maheshwari JG, Chikkappa G. Antileukemia effect of resveratrol. Leuk Lymphoma 2002; 43:983–987.

Turner RT, Evans GL, Zhang M, Maran A, Sibonga JD. Is resveratrol an estrogen agonist in growing rats? Endocrinology 1999; 140:50–54.

von Knethen A, Callsen D, Brune B. Superoxide attenuates macrophage apoptosis by NF-kappa B and AP-1 activation that promotes cyclooxygenase-2 expression. J Immunol 1999; 163:2858–2866.

Wadsworth TL, Koop DR. Effects of the wine polyphenolics quercetin and resveratrol on pro- inflammatory cytokine expression in RAW 264.7 macrophages. Biochem Pharmacol 1999; 57:941–949.

Whitehead TP, Robinson D, Allaway S, Syms J, Hale A. Effect of red wine ingestion on the antioxidant capacity of serum. Clin Chem 1995; 41:32–35.

Wilson T, Knight TJ, Beitz DC, Lewis DS, Engen RL. Resveratrol promotes atherosclerosis in hypercholesterolemic rabbits. Life Sci 1996; 59:L15–L21.

23

Pharmacological and Physiological Effects of Ginseng

An-Sik Chung and Kyung-Joo Cho
Korea Advanced Institute of Science and Technology
Daejeon, South Korea

Jong Dae Park
KT & G Central Research Institute
Daejeon, South Korea

I. INTRODUCTION

Ginseng is a medicinal plant widely used for the treatment of various diseases such as cancer, diabetes, and cardiovascular diseases, as well as for improving immune function and vitality. In this chapter, we review recent studies on the effects of ginseng on various diseases, particularly on diabetes, hypertension, and cancer. Ginseng improves glucose homeostasis and insulin sensitivity. It exerts cytotoxic and antimetastatic activities against various kinds of cancer cell lines, and induces differentiation or apoptosis of several cancer cells. Furthermore, ginseng has been reported to have an antineoplastic effect by enhancing immune function. An antihypertensive effect of ginseng is shown to occur by the enhanced synthesis and release of nitric oxide (NO). In addition, ginseng exerts antiatherosclerotic and antiplatelet effects. This chapter provides useful information on the pharmacological and clinical usage, and also suggests a method to conduct further study on ginseng to identify its potential effects.

The root of *Panax ginseng* C. A. Meyer, known as Korean ginseng, has been a valuable and important folk medicine in East Asian countries, including China, Korea, and Japan, for about 2000 years. Panax is derived from the word "panacea," which means a cure-all for diseases and a source of longevity as well as physical strength and resistance. As the use of traditional Chinese herbs for medicinal and dietary purposes becomes increasingly popular in Western countries, sales of *P. ginseng* are increasing in North America and Europe as well as other parts of the world.

Active constituents found in most ginseng species include ginsenosides, polysaccharides, peptides, polyacetylenic alcohols, and fatty acids (1). The major active components in *P. ginseng* are the ginsenosides, a group of saponins with triterpenoid dammarane structure (2). More than 30 ginsenosides have been isolated (3), and novel structures continue to be identified, particularly from *Panax quinquefolius* and *Panax japonica* as well as *P. ginseng* berry (4,5). Pharmacological effects of ginseng have been demonstrated in cancer, diabetes, and the cardiovascular, immune, and central nervous systems including antistress and antioxidant activity (6). This review focuses on the effects of ginseng on diabetes, anticancer activity, and the immune, and cardiovascular systems.

II. STRUCTURAL PROPERTY OF GINSENG

Ginsenosides, known as saponins, are the major components of ginseng (Fig. 1). Ginsenosides have a steroidal skeleton with a modified side chain at C-20 (7,8). They differ from one another by the type of sugar moieties, their number, and their site of attachment. Among the saponins, the genuine sapogenins 20(S)-protopanaxa-diol and -triol have been identified as 20(S) 12β-hydroxyl- and 20(S) 6α, 12β-dihydroxy-dammarenediol-II, respectively (9). Some partly deglycosylated saponins such as ginsenoside Rh_1, Rh_2, and Rg_3 are obtained from red ginseng as artifacts produced during steaming. Stepwise deglycosylated compounds such as compound K and 20(S)-protopanaxadiol can be generated through metabolic transformation by human intestinal bacteria. Ginsenoside Rg_1 is converted into 20(S)-protopanaxatriol via ginsenoside Rh1. The binding of the sugar has been shown to influence biological activity. Rh_1 and Rh_2 are structurally similar, but have different activity. Ginsenoside Rh_2 has been shown to decrease growth of B16-BL6 melanoma cells, and stimulates melanogenesis and cell-to-cell adhesiveness. However, Rh_1 has no effect on cell growth and cell-to-cell adhesiveness, but stimulates melanogenesis (10). Although both Rh_2 and Rh_3 induce differentiation of promyelocytic leukemia HL-60 cells into morphological and

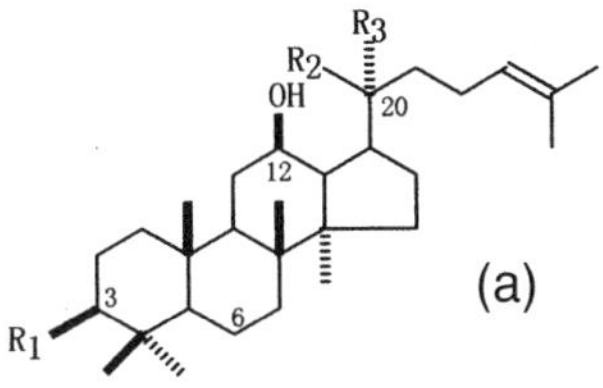

	R_1	R_2	R_3
Ginsenoside-Rb_1	O-glc(2→1)glc	O-glc(6→1)glc	CH_3
Ginsenoside-Rb_2	O-glc(2→1)glc	O-glc(6→1)arap	CH_3
Ginsenoside-Rc	O-glc(2→1)glc	O-glc(6→1)araf	CH_3
Ginsenoside-Rd	O-glc(2→1)glc	O-glc	CH_3
20(S)-Ginsenoside-Rg_3	O-glc(2→1)glc	OH	CH_3
20(R)-Ginsenoside-Rg_3	O-glc(2→1)glc	CH_3	OH

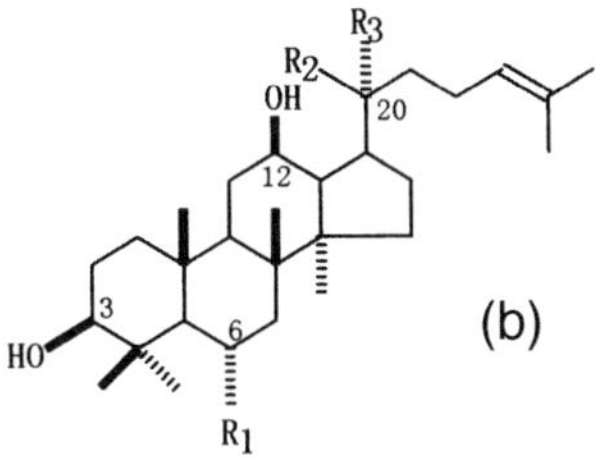

	R_1	R_2	R_3
Ginsenoside-Re	O-glc(2→1)rha	O-glc	CH_3
Ginsenoside-Rg_1	O-glc	O-glc	CH_3
20(S)-Ginsenoside-Rg_2	O-glc(2→1)rha	OH	CH_3
20(R)-Ginsenoside-Rg_2	O-glc(2→1)rha	CH_3	OH
20(S)-Ginsenoside-Rh_1	O-glc	OH	CH_3

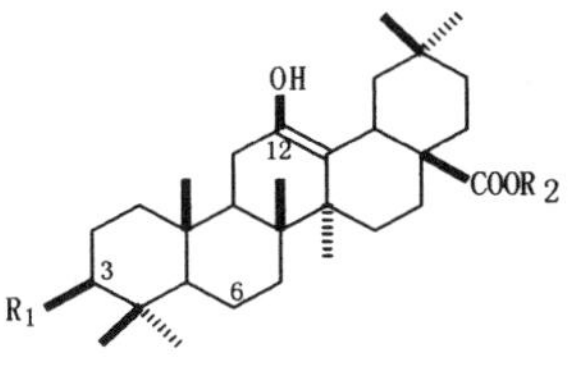

(c)

	R_1	R_2
Ginsenoside Ro	O-glcUA(2→1)rha	O-glc

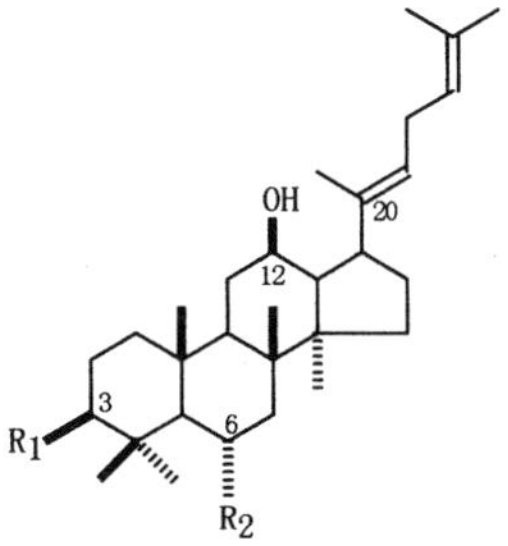

(d)

	R_1	R_2
Ginsenoside Rh_3	O-glc	H
Ginsenoside Rh_4	OH	O-glc
Ginsenoside Rg_5	O-glc(2→1)glc	H

FIGURE 1 Structure of ginsenosides.

functional granulocytes, the potency of Rh_2 is higher (11). Another factor that contributes to structural difference between ginsenosides is stereochemistry at C-20. Although both 20(S)- and 20(R)-ginsenoside Rg_2 inhibit acetycholine-evoked secretion of catecholamines from cultured bovine adrenal chromaffin cells, the 20(S) isomer has a greater inhibitory effect (12). Structural changes after oral administration also contribute to diversity. Certain ginsenosides such as Rb_1 and Rg_1 are poorly absorbed after injection (13). Rb_1 was hydrolyzed to compound K by intestinal flora (14); compound K was shown to increase the cytotoxicity of antineoplastic drugs (15) and to induce apoptosis in B16-BL6 melanoma cells (16).

The other major bioactive ingredient of ginseng is polysaccharide. Acidic polysaccharides found in ginseng such as ginsan (17,18), ginsenan S-IA, and ginsenan S-IIA (19) have been reported to have potential immunological activities. Ginseng's immunomodulatory effects may be one of its antitumor mechanisms. Ginseng polysaccharide GH1 reduces blood glucose and liver glycogen of mice (20). A high-output inducible nitric oxide synthase (iNOS) was shown in female BALB/c mice administered intraperitoneally (i.p.) with acidic polysaccharide from ginseng (21). Rhamnogalacturonan II from the leaves of *P. ginseng* C. A. Meyer acts as a macrophage Fc receptor expression-enhancing polysaccharide (22).

These structure-activity relationships are useful for understanding previously identified, bioactive components of ginseng, and to isolate and develop new therapeutic ingredients of ginseng.

III. REDUCTION OF BLOOD GLUCOSE LEVEL AND IMPROVEMENT OF DIABETES TREATMENT

Diabetes, affecting almost 3% of the world's population, is one of the major global health problems. In particular, there is a high incidence among the elderly population. It has been shown that the root of *P. ginseng* and other ginseng species has antihyperglycemic activity in vitro (23,24) and in vivo (25–28). More than 90% of patients with diabetes have type 2 diabetes, which is related to aging and diet. Although type 2 diabetes is more common and has serious complications, even reducing life expectancy by 8–10 years (29), most in vivo animal studies using ginseng have been conducted using type 1 rather than type 2 diabetes models. In this study, we focus on the effects of ginseng on type 2 diabetes.

The root of *P. ginseng* has been used to improve glucose homeostasis and insulin sensitivity (30) and clinically to treat type 2 diabetes (2,31). It has been observed that blood glucose level falls significantly in genetically obese diabetic mice after treatment with a single 90 mg/kg ginseng root extract at an i.p. dose (28). It has also been demonstrated that 3 g of American ginseng root given 40 min before a test meal significantly lowered blood glucose level in nondiabetic subjects and type 2 diabetic patients (32). Oral administration of *P. ginseng* root to diabetic KKAy mice for 4 weeks reduced blood glucose levels similar to that of an insulin sensitizer (rosiglitazone)-treated group (33). Moreover, ginseng therapy for type 2 diabetes elevates mood, improves psychophysical performance, and reduces fasting blood glucose and body weight. A 200-mg dose of ginseng improves glycated hemoglobin, serum lipid, amino-terminal propeptide concentration, and physical activity. These observations suggest that ginseng is beneficial for patients with type 2 diabetes and to prevent development of diabetes in nondiabetic subjects.

The main component of *P. ginseng* is ginsenosides (ginseng saponins). Ginsenoside Rb_2 was found to be the most effective component of ginsenosides for streptozotocin-diabetic rats (27). Rats treated with ginsenoside Rb_2 had a significant decrease in blood glucose levels with increased activity of glucokinase and decreased activity of glucose-6-phosphatase. Recently, antihyperglycemic and antiobese effects of *P. ginseng* berry extract have been demonstrated, and its major constituent, ginsenoside Re, has been observed (5). Treatment with the berry extract by daily i.p. injection for 12 days in obese diabetic C56BL/6J mice reduced glucose to levels similar to normal control value; after treatment the mice also had significantly improved glucose tolerance. The improvement of blood glucose level in the extract-treated *ob/ob* mice is associated with a significant reduction in serum insulin level in fed and fasting mice. A hyperinsulinemic-euglycemic clamp study revealed more than a twofold increase in the rate of insulin-stimulated glucose disposal in treated *ob/ob* mice. In addition, the extract-treated *ob/ob* mice lost a significant amount of weight, which was associated with a significant reduction in food intake and very significant increase in energy expenditure and body temperature.

Several studies have investigated the mechanism responsible for the antidiabetic effect of *P. ginseng*. Postulated mechanisms of lowering blood glucose by ginseng are as follows.

A. Modulation of Insulin Secretion

Some ginseng fractions have been observed to increase the blood insulin level and glucose-stimulated insulin secretion in alloxan-induced diabetic mice (24). This effect may also be mediated by increased NO synthesis of ginseng. Recently, it has been shown that NO stimulates glucose-dependent secretion of insulin in rat pancreatic islet cells (34).

B. Modulation of Digestion and Absorption of Carbohydrates

An inhibition of neuronal discharge frequency from the gastric compartment of the brain stem in rats has been observed (35), and inhibition of gastric secretion by Asian ginseng has also been observed in rats (36). The antidiabetic effect of ginseng root has also been shown to block intestinal glucose absorption and inhibit hepatic glucose-6-phosphatase activity (33). These results suggest that ginseng triggers digestion of food and decreases the rate of carbohydrate absorption into the portal hepatic circulation.

C. Control of Blood Glucose Level

Two recent epidemiological cohort studies found that a reduction in dietary glycemic index (GI, an indicator of carbohydrate's ability to raise blood glucose level) between the highest and lowest quintiles decreases the risk of developing diabetes (37,38). The difference in GI between these quintiles for nondiabetic subjects and for subjects with type 2 diabetes has been observed after oral administration of ginseng before oral glucose administration (32). It has been suggested that ginseng is useful for healthy people to prevent diabetes, and for type 2 diabetes patients to improve glycemic control (39). More studies are required to confirm that ginseng administration decreases the GI. If this is the case, ginseng may be useful in the conventional treatment of diabetes. Before ginseng's therapeutic benefit in these areas is claimed, studies of the efficacy of long-term administration using hemoglobin A1c (HbA1c) as a surrogate end-point marker and dose response are required.

D. Effect on Glucose Transport

P. ginseng has been shown to increase both glucose transporter-2 protein in the liver of normal and hyperglycemic mice (40) and glucose uptake into sheep erythrocytes in a dose-dependent manner (41). Recently, it has been shown that insulin-stimulated glucose uptake in rat skeletal muscles and adipose tissue is NO-dependent (42). Evidence suggests that ginseng can increase NO. Increased NO synthesis by ginseng in the endothelium of the lungs, heart, and kidney and in the corpus cavernosum has been detected (3).

E. Regulation of Adipogenic Transcription Factor Peroxisome Proliferator Activated Receptor-γ

Treatment with white ginseng rootlet in KKAy mice has been shown to increase peroxisome proliferator activated receptor-γ (PPARγ) (33), a pivotal regulator of adipocyte differentiation. Pharmaceutical ligands for PPARγ, including the thiazolidinedione (TZD) class of drugs, are potent insulin sensitizers that impact whole-body glucose utilization (43,44).

IV. ANTICARCINOGENIC ACTIVITY

The main weapons in the war against cancer have been early detection and surgical removal, radiotherapy, chemotherapy, and attempts to develop gene therapy. However, the result have been less than ideal, and the dominant strategy is now changing from therapeutic approaches to prevention of cancer by identifying effective natural products as chemopreventive agents. One promising candidate with cancer-preventive effects is ginseng. Its usefulness as an anticarcinogen has been shown by extensive preclinical and epidemiological studies. The following details anticarcinogenic effects of ginseng based on its diverse mechanisms.

A. Effects on Tumor Cell Cytotoxicity and Differentiation

Saponin and nonsaponin compounds have been reported to show cytotoxic activities against various kinds of cancer cell lines in culture. The major active components are ginsenoside Rh_2, a peculiar component of red ginseng, and also polyacetylenes, panaxydol, panaxynol, and panaxytriol. In addition, acetylpanaxydol and panaxydolchlorohydrin, showing cytotoxicity against lymphoid leukemia L1210, have been isolated from Korean ginseng root (45). The critical early even in the cytotoxicity of panaxytriol was identified as ATP depletion resulting from a direct inhibition of mitochondrial respiration (46). Further experimental evidence suggested that polyacetylenes inhibited the synthesis of macromolecules such as DNA, RNA, and protein in L1210 cells, resulting in cytotoxicity (17).

Ginseng was found to have the ability to induce the transformation of neoplastic cells into normal cells. Ginsenoside Rh_2 inhibited the growth and colony-forming ability of Morris hepatoma cells in soft agar suspension culture, and stimulated serum protein synthesis of these cells, thus converting the cell characteristics both functionally and morphologically to those resembling original normal liver cells, a process known as "redifferentiation or reverse transformation" (47). Similarly, ginsenosides Rh1 and Rh2 have been shown to cause differentiation of F9 teratocarcinoma stem cells via binding to a steroid receptor (48). Accordingly, recent studies on therapy for various types of cancers have focused on drugs that induce differentiation of maturation-resistant cells causing the related disease. Furthermore, ginsenoside Rh_2 has been found to significantly induce B16 cell differentiation and to increase melanin synthesis in B16 cells (49).

B. Antimetastatic Effect and Inhibitory Activity on Multidrug Resistance (MDR)

Generally, primary tumors are not fatal. Instead, most cancer patients succumb to metastases—multiple, widespread tumor colonies established by malignant cells that detach themselves from the original tumor and travel through the body, often to distant sites. Some invading cells penetrate body cavities, the blood, lymph, or spinal fluids and are then released (50). Ginseng saponin has recently received a great deal of attention for its effects in inhibiting invasion and metastasis of cancer cells. 20(R)- and 20(S)-ginsenoside Rg_3 was found to inhibit the lung metastasis of tumor cells such as B16-

BL-6 melanoma and colon 26M3.1, when they were orally administered at a dose of 100–1000 μg per mouse. The mechanism of their antimetastatic effect is considered to be related to inhibition of the adhesion and invasion of tumor cells, and also to antiangiogenesis activity (51). Glucocorticoid receptor-induced downregulation of matrix metalloproteinase (MMP)-9 by panaxadiol and panaxatriol appear to be associated with the reduced invasive capacity of HT1080, a highly metastatic human fibrosarcoma cell line (52). Multiple administration of ginsenoside Rb_2 after the intravenous inoculation of B16-BL6 melanoma cells resulted in significant inhibition of tumor-associated angiogenesis responsible for the inhibition of lung tumor metastasis (53). Ginsenoside Rb2 has been reported to inhibit invasion to the basement membrane via MMP-2 suppression in some endometrial cancers such as HHUA and HEC-1-A cells, and is projected for use as a medicine for inhibition of secondary spreading of uterine endometrial cancers (54). It was shown that ginsenoside Rg_3 inhibited experimental pulmonary metastasis by highly metastatic mouse melanoma B16FE7 cells, which was mediated by inhibiting the 1-oleoyl-lysophosphatidic acid (LPA)-triggered rise of intracellular Ca^{2+} (55). While these results suggest the usefulness of ginsenoside Rg_3 in preventing cancer spread, further in vivo studies are necessary to clarify te antimetastatic effects of ginseng.

One of the major side effects to the effective treatment of human malignancies is the acquisition of broad anticancer drug resistance by tumor cells. This phenomenon has been termed "multidrug resistance (MDR)." Therefore, development of new modulators for the inhibition of drug resistance is required. MDR inhibitory activity was determined by measuring cytotoxicity to MDR cells using MDR human fibrocarcinoma KB V20C, which is resistant to 20 nM of vincristine and expresses a high level of *mdr1* gene. 20(S)-Ginsenoside Rg_3, saponin of red ginseng, was found to have the most potent inhibitory activity on MDR, and its ID_{50} (dose for 50% inhibition) was 8.2×10^{-5} M. In cytotoxicity assays, ginsenoside Rg_3 did not affect the growth of normal cells. Moreover, ginsenoside Rg_3 (40 mg/kg, i.p.) potentiated adriamycin chemotherapy in P388/ADR BDF1 mice expressing MDR. Ginsenoside Rg_3 appears to compete with vincristine for binding to p-glycoprotein (Pgp) and blocks the efflux of anticancer drugs (56). It is also reported that quasipanaxatriol, 20(S)-protopanaxatriol, ginsenoside Rh_2, and compound K, the metabolic final product of protopanaxadiol saponin, greatly enhanced the cytotoxicity of the anticancer drugs in P388/ADM cells (adriamycin-resistant P388 leukemia cells) (15). The reversal of daunomycin resistance in P388/ADM by quasipanaxatriol with a double bond introduced at C-20 of protopanxatriol was found to show effective accumulation of drugs mediated by daunomycin-efflux blockage. These results suggest that further clinical trials of ginseng components in reversal of Pgp-associated MDR are highly feasible.

C. Anticarcinogenic Activities and Synergistic Effects in Combination with Chemical Therapeutic Agents

Several investigations were carried out to evaluate the inhibitory or preventive effects of ginseng on carcinogenesis induced by various chemical carcinogens. The prolonged administration of Korean red ginseng extract inhibited the incidence and the proliferation of tumors induced by 7,12-dimethylbenz (a) anthracene (DMBA), urethane, and aflatoxin B1 (57). The chemopreventive potential of ginseng was evaluated using DMBA-induced skin tumorigenesis (papillomagenesis) in male Swiss albino mice. There was a marked reduction not only in tumor incidence but also in cumulative tumor frequency at the initiation phase of tumorigenesis, with a small reduction at the promotional stage, suggesting the anticarcinogenic activities of ginseng (58). Ginsenosides Rg_3 and Rg_5 were found to show statistically significant reduction of lung tumor incidence in a newly established 9-week, medium-term anticarcinogenicity test model of lung tumors in mice, and ginsenoside Rh_2 showed a tendency to decrease the incidence, indicating that these ginsenosides are active anticarcinogenic compounds (59). The inhibitory effects of ginseng on the development of 1,2-dimethylhydrazine (DMH)-induced aberrant crypt foci (ACF) in the colon were investigated in rats. Dietary administration of red ginseng in combination with DMH suppressed colon carcinogenesis in rats associated partly with inhibition of cell proliferation, acting on ACF in the colonic mucosa (60). In addition, an anticarcinogenic effect of red ginseng on the development of liver cancer induced by diethylnitrosamine (DEN) in rats was identified in preventive and curative groups (61).

More recently, it has been reported that less glycosylated protopanaxadiol derivatives are effective in cancer prevention and some oleanane-type pentacyclic triterpenoid compounds show anticarcinogenic activities in two-stage anticancer promotion experiments in vitro and in vivo (9). Ginsenoside Rh_2 has been described to have diverse effects on the expression of the transformed phenotype in BALB/c 3T3 cells, and augments the metastatic potential in an experimental metastasis assay (62). The estrogenic potential of American ginseng extract to induce the expression of pS2, an estrogen-regulated gene, was evaluated in breast cancer cell lines MCF-7, T-47D, and BT-20. It was found that American ginseng exhibits estrogen-like effects on estrogen-receptor-positive breast cancer cells by inducing pS2 expression, suggesting that it may play a protective role against breast cancer (63). This is further supported by the observation that American ginseng inhibits breast cancer cell growth by transcriptional activation of the p21 gene, a universal cell cycle inhibitor, independent of p53 (64). It is also reported that concurrent use of American ginseng extract and breast cancer therapeutic agents results in a significant suppression of cancer cell growth, suggesting its synergistic effects on breast cancer therapeutics (65).

D. Antitumor Activities of Ginsenosides

Oral administration of ginsenoside Rh_2 has been reported to have an inhibitory effect on tumor growth in nude mice bearing human ovarian cancer cells (HRA), resulting in remarkable retardation of the tumor growth. In particular, tumor growth in mice treated with 15, 30, and 120 μM of Rh_2 was significantly inhibited, compared to that in CDDP (cis-diaminedichloroplatinum) (II)-treated mice as well as in untreated mice (66). Further investigation showed that p.o. but not i.p. treatment with ginsenoside Rh_2 resulted in induction of apoptosis in the tumors in addition to augmentation of the natural killer activity in spleen cells from tumor-bearing nude mice, suggesting that an evaluation of the treatment of recurrent or refractory ovarian tumors is warranted (67).

E. Immunomodulatory Antitumor Activities of Ginseng Polysaccharide

It has long been reported that ginseng strengthens the resistance of an organism to harmful physical, chemical, and biological stresses. This capability is related to its regulation of the immune system, which plays an important role in the protective mechanism of the body. Recently, an acidic polysaccharide named ginsan has been isolated from white ginseng, peeled dried ginseng, and identified as an ideal nontoxic antineoplastic immunostimulator. It acts by activating multiple effector arms of the immune system and killer cells ($Thyl^+$, $AsGM1^+$, $CD8^+$) (68). Ginsan has been found to generate LAK cells from both NK and T cells by endogenously producing multiple cytokines, contributing to its effectiveness in the immunoprevention and immunotherapy of cancer (17). More recently, red ginseng acidic polysaccharide (RGAP) has also been isolated from Korean red ginseng. Having different chemical molar composition from ginsan, it is reported to have immunomodulatory antitumor activity. RGAP was found to induce inducible nitric oxide synthase (iNOS) in mice resulting in NO secretion (21). Peritoneal macrophages from RGAP-treated mice exhibited potent tumoricidal activities toward P815 and WEHI 164 tumor cells. In addition, treatment of RGAP in vivo stimulated tumoricidal activities of natural killer (NK) cells and showed increased life span of sarcoma 180–bearing mice together with decreased tumor weight of B16 tumor–bearing mice. These results suggest that activation of macrophages and NK cells serve to enhance in vivo antitumor activities of RGAP (69). GFP, a more active fraction of RGAP, increased the survival rates of male ICR mice transplanted with sarcoma 180 10 times higher than RGAP, and showed more potent tumoricidal activities of NK cells than RGAP. Recently, it has also been demonstrated that polysaccharide fraction of American ginseng, *P. quinquefolius*, exerts TNF-α-stimulating activity on macrophages, and is found to contain glucose, galactose, arabinose, rhamnose, and mannose (70). These results suggest that clinical trials of these ginseng polysaccharides in immunotherapy against cancer are highly feasible.

F. Induction of Apoptosis by Ginsenosides

Apoptosis is responsible for a pathological mechanism related to human diseases such as cancer, autoimmune disease, viral infection, and neurodegenerative disorder (71). Ginsenoside Rh_2 has been shown to arrest cell cycle at the G1 phase and to prolong the S phase (72,73). It was reported that ginsenoside Rh_2 induced apoptosis through protein kinase C in human neuroblastoma SK-N-BE (2) and rat glioma C6Bu-1 cells (17). In addition, ginsenoside Rh_2 has been shown to induce apoptosis independently of Bcl-2, Bcl-x_L, or Bax in C6Bu-1 cells (74). In a parallel study, it was found that ginsenoside Rh_2–induced cell death was mediated by the generated reactive oxygen species and activation of the caspase pathway in a Bcl-x_L-independent manner (75). These reports demonstrate that the induction of apoptosis by ginseng may be one of its anticarcinogenic mechanisms.

As described above, the protective influence of ginseng against cancer has been shown by extensive preclinical and epidemiological studies; however, these effects need to be carefully investigated by scientific clinical trials focusing on the major cancer killers such as stomach, lung, liver, and colorectal cancers.

V. ANTIHYPERTENSIVE EFFECTS

High blood pressure is associated with decreased life expectancy and increased risk of stroke, coronary heart disease, and other end-organ diseases such as renal failure. Ginseng contains active compounds that normalize blood pressure. The effect of a certain drug on blood pressure can be analyzed by investigating the effect of the drug on the smooth muscle of blood vessels. It is well established that blood vessel smooth muscle tone is regulated by the available intracellular Ca^{2+} concentration, which in turn is profoundly influenced by interaction of the cellular membrane and sarcoplasmic reticulum in the smooth muscle. It was found that both protopanxatriol and protopanaxadiol saponins inhibit Ca^{2+} binding to the cellular membrane; protopanaxatriol is approximately 180% more potent than protopanaxadiol ginsenosides (76). It was reported that ginseng induced no significant change in blood pressure in subjects with normal blood pressure, but had a normalizing effect on subjects with abnormal blood pressure (77). It has recently been reported that vasodilation and protective effects of ginsenoside Rg1 against free radical injury might be related to enhanced synthesis and release of NO, demonstrating the usefulness of ginseng in treatment of pulmonary and systemic hypertension (78). The detailed mechanism and evidence of antihypertensive effects of ginseng are as follows.

A. Endothelium-Dependent Vasorelaxation of Ginsenosides

Endothelium plays an important role in regulating vascular tone by releasing several vasoactive autacoids, including prostacyclin, endothelium-derived relaxing factor (EDRF), and endothelium-derived hyperpolarizing factor (EDHF) (79). EDRF has been identified as NO, which is produced from L-arginine by NOS (80). NO relaxes blood vessels mostly by stimulating soluble guanylyl cyclase, which leads to an increased production of cGMP in vascular smooth muscle (81). Ginsenosides have been found to lower blood pressure in a dose-dependent manner in rats at doses of 10–100 mg/kg. This effect is mediated by release of endothelium-derived NO, enhancing the accumulation of cGMP (82). Recently, it has also been reported that ginseng can improve vascular endothelial dysfunction in patients with hypertension, possibly by increasing synthesis of NO. Protopanaxatriol and its purified ginsenosides Rg_1 and Re caused endothelium-dependent relaxation, which is associated with the formation of cGMP. In contrast, protopanaxadiol or ginsenosides Rg_1 and Re did not affect vascular tone or production of cGMP in rat aorta. Moreover, ginsenosides Rg_1 and Re were less effective endothelium-dependent vasodilators than total ginsenosides and protopanaxatriol (83). Ginsenoside Rg_3 belongs to the protopanaxadiol group of red ginseng, steamed and dried ginseng. Present findings indicate that ginsenoside Rg_3 effectively stimulates NO formation in endothelial cells, which accounts for the endothelim-dependent relaxation and production of cGMP in the rat aorta. Ginsenoside Rg_3–induced endothelium-dependent relaxation was markedly inhibited by a nonselective K^+ channel blocker, but not by an ATP-sensitive K^+ channel blocker (84). These findings show that ginsenoside Rg_3 activates tetraethylammonium-sensitive K^+ channels in endothelial cells, which presumably leads to an influx of Ca^{2+} and the subsequent activation of the endothelial NOS (eNOS) (85).

To investigate the effects of red ginseng on blood pressure, change of blood pressure and heart rate after intravenous injection of red ginseng was studied in conscious normotensive and one-kidney, one-clip Goldblatt hypertensive rats. Experimental evidence indicates that the NO-releasing effect of red ginseng, like other NO donors, partly contributes to hypotensive effects (86). Clinical study has been performed to estimate the effect of Korean red ginseng on vascular endothelial cell dysfunction in patients with hypertension. To assess the function of the vascular endothelial cell, changes of forearm blood flow to infusion of acetylcholine, sodium nitroprusside, and bradykinin in incremental doses were measured by venous occlusion plethysmography. In the ginseng-treated hypertensive group, forearm blood flows at the highest dose of acetylcholine and bradykinin were significantly higher than those of the nontreated hypertensive group. It was found that Korean red ginseng could improve the vascular endothelial dysfunction in patients with hypertension possibly by increasing NO synthesis (87). These results support the claim that ginseng has pharmacological activities on circulatory diseases including hypertension.

B. Antiatherosclerosis and Antiplatelet Effects of Ginsenosides

Endothelial cell damage is considered to be the initial step in the genesis of thrombosis and arteriosclerosis, the common precursors of cardiovascular disoders. Platelet hyperfunction, such as enhanced platelet aggregation associated with overproduction of thromboxane A_2 (TXA_2), a potent platelet aggregative and vasoconstrictive substance, has been frequently encountered in patients with cardiovascular thrombotic diseases. Prostaglandin I_2 (PGI_2), a potent antiplatelet aggregative and vasodilatatory substance produced in vascular walls, is also reported to synthesize less in patients with atherosclerotic changes than in normal subjects. Panaxynol was found to markedly inhibit the aggregation of platelets induced by collagen, arachidonic acid, and platelet-activating factor (PAF), while ginsenosides had no significant effect on the aggregation. It was suggested that panaxynol is the most potent antiplatelet agent in ginseng and its mechanism of action is chiefly due to the inhibition of thromboxane formation (88). In addition, it was reported that panaxynol inhibited the aggregation, release, and thromboxane formation in rabbit platelets, while ginsenosides Ro, Rg_1, and Rg_2 suppressed only the release (89). It has also been demonstrated that ginsenoside Rg_1 inhibited platelet activation induced by TXA_2 through inhibition of TXA_2-induced Ca^{2+} mobilization, and ginsenoside Rg_3 induced TXA_2-induced platelet aggregation. Ginsenoside Rc was shown to stimulate in vitro PGI_2 formation by cultured rat vascular smooth muscle cells through enhanced gene expression of cyclooxygenase (90). These results suggest that ginsenoside Rg_1 and Rg_3, which have antiplatelet and antiatherosclerotic effects, may have clinical potential for the prevention and the treatment of certain thrombotic and atherosclerotic disorders. Furthermore, American ginseng extract was proved to be associated with the inhibition of thrombin-induced endothelin release due to NO release (91). This result suggests that American ginseng may play a therapeutic role in facilitating the hemodynamic balance of vascular endothelial cells.

VI. SUMMARY AND FUTURE WORK

For centuries, ginseng has been a highly valued herb in the East. Recently, many clinical trials using ginseng have been undertaken in Western countries as well as in East Asia. In this chapter, we have summarized the diverse pharmacological and physiological effects of ginseng on various diseases such as diabetes, cancer, and cardiovascular diseases. However, although there is a wealth of evidence suggesting that ginseng can be useful for the treatment of various diseases, a great deal of vital research remains to be solved. First, numerous experiments reported have been performed in animal models instead of humans. Therefore, a large-scale, controlled clinical study is needed to validate these results in terms of their applicability to humans. Second, there is still little evidence on ginseng's effectiveness at molecular levels. Understanding of molecular regulation of ginseng is necessary to apply it clinically, and also to discover new therapeutic effects. Third, the standardization of ginseng extract to yield constant results in the treatment of ginseng to cells, animals, and human is also urgently needed.

ACKNOWLEDGMENT

This work was supported by the Aging and Apoptosis Research Center Program Grant (R11-079) from the Korea Science and Engineering Foundation.

REFERENCES

1. Lee FC. Facts About Ginseng, The Elixir of Life. Elizabeth, NJ: Hollyn International Corp, 1992.
2. Huang KC. The Pharmacology of Chinese Herbs. Boca Raton, FL: CRC Press, 1999.
3. Gillis CN. *Panax ginseng* pharmacology: a nitric oxide link? Biochem Pharmacol 1997; 54(1):1–8.
4. Yoshikawa M, Murakami T, Yashiro K, Yamahara J, Matsuda H, Saijoh R, Tanaka O. Bioactive saponins and glycosides. XI. Structures of new dammarane-type triterpene oligoglycosides, quinquenosides II. I, IV. III, and V, from Amer-

ican ginseng, the roots of *Panax quinquefolium* L. Chem Pharm Bull (Tokyo) 1998; 46:647–654.

5. Attele AS, Zhou YP, Xie JT, Wu JA, Zhang L, Dey L, Pugh W, Rue PA, Polonsky KS, Yuan CS. Antidiabetic effects of *Panax ginseng* berry extract and the identification of an effective component. Diabetes 2002; 51(6):1851–1858.
6. Jung NP, Jin SH. Studies on the physiological and biochemical effect of Korean ginseng. Korean J Ginseng Sci 1996; 20(4):431–471.
7. Huang KC. The Pharmacology of Chinese Herbs. Boca Raton, FL: CRC Press, 1999.
8. Shibata S, Tanaka O, Shoji J, Saito H. Chemistry and pharmacology of *Panax*. In: Wagner H, Hikino H, Farnsworth NR, eds. Economic and Medicinal Plant Research. New York: Academic Press, 1995:217–284.
9. Shibata S. Chemistry and cancer preventing activities of ginseng saponins and some related triterpenoid compounds. J Korean Med 2001; 16:S28–37.
10. Odashima S, Ohta T, Kohno H, Matsuda T, Kitagawa I, Abe H, Arichi S. Control of phenotypic expression of cultured B16 melanoma cells by plant glycosides. Cancer Res 1985; 45(6):2781–2784.
11. Kim YS, Kim DS, Kim SI. Ginsenoside Rh2 and Rh3 induce differentiation of HL-60 cells into granulocytes: modulation of protein kinase C isoforms during differentiation by ginsenoside Rh2. Int J Biochem Cell Biol 1998; 30(3):327–338.
12. Kudo K, Tachikawa E, Kashimoto T, Takahashi E. Properties of ginseng saponin inhibition of catecholamine secretion in bovine adrenal chromaffin cells. Eur J Pharmacol 1998; 341(2-3):139–144.
13. Odani T, Tanizawa H, Takino Y. Studies on the absorption, distribution, excretion and metabolism of ginseng saponins. III. The absorption, distribution and excretion of ginsenoside Rb1 in the rat. Chem Pharm Bull (Tokyo) 1983; 31(3):1059–1066.
14. Karikura M, Miyase T, Tanizawa H, Taniyama T, Takino Y. Studies on absorption, distribution, excretion and metabolism of ginseng saponins. VII. Comparison of the decomposition modes of ginsenoside-Rb1 and -Rb2 in the digestive tract of rats. Chem Pharm Bull (Tokyo) 1991; 39(9):2357–2361.
15. Hasegawa H, Sung JH, Matsumiya S, Uchiyama M, Inouye Y, Kasai R, Yamasaki K. Reversal of daunomycin and vinblastine resistance in multidrug-resistant P388 leukemia in vitro through enhanced cytotoxicity by triterpenoids. Planta Med 1995; 61(5):409–413.
16. Wakabayashi C, Murakami K, Hasegawa H, Murata J, Saiki I. An intestinal bacterial metabolite of ginseng protopanaxadiol saponins has the ability to induce apoptosis in tumor cells. Biochem Biophys Res Commun 1998; 246(3): 725–730.
17. Kim KH, Lee YS, Jung IS, Park SY, Chung HY, Lee IR, Yun YS. Acidic polysaccharide from *Panax ginseng*, ginsan, induces Th1 cell and macrophage cytokines and generates LAK cells in synergy with rIL-2. Planta Med 1998; 64(2):110–115.

18. Shin JY, Song JY, Yun YS, Yang HO, Rhee DK, Pyo S. Immunostimulating effects of acidic polysaccharides extract of *Panax ginseng* on macrophage function. Immunopharmacol Immunotoxicol 2002; 24(3):469–482.
19. Tomoda M, Hirabayashi K, Shimizu N, Gonda R, Ohara N, Takada K. Characterization of two novel polysaccharides having immunological activities from the root of *Panax ginseng*. Biol Pharm Bull 1993; 16(11):1087–1090.
20. Yang M, Wang BX, Jin YL, Wang Y, Cui ZY. Effects of ginseng polysaccharides on reducing blood glucose and liver glycogen. Zhongguo Yao Li Xue Bao 1990; 11(6):520–524.
21. Park KM, Kim YS, Jeong TC, Joe CO, Shin HJ, Lee YH, Nam KY, Park JD. Nitric oxide is involved in the immunomodulating activities of acidic polysaccharide from *Panax ginseng*. Planta Med 2001; 67(2):122–126.
22. Shin KS, Kiyohara H, Matsumoto T, Yamada H. Rhamnogalacturonan II from the leaves of *Panax ginseng* C. A. Meyer as a macrophage Fc receptor expression-enhancing polysaccharide. Carbohydr Res 1997; 300(3):239–249.
23. Kimura M. Hypoglycemic component in ginseng radix and its insulin release. Proc. 3rd Intern. Ginseng Symp. Seoul, Korea. Korean Ginseng Research Institute, 1980.
24. Kimura M, Waki I, Chujo T, Kikuchi T, Hiyama C, Yamazaki K, Tanaka O. Effects of hypoglycemic components in ginseng radix on blood insulin level in alloxan diabetic mice and on insulin release from perfused rat pancreas. J Pharmacobiodyn 1981; 4(6):410–417.
25. Kimura M, Waki I, Tanaka O, Nagai Y, Shibata S. Pharmacological sequential trials for the fractionation of components with hypoglycemic activity in alloxan diabetic mice from ginseng radix. J Pharmacobiodyn 1981; 4(6):402–409.
26. Kimura M, Suzuki J. The pattern of action of blended Chinese traditional medicines to glucose tolerance curves in genetically diabetic KK-CAy mice. J Pharmacobiodyn 1981; 4(12):907–915.
27. Yokozawa T, Kobayashi T, Oura H, Kawashima Y. Studies on the mechanism of the hypoglycemic activity of ginsenoside-Rb2 in streptozotocin-diabetic rats. Chem Pharm Bull (Tokyo) 1985; 33(2):869–872.
28. Kimura I, Nakashima N, Sugihara Y, Fu-jun C, Kimura M. The antihyperglycaemic blend effect of traditional chinese medicine byakko-ka-ninjin-to on alloxan and diabetic KK-CA(y) mice. Phytother Res 1999; 13(6):484–488.
29. Astrup A, Finer N. Redefining type 2 diabetes: "diabesity" or "obesity dependent diabetes mellitus"? Obes Rev 2000; 1(2):57–59.
30. Sonnenborn U, Proppert Y. Ginseng (*Panax ginseng* C. A. Meyer). Zschr Phytother 1990; 11:35–49.
31. Bensky D, Gamble A. Chinese Herbal Medicine Materia Medica. Seattle, WA: Eastland Press, 1993.
32. Vuksan V, Sievenpiper JL, Koo VY, Francis T, Beljan-Zdravkovic U, Xu Z, Vidgen E. American ginseng (*Panax quinquefolius* L) reduces postprandial glycemia in nondiabetic subjects and subjects with type 2 diabetes mellitus. Arch Intern Med 2000; 160(7):1009–1013.
33. Chung SH, Choi CG, Park SH. Comparisons between white ginseng radix and

rootlet for antidiabetic activity and mechanism in KKAy mice. Arch Pharm Res 2001; 24(3):214–218.

34. Spinas GA, Laffranchi R, Francoys I, David I, Richter C, Reinecke M. The early phase of glucose-stimulated insulin secretion requires nitric oxide. Diabetologia 1998; 41(3):292–299.
35. Yuan CS, Wu JA, Lowell T, Gu M. Gut and brain effects of American ginseng root on brainstem neuronal activities in rats. Am J Chin Med 1998; 26(1):47–55.
36. Suzuki Y, Ito Y, Konno C, Furuya T. Effects of tissue cultured ginseng on gastric secretion and pepsin activity. Yakugaku Zasshi 1991; 111(12):770–774.
37. Salmeron J, Manson JE, Stampfer MJ, Colditz GA, Wing AL, Willett WC. Dietary fiber, glycemic load, and risk of non-insulin-dependent diabetes mellitus in women. JAMA 1997; 277(6):472–477.
38. Salmeron J, Ascherio A, Rimm EB, Colditz GA, Spiegelman D, Jenkins DJ, Stampfer MJ, Wing AL, Willett WC. Dietary fiber, glyemic load, and risk of NIDDM in men. Diabetes Care 1997; 20(4):545–550.
39. Group UPDSU. Intensive blood-glucose control with sulphonylureas or insulin compared with conventional treatment and risk of complications in patients with type 2 diabetes (UKPDS 33). Lancet 1998; 352(9131):837–853.
40. Lee FC. Facts About Ginseng, The Elixir of Life. Elizabeth, NJ: Hollyn International, 1992.
41. Hasegawa H, Matsumiya S, Murakami C, Kurokawa T, Kasai R, Ishibashi S, Yamasaki K. Interactions of ginseng extract, ginseng separated fractions, and some triterpenoid saponins with glucose transporters in sheep erythroytes. Planta Med 1994; 60(2):153–157.
42. Roy D, Perreault M, Marette A. Insulin stimulation of glucose uptake in skeletal muscles and adipose tissues in vivo is NO dependent. Am J Physiol 1998; 274(4 Pt 1):E692–E699.
43. Debril MB, Renaud JP, Fajas L, Auwerx J. The pleiotropic functions of peroxisome proliferator-activated receptor gamma. J Mol Med 2001; 79(1):30–47.
44. Spiegelman BM. PPAR-gamma: adipogenic regulator and thiazolidinedione receptor. Diabetes 1998; 47(4):507–514.
45. Ahn BZ, Kim SI, Lee YH. Acetylpanaxydol and panaxydolchlorohydrin, two new polyenes from Korean ginseng with cytotoxic activity against L1210 cells. Arch Pharm 1989; 322(4):223–226.
46. Matsunaga H, Saita T, Nagumo F, Mori M, Katano M. A possible mechanism for the cytotoxicity of a polyacetylenic alcohol, panaxytriol: inhibition of mitochondrial respiration. Cancer Chemother Pharmacol 1995; 35(4):291–296.
47. Odashima S, Ota T, Fujikawa-Yamamoto K, Abe H. Induction of phenotypic reverse transformation by plant glycosides in cultured cancer cells. Gan To Kagaku Ryoho 1989; 16(4 Pt 2-2):1483–1489.
48. Lee YH, Kim SI, Lee SK, Chung HY, Kim KW. Differentiation mechanism of ginsenosides in cultured murine F9 teratocarcinoma stem cells. Proceedings of the 6th Intl. Ginseng Symposium, 1993:127–131.
49. Xia LJ, Han R. Differentiation of B16 melanoma cells induced by ginsenoside Rh2. Yao, Xue Xue Bao 1996; 31(10):742–745.

50. Friedberg EC. Cancer Biology. New York: W. H. Freeman and Company, 1986: 138–148.
51. Mochizuki M, Yoo YC, Matsuzawa K, Sato K, Saiki I, Tono-oka S, Samukawa K, Azuma I. Inhibitory effect of tumor metastasis in mice by saponins, ginsenoside-Rb2, 20(R)- and 20(S)-ginsenoside-Rg3, of red ginseng. Biol Pharm Bull 1995; 18(9):1197–1202.
52. Park MT, Cha HJ, Jeong JW, Kim SI, Chung HY, Kim ND, Kim OH, Kim KW. Glucocorticoid receptor-induced down-regulation of MMP-9 by ginseng components, PD and PT contributes to inhibition of the invasive capacity of HT1080 human fibrosarcoma cells. Mol Cells 1999; 9(5):476–483.
53. Sato K, Mochizuki M, Saiki I, Yoo YC, Samukawa K, Azuma I. Inhibition of tumor angiogenesis and metastasis by a saponin of *Panax ginseng*, ginsenoside-Rb2. Biol Pharm Bull 1994; 17(5):635–639.
54. Fujimoto J, Sakaguchi H, Aoki I, Toyoki H, Khatun S, Tamaya T. Inhibitory effect of ginsenoside-Rb2 on invasiveness of uterine endometrial cancer cells to the basement membrane. Eur J Gynaecol Oncol 2001; 22(5):339–341.
55. Shinkai K, Akedo H, Mukai M, Imamura F, Isoai A, Kobayashi M, Kitagawa I. Inhibition of in vitro tumor cell invasion by ginsenoside Rg3. Jpn J Cancer Res 1996; 87(4):357–362.
56. Park JD, Kim DS, Kwon HY, Son SK, Lee YH, Baek NI, Kim SI, Rhee DK. Effects of ginseng saponin on modulation of multidrug resistance. Arch Pharm Res 1996; 19(3):213–218.
57. Yun TK, Yun YS, Han IW. Anticarcinogenic effect of long-term oral administration of red ginseng on new born mice exposed to various chemical carcinogens. Cancer Detect Prev 1983; 6(6):515–525.
58. Kumar A. Chemopreventive action of ginseng on DMBA-induced papillomagenesis in the skin of mice. Proceedings of the 6th Intl. Ginseng Symposium, 1993:66–68.
59. Yun TK, Lee YS, Lee YH, Kim SI, Yun HY. Anticarcinogenic effect of *Panax ginseng* C. A. Meyer and identification of active compounds. J Korean Med 2001; 16 (suppl):S6–18.
60. Fukushima S, Wanibuchi H, Li W. Inhibition by ginseng of colon carcinogenesis in rats. J Korean Med Sci 2001; S75–80.
61. Wu XG, Zhu DH, Li X. Anticarcinogenic effect of red ginseng on the development of liver cancer induced by diethylnitrosamine in rats. J Korean Med 2001; 16(suppl):S61–S65.
62. Tatsuka M, Maeda M, Ota T. Anticarcinogenic effect and enhancement of metastatic potential of BALB/c 3T3 cells by ginsenoside Rh(2). Jpn J Cancer Res 2001; 92(11):1184–1189.
63. Duda RB, Taback B, Kessel B, Dooley DD, Yang H, Marchiori J, Slomovic BM, Alvarez JG. pS2 expression induced by American ginseng in MCF-7 breast cancer cells. Ann Surg Oncol 1996; 3(6):515–520.
64. Duda RB, Kang SS, Archer SY, Meng S, Hodin RA. American ginseng transcriptionally activates p21 mRNA in breast cancer cell lines. J Korean Med Sci 2001; 16:S54–S60.

65. Duda RB, Zhong Y, Navas V, Li MZ, Toy BR, Alavarez JG. American ginseng and breast cancer therapeutic agents synergistically inhibit MCF-7 breast cancer cell growth. J Surg Oncol 1999; 72(4):230–239.
66. Tode T, Kikuchi Y, Hirata J, Kita T, Imaizumi E, Nagata I. Inhibitory effects of oral administration of ginsenoside Rh2 on tumor growth in nude mice bearing serious cyst adenocarcinoma of the human ovary. Nippon Sanka Fujinka Gakkai Zasshi 1993; 45(11):1275–1282.
67. Nakata H, Kikuchi Y, Tode T, Hirata J, Kita T, Ishii K, Kudoh K, Nagata I, Shinomiya N. Inhibitory effects of ginsenoside Rh2 on tumor growth in nude mice bearing human ovarian cancer cells. Jpn J Cancer Res 1998; 89(7):733–740.
68. Lee YS, Chung IS, Lee IR, Kim KH, Hong WS, Yun YS. Activation of multiple effector pathways of immune system by the antineoplastic immunostimulator acidic polysaccharide ginsan isolated from *Panax ginseng*. Anticancer Res 1997; 17(1A):323–331.
69. Kim YS, Park KM, Shin HJ, Song KS, Nam KY, Park JD. Anticancer activities of red ginseng acidic polysaccharide by activation of macrophages and natural killer cells. Yakhak Hoeji 2002; 46(2):113–119.
70. Assinewe VA, Amason JT, Aubry A, Mulln J, Lemaire I. Extractable polysaccharides of *Panax quinquefolius* L. (North American ginseng) root stimulate TNFalpha production by alveolar macrophages. Phytomedicine 2002; 9(5):398–404.
71. Thompson CB. Apoptosis in the pathogenesis and treatment of disease. Science 1995; 267(5203):1456–1462.
72. Fujikawa-Yammamoto K, Ota T, Odashima S, Abe H, Arichi S. Different response in the cell cycle of tumor cells to ginsenoside Rh2. Cancer J 1987; 1:349–352.
73. Lee KY, Park JA, Chung E, Lee YH, Kim SI, Lee SK. Ginsenoside-Rh2 blocks the cell cycle of SK-HEP-1 cells at the G1/S boundary by selectively inducing the protein expression of p27kip1. Cancer Lett 1996; 110(1-2):193–200.
74. Kim HE, Oh JH, Lee SK, Oh YJ. Ginsenoside RH-2 induces apoptotic cell death in rat C6 glioma via a reactive oxygen- and caspase-dependent but Bcl-X(L)-independent pathway. Life Sci 1999; 65(3):PL33–40.
75. Kim YS, Jin SH, Lee YH, Kim SI, Park JD. Ginsenoside Rh2 induces apoptosis independently of Bcl-2, Bcl-xL or Bax in C6Bu-1 cells. Proceedings of '99 Korea-Japan Ginseng symposium, 1999:150–162.
76. Lee KS. Effect of ginseng saponin on the vascular smooth muscle. Proceeding of the 3rd Intl Ginseng Symposium, 1980:71–76.
77. Yammamoto M. Effects of administration of red ginseng on hypertension, normotension and hypotension. Ginseng Rev 1992; 9:15–20.
78. Gillis CN, Kim HY, Chen X, Park H. Pulmonary vascular effects of ginsenosides. Proc. of 6th Intl' Ginseng Symp, 1993:36–39.
79. Vane JR, Anggard EE, Botting RM. Regulatory functions of the vascular endothelium. N Engl J Med 1990; 323(1):27–36.
80. Palmer RM, Ashton DS, Moncada S. Vascular endothelial cells synthesize nitric oxide from L-arginine. Nature 1988; 333(6174):664–666.

81. Rapoport RM, Murad F. Agonist-induced endothelium-dependent relaxation in rat thoracic aorta may be mediated through cGMP. Circ Res 1983; 52(3):352–357.
82. Kim ND, Kang SY, Schini VB. Ginsenosides evoke endothelium-dependent vascular relaxation in rat aorta. Gen Pharmacol 1994; 25(6):1071–1077.
83. Kang SY, Schini-Kerth VB, Kim ND. Ginsenosides of the protopanaxatriol group cause endothelium-dependent relaxation in the rat aorta. Life Sci 19; 56:(1995) 1577–1586.
84. Kim ND, Kang SY, Park JH, Schini-Kerth VB. Ginsenoside Rg3 mediates endothelium-dependent relaxation in response to ginsenosides in rat aorta: role of K+ channels. Eur J Pharmacol 1999; 367(1):41–49.
85. Kim ND, Kang SY, Kim MJ, Park JH, Schini-Kerth VB. The ginsenoside Rg3 evokes endothelium-independent relaxation in rat aortic rings: role of K+ channels. Eur J Pharmacol 1999; 367(1):51–57.
86. Jeon BH, Kim CS, Park KS, Lee JW, Park JB, Kim KJ, Kim SH, Chang SJ, Nam KY. Effect of Korea red ginseng on the blood pressure in conscious hypertensive rats. Gen Pharmacol 2000; 35(3):135–141.
87. Sung J, Han KH, Zo JH, Park HJ, Kim CH, Oh BH. Effects of red ginseng upon vascular endothelial function in patients with essential hypertension. Am J Chin Med 2000; 28(2):205–216.
88. Teng CM, Kuo SC, Ko FN, Lee JC, Lee LG, Chen SC, Huang TF. Antiplatelet actions of panaxynol and ginsenosides isolated from ginseng. Biochim Biophys Acta 1989; 990(3):315–320.
89. Kuo SC, Teng CM, Lee JC, Ko FN, Chen SC, Wu TS. Antiplatelet components in *Panax ginseng*. Planta Med 1990; 56(2):164–167.
90. Hirai A. Studies on the mechanisms of anti-platelet and anti-atherosclerotic effects of Korean red ginseng: focusing on arachidonic acid cascade. Proceedings of '99 Korea-Japan Ginseng Symposium, 1999:16–31.
91. Yuan CS, Attele AS, Wu JA, Lowell TK, Gu Z, Lin Y. *Panax quinquefolium* L. inhibits thrombin-induced endothelin release in vitro. Am J Chin Med 1999; 27(3-4):331–338.

24

Antioxidant Activities of Prickly Pear (*Opuntia ficus indica*) Fruit and Its Betalains

Betanin and Indicaxanthin

Maria A. Livrea and Luisa Tesoriere
University of Palermo
Palermo, Italy

I. INTRODUCTION

The importance of diet in reducing the incidence of chronic and degenerative diseases such as cancer and cardiovascular disease is well recognized (1,2). Epidemiological evidence, especially regarding the Mediterranean population (3,4), pointed out on the importance of herbs, fruits, grains, and vegetables. Among other components such as fiber and micronutrients, antioxidants in these foods are thought to be active agents responsible for some of the beneficial effects. Some of the dietary antioxidants are essential nutrients, such as vitamin E, C, and A, and minerals such as Cu, Mn, Zn, and Se, which are cofactors of antioxidant enzymes. In addition, fruits, vegetables, and herbs are particularly rich sources of other nonnutrient antioxidants, including a vast array of phytochemicals (5,6), from carotenoids and bioflavonoids to phytosterols and terpenoids. Other compounds such as betalains, less common in edible species, have more recently been studied (7–10).

The prickly pear cactus, or nopal, is a member of the Cactaceae family widely distributed in Mexico, much of Latin America, South Africa, and the Mediterranean area (11). The metabolism of its crassulacean acid gives this plant a high potential of biomass with low water consumption (12), favoring its growth under semiarid conditions. About 1500 species are in the genus *Opuntia*, many of which produce edible fruit.

Prickly pear has long been known in traditional medicine for treating a number of pathologies from ulcer, fatigue, and dyspnea to glaucoma, liver conditions, and wounds (11,13). Studies with different models and several experimental conditions provided some scientific basis for the popular use of this plant. Various preparations from fleshy stems (cladodes) have been tested for treatment of diabetes symptomatology in animal models (14,15), or in humans (16). The mechanism for this action is still unknown; some results, however, preclude a role for dietary fiber (15). Other studies revealed beneficial effects against ethanol-induced ulcer (17), in the treatment of benign prostatic hypertrophy (18,19), and in hypercholesterolemia in humans (20) and guinea pigs (21). Diuretic activity of cladode, flower, and fruit infusions has been shown in rats (22). Obviously, other investigations are required to gain insight into the active agents in this plant and the mechanisms involved in all the observed effects.

Cladodes of prickly pear are rich in proteins, carbohydrates, minerals, and vitamins, so Mexicans eat the young pads of the plant, also known as nopalitos, cooked as vegetables. In the industrialized countries of the Mediterranean area, cladodes are not a common nutritional source for humans, but the peeled fruits are usually consumed.

The Sicilian cultivars of prickly pear [*Opuntia ficus indica* (L.) Mill.] are characterized by yellow, red, and white fruits, due to the combination of two betalain pigments, the purple-red betanin and the yellow-orange indicaxanthin (23,24). The composition and nutritional properties of the prickly pear fruit have long been reported (11,25–29). In contrast, though it was known that the fruit contains vitamin C (29,30), investigations on other antioxidant components, and on its antioxidant capacities, have started only recently. Antioxidant nutrients have been researched in the authors' laboratory, and antioxidant activities of the fruit extracts and of the purified betalains have been evaluated in a number of models in vitro (9,10). In addition, the effects of the regular ingestion of prickly pear fruits on redox balance and bioavailability of betalain components in healthy humans have been investigated (31). This chapter summarizes findings to date, with special emphasis on betanin and indicaxanthin, the characteristic pigments. These phytochemicals, poorly studied until recently, have appeared as important functional components whose antioxidant activity may be a matter of future development.

II. BETALAIN PIGMENTS

A. Chemistry

Betalains are vacuole pigments restricted to flowers and fruits of 10 families of Cariophyllalae plants and to a few superior fungi of the the genus *Amanita* of the Basidiomycetes (32). Beet (*Beta vulgaris*) and prickly pear cactus are the only foods containing betalains (33,34). Betalains constitute a class of cationized nitrogenous compounds, the colors of which range from the yellow betaxanthins to the violet-red betacyanins. The betaxanthins are conjugates of betalamic acid with amino acids or the corresponding amines (including dopamine), while almost all betacyanins are derivatives of betanidin, the conjugate of betalamic acid with cyclodopa. The hydroxyl groups at the C5 and C6 position of cyclodopa can be esterified with either a carbohydrate or a carbohydrate derivative to form various betacyanins (Scheme 1). Tyrosinase and Dopa dioxygenase are the only enzymes involved in the synthesis of Dopa, cyclodopa, and betalamic acid, to form the basic skeleton of betalains in plant tissues (35–38), whereas the condensation process of betalamic acid with cyclodopa or amino acids/amines appears as a nonenzymatic reaction (39,40). Glucosyl transferase is involved in the attachment of glucose to betanidine (41).

B. Betanin and Indicaxanthin from Prickly Pear Fruit

The structure of the major betalains occurring in the fruits of *O. ficus indica* is shown in Figure 1. They are the betacyanin betanin (5-*O*-glucose betanidine) and the betaxanthin indicaxanthin, the adduct of betalamic acid with proline (9,23,24,42–44). Minor amounts of a few other betacyanins and betaxanthins have been found (44).

Betalains possess high molar absorption coefficients in visible light (33,45), which allows their detection in extracts from various vegetal sources. Indicaxanthin (MW 309) has a clear absorbance peak at 482 nm (A_{482} = 42,600). Betanin (MW 565) shows an absorbance peak at a wavelength of 536 nm (A_{536} = 65,000); however, it also absorbs at 482 nm (Fig. 2). Owing to the overlapping of betanin absorbance on the absorbance of indicaxanthin (calculated betanin A_{482} = 30,900) (9), the indicaxanthin concentration in crude extracts containing both pigments should be measured according to the following equation:

$$[\text{Indicaxanthin}](\mu\text{M}) = 23.8\ A_{482} - 7.7\ A_{536}$$

This was applied to investigate the amounts of both betalains in methanolic extracts from fruit of the white, yellow, and red Sicilian cultivars of prickly pear (9).

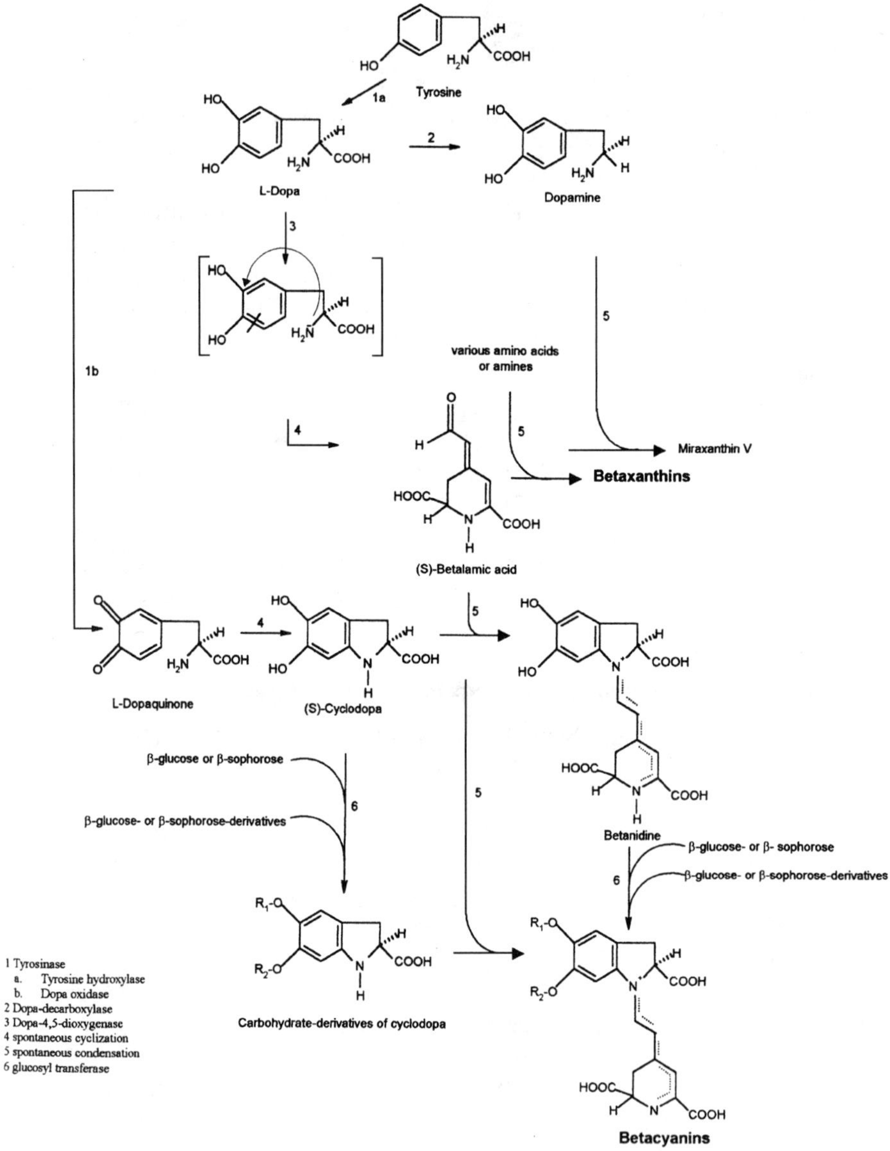

SCHEME 1 Biosynthetic pathway of betaxanthins and betacyanins.

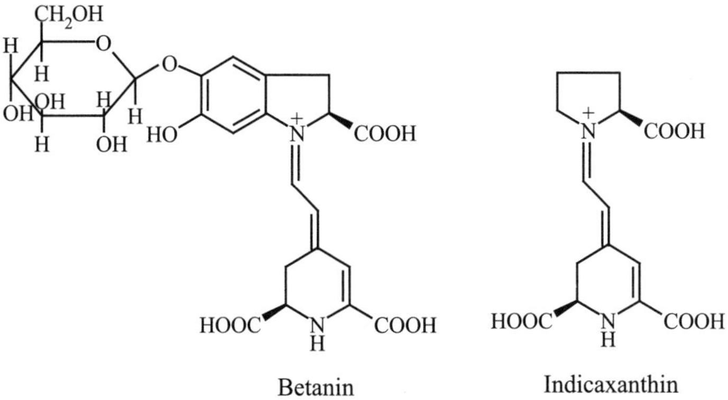

FIGURE 1 Structure of betanin and indicaxanthin.

Simple chromatographic methods have been described to isolate and purify the two major pigments from the fruit of prickly pear (9,42–44).

C. Redox Potential

The oxidation potentials of betanin and indicaxanthin have been evaluated by cyclic voltammetry (9). The cyclic voltammogram showed two and three anodic waves for indicaxanthin and betanin, respectively, indicating that both

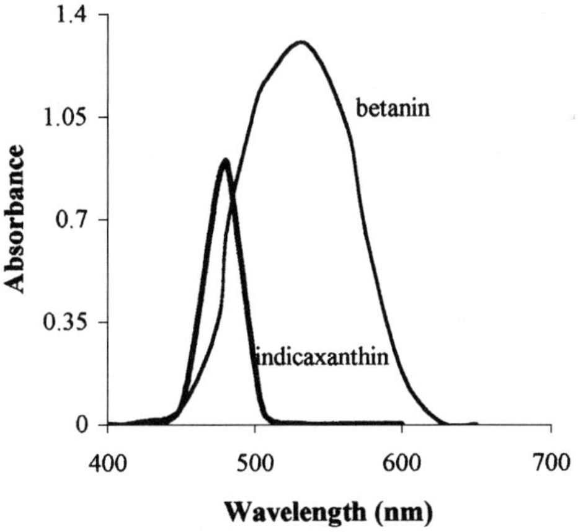

FIGURE 2 Visible-light absorption spectra of indicaxanthin and betanin.

are able to donate their electrons. Three peak potentials of 404, 616, and 998 mV, and two peak potentials of 611 and 895 mV have been calculated for betanin and indicaxanthin, respectively, from the differential pulse voltammogram (Fig. 3).

D. Safety

Betalains are important natural pigments for industry. They have been exploited as colorants in processed food (46–48), cosmetics, and pharmaceutical products. To this end, the safety of these compounds has been tested. Studies carried out to determine decomposition and stability (49,50), mutagenicity (48,51,52), and toxicological and toxicokinetic effects (53) showed that these pigments are not harmful. Some in vivo studies in rats indicated that betalains did not have toxic effects with any of the doses tested, up to 5 g/kg body weight (53).

In the authors' laboratory the potential prooxidant activity of the pure betanin and indicaxanthin was tested in a model of copper-stimulated oxidation of human LDL (10). Neither betalain showed adverse effects when assayed in a concentration range of 0.05–50 μM. Rather, both compounds were able to decrease dose-dependently the conjugated diene lipid hydro-

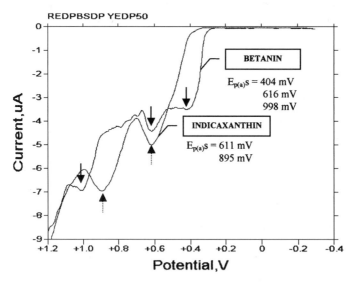

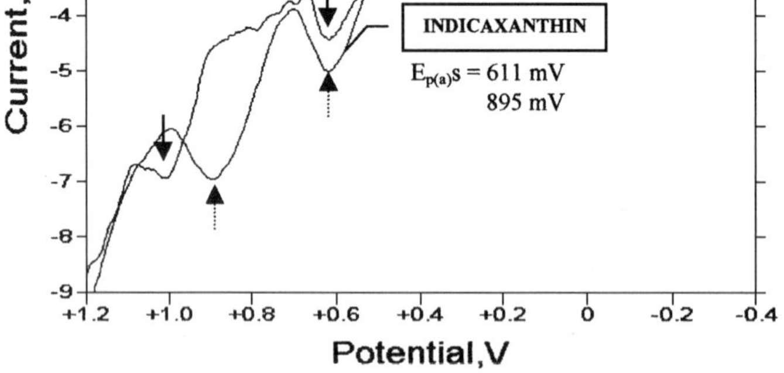

FIGURE 3 Differential pulse voltammetry of betanin and indicaxanthin. The arrows represent the $E_{p(a)}$ of the anodic waves. (Modified from Ref. 9.)

peroxides formed in 120 min, with indicaxanthin more effective than betanin in the range 0.05–1.0 μM. Above 1.0 μM both betalains completely inhibited LDL lipid oxidation for the period of observation.

III. ANTIOXIDANT COMPOSITION OF FRUITS OF *O. FICUS INDICA*

Organic extracts in dichloromethane (DCM) and aqueous extracts in methanol of the yellow, red, and white fruits from Sicilian cultivars of *O. ficus indica* have been analyzed for lipid-soluble and water-soluble antioxidants, respectively (54). Very limited amounts of lipophilic antioxidant vitamins have been found, α-tocopherol, *trans*-β-Carotene, and retinyl palmitate representing the major compounds, with minor variations among the cultivars. Retinyl oleate and *trans*-retinol are absent. In contrast, all cultivars are a good source of vitamin C (Table 1). Negligible amounts of flavonols (237 ± 20 ng/100 g fruit pulp) have been found in the aqueous extracts from the red fruit only (9).

Betalains have been measured in the three cultivars. According Butera et al. (9), the yellow cultivar has the highest content of betalains, indicaxanthin accounting for 89% of the pigments. Betanin is mostly concentrated in the red cultivar, which accounts for 66% of betalains. Finally, the white cultivar, which exhibits the lowest amount of betalain pigments, contains almost exclusively indicaxanthin (Table 2). Other researchers (42,43), who investigated betalains in the red and yellow cultivars, have reported quite different values (Table 2). As observed (9), overestimation of indicaxanthin due to biased spectrophotometric evaluation of crude extracts, and/or different cultivars, may account for the discrepancy.

TABLE 1 Major Antioxidant Vitamins in Prickly Pear Fruit from Yellow, Red, and White Cultivars

Cultivar	α-Tocopherol (μg/100 g edible pulp)	β-Carotene (μg/100 g edible pulp)	Retinyl palmitate (μg/100 g edible pulp)	Ascorbic acid (mg/100 g edible pulp)
Yellow	66 ± 5.8	1.1 ± 0.09	0.13 ± 0.01	30 ± 2.8
Red	69 ± 7.0	2.7 ± 0.22	0.44 ± 0.05	29 ± 1.7
White	65 ± 5.2	1.2 ± 0.1	0.11 ± 0.02	28 ± 2.5

Each value is the mean ± SD of four determinations on different lots of fruits.

TABLE 2 Indicaxanthin and Betanin in *O. ficus indica*

	Content (mg/100 g edible pulp)	
Cultivar	Indicaxanthin	Betanin
Yellow	8.42 ± 0.51[a]	1.04 ± 0.12[a]
	25[b]	Not detectable[b]
Red	2.61 ± 0.30[a]	5.12 ± 0.51[a]
	30[b]	19[b]
	40[c]	14[c]
White	5.86 ± 0.49[a]	0.10 ± 0.02[a]

[a] *Source*: From Ref. 9.
[b] *Source*: From Ref. 43.
[c] *Source*: From Ref. 42.

IV. ANTIOXIDANT ACTIVITIES OF FRUITS OF *O. FICUS INDICA*

A. In Vitro Studies

1. Chemical Models

The decolorization of the 2,2′-azino-bis(3-ethylbenzthiazoline-6-sulfonic acid) (ABTS) radical cation is an accurate assay for screening the antioxidant activities of either lipophilic substances or food extracts (55). The total antioxidant capacity of either the DCM lipophilic extracts or the methanolic hydrophilic extracts from fruits of the yellow, red, and white Sicilian cultivars of prickly pear has been evaluated by the reaction with the ABTS radical cation, generated by reacting ABTS with potassium persulfate (9), and expressed as Trolox equivalents. Because of the low amount of lipophilic antioxidants, the organic extracts of the prickly pear fruits exhibit a modest radical-scavenging activity, when compared, for example, to extracts from tomato (55), a good source of carotenoids (Table 3). The activity of the extract from the red fruit appears higher than the activity of the yellow and white ones, possibly as a reflection of the relatively higher content of β-carotene. In contrast, the water-soluble extracts from prickly pear fruits appear very active, as compared with a number of other fruits (Table 3). The total antioxidant capacity is higher than that reported for pear, apple, tomato, banana, and white grape, and of the same order of pink grapefruit, red grape, and orange (56). The extract from the yellow fruit is the most effective among the three cultivars. Considering its antioxidant potential evaluated in the ABTS test (57), vitamin C, which occurs in approximately the same amount in the three cultivars of prickly pear, may account for no more than 40% of

TABLE 3 Total Antioxidant Activity (TAA) of Lipophilic and Water-Soluble Extracts *of O. ficus indica* and Other Fruits

	Lipophilic extract (mmol Trolox equivalent/kg dry wt)	Water-soluble extract (μmol Trolox equivalent/g edible pulp)
Prickly pear		
Yellow	0.010 ± 0.002[a]	5.31 ± 0.49[a]
Red	0.016 ± 0.002[a]	4.20 ± 0.51[a]
White	0.011 ± 0.001[a]	4.36 ± 0.41[a]
Pear		1.34 ± 0.06[b]
Tomato	5.72 ± 0.21[c]	1.89 ± 0.12[c]
Apple		2.18 ± 0.35[b]
Banana		2.21 ± 0.19[b]
Grape		
White		4.46 ± 1.06[b]
Red		7.39 ± 0.48[b]
Grapefruit		
Pink		4.83 ± 0.18[b]
Orange		7.50 ± 1.01[b]

[a] *Source*: From Ref. 9.
[b] *Source*: From Ref. 57.
[c] *Source*: From Ref. 55.

the evaluated antioxidant capacity of the extracts, which has suggested that other hydrophilic constituents, possibly betalain pigments, may act as efficient radical scavengers (9). This seemed to somewhat explain the activity of the extract from the yellow fruit, which contains the highest amounts of betalains (9).

In addition to the activity measured in fruits, ethanol extracts of stems of *O. ficus indica* var. Saboten were found to have radical-scavenging activity in a number of assays generating radicals such as 2,2-diphenyl-1-picrylhydrazyl (DPPH), superoxide anions, and hydroxyl radicals (58). In light of the high amount of phenolics in the stems (180.3 mg/g lyophilized extract), these substances have been suggested to be the active components.

2. Biological Models

Methanolic extracts from the fruits of the yellow, red, and white cultivars of prickly pear have been found capable of preventing lipid oxidation stimulated by organic hydroperoxide in human red blood cells, and by either copper or 2,2′-azobis(2-amidinopropaane) hydrochloride (AAPH) in human low-density lipoproteins (9). Extracts from 0.5–5 mg of fruit pulp dose-dependently inhibited malondialdehyde formation in red blood cells (Fig. 4). With reference to the antioxidant activity of α-tocopherol, the white cultivar has been the most effective at inhibiting lipid oxidation, the extract from 1 mg pulp being as effective as 0.2 μM α-tocopherol. Comparable amounts of extracts from the red and yellow cultivars showed an antioxidant activity equivalent to that of 0.13 μM α-tocopherol (9).

Methanolic extracts of fruit pulp markedly elongated, in a dose-dependent fashion, the period preceding the formation of conjugated diene lipid hydroperoxides of human LDL, submitted to either metal-dependent or -independent oxidation (Fig. 5). As already observed with the red blood cell oxidation model, the extract from the white cultivar was the most effective in both LDL models, followed by the red and the yellow ones.

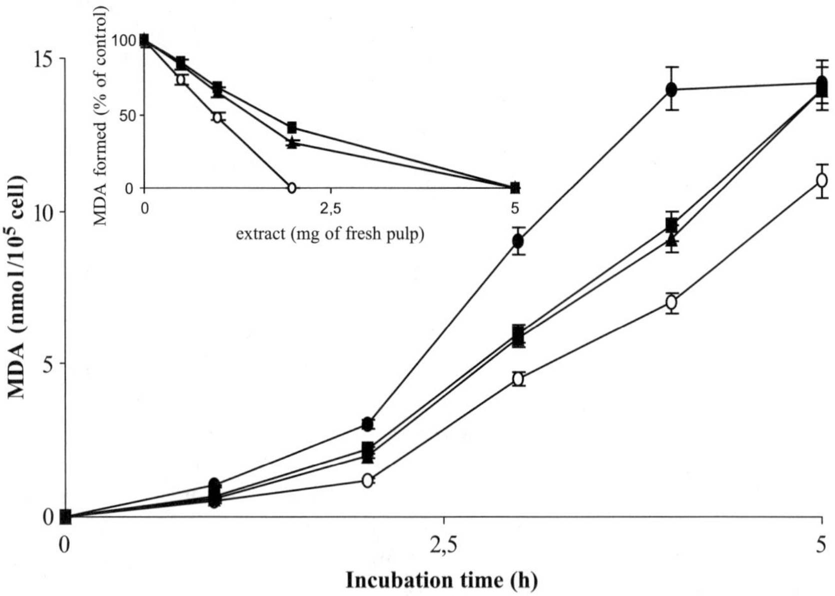

FIGURE 4 Inibitory effect of methanolic extracts from 1 mg fresh pulp of *O. ficus indica* on MDA formation, in *tert*-butyl hydroperoxide-treated RBCs. Human RBCs (HT 1%) were incubated with 50 μM *tert*-butyl hydroperoxide at 37°C either in the absence (●) or in the presence of methanolic extract of edible pulp from white (○), yellow (▲), and red (■) cultivars. Inset. Dose-dependent inhibitory effect of methanolic extracts on MDA formation, after 4-hr incubation.

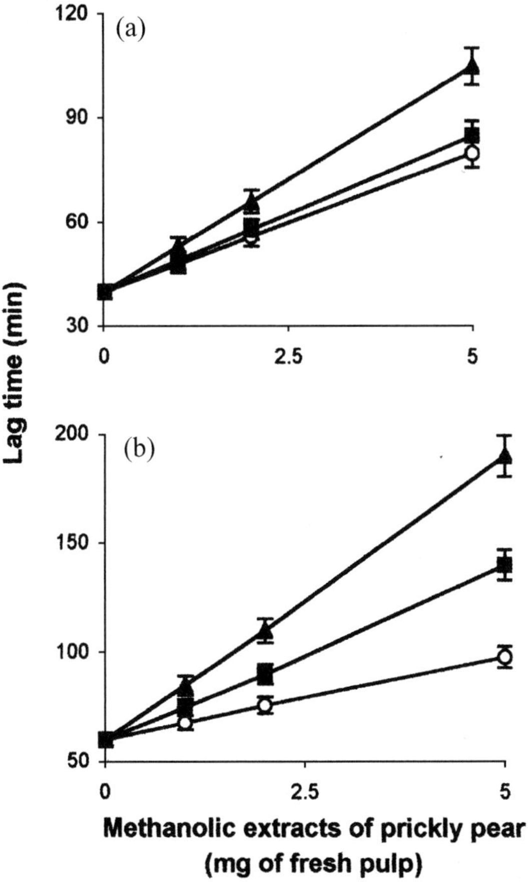

FIGURE 5 Elongation of the lag period during the Cu^{2+}- (a) or AAPH- (b) induced oxidation of human LDL by methanolic extracts of prickly pear. ▲, yellow cultivar; ■, red cultivar; ○, white cultivar.

While taking into consideration the contribution of vitamin C, the involvement of the betalain pigments in the observed antioxidant activity of the extracts has been suggested on the basis of the measured redox potential of betanin and indicaxanthin (9). In addition, it has been pointed out that the extract from the white fruit, in which betanin is virtually absent, has the highest activity in all models of lipid oxidation. This can be an indication that, in addition to betacyanins (8), indicaxanthin may act as an antioxidant compound in biological environments.

B. In Vivo Studies with Humans

A strong protection of the body's antioxidant system, and reduction of oxidative stress by regular ingestion of prickly pear, has recently been observed in an in vivo study in which eight healthy volunteers, aged 20–55, received six fruits per day (400 g edible pulp), for 2 weeks during which they were allowed to eat according to their usual diet, with the exception of fruits (31). Plasma measurements, before and after the 2-week trial, have shown a very marked elevation of vitamin C and vitamin E, with a concomitant decrease of markers of oxidative stress such as malondialdehyde and isoprostans (8-epi-$PGF_{2\alpha}$). The mechanism underlying these effects is still unclear. The observed increase of the plasma vitamins cannot be accounted for by the amount of vitamins introduced with the fruit. This suggests that other bioavailable components may protect the whole-body redox system.

With focus on the betalain components, recent observations in the authors' laboratory with eight human volunteers showed that both indicaxanthin and betanin from prickly pear are absorbed, with a plasma peak of indicaxanthin markedly higher than betanin (Table 4). A single ingestion of 500 g fresh pulp (eight fruits) was followed by a progressive increase of the plasma levels of betanin and indicaxanthin, with a maximum level at 3 hr, followed by a decrease during the following 5 hr. Since the intake represented 27 μmoles of betanin (15.4 mg) and 89 μmoles of indicaxanthin (27.5 mg), it has been calculated that the plasma peak of the two substances (5 μM and 0.1 μM for indicaxanthin and betanin, respectively) accounts for 14% and 1% of the amount assumed with the fruits. Bioavailability of betanin in humans has also been demonstrated in a study with four volunteers who consumed 300 mL of red beet juice containing 120 mg of pigment (8). The betacyanin was identified in the urine after 2–4 hr, the escreted amount accounting for 0.5–0.9% of that ingested.

Both LDL and red blood cells, isolated 3 hr after the ingestion of 500 g fresh fruit pulp, revealed the presence of indicaxanthin and betanin (Table 4).

TABLE 4 Occurrence of Betalains in Humans 3 hr After the Ingestion of 500 g Prickly Pear Pulp

	Plasma (μM)	Red blood cells (nmoles/4.5 × 10^9 RBCs)	LDL (nmoles/mg LDL prot)
Indicaxanthin	5 ± 0.8 (8)	0.5 ± 0.01 (8)	0.1 ± 0.005 (6)
Betanin	0.1 ± 0.02 (8)	(7.5 ± 0.3) × 10^{-3} (8)	(2 ± 0.27) × 10^{-3} (6)

Values are the mean ± SD of (*n*) samples, contributed by different volunteers, analyzed in duplicate.

Concomitantly, a marked increase in the resistance of LDL to the copper-induced lipid oxidation, and a significant decrease in the susceptibility of red blood cells to the cumene-hydroperoxide-induced oxidative hemolysis, were measured. Although the antioxidant activity of other yet-unidentified compounds cannot be ruled out, the above results suggest that betalain pigments may be involved.

Metabolic products from betalains, eventually circulating in blood or excreted in urine or through the gastrointestinal tract, have not been researched yet. This could be an interesting area of future investigation to disclose reactions, eventual sites of activities, and possibly other nonantioxidant effects of these substances. Recent research now indicates that other phytochemicals such as flavonoids may be involved in biochemical activities independent of, or only partly related to, antioxidant activity, including signal transduction and modulation of enzyme activities (59,60).

It may also be mentioned that the regular ingestion of broiled edible cladodes of prikly pear (*Opuntia robusta*) has been shown able to significantly reduce the in vivo oxidation injury in patients suffering from familial hypercholesterolemia (61). Other components, possibly flavonoids, may be the effective compounds in the stems (58).

V. RADICAL-SCAVENGING AND ANTIOXIDANT ACTIVITIES OF PURIFIED BETALAINS

A. In Vitro Studies

1. Chemical Models

The antiradical activity of betalains has recently been investigated in a few studies (7–9). Betacyanins such as betanin (7,9) and betanidin (7), as well as betaxanthins such as indicaxathin (9) and vulgaxanthin (7), have been found capable of reducing the cation radical from ABTS, generated either by horseradish peroxidase/hydrogen peroxide–mediated oxidation (7) or by reaction with potassium persulfate (9). When expressed as trolox equivalents, betanin has appeared very effective (9), with an antiradical activity higher than the two betaxanthins with both experimental sets (7,9) (Table 5). This appears in accordance with the redox potential of indicaxanthin and betanin. By considering the phenolic hydroxyl group, the higher scavenging capacity of betanin has been explained by the ease with which it is possible to withdraw an electron from the betacyanin, and by the stability of the resulting delocalized radical (7). In contrast, the electron abstracted from the betaxanthins could only be from the π-orbitals, this loss being hindered by the positive charge of the N-atom. It should be mentioned that according to the ABTS assay, betanin is much more effective than a number of polyphenol com-

TABLE 5 Antiradical Activity of Betalains and Betalamic Acid Toward $ABTS^+$ Radical

	Trolox equivalents	Rate of $ABTS^+$ radical disappearance (μmoles $ABTS^+$ radical/first min)
Betanin	20.0 ± 0.5[a,b]	45.5[c]
Indicaxanthin	1.76 ± 0.1[a,b]	
Vulgaxanthin I		4.2[c]
Betalamic acid[d]	33 ± 1.0[a]	

[a] Each value is the mean ± SD of four determinations performed in duplicate.
[b] *Source*: From Ref. 9.
[c] Calculated from Ref. 7. Betanin and vulgaxanthin I were assayed at 12 μM, while $ABTS^+$ radical was 70 μM. (7).
[d] Prepared according to Ref. 44.

pounds (62). Betalamic acid shows a high radical-scavenging activity (Table 5), suggesting that the products of betalain hydrolysis may have antioxidant activity.

The activity of betalains in reducing the formation of lipoperoxyl radicals has also been reported. Linoleate peroxidation by cyt c was inhibited by betanin and betanidin, with IC_{50} of 0.4 and 0.8 μM, respectively, and by vulgaxanthin, with IC_{50} around 1.0 μM (8). In comparison, vitamin E inhibited lipid oxidation with IC_{50} of 5 μM (8), indicating a relatively higher antioxidant potential of betalains in this system. Oxidation of linoleic acid was also inhibited by betanidin and betanin, when the lipid oxidation was stimulated by H_2O_2-activated metmyoglobin, or by lipoxygenase. In the latter assays the IC_{50} for betanidin and betanin were 0.3 and 0.6 μM, respectively (8). Interestingly, monoelectronic redox reactions between betanin and the oxoferryl catalytic forms of horseradish peroxidase have been shown (63). Such an activity could also be considered in the above-reported reactions in which activated heme proteins are involved (8), as well as to explain why either betanin or betanidin was able to inhibit the decomposition of the myoglobin heme during the oxidation of linoleate (8).

The antioxidant activity of nine betalains has been studied, and the relationship between the structure and antioxidant activity was examined, with the linetol peroxidation model (64). Betaxanthins were shown to have the highest antioxidant activity in this system.

B. Biological Models

The positive charge of betalains could favor interactions with polar head groups of lipids and/or polar sites on the protein surface. Ex vivo plasma spiking of pure either betanin or indicaxanthin has been performed to provide evidence that both betalains can bind to human LDL in a saturable fashion, with a maximum binding of 0.5 nmoles/mg LDL protein (10). The betanin- as well as the indicaxanthin-enriched LDL has been shown more resistant than the homologous native LDL to copper-induced oxidation, as assessed by elongation of the lag period (Fig. 6). In addition, indicaxanthin-enriched LDL has appeared much more resistant than betanin-enriched LDL in this system, possibly as the result of synergistic interactions of indicaxanthin with the LDL vitamin E (10). Consumption of vitamin E was not varied by betanin. In contrast, indicaxanthin prevented vitamin E consumption at the beginning of LDL oxidation, and prolonged the time of its utilization (Fig. 6).

The affinity of betacyanins for microsomal membranes has been demonstrated by evaluating the rate of migration of these compounds through a dialysis tube, either in the absence or in the presence of microsomes (8).

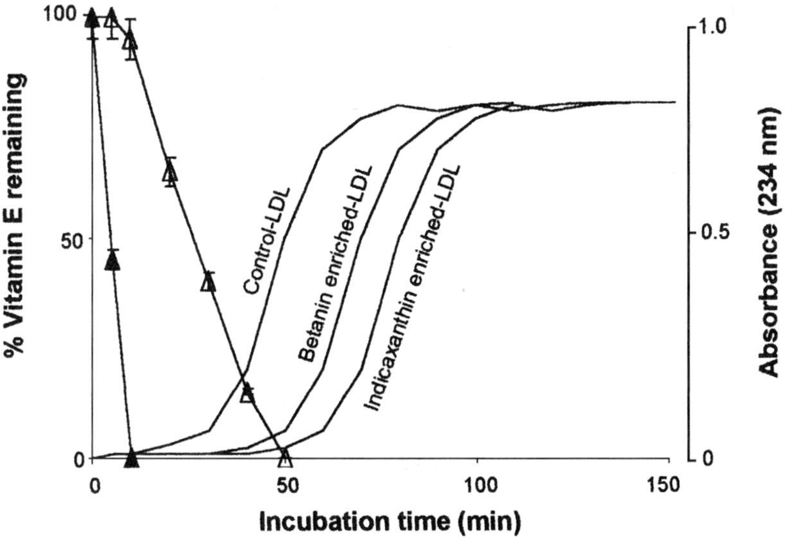

FIGURE 6 Oxidation of human control-LDL, betanin- and indicaxanthin-enriched LDL, and time course of vitamin E consumption in either control- or betanin-enriched LDL (closed triangle) and in indicaxanthin-enriched LDL (open triangle).

In addition, it has been shown that the oxidation of microsomal lipids by either $FeCl_2$/ascorbate or H_2O_2-activated myoglobin was reduced by variable concentrations of betanin (8). However, because of its electron-donating capability, low amounts of betanin (<12.5 μM) were prooxidant in the system catalyzed by iron/ascorbate, as a result of the reduction of ferric to ferrous ions. At high concentrations (25 μM) the antioxidant works also with lipoperoxyl radicals, thus preventing lipid oxidation (8).

VI. CONCLUSIONS

Phytochemicals and phytomedicines are now an expanding research field. A great number of active agents occurring in plants and herbs have been discovered, which is fundamental to finding rationale for the health effects of these herbs, in many cases used for centuries as traditional remedies. The knowledge of the mechanisms and molecular basis of action is the final objective to understand the mode of action of the discovered principles. Many antioxidant substances are listed among the phytochemicals occurring in a varieties of plants and herbs, which have been supposed to have a role in the biochemical potential of these plants and herbs.

Studies of the antioxidant properties of prickly pear are very recent, and results obtained so far, while exciting, now generate new questions. In vivo studies in healthy humans showed a strong protection of the body antioxidant system, and a marked reduction of plasma levels of markers of oxidative stress, by regular consumption of moderate amounts of prickly pear fruits. Betanin and indicaxanthin, two bioavailable, apparently very potent antiradical and antioxidant pigments with proved activity in biological environments, occur in the fruits. However, distinguishing protective effects of food rich in antioxidants from direct effects of the antioxidants themselves is essential. At present it is not possible to assess to what extent, and how, these betalain pigments may be involved in the in vivo observed effects, and the molecular mechanism underlying these effects is unclear. Cytoprotective effects of phytochemicals can be related to their reducing properties, as well as to their influence on intracellular redox status. However, other biochemical activities independent of conventional hydrogen-donating/free-radical-scavenging activity should be considered, and deserve future research.

REFERENCES

1. Rice-Evans CA, Miller NJ. Antioxidants: the case of fruit and vegetables in the diet. Br Food J 1985; 97:35–40.

2. Ames B, Shigenaga MK, Hagen TM. Oxidants, antioxidants and the degenerative disease of aging. Proc Natl Acad Sci USA 1993; 90:7915–7922.
3. Willett WC, Sacks F, Trichopoulou A, Drescher G, Ferro-Luzzi A, Helsing E, Trichopoulous D. Mediterranean diet pyramid: a cultural model for healthy eating. Am J Clin Nutr 1995; 61(suppl 6):1402S–1406S.
4. Kushi LH, Lenart EB, Willett WC. Health implication of Mediterranean diets in light of contemporary knowledge. 1. Plant foods and dairy products. Am J Clin Nutr 1995; 61(suppl 6):1407S–1415S.
5. Lin RI-S. Phytochemical and antioxidants. In: Goldberg IE, ed. Functional Foods. New York: Chapman & Hall, 1995:393–441.
6. Cao G, Sofic E, Prior RL. Antioxidant and prooxidant behavior of flavonoids: structure-activity relationships. Free Rad Biol Med 1997; 22:749–760.
7. Escribano J, Pedreno MA, Garcia-Carmona F, Munoz R. Characterization of the antiradical activity of betalains from *Beta vulgaris* L. roots. Phytochem Anal 1998; 9:124–127.
8. Kanner J, Harel S, Granit R. Betalains—a new class of dietary cationized antioxidants. J Agric Food Chem 2001; 49:5178–5185.
9. Butera D, Tesoriere L, Di Gaudio F, Bongiorno A, Allegra M, Pintaudi AM, Kohen R, Livrea MA. Antioxidant activities of sicilian prickly pear (*Opuntia ficus indica*) fruit extracts and reducing properties of its betalains: betanin and indicaxantin. J Agric Food Chem 2002; 50:6895–6901.
10. Tesoriere L, Butera D, D'Arpa D, Di Gaudio F, Allegra M, Gentile C, Livrea MA. Increased resistance to oxidation of betalain-enriched human low density lipoproteins. Free Radic Res 2003; 37:689–696.
11. Muñoz de Chavez M, Chavez A, Valles V, Roldan JA. The Nopal: a plant of manifold qualities. In: Simopoulos AP, ed. World Review of Nutrition and Dietetics. Vol. 77. Basel, Switzerland: Karger, 1995:109–134.
12. De Cortazar VG, Nobel PS. Biomass and fruit production for the prickly pear cactus, *Opuntia ficus indica*. J Am Soc Hortic Sci 1992; 117:558–562.
13. Hegwood DA. Human health discoveries with *Opuntia* sp. (prickly pear). HortScience 1990; 25:1515–1516.
14. Ibanez-Camacho R, Meckes-Lozoya M, Mellado-Campos V. The hypoglycemic effect of *Opuntia streptacantha* studied in different animal experimental models. J Ethnopharmacol 1983; 7:175–181.
15. Trejo-Gonzales A, Gabriel-Ortiz G, Puebla-Perez AM, Huizar-Contreras MD, Munguia-Mazariegos MR, Mejia-Arreguin S, Calva E. A purified extract from prickly pear cactus (*Opuntia fuliginosa*) controls experimentally induced diabetes in rats. J Ethnopharmacol 1996; 55:27–33.
16. Frati AC, Gordillo BE, Altamirano P, Ariza CR, Cortes-Franco R, Chavez-Negrete A, Islas-Andrade S. Influence of nopal intake upon faasting glicemia in type II diabetics and healthy subjects. Arch Invest Med (Mex) 1991; 22: 51–56.
17. Galati EM, Monforte MT, Tripodo MM, d'Aquino A, Mondello MR. Antiulcer activity of *Opuntia ficus indica* (L.) Mill. (Cactaceae): ultrastructural study. J Ethnopharmacol 2001; 76:1–9.

18. Palevitch D, Earon G, Levin I. Treatment of benign prostatic hypertrophy with *Opuntia ficus indica* (L.) Miller. J Herbs Spices Med Plants 1993; 2:45–49.
19. Jonas A, Rosenblat G, Krapf D, Bitterman W, Neeman I. Cactus flower extracts may prove beneficial in benign prostatic hyperplasia due to inhibition of 5alpha reductase activity, aromatase activity and lipid peroxidation. Urol Res 1998; 26:265–270.
20. Cardenas Medellin ML, Serna Saldivar SO, Velazco de la Garza J. Effect of raw and cooked nopal (*Opuntia ficus indica*) ingestion on growth and profile of total cholesterol, lipoprotein, and blood glucose in rats. Arch Latinoam Nutr 1998; 48:316–323.
21. Fernandez ML, Lin EC, Trejo A, McNamara DJ. Prickly pear (*Opuntia* sp.) pectin reverses low density lipoprotein receptor suppression induced by a hypercholesterolemic diet in guinea pigs. J Nutr 1992; 122:2330–2340.
22. Galati EM, Tripodo MM, Trovato A, Miceli N, Manforte MT. Biological effect of *Opuntia ficus indica* (L.) Mill. (Cactaceae) waste matter. Note I: diuretic activity. J Ethnopharmacol 2002; 79:17–21.
23. Piattelli M, Minale L. Pigments of centrospermae I. Betacyanins from *Phyllocactus hybridus hort.* and *Opuntia* ficus-indica Mill. Phytochemistry 1964; 3:307–311.
24. Piattelli M, Minale L, Prota G. Isolation structure and absolute configuration of indicaxanthin. Tetrahedron 1964; 20:2325–2329.
25. Gurrieri S, Miceli L, Lanza CM, Tomaselli F, Bonomo RP, Rizzarelli E. Chemical characterization of Sicilian prickly pear (*Opuntia ficus indica*) and perspectives for the storage of its juice. J Agric Food Chem 2000; 48:5424–5431.
26. Sawaya WN, Khatchadourian HA, Safi WM, Al Muhammad HN. Chemical characterization of prickly pear pulp, *Opuntia ficus indica*, and the manufacturing of prickly pear jam. J Food Technol 1983; 18:183–193.
27. Sepulveda E, Saenz C. Caracteristicas quimicas y fisicas de pulpa de tuna (*Opuntia ficus indica*). Rev Agroquim Tecnol Aliment 1990; 30:551–555.
28. Joubert E. Processing of the fruit of five prickly pear cultivar crown in South Africa. Int J Food Sci Technol 1993; 28:377–387.
29. El Kossori RL, Villaume C, El Boustani E, Sauvaire Y, Mejean L. Composition of pulp, skin and seeds of prickly pears fruit (*Opuntia ficus indica* sp.). Plant Foods Hum Nutr 1998; 52:263–270.
30. El moghazy AM, El-Sayyad SM, Abdel-Beky AM, Bechait EY. A phytochemical study of *Opuntia ficus indica* (L.) Mill cultivated in Egypt. J Pharmacol Sci 1982; 23:224–254.
31. Tesoriere L, Livrea MA. Antioxidant activities of Sicilian prickly pear (*Opuntia ficus indica*) and its betalains: betanin and indicaxantin. Ital J Biochem 2002; 51:R.35.
32. Waterman PG. Alkaloid chemosystematics. In: Cordell GA, ed. The Alkaloids—Chemistry and Pharmacology. Vol. 50. San Diego, CA: Academic Press, 1988:537–565.
33. Schwartz SJ, von Elbe JH. Quantitative determination of individual betacyanin pigments by high-performance liquid chromatography. J Agric Food Chem 1980; 28:540–543.

34. Jackman RL, Smith JL. Anthocyanins and betalains. In: Heandry GAF, Houghton JD, eds. Natural Food Colorants. London: Chapman & Hall, 1996:244–309.
35. Mueller LA, Hinz U, Zryd J-P. Characterization of a tyrosinase from *Amanita muscaria* involved in betalain biosynthesis. Phytochemistry 1996; 42:1511–1515.
36. Steiner U, Schliemann W, Böhm H, Strack D. Tyrosinase involved in betalain biosynthesis of higher plants. Planta 1999; 208:114–124.
37. Hinz UG, Fivaz J, Girod G-A, Zryd J-P. The gene coding for the DOPA dioxygenase involved in betalain biosynthesis in *Amanita muscaria* and its regulation. Mol Gen Genet 1997; 256:1–6.
38. Mueller LA, Hinz U, Zryd J-P. The formation of betalamic acid and muscaflavin by recombinant DOPA-dioxygenase from *Amanita*. Phytochemistry 1997; 44: 567–569.
39. Trezzini G-P, Zryd J-P. *Portulaca grandiflora*: a model system for the study of the biochemistry and genetics of betalain biosynthesis. Acta Horticult 1990; 280:581–585.
40. Terradas F, Wyler H. 2,3- and 4,5-Secodopa, the biosynthetic intermediates generated from L-Dopa by an enzyme system extracted from the fly agaric, *Amanita muscaria* L., and their spontaneous conversion to muscaflavin and betalamic acid, respectively, and betalains. Helv Chim Acta 1991; 74:124–140.
41. Vogt T, Grimm R, Strack D. Cloning and expression of a cDNA encoding betanidin glucosyltransferase, a betanidin- and flavonoid-specific enzyme with high homology to inducible glucosyltransferases from the Solanaceae. Plant J 1999; 19:509–519.
42. Forni E, Polesello A, Montefiori D, Maestrelli A. High-performance liquid chromatographic analysis of the pigments of blood-red prickly pear (*Opuntia ficus indica*). J Chromatogr 1992; 593:177–183.
43. Fernandez-Lopez JA, Almela L. Application of high-performance liquid chromatography to the characterization of the betalain pigments in prickly pear fruits. J Chromatogr 2001; 913:415–420.
44. Stintzing FC, Schieber A, Carle R. Identification of betalains from yellow beet (*Beta vulgaris* L.) and cactus pear [*Opuntia ficus-indica* (L.) Mill.] by high-performance liquid chromatography-electrospray ionization mass spectrometry. J Agric Food Chem 2002; 50:2302–2307.
45. Clement JS, Mabry TJ. Pigment evolution in the caryophyllales: a systematic overview. Bot Acta 1996; 109:360–367.
46. Saguy I, Kopelman IJ, Mizrahi S. Thermal kinetic degradation of betanin and betalamic acid. J Agric Food Chem 1978; 26:360–368.
47. von Elbe JH, Klement JT, Amundson CH, Cassens RG, Lindsay RC. Evaluation of betalain pigments as sausage colorants. J Food Sci 1974; 39:128–132.
48. von Elbe JT, Schwartz SJ. Absence of mutagenic activity and a short term toxicity study of beet pigments as food colorants. Arch Toxicol 1981; 49:93–98.
49. Patkai G, Barta J. Decomposition of anticardinogen factors of the beetroot durino juice and nectar productions. Cancer Lett 1997; 114:105–106.
50. Reynoso R, Garcia FA, Morales D, de Mejia Gonzales E. Stability of betalain pigments from a Cactacea fruit. J Agric Food Chem 1997; 45:2884–2889.

51. Haveland-Smith RB. Evaluation of the genotoxicity of some natural food colours using bacterial assays. Mutat Res 1981; 91:285–289.
52. Schwartz SJ, von Elbe JH, Pariza MW, Goldsworthy T, Pitot HC. Inability of red beet betalain pigments to initiate or promote hepatocarcinogenesis. Food Chem Toxicol 1983; 21:531–535.
53. Reynoso RC, Giner TV, de Mejia Gonzales E. Safety of a filtrate of fermented Garambullo fruit: biotransformation and toxicity studies. Food Chem Toxicol 1999; 37:825–830.
54. Livrea MA, Tesoriere L, Butera D, Di Gaudio F, Scaglione C, Allegra M, Bongiorno A. Antioxidants and antioxidant activity of Sicilian prickly pear (*Opuntia ficus indica*) fruit extracts. Proceedings of the 11th Biennial Meeting of the Society for Free Radical Research International, Paris, France, Monduzzi Editore, July 16–20, 2002.
55. Pellegrini N, Re R, Yang M, Rice-Evans C. Screening of dietary carotenoids and carotenoid-rich fruit extracts for antioxidant activities applying 2,2′-azinobis (3-ethylenebenzothiazoline-6-sulfonic cid) radical cation decolorization assay. Meth Enzymol 1999; 299:379–389.
56. Rice-Evans C, Miller NJ. Total antioxidant status in plasma and body fluids. Meth Enzymol 1994; 234:279–293.
57. Wang H, Cao G, Prior RL. Total antioxidant capacity of fruits. J Agric Food Chem 1996; 44:701–705.
58. Lee J-C, Kim H-R, Jang Y-S. Antioxidant propertiy of an ethanol of the stem of *Opuntia ficus-indica* var. Saboten. J Agric Food Chem 2002; 50:6490–6496.
59. Zhang LX, Cooney RV, Bertram JS. Carotenoids up-regulate connexin43 gene expression independent of their provitamin A or antioxidant properties. Cancer Res 1992; 52:5707.
60. Azzi A, Ricciarelli R, Zingg JM. Non-antioxidant molecular functions of alpha-tocopherol (vitamin E). FEBS Lett 2002; 519:8–10.
61. Budinsky A, Wolfram R, Oguogho A, Efthiniou Y, Stomatopoulos Y, Sinzinger H. Regular ingestion of *Opuntia robusta* lowers oxidation injury. Prostagland Leukot Essent Fatty Acids 2001; 65:45–50.
62. Rice-Evans CA, Miller N, Paganga G. Antioxidant properties of phenolic compounds. Trends Plant Sci 1997; 2:152–159.
63. Martínez Parra J, Munoz R. An approach to the characterization of betanine oxidation catalyzed by horseradish peroxidase. J Agric Food Chem 1997; 45: 2984–2988.
64. Zakharova NS, Petrova T.A. Relationship between the structure and antioxidant activity of various betalains. Prikl Biochim Microbiol 1998; 34:199–202.

25

Antioxidant Activity and Antigenotoxicity of *Cassia tora*

Gow-Chin Yen and Chi-Hao Wu
National Chung Hsing University
Taichung, Taiwan

I. INTRODUCTION

Herbal medicines are increasingly used in both Western and Chinese societies. The Chinese herb Jue-ming-zi, which is the seed of the plant *Cassia tora* L. (Leguminosae), has been reported to have hypotensive, antibacterial, antiviral, antifungal, antihepatotoxic activity, etc. The herb *C. tora* contains a variety of bioactive phenolic substances, including chrysophanol, emodin, rhein, etc., which are mainly responsible for the pharmacological action ascribed to them. In addition, many recent studies have suggested that *Cassia* seed has potential antioxidant and antimutagenic activity, and these biological effects of *C. tora* decreased with higher roasting temperature or longer roasting time. In this chapter, we review the recent studies on the antioxidant activity and antigenotoxicity of *C. tora*.

Much attention has been focused on the nutraceuticals and their roles in human health. Several epidemiological studies have shown an association between a diet rich in fresh fruit and vegetables and a decreased risk of cardiovascular diseases, stroke, and certain forms of cancer (1,2). The close relationship between antioxidant activity and antimutagenicity has been demonstrated (3). It is now widely accepted that the use of naturally occurring antioxidants or antimutagens in everyday life will be the most effective procedure for promoting human health. Such compounds include vitamins, trace elements, and a variety of other substances with antioxidant properties. Polyphenols, isoflavones, catechins, and several other components found in higher plants are known to protect against the deleterious effect of reactive oxygen species (4). Hertog and Hollman (5) have suggested that diets rich in phenolic compounds are associated with longer life expectancy. These compounds have also been found to have various health-related properties because of their antioxidant activities. These properties include anticancer, antiviral, and anti-inflammatory activities, effects on capillary fragility, and an ability to inhibit human platelet aggregation (6).

The Chinese herb Jue-ming-zi has been used in many traditional Chinese medical prescriptions. *C. tora* was first recorded in *Shen-Nung-Pen-Tsao-Ching* as upper category, and in the successive *Pen-Tsao* of descending dynasties. It is used to remove "heat" from the liver and improve visual acuity, to moisten the supposedly dry digestive apparatus, and to facilitate bowel movement as a laxative. Previous studies on *C. tora* show its therapeutic effects on hypertension (7,8), on hypercholesterolemia (9,10), as an antihepatotoxin (11), an antimicrobial (12–14), on blood platelet coagulation (15), on the eyes, and in constipation (16). This herb has been reported to contain many active substances, including chrysophenol, emodin, rhein, etc. (17). Recently many researchers have studied the antioxidant activity and antigenotoxicity of *C. tora*. Choi et al. (18) reported that anthraquinone aglycons and naphthopyrone glycosides from *C. tora* had inhibitory activity against aflatoxin B_1 in the Ames test. Furthermore, anthraquinone compounds isolated from roasted *C. tora* have antimutagenicity (19). Wu and Yen (20) indicated that the antimutagenicity of extracts of *C. tora* was due to a desmutagenic action, but not a biomutagenic action. The mechanism of *Cassia* seed to suppress B[a]P genotoxicity in cells was to interfere with CYP-450 enzyme activation, and the key was suppressing NADPH CYP-450 reductase (21). Su (22) and Kim et al. (23) reported that methanolic extract from *C. tora* had a strong antioxidant activity on lipid peroxidation. *Cassia* extracts were also found to promote hepatic enzymes in rats with ethanol-induced hepatotoxicity, including catalase, superoxide dismutase, and glutathione peroxidase (10). Yen et al. (24) also indicated tha the antioxidant activity of methanolic extracts from *C. tora* L. was stronger than that of *Cassia occidentalis* L., and they also identified an antioxidative compound as emodin from *C. tora* L. The methanolic extracts of *C. tora*, containing anthraquinones, were also found to be effective peroxynitrile scavengers in vitro (25,26).

The commercial products of *C. tora* include both unroasted and roasted samples, and the laxative effect was found to be higher in unroasted *C. tora* than in the roasted product. Roasted *C. tora* has a special flavor and color, and it is popularly used to make a health drink. Zhang et al. (27) reported that some components, for example chrysophanol, in *C. tora* decreased after the roasting process. Moreover, the antihepatotoxic effect of *C. tora* decreased with an increase roasting temperature (28). In view of this, the biological activity of *C. tora* might be influenced by the roasting treatment. Thus, apart from the traditional pharmacological effects, the influence of roasting temperature on the chemical constituents and bioactive effects of seed of *C. tora* are discussed here. Also, other and more specific biological activity will be discussed.

II. EVALUATION OF ANTIOXIDANT ACTIVITY OF *C. TORA* WITH ROASTING

A. Scavenging Activity on DPPH Radical, Superoxide Anion, and Hydroxyl Radical

Free radicals are produced in cells by cellular metabolism and by exogenous agents. The extracts of *C. tora*, especially roasted and unroasted samples, were evaluated for their free-radical, 2,2-diphenyl-1-piperylhydrazyl radical ($DPPH^{\bullet}$), superoxide, and hydroxyl radical scavenging activities. Choi et al. (29) found that the methanolic extracts of the seed of *C. tora* have a scavenging activity on the DPPH radical. 2-Hydroxyemodin cassiaside and rubrofusarin gentiobioside were isolated from methanolic extract as antioxidant substances on DPPH radical.

Superoxide anion ($O_2^{\bullet}$), the one-electron reduced form of molecule oxygen, acts as an oxidizing or reducing agent and is capable of decomposing to form stronger oxidative species, such as singlet oxygen, hydroxyl radical, and hydrogen peroxide, that initiate the peroxidation of lipid and eventually lead to membrane damage (30). Water extracts of *C. tora* prepared under different roasting temperatures scavenge superoxide anion generated in the phenazine methosulfate–NADH system in a dose-dependent manner (31). The scavenging effects of extracts were in the following order: unroasted > 150°C roasted > 200°C roasted > 250°C roasted.

Yen and Chung (32) investigated the hydroxyl-radical-scavenging activity of extracts from *C. tora* using spin-trapping agent detected by EPR spectrometer. The hydroxyl radical rapidly reacted with the nitrone spin trap 5,5-dimethylpyrrolidine *N*-oxide (DMPO). Signal intensity of the DMPO-OH adduct decreased when the concentration of unroasted *C. tora* extracts was increased. The scavenging effects of water extracts from *C. tora* on hydroxyl radical were similar to the trend of scavenging action of superoxide anion. This trend is in agreement with the Finding that the antioxidant activity of the extracts of unroasted samples was greater than that of roasted samples (33). The scavenging activity of *C. tora* on both hydroxyl radical and superoxide anion decreased with increasing roasting.

B. Enzymatic and Nonenzymatic Lipid Peroxidation Systems

It is now clear that oxygen species such as superoxide anion hydroxyl radical, hydrogen peroxide, and other free radicals are proposed as agents that attack polyunsaturated fatty acid in the cell membranes giving rise to lipid peroxidation (34). *C. tora* has been reported to have antioxidant properties in vitro that act as reducing agents, hydrogen donors, free-radical quenchers, and metal ion chelators (32). In view of this, Yen and Chung (33) evaluated the antioxidant properties of water extracts from *C. tora* prepared under different roasting temperatures on enzymatic microsomes and nonenzymatic lipid peroxidation systems. Their study shows that unroasted *C. tora* extracts had a greater inhibition effect on peroxidation of linoleic acid than that of α-tocopherol (82%). The extracts from *C. tora* roasted at 170 °C for 80 min and at 200 °C for 5 min showed equal inhibition effects on peroxidation of linoleic acid. This means that the antioxidant activity of *C. tora* was reduced by higher roasting temperature and longer roasting periods. The extracts of unroasted *C. tora* also had good antioxidant activity in the liposome peroxidation system induced by the Fenton reaction as well as in the enzymatic microsome peroxidation system. This suggests that the oxidation of biological membrane in vivo may be inhibited. The antioxidant activity of roasted *C. tora* extracts decreased compared with that of the unroasted sample. These results might be caused by several factors, including (1) the reduction of phenolic content in *C. tora* as a result of roasting and (2) the degradation of Maillard reaction products during overroasting, making them oxidation products without antioxidant activity.

Salah et al. (35) demonstrated that quercetin has better antioxidant activity than rutin in a biomembrane system. The reason may be that quercetin rather than rutin interacts with that bilayer membrane of phospholipid. Therefore, the antioxidant activity of antioxidants in a membrane system depends on their ability not only to donate a hydrogen atom but also to incorporate into the membrane. α-Tocopherol scavenges the peroxyl radicals formed from the lipid peroxidation in the inner membrane (36). Therefore, it can be predicted that there are some water-insoluble components in *C. tora* that could be incorporated into the membrane to afford antioxidant activity.

C. Hydrogen-Peroxide-Induced Oxidative DNA Damage in Human Lymphocytes

Hydrogen peroxide is a well-known ROS produced intracellular during physiological and pathological processes, and causes oxidative DNA damage in cells. (37) As mentioned earlier, several noncell studies have demonstrated that *Cassia* seed was capable of reducing lipid peroxidation caused by ROS. The effect of *C. tora* on hydrogen-peroxide-induced oxidative DNA damage in human lymphocytes was assessed using single-cell gel electropheresis (comet assay). Water extracts of *C. tora* prepared under different roasting temperatures have the ability to suppress the oxidative DNA damage induced by H_2O_2, albeit to different extents (38). The protective effects of extracts of *C. tora* were significantly decreased with an increasing roasting temperature. The lower activity of certain samples, such as those roasted at 150 °C and 250 °C, may be due to low concentration of active phenolic antioxidants that degraded after overroasting.

III. EVALUATION OF ANTIGENOTOXIC ACTIVITY OF *C. TORA* WITH ROASTING

A. Effects of *C. Tora* on B[a]P-Induced DNA Damage in HepG2 Cell Line

Single-cell gel electrophoresis (comet assay) is a rapid and sensitive method for the detection of DNA damage in individual cells, especially for detecting oxidative DNA strand breaks (39). In this assay, under alkaline conditions, DNA loops containing breaks lose supercoiling, unwind, and are released from the nucleus forming a "comet tail" after gel electrophoresis. DNA strand breaks are thus visualized by the comet assay and computer analysis or by visual grading. Recently, it also has beenused to detect the effect of dietary components on genotoxicity of mammalian cells (40). Benzo[a]pyrene (B[a]P), a polycyclic aromatic hydrocarbon (PAH), is often observed in cigarette smoke, the surface of meat roasted with charcoal, or the incompletely combusted exhaust gas emitted from mills or automobiles (41). Most people are exposed to extremely low dosages of B[a]P or other PAHs in the environment. With the comet assay, severe DNA breaking was found after C57BL/6 rat feeding with B[a]P (42). Since evaluation of DNA damage with the comet assay is considered to be a good index for cancer risk for bioorganisms, the effects of water extracts from *C. tora* treated with different degrees of roasting on B[*a*]P-induced DNA damage in HepG2 were investigated (21). *C. tora* alone showed neither cytotoxic nor genotoxic effect toward HepG2 cells. B[a]P-induced DNA damage in HepG2 cells could be reduced by *C. tora* in a dose-dependent manner. The inhibitory effects of *C. tora* on DNA damage were in the order: unroasted (72%) > roasted at 150 °C (60%) > roasted at 250 °C (23%), at a concentration of 1 mg/mL. Unroasted samples exhibited the best inhibitory effect. The higher degrees of roasting resulted in less protecting effects.

Choi et al. (18) demonstrated the antimutagenicity of methanolic extract of *C. tora* against AFB1 in the *Salmonella typhimurium* assay. It has also been reported that *C. tora* had a marked and dose-dependent inhibition effect on the Aroclor 1254-hepatic S9-mediated mutagenicity of IQ, Trp-P-1, Glu-P-1, and B[a]P (20,31). In addition, unroasted *C. tora* extract could have direct interaction with various mutagens to reduce the biological function of mutagenicity (20).

B. Interference with CYP-450 Enzyme Activation

1. CYP-450 1A

Ferguson (43) indicated that the best way for antimutagenicity to suppress the toxicity or mutagenicity of a genotoxin was to affect its metabolism and block its activation. There are many metabolism possibilities after B[a]P enters the bioorganism: the main way is through CYP-450 1A1 activation to produce (-)-*trans*-7,8-dihydroxy-7,8-dihydro-benzo[a]pyrene, and then further through epoxidation to form the final carcinogens benzo[a]pyrene-7,8-diol-9,10-epoxide (BPDE) (44). The HepG2 cell, derived from human hepatoma, retains the characteristics of general normal liver cells and also has all the metabolizing enzymes that activate B[a]P (45). In general, ethoxyresorufin *O*-deethylase (EROD) activity was used as a measure of CYP 1A1 activity (46). Wu et al. (21) reported that the inhibitory effects of *C. tora* on B[a]P-mediated DNA damage were correlated with the inhibition of CYP 1A1-linked EROD activity in the HepG2 cell line. The correlation (r) between the suppressing effects and antigenotoxicity of *C. tora* was: unroasted (0.88), roasted at 150°C (0.94), and roasted at 250°C (0.96). In addition, similar inhibition of *C. tora* was seen on EROD activity in the Ames test using rat hepatic microsomes (S9) as the metabolizing activation system (20). Inferring from this, HepG2 cell DNA damage induced by B[a]P and suppressed by *C. tora* may be through-interference with CYP-450 1A1 enzyme activation.

Hao et al. (47) showed that the mechanism of 17 natural and synthetic anthraquinones, such as chrysophanol, emodin, rhein, etc., to suppress IQ mutagenicity were to interfere with CYP-450 enzyme activation by S9 mix. Antimutagens such as green tea or pine cone extracts were related to their suppressing activation enzymes in a similar system (48,49).

2. NADPH CYP-450 Reductase

NADPH CYP-450 reductase is the carrier of electrons to CYP-450; the monooxygenase can function only while the cytochrome can accept electrons smoothly. Sipes and Gandolfi (50) indicated that suppressing NADPH CYP-450 reductase was an effective mechanism for interfering with the progression of cancer. Many antimutagens, such as extracts of pine nuts (49), chlorophyll

(51), menadione (52), and (+)-catechin (53), could interfere with electron transport. As stated earlier, the major mechanism in forming antigenotoxicity of *C. tora* is suppression of B[a]P activation. Therefore, if NADPH CYP-450 reductase is inhibited, EROD activity would surely be affected. NAPPH CYP-450 reductase activities of HepG2 cells treated with water extracts of unroasted and 150°C-roasted *C. tora* were both suppressed in a dose-dependent manner (21). Overroasting (roasted at 250°C) of *Cassia* extract had no effect on reductase activity.

C. Induction of Phase II Detoxification Enzymes

Prestera and Talalay (54) suggested that evaluating the ability to promote phase II detoxification enzymes would be one of the indexes for detecting antimutagenicity and anticancer action of substances. It was known that B[a]P exerted its detoxification functions through GST (55). Therefore, exploring the effects of *C. tora* on GST activity of mammalian cells might reveal their function in lessening the genotoxicity of B[a]P. In the HepG2 cell line, unroasted and 150°C-roasted *C. tora* promoted enzyme activation (21). These two water extracts increased the enzyme activity by 1.26 and 1.35 times, respectively. Induction of the 250°C-roasted sample on GST activity was not significant. The result suggested that promoting GST activity of water extracts from unroasted and 150°C-roasted *C. tora* might be another reacting mechanism of antigenotoxicity compare with suppressing EROD.

Further investigation by Choi et al. (10) has demonstrated that ethanolic extract of *C. tora* was able to reduce levels of hepatic enzymes of ethanol-treated rats, including superoxide dismutase, catalase, and glutathione peroxide. Glutathione levels were higher in rats fed *Cassia* ethanolic extract than the depleted levels observed in rats treated with ethanol. Therefore, the enhancement of antioxidant and phase II detoxification enzyme activities may be responsible in part for the chemopreventive effects of *C. tora* against reactive oxygen species and carcinogens. The balance between the phase I mutagen-activating enzymes and the phase II detoxifying enzymes could be important in preventing the risk of developing chemically induced cancer.

IV. CHANGES IN ACTIVE COMPOUNDS OF *C. TORA* WITH ROASTING

A. Total Phenolic Compounds

C. tora contains many phenolic compounds, such as emodin, rhein, chrysophanol, and obtusin, some of which belong to anthraquinones (56). Some anthraquinones have been reported to have antioxidant activity (57). The total polyphenols in extracts of *C. tora* decreased significantly ($p > 0.05$) during roasting. The amount of polyphenols in extracts of *C. tora* decreased from 180.64 mg/g (unroasted) to 103.55 mg of gallic acid/g extracts of *C. tora* after roasting at 250°C. This means that polyphenols were degraded during the roasting process. The decrease of polyphenol contents in *C. tora* after roasting is correlated to the decrease in antioxidant activity. Therefore, it can be suggested that the decrease in antioxidant activity of extracts of roasted *C. tora* was related to the decrease in polyphenols.

B. Anthraquinones: Characteristic and Content in *Cassia* Extracts

Anthraquinones have been reported to be the main active components in *C. tora*, including aloe-emodin, anthrone, aurantiobtusin, chrysophanol, emodin, obtusifolin, physcion, rhein, etc. (17,56). The basic chemical structures of anthraquinones are shown in Fig. 1. The anthraquinones, with two ketone groups added at position C9 and position C10, occur naturally in plants. Total anthraquinones, including free anthraqinones (anthraquinones aglycon) and bound anthraquinones (anthraquinones *O*-glycosides), were deter-

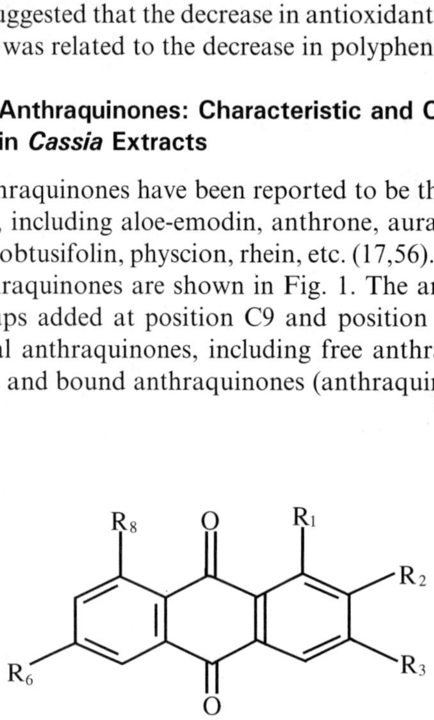

Anthraquinone	R_1=R_2=R_3=R_6=R_8=H
Alizarin	R_1=R_2=OH, R_3=R_6=R_8=H
Aloe-emodin	R_1=R_8=OH, R_2=R_6=H, R_3=CH_2OH
Chrysophanol	R_1=R_8=OH, R_2=R_6=H
Emodin	R_1=R_6=R_8=OH, R_2=H, R_3=CH_3
Rhein	R_1=R_8=OH, R_2=R_6=H, R_3=COOH

FIGURE 1 Basic chemical structures of anthraquinones.

mined by Yen and Chung (32). Their results showed that the total content of anthraquinones in extracts of *C. tora* were degraded by thermal treatment, in the order of unroasted (88.2 mg/g) > 150°C-roasted (70.7 mg/g) > 200°C-roasted (26.9 mg/g) > 250°C-roasted (14.9 mg/g). The data also indicate that most of the anthraquinones in extracts of *C. tora* are in a bound form and contain glycosides. This is in agreement with the studies of Fairbirn and Moss (58), who reported that the anthraquinones in *Cassia* plants are partly free but mostly are present as glycosides (with aglycon occurring usually as a reduced form, e.g., anthrones).

The individual anthraquinone content in extracts of *C. tora* was also measured by Wu (31) using HPLC. Three anthraquinones, chrysophenol, emodin and rhein, have been detected in extracts of *C. tora* under experimental conditions. The unroasted sample contains the highest anthraquinones content; the content of rhein, chrysophanol, and emodin was 10.4, 0.6, and 0.3 mg/g *Cassia* extract, respectively. The anthraquinone content decreased with increased roasting temperature. It is noted that the extracts of *C. tora* prepared by roasting at 250°C did not show any detectable anthraquinones. Zhang et al. (27) indicated that anthraquinones in *C. tora* were degraded to a free form (aglycon) by roasting. The content of these three anthraquinones has only one-eighth of the total content of anthraquinones compared with the results reported by the Yen and Chung (32). Most individual anthraquinones or anthrones have shown antioxidant activity in linoleic acid peroxidation systems (57). Thus, the decrease in antioxidant activity of roasted *C. tora* was related to the decrease in anthraquinones.

V. ANTIGENOTOXICITY OF CHRYSOPHANOL, EMODIN, AND RHEIN

Natural herbs contain a large number of potential anticancer materials. For example, within *Rhei rhizoma*, *Scutellariae radix*, and *Rehmanniae radix*, there is antimutagenicity that suppresses B[a]P (59). The major active components in *Cassia* seed are probably a derivative of anthraquinones (AQ) (17,56); and its mechanism was considered as suppressing exogenic activation enzymes (47).

As for DNA damage induced by B[a]P in HepG2 cells, chrysophanol had 78% inhibitory effect, as well as rhein (71%), at a concentration of 100 μM. Emodin, which suppressed B[a]P the most, had 86% protective effect at the same dose. There is neither cell toxicity nor genotoxicity in selected concentrations (1–100 μM) of chrysophanol, emodin, and rhein on HepG2 cells (21). On the basis of these results, the intensity of antigenotoxicity of *C. tora* might relate to the change in anthraquinone quantity. In the meantime, samples roasted at 250°C contain no 1,8-HQ compounds, but still show protection of 23%, indicating that there may be other active components in *Cassia* seeds that are worthy of being explored.

It is also interesting that anthraquinones in *C. tora* showed genotoxicity in some in vitro assays. Chrysophanol, emodin, etc., upon metabolism by rat liver microsome enzyme (CYP-450), might give products with genotoxicity (60) and show mutagenicity in various bacterial and cell test systems (61,62). On the contrary, Mengs et al. (63), in an internal experiment, indicated that when a rat was fed the highest suggested daily intake of 2000 mg/kg of emodin and then the emodin amount in the rat's internal plasma was measured, emodin reached 190 μg/mL, the highest in plasma (about 700 μM in this experiment). This is 10 times or more than the genotoxicity produced in the studies of Westendorf et al. (62). Nevertheless, no cytotoxicity or micronucleus caused by emodin was discovered in the study. Heidemann et al. (64) also pointed out that rhein and aloe-emodin have no mutagenic or carcinogenic reactions. The U.S. National Toxicology Program conducted rat internal tests on subacute toxicity and mutagenicity of 30 suspected mutagenic chemical materials in 1996. Anthraquinone and emodin were categorized as probable noncarcinogens and possible noncarcinogens; i.e., they had no unfavorable mutagenic actions on developing animals (65).

VI. OTHER BIOLOGICAL EFFECTS OF *C. TORA*

A. Hypotensive Effect

Aqueous and methanol extracts from *Cassia* seeds elicit hypotensive effects on anesthetized rats. Experimental results indicate that the hypotensive effect of the *C. tora* extract possibly involves a vagal reflex that reciprocally alters the vasomotor tone of the centrally emanating sympathetic nervous system. It is shown that the capacity of *C. tora* extracts to reduce blood pressure is significantly reduced in vagotomized rats and that hypotensive effects are greatly antagonized in rats whose sympathetic nervous systems are interrupted by transection of the spinal cord. Phytochemical studies also show that the active hypotensive principles are derived from the kernel of the seed and consist of mainly glycosides (7,8).

B. Lipid-Lowering Effect

Ha et al. (9) investigated the lipid-lowering effect of *C. tora* ethanol extacts in rats fed a high-cholesterol diet. Rats were fed either normal diets or diets high in cholesterol (10 g/kg diet), supplemented with *C. tora* ethanolic extract (0, 0.25, or 0.5%) for 4 weeks. Liver triglyceride and cholesterol contents were raised in the high-cholesterol groups and were significantly reduced in the groups fed *C. tora*. Serum levels of HDL cholesterol were slightly increased by consumption of *C. tora*. The results showed that ethanol extracts of *C. tora* may exert a lipid-lowering effect in rats fed high-cholesterol diets. Furthermore, Choi et al. (10) indicated that ethanol-treated rats fed with 200 or 400 mg/kg body wt./day *Cassia* ethanolic extract had a hypolipemic effect compared with rats treated with ethanol alone.

C. Antiplasmodial Effect

Plant extract of *C. tora* had antiplasmodial activity in vitro against *Plasmodium falciparum* 3D7 and Dd2, and had an IC_{50} value less than 5 μg/mL on both tested strains (12). The effect of *Cassia* extracts on lymphocyte proliferation showed low toxicity to the human cells. This plant has been subjected to long-term clinical trials in folk medicine and is a promising plant.

D. Antifungal Activity

An antifungal principle of defatted seed powder of *C. tora* was isolated by extraction of the powder with benzene. Besides chrysophanol and other hydroanthroquinone derivatives, the major antifungal compound was identified as chrysophanic acid-9-anthrine. This compound was active against *Trichophyton rubrum*, *T. mentagrophytes*, *Microsporum canis*, *M. gypseum*, and *Geotrichum candidum* in broth in the presence of 100 μg/mL L-ascorbic acid as antioxidant (13).

VII. ANTIBACTERIAL EFFECT

Thirteen phenolic glycosides including six new compounds were isolated from seeds of *C. tora*. The structures of the new compounds, rubrofusarin triglucoside, nor-rubrofusarin gentiobioside, demethylflavasperone gentiobioside, torachrysone gentiobioside, torachrysone tetraglucoside, and torachrysone apioglucoside, were deduced on the basis of spectroscopic and chemical evidence. The effect of the phenolic glycosides, their aglycones, and several other compounds structurally related to the on *Escherichia coli* K12, *Pseudomonas aeruginosa* PAO1, and some strains of *Staphylococcus aureus* were then examined. Among them, torachrysone, toralactone, aloe-emodin, rhein, and emodin showed noticeable antibacterial effects on four strains of methicillin-resistant *Staph. aureus* with a minimum inhibitory concentration of 2–64 μg/mL. On the other hand, the phenolic compounds tested did not show strong antibacterial effects on *E. coli* and *Ps. aeruginosa* (14).

A. Antihepatotoxic Effect

Two new naphtho-pyrone glycosides, 9-[(beta-D-glucopyranosyl-(1-6)-*O*-beta-D-glucopyranosyl)oxy]-10-hydroxy-7-methoxy-3-methyl-1H-naphtho[2,3-c]pyran-1-one and 6-[(alpha-apiofuranosyl-(1—6)-*O*-beta-D-glucopyranosyl)oxyl-rubrofusarin, together with cassiaside and rubrofusarin-6-beta-gentiobioside, were isolated from the seeds of *C. tora* L. Their structures were deduced on the basis of chemical and spectral data. The naphtho-gamma-pyrone glycosides were found to have significant hepatoprotective effects against galactosamine damage, which were higher than that of silybin from *Silybum marianum* (11).

VIII. CONCLUSIONS

Herbs have been used as food and for medicinal purposes for centuries. The Chinese herb *C. tora* has been reported to have hypotensive, hypolipemic, antibacterial, antiviral, antifungal, and antihepatotoxic activity. The commercial products of *C. tora* include both unroasted and roasted samples, and the biological effects were found to be higher with unroasted *C. tora* than with the roasted product. Roasted *C. tora* has a special flavor and color, and it is popularly used to make a health drink. *C. tora* contains a variety of bioactive phenolic substances, including chrysophanol, emodin, rhein, etc., which are mainly responsible for the pharmacological action ascribed to them.

The extracts of *C. tora* scavenge hydrogen peroxide, superoxide anion, and hydroxyl radicals, inhibit lipid peroxidation, and suppress DNA damage in human lymphocytes induced by hydrogen peroxide. The unroasted *C. tora* extract has greater antioxidant activity than roasted samples. Higher roasting temperature and longer roasting periods reduced the antioxidant activity of *C. tora*. The extracts of *C. tora* reacted under the HepG2 cell cultivating model of nonexogenic enzyme have suppressive effects for the DNA damage induced by B[a]P. The inhibitory effects of *C. tora* on DNA damage are similar to the trend of its antioxidant properties, and decreased with increasing roasting temperature. The mechanism involved in antigenotoxicity includes suppressing EROD, NADPH CYP-450 reductase in cells and promoting GST activity. Overall, the biological activities of extracts from roasted *C. tora* decreased as compared with that of unroasted samples. This result might be caused by the reduction of phenolics and anthraquinones in *C. tora* as a result of roasting.

REFERENCES

1. Stampfer MJ, Henneekens CH, Manson JE, Colditz GA, Rosner B, Willet WC. Vitamin E consumption and the risk of coronary disease in women. N. Engl J Med 1993; 328:1444–1449.
2. Saija A, Scalese M, Lanza M, Marzullo D, Bonina F, Castelli F. Flavonoids as antioxidant agents: importance of their interaction with biomembranes. Free Rad Bio Med 1995; 19:481–486.

3. Yen GC, Chen HY. Antioxidant activity of various tea extracts in relation to their antimutagenicity. J Agric Food Chem 1995; 43:27–32.
4. Shahidi F, Ho CT. Phytochemicals and Phytopharmaceuticals. Champaign, IL: AOCS Press; 2000.
5. Hertog MGL, Hollman PCH. Potential health effects of the dietary flavonoid quercetin. Eur J Clin Nutr 1996; 50:63–66.
6. Benavente-Garcisa O, Castillo J, Marin FR, Ortuno A, Rio JAD. Use and properties of citrus flavonoids. J Agric Food Chem 1997; 45:4505–4515.
7. Koo A, Chan WS, Li KM. Extraction of hypotensive principles from seeds of *Cassia tora*. Am J Chin Med 1976; 4:245–248.
8. Koo A, Chan WS, Li KM. A possible reflex mechanism of hypotensive action of extract from *Cassia tora* seeds. Am J Chin Med 1976; 4:249–255.
9. Ha TY, Cho IJ, Seong KS, Lee SH. Effect of *Cassia tora* ethanol extract on the lipid levels of serum and liver in rats fed high cholesterol diet. J Korean Soc Food Sci Nutr 2002; 30:1171–1176.
10. Choi HS, Cha SS, Na MS, Shin KM, Lee MY. Effect of the ethanol extracts of *Cassia tora* L. of antioxidative compounds and lipid metabolism in hepatoxicity of rats-induced by ethanol. J Korean Soc Food Sci Nutr 2002; 30:1177–1183.
11. Wong SM, Wong MM, Seligmann O, Wagner H. New antihepatotoxic naphthopyrone glycosides from the seeds of *Cassia tora*. Planta Med 1989; 55:276–280.
12. El-Tahir A, Satti GM, Khalid SA. Antiplasmodial activity of selected Sudanese medicinal plants with emphasis on *Acacia nilotica*. Phytother Res 1999; 13(6): 474–478.
13. Acharya TK, Chatterjee IB. Isolation of chrysophanic acid-9-anthrone, the major antifungal principle of *Cassia tora*. Lloydia 1975; 38:218–220.
14. Hatano T, Uebayashi H, Ito H, Shiota S, Tsuchiya T, Yoshida T. Phenolic constituents of *Cassia* seeds and antibacterial effect of some naphthalenes and anthraquinones on methicillin-resistant *Staphylococcus aureus*. Chem Pharm Bull (Tokyo) 1999; 47:1121–1127.
15. Yun-Choi HS, Kim JH, Takido M. Potential inhibitors of platelet aggregation from plant sources. V. Anthraquinones from seeds of *Cassia obtusifolia* and related compounds. J Nat Prod 1990; 53:630–633.
16. Elujoba AA, Ajulo OO, Iweibo GO. Chemical and biological analyses of Nigerian *Cassia* species for laxative activity. J Pharm Biomed Anal 1989; 7:1453–1457.
17. Huang KC. The Pharmacology of Chinese Herbs. Boca Raton FL: CRC Press, 1993:103.
18. Choi JS, Lee HJ, Park KY, Ha JO, Kang SS. In vitro antimutagenic effects of anthraquinone aglycones and naphthopyrone glycosides from *Cassia tora*. Planta Med 1997; 63:11–14.
19. Choi JS, Lee HJ, Park KY, Jung GO. In vitro antimutagenic effects of alaternin and isorubrofusarin gentiobioside from roasted *Cassia tora*. Planta Med 1997; 63:100–104.

20. Wu CH, Yen GC. Inhibitory effect of water extracts from *Cassia tora* L. on the mutagencicity of benzo[a]pyrene and 2-amino-3-methylimidazo[4,5-f]quinoline. J Chin Agric Chem Soc 1999; 37:263–275.
21. Wu CH, Hsieh CL, Song TY, Yen GC. Inhibitory effects of *Cassia tora* L. on benzo[a]pyrene-mediated DNA damage toward HepG2 cells. J Agric Food Chem 2001; 49:2579–2586.
22. Su JD. Investigation of antioxidative activity and tocopherol contents on Chinese crude drugs of fruits and seeds. Food Sci (Chinese) 1992; 19:12–24.
23. Kim SY, Kim JH, Kim SK, Oh MJ, Jung MY. Antioxidant activities of selected Oriental herb extracts. J. Am Oil Chem Soc 1994; 71:633–640.
24. Yen GC, Chen HW, Duh PD. Extraction and identification of an antioxidative component from Jue Ming Zi (*Cassia tora* L.). J Agric Food Chem 1998; 46:820–824.
25. Choi JS, Chung HY, Jung HA, Park HJ, Yokozawa T. Comparative evaluation of antioxidant potential of alaternin (2-hydroxyemodin) and emodin. J Agric Food Chem 2000; 48:6347–6351.
26. Park YB, Lee TG, Kim OK, Do JR, Yeo SG, Park YH, Kim SB. Characteristics of nitrite scavenger derived from seeds of *Cassia tora* L. Korea J Food Sci Technol 1995; 27:124–128.
27. Zhang Q, Zhou Z, Yin J, Xiong Y, Wang Y, Sun J. Influence of temperature on the chemical constituents and pharmacological effects of semen cassiae. Zhongguo Zhong Yao Za Zhi 1996; 21:663–665.
28. Zhang Q, Yin J, Zhang J. Comparison of contents of some active components between crude and processed seeds of sickle senna (*Cassia tora*) and their decoctions by HPLC. Chin Herb 1996; 27:79–81.
29. Choi JS, Lee HJ, Kang SS. Alaternin, cassiaside and rubrofusarin gentiobioside, radical scavenging principles from the seeds of *Cassia tora* on 1,1-diphenyl-2-picrylhyrazyl (DPPH) radical. Arch Pharm Res 1994; 17:462–466.
30. Halliwell B, Gutteridge JMC. Oxygen is poisonous—an introduction to oxygen toxicity and free radicals. In: Halliwell B, Gutteridge JMC, eds. Free Radicals in Biology and Medicine. Oxford: Clarendon Press, 1999:1–21.
31. Wu CH. Antimutagenicity of water extracts from *Cassia tora* L. prepared under different degrees of roasting and their protective effects on DNA damage. Master's thesis. National Chung Hsing University, Taiwan, 1999.
32. Yen GC, Chung DY. Antioxidant effects of extracts from *Cassia tora* L. prepared under different degrees of roasting on the oxidative damage to biomolecules. J Agric Food Chem 1999; 47:1326–1332.
33. Yen GC, Chung DY. Antioxidant properties of water extracts from *Cassia tora* L. in relation to the degree of roasting. J Agric Food Chem 2000; 48:2760–2765.
34. Halliwell B, Gutteridge JMC. Role of free radicals and catalytic metal ions in human disease: an overview. Methods Enzymol 1990; 186:1–85.
35. Salah N, Miller NJ, Paganga G, Tijburg L, Bolwell GP, Rice-Evans C. Polyphenolic flavonols as scavenger of aqueous phase radicals and as chain-breaking antioxidants. Arch Biochem Biophys 1995; 2:339–346.

36. Ratty AK, Sunamoto J, Das NP. Interaction of flavonoids with 1,1-diphenyl-2-picrydrazyl free radical, liposomal membranes and soybean lipoxygenase-1. Biochem Pharmocol 1988; 37:989–995.
37. Anderson D, Yu T, Phillips BJ, Schmezer P. The effect of various antioxidants and other modifying agents on the oxygen-radical-generated DNA damage in human lymphocytes in the comet assay. Mutat Res 1994; 307:261–271.
38. Yen GC, Chuang DY, Wu CH. Effect of roasting process on the antioxidant properties of *Cassia tora* L. In: Morello MJ, Shahidi F, Ho CT, eds. Free Radicals in Food: Chemistry Nutrition and Health Effects. ACS Symposium Series No. 807. Washington DC, 2002:201–212.
39. Fairbairn DW, Olive PL, O'Neill KL. The comet assay: a comprehensive review. Mutat Res 1995; 339:37–59.
40. Duthie SJ, Johnson W, Dobson VL. The effect of dietary flavonoids on DNA damage (strand breaks and oxidised pyrimidines) and growth in human cells. Mutat Res 1997; 390:141–151.
41. Lijinsky W. The formation and occurrence of polynuclear aromatic hydrocarbons associated with food. Mutat Res 1991; 259:251–261.
42. Vaghef H, Wusen A-C, Hellman B. Demonstration of benzo[a]pyrene-induced DNA damage in mice by alkaline single cell gel electrophoresis: evidence for strand breaks in liver but not in lymphocytes and bone marrow. Pharmacol Toxicol 1996; 78:37–43.
43. Ferguson LR. Antimutagens as cancer chemopreventive agents in the diet. Mutat Res 1994; 307:395–410.
44. Dipple A, Cheng SC, Bigger CAH, Pariza MW, Felton JS, Aeschbacher HU, Sato S. Polycyclic aromatic hydrocarbon carcinogens. In: Pariza MW, Pariza JS, Felton HU, eds. Mutagens and Carcinogens in the Diet. New York: Wiley-Liss Inc, 1990:109–127.
45. Diamond L, Kruszewski F, Aden DP, Knowles BB, Baird WM. Metabolic activation of benzo[a]pyrene by a human hepatoma cell line. Carcinogenesis 1980; 1:871–875.
46. Grant MH, Duthie SJ, Gray AG, Burke MD. Mixed function oxidase and udp-glucuronyltransferase activities in the human Hep G2 hepatoma cell line. Biochem Pharmacol 1988; 37:4111–4116.
47. Hao NJ, Huang MP, Lee H. Structure-activity relationships of anthraquinones as inhibitors of 7-ethoxycoumarin *O*-deethylase and mutagenicity of a-amino-3-methylimidazo[4,5-f]quinoline. Mutat Res 1995; 328:183–191.
48. Chen HY, Yen GC. Possible mechanisms of antimutagens by various teas as judged by their effects on mutagenesis by 2-amino-3-methylimidazo[4,5-f]quinoline and benzo[a]pyrene. Mutat Res 1997; 393:115–122.
49. Lee H, Aoki K, Sakagami H, Yoshida T, Kuroiwa Y. Interaction of pine cone extract fraction-VI with mutagens. Mutat Res 1993; 297:53–60.
50. Sipes IG, Gandolfi AJ. Biotransformation of toxicants. In: Klaassen CD, Amdur MO, Doull J, eds. Casarett and Doull's Toxicology. 3rd ed. New York: Macmillan, 1986:64–98.
51. Tachino N, Guo D, Dashwood WM, Yamane S, Larsen R, Dashwood R.

Mechanisms of the in vitro antimutagenic action of chlorophyllin against benzo[a]pyrene: studies of enzyme inhibition, molecular complex formation and degradation of ultimate carcinogen. Mutat Res 1994; 308:191–203.
52. Sadowski IJ, Wright JA, Ollmann D, Israels LG. Menadione inhibition of benzo[a]pyrene metabolism in whole cells, microsomes and reconstituted system. Int J Biochem 1986; 18:565–568.
53. Stelle CM, Lalies M, Ioannides C. Inhibition of the mutagenicity of aromatic amines by the plant flavonoid (+)-catechin. Cancer Res 1985; 45:3573–3577.
54. Prestera T, Talalay P. Electrophile and antioxidant regulation of enzymes that detoxify carcinogens. Proc Natl Acad Sci USA 1995; 92:8965–8969.
55. Swedmark S, Romert L, Morgensterm R, Jenssen D. Studies on glutathione transferase belonging to class pi in cell line with different capabilities for conjugation (+)-7β,8δ-dihydroxy-9δ,10δ-oxy-7,8,9,10-tetrahydrobenzo[a]pyrene. Carcinogenesis 1992; 13:1719–1723.
56. Duke JA. Handbook of Phytochemical Constituents of GRAS Herbs and Other Economic Plants. Boca Raton FL: CRC Press, 1992:143–144.
57. Yen GC, Duh PD, Chuang DY. Antioxidant activity of anthraquinones and anthrone. Food Chem 2000; 70:437–441.
58. Fairbirn JW, Moss MJR. Relative purgative activities of 1,8-dihydroxyanthracene derivaties. J Pharm Pharmacol 1970; 32:584–593.
59. Sakai Y, Nagase H, Ose Y, Sato T, Kawai M, Miizuno M. Effects of medical plant extracts from Chinese herbal medicines on the mutagenic activity of benzo[a]pyrene. Mutat Res 1988; 206:327–334.
60. Mueller SO, Stopper H, Dekant W. Biotransformation of the anthraquinones emodin and chrysophanol by cytochrome p450 enzyme. Drug Metab Dispos 1998; 26:540–546.
61. Tikkanen L, Matsushima T, Natori S. Mutagenicity of anthraquinones in the *Salmonella* preincubation test. Mutat Res 1983; 116:297–304.
62. Westendorf J, Marquardt H, Poginsky B, Dominiak M, Schmidt J, Marquardt H. Genotoxicity of naturally occurring hydroxyanthraquinones. Mutat Res 1990; 240:1–12.
63. Mengs U, Krumbiegel G, Volkner W. Lack of emodin genotoxicity in the mouse micronucleus assay. Mutat Res 1997; 393:289–293.
64. Heidemann A, Volkner W, Mengs U. Genotoxicity of aloe emodin in vitro and in vivo. Mutat Res 1996; 367:123–133.
65. Ashby J. Prediction of rodent carcinogenicity for 30 chemicals. Environ Health Perspect 1996; 104:1101–1104.

26

Sho-saiko-to

Ichiro Shimizu
Tokushima University School of Medicine
Tokushima, Japan

I. INTRODUCTION

The Chinese herbal medicine Sho-saiko-to, a mixture of seven herbal preparations, is an officially approved prescription drug in Japan and is widely administered in Japan to patients with chronic hepatitis C virus (HCV) infection. The most common cause of hepatic fibrosis is chronic HCV infection, the characteristic feature of which is hepatic steatosis. Hepatic steatosis leads to an increase in lipid peroxidation in hepatocytes, which in turn leads to the activation of hepatic stellate cells (HSCs). HSCs are also thought to be the primary target cells of inflammatory stimuli, and produce collagen. Tests indicate that Sho-saiko-to improves liver function, and a prospective study reported a reduced incidence of hepatocellular carcinoma in patients with HCV-related cirrhosis. However, little information is available concerning the mechanism by which Sho-saiko-to protects against hepatic fibrosis and carcinoma. Several laboratories, including ours, have demonstrated the preventive and therapeutic effects of Sho-saiko-to on experimental hepatic fibrosis, as well as its inhibitory effect on the activation of HSCs. We provided evidence that Sho-saiko-to functions as a potent fibrosuppressant via the inhibition of oxidative stress in hepatocytes and

HSCs, and that its active components are baicalin and baicalein. In addition, Sho-saiko-to has anticarcinogenic properties in that it inhibits chemical hepatocarcinogenesis in animals, inhibits the proliferation of hepatoma cells by inducing apoptosis, and arrests the cell cycle. Among the active components of Sho-saiko-to, baicalin, baicalein, and saikosaponin-a have the ability to inhibit cell proliferation. It should be noted that baicalin and baicalein are flavonoids, the chemical structures of which are very similar to those of silybinin and quercetin, which show antifibrogenic activities. This may provide valuable information on the search for novel antifibrogenic agents.

Herbal medicines have been used in China for thousands of years. Their principles are based on clinical experience and practice, but the effective ingredients in most of these medications have not been identified. Chinese herbal medicines have now attracted the attention of practitioners of Western medicine, and are being manufactured in Japan in uniform quality and in sufficient quantities for use as drugs for hospital use. Among these, the herbal medicine Sho-saiko-to, or Xiao-Chai-Hu-Tang (Chinese name), which has been used in the treatment of pyretic diseases in China, is an officially approved prescription drug in Japan. Sho-saiko-to is the most commonly administered drug in Japan to outpatients with chronic liver diseases, especially those with chronic HCV infection, chronic hepatitis C (1,2), and cirrhosis (3). HCV infections are widespread throughout the world, and are recognized as a major causative factor in chronic hepatitis, cirrhosis, and hepatocellular carcinoma (HCC) (4 5). In fact, the World Health Organization reported that up to 3% of the world's population is infected with HCV, suggesting that more than 170 million chronic carriers are currently at risk for developing cirrhosis and HCC (6).

The usual daily dose of Sho-saiko-to is 7.5 g, administered orally in three equal doses. Seven and one-half grams of Sho-saiko-to contains 4.5 g of dried Sho-saiko-to extract, which is prepared from boiled water extracts of seven herbs: 7.0 g of *Bupleurum* root, 5.0 g of *Pinellia* tuber, 3.0 g of *Scutellaria* root, 3.0 g of jujube fruit, 3.0 g of ginseng root, 2.0 g of glycyrrhiza root, and 1.0 g of ginger rhizome (Table 1). For the putative major active ingredients, the approximate concentrations of the components in 50 mg/mL of the ethanol extract of Sho-saiko-to have been determined to be baicalin: 1.75 mg/mL (3.5%), glycyrrhizin: 500 μg/mL (1%), baicalein: 150 μg/mL (0.3%), each of saikosaponin-a, -c, and -d, and ginsenoside Rb_1 and ginsenoside Rg_1: 100 μg/mL (0.2%), wogonin: 20 μg/mL (0.04%), and viscidulin III: less than 50 μg/mL (<0.1%) (Table 1) (7).

Sho-saiko-to has been shown to improve liver function (1,2), as well as to alleviate the subjective symptoms associated with chronic liver diseases, such as digestive discomfort. In a double-blind, multicenter clinical trial, Sho-saiko-to was shown to lower the serum levels of aspartate aminotransferase

TABLE 1 Main Active Ingredients of 7.5 g Sho-saiko-to

Herbal components	Amount (g)	Main active ingredients	Approximate concentration (%)
Bupleurum root	7.0	Saikosaponin-a	0.2
		Saikosaponin-b_1, -b_2	
		Saikosaponi-c	0.2
		Saikosaponi-d	0.2
Pinellia tuber	5.0	Ephedrine	
Scutellaria root	3.0	Baicalin	3.5
		Baicalein	0.3
		Wogonin	0.04
		Viscidulin III	<0.1
Jujube fruit	3.0	Cyclic AMP	
Ginseng root	3.0	Ginsenoside Rb_1	0.2
		Ginsenosid g_1	0.2
Glycyrrhiza root	2.0	Glycyrrhizin	1
		Liquiritin	
Ginger rhizome	1.0	6-Gingerol	
		6-Shogaol	
		Zingerone	

(AST), alanine aminotransferase (ALT), and gamma-glutamyl transpeptidase (gamma-GTP) (1), in patients with chronic hepatitis. As shown in Figure 1, in addition to serum ALT levels, serum concentrations of hepatic fibrogenesis markers of the 7S domain of type IV collagen (7S-IV) and the amino terminal propeptide of type III procollagen (P-III-P) were significantly attenuated by Sho-saiko-to in chronic hepatitis C patients with fibrosis of Stages 0–3. Hepatic fibrosis, or the deposition of extracellular matrix (ECM), is classified on a scale of 0–4: 0, no fibrosis; 1, portal fibrosis without septa; 2, few septa; 3, numerous septa without cirrhosis; 4, cirrhosis. Hepatic fibrosis is often associated with inflammation and cell death, which accompanies the repair processes, and is a consequence of severe liver damage that occurs in many patients with chronic liver diseases, including chronic HCV infection. The main origin of the abnormal ECM proteins is a cell known as the hepatic stellate cell (HSC) (also known as the fat-storing cell, lipocyte, or the Ito cell). HSCs are located in the space of Disse in close contact with hepatocytes and sinusoidal endothelial cells. Their three-dimensional structure consists of the cell body and several long and branching cytoplasmic processes (8). It is now evident that HSCs undergo proliferation and transformation under inflammatory stimuli into α-smooth muscle actin (alpha-SMA)-positive myofibroblast-like cells, which are referred to as activated cells, and serve as the origin

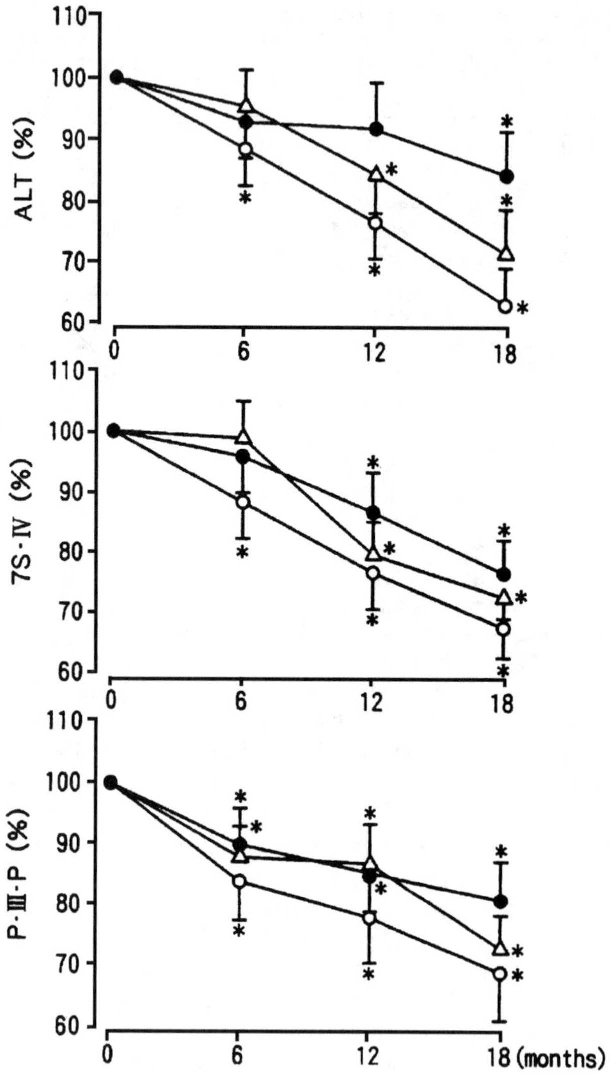

FIGURE 1 Changes in individual percentages of the initial values for serum levels of ALT and hepatofibrogenesis markers of 7S domain of type IV collagen (7S-IV) and amino-terminal propeptide of type II procollagen (P-III-P) after administration of Sho-saiko-to to chronic hepatitis C patients with fibrosis of stages 0–1 (○, $n = 10$), 2 (△, $n = 8$), and 3, (●, $n = 8$). Values are expressed as mean percentages (± SD) of each initial value before treatment. $^{*}p < 0.05$.

of much of the collagen hypersecretion and nodule formation that occurs during hepatic fibrosis and cirrhosis (9,10).

Furthermore, in a prospective study, Sho-saiko-to inhibited the development of HCC in patients with cirrhosis (3). Although Sho-saiko-to is widely used in the treatment of chronic hepatitis C and cirrhosis, little is known about the mechanism by which it protects against hepatic fibrosis and carcinoma. This chapter summarizes our current knowledge of the biological functions of Sho-saiko-to as it relates to fibrogenesis and carcinogenesis in the liver.

II. HEPATOCYTE INJURY INDUCED BY HCV INFECTION

During the course of a chronic HCV infection, hepatocytes are continuously damaged and replicated, and hepatic fibrosis appears to progress, whereas the frequencies of genetic alteration also probably increase. It is generally accepted that multiple genetic alteration, induced by mutations, is an important factor in carcinogenesis. Therefore, continuous cell death and replication and multiple genetic alteration may lead to the development of cirrhosis and HCC (Fig. 2). However, the mechanisms by which HCV induces liver injury and hepatocyte death remain, to a great extent, ambiguous.

Cytotoxic T lymphocytes (CTLs) are not only thought to be a major host defense against viral infection, but have been implicated in immunopathogenesis as well. Two pathways, the perforin and Fas/Fas ligand pathways, have been proposed to account for all cytolytic activity of CTLs (11), although tumor necrosis factor-α (TNF-α), a proinflammatory cytokine, is released by all HCV-specific CTL clones studied to date (12) and may also contribute to the cytotoxicity of CTLs (13). The core protein of HCV has been recognized as a target for CTLs (14–16). Viral proteins have various accessory functions that target host proteins and thus alter normal cellular growth properties, affecting many signal pathways. A few examples of signaling molecules, such as the nuclear factor-κB (NF-κB) and activator protein 1 (AP-1), have been reported to be activated by HCV proteins. The NF-κB pathway plays an important role in the cellular response to a variety of extracellular stimuli, including TNF-κ and interleukin-1 (IL-1). Because the HCV core protein binds both the TNF receptor and p53 (17,18), induction of NF-κB by HCV proteins may either cause or suppress hepatocyte death and, on other occasions, may promote cellular proliferation, thus contributing to liver injury or tumorigenesis induced by HCV. Likewise, the activation of AP-1, a transcription factor that regulates a number of genes involved in the control of cellular growth, by viral proteins presumably would promote oncogenesis and a myriad of other effects. Our preliminary study demonstrated that prooxidants induce the activation both of AP-1 and NF-κB with

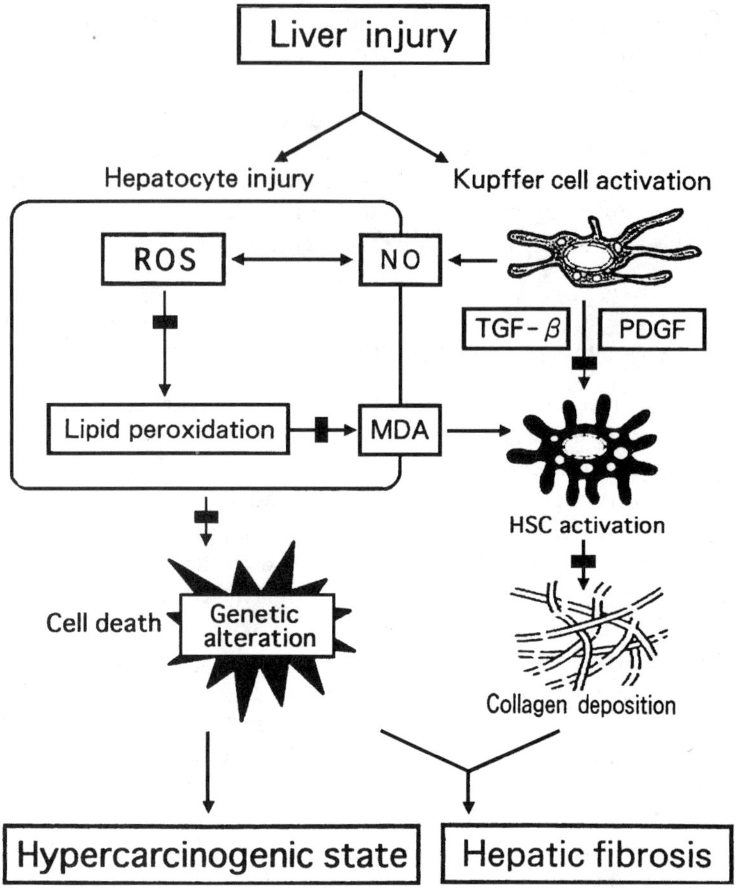

FIGURE 2 A working hypothesis regarding the role of ROS generation in stimulating hepatic fibrogenesis and carcinogenesis. Black boxes indicate the putative suppression site by Sho-saiko-to. ROS, reactive oxygen species; NO, nitric oxide; MDA, malondialdehyde; TGF, transforming growth factor; PDGF, platelet-derived growth factor; HSC, hepatic stellate cell.

degradation of IκB-κ, an inhibitory subunit of NF-κB, in cultured rat hepatocytes, and that Sho-saiko-to inhibited the oxidative-stress-induced activation of NF-κB and AP-1 in a dose-dependent manner (Fig. 3). In addition, oxidative stress was observed to induce early apoptosis, by decreasing the expression of antiapoptotic proteins Bcl-2 and Bcl-XL, and by increasing the expression of proapoptotic protein Bad in cultured rat hepatocytes, whereas Sho-saiko-to was found to suppress oxidative-stress-induced

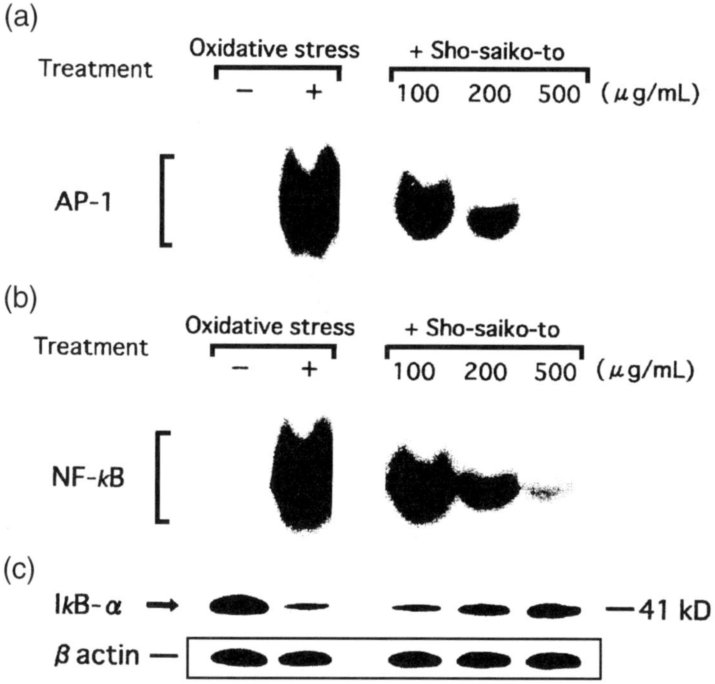

FIGURE 3 Sho-saiko-to prevents oxidative stress-induced activation of AP-1 (a) and NF-κB (b) by blocking the degradation of IκB-α (c) in cultured rat hepatocytes in a dose-dependent manner. Cells were incubated with 100 μmol/L of ferric nitrilotriacetate solution (oxidative stress) in the presence or absence of Sho-saiko-to at the indicated dose. Whole-cell extracts were measured for DNA-binding activities of AP-1 and NF-κB by electrophoretic mobility shift assay, and analyzed by Western blotting using the antibody of IκB-α, an inhibitory subunit of NF-κB.

early apoptosis by modulating Bcl-2 family protein expression (I. Shimizu, unpublished data, 2000).

Sho-saiko-to has also been reported to modulate in vitro cytokine production in peripheral blood mononuclear cells, downregulating the synthesis of IL-4 and -5 in favor of IL-10 in patients with chronic hepatitis C. IL-10 production in mononuclear cells of hepatitis C patients was reported to be lower than that of healthy subjects (19). IL-10 would be expected to have an effective activity for inflammatory bowel disease (20), endotoxin shock (21), and experimental liver injury (M. Tanaka, unpublished data, presented at the 37th annual meeting of the Japanese Society of Gastroenterology, 1995).

These findings suggest that Sho-saiko-to may play a role in the repair of abnormalities in the cytokine production system in patients with chronic HCV infection.

Parenchymal cell membrane damage could result in the release of oxygen-derived free radicals and other reactive oxygen species (ROS) derived from lipid peroxidative processes, which represent a general feature of sustained inflammatory response and liver injury, once the antioxidant mechanisms have been depleted (22). Many cells have their own unique enzymatic defense systems against oxidative stress, including the production of superoxide dismutase (SOD) and glutathione peroxidase (GPx). In addition, histopathological studies associated with chronic HCV infection showed fatty changes in 31–72% of patients (23–25), indicating that hepatic steatosis is a characteristic feature of chronic HCV infection. It has been suggested that hepatic steatosis may reflect a direct cytopathic effect of HCV and may play a role in the progression of the disease. In support of these proposals, a transgenic mouse model, which expresses the HCV core gene, was observed to develop progressive hepatic steatosis and HCC (26,27). It is conceivable that followig hepatocyte injury, hepatic steatosis leads to an increase in lipid peroxidation, which might contribute to HSC proliferation and transformation by releasing soluble mediators (28,29), and, thus, induce hepatic fibrosis.

We previously reported that, in two rat models of hepatic fibrosis, hepatic concentrations of malondialdehyde (MDA), an end product of lipid peroxidation, in Sho-saiko-to-fed animals were significantly lower than in those fed a basal diet, and that Sho-saiko-to inhibited the prooxidant-enhanced lipid peroxidation in cultured rat hepatocytes, and inhibited lipid peroxidation induced in rat liver mitochondria by Fe^{2+}/adenosine 5′-diphosphate (7). In addition, we observed that Sho-saiko-to scavenges the free radical 1,1-diphenyl-2-picrylhydrazyl (DPPH) (7). Free radicals, generated mainly by Kupffer cells, are thought to cause tissue injury by initiating lipid peroxidation and inducing irreversible modifications of cell membrane structure and function (30). In an animal model of endotoxemia, preadministration of Sho-saiko-to was found to significantly increase the activity of SOD and GPx, suggesting that Sho-saiko-to acts by protecting against plasma membrane damage by ROS such as free radicals (31).

III. EFFECTS OF SHO-SAIKO-TO ON HEPATIC FIBROSIS

In the injured liver, HSCs in the space of Disse are generally thought to be the primary target cells for inflammatory stimuli (32), and to produce ECM components, while in intact liver lobules they function as the primary storage area for retinoids (33). It has been shown that the activation of HSCs in injured livers leads to their proliferation and transformation into myofibroblast-like cells. This is accompanied by a loss of cellular retinoid, and the synthesis of α-SMA and large quantities of the major components of the ECM, including collagen types I, III, and IV, fibronectin, laminin, and proteoglycans. α-SMA is an activation marker of HSCs. It has been shown that, in vivo, HSCs express the genes that encode for enzymes such as matrix metalloproteinase (MMP)-1, which catalyzes the digestion of native fibrillar collagen types I and III, and MMP-2, which acts on denatured collagen types I and III and native collagen type IV, as well as a tissue inhibitor of metalloproteinase (TIMP)-1 (34). The net effect of the production of proteins involved in matrix synthesis and degradation could be reduced matrix degradation, which could account for the marked increases in matrix deposition and nodule formation observed during hepatic fibrosis and cirrhosis (9,35).

Several reports concerning the role of Sho-saiko-to with respect to the prevention and treatment of experimental liver damage induced in rats by D-galactosamine (36), carbon tetrachloride (37), dimethylnitrosamine (DMN) (38), and pig serum (PS) (38) have appeared. Although the mechanism by which Sho-saiko-to prevents hepatic fibrosis is not at present clear, it has been reported that the preadministration of this herbal medicine protects the liver plasma membrane and HSCs against injury (31). Moreover, Sho-saiko-to was reported to prevent the development of hepatic fibrosis by the inhibition of HSC activation in a different animal model, the choline-deficient rat (39). We confirmed the preventive and therapeutic effects of Sho-saiko-to on rat experimental hepatic fibrosis induced by DMN and PS (7). The rats were fed a basic diet that contained Sho-saiko-to for 2 weeks prior to the induction of hepatic fibrosis, or during the last 2 weeks of treatment. Sho-saiko-to suppressed the induction of hepatic fibrosis, maintained hepatic retinoid stores, and reduced hepatic collagen levels and the hepatic expression of α-SMA and type I collagen. In addition, when incubated with cultured rat HSCs, the presence of Sho-saiko-to led to an increase in lipid droplets, which include retinoid and occupy the cytoplasmic space, and inhibit type I collagen production, α-SMA expression, cell spreading, and DNA synthesis. Furthermore, Sho-saiko-to was reported to induce the arrest at the G_0/G_1 phase in the cell cycle of HSCs (40). These findings suggest that the antifibrogenic activities of Sho-saiko-to are associated with the regulation of ECM proteins including type I collagen and α-SMA expression, retinoid disappearance, as well as HSC proliferation.

In investigating the mechanism by which Sho-saiko-to inactivates HSCs, Kakumu et al. showed that Sho-saiko-to enhanced the in vitro production of interferon (IFN)-γ and antibodies to the hepatitis B core and e antigens, produced by peripheral blood mononuclear cells from patients with chronic hepatitis (41). IFN-γ is a potent cytokine with immunomodulatory and antiproliferative properties, which inhibits HSC activation and ECM production in in vivo models of hepatic schistosomiasis and carbon tetrachloride-, DMN-, and PS-induced hepatic fibrosis (42–46). Oxidative stress (10,47), including the generation of ROS, has also been implicated as a cause of hepatic fibrosis (Fig. 2). There is evidence that the products of lipid peroxidation modulate collagen gene expression (34,48), suggesting that lipid peroxidation is a link between liver tissue injury and fibrosis (22,49). It has been reported that paracrine stimuli derived from hepatocytes undergoing oxidative stress induce HSC proliferation and collagen synthesis (50). HSCs have also been shown to be activated by the generation of free radicals with Fe^{2+}/ascorbate (29) and by MDA and 4-hydroxynonenal (47,51), aldehydic products of lipid peroxidation, and antioxidants such as α-tocopherol were observed to inhibit HSC activation (29). We also reported that Sho-saiko-to supplementation led to a dose-dependent suppression in oxidative stress in cultured rat HSCs in parallel with the inhibition of the type I collagen production (7). In hepatic fibrosis, Sho-saiko-to may exert its suppressive effects, at least in part, by acting as an antioxidant, and/or by stimulating IFN-γ.

Inflammatory cells, such as Kupffer cells and invading mononuclear cells, which release cytokines, transforming growth factor-β_1 (TGF-β_1), and platelet-derived growth factor (PDGF), may also contribute to the fibrogenic response to liver injury. Although the precise nature of the Kupffer-cell-derived factors that induce HSC activation is currently poorly understood, it has been shown, for example, that TGF-β_1 and PDGF activate cultured HSCs (52,53). HSCs also produce and respond to TGF-β_1 in an autocrine manner with increased collagen expression. These findings suggest that these growth factors may act as paracrine and autocrine (i.e., from HSCs) mediators that trigger the transformation of HSCs in vivo. PDGF is a major mitogen that drives HSC proliferation (54). Importantly, TGF-β_1 is a key fibrogenic mediator that is capable of enhancing ECM deposition and inhibiting MMP activity (55). It is also noteworthy that TGF-β is an inhibitor of the proliferation of hepatocytes (56), and that, at higher concentrations, TGF-β induces oxidative stress leading to hepatocyte apoptosis (56). A preliminary report concluded that Sho-saiko-to inhibited the PDGF-induced proliferation of HSCs (40) (Fig. 2).

Because of their anatomical location, their ultrastructural features, and similarities with pericytes that regulate blood flow in other organs, it has been proposed that HSCs function as liver-specific pericytes (57). Previous studies have shown that the contraction and relaxation of HSCs regulate hepatic sinusoidal blood flow (57,58). Two vasoregulatory compounds with obvious effects on HSCs include endothelin (ET)-1 and nitric oxide (NO) (59–61). Experimental evidence suggests that ET-1 is a potent vasoconstrictor in the liver microcirculation in vivo, acting at both the sinusoidal and extrasinusoi-

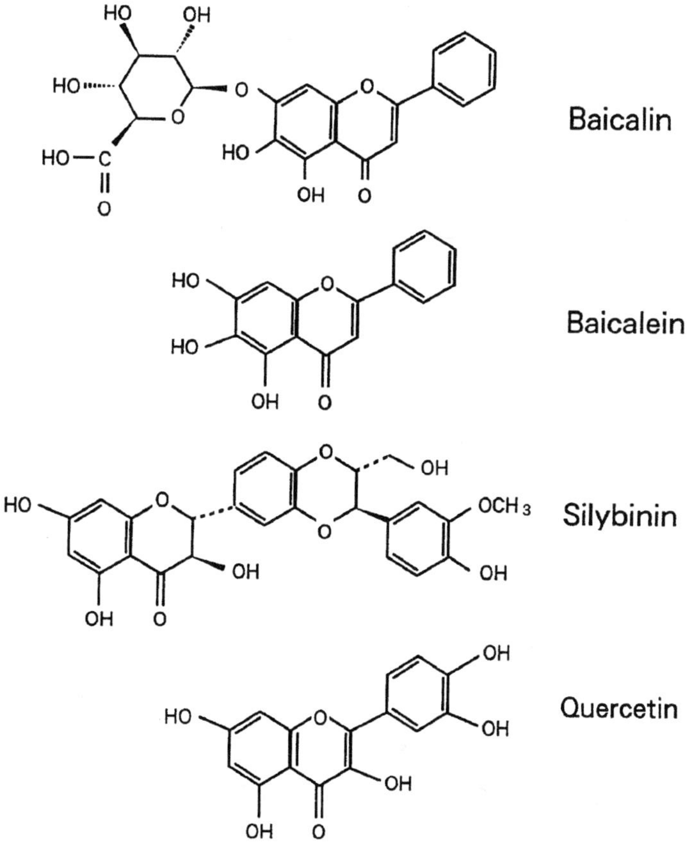

FIGURE 4 Comparison of the chemical structure of baicalin, baicalein, silybinin, and quercetin. Each of these molecules contain a 2-phenyl-1-benzopyrane-4-one (flavone) structure.

dal sites (62), and that exogenous NO prevents ET-induced contraction as well as causing precontracted cells to relax (63). HSCs and sinusoidal endothelial cells produce NO in response to various stimuli in the presence and absence of endotoxins (64 65). It should be pointed out that Sho-saiko-to upregulates the inducible NO synthase in hepatocytes, when cultured in the presence of IFN-γ (66).

In our study, among the herbal components of Sho-saiko-to, the *Scutellaria* root extract actively inhibited superoxide anion production (7). Superoxide anion is generated in reperfusion-induced oxidative stress and liver inflammation, and is closely related to membrane injury by lipid peroxidation (67). The antioxidant activity of *Scutellaria* root was due to the action of baicalin, baicalein, and viscidulin III, all of which showed antioxidative effects. These findings are consistent with previously reported data (68). However, because an ethanol extract of Sho-saiko-to contains approximately 3.5% baicalin, 0.3% baicalein, and <0.1% viscidulin III (Table 1), the antioxidant action of Sho-saiko-to may be largely dependent on the action of the two flavonoids, baicalin and baicalein (Fig. 4). These flavonoids have been shown to suppress the proliferation of HSCs (69) and vascular smooth muscle cells (70,71). It is noteworthy that the chemical structures of the flavonoids are very similar to those of silybinin and quercetin (72). Each molecule contains a 2-phenyl-1-benzophyrane-4-one (flavone) structure (72). Silybinin (73) and quercetin (74) have been reported to have antifibrogenic properties; silybinin acts as an oxygen radical scavenger (73), affecting the lipid profile of hepatocyte membranes (75), inhibits the proliferation of HSCs in vitro, and retards collagen accumulation in chronic bile duct ligated rats (73); and quercetin suppresses the proliferation and α-SMA expression of HSCs and interferes with PDGF-induced signal transduction (74). In addition, some positive clinical trials involving silymarin have been reported. The latter is prepared as a standardized extract from milk thistle, the principle active component of which is the silybinin, comprising 60–70% of the silymarin (76,77). However, the latest results of a randomized controlled trial indicate that silymarin had no effect on survival and the clinical course in alcoholic patients with cirrhosis (78).

IV. EFFECTS OF SHO-SAIKO-TO ON HEPATIC CARCINOGENESIS

HCC is, worldwide, one of the most common malignancies, especially in Southeast Asia. Based on clinical information, as a causative agent, HCV is more common than HBV in both Japan and Western countries. The incidence of HCC has been shown to be higher in patients with chronic HCV infection than for those with chronic HBV infection (79). In chronic hepatitis B, a resolution of the disease can frequently be seen after the inactivation of viral replication (4), which probably contributes to a lower incidence of HCC. In contrast, HCV multiplication is sustained throughout the course of a typical infection (80,81). When hepatocytes are continuously damaged and replicated, as is the case for HCV-infected patients with cirrhosis, the frequencies of genetic alteration also probably increase along with hepatic fibrosis, leading to the development of cirrhosis and HCC (Fig. 2). It is generally accepted that multiple genetic alteration is important in carcinogenesis. The HCC occurrence rate in patients with HCV-related cirrhosis has been reported to increase steadily, with a yearly incidence of 1.4–7% (82–84).

In a prospective, randomized, and controlled trial, Sho-saiko-to acted as a chemopreventive drug, preventing the development of HCC in patients with cirrhosis, particularly those with HCV infection, but not HBV infection (3). It should also be pointed out that Sho-saiko-to protects against liver injury from oxidative stress including ROS generation and lipid peroxidation, which may ultimately lead to a decrease in genetic alteration as well as stopping or slowing the progression of hepatic fibrosis to cirrhosis (Fig. 2). As a result, Sho-saiko-to might exert its anticarcinogenic role in the liver. Furthermore, Sho-saiko-to has been shown to have antitumor activity; Sho-saiko-to was reported to inhibit the development of preneoplastic and neoplastic lesions of the liver in rats treated with *N*-nitrosomorpholine (85), 2-acetylaminofluorene (86), diethylnitrosamine (87), and a choline-deficient diet (39); and Sho-saiko-to cured mice in which Ehrlich tumors had been transplanted (88), and showed an antimetastatic effect on Lewis lung carcinoma in mice (89). A recent report showed that Sho-saiko-to is able to scavenge hydroxyl radicals in a dose-dependent manner and might prevent hepatocarcinogenesis in association with the inhibition of 8-hydroxy-2′-deoxyguanosine production, which is a DNA adduct associated with ROS and is known to be a parameter of genetic risk for carcinogenesis in the liver (87). In addition, Sho-saiko-to suppressed the proliferation of the human HCC cell line KIM-1 by inducing apoptosis and arrest at the G_0/G_1 phase (90). An in vitro study also demonstrated that Sho-saiko-to stimulated the release of TNF-α and granulocyte-colony-stimulating factor (G-CSF) in peripheral blood mononuclear cells of HCC patients with HCV-related cirrhosis (91). In addition to its activation of inflammatory cells, TNF-α is in functions such as immune response regulation, antiviral activities, and antitumor effects. G-CSF is recognized to be of benefit in the treatment of neutropenia. Thus, Sho-saiko-to may play a role in biological defense mechanisms in HCC patients.

In a study of the antitumor activity of the active components of Sho-saiko-to, saikosaponin-a and ginsenoside Rb1 showed an antimutagenic effect on mutagenesis induced by a direct-acting mutagen, 2-(2-furyl)-3-(5-nitro-2-furyl) acrylamide (92). Okita et al. reported that baicalein, baicalin, saikosaponin-a, and glycyrrhizin inhibited the proliferation of the human HCC cell line HuH-7 and decreased the production of α-fetoprotein by cells (93). Motoo and Sawabu also reported that, among the active components of Sho-saiko-to, baicalein, baicalin, and saikosaponin-a and -d were active in inhibiting cell growth and DNA synthesis in human HCC cells (Hep-G_2 and PLC/PRF/5) (94). Flavonoids, including baicalein and baicalin, have been shown to inhibit the nuclear enzyme topoisomerase II, which alters the topological state of DNA through a concerted breaking and rejoining of the DNA strands (95). Some antitumor drugs are known to induce apoptosis via the inhibition of topoisomerase II (96,97). However, the mode of cell death induced by baicalein was found to differ, depending on the HCC cell line, with apoptosis induced in KIM-1 cells, and necrosis in HuH-7 and HLF cells (98). Baicalin has been reported to act as a prooxidant and to induce caspase-3 activation and apoptosis via the mitochondrial pathway (99). Although Sho-saiko-to and the flavonoids baicalein and baicalin appeared to play a cytoprotective role in hepatocytes, they also may induce apoptosis in hepatoma cells. The different action between hepatocytes and hepatoma cells remains to be elucidated.

V. CONCLUSION

Although herbal medicines are thought to be safe drugs, a complicating factor, which has caused physicians and patients to lose confidence in the safety of Sho-saiko-to, is the development of severe interstitial pneumonia associated with its use, particularly when it is used in combination with IFN in treating some Japanese patients with chronic hepatitis C. Interstitial pneumonia is also induced by G-CSF, whereas Sho-saiko-to induced G-CSF production in peripheral blood mononuclear cells in patients with chronic hepatitis C (100). These findings suggest that Sho-saiko-to, when used in combination with IFN, may be a cause of interstitial pneumonia. In any case, it should be noted that Sho-saiko-to may have beneficial effects, not only on hepatic fibrosis, but also on HCC development in patients with chronic liver disease.

Since Sho-saiko-to has been showed to have a stronger antiproliferative effect than any one of its active ingredients, these effects are difficult to explain, based on a single ingredient, and the combination of several ingredients may possess synergistic or additive effects. However, the striking similarity in chemical structures of the flavonoids baicalein and baicalin, which are mainly responsible for the antioxidant activity of Sho-saiko-to, and silybinin and quercetin, which have antifibrogenic properties in vitro and in animal models of hepatic fibrosis, is an important lead in the search for novel antifibrogenic drugs (72,101).

REFERENCES

1. Hirayama C, Okumura M, Tanikawa K, Yano M, Mizuta M, Ogawa N. A multicenter randomized controlled clinical trial of Sho-saiko-to in chronic active hepatitis. Gastroenterol Jpn 1989; 24:715–719.
2. Tajiri H, Kozaiwa K, Ozaki Y, Miki K, Shimuzu K, Okada S. Effect of Sho-saiko-to (Xiao-Chai-Hu-Tang) on HBeAg clearance in children with chronic

hepatitis B virus infection and with sustained liver disease. Am J Chin Med 1991; 19:121–129.

3. Oka H, Yamamoto S, Kuroki T, Harihara S, Marumo T, Kim SR, Monna T, Kobayashi K, Tango T. Prospective study of chemoprevention of hepatocellular carcinoma with Sho-saiko-to (TJ-9). Cancer 1995; 76:743–749.
4. Takano S, Yokosuka O, Imazeki F, Tagawa M, Omata M. Incidence of hepatocellular carcinoma in chronic hepatitis B and C: a prospective study of 251 patients. Hepatology 1995; 21:650–655.
5. Shiratori Y, Shiina S, Imamura M, Kato N, Kanai F, Okudaira T, Teratani T, Tohgo G, Toda N, Ohashi M. Characteristic difference of hepatocellular carcinoma between hepatitis B- and C-viral infection in Japan. Hepatology 1995; 22:1027–1033.
6. WHO. Hepatitis C: global prevalence. Wkly Epidemiol Rec 1997; 72:341–344.
7. Shimizu I, Ma Y-R, Mizobuchi Y, Liu F, Miura T, Nakai Y, Yasuda M, Shiba M, Horie T, Amagaya S, Kawada N, Hori H, Ito S. Effects of Sho-saiko-to, a Japanese herbal medicine, on hepatic fibrosis in rats [see comments]. Hepatology 1999; 29:149–160.
8. Wake K. Cell-cell organization and functions of "sinusoids" in liver microcirculation system. J Electron Microsc 1999; 48:89–98.
9. Gressner AM, Bachem MG. Cellular sources of noncollagenous matrix proteins: role of fat-storing cells in fibrogenesis. Semin Liver Dis 1990; 10:30–46.
10. Shimizu I. Antifibrogenic therapies in chronic HCV infection. Curr Drug Targets Infect Disord 2001; 1:227–240.
11. Kagi D, Vignaux F, Ledermann B, Burki K, Depraetere V, Nagata S, Hengartner H, Golstein P. Fas and perforin pathways as major mechanisms of T cell-mediated cytotoxicity. Science 1994; 265:528–530.
12. Koziel MJ, Dudley D, Afdhal N, Grakoui A, Rice CM, Choo QL, Houghton M, Walker BD. HLA class I–restricted cytotoxic T lymphocytes specific for hepatitis C virus. Identification of multiple epitopes and characterization of patterns of cytokine release. J Clin Invest 1995; 96:2311–2321.
13. Braun MY, Lowin B, French L, Acha-Orbea H, Tschopp J. Cytotoxic T cells deficient in both functional fas ligand and perforin show residual cytolytic activity yet lose their capacity to induce lethal acute graft-versus-host disease. J Exp Med 1996; 183:657–661.
14. Shimizu I, Yao D-F, Horie C, Yasuda M, Shiba M, Horie T, Nishikado T, Meng XY, Ito S. Mutations in a hydrophilic part of the core gene of hepatitis C virus in patients with hepatocellular carcinoma in China. J Gastroenterol 1997; 32:47–55.
15. Horie T, Shimizu I, Horie C, Yogita S, Tashiro S, Ito S. Mutations of the core gene sequence of hepatitis C virus isolated from liver tissues with hepatocellular carcinoma. Hepatol Res 1999; 13:240–251.
16. Kato N, Yoshida H, Kioko Ono-Nita S, Kato J, Goto T, Otsuka M, Lan K, Matsushima K, Shiratori Y, Omata M. Activation of intracellular signaling by hepatitis B and C viruses: C-viral core is the most potent signal inducer. Hepatology 2000; 32:405–412.

17. Zhu N, Khoshnan A, Schneider R, Matsumoto M, Dennert G, Ware C, Lai MM. Hepatitis C virus core protein binds to the cytoplasmic domain of tumor necrosis factor (TNF) receptor 1 and enhances TNF-induced apoptosis. J Virol 1998; 72:3691–3697.
18. Lu W, Lo SY, Chen M, Wu K, Fung YK, Ou JH. Activation of p53 tumor suppressor by hepatitis C virus core protein. Virology 1999; 264:134–141.
19. Yamashiki M, Nishimura A, Suzuki H, Sakaguchi S, Kosaka Y. Effects of the Japanese herbal medicine "Sho-saiko-to" (TJ-9) on in vitro interleukin-10 production by peripheral blood mononuclear cells of patients with chronic hepatitis C. Hepatology 1997; 25:1390–1397.
20. Kuhn R, Lohler J, Rennick D, Rajewsky K, Muller W. Interleukin-10-deficient mice develop chronic enterocolitis. Cell 1993; 75:263–274.
21. Howard M, Muchamuel T, Andrade S, Menon S. Interleukin 10 protects mice from lethal endotoxemia. J Exp Med 1993; 177:1205–1208.
22. Houglum K, Filip M, Witztum JL, Chojkier M. Malondialdehyde and 4-hydroxynonenal protein adducts in plasma and liver of rats with iron overload. J Clin Invest 1990; 86:1991–1998.
23. Scheuer PJ, Ashrafzadeh P, Sherlock S, Brown D, Dusheiko GM. The pathology of hepatitis C. Hepatology 1992; 15:567–571.
24. Bach N, Thung SN, Schaffner F. The histological features of chronic hepatitis C and autoimmune chronic hepatitis: a comparative analysis. Hepatology 1992; 15:572–577.
25. Lefkowitch JH, Schiff ER, Davis GL, Perrillo RP, Lindsay K, Bodenheimer HC Jr, Balart LA, Ortego TJ, Payne J, Dienstag JL. Pathological diagnosis of chronic hepatitis C: a multicenter comparative study with chronic hepatitis B. The Hepatitis Interventional Therapy Group. Gastroenterology 1993; 104:595–603.
26. Moriya K, Yotsuyanagi H, Shintani Y, Fujie H, Ishibashi K, Matsuura Y, Miyamura T, Koike K. Hepatitis C virus core protein induces hepatic steatosis in transgenic mice. J Gen Virol 1997; 78(pt 7):1527–1531.
27. Moriya K, Fujie H, Shintani Y, Yotsuyanagi H, Tsutsumi T, Ishibashi K, Matsuura Y, Kimura S, Miyamura T, Koike K. The core protein of hepatitis C virus induces hepatocellular carcinoma in transgenic mice. Nat Med 1998; 4:1065–1067.
28. Gressner AM, Lotfi S, Gressner G, Lahme B. Identification and partial characterization of a hepatocyte-derived factor promoting proliferation of cultured fat-storing cells (parasinusoidal lipocytes). Hepatology 1992; 16:1250–1266.
29. Lee KS, Buck M, Houglum K, Chojkier M. Activation of hepatic stellate cells by TGF alpha and collagen type I is mediated by oxidative stress through c-myb expression. J Clin Invest 1995; 96:2461–2468.
30. Sevanian A, Wratten ML, McLeod LL, Kim E. Lipid peroxidation and phospholipase A2 activity in liposomes composed of unsaturated phospholipids: a structural basis for enzyme activation. Biochim Biophys Acta 1988; 961:316–327.
31. Sakaguchi S, Tsutsumi E, Yokota K. Preventive effects of a traditional Chinese

medicine (Sho-saiko-to) against oxygen toxicity and membrane damage during endotoxemia. Biol Pharm Bull 1983; 16:782–786.
32. Pinzani M. Novel insights into the biology and physiology of the Ito cell. Pharmacol Ther 1995; 66:387–412.
33. Hendriks HF, Verhoofstad WA, Brouwer A, de Leeuw AM, Knook DL. Perisinusoidal fat-storing cells are the main vitamin A storage sites in rat liver. Exp Cell Res 1985; 160:138–149.
34. Iredale JP, Murphy G, Hembry RM, Friedman SL, Arthur MJ. Human hepatic lipocytes synthesize tissue inhibitor of metalloproteinases-1. Implications for regulation of matrix degradation in liver. J Clin Invest 1992; 90:282–287.
35. Friedman SL. Cellular sources of collagen and regulation of collagen production in liver. Semin Liver Dis 1990; 10:20–29.
36. Ymamoto K, Araki N, Ogawa K. Ultrastructural and utlaracytochemical examination of the effects of preadministration of Xiao-Chai-Hu-Tang on hepatic disorders induced by D-galactosamine HCl. Acta Histochem Cytochem 1985; 18:403–418.
37. Amagaya S, Hayakawa M, Ogihara Y, Fujiwara K. Effects of Sho-saiko-to and Dai-saiko-to on carbon tetrachloride-induced hepatic injury in rats. J Med Pharm Soc Wakan-Yaku 1988; 5:129–136.
38. Amagaya S, Hayakawa M, Ogihara Y, Fujiwara K. Effects of Sho-saiko-to and Dai-saiko-to on experimental hepatic fibrosis in rats. J Med Pharm Soc Wakan-Yaku 1988; 5:137–145.
39. Sakaida I, Matsumura Y, Akiyama S, Hayashi K, Ishige A, Okita K. Herbal medicine Sho-saiko-to (TJ-9) prevents liver fibrosis and enzyme-altered lesions in rat liver cirrhosis induced by a choline-deficient L-amino acid–defined diet. J Hepatol 1998; 28:298–306.
40. Kayano K, Sakaida I, Uchida K, Okita K. Inhibitory effects of the herbal medicine Sho-saiko-to (TJ-9) on cell proliferation and procollagen gene expressions in cultured rat hepatic stellate cells. J Hepatol 1998; 29:642–649.
41. Kakumu S, Yoshioka K, Wakita T, Ishikawa T. Effects of TJ-9 Sho-saiko-to (kampo medicine) on interferon gamma and antibody production specific for hepatitis B virus antigen in patients with type B chronic hepatitis. Int J Immunopharmacol 1991; 13:141–146.
42. Czaja MJ, Weiner FR, Takahashi S, Giambrone MA, van der Meide PH, Schellekens H, Biempica L, Zern MA. Gamma-interferon treatment inhibits collagen deposition in murine schistosomiasis. Hepatology 1989; 10:795–800.
43. Rockey DC, Maher JJ, Jarnagin WR, Gabbiani G, Friedman SL. Inhibition of rat hepatic lipocyte activation in culture by interferon-gamma. Hepatology 1992; 16:776–784.
44. Rockey DC, Chung JJ. Interferon gamma inhibits lipocyte activation and extracellular matrix mRNA expression during experimental liver injury: implications for treatment of hepatic fibrosis. J Invest Med 1994; 42:660–670.
45. Baroni GS, D'Ambrosio L, Curto P, Casini A, Mancini R, Jezequel AM, Benedetti A. Interferon gamma decreases hepatic stellate cell activation and extracellular matrix deposition in rat liver fibrosis. Hepatology 1996; 23:1189–1199.

46. Sakaida I, Uchida K, Matsumura Y, Okita K. Interferon gamma treatment prevents procollagen gene expression without affecting transforming growth factor-beta1 expression in pig serum-induced rat liver fibrosis in vivo. J Hepatol 1998; 28:471–479.
47. Parola M, Pinzani M, Casini A, Albano E, Poli G, Gentilini P, Dianzani MU. Stimulation of lipid peroxidation or 4-hydroxynonenal treatment increases procollagen (I) gene expression in human liver fat-storing cells. Biochem Biophys Res Commun 1993; 194:1044–1050.
48. Houglum K, Brenner DA, Chojkier M. D-Alpha-tocopherol inhibits collagen alpha 1(I) gene expression in cultured human fibroblasts: modulation of constitutive collagen gene expression by lipid peroxidation. J Clin Invest 1991; 87:2230–2235.
49. Bedossa P, Houglum K, Trautwein C, Holstege A, Chojkier M. Stimulation of collagen alpha1(I) gene expression is associated with lipid peroxidation in hepatocellular injury: a link to tissue fibrosis? Hepatology 1994; 19:1262–1271.
50. Baroni GS, D'Ambrosio L, Ferretti G, Casini A, Sario AD, Salzano R, Ridolfi F, Saccomanno S, Jezequel AM, Benedetti A. Fibrogenic effect of oxidative stress on rat hepatic stellate cells. Hepatology 1998; 27:720–726.
51. Baraona E, Liu W, Ma XL, Svegliati BG, Lieber CS. Acetaldehyde-collagen adducts in *N*-nitrosodimethylamine-induced liver cirrhosis in rats. Life Sci 1993; 52:1249–1255.
52. Pinzani M, Gesualdo L, Sabbah GM, Abboud HE. Effects of platelet-derived growth factor and other polypeptide mitogens on DNA synthesis and growth of cultured rat liver fat-storing cells. J Clin Invest 1989; 84:1786–1793.
53. Matsuoka M, Tsukamoto H. Stimulation of hepatic lipocyte collagen production by Kupffer cell–derived transforming growth factor beta: implication for a pathogenetic role in alcoholic liver fibrogenesis. Hepatology 1990; 11:599–605.
54. Friedman SL, Arthur MJ. Activation of cultured rat hepatic lipocytes by Kupffer cell conditioned medium: direct enhancement of matrix synthesis and stimulation of cell proliferation via induction of platelet-derived growth factor receptors. J Clin Invest 1989; 84:1780–1785.
55. Casini A, Pinzani M, Milani S, Grappone C, Galli G, Jezequel AM, Schuppan D, Rotella CM, Surrenti C. Regulation of extracellular matrix synthesis by transforming growth factor *f*À1 in human fat-storing cells. Gastroenterology 1993; 105:245–253.
56. Sanchez A, Alvarez AM, Benito M, Fabregat I. Apoptosis induced by transforming growth factor-beta in fetal hepatocyte primary cultures: involvement of reactive oxygen intermediates. J Biol Chem 1996; 271:7416–7422.
57. Pinzani M, Failli P, Ruocco C, Casini A, Milani S, Baldi E, Giotti A, Gentilini P. Fat-storing cells as liver-specific pericytes: spatial dynamics of agonist-stimulated intracellular calcium transients. J Clin Invest 1992; 90:642–646.
58. Bataller R, Gines P, Nicolas JM, Gorbig MN, Garcia-Ramallo E, Gasull X, Bosch J, Arroyo V, Rodes J. Angiotensin II induces contraction and proliferation of human hepatic stellate cells. Gastroenterology 2000; 118:1149–1156.

59. Rockey DC, Housset CN, Friedman SL. Activation-dependent contractility of rat hepatic lipocytes in culture and in vivo. J Clin Invest 1993; 92:1795–1804.
60. Sakamoto M, Ueno T, Kin M, Ohira H, Torimura T, Inuzuka S, Sata M, Tanikawa K. Ito cell contraction in response to endothelin-1 and substance P. Hepatology 1993; 18:978–983.
61. Rockey D. The cellular pathogenesis of portal hypertension: stellate cell contractility, endothelin, and nitric oxide. Hepatology 1997; 25:2–5.
62. Bauer M, Zhang JX, Bauer I, Clemens MG. ET-1 induced alterations of hepatic microcirculation: sinusoidal and extrasinusoidal sites of action. Am J Physiol 1994; 267:G143–G149.
63. Rockey DC, Chung JJ. Inducible nitric oxide synthase in rat hepatic lipocytes and the effect of nitric oxide on lipocyte contractility. J Clin Invest 1995; 95:1199–1206.
64. Helyar L, Bundschuh DS, Laskin JD, Laskin DL. Induction of hepatic Ito cell nitric oxide production after acute endotoxemia. Hepatology 1994; 20:1509–1515.
65. Shah V, Haddad FG, Garcia-Cardena G, Frangos JA, Mennone A, Groszmann RJ, Sessa WC. Liver sinusoidal endothelial cells are responsible for nitric oxide modulation of resistance in the hepatic sinusoids. J Clin Invest 1997; 100:2923–2930.
66. Hattori Y, Kasai K, Sekiguchi Y, Hattori S, Banba N, Shimoda S. The herbal medicine Sho-saiko-to induces nitric oxide synthase in rat hepatocytes. Life Sci 1995; 56:L143–L148.
67. Comporti M. Lipid peroxidation and cellular damage in toxic liver injury. Lab Invest 1985; 53:599–623.
68. Yoshino M, Ito M, Okajima H, Haneda M, Murakami K. Role of baicalein compounds as antioxidant in the traditional herbal medicine. Biomed Res 1997; 18:349–352.
69. Inoue T, Jackson EK. Strong antiproliferative effects of baicalein in cultured rat hepatic stellate cells. Eur J Pharmacol 1999; 378:129–135.
70. Huang HC, Wang HR, Hsieh LM. Antiproliferative effect of baicalein, a flavonoid from a Chinese herb, on vascular smooth muscle cell. Eur J Pharmacol 1994; 251:91–93.
71. Dethlefsen SM, Shepro D, D'Amore PA. Arachidonic acid metabolites in bFGF-, PDGF-, and serum-stimulated vascular cell growth. Exp Cell Res 1994; 212:262–273.
72. Geerts A, Rogiers V. Sho-saiko-to: the right blend of traditional Oriental medicine and liver cell biology. Hepatology 1999; 29:282–284.
73. Boigk G, Stroedter L, Herbst H, Waldschmidt J, Riecken EO, Schuppan D. Silymarin retards collagen accumulation in early and advanced biliary fibrosis secondary to complete bile duct obliteration in rats. Hepatology 1997; 26:643–649.
74. Kawada N, Seki S, Inoue M, Kuroki T. Effect of antioxidants, resveratrol, quercetin, and *N*-acetylcysteine, on the functions of cultured rat hepatic stellate cells and Kupffer cells. Hepatology 1998; 27:1265–1274.
75. Pietrangelo A, Borella F, Casalgrandi G, Montosi G, Ceccarelli D, Gallesi D,

Giovannini F, Gasparetto A, Masini A. Antioxidant activity of silybin in vivo during long-term iron overload in rats. Gastroenterology 1995; 109:1941–1949.
76. Salmi HA, Sarna S. Effect of silymarin on chemical, functional, and morphological alterations of the liver: a double-blind controlled study. Scand J Gastroenterol 1982; 17:517–521.
77. Ferenci P, Dragosics B, Dittrich H, Frank H, Benda L, Lochs H, Meryn S, Base W, Schneider B. Randomized controlled trial of silymarin treatment in patients with cirrhosis of the liver. J Hepatol 1989; 9:105–113.
78. Pares A, Planas R, Torres M, Caballeria J, Viver JM, Acero D, Panes J, Rigau J, Santos J, Rodes J. Effects of silymarin in alcoholic patients with cirrhosis of the liver: results of a controlled, double-blind, randomized and multicenter trial. J Hepatol 1998; 28:615–621.
79. Kasahara A, Hayashi N, Mochizuki K, Takayanagi M, Yoshioka K, Kakumu S, Iijima A, Urushihara A, Kiyosawa K, Okuda M, Hino K, Okita K. Risk factors for hepatocellular carcinoma and its incidence after interferon treatment in patients with chronic hepatitis C. Osaka Liver Disease Study Group. Hepatology 1998; 27:1394–1402.
80. Hagiwara H, Hayashi N, Mita E, Naito M, Kasahara A, Fusamoto H, Kamada T. Quantitation of hepatitis C virus RNA in serum of asymptomatic blood donors and patients with type C chronic liver disease. Hepatology 1993; 17:545–550.
81. Yokosuka O, Omata M, Imazeki F, Ito Y, Okuda K. Hepatitis B virus RNA transcripts and DNA in chronic liver disease. N Engl J Med 1986; 315:1187–1192.
82. Oka H, Kurioka N, Kim K, Kanno T, Kuroki T, Mizoguchi Y, Kobayashi K. Prospective study of early detection of hepatocellular carcinoma in patients with cirrhosis. Hepatology 1990; 12:680–697.
83. Ikeda K, Saitoh S, Koida I, Arase Y, Tsubota A, Chayama K, Kumada H, Kawanishi M. A multivariate analysis of risk factors for hepatocellular carcinogenesis: a prospective observation of 795 patients with viral and alcoholic cirrhosis. Hepatology 1993; 18:47–53.
84. Fattovich G, Giustina G, Degos F, Tremolada F, Diodati G, Almasio P, Nevens F, Solinas A, Mura D, Brouwer JT, Thomas H, Njapoum C, Casarin C, Bonetti P, Fuschi P, Basho J, Tocco A, Bhalla A, Galassini R, Noventa F, Schalm SW, Realdi G. Morbidity and mortality in compensated cirrhosis type C: a retrospective follow-up study of 384 patients. Gastroenterology 1997; 112:463–472.
85. Tatsuta M, Iishi H, Baba M, Nakaizumi A, Uehara H. Inhibition by Xiao-Chai-Hu-Tang (TJ-9) of development of hepatic foci induced by *N*-nitrosomorpholine in Sprague-Dawley rats. Jpn J Cancer Res 1991; 82:987–992.
86. Okita K, Kurokawa F, Yamazaki T, Furukawa T, Li Q, Murakami T, Takahashi M. The use of Sho-saiko-to (TJ-9) for chemoprevention of chemical hepatocarcinogenesis in rats and discussion of its possible pharmacological action. Transgenica 1994; 1:39–44.
87. Shiota G, Maeta Y, Mukoyama T, Yanagidani A, Udagawa A, Oyama K, Yashima K, Kishimoto Y, Nakai Y, Miura T, Ito H, Murawaki Y, Kawasaki

H. Effects of Sho-Saiko-to on hepatocarcinogenesis and 8-hydroxy-2′-deoxyguanosine formation. Hepatology 2002; 35:1125–1133.

88. Haranaka K, Satomi N, Sakurai A, Haranaka R, Okada N, Kobayashi M. Antitumor activities and tumor necrosis factor producibility of traditional Chinese medicines and crude drugs. Cancer Immunol Immunother 1985; 20:1–5.
89. Ito H, Shimura K. Effects of a blended Chinese medicine, Xiao-Chai-Hu-Tang, on Lewis lung carcinoma growth and inhibition of lung metastasis, with special reference to macrophage activation. Jpn J Pharmacol 1986; 41:307–314.
90. Yano H, Mizoguchi A, Fukuda K, Haramaki M, Ogasawara S, Momosaki S, Kojiro M. The herbal medicine Sho-saiko-to inhibits proliferation of cancer cell lines by inducing apoptosis and arrest at the G0/G1 phase. Cancer Res 1994; 54:448–454.
91. Yamashiki M, Nishimura A, Nomoto M, Suzuki H, Kosaka Y. Herbal medicine "Sho-saiko-to" induces tumour necrosis factor-alpha and granulocyte colony-stimulating factor in vitro in peripheral blood mononuclear cells of patients with hepatocellular carcinoma. J Gastroenterol Hepatol 1996; 11:137–142.
92. Ohtsuka M, Fukuda K, Yano H, Kojiro M. Effects of nine active ingredients in Chinese herbal medicine Sho-saiko-to on 2-(2-furyl)-3-(5-nitro-2-furyl)acrylamide mutagenicity. Jpn J Cancer Res 1995; 86:1131–1135.
93. Okita K, Li Q, Murakami T, Takahashi M. Antigrowth effects with components of Sho-saiko-to (TJ-9) on cultured human hepatoma cells. Eur J Cancer Prev 1993; 2:169–176.
94. Motoo Y, Sawabu N. Antitumor effects of saikosaponins, baicalin and baicalein on human hepatoma cell lines. Cancer Lett 1994; 86:91–95.
95. Austin CA, Patel S, Ono K, Nakane H, Fisher LM. Site-specific DNA cleavage by mammalian DNA topoisomerase II induced by novel flavone and catechin derivatives. Biochem J 1992; 282(pt 3):883–889.
96. Walker PR, Smith C, Youdale T, Leblanc J, Whitfield JF, Sikorska M. Topoisomerase II–reactive chemotherapeutic drugs induce apoptosis in thymocytes. Cancer Res 1991; 51:1078–1085.
97. Stevnsner T, Bohr VA. Studies on the role of topoisomerases in general, gene- and strand- specific DNA repair. Carcinogenesis 1993; 14:1841–1850.
98. Matsuzaki Y, Kurokawa N, Terai S, Matsumura Y, Kobayashi N, Okita K. Cell death induced by baicalein in human hepatocellular carcinoma cell lines. Jpn J Cancer Res 1996; 87:170–177.
99. Ueda S, Nakamura H, Masutani H, Sasada T, Takabayashi A, Yamaoka Y, Yodoi J. Baicalin induces apoptosis via mitochondrial pathway as prooxidant. Mol Immunol 2001; 38:781–791.
100. Yamashiki M, Nishimura A, Nobori T, Nakabayashi S, Takagi T, Inoue K, Ito M, Matsushita K, Ohtaki H, Kosaka Y. In vitro effects of Sho-saiko-to on production of granulocyte colony-stimulating factor by mononuclear cells from patients with chronic hepatitis C. Int J Immunopharmacol 1997; 19:381–385.
101. Blendis L, Bomzon A, Wong F. Herbal remedies for the liver: myths, proofs, and treatments. Gastroenterology 1999; 117:1250–1251.

27

Licorice Root Flavonoid Antioxidants Reduce LDL Oxidation and Attenuate Cardiovascular Diseases

Michael Aviram
Technion-Israel Institute of Technology
Haifa, Israel

Jacob Vaya
Tel-Hai Academic College
and MIGAL-Galilee Technology Center
Kiryat Shmona, Israel

Bianca Fuhrman
Rambam Medical Center
Haifa, Israel

I. ATHEROGENIC MODIFICATIONS OF LDL AND ATHEROSCLEROSIS

Atherosclerosis is the leading cause of morbidity and mortality among people with a Western lifestyle. The early atherosclerotic lesion is characterized by the accumulation of arterial foam cells derived mainly from cholesterol-loaded macrophages (1,2). Most of the accumulated cholesterol in foam cells originates from plasma low-density lipoprotein (LDL), which is internalized into the cells via the LDL receptor. Native LDL, however, does not induce cellular cholesterol accumulation, because the LDL receptor activity is down regulated by the cellular cholesterol content (3,4). LDL has to undergo some modifications, such as aggregation or oxidation, to be taken up by macrophages at enhanced rate via the macrophage scavenger receptors pathway, which, unlike the LDL receptor, are not subjected to downregulation by cellular cholesterol (5–7). The underlying mechanisms leading to the formation of atherosclerotic lesion are complicated and represent the outcome of multiple interactive processes (8–10).

Atherosclerosis is related to inflammatory conditions, which are initiated by lipoprotein invasion into the artery wall (11). Elevated plasma levels of LDL, a major risk factor for cardiovascular disease, is associated with increased adherence of circulating monocytes to arterial endothelial cells, and to increased rate of LDL infiltration into the intima. When LDL particles are entrapped in the artery, they can undergo progressive oxidation followed by a rapid internalization via the macrophage scavenger receptors, leading to foam cell formation. The atherogenicity of LDL in the arterial wall depends on the content of LDL, which is focally retained in the intima. The "response to retention" hypothesis of atherosclerosis supports subendothelial retention of atherogenic lipoproteins as the central pathological process in atherogenesis (12–14). This theory points to the retention of LDL as a prerequisite step to oxidative modification of the lipoprotein. Lipoprotein retention in the artery wall was suggested to be a more important as a risk factor for atherosclerosis than the rate of LDL transport into the artery wall (15,16). Retention of LDL in the intima involves its binding to arterial proteoglycans, and the association of LDL with such proteoglycans depends on structural properties of the LDL, such as its size and density (12,17,18). Proteoglycan-bound LDL forms aggregates (18), and aggregated LDL is avidly taken up by macrophages, as well as by smooth muscle cells (19), leading to foam cell formation (20–22). Retention and aggregation of LDL in the arterial wall are key events in atherogenesis, and aggregated LDL exists in atherosclerotic lesions (23). In vitro, LDL aggregation can be induced by phospholipase C, by sphingomyelinase (SMase), or even by mechanical vortexing (24,25). Aggregation of LDL stimulates its uptake by macrophages independently of the LDL receptor pathway, thus converting macrophages into foam cells (26). Recently, it was demonstrated that extensive oxidation of LDL leads to its aggregation (27–29). On the other hand, adherence of LDL to arterial proteoglycans increases the susceptibility of LDL to oxidation (18,30).

The "oxidative modification of lipoproteins" hypothesis of atherosclerosis proposes that LDL oxidation plays a pivotal role in early atherogenesis (31–40). This hypothesis is supported by evidence that LDL oxidation occurs in vivo (36,41) and contributes to the clinical manifestation of atherosclerosis.

The uptake of oxidized LDL (Ox-LDL) via scavenger receptors promotes cholesterol accumulation and foam cell formation (57,39,42). In addition, Ox-LDL atherogenicity is related to recruitment of monocytes into the intima (43), to stimulation of monocyte adhesion to the endothelium (44), and to Ox-LDL cytotoxicity toward arterial cells (45,46).

Oxidation of LDL involves free radicals attack on the lipoprotein components including cholesterol, phospholipids, fatty acids, and apolipoprotein B-100. LDL oxidation results first in the consumption of its antioxidants (mainly vitamin E and carotenoids), and in a substantial loss of polyunsaturated fatty acids and of cholesterol, which is converted to oxysterols. A predominant oxysterol formed at early stages of oxidation is 7-hydroperoxycholesterol, and at later stages, 7-ketocholesterol is formed (47). Both of these oxysterols are formed as a result of an oxygenation at the 7-position. The polyunsaturated groups of the esterified cholesteryl esters and of phospholipids are also major targets for oxidation. The primary products formed are hydroperoxides, which can undergo subsequent reduction to hydroxides and aldehydes. Nonenzymatic peroxidation of arachidonic acid results in the formation of isoprostanes and epoxyisoprostanes (48). In the presence of transition metal ions, acyl hydroperoxides also undergo carbon-carbon bond cleavage to form reactive short-chain aldehydes.

During oxidation of LDL, apolipoprotein B-100 also undergoes direct and indirect modifications. Direct attack of oxidants can oxidize amino acid side chains and fragment the polypeptide backbone. Reactive lipid peroxidation products, such as short-chain aldehydes, can form stable adducts with amino acid residues in the apolipoprotein B-100 (49), which can then lead to intermolecular cross-linking and to aggregation of lipoprotein particles (50). Enrichment of LDL with lipid hydroperoxides appears to be an important first step in LDL oxidation. After depletion of LDL antioxidants, transition metal ions catalyze propagation reactions, breakdown of lipid hydroperoxides, and the formation of reactive products, such as malondialdehyde and hydroxynonenal, which are responsible for apolipoprotein B-100 modification. All these reactions result in changes in the LDL structure and the oxidatively modified LDL cannot bind to the LDL receptor anymore, but interacts with the macrophage scavenger receptors, leading to the accumulation of cholesterol and oxidized lipids and to foam cell formation.

II. MACROPHAGE-MEDIATED OXIDATION OF LDL

The process of LDL oxidation is unlikely to occur in plasma because plasma has high concentrations of antioxidants and of metal ions chelators. It is more likely to occur within the artery wall, an environment depleted of antioxidants, and therefore the LDL is exposed there to oxidative stress. The identity of the cells responsible for the oxidation of LDL along atherogenesis in the arterial wall is uncertain. Monocyte-derived macrophages are likely candidates to induce the oxidation of LDL during early atherogenesis, because they are prominent in arterial lesions, and because they generate reactive oxygen and nitrogen (51,52). Macrophage-mediated oxidation of LDL is considerably affected by the oxidative state in the cells, which depends on the balance between cellular oxygenases and macrophage-associated antioxidants (53).

Macrophage binding of LDL to the LDL receptor initiates the activation of cellular oxygenases (54,55). LDL oxidation by arterial wall cells was suggested to involve the activation of macrophage 15-lipoxygenase and nicotinamide adenine dinucleotide phosphate (NADPH) oxidase (55,56). When NADPH oxidase is activated, the cytosolic components of the NADPH oxidase complex, P-47 and P-67, translocate to the plasma membrane, where they form, together with the membrane-bound cytochrome b558, the active NADPH oxidase complex. Both phospholipase A_2 and phospholipase D can induce macrophage NADPH oxidase-dependent oxidation of LDL (57). On the other hand, macrophage antioxidants also contribute to the extent of cell-mediated oxidation of LDL. Cellular reduced glutathione (GSH) is a potent antioxidant (58,59), and an inverse relationship was shown between the extent of macrophage-mediated oxidation of LDL and the cellular reduced glutathione content (59).

Macrophage-mediated oxidation of LDL can also result from an initial cellular lipid peroxidation. When cultured macrophages were exposed to ferrous ions, cellular lipid peroxidation took place (60,61). These "oxidized macrophages" could easily oxidize the LDL lipids, even in the absence of any added transition metal ions. LDL oxidation by oxidized macrophages can also result from the transfer of peroxidized lipids from the cell membranes to LDL particle.

III. PARAOXONASE AND LDL OXIDATION

Human serum paraoxonase (PON1) is an esterase that is physically associated with HDL, and is also distributed in tissues such as liver, kidney, and intestine (62,63). Activities of serum PON1 that are routinely measured include hydrolysis of organophosphates, such as paraoxon (the active metabolite of the insecticide parathion), hydrolysis of arylesters, such as phenyl acetate, and lactonase activities. Human serum paraoxonase activity has been shown to be inversely related to the risk of cardiovascular disease (64–66), as shown in atherosclerotic, hypercholesterolemic, and diabetic patients (67–69). HDL-associated PON1 has recently been shown to protect LDL, as well as the HDL particle itself, against oxidation induced by either copper ions or free radical generators (70,71), and this effect could be related to the hydrolysis of specific lipoprotein's oxidized lipids such as cholesteryl linoleate hydroperoxides or some specific oxidized phospholipids. Protection of HDL from oxidation by PON1 was shown to preserve the antiatherogenic effect of HDL in reverse cholesterol transport, as shown by its beneficial effect on HDL-mediated macrophage cholesterol efflux (70). These effects of PON 1 may be relevant to its beneficial properties against cardiovascular disease (63–65). Antioxidants were shown to preserve PON1's activity as they decrease the formation of lipid peroxides, which can inactivate PON1 (72).

IV. FLAVONOIDS AND CARDIOVASCULAR DISEASE

Dietary consumption of flavonoids was shown to be inversely related to morbidity and mortality from coronary heart disease (73–75). Flavonoids compose the largest and most studied group of plant phenols. Over 4000 different flavonoids have been identified to date. They are usually found in plants as glycosides, and large compositional differences exist between different types of plants, even between different parts of the same plant.

Flavonoids are grouped into anthocyanins and anthoxantins. Anthocyanins are glycosides of anthocyanidin, and they are the most important group of water-soluble plant pigments, responsible for the red, blue, and purple colors of flowers and fruits. Anthoxantins are colorless or colored white to yellow, and include flavonols, flavanols, flavones, flavans, isoflavones, and isoflavans.

Flavonoids are powerful antioxidants, and their activity is related to their chemical structures (76–78). Plant flavonoids can act as potent inhibitors of LDL oxidation, via several mechanisms, including scavenging of free radicals, chelation of transition metal ions, and preservation of serum paraoxonase (PON1) activity (and as a result hydrolysis of LDL-associated lipid peroxides).

Flavonoids are also quite suitable for protecting cell membranes from free-radical-induced oxidation, since they are both lipophilic and hydrophilic, thus resulting in a reduced cell-mediated oxidation of LDL. Being partly inside and partly outside of the cells' plasma membrane, flavonoids can scavenge free radicals that are generated within the cells, as well as free radicals that attack the cell from the outside.

V. LICORICE, LDL OXIDATION, AND ATHEROSCLEROSIS

Glycyrrhiza glabra, the licorice plant, has been known as a healthy nutrient for more than 3000 years. The licorice roots have long been used as flavoring and sweetening agents. Licorice root has also been used medicinally for a wide range of therapeutics, such as antibacterial, antiviral, anti-inflammatory, antiallergic, and antihepatotoxic. Minor components of licorice, mostly flavonoids from the isoflavan and chalcon subclasses, were shown to have potent antioxidative properties.

VI. CHARACTERIZATION OF ANTIOXIDANT CONSTITUENTS FROM LICORICE ROOTS

Licorice root contains flavonoids with biological activities, several of which were isolated and purified. Licochalcone B and D, isolated from the roots of *Glycyrrhiza inflata*, were shown to inhibit superoxide anion production in the xantine/xantine oxidase system (79), and to have free-radical-scavenging activity toward the DPPH (1,1-diphenyl-2-picrylhydrazyl) radical. These phenolic compounds were also shown to be effective in protecting biological systems against various oxidative processes. They inhibit mitochondrial lipid peroxidation induced by Fe(III)-ADP/NADH, scavenge superoxide anions in microsomes, and protect red blood cells against oxidative hemolysis (79). Other antioxidant constituents that were isolated from licorice were identified as the isoflavans glabridin, hispaglabridin A, hispaglabridin B, 4-*O*-methyl glabridin, and two chalcones; isoprenylchalcone and isoquitirigenin (80). Among these compounds, glabridin was the major flavonoid in the licorice root extract (5 g/kg of root).

Possible antiatherogenic effects of licorice are illustrated in Figure 1. Upon LDL incubation with glabridin, the latter was shown to bind to the LDL, and subsequently, to protect it from oxidation (80–82).

Glabridin inhibited AAPH-induced LDL oxidation in a dose-dependent manner, as shown by the inhibition of cholesteryl linoleate hydroperoxide (CL-OOH) formation, as well as by the inhibition of lipid peroxide and aldehyde formation. Addition of glabridin (30 μM) to LDL that was incubated with AAPH or with copper ions also inhibited the formation of oxysterols (7-hydroxycholesterol, 7-ketocholesterol, and 5, 5- epoxycholesterol) by 65%, 70%, and 45%, respectively. Glabridin inhibited the consumption of β-carotene and that of lycopene by 41% and 50%, respectively, after 1 hr of LDL oxidation in the presence of AAPH, but failed to protect vitamin E, the major LDL-associated antioxidant, from oxidation (82) (Fig. 2).

Glabridin was also found to preserve the arylesterase activity of human serum paraoxonase (PON1), including its ability to hydrolyze oxidized LDL (Ox-LDL) cholesteryl linoleate hydroperoxides (72), since PON1 was found to be more potent in reducing the amount of cholesteryl linoleate hydroperoxides when added to Ox-LDL in the presence of glabridin, in comparison to its effects in the absence of glabridin.

Glabridin was also shown to accumulate in macrophages in a dose- and time-dependent process, and in parallel, in glabridin-enriched cells,

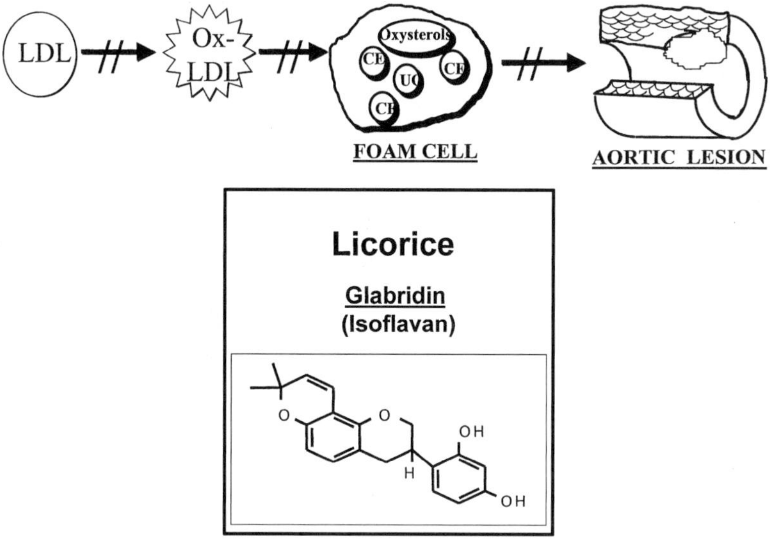

FIGURE 1 Antiatherogenic effects of licorice flavonoids. Dietary consumption of nutrients rich in flavonoids inhibits LDL oxidation, foam cell formation, and the development of aortic atherosclerotic lesions. The major licorice flavonoid, the isoflavan glabridin, is shown, along with its chemical structure. CE, cholesteryl ester; Ox-LDL, oxidized LDL; UC, unesterified cholesterol.

macrophage-mediated oxidation of LDL was inhibited by up to 80% compared with control cells (Fig. 3a). These effects could be related to glabridin-mediated inhibition of superoxide anion release from macrophages in response to phorbol 12-myristate 13-acetate (PMA) (Fig. 3b), to inhibition of the translocation of P-47 (a cytosolic component of NADPH oxidase) to the plasma membrane, and to a reduction in cellular protein kinase C activity (83) (Fig. 3c), which is required for P-47 phosphorylation and activation. Thus, glabridin-induced inhibition of P-47 phosphorylation may be the primary event responsible for its inhibitory effect on NADPH oxidase-induced macrophage-mediated oxidation of LDL. All the above inhibitory effects of glabridin on the events related to cell-mediated oxidation of LDL required the hydroxyl groups on the isoflavan B ring (81).

The protective capabilities of licorice crude extract, and of its main isolated flavonoid, the isoflavan glabridin, against LDL atherogenic modifications, including LDL oxidation, LDL retention, and LDL aggregation, were also investigated ex vivo in humans, and in the atherosclerotic apolipoprotein E–deficient (E^0) mice.

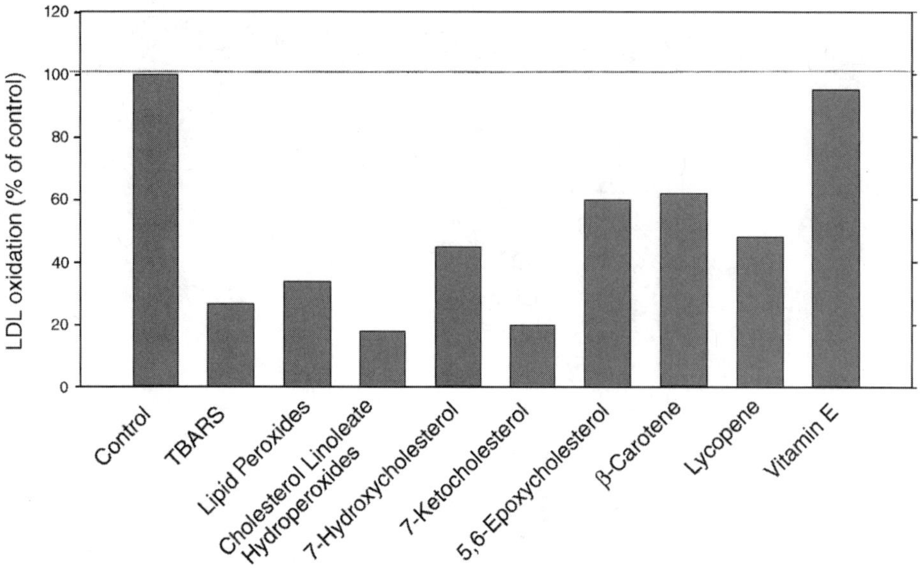

FIGURE 2 The antioxidative effect of glabridin on LDL endogenous constituents during AAPH-induced LDL oxidation. LDL (100 mg of protein/L) was incubated for 3 hr at 37°C with 5 mM AAPH in the presence of 30 μg/mL of glabridin. The extent of LDL oxidation was measured as formation of thiobarbituric acid reactive substances (TBARS), lipid peroxides, cholesteryl linoleate hydroperoxide (CLOOH), 7-hydroxycholesterol, 7-ketocholesterol, and 5,6-epoxycholesterol. It was also analyzed as the consumption of LDL-associated β-carotene, lycopene, and vitamin E. Results are expressed as % of control, relative to LDL incubated with AAPH in the absence of glabridin.

VII. THE ANTIOXIDATIVE PROPERTIES OF LICORICE CONSUMPTION IN HUMANS

Evaluation of the protective effect of licorice root extract on the resistance of LDL to ex vivo oxidation was studied in normolipidemic human subjects (84), as well as in hypercholesterolemic patients (85). LDL, which was isolated from the plasma of 10 healthy volunteers after consumption of 100 mg of licorice root ethanolic extract per day, for a period of 2 weeks, was more resistant to copper-ion-induced oxidation, as well as to AAPH-induced oxidation, by 44% and by 36%, respectively, in comparison to LDL isolated prior to licorice supplementation.

Supplementation of licorice root extract (0.1 g/day) to hypercholesterolemic patients for a period of 1 month was followed by an additional 1 month of placebo consumption (85). Licorice consumption resulted in a

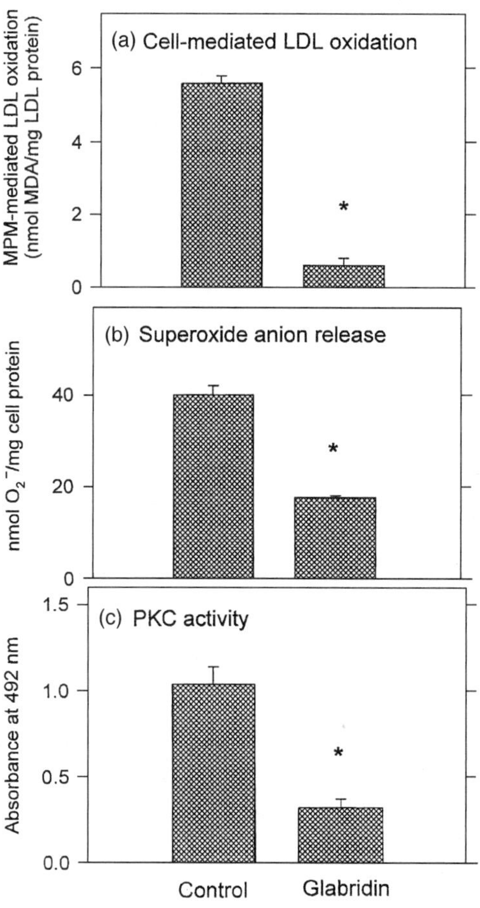

FIGURE 3 Glabridin inhibits macrophage-mediated oxidation of LDL. (a) Mouse peritoneal macrophages (MPM), harvested from E° mice that consumed placebo (control) or glabridin, were incubated with LDL (100 μg of protein/mL) for 6 hr under oxidative stress (in the presence of 2 μM $CuSO_4$). The extent of LDL oxidation was measured directly in the medium by the TBARS assay. Results are expressed as mean ± SD ($n = 3$). (b) Superoxide anion release: Glabridin enrichment of macrophages decreases superoxide anion release in response to PMA. MPM from control mice were incubated with ethanol (0.2%, control) or with 20 μM of glabridin (in 0.2% ethanol) for 2 hr at 37°C. Then, the amount of superoxide anion release to the medium in response to 50 ng/mL of PMA was determined. Results are expressed as mean ± SD ($n = 3$). (c) PKC activity: Glabridin inhibits protein kinase C (PKC) in macrophages. Macrophage PKC activity was measured in the cytosolic fraction from macrophages that were enriched with glabridin in comparison to control macrophages. Results are expressed as mean ± SD ($n = 3$). $^*p < 0.01$ (vs. placebo).

moderate reduction in the patients' plasma susceptibility to lipid peroxidation (by 19%), and in a marked reduction in the susceptibility of the patients' plasma LDL to oxidation (by 55%), as shown by a prolongation of the lag time required for the initiation of LDL oxidation by 55%, in comparison to the lag time of LDL isolated from plasma derived before licorice extract consumption (Fig. 4a). This effect was even partially sustained after an additional 1 month of placebo supplementation, since LDL derived after this period was still less susceptible to copper-ion-induced lipid peroxidation, as

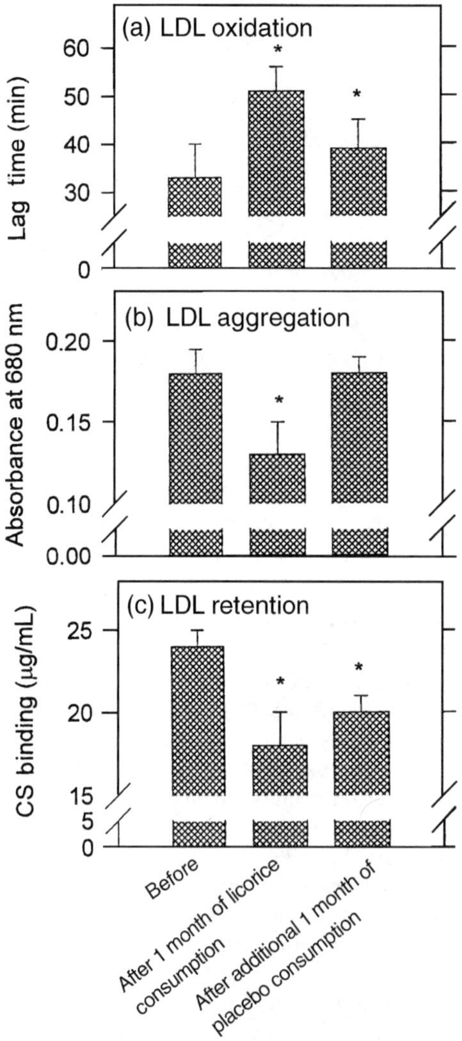

demonstrated by an 18% increment in the lag time in comparison to the baseline lag time (before licorice administration).

Atherogenicity of LDL is attributed not only to its oxidative modification, but also to its aggregation. Upon analyzing the susceptibility to aggregation of LDL isolated from hypercholesterolemic patients who consumed licorice extract for 1 month, a significant ($p < 0.01$) reduction of 28% in LDL aggregation was observed (Fig. 4b). After an additional 1 month of placebo consumption, LDL aggregation rates returned toward baseline values.

Retention of LDL, which is an early step in atherogenesis, was measured by analysis of LDL binding to the proteoglycan chondroitin sulfate (CS). Following licorice consumption, LDL CS binding ability was significantly reduced by 25% and this effect was partly sustained for the additional 1 month of placebo consumption (Fig. 4c).

Licorice extract supplementation also resulted in a 10% reduction in the patients' systolic blood pressure, which was sustained for an additional month (during the placebo consumption). Thus, dietary consumption of licorice root extract by hypercholesterolemic patients may act as a moderate hypotensive nutrient and as a potent antioxidant agent, which confer its beneficial health benefit against cardiovascular disease.

VIII. THE EFFECT OF LICORICE CONSUMPTION BY MICE ON LDL OXIDATION, MACROPHAGE FOAM CELL FORMATION, AND ATHEROSCLEROSIS

Dietary supplementation of licorice (200 μg/day/mouse) to apolipoprotein E–deficient (E°) mice for 6 weeks resulted in an 80% reduction in the suscep-

FIGURE 4 The effect of licorice extract supplementation to hypercholesterolemic patients on the susceptibility of their LDL to atherogenic modifications: oxidation (a), aggregation (b), or retention (c). LDL was isolated from hypercholesterolemic patients before, after 1 month of licorice extract supplementation, and after an additional 1 month of placebo supplementation. (a) LDL oxidation: LDL (100 mg of protein/L) was incubated with 5 μmol/L $CuSO_4$ for 3 hr at 25°C. The formation of conjugated dienes was kinetically monitored at 234 nm and the lag time was measured. (b) LDL aggregation: The extent of LDL aggregation induced by vortexing was kinetically monitored at 680 nm, and results are given after 60 sec of vortexing. (c) LDL CS binding ability: LDL (200 mg of lipoprotein protein/L) was incubated with chondroitin sulfate (CS, 100 mg/L) for 30 min at 37°C. LDL was then precipitated, and the LDL-associated glycoseaminoglycan (GAG) content was determined in the precipitate. Results are expressed as mean ± SEM. *$p < 0.01$ (vs. baseline at study entry).

tibility of their LDL to copper-ion-induced oxidation, in comparison to LDL isolated from placebo-treated mice (84).

Administration of purified glabridin to E° mice in their drinking water was followed by analysis of its antioxidative effect against ex vivo LDL oxidation (84). GC-MS analysis of the LDL derived from E° mice after consumption of glabridin revealed that glabridin was absorbed, and bound to the LDL particle. Whereas no glabridin could be detected in LDL from control mice, LDL from mice that consumed glabridin (20 μg/day/mouse) contained about 2 nmol of glabridin/mg LDL protein. LDL derived from E° mice after consumption of 20 μg glabridin/day/mouse for 6 weeks was significantly more resistant to copper-ion-induced oxidation (by 22%) than LDL derived from placebo-treated mice. Administration of glabridin (25 μg/

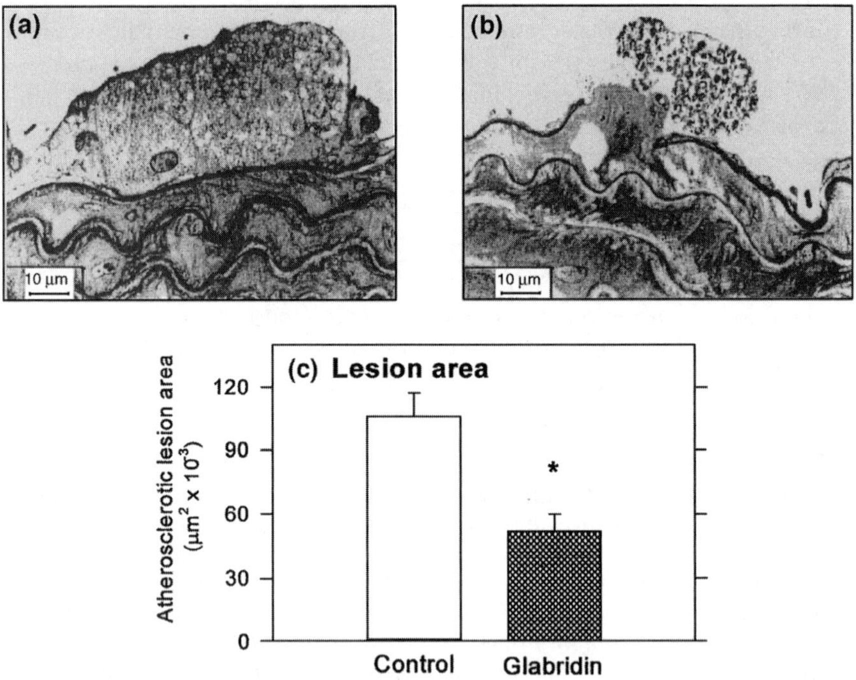

FIGURE 5 Effects of glabridin consumption by E^0 mice, on the size of their aortic arch atherosclerotic lesion area. Photomicrographs of a typical atherosclerotic lesion of the aortic arch following treatment with placebo (a) or glabridin (b). The sections were stained with alkaline toludine blue. All micrographs are at the same magnification. (c) The lesion area is expressed in square micrometers ± SD. $^*p < 0.01$ vs. placebo.

day/mouse) to E° mice for 3 months also reduced (by 50%) an additional atherogenic modification of LDL, i.e., its susceptibility to aggregation induced by vortexing (86). Most important, inhibition of atherogenic modifications of LDL (oxidation and aggregation) in E° mice following glabridin consumption was associated with a substantial reduction in macrophage foam cell formation and in the development of the atherosclerotic lesion area (Fig. 5).

IX. SUMMARY

The beneficial health effects attributed to the consumption of fruits and vegetables are related, at least in part, to their antioxidant activity. Of special

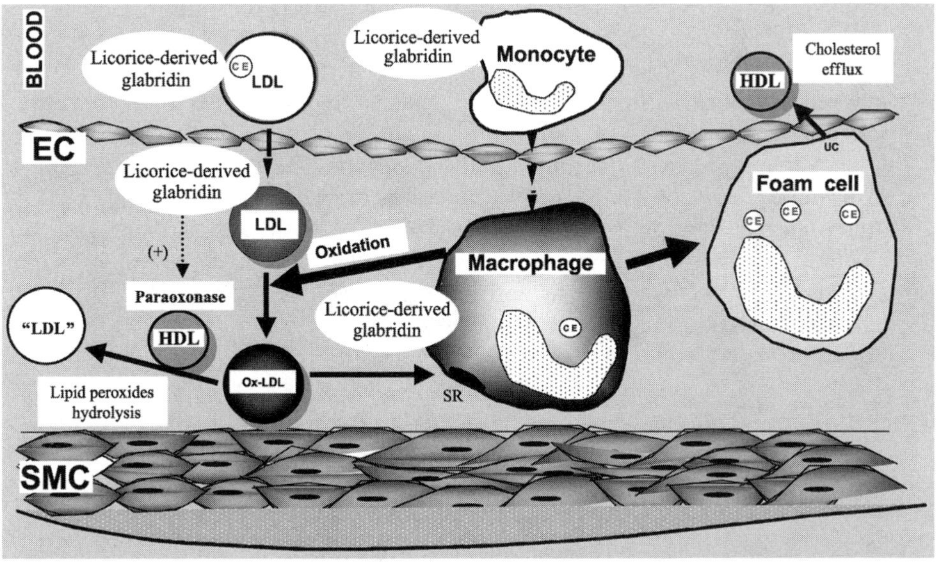

FIGURE 6 Major pathways by which licorice flavonoids inhibit LDL cholesterol oxidation and atherosclerosis. Licorice-derived flavonoids affect LDL directly by interacting with the lipoprotein and inhibiting LDL oxidation. Licorice flavonoids can also protect LDL indirectly, by their accumulation in the arteries and protection of arterial macrophages against oxidative stress. The latter effect is associated with inhibition of the formation of "oxidized macrophages" and reduction in the capacity of macrophages to oxidize LDL. In addition, licorice-derived glabridin preserves paraoxonase activity, thereby increasing the hydrolysis of lipid peroxides in lipopoteins and in atherosclerotic lesion, leading to attenuation in the progression of atherosclerosis.

interest is the inverse relationship between intake of dietary nutrients rich in polyphenols and cardiovascular diseases. This effect is attributed to the polyphenols' capability to inhibit LDL oxidation, macrophage foam cell formation, and atherosclerosis. Our current view on the major pathways by which licorice flavonoids protect LDL against oxidative modifications, and thereby reduce macrophage foam cell formation and the development of advanced atherosclerosis, are summarized in Figure 6. Licorice-derived glabridin can protect LDL against cell-mediated oxidation via two major pathways, including a direct interaction with the lipoprotein and/or an indirect effect through accumulation in arterial macrophages. Licorice-derived glabridin was shown to reduce the capacity of macrophages to oxidize LDL, owing to its binding to LDL and inhibition of its oxidation [by scavenging reactive oxygen species (ROS) and reactive nitrogen species (RNS)], also owing to its accumulation in arterial macrophages, followed by inhibition of macrophage lipid peroxidation and the formation of lipid-peroxide-rich macrophages. Furthermore, licorice-derived glabridin was shown to preserve serum paraoxonase (PON1) activity, resulting in PON1-induced hydrolysis of lipid peroxides in oxidized lipoproteins and in atherosclerotic lesion.

All these antioxidative and antiatherosclerotic effects of licorice-derived glabridin were demonstrated in vitro, as well as in vivo (in humans and in the atherosclerotic apolipoprotein E–deficient mice). We conclude that licorice is a source of some potent nutrients, which can attenuate the development of atherosclerosis secondary to its antioxidatie properties against lipid peroxidation in cells and in lipoproteins (87–89).

REFERENCES

1. Schaffner T, Taylor K, Bartucci EJ, Fischer-Dzoga K, Beenson JH, Glagov S, Wissler R. Arterial foam cells with distinctive immunomorphologic and histochemical features of macrophages. Am J Pathol 1980; 100:57–80.
2. Gerrity RG. The role of monocytes in atherogenesis. Am J Pathol 1981; 103: 181–190.
3. Goldstein JL, Brown MS. Regulation of the mevalonate pathway. Nature 1990; 343:425–430.
4. Brown MS, Goldstein JL. A receptor-mediated pathway for cholesterol homeostasis. Science 1986; 232:34–47.
5. Steinberg D, Parthasarathy S, Carew TE, Khoo JC, Witztum JL. Beyond cholesterol: modifications of low-density lipoprotein that increase its atherogenicity. N Engl J Med 1989; 320:915–924.
6. Aviram M. Modified forms of low density lipoprotein and atherosclerosis. Atherosclerosis 1993; 98:1–9.

7. Aviram M. Beyond cholesterol: modifications of lipoproteins and increased atherogenicity. In: Neri Serneri GG, Gensini GF, Abbate R, Prisco D, eds. Atherosclerosis Inflammation and Thrombosis. Florence, Italy: Scientific Press, 1993:15–36.
8. Aviram M, Rosenblat, M. Oxidative stress in cardiovascular diseases: role of oxidized lipoproteins in macrophage foam cell formation and atherosclerosis. In: Fuchs J, Podda M, Packer L, eds. Redox Genome Interactions in Health and Disease. New York: Marcel Dekker, 2004:557–590.
9. Aviram M. Review of human studies on oxidative damage and antioxidant protection related to cardiovascular disease. Free Rad Res 2000; 33:S85–S97.
10. Aviram M. Macrophage foam cell formation during early atherogenesis is determined by the balance between pro-oxidants and antioxidants in arterial cells and blood lipoproteins. Antiox Redox Signal 1999; 1:585–594.
11. Ross R. Atherosclerosis: an inflammatory disease. N Engl J Med 1999; 340:115–126.
12. Williams KJ, Tabas I. The response-to-retention hypothesis of early atherogenesis. Arterioscler Thromb Vasc Biol 1995; 15:551–561.
13. Williams KJ, Tabas I. The response-to-retention hypothesis of atherogenesis reinforced. Curr Opin Lipidol 1998; 9:471–474.
14. Nordestgaard BG. The vascular endothelial barrier-selective retention of lipoproteins. Curr Opin Lipidol 1996; 7:269–273.
15. Schwenke DC, Carew TE. Initiation of atherosclerotic lesions in cholesterol-fed rabbits. I. Focal increases in arterial LDL concentrations precede development of fatty streak lesions. Arteriosclerosis 1989; 9:895–907.
16. Schwenke DC, Carew TE. Initiation of atherosclerotic lesions in cholesterol-fed rabbits II: selective retention of LDL vs. selective increase in LDL permeability in susceptible sites of arteries. Arteriosclerosis 1989; 9:908–918.
17. Carmena R, Ascaso JF, Camejo G, Varela G, Hurt-Camejo E, Ordovas JM, Bergstom M, Wallin B. Effect of olive and sunflower oils on low density lipoprotein level, composition, size, oxidation, and interaction with arterial proteoglycans. Atherosclerosis 1996; 125:243–255.
18. Camejo G, Hurt-Camejo E, Olson U, Bonders G. Proteoglycans and lipoproteins in atherosclerosis. Curr Opin Lipidol 1993; 4:385–391.
19. Ismail NA, Alavi MZ, Moore S. Lipoprotein-proteoglycan complexes from injured rabbit aortas accelerate lipoprotein uptake by arterial smooth muscle cells. Atherosclerosis 1994; 105:79–87.
20. Kostner GM, Bihari-Varga M. Is the atherogenicity of Lp(a) caused by its reactivity with proteoglycans? Eur Heart J 1990; 11(suppl E):184–189.
21. Vijayagopal P, Srinivasan SR, Radhakrishnamurthy B, Berenson GS. Lipoprotein-proteoglycan complexes from atherosclerotic lesions promote cholesteryl ester accumulation in human monocyte/macrophages. Arterioscler Thromb 1992; 12:237–249.
22. Hurt E, Bonders G, Camejo G. Interaction of LDL with human arterial proteoglycans stimulates its uptake by human monocyte-derived macrophages. J Lipid Res 1990; 31:443–454.

23. Aviram M, Maor I, Keidar S, Hayek T, Oiknine J, Bar-El Y, Adler Z, Kertzman V, Milo S. Lesioned low density lipoprotein in atherosclerotic apolipoprotein E-deficient transgenic mice and in humans is oxidized and aggregated. Biochem Biophys Res Commun 1995; 216:501–513.
24. Pentikainen MO, Lethonen EM, Kovanen PT. Aggregation and fusion of modified low density lipoprotein. J Lipid Res 1996; 37:2638–2649.
25. Schissel SL, Tweedie-Hardman J, Rapp JH, Graham G, Williams KJ, Tabas I. Rabbit aorta and human atherosclerotic lesion hydrolyze the sphingomyelin of retained low-density lipoprotein: proposed role for arterial-wall sphingomyelinase in subendothelial retention and aggregation of atherogenic lipoproteins. J Clin Invest 1996; 98:1455–1464.
26. Zhang WY, Gaynor PM, Kruth HS. Aggregated low density lipoprotein induces and enters surface-connected compartments of human monocyte-macrophages: uptake occurs independently of the low density lipoprotein receptor. J Biol Chem 1997; 272:31700–31706.
27. Hoff HF, O'Neil Y. Lesion-derived low density lipoprotein and oxidized low density lipoprotein share a lability for aggregation, leading to enhanced macrophage degradation. Arterioscler Thromb Vasc Biol 1991; 11:1209–1222.
28. Hoff HF, Whitaker TE, O'Neil Y. Oxidation of low density lipoprotein leads to particle aggregation and altered macrophage recognition. J Biol Chem 1992; 267:602–609.
29. Maor I, Hayek T, Coleman R, Aviram M. Plasma LDL oxidation leads to its aggregation in atherosclerotic apolipoprotein E–deficient mice. Arterioscler Thromb Vasc Biol 1997; 17:2995–3005.
30. Hurt-Camejo E, Camejo G, Rosengren B, Lopez F, Ahlstrom C, Fager G, Bondjers G. Effect of arterial proteoglycan and glycosaminoglycans on low density lipoprotein oxidation and its uptake by human macrophages and arterial smooth muscle cells. Arterioscler Thromb 1992; 12:569–583.
31. Jialal I, Devaraj S. The role of oxidized low density lipoprotein in atherogenesis. J Nutr 1996; 126:1053S–1057S.
32. Steinberg D. Low density lipoprotein oxidation and its pathobiological significance. J Biol Chem 1997; 272:20963–20966.
33. Berliner JA, Heinecke JW. The role of oxidized lipoproteins in atherosclerosis. Free Rad Biol Med 1996; 20:707–727.
34. Aviram M. Oxidative modification of low density lipoprotein and atherosclerosis. Isr J Med Sci 1995; 31:241–249.
35. Witztum JL, Steinberg D. Role of oxidized low density lipoprotein in atherogenesis. J Clin Invest 1991; 88:1785–1792.
36. Aviram M. Interaction of oxidized low density lipoprotein with macrophages in atherosclerosis and the antiatherogenicity of antioxidants. Eur J Clin Chem Clin Biochem 1996; 34:599–608.
37. Kaplan M, Aviram M. Oxidized low density lipoprotein: atherogenic and proinflammatory characteristics during macrophage foam cell formation: an inhibitory role for nutritional antioxidants and serum paraoxonase. Clin Chem Lab Med 1999; 37:777–787.

38. Parthasarathy S, Santanam N, Auge N. Oxidized low-density lipoprotein, a two-faced janus in coronary artery disease? Biochem Pharmacol 1998; 56:279–284.
39. Parthasarathy S, Rankin SM. The role of oxidized LDL in atherogenesis. Prog Lipid Res 1992; 31:127–143.
40. Aviram M. Antioxidants in restenosis and atherosclerosis. Curr Interven Cardiol Rep 1999; 1:66–78.
41. Herttuala SY. Is oxidzed low density lipoprotein present in vivo? Curr Opin Lipidol 1998; 9:337–344.
42. Aviram M. The contribution of the macrophage receptor for oxidized LDL to its cellular uptake. Biochem Biophys Res Commun 1991; 179:359–365.
43. Kim JA, Territo MC, Wayner E, Carlos TM, Parhami F, Smith CW, Haberland ME, Fogelman AM, Berliner JA. Partial characterization of leukocyte binding molecules on endothelial cells induced by minimally oxidized LDL. Arterioscler Thromb 1994; 14:427–433.
44. Khan NBV, Parthasarathy S, Alexander RW. Modified LDL and its constituents augment cytokine-activated vascular cell adhesion molecule-1 gene expression in human vascular endothelial cells. J Clin Invest 1995; 95:1262–1270.
45. Rangaswamy S, Penn MS, Saidel GM, Chisolm GM. Exogenous oxidized low density lipoprotein injures and alters the barrier function of endothelium in rats in vivo. Circ Res 1997; 80:37–44.
46. Penn MS, Chisolm GM. Oxidized lipoproteins, altered cell function and atherosclerosis. Atherosclerosis 1994; 108:S21–S29.
47. Brown AJ, Leong SL, Dean RT, Jessup W. 7-Hydroxycholesterol and its products in oxidized low density lipoprotein and human atherosclerotic plaque. J Lipid Res 1997; 38:1730–1745.
48. Lynch SM, Morrow JD, Roberts LJ II, Frei B. Formation of non-cyclooxygenase-derived prostanoids (F2-isoprostanes) in plasma and low density lipoprotein exposed to oxidative stress in vitro. J Clin Invest 1994; 93:998–1004.
49. Slatter DA, Paul RG, Murray M, Bailey AJ. Reactions of lipid derived malondialdehyde with collagen. J Biol Chem 1999; 274:19661–19669.
50. Jessup W, Mander EL, Dean RT. The intracellular storage and turnover of apolipoprotein B of oxidized LDL in macrophages. Biochim Biophys Acta 1992; 1126:167–177.
51. Chisolm GM, Hazen ST, Fox PL, Catchard MK. The oxidation of lipoproteins by monocyte-macrophages. J Biol Chem 1999; 274:25959–25962.
52. Parthasarathy S, Printz DJ, Boyd D, Joy L, Steinberg D. Macrophage oxidation of low density lipoprotein generates a modified form recognized by the scavenger receptor. Arteriosclerosis 1986; 6:505–510.
53. Aviram M, Fuhrman B. LDL oxidation by arterial wall macrophages depends on the antioxidative status in the lipoprotein and in the cells: role of prooxidants vs. antioxidants. Mol Cell Biochem 1998; 188:149–159.
54. Aviram M, Rosenblat M. Macrophage mediated oxidation of extracellular low density lipoprotein requires an initial binding of the lipoprotein to its receptor. J Lipid Res 1994; 35:385–398.

55. Aviram M, Rosenblat M, Etzioni A, Levy R. Activation of NADPH oxidase is required for macrophage-mediated oxidation of low density lipoprotein. Metabolism 1996; 45:1069–1079.
56. Herttuala YS, Rosenfeld ME, Parthasarathy S, Glass CK, Sigal E, Witztum JL, Steinberg D. Colocalization of 15-lipoxygenase mRNA and protein with epitopes of oxidized low density lipoprotein in macrophage-rich areas of atherosclerotic lesions. Proc Natl Acad Sci USA 1990; 87:6959–6963.
57. Aviram M, Kent UM, Hollenberg PF. Microsomal cytochrom P450 catalyze the oxidation of low density lipoprotein. Atherosclerosis 1999; 143:253–260.
58. Meister A, Anderson ME. Glutathione. Annu Rev Biochem 1983; 52:711–760.
59. Rosenblat M, Aviram M. Macrophage glutathione content and glutathione peroxidase activity are inversely related to cell-mediated oxidation of LDL. Free Rad Biol Med 1997; 24:305–313.
60. Fuhrman B, Oiknine J, Aviram M. Iron induces lipid peroxidation in cultured macrophages, increases their ability to oxidatively modify LDL and affect their secretory properties. Atherosclerosis 1994; 111:65–78.
61. Fuhrman B, Oiknine J, Keidar S, Kaplan M, Aviram M. 1997 Increased uptake of low density lipoprotein (LDL) by oxidized macrophages is the result of enhanced LDL receptor activity and of progressive LDL oxidation. Free Rad Biol Med 1994; 23:34–46.
62. Mackness MI, Mackness B, Durrington PN, Connelly PW, Hegele RA. Paraoxonases biochemistry, genetics and relationship to plasma lipoproteins. Curr Opin Lipidol 1996; 7:69–76.
63. La Du BN, Adkins S, Kuo CL, Lipsig D. Studies on human serum paraoxonase/arylesterase. Chem Biol Interact 1993; 87:25–34.
64. Aviram M. Does paraoxonase play a role in susceptibility to cardiovascular disease? Mol Med 1999; 5:381–386.
65. Aviram M. Paraoxonase protects lipoproteins from oxidation and attenuates atherosclerosis. Ateroscleroza 2000; 4:3–7.
66. La Du BN, Aviram M, Billecke S, Navab M, Primo-Parmo S, Sorenson RC, Standiford TJ. On the physiological role(s) of the paraoxonases. Chem Biol Interact 1999; 119/120:379–388.
67. Mackness MI, Harty D, Bhatnagar D, Winocour PH, Arrol S, Ishola M, Durrington PN. Serum paraoxonase activity in familial hypercholesterolaemia and insulin-dependent diabetes mellitus. Atherosclerosis 1991; 86:193–197.
68. Abbott CA, Mackness MI, Kumar S, Boulton AJ, Durrington PN. Serum paraoxonase activity, concentration, and phenotype distribution in diabetes mellitus and its relationship to serum lipids and lipoproteins. Arterioscler Thromb Vasc Biol 1995; 15:1812–1818.
69. Garin MC, James RW, Dussoix P, Blanche H, Passa P, Froguel P, Ruiz J. Paraoxonase polymorphism Met-Leu54 is associated with modified serum concentrations of the enzyme: a possible link between the paraoxonase gene and increased risk of cardiovascular disease in diabetes. J Clin Invest 1997; 99:62–66.
70. Aviram M, Rosenblat M, Bisgaier CL, Newton RS, Primo-Parmo SL, La Du

BN. Paraoxonase inhibits high density lipoprotein (HDL) oxidation and preserves its functions: a possible peroxidative role for paraoxonase. J Clin Invest 1998; 101:1581–1590.
71. Aviram M, Billecke S, Sorenson R, Bisgaier C, Newton R, Rosenblat M, Erogul J, Hsu C, Dunlp C, La Du BN. Paraoxonase active site required for protection against LDL oxidation involves its free sulfhydryl group and is different from that required for its arylesterase/paraoxonase activities: selective action of human paraoxonase allozymes Q and R. Arterioscler Thromb Vasc Biol 1998; 18:1617–1624.
72. Aviram M, Rosenblat M, Billecke S, Erogul J, Sorenson R, Bisgaier CL, Newton RS, La Du B. Human serum paraoxonase (PON 1) is inactivated by oxidized low density lipoprotein and preserved by antioxidants. Free Rad Biol Med. 1999; 26:892–904.
73. Fuhrman B, Aviram M. Anti-atherogenicity of nutritional antioxidants. IDrugs 2001; 4:82–92.
74. Hertog MG, Kromhout D, Aravanis C, Blackburn H, Buzina R, Fidanza F, Giampaoli S, Jansen A, Menotti A, Nedeljkovic S. Flavonoid intake and long-term risk of coronary heart disease and cancer in the seven countries study. Arch Intern Med 1995; 155:381–386.
75. Aviram M, Fuhrman, B. Effects of flavonoids on the oxidation of LDL and atherosclerosis. In: Rice-Evans C, Packer L, eds. Flavonoids in Health and Disease. 2d ed. New York: Marcel Dekker, 2003:165–203.
76. Rice-Evans CA, Miller NJ, Bolwell PG, Bramley PM, Pridham JB. The relative antioxidant activities of plant-derived polyphenolic flavonoids. Free Rad Res 1995; 22:375–383.
77. Rice-Evans CA, Miller NJ, Paganga G. Structure-antioxidant activity relationships of flavonoids and phenolic acids. Free Rad Biol Med 1996; 20:933–956.
78. Van Acker SABE, Van-den Berg DJ, Tromp MNJL, Griffioen DH, van Bennekom WP, Van der Vijgh WJF, Bast A. Structural aspects of antioxidants activity of flavonoids. Free Rad Biol Med 1996; 20:331–342.
79. Haraguchi H, Ishikawa H, Mizutani K, Tamura Y, Kinoshita T. Antioxidative and superoxide scavenging activities of retrochalcones in *Glycyrrhiza inflata*. Bioorg Med Chem 1998; 6:339–347.
80. Vaya J, Belinky PA, Aviram M. Antioxidant constituents from licorice roots: isolation, structure elucidation and antioxidative capacity toward LDL oxidation. Free Rad Biol Med 1997; 23:302–313.
81. Belinky PA, Aviram M, Mahmood S, Vaya J. Structural aspects of the inhibitory effect of glabridin on LDL oxidation. Free Rad Biol Med 1998; 24:1419–1429.
82. Belinky PA, Aviram M, Fuhrman B, Rosenblat M, Vaya J. The antioxidative effects of the isoflavan glabridin on endogenous constituents of LDL during its oxidation. Atherosclerosis 1998; 137:49–61.
83. Rosenblat M, Belinky P, Vaya J, Levy R, Hayek T, Coleman R, Merchav S, Aviram M. Macrophage enrichment with the isoflavan glabridin inhibits NADPH oxidase-induced cell mediated oxidation of low density lipoprotein. J Biol Chem 1999; 274:13790–13799.

84. Fuhrman B, Buch S, Vaya J, Belinky PA, Coleman R, Hayek T, Aviram M. Licorice extract and its major polyphenol glabridin protect low-density lipoprotein against lipid peroxidation: in vitro and ex vivo studies in humans and in atherosclerotic apolipoprotein E-deficient mice. Am J Clin Nutr 1997; 66:267–275.
85. Fuhrman B, Volkova N, Kaplan M, Presser D, Attias J, Hayek T, Aviram M. Antiatherosclerotic effects of licorice extract supplementation to hypercholesterolemic patients: increased resistance of their LDL to atherogenic modifications, reduced plasma lipids levels, and decreased systolic blood pressure. Nutrition 2002; 18:268–273.
86. Aviram M, Fuhrman B. Polyphenolic flavonoids inhibit macrophage-mediated oxidation of LDL and attenuate atherogenesis. Atherosclerosis 1998; 137 (suppl):45–50.
87. Fuhrman B, Aviram M. Flavonoids protect LDL from oxidation and attenuate atherosclerosis. Curr Opin Lipidol 2001; 12:41–48.
88. Fuhrman B, Aviram M. Polyphenols and flavonoids protect LDL against atherogenic modifications. 2d ed. Handbook of Antioxidants: Biochemical, Nutritional and Clinical Aspects. 2001: 303–336.
89. Vaya J, Aviram M. Nutritional antioxidants: mechanisms of action, analyses of activities and medical application. Curr Med Chem Imm Endocr Metab Agents 2001; 1:99–117.

28

Estrogen-Like Activity of Licorice Root Extract and Its Constituents

Jacob Vaya
Tel-Hai Academic College, Upper Galilee
and MIGAL-Galilee Technology Center
Kiryat Shmona, Israel

Snait Tamir
Tel-Hai Academic College
Upper Galilee, Israel

Dalia Somjen
The Tel-Aviv Sourasky Medical Center
Tel-Aviv, Israel

I. INTRODUCTION

A. Estrogens

Estrogens are steroid hormones that exhibit a broad range of physiological activities. 17β-Hydroxyestradiol is the female sex hormone active in developing the mammary gland and the uterus, maintaining pregnancy, relieving menopausal symptoms, and preventing cardiovascular and bone diseases (1). An apparent consequence of estrogen is the increase in short-term menopausal symptoms including vasomotor hot flashes, urogenital atrophy, and psychological functioning. A hot flash is the classic sign of menopause and the primary clinical symptom experienced by women during this transitional stage (2).

Estrogen is beneficial in reducing the risk of cardiovascular disease (3–5). The incidence of heart disease among premenopausal women is low compared with men, whereas the incidence among postmenopausal women approaches that of men. The administration of estrogen to postmenopausal women decreases the incidence of heart disease (6). This protective effect of estrogen may partly be attributed to its influence in decreasing the ratio between LDL and HDL (7), to reduction of thrombus formation, and to improvement in vascular compliance. Secondary prevention trials, conducted on women with established coronary heart disease, failed to confirm the benefits of hormone replacement therapy (HRT) (8). A randomized controlled trial by the Women's Health Initiative begun in 1993 and involving 16,608 participants who were undergoing HRT of estrogen plus progestin, was terminated before it reached its end, owing to a 26% increase in invasive breast cancer and, surprisingly, to an increase in the risk of heart attack (strokes, blood clots) among those taking the hormone regimen, compared with women taking a placebo (9).

Estrogen is known to be involved in osteoporosis (10), which affects more than 25 million women, causing some 250,000 hip fractures annually. Osteoporosis is characterized by a reduction in bone mineral density to the extent that a fracture may occur after minimal trauma. However, estrogen can also stimulate malignant growths and in this way contributes to the development of estrogen-dependent tumors such as breast and uterus cancer (11). Breast cancer is the most common malignancy among women in Western society and is the leading cause of death among American women aged between 40 and 55 years.

The mechanism of estrogen action includes binding to the estrogen receptor in the target cell. The estrogen receptor complex is then translocated from the cytosol to the cell nucleus, where it binds to the DNA, and modulates the transcription rate of certain specific genes in the nucleus of the target cells. At present two estrogen receptors (ERs) are known, ERα and ERβ, which have different structure and tissue distributions (12). The biological effect of an ER ligand in a specific tissue is determined by the expression of ERα and ERβ in that tissue. It was demonstrated that oxidative stress induced by H_2O_2, Fe^{2+}, AAPH, and activated macrophages affect the expression of ERα and ERβ differently, demonstrating cell-specific response, which can be blocked by antioxidants (13). The two key events controlling the tissue selectivity of an estrogen are the receptor's shape and the interaction with adaptor proteins (14,15). Compounds known as selective estrogen receptor modulators (SERMS) function as estrogen antagonists in some tissues and as agonists in others. For example, tamoxifen, an antagonist in breast tissue, is used to treat breast cancer and acts as an estrogen agonist in bone (16), whereas raloxifene functions as an agonist in the bone, breast, and cardiovascular system but not in the uterus (17,18). This discrepancy led to a search for new therapeutic agents such as phytoestrogens that would mimic specific activities of estrogen. Thus, compounds that inhibit the estrogen receptor in breast tissue or function like estrogen in nonreproductive tissues (such as bone and cardiovascular tissues) may be of therapeutic use.

B. Studies on Structure-Activity Relationships

Several studies have been carried out on the relationship between the structure of compounds and their estrogen-like activity (12,19). Although it is expected that the binding affinity of the ligand to the ER does not accurately indicate the biological activity of the ligand in vivo, receptor binding is still a requisite for the stimulation of biological activity. Wiese et al. (20) evaluated 42 analogs of estradiol for their ER-binding affinity and toxicity to breast cancer cell lines, correlating the structure of these compounds with the above activities by means of three-dimensional quantitative structure activity (QSAR), employing a comparative molecular field analysis (CoMFA). They concluded that additional structural characteristics to those responsible for tight receptor binding must be present to induce an optimal mitogenic response, such as steric factor interference in specific zones and electronegative and electropositive properties near position 3. Sadler et al. (21) used the CoMFA method, which can visualize the steric and electrostatic features of the ligands corresponding to ER-binding affinity. Using the above technique, 30 compounds sharing the transstilbene structure were examined and results were compared to information from the ER-binding affinities of substituted estradiol analogs. This study demonstrated the importance of hydroxy substituents in nonsteroidal ligands that mimic the 3-OH and 17-OH of estradiol to obtain a high binding affinity. Grese et al. (22) examined a series of raloxifene analogs in vitro and in vivo in which the 2-arylbenzothiophene substructure had been modified, measuring the reduction of serum cholesterol, uterine weight gain, and uterine eosinophil peroxidase activity in an ovariectomized (OVX) rat model. In this study, they showed the importance of highly electronegative 4′-substituents, such as hydroxy or fluoro attached to the raloxifene molecule, in their ability to bind to the receptor. They also showed that increasing steric bulk at position 4′ led to increased uterine stimulation in vivo and that additional substitutions at the 4-, 5-, or 7-positions of the benzothiophene moiety resulted in reduced biological activity, while an additional substitution of the 2-aryl moiety had little effect.

Shiau et al. (23) investigated the crystal structure of the human LBD complex with an agonist (diethylstilbestrol), together with a peptide derived from an ERα coactivator and the crystal structure of LBD with an antagonist (4-hydroxy tamoxifen). They showed that the peptide binds as a short α helix to a hydrophobic groove on the LBD surface in the complex with the agonist, while the binding of the antagonist promotes a helix 12 conformation, inhibiting the binding of a coactivator. They concluded that two effects occur when the antagonist binds to LBD: a change in the position of the helix 12 so that it occupies part of the coactivator-binding groove, and a change in LBD conformation resulting from the interaction with the antagonist that stabilizes this conformation. These data suggest that the ligand structure will have a direct effect on the complex ER-ligand structure, which dictates the specific biological activities. Thus a search for natural and synthetic ligands that form complexes leading to tissue-specific beneficial effects is desired.

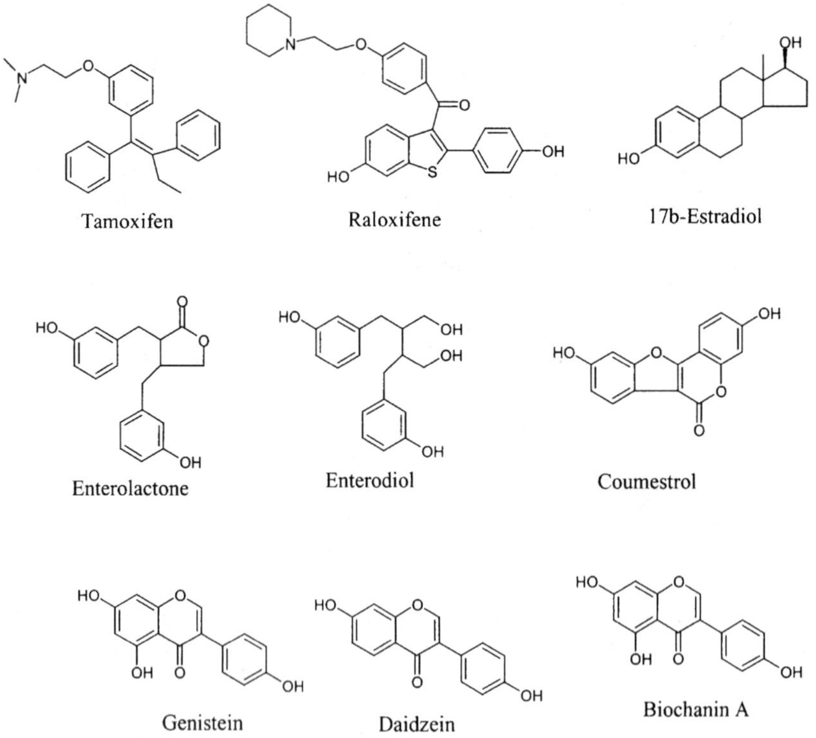

Figure 1 Structures of several phytoestrogens, tamoxifen, raloxifene, and estradiol.

C. Phytoestrogens

Phytoestrogens are naturally occurring ligands for the estrogen receptor that are derived from plants. They are part of the human diet and exhibit estrogen-like activity (24,25). Phytoestrogens include the subclasses of lignans, coumestans, isoflavones, and isoflavans (Fig. 1) that are widely distributed in oilseeds (flax, cereals), vegetables, soybeans, and roots. The main mammalian lignans are enterolactone (II) and enterodiol (III) (26), and of coumestan, coumestrol. The major food-active isoflavonoids are genistein (IV) and daidzein (V) (27) while the major isoflavan is glabridin (28). Epidemiological evidence indicates that soy intake (rich in isoflavonoids) is associated with lower breast cancer risk in women (29,30). Genistein is reported to prevent cancellous bone loss and to maintain or increase bone density in postmenopausal women (31,32). The effects of different phytoestrogens in a wide range of concentrations on estrogen receptor binding, PS2 induction (estrogen-regulated antigen), and cell proliferation rate in human breast cancer cells were compared to the effects of estradiol. Phytoestrogens were shown to have weak estrogenic activity, ranging from 500 to 15,000 times less than estradiol (33,34).

II. ESTROGEN-LIKE ACTIVITY OF LICORICE ROOT EXTRACT

The phytoestrogenic activity of licorice root extract (*Glycyrrhiza glabra* L.) was tested among 150 other herbal extracts exerting a high ER-binding affinity (35) while others reported that it showed a low binding affinity (36). Licorice root extract in combination with a mixture of other herbal extracts was reported to exert potent estrogenic activity in vitro in animals and in patients

TABLE 1 The Effect of Licorice Extract on the Induction of CK Activity in Various Female Rat Tissue

	Control	Estradiol (0.5 μg)	Licorice extract (25 μg)	Glabridin (25 μg)
Epiphysis	1 + 0.07	1.42 + 0.12	1.18 + 0.13	1.46 ± 0.09
Diaphysis	1 + 0.30	1.99 + 0.10	4.17 + 0.07	3.41 ± 0.19
Uterus	1 + 0.25	2.15 + 0.14	1.36 + 0.10	2.30 ± 0.19
Aorta	1 + 0.25	1.7 + 0.20	1.42 + 0.18	1.42 ± 0.09
Left ventricle	1 + 0.15	1.74 + 0.17	1.38 + 0.07	2.26 ± 0.24
Pituitary	1 + 0.16	2 – 0.20	3.68 + 0.09	2.15 ± 0.23

The effect of licorice extract, glabridin, and estradiol feeding on the induction of creatine kinase activity in ovariectomized female rat tissues. Rats were fed with 0.5 μg/day/rat of estradiol, 25 μg/day/rat of licorice extract, or 25 μg/day/rat of glabridin for 4 weeks. CK activity was tested in various selected tissues.

TABLE 2 Histomorphometric Analysis of OVX Bone Tissues of Female Rats Fed with Licorice Extract, Glabridin, or Estradiol for 4 Weeks

	Control	Estradiol	Licorice	Glabridin
Total bone volume (%)	35.6 ± 6.7	40.5 ± 4.8	37.0 ± 8.0	40.4 ± 3.3
Cartilage (width, μm)	24.2 ± 6.7	28.6 ± 9.3	21.3 ± 7.0	33.2 ± 7.3
Growth plate (height, μm)	18.1 ± 0.7	20.0 ± 2.3	22.3 ± 2.8	20.8 ± 1.4
Width of trabecules (μm)	4.2 ± 0.9	5.0 ± 0.7	4.8 ± 0.8	5.4 ± 1.2

The effect of licorice extract, glabridin, and estradiol feeding on bone volume, cartilage, epiphysal growth plate, and the trabecules was tested in ovariectomized females. Rats were fed with 0.5 μg/day/rat of estradiol, 25 μg/day/rat of licorice extract, or 25 μg/day/rat of glabridin for 4 weeks. The histomorphometric changes in the tested tissues are summarized.

with prostate cancer (37), which was attributed to licochalcone A present in the extract. The estrogen-like effects of licorice extract in vivo were tested in our laboratory (38). Ovariectomized female rats fed with licorice extract (25 μg/day/rat) or estradiol (0.5 μg/day/rat) for 4 weeks showed a significant increase in creatine kinase (CK) activity in the epiphysis, diaphysis, left ventricle of the heart, aorta, uterus, and pituitary gland (Table 1). CK activity is known to be induced by estrogens in vivo and in vitro (39,40), and can therefore be used as an ER-response marker. These results showed that at 0.5 μg/day/rat, estradiol stimulated CK activity at the same level as licorice extract at 25 μg/day/rat only in diaphyseal bone and the pituitary gland. A histomorphometric analysis of the diaphysis and epiphysis of the femoral bone showed similar effects of licorice and estradiol on the bone's tracular volume and trabecular width, but not on the cartilage width or the growth plate height (Table 2). These results suggest that licorice extract is as active as estradiol in some parameters and may be safer for use. Additional in vivo experiments exceeding 1 month may better clarify the licorice extract potential.

III. ESTROGEN-LIKE ACTIVITY OF LICORICE ROOT CONSTITUENTS

Licorice root constituents were isolated from the aqueous extract, such as glycyrrhizin and its glycone, glycyrrhetinic acid, and were used in the treatment of hyperlipemia, atherosclerosis, viral diseases, and allergic inflammation (41). The organic extract of licorice root (acetone or ethanol) is known to contain isoflavans, isoflavene, and chalcones (Fig. 2) such as glabridin,

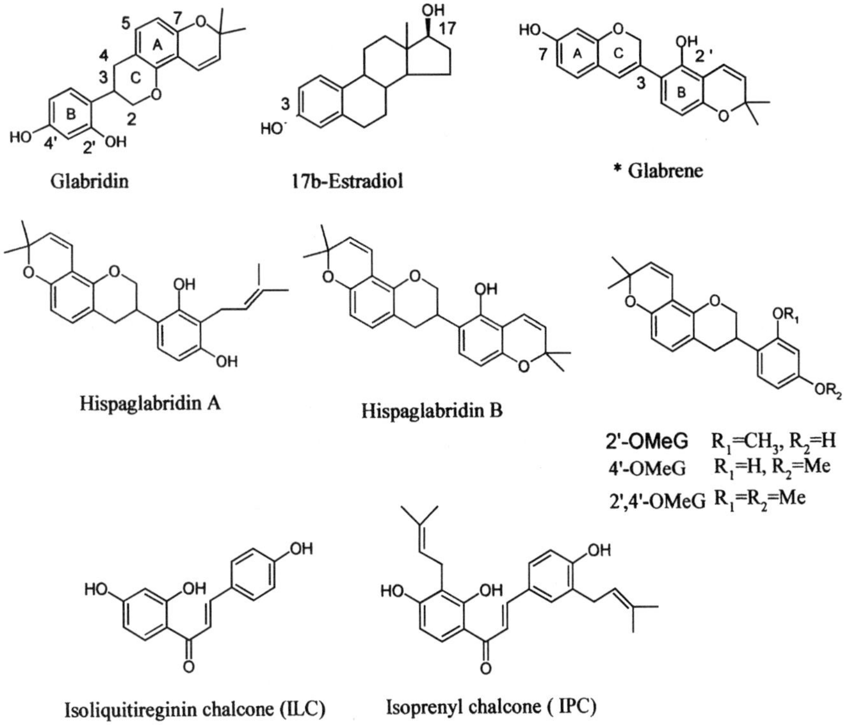

FIGURE 2 The structure of licorice constituents and estradiol. 2′-*O*-Methyl glabridin (2′-OMeG), and 2′,4′-*O*-Dimethtyl glabridin (2′,4′-OMeG) were synthesized from glabridin. *A revised structure for glabrene was assigned by Kinoshita, Tamura, et al. (1997) (74).

glabrol, glabrene, 3-hydroxyglabrol, 4′-*O*-methylglabridin (4′-OMeG), hispaglabridin A (hisp A), hispaglabridin B (hisp B), isoprenylchalcone derivative (IPC), isoliquitireginin chalcone (ILC), and formononetin (28,42,43). Licorice root is one of the richest sources of a unique subclass of the flavonoid family, the isoflavans. We recently showed that glabridin, the major compound of this class having diverse biologically activities (see Aviram et al., in this book) and which is present in the extract in more than 10% w/w, also exhibits estrogen-like activity (38,44). The isoflavans contain ring A fused to ring C connected to ring B through carbon 3 (Fig. 2). Several functional groups, mainly hydroxyl, may be attached to this basic skeleton. The heterocyclic ring C of the isoflavans does not contain a double bond between carbon 2 and 3, or a carbonyl group attached to carbon 4. This structure does not allow a conjugation of the double bonds between rings A and B.

The similarity of the glabridin structure and lipophilicity to that of estradiol (Fig. 2) encouraged us to investigate the subclass of isoflavans as a possible candidate for mimicking estrogen activity. In vivo studies testing the effects of licorice extract suggested that there may be more compounds in the extract contributing to its estrogen-like activity. This led us to identify other active constituents, such as glabrene and chalcones.

A. Glabridin

Among the licorice constituents isolated and tested, the most active phytoestrogen in vitro and in vivo is glabridin (38,44). Several features are common to the structures of glabridin and estradiol (Fig. 2). Both have an aromatic ring substituted with a hydroxyl group at para (glabridin) or position 3 (estradiol), with three additional fused rings of a phenanthrenic shape. Both are relatively lipophilic, containing a second hydroxyl group, although not at the same position (17β in estradiol and 2′ in glabridin).

1. Binding of Glabridin to the ERα

Glabridin binds the ER with IC_{50} of 5 μM (44) and with approximately the same affinity as genistein, the best known phytoestrogen (33), 10^4 times lower than estradiol (45) (Fig. 3).

2. Effect of Glabridin on Breast Cancer Cells

Glabridin stimulated growth over a range of 0.1–10 μM, reaching a maximum level at about 10 μM; at a higher level (15 μM), it inhibited cell growth (44) (Fig. 4). Growth stimulation of ER(+) cells by glabridin closely correlated to its binding affinity to ER. The concentrations at which the proliferative effects of glabridin were observed are well within the reported in vitro range of other phytoestrogens, such as genistein, daidzein, and resveratrol from grapes (45–48).

Using human breast cancer cells that do not express active ERs (MDA-MB-468) and cells that express active ERs (T47D) confirmed that this cell growth inhibition at a high concentration exhibits ER-independent behavior.

3. Effect of Glabridin on Cardiovascular Cells

Animal and human studies indicate that estrogens are protective against coronary atherosclerosis (4). Since endothelial and vascular smooth muscle cells are involved in vascular injury and atherogenesis, the potential modulation of such processes by estrogen and estrogen-like compounds is of obvious interest. Glabridin as an estradiol-induced, dose-dependent increase of DNA synthesis of human endothelial cells (ECV304) had a biphasic effect on the smooth human primary vascular smooth muscle cells (VSMC) (Table 3) (49).

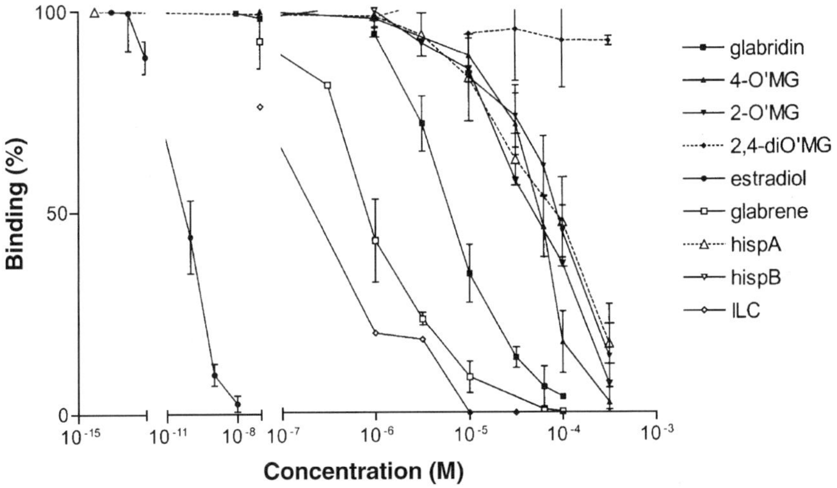

FIGURE 3 The binding of estradiol and licorice constituents to human estrogen receptor α (ERα). Competition of isolated licorice constituents for estrogen receptor with [^{3}H] labeled. 17β-Estradiol was tested in human breast cancer cells (T-47D). The cells were incubated with [^{3}H] 17β-estradiol and increasing concentrations of the tested compounds. 17β-Estradiol and 0.1% ethanol were used as controls. Radioactivity in cells' nuclei was counted and ploted as % of control. Values are means ± SD of >3 experiments.

The inhibition of VSMC proliferation and the induction of ECV304 cell proliferation by either estradiol or glabridin, which are estrogen-mimetic, are beneficial in preventing atherosclerosis.

4. In Vivo Effects of Glabridin on Female Rat Tissues

Ovariectomized female rats fed with estradiol or glabridin for 4 weeks (Table 1) showed that 0.5 μg/day/rat of estradiol stimulated CK activity at the same level as 25 μg/day/rat of glabridin in all tissues tested. The histomorphological analysis suggests that glabridin is slightly more active than the licorice extract and is similar to estradiol (Table 2). The above effects of glabridin on estrogen-responsive tissues suggest that it has the potential to mimic the beneficial activities of estrogen in bone and cardiovascular tissues, but also has a hazardous influence on the uterus.

B. Glabrene and Other Constituents from the Licorice Root

Glabrene, an isoflavene and ILC that was isolated from organic extract, binds to the human estrogen receptor with about the same affinity as glabridin and

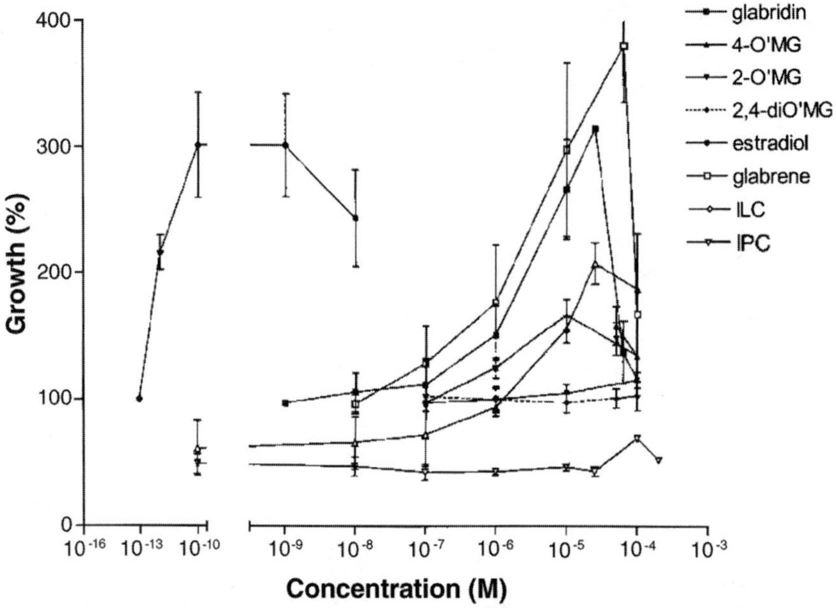

FIGURE 4 The effects of licorice constituents on the growth of estrogen-responsive human breast cancer cells. T-47D cells were incubated with increasing concentrations of 17β-estradiol or the isolated licorice constituents for 7 days. Proliferation was tested using the XTT cell proliferation reagent. Results are presented as the % of controls (0.1% ethanol). Values are means ± SD of >3 experiments.

TABLE 3 The Effect of Estradiol and Glabridin on Human Endothelial Cells and on Vascular Smooth Muscle Cells

Cells		ECV304	VSMC
Estradiol	0.3 nM	1.77 + 0.16	3.28 + 0.09
	30 nM	2.44 + 0.11	0.53 + 0.19
Glabridin	30 nM	1.52 + 0.20	2.37 + 0.10
	300 nM	3.34 + 0.30	0.89 + 0.22
	3 μM	8.72 + 0.28	0.40 + 0.22

Human endothelial cells (ECV304) and human primary vascular smooth muscle cells (VSMC) were exposed to increasing concentrations of glabridin. DNA synthesis was tested using ^{3}H-thymidine incorporation. Results are presented as an increased fold of control.

genistein. The hisp A and B, two additional isoflavans in the licorice root, were barely active, whereas IPC, another chalcone, was totally inactive. Glabrene and ILC showed ER-regulated growth-promoting effects such as glabridin (Fig. 4) and genistein. Glabrene produced dose-dependent transcriptional activation with half-maximal induction at 1 μM, corresponding to the concentration required for the inhibition of estradiol binding, and showed a maximum induction level similar to that achieved by 10 nM of estradiol. The administration of 25 μg/day/rat glabrene resulted in a similar effect to that of 5 μg/rat of estradiol in specific skeletal and cardiovascular tissues.

Glabrene, glabridin, and genistein all exhibited phytoestrogenic activity and are characterized by the connection of ring B to position 3 of the isoflavan and isoflavone, respectively. On the other hand, many compounds have a flavonol or flavonone structure whereby ring B is attached to carbon 2, and are not active as phytoestrogens, such as quercetin, catechin, apigenin, etc. (reviewed in Ref. 50). This may emphasize the importance of the former structure for performing phytoestrogenic activity. Results also show that the glabrene structure, having a double bond between carbons 3 and 4, resembles that of trans-diphenyl stilbene, a structure critical for the antagonistic and agonistic activities of the two drugs, tamoxifen and raloxifene (Fig. 1). However, glabridin lacks this double bond in ring C but nonetheless demonstrated phytoestrogenic activity in vitro and in vivo, which may suggest that conjugated double bonds between ring A to ring B are not essential for this activity. This phenomenon could be explained by the effect of ring C on the isoflavans stracture, which fixed the position of rings A and B, similar to the effect of the double bond in trans-stilbene, thus enabling them to bind efficiently to the ER. Both chalcones of the licorice constituents tested, ILC and IPC, contain an α, β double bond, a hydroxyl at position 2′ (with two additional hydroxyls at positions 4 and 4′). However, only ILC, which does not contain the isoprenyl group, binds to the ER, whereas IPC, containing two isoprenyl groups, was totally inactive.

IV. THE EFFECT OF GLABRIDIN DERIVATIVES ON THEIR ER BINDING

Glabridin, which contains two hydroxyl groups at positions 2′ and 4′, has a higher affinity to ER and a stronger effect on cell growth stimulation than 2′-*O*-MeG and 4′-*O*-MeG. 2′,4′-*O*-MeG did not bind to the human estrogen receptor and showed no proliferative activity. This suggests that when both hydroxyl groups are free, binding and cell growth promotion are more pronounced. Previous reports on the involvement of the two hydroxyl groups of estradiol in binding to the human estrogen receptor showed that both hydroxyl groups 3 and 17β are required for binding (20,51). In glabridin, hydroxyl 4′ may play the same role as hydroxyl 3 of estradiol, forming hydrogen bonds with Arg 394 and Glu 353 in the binding site. Glabridin lacks the additional hydroxyl group of estradiol at position 17β but has ether oxygen in a parallel position (the γ-pyran ring), which could contribute to the interaction to histidin 524 in the ligand-binding domain.

V. EFFECTS OF LICORICE CONSTITUENTS ON CELL PROLIFERATION

In contrast to the ER-regulated growth-promoting phytoerogenic effects of glabridin and glabrene in concentrations ranging from 100 nM to 10 μM, higher concentrations abruptly inhibited the proliferation of ER-positive and ER-negative breast cancer cells. The most plausible explanation for this biphasic effect of glabridin and glabrene on human breast cancer cells is that it mediates its actions, not only via the ER as an estrogen agonist, but also by interacting at higher concentrations with other ER-independent cellular mechanisms to inhibit cell proliferation induced by glabridin via ER pathways. Antiproliferative effects of genistein were also observed in other non-breast carcinoma cell lines (52). The inhibited growth of ER-negative cells by glabridin supports the hypothesis that the actions of phytoestrogen on cell growth inhibition occur via different molecular mechanisms (53–55).

VI. DIFFERENTIAL EFFECTS OF GLABRIDIN AND GLABRENE ON ERα AND ERβ EXPRESSIONS

Estrogen is known to offer protection from coronary artery disease in postmenopausal women, to be involved in Alzheimer's disease, and to inhibit oxidative stress-induced nerve cell death and apoptosis, which are implicated in a variety of pathologies including strokes and Parkinson's disease. The existence of estrogen receptors in these cells and tissues, and the possibility that some of these estrogen effects are ER-dependent, led to the investigation of whether phytoestrogens, known to bind the estrogen receptor and exhibiting some estrogen-like activities, can also regulate the expression of ERs.

Results showed that the phytoestrogens glabridin and glabrene promoted ERα and ERβ expressions differently and in a cell-specific manner. ERβ was significantly increased in human breast cancer cells only after being exposed to estradiol and glabridin (two- to fourfold increase), while vitamin D and glabrene inhibited ERβ expression in these cells. On the other hand, ERα was significantly increased in all treatments (estradiol, fourfold; vitamin D, threefold; and glabridin, sixfold). Estradiol treatment inhibited ERβ in colon and melanoma cells, while glabrene significantly increased ERβ (two- to threefold). Glabridin had no significant effect in these cell lines, which only exhibited ERβ. Vitamin D showed the same effect as estradiol on ERβ inhibition in colon cells but had the same stimulating effect on ERβ (twofold) as glabrene in melanoma cells (unpublished data).

These data suggest that phytoestrogens not only mimic the estradiol function as physiological regulators of ERα and ERβ expressions but also present tissue selectivity. They may also suggest that treatment using both estradiol and specific phytoestrogens may increase tissue sensitivity to estradiol, enabling fewer hormones to be used, thus leading to favorable effects of estradiol and a reduction in the deleterious effects. All of this may provide new insight into the ER-dependent protective action of estrogen and phytoestrogens in various postmenopausal diseases and contribute to the development of novel therapeutic treatment strategies.

VII. LICORICE CONSTITUENTS INHIBIT SEROTONIN REUPTAKE—A POTENTIAL NATURAL TREATMENT FOR POSTMENOPAUSAL DEPRESSION

An increase in the prevalence of depressive symptoms in women undergoing menopause can be related to fluctuating estrogen levels (56). Depression in women seems to increase with a change in hormone levels (57). The serotonergic system appears to play a major role in depression, although other neurotransmitters are also involved (2,58,59).

Serotonin is a neurotransmitter in the central and peripheral nervous systems (60). Serotonin inactivation following its release is controlled by a specific reuptake of the transmitter from the synaptic cleft into the presynaptic nerve terminal by the plasma membrane 5HT transporter (SERT3). Selective blockage of central nervous system SERTs in humans is the initial step in the pharmacological improvement of a wide variety of disorders, including major depression (59). The ability of steroids to modulate 5HT transport was investigated, and it has been shown that estradiol exhibits a nongenomic, possibly allosteric, inhibition of 5-HT serotonin transport (61). Glabridin and 4′-OMeG were found to be the most effective inhibitors (60% inhibition) of licorice constituents of 5-HT uptake, expressing a slightly higher activity than that of glabrene (47% inhibition). The 2′-OMeG was totally inactive, proving the importance of hydroxyl 2′ for the serotonin reuptake inhibition (62).

VIII. WHITENING EFFECT OF LICORICE EXTRACT AND ITS CONSTITUENTS

The color of mammalian skin and hair is determined by a number of factors, the most important of which is the degree and distribution of melanin pigmentation. Melanin protects the skin from ultraviolet (UV) lesion by absorbing the ultraviolet sunlight and removing reactive oxygen species (ROS). Various dermatological disorders arise from the accumulation of an excessive amount of epidermal pigmentation (melasma, age spots, actinic damage sites). Melanin is formed through a series of oxidative reactions involving the conversion of the amino acid tyrosine in the presence of the enzyme tyrosinase to dihydroxyphenylalanine (DOPA) and then to dopaquinone. Subsequently, dopaquinone is converted to melanin by nonenzymatic reactions. Compounds may inhibit melanin biosynthesis through different mechanisms such as the absorption of UV light, the inhibition and proliferation of melanocyte metabolism (63,64), or the inhibition of tyrosinase, the major enzyme in melanin biosynthesis. Existing inhibitors suffer from several drawbacks such as low activity (kojic acid), high cytotoxicity, and mutagenicity (hydroquinone) or poor skin penetration (arbutin). Therefore, new depigmentation agents are needed that have improved properties. Yokota et al. (65) investigated the inhibitory effect of glabridin on melanogenesis in vitro in cell culture and found that glabridin inhibits tyrosinase activity at concentrations of 0.1–1.0 μg/mL; in vivo it prevented UVB-induced pigmentation on guinea pig skins by topical applications of 0.5% glabridin. In our laboratory, the effects of other constituents of licorice extract were tested for their tyrosinase inhibitory activity using L-DOPA and L-tyrosine as substrates, and melanin biosynthesis using human melanocytes (66). Glabrene (IC_{50} = 16 μg/mL) proved to be active while hisp A and hisp B were not. The inactivity of hisp A could be attributed to the presence of the isoprenyl groups, which may prevent interaction with the enzyme owing to the steric effect. The inactivity of hisp B may be due to the absence of two free hydroxyl groups at positions 2′ and 4′, as was found in glabridin. The importance of both hydroxyl groups is supported by the inactivation of the 2′-*O*-MeG and 4′-*O*-MeG.

IX. SUMMARY

Although licorice has been known to be a useful medicinal plant for the past 3000 years, it is still luring investigators to explore new medicinal properties of this plant. In a separate chapter, Aviram et al. review the therapeutic effects of licorice extract and its major antioxidant constituents of glabridin on atherosclerosis via inhibition of the LDL oxidation molecular mechanism. The second part of the chapter reviews the potential of licorice extract and its constituents as HRT for postmenopausal women. The licorice extract and its constituents were found to bind to estrogen receptors, affect endothelial and smooth muscle cells known to have a role in cardiovascular diseases, inhibit a decrease in bone mass, affect the expression of estrogen receptors α and β, and inhibit serotonin reuptake, which may be beneficial for reducing postmenopausal hot flashes and depression. In the last part of the chapter, the depigmentation effect of the licorice extract and its constituents via the inhibition of tyrosinase, the major enzyme in the biosynthesis of melanin, is discussed.

Are the above activities just random phenomena or do they have something in common? The inhibition of LDL oxidation, the estrogen agonistic activities, and the inhibition of serotonin reuptake may all be related to the antioxidant properties of the extract and its constituents (see references in Aviram chapter). Antioxidants are known to increase LDL susceptibility and prevent atherosclerosis, and are potential therapeutic agents for ROS/RNS-related diseases (67). All of the phytoestrogens known in the literature (lignans, coumestans, isoflavones, and isoflavans) have antioxidant activity, including the female hormone, the estradiol itself (68). The molecular mechanism that relates the antioxidant activity of a compound to its estrogen-like activity is not yet clear. A possible mechanism that relates antioxidants to phytoestrogens may result from the known effects of antioxidants on the level and type of ROS/RNS associated with the induction of ERs (13,69). The molecular relationship between serotonin reuptake and antioxidant activity is unclear and has been only slightly investigated (70). The natural serotonin reuptake inhibitors that were found in our laboratory are isoflavans, which are also known to be antioxidants.

The relationship between tyrosinase inhibitors and antioxidants may be explained by the fact that many of the tyrosinase inhibitors contain phenolic hydroxyl(s) (hydroquinone, resveratrol derivatives, galic acid), which is one of the main features of antioxidant activity (donation of an electron or hydrogen atom) (71). The other group of tyrosinase inhibitors are able to form complexes with transition metal ions such as copper ion (oxalic acid, kojic acid), an additional mechanism by which antioxidants may exert their activity. Tyrosinase is an enzyme containing copper ions in its active site, and one of the suggested mechanisms for its inhibition is by chelating the ion. Antioxidants or compounds with redox properties can prevent or delay pigmentation by different mechanisms: by scavenging reactive oxygen and nitrogen species (ROS and RNS), known to induce melanin synthesis (72), or by reducing *o*-quinones or other intermediates in the melanin biosynthesis, and thus delaying oxidative polymerization (73).

The chemical structure of isoflavans found to be important in all of the biological activities tested—inhibition of LDL oxidation, binding to ERs, effect on human breast cancer cell proliferation, inhibition of serotonin reuptake and tyrosinase inhibition—is the presence of free hydroxyl at the 2′ position of ring B. Additional knowledge of structure-activity relationships between natural compounds and their specific bioactivity could shed some light on the mechanisms by which these compounds manifest different activities in different target cells, and may contribute to the development of novel therapeutic treatment strategies. In the case of estrogen-like compounds, this knowledge will contribute to the design and development of new HRT agents that have beneficial effects on bone and cardiovascular tissue and block the deleterious effect of estrogen on breast and uterus cancer.

REFERENCES

1. Korach KS. Insights from the study of animals lacking functional estrogen receptor. Science 1994; 266:1524–1527.
2. Barton D, Loprinzi C, Wahner-Roedler D. Hot flashes: aetiology and management. Drugs Aging 2001; 18:597–606.
3. Seed M. Sex hormones, lipoproteins, and cardiovascular risk. Atherosclerosis 1991; 90:1–7.
4. Iafrati MD, Karas RH, Aronovitz M, Kim S, Sullivan TR Jr, Lubahn DB, O'Donnell TF Jr, Korach KS, Mendelsohn ME. Estrogen inhibits the vascular injury response in estrogen receptor alpha-deficient mice. Nat Med 1997; 3:545–548.
5. Sourander L, Rajala T, Raiha I, Makinen J, Erkkola R, Helenius H. Cardiovascular and cancer morbidity and mortality and sudden cardiac death in postmenopausal women on oestrogen replacement therapy (ERT). Lancet 1998; 352: 1965–1969.
6. Stampfer MJ, Colditz GA, Willett WC, Manson JE, Rosner B, Speizer FE, Hennekens CH. Postmenopausal estrogen therapy and cardiovascular disease: ten-year follow-up from the nurses' health study. N Engl J Med 1991; 325:756–762.
7. Shewmon DA, Stock JL, Rosen CJ, Heiniluoma KM, Hogue MM, Morrison A, Doyle EM, Ukena T, Weale V, Baker S. Tamoxifen and estrogen lower circulating lipoprotein(a) concentrations in healthy postmenopausal women. Arterioscler Thromb 1994; 14:1586–1593.
8. Herrington DM, Reboussin DM, Brosnihan KB, Sharp PC, Shumaker SA, Snyder TE, Furberg CD, Kowalchuk GJ, Stuckey TD, Rogers WJ, Givens DH, Waters D. Effects of estrogen replacement on the progression of coronary-artery atherosclerosis. N Engl J Med 2000; 343:522–529.
9. Rossouw JE, Anderson GL, Prentice RL, LaCroix AZ, Kooperberg C, Stefanick ML, Jackson RD, Beresford SA, Howard BV, Johnson KC, Kotchen JM, Ockene J. Risks and benefits of estrogen plus progestin in healthy postmenopausal women: principal results from the Women's Health Initiative randomized controlled trial. JAMA 2002; 288:321–333.
10. Ettinger B, Genant HK, Cann CE. Long-term estrogen replacement therapy prevents bone loss and fractures. Ann Intern Med 1985; 102:319–324.
11. Russo IH, Russo J. Role of hormones in mammary cancer initiation and progression. J Mammary Gland Biol Neoplasia 1998; 3:49–61.
12. Katzenellenbogen BS, Sun J, Harrington WR, Kraichely DM, Ganessunker D, Katzenellenbogen JA. Structure-function relationships in estrogen receptors and the characterization of novel selective estrogen receptor modulators with unique pharmacological profiles. Ann NY Acad Sci 2001; 949:6–15.

13. Tamir S, Izrael S, Vaya J. The effect of oxidative stress on ERalpha and ERbeta expression. J Steroid Biochem Mol Biol 2002; 81:323–332.
14. Horwitz KB, Jackson TA, Bain DL, Richer JK, Takimoto GS, Tung L. Nuclear receptor coactivators and corepressors. Mol Endocrinol 1996; 10:1167–1177.
15. Smith CL, Nawaz Z, O'Malley BW. Coactivator and corepressor regulation of the agonist/antagonist activity of the mixed antiestrogen, 4-hydroxytamoxifen. Mol Endocrinol 1997; 11:657–666.
16. Pritchard KI. Breast cancer prevention with selective estrogen receptor modulators: a perspective. Ann NY Acad Sci 2001; 949:89–98.
17. Somjen D, Waisman A, Kaye AM. Tissue selective action of tamoxifen methiodide, raloxifene and tamoxifen on creatine kinase B activity in vitro and in vivo. J Steroid Biochem Mol Biol 1996; 59:389–396.
18. Yang NN, Bryant HU, Hardikar S, Sato M, Galvin RJ, Glasebrook AL, Termine JD. Estrogen and raloxifene stimulate transforming growth factor-beta 3 gene expression in rat bone: a potential mechanism for estrogen- or raloxifene-mediated bone maintenance. Endocrinology 1996; 137:2075–2084.
19. Egner U, Heinrich N, Ruff M, Gangloff M, Mueller-Fahrnow A, Wurtz JM. Different ligands-different receptor conformations: modeling of the hER alpha LBD in complex with agonists and antagonists. Med Res Rev 2001; 21:523–539.
20. Wiese TE, Polin LA, Palomino E, Brooks SC. Induction of the estrogen specific mitogenic response of MCF-7 cells by selected analogues of estradiol-17 beta: a 3D QSAR study. J Med Chem 1997; 40:3659–3669.
21. Sadler BR, Cho SJ, Ishaq KS, Chae K, Korach KS. Three-dimensional quantitative structure-activity relationship study of nonsteroidal estrogen receptor ligands using the comparative molecular field analysis/cross-validated r2-guided region selection approach. J Med Chem 1998; 41:2261–2267.
22. Grese TA, Cho S, Finley DR, Godfrey AG, Jones CD, Lugar CW 3rd, Martin MJ, Matsumoto K, Pennington LD, Winter MA, Adrian MD, Cole HW, Magee DE, Phillips DL, Rowley ER, Short LL, Glasebrook AL, Bryant HU. Structure-activity relationships of selective estrogen receptor modulators: modifications to the 2-arylbenzothiophene core of raloxifene. J Med Chem 1997; 40:146–167.
23. Shiau AK, Barstad D, Loria PM, Cheng L, Kushner PJ, Agard DA, Greene GL. The structural basis of estrogen receptor/coactivator recognition and the antagonism of this interaction by tamoxifen. Cell 1998; 95:927–937.
24. Cassidy A, Bingham S, Carson J, Setchell KDR. Biological effects of plant estrogens in premenopausal women. FASEB J 1993; 7(3 Pt II):5000.
25. Tham DM, Gardner CD, Haskell WL. Clinical review 97: Potential health benefits of dietary phytoestrogens: a review of the clinical, epidemiological, and mechanistic evidence. J Clin Endocrinol Metab 1998; 83:2223–2235.
26. Liggins J, Grimwood R, Bingham SA. Extraction and quantification of lignan phytoestrogens in food and human samples. Anal Biochem 2000; 287:102–109.
27. Wiseman H. The therapeutic potential of phytoestrogens. Expert Opin Invest Drugs 2000; 9:1829–1840.
28. Vaya J, Belinky PA, Aviram M. Antioxidant constituents from licorice roots: isolation, structure elucidation and antioxidative capacity toward LDL oxidation. Free Rad Biol Med 1997; 23:302–313.

29. Lee HP, Gourley L, Duffy SW, Esteve J, Lee J, Day NE. Dietary effects on breast-cancer risk in Singapore [see comments]. Lancet 1991; 337:1197–1200.
30. Fournier DB, Erdman JW Jr, Gordon GB. Soy, its components, and cancer prevention: a review of the in vitro, animal, and human data. Cancer Epidemiol Biomarkers Prev 1998; 7:1055–1065.
31. Valente M, Bufalino L, Castiglione GN, D'Angelo R, Mancuso A, Galoppi P, Zichella L. Effects of 1-year treatment with ipriflavone on bone in postmenopausal women with low bone mass. Calcif Tissue Int 1994; 54:377–380.
32. Arena S, Rappa C, Del Frate E, Cenci S, Villani C. A natural alternative to menopausal hormone replacement therapy: phytoestrogens. Minerva Ginecol 2002; 54:53–57.
33. Zava DT, Blen N, Duwe G. Estrogenic activity of natural and synthetic estrogens in human breast cancer cells in culture. Environ Health Perspect 1997; 105(suppl 3):637–645.
34. Bingham SA, Atkinson C, Liggins J, Bluck L, Coward A. Phyto-oestrogens: where are we now? Br J Nutr 1998; 79:393–406.
35. Zava DT, Dollbaum CM, Blen M. Estrogen and progestin bioactivity of foods, herbs, and spices. Proc Soc Exp Biol Med 1998; 217:369–378.
36. Liu J, Burdete JE, Xu H, Gu C, van Breemen RB, Bhat KP, Booth N, Constantinou AI, Pezzuto JM, Fong HH, Farnsworth NR, Bolton JL. Evaluation of estrogenic activity of plant extracts for the potential treatment of menopausal symptoms. J Agric Food Chem 2001; 49:2472–2479.
37. Rafi MM, Rosen RT, Vassil A, Ho CT, Zhang H, Ghai G, Lambert G, DiPaola RS. Modulation of bcl-2 and cytotoxicity by licochalcone-A, a novel estrogenic flavonoid. Anticancer Res 2000; 20:2653–2658.
38. Tamir S, Eizenberg M, Somjen D, Izrael S, Vaya J. Estrogen-like activity of glabrene and other constituents isolated from licorice root. J Steroid Biochem Mol Biol 2001; 78:291–298.
39. Malnick SD, Shaer A, Soreq H, Kaye AM. Estrogen-induced creatine kinase in the reproductive system of the immature female rat. Endocrinology 1983; 113: 1907–1909.
40. Somjen D, Waisman A, Weisman J, Kaye AM. Nonhypercalcemic analogs of vitamin D stimulate creatine kinase B activity in osteoblast-like ROS 17/2.8 cells and up-regulate their responsiveness to estrogens. Steroids 1998; 63:340–343.
41. Kimura Y, Okuda T, Okuda H. Effects of flavonoids from licorice roots (*Glycyrrhiza inflata* Bat.) on arachidonic acid metabolism and aggregation in human platelets. Phyt Res 1993; 7:341–347.
42. Saitoh T, Kinoshita T. New isoflavane and flavanone from licorice root. Chem Pharm Shibata, S Bull 1976; 24:752–755.
43. Mitscher LA, Park YH, Clark D, Beal JL. Antimicrobial agents from higher plants: antimicrobial isoflavonoids and related substances from *Glycyrrhiza glabra* L. var. typica. J Nat Prod 1980; 43:259–269.
44. Tamir S, Eizenberg M, Somjen D, Stern N, Shelach R, Kaye A, Vaya J. Estrogenic and antiproliferative properties of glabridin from licorice in human breast cancer cells. Cancer Res 2000; 60:5704–5709.

45. Wang C, Kurzer MS. Phytoestrogen concentration determines effects on DNA synthesis in human breast cancer cells. Nutr Cancer 1997; 28:236–247.
46. Gehm BD, McAndrews JM, Chien PY, Jameson JL. Reveratrol, a polyphenolic compound found in grapes and wine, is an agonist for the estrogen receptor. Proc Natl Acad Sci USA 1997; 94:14138–14143.
47. Breinholt V, Larsen JC. Detection of weak estrogenic flavonoids using a recombinant yeast strain and a modified MCF7 cell proliferation assay. Chem Res Toxicol 1998; 11:622–629.
48. Hsieh CY, Santell RC, Haslam SZ, Helferich WG. Estrogenic effects of genistein on the growth of estrogen receptor-positive human breast cancer (MCF-7) cells in vitro and in vivo [published erratum appears in Cancer Res 1999 Mar 15; 59(6):1388]. Cancer Res 1998; 58:3833–3838.
49. Somjen D, Kohen F, Jaffe A, Amir-Zaltsman Y, Knoll E, Stern N. Effects of gonadal steroids and their antagonists on DNA synthesis in human vascular cells. Hypertension 1998; 32:39–45.
50. Vaya J, Tamir S. The relation between the chemical structure of flavonoids and their estrogen-like activities. Curr Med Chem. In press.
51. Brzozowsk AM, Pike AC, Dauter Z, Hubbard RE, Bonn T, Engstrom O, Ohman L, Greene GL, Gustafsson JA, Carlquist M. Molecular basis of agonism and antagonism in the oestrogen receptor. Nature 1997; 389:753–758.
52. Zhou JR, Mukherjee P, Gugger ET, Tanaka T, Blackburn GL, Clinton SK. Inhibition of murine bladder tumorigenesis by soy isoflavones via alterations in the cell cycle, apoptosis, and angiogenesis. Cancer Res 1998; 58:5231–5238.
53. Peterson G, Barnes S. Genistein inhibits both estrogen and growth factor-stimulated proliferation of human breast cancer cells. Cell Growth Differ 1996; 7:1345–1351.
54. Shao ZM, Alpaugh ML, Fontana JA, Barsky SH. Genistein inhibits proliferation similarly in estrogen receptor-positive and negative human breast carcinoma cell lines characterized by P21WAF1/CIP1 induction, G2/M arrest, and apoptosis. J Cell Biochem 1998; 69:44–54.
55. Shao ZM, Wu J, Shen ZZ, Barsky SH. Genistein exerts multiple suppressive effects on human breast carcinoma cells. Cancer Res 1998; 58:4851–4857.
56. Archer JS. NAMS/Solvay Resident Essay Award. Relationship between estrogen, serotonin, and depression. Menopause 1999; 6:71–78.
57. Avis NE, Crawford S, Stellato R, Longcope C. Longitudinal study of hormone levels and depression among women transitioning through menopause. Climacteric 2001; 4:243–249.
58. Fuller RW. Uptake inhibitors increase extracellular serotonin concentration measured by brain microdialysis. Life Sci 1994; 55:163–167.
59. Barker EL, Blakely RD. Norepinephrine and serotonin transporter: molecular targets of antidepressant drugs. In: Bloom FE, Kupfer DJ, eds. Psychopharmacology: The Fourth Generation of Progress. New York: Raven, 1995:321–333.
60. Fozzard J. Peripheral actions of 5-hydroxytryptamine. In: Fozzard J. ed. Peripheral Actions of 5-Hydroxytryptamine. New York: Oxford University Press, 1989.

61. Chang AS, Chang SM. Nongenomic steroidal modulation of high-affinity serotonin transport. Biochim Biophys Acta 1999; 1417:157–166.
62. Ofir R, Tamir S, Khatib S, Vaya J. Inhibition of serotonin reuptake by licorice constituents. J Mol Neurosci 2003; 20:135–140.
63. Seiberg M, Paine C, Sharlow E, Andrade-Gordon P, Costanzo M, Eisinger M, Shapiro SS. Inhibition of melanosome transfer results in skin lightening. J Invest Dermatol 2000; 115:162–167.
64. Seiberg M, Paine C, Sharlow E, Andrade-Gordon P, Costanzo M, Eisinger M, Shapiro SS. The protease-activated receptor 2 regulates pigmentation via keratinocyte-melanocyte interactions. Exp Cell Res 2000; 254:25–32.
65. Yokota T, Nishio H, Kubota Y, Mizoguchi M. The inhibitory effect of glabridin from licorice extracts on melanogenesis and inflammation. Pigment Cell Res 1998; 11:355–361.
66. Nerya O, Vaya J, Musa R, Izrael S, Ben-Arie R, Tamir S. Glabrene and isoliquiritigenin as tyrosinase inhibitors from licorice roots. J Agric Food Chem 2003; 51:1201–1207.
67. Castro L, Freeman BA. Reactive oxygen species in human health and disease. Nutrition 2001; 17:161, 163–165.
68. Yen CH, Hsieh CC, Chou SY, Lau YT. 17Beta-estradiol inhibits oxidized low density lipoprotein-induced generation of reactive oxygen species in endothelial cells. Life Sci 2001; 70:403–413.
69. Hensley K, Robinson KA, Gabbita SP, Salsman S, Floyd RA. Reactive oxygen species, cell signaling, and cell injury. Free Rad Biol Med 2000; 28:1456–1462.
70. Jiang XR, Wrona MZ, Dryhurst G. Tryptamine-4,5-dione, a putative endotoxic metabolite of the superoxide-mediated oxidation of serotonin, is a mitochondrial toxin: possible implications in neurodegenerative brain disorders. Chem Res Toxicol 1999; 12:429–436.
71. Kubo I, Kinst-Hori I, Kubo Y, Yamagiwa Y, Kamikawa T, Haraguchi H. Molecular design of antibrowning agents. J Agric Food Chem 2000; 48:1393–1399.
72. Seo SY, Sharma VK, Sharma N. Mushroom tyrosinase: recent prospects. J Agric Food Chem 2003; 51:2837–2853.
73. Karg E, Odh G, Wittbjer A, Rosengren E, Rorsman H. Hydrogen peroxide as an inducer of elevated tyrosinase level in melanoma cells. J Invest Dermatol 1993; 100:209S–213S.
74. Kinoshita T, Tamura Y. Chemical studies on *Glycyrrhiza glabra* (licorice): isolation of two new 3-arylcoumarins and revised structure of an isoflav-3-ene glabrene. Nat Prod Lett 1997; 9:289–296.

29

Protection of Oxidative Brain Injury by Chinese Herbal Medicine

Shengmai San as a Model Formula for Antioxidant-Based-Compounds Therapy of Oxidative Stress-Related Diseases

Tetsuya Konishi, Haruyo Ichikawa, and Hiroshi Nishida

Niigata University of Pharmacy and Applied Life Sciences
Niigata, Japan

XueJiang Wang

Capital University of Medical Sciences
Beijing, China

I. INTRODUCTION

Oxidative stress is implicated in many diseases related to lifestyle and aging. Therefore, antioxidant protection attracts much attention against these diseases (1–3). The brain is essentially vulnerable against oxidative abuse because of its poor anitoxidant defense including low level of antioxidant small molecules and also antioxidant enzymes (4). Moreover, the tissue is rich in sensitive cellular components toward oxidative abuse such as polyunsaturated fatty acids and catecholamine. Indeed accumulated oxidative injury of cellular components results in many brain disorders including Alzheimer's and Parkinson's diseases. Therefore, protection of cerebral oxidative injury is important for the quality of life in our society. The antioxidant approach is attractive for the treatment of cerebral disorders including dementia, and many trials have been reported to prevent cerebral oxidative tissue injury using natural and artificial small antioxidants such as vitamins E, lazaroid, and lipoic acid, as well as antioxidant enzymes (5–7).

However, this approach is complicated, because the tissue-damaging process initiated by free radicals is not simple but involves several complex steps such as Ca^{2+} release in cytoplasm, membrane potential dissipation, free iron release, etc. (1). At the same time, the cellular repair system operates to prevent further progression of tissue injury. In this sense, combination therapy would be a more promising approach to treat these complex pathological conditions in that prevention and repair of radical-initiated tissue damages are modulated by the combined effects of antioxidants and other components in a complex formula that modulates cellular function.

II. TRADITIONAL CHINESE HERBAL MEDICINE AS A MODEL OF ANTIOXIDANT-BASED-COMPOUNDS FORMULA

In this sense, traditional Chinese herbal medicine (TCM) is interesting because herbs have been used to treat many complex disorders such as diabete mellitus, cancer, and others for which Western medicine may not have an appropriate diagnostic name. TCM is usually prescribed with several herbal constituents having different functions and the synergistic action exhibited by the multicomponent formula is effective for the management of many complicated diseases (8). Moreover, their therapeutic strategy is modulation of the inherent potential to recover the distorted balance of the physical condition (disease condition) by either suppressing or stimulating physiological reactions with a multifunctional-compound formula comprising several herbal components. It is also known that free-radical or reactive oxygen species (ROS) are exclusively involved in the pathogenesis of such disorders for which the Chinese herbal medicines are effectively applied. Therefore, antioxidant TCM is an attractive model for study of the antioxidant-based-compounds therapy of disorders related to oxidative stress. In this chapter, we discuss results obtained in the study of the preventive effect of Shengmai San (SMS), a traditional Chinese herbal prescription, on cerebral oxidative injury in rats.

III. ANTIOXIDANT POTENTIAL OF SMS DETERMINED IN VITRO

SMS, a famous Chinese medicinal formula that has been used for more than 800 years in China, is comprised of three herbal components, *Panax ginseng*, *Shisandra chinensis*, and *Ophiopogon japonicus* (9). Traditionally, SMS is used for the treatment of excess loss of essence qi and body fluid that threatens heart failure. It can restore blood volume and prevent myocardial infarction. SMS is also prescribed for patients with coronary heart disease and various cardiovascular disorders.

Ancient TCM theory states that the physical condition of the human body is controlled by the interaction of five elemental organs, heart, liver, kidney, lung, and spleen, although the nature of these organs is not the same as understood in Western medicine. The brain was not classified in the five elemental organs but its function is considered strictly related to liver, kidney, and heart functions. Therefore, it is worth examining protective effects on cerebral oxidative damage by TCM prescriptions that have been used for treating complex diseases, especially related to heart, lung, or kidney failure. In this sense, it is interesting to study the effect of SMS on cerebral oxidative injury.

We first examined the antioxidant property of SMS by five different antioxidant assays in vitro and the antioxidant activity was compared using Trolox as the reference antioxidant in each antioxidant assays. (Table 1). Interestingly, SMS was found to have extremely strong hydroxyl-radical-scavenging activity. This characteristic was emphasized when the antioxidant activity was compared with those determined for four typical TCM or Kampo (Japanese traditional herbal prescriptions) formulations that have been tested for post stroke treatment or dementia: Cho-To-San, Zokumei-To, Ryou-Kei-Jutsu-Kan-To, and Keishi-Bukuryo-Gan + Yokuinin. All these prescriptions commonly had stronger scavenging activity toward superoxide radical than

TABLE 1 Antioxidant Potential of SMS as Trolox Equivalent Determined by Several In Vitro Assay Systems

Antioxidant assay	SMS IC_{20} as Trolox equivalent (μM)
TBARS formation	5
DPPH quenching	3.2
Crocin bleaching test	1.1
Superoxide radical scavenging	200
Hydroxyl radical scavenging	0.4

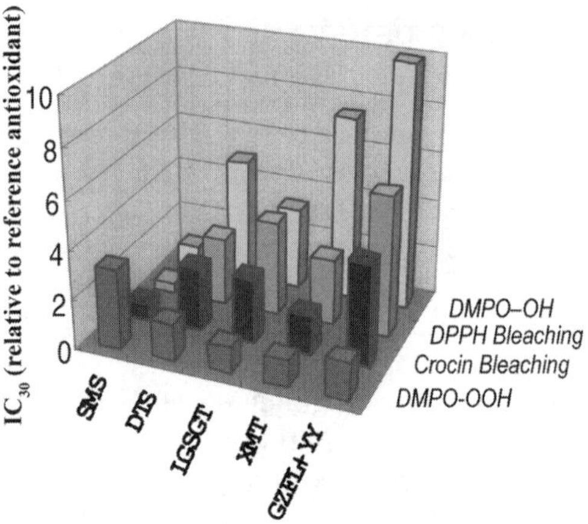

FIGURE 1 Relative antioxidant activity of brain-directed TCM formulations. SMS, Shengmai San; DTS, Cho-To-San; LGSGT, Rei-Kei-Jutsu-Kan-To; XMT, Zokumei-To; GZFL + YY, Keishi-Bukuryou-Gan + Yokuinin.

to other radicals but SMS did not. In contrast, SMS had strong hydroxyl-radical-scavenging potential (Fig. 1).

IV. PREVENTION OF CEREBRAL OXIDATIVE INJURY PRODUCED BY ISCHEMIA REPERFUSION BY SMS

When the SMS was administered to rats either before or after cerebral ischemia reperfusion, oxidative damage in the brain was markedly prevented as evaluated by two biochemical indications, thiobarbiturate reactive substance (TBARS) formation and glutathione peroxidase (GPX) activity (10,11).

The same protective effect of SMS was shown against brain oxidative damage in mice as well as in rats. Figure 2 shows the preventive effect of SMS on brain oxidative injury induced by ischemia reperfusion in C57BL/6 mice. The mice were administered SMS directly into the duodenum 2 hr before ischemia produced by the occlusion of both right and left common carotid arteries exposed through a middle skin incision for 85 min. At the end of the ischemic period, carotid arteries were declamped to allow blood reperfusion for 45 min. The both TBARS formation and GPX activity were measured in isolated brain homogenate. After the ischemia reperfusion, TBARS formation was increased to approximately 260% of untreated control but the formation was almost completely inhibited by the administration of SMS

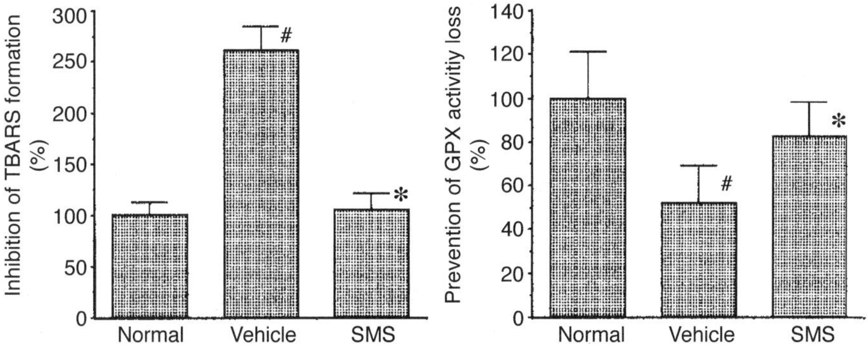

FIGURE 2 Inhibitory effects of SMS on TBARS formation and GPX activity loss in mouse brain after ischemia-reperfusion.

prior to ischemia treatment. GPX activity, on the other hand, decreased to approximately 46% of vehicle control after ischemia reperfusion but this decline was also effectively prevented by SMS preadministration (recovered to 84% of control). This SMS effect was completely dose-dependent for both the inhibition of TBARS formation and GPX activity loss; furthermore, TTC (2,3,5-trimethyl tetrazolium chloride) staining of the brain slices confirmed the preventive effect of SMS on cerebral oxidative injury caused by ischemia reperfusion (11) (Fig. 3). Recently, we also studied the effect of SMS on

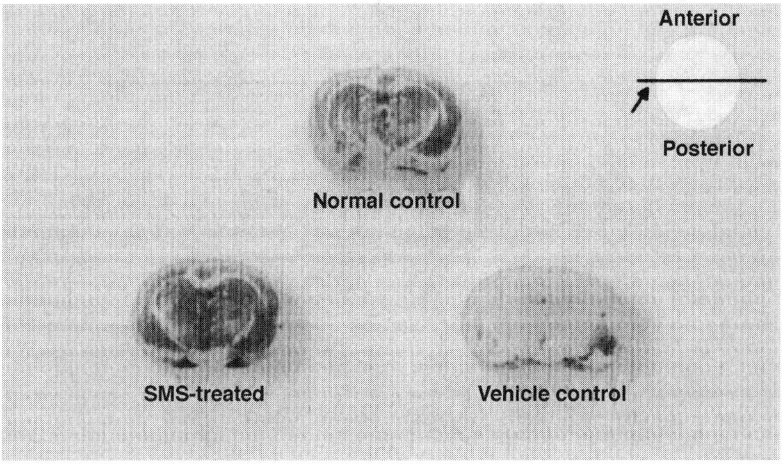

FIGURE 3 Protective effect of SMS against cerebral ischemia-reperfusion injury in rats evaluated by TTC staining.

cerebral oxidative damage caused by MPTP (1-methyl-4-phenyl-1,2,3,6-tetrahydropyridine) administration in a Parkinson's disease model in mice and found that the oxidative injury in the substantia nigra was sufficiently inhibited by orally administered SMS (12).

V. SMS MODULATES CELLULAR ANTIOXIDANT POTENTIAL THROUGH INDUCTION OF GPX

GPX is an enzyme participating in the capture of H_2O_2 and hydroperoxides produced in the cell. Therefore, the change in the activity reflects more or less overall tissue damage or cellular potential of antioxidant defense. Thus the preventive effect of SMS on GPX activity loss was further studied by the immunohistchemical method in culture cells using anti-GPX monoclonal antibody conjugated with FITC fluoroprobe. As shown in Figure 4, GPX activity was significantly induced by incubating cells with SMS prior to H_2O_2 stress, although H_2O_2 also induced GPX, as was reported elsewhere (13). This SMS-dependent enhancement of GPX activity was also confirmed by RT-

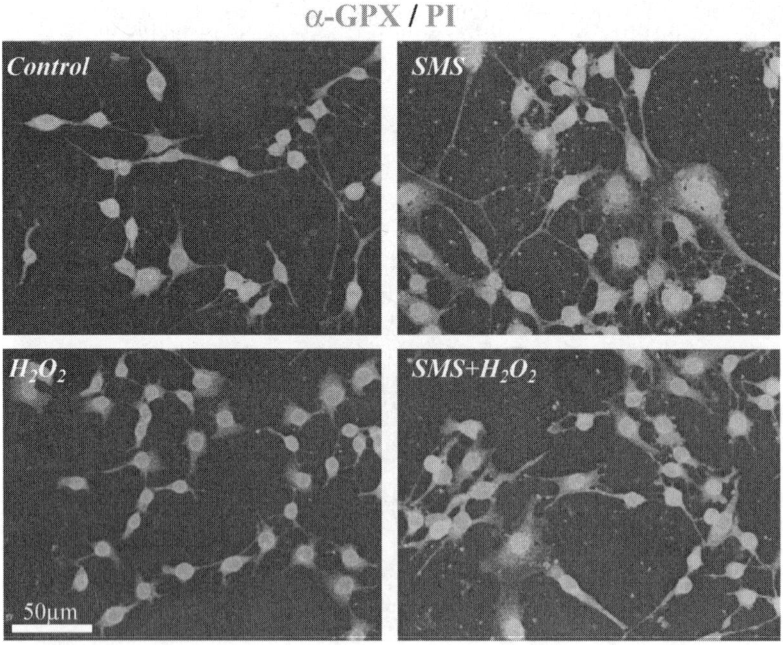

FIGURE 4 SMS and H_2O_2-dependent expression of GPX. PI stain for nucleus; α-GPX stain for GPX.

PCR at the transcriptional level (unpublished data), indicating that the protective action of SMS against oxidative abuse in the brain is due not only to its strong hydroxyl-radical-scavenging activity but also to its role as cell functional modulator.

VI. CONCLUSION

Our recent studies reveled that the component herbs in SMS contributing to the antioxidant property and GPX preservation are *Shisandra* and *Ophiopogon*, respectively. Ginseng seems to act as organizer in this formula (11,14). Although the importance of *Shisandra* as antioxidant has been suggested elesewhere (15,16) as well as in our study, the antioxidant property of other components in SMS are still in discussion. On the other hand, previous studies indicated that ginseng saponins improve brain functions such as learning ability or dementia (17). Thus it is not unexpected that SMS was active in preventing oxidative damage in the brain, as shown above, although it was primarily prescribed for treating coronal heart failure by replenishing the qi (vital energy), stimulating the pulse, and stimulating the circulation of body fluids. Further analysis of the functional roles of each component herb and their synergism will help our understanding of the basic principle underlying the mechanism of action of the complex herbal formula suitable for prevention and repair of cerebral oxidative injury.

We have also reported the similar protective effect of another TCM formula, Qizhu Tang (QZT), on cerebral oxidative injury in rats, which comprises four herbal components, *Rhizoma atractyloidis*, *Poria*, *Radix notoginseng*, and *Radix astragali* (18). QZT was traditionally prescribed for treating syndromes related to qi depression in the spleen and stomach, and is also used for enhancing the immune system of the body. Although the herbal composition of QZT is completely different from SMS, QZT was found to have the same strong hydroxyl-radical-scavenging activity as SMS (18). It is thus accurate to say that reevaluation of hydroxyl-radical-scavenging activity of the TCM formulations prescribed for qi stimulation will be important to find the model formula for antioxidant-based-compounds therapy of brain oxidative stress.

REFERENCES

1. Liu J, Mori A. Stress, aging, and brain oxidative damage. Neurochem Res 1999; 24:1479–1497.
2. Laight DWM, Carrier J, Anggard EE. Antioxidants, diabetes and endothelial dysfunction. Cardiovasc Res 2000; 47:457–464.

3. Halliwell B. Reactive oxygen species and the central nervous system. J Neurochem 1992; 59(5):1609–1623.
4. Buoonocore G, Perrone S, Bracci R. Free radicals and brain damage in the newborn. Biol Neonate 2001; 79:180–186.
5. Behl C. Vitamin E and other antioxidants in neuroprotection. Int J Vitam Nutr Res 1999; 69:213–219.
6. Hall ED, Pazara EK, Braughler JM. Nonsteroidal lazaroid U78517F in models of focal and global ischemia. Stroke 1990; 21:III83–III87.
7. Halliwell B, Gutteridge JMC. Lipid peroxidation, oxygen radicals, cell damage and antioxidant therapy. Lancet 1984; 1:1396–1398.
8. Cheng J-T. Review: Drug therapy in Chinese traditional medicine. J Clin Pharmacol 2000; 40:445–450.
9. Rong Y, Wen W, Fu L, Han Y. Protective effect of Sheng Mai San on adriamycin-induced cardiotoxicity—an experimental study. J Shanghai Second Med Univ 1989; 3:39–43.
10. Wang X-J, Magara T, Konishi T. Prevention and repair of cerebral ischemia-reperfusion injury by Chinese herbal medicine. Shengmai San, in rats. Free Rad Res 1999; 31:449–455.
11. Ichikawa H, Konishi T. In vitro antioxidant potentials of traditional Chinese medicine, Shengmai San and their relation to in vivo protective effect on cerebral oxidative damage in rats. Biol Pharm Bull 2002; 25:898–903.
12. Bin Xu, Konishi T, Traditional Chinese medicine (TCM) protects against MPTP-induced oxidative damage in C57BL/6 mice. 123th Japan Pharm. Soc. Congress, 2002.
13. Rohrdanz E, Schmuck G, Ohler S, Tran-Thi Q-H, Kahl R. Changes in antioxidant enzyme expression in response to hydrogen peroxidase in rat astroglial cells. Arch Toxicol 2001; 75:150–158.
14. Ichikawa H, Wang X-J, Konishi T. Role of component herbs in antioxidant activity of Shengmai San, a traditional Chinese medicine preventing cerebral oxidative damage. Am J Chin Med 2003; 31:509–521.
15. Ko K-M, Y K-P, P K-M-T, Che C-T, Ng K-H, K Y-C. *Schisandra chinensis*–derived antioxidant activities in "Sheng Mai San," a compound formulation, in vivo and in vitro. Phytother Res 1995; 9:203–206.
16. Li PC, Poon MKT, Ko KM. *Schisandra chinensis*–dependent myocardial protective action of Sheng-Mai-San in rats. Am J Chin Med 1996; 24:255–262.
17. Gillis CN. *Panax ginseng* pharmacology: a nitric oxide link? Biochem Pharmacol 1997; 54:1–8.
18. Wang X-J, Ichikawa H, Konishi T. Antioxidant potential of Qizhu Tang, a Chinese herbal medicine, and the effect on cerebral oxidative damage after ischemia-reperfusion in rat. Biol Pharm Bull 2001; 24:558–563.

30

Eurycoma longifolia Jack (Tongkat Ali)

Hooi Hoon Ang
University Science Malaysia
Minden, Penang, Malaysia

I. TRADITIONAL MEDICINE

According to the World Health Organization (WHO), up to 80% of people in the developing world use traditional medicine as part of their primary health care, and therefore, it is becoming increasing popular in countries in the North, too. Traditional medicine incorporates plants, animals, and mineral-based medicines, spiritual therapies, as well as manual techniques or exercise (1).

In Ethiopia, 90% of the population uses traditional medicine for primary health care; in Benin, India, and Rwanda, the figure is 70%. However in the West, concern about the effects of chemical medicines and a need for more personalized health care and greater access to information about health promote the use of complementary and alternative medicines. The United Nations health agency said 70% of people in Canada, 49% in France, and 42% in the United States had used alternative medicine at least once. The global market for traditional therapies is US$60 billion (RM 228 billion) a year (1).

In Malaysia, the demand for herbs and plant-based medicines grew 450% to RM 4.5 billion in 2001 from RM 1 billion in 1998. Malaysia's sales of herbal-based products average about RM 1.5 billion a year, with most exports going to China, Indonesia, and India. Demand is growing at an annual rate of 20% with export value at RM 38 million in 1994 and RM 60 million in 1996 (2).

II. SIMAROUBACEAE

The Simaroubaceae, as defined in *Engler's Syllabus* (3), consist of six subfamilies with 32 genera and over 170 arboreous or shrubby species. The largest genus is *Picramnia* with ca. 40 species native to the New World tropics. Indeed the entire family is of pantropical occurrence with the exception of the genera *Picrasma* and *Ailanthus*, which extend to temperate Asia (4). The genera of Simaroubaceae are mostly well defined, but the family is only loosely knit (5). However, only eight genera and 10 species are found in Malaysia (6). An example of a plant found in Malaysia from this family is *Eurycoma longifolia* Jack and a detailed description of this tree is given (7,8).

III. HABITAT *E. LONGIFOLIA* JACK

E. longifolia Jack is a tall, slender shrub-tree, up to 10 m high, often unbranched with reddish-brown petioles (9). It is found on the acid (10) and sandy soil in primary and secondary, evergreen and mixed deciduous forests in Southeast Asia, viz. Burma, Indochina, Thailand, Malaysia, Indonesia, Borneo, and the Philippines. It inhabits the understory in the lowland forests at up to 500 m above sea level (6,11).

A. National Name

It is known as *tongkat Ali*, or Ali's walking stick, *penawar bisa*, or *bedara pahit* in Malaysia (12,13), *Pasak Bumi* in Indonesia (12,13), *Plalaiphuak* in Thailand (14), and *cay ba binh* (tree that cures hundreds of diseases) in Vietnam (15). In Vietnam, it is found in Bien-Hoa, Trang-Bom, and Dinh-Quan (16) and its bark is used in the Vietnamese pharmacopeia (15,16).

B. Uses Described in Folk Medicine

The bark is very bitter and is prescribed for indigestion, as a vermifuge, and it is used as a medication for lumbago in South Vietnam (15). In Cambodia, the roots are used as antidotal, and in jaundice, dropsy, and cachexia. The whole plant is very bitter and supposed to be a febrifuge (15). The fruits and flowers are antidysenteric (10,15).

In Malaysia, the roots are used to cure boils (10,17,18), wounds, ulcers (10,18,19), fever, as a tonic after birth (10,18), and for intestinal worms (10). They are also used as a paste to relieve headache (10), stomachache (10), pain caused by syphilis (10,19), and bleeding gums (10,20). In Sabah and Kalimantan, a decoction of the bark is drunk to relieve pain in the bones and a decoction of the leaves is used for washing itches (10).

In addition to the above uses described in folk medicine, this plant is a symbol of man's ego and strength because it has been claimed by the Malaysians to improve strength and power during sexual activities; it increases male virility and sexual prowess (11,13). It is usually taken as a decoction of the roots in water.

Thus, this tree has long captured the Malaysian market and currently, there are about 200 tongkat Ali products, most of them emphasizing its aphrodisiac properties (21). As such, the above claim has one way or another been responsible for the uncontrolled and excessive harvesting of the tree in the Malaysian jungles (22).

In Indonesia, people from Sumatra and Kalimantan also used the roots as an antipyretic; in Lampung and Belitung, it is used for dysentery. However, in Riau, people living in the surrounding forests drink a decoction of the roots or stems to cure malaria. Currently, it is mostly known as aphrodisiac (10). One of the most unique uses is by the Sakai ethnic group in Sumatra, which employs this tree as an amulet to protect people from the smallpox virus (10).

Furthermore, in Jambi and Riau, there is often much superstition pertaining to the harvesting of this plant or its parts. It is emphasized that harvesting must be conducted quietly and respectfully, and a failure to do so will result in loss of the plant's benefits. Thus, it is believed that the highest benefits will be obtained if the harvester's back is turned while he is pulling the tree (10).

IV. PRODUCTION OF TONGKAT ALI

It is found that this crop grows well in deep sandy loams mixed with plenty of organic matter. The plants are propagated usually from seeds (fresh seeds collected from tree burst fruits) that take about a week to germinate. The seedlings will then grow to a height of 10–15 cm after 2 months and at this stage, they can be removed from the nursery bed and potted, then later transferred to permanent positions when they are 6 months old. Intercropping tongkat Ali with other grown timber species is recommended especially in the early stages of growth to enhance its growth rate as the young plants cannot withstand full sunlight (14,21). It has been reported that in cultivation of tongkat Ali, the most susceptible pest is the caterpillar *Atteva scrodoxa* (21).

At present, researchers at FRIM (Forest Research Institute Malaysia), Kuala Lumpur, Malaysia are working on several methods of cultivating tongkat Ali. Tissue culture has several advantages, as it has been shown to produce taproots, unlike planting from cuttings, which tend to produce only fibrous roots, which do not contain the active ingredients (23).

A. Harvest

Tongkat Ali plants can be harvested after a period of at least 5 years. The whole plant is pulled out to obtain its taproot, which has medicinal values (14). The taproot is cylindrical, usually not branched, yellowish-white in color, and very bitter (9).

B. Postharvest Handling

Roots are collected and then other foreign substances are removed. They are thoroughly washed, cut into cylindrical segments, and dried in the sun (14).

V. SCIENTIFIC INVESTIGATIONS

A. Phytochemistry

The immense and diverse therapeutic uses described in folk medicine have prompted numerous scientists to carry out scientific investigations pertaining to both the phytochemistry and the biological effects of tongkat Ali, for the past 40 years.

Scientific investigations on this plant showed that it contains a series of quassinoids (16,24–45) that are responsible for the bitter taste, tirucallane-type triterpenes (36), squalene derivatives (46–48), biphenylneolignans (49), canthin-6-one (28,33,50), and β-carboline alkaloids (33,50).

One of the these scientific investigations revealed unique structural features with eurycolactone A (C_{18} quassinoid), which as a novel carbon framework, eurycolactone B (C_{18} quassinoid), which is the first halogenated quassinoid separated from plant sources, and eurycolactone C (C_{18} quassinoid), which is a quassinoid with an unusual structure having a lactone A ring (42).

A further extremely interesting and important feature of eurycolactones A–D is that these quassinoids were found to be very similar to two previously isolated quassinoids, laurycolactone B and 5,6-dehydroeurycomalactone. Therefore, some biosynthetic relationships among these six quassinoids were suggested (42,44).

An extremely interesting compound is eurycolactone A, which is apparently an intermediate key structure between C_{18} and C_{19} quassinoids.

Therefore, a possible biogenetic pathway for laurycolactone B and eurycolactones A–D from 5,6-dehydroeurycomalactone is speculated. 5,6-Dehydroeurycomalactone is oxidized to a triketone, which is then converted to an intermediate via a benzilic-acid-type rearrangement, which via oxidative decarboxylation produces laurycolactone B (42).

Methylation of the intermediate produces eurycolactone A, chlorination of laurycolactone B affords eurycolactone B, oxidation of laurycolactone B involving a Baeyer-Villiger-type rearrangement produces eurycolactone C and finally, hydrogenation of laurycolactone B produces eurycolactone D (42,44).

B. Biological Activities

So far, quassinoids from this plant have been reported to exhibit a wide range of activities in animals, both in vivo and in vitro (28,30–34,36–42,45,51,52).

Detailed investigations on this plant showed that some of the quassinoids, one of the major bioactive groups in this plant, had antimalarial activities against drug-resistant Malaysian and non-Malaysian *Plasmodium falciparum* isolates, and some were found to have favorable potency compared to chloroquine (28,30,32 33,41,45,51). Most of the above isolates were cultured in vitro following the method of Trager and Jensen (53,54).

In addition, some of the above quassinoids were found to have antiulcer (34), antipyretic (40), and antischistosomal (45) properties. In addition, some of these quassinoids, squalenes, and the tirucallane-type triterpenes had cytotoxicity activities against cancer cells (31,33,36–39,42,45–49).

In contrast, a recent investigation revealed that some of the above quassinoids had plant-growth-inhibitory activities (43) and this may be useful as a preliminary screening method for finding valuable quassinoids with medicinal activities (43).

Therefore, it is suggested that this plant has high medicinal values owing to the occurrence of a variety of quassinoids.

VI. TONGKAT ALI AND APHRODISIAC PROPERTY: FACT OR FOLKLORE?

The possibility of bioactive aphrodisiacs, substances that stimulate sexual desire and that may be derived from animals, minerals, and plants (55), has been attractive throughout recorded history and the passion of man since time immemorial.

Most of these ideas originated from the ancient belief in the therapeutic efficacy of "signature"—the notion that plants or animal organs resembling the genitalia would impart sexual powers. As such, among them are rhinoceros horn and reindeer antler, which have been extensively used by men to enhance sexual drive, based on the association between their shapes and the erect penis.

Reindeer shed their antlers annually; collected shedded antlers are imported from Canada, Finland, Norway, and Sweden into Japan for aphrodisiac purpose. Although the fresh antlers are supposed to be more powerful, removal of live antlers from the animals is forbidden in Scandinavia. Therefore, live reindeers have been imported to provide the best possible aphrodisiac quality (56).

Rhinoceros horn is considered a panacea in East Asia and the horns are widely used to increase male sexual capacity including the capacity for erection. Chemical analysis of powdered horn extracts reveals only polypeptides, sugars, phosphorus, ethanolamine, and free amino acids such as aspartic acid, threonine, ornithine, lysine, histidine, and arginine (which has been suggested to increase the intensity of sensation during sex) (57). Rhinoceros horn is, after all, only a modified epidermis.

Mylabris, an alcoholic extract from the dried bodies of China blister beetles (*Pan mao*), or Spanish fly (the generic name for a variety of species of beetles including *Cantharis vesicatoria*, *Lytta vesicatoria*, *Epicauta funebris*, and *Mylabris phalerata*), is used in China today as an aphrodisiac and to induce abortions. The active principle, called cantharidin, is a potent vesicant with an estimated fatal dose in humans of 32 mg. It causes irritation of the urethra, resulting in priapism (58).

Other popular aphrodisiacs include lion-tailed macaque (59), tiger penis, bear paws, and snake bile (60).

The study of plants exhibiting aphrodisiac property is becoming more important because of international pressure against the slaughter of animals since this eventually will cause many animals to become endangered or extinct.

Punica granatum has been a symbol of love, fertility, and immorality in Oriental regions (61). The yohimbine-rich bark of *Corynanthe yohimbe*, indigenous to West Africa, has been employed for centuries as an aphrodisiac (62). It contains the indole alkaloid, which has been used as a sexual stimulant for domestic animals and, more recently, to treat impotence in men (63–66).

Chelidonium majus, *Heracleum sphondylium*, and *Satureja montana* have been formulated into topical preparations by the European community for vaginal douches to increase sexual desire in women (67). Similarly, Hindu medicine still claims that *Aristolochia indica*, *Crocus sativus*, *Alpinia galanga*, and *Allium cepa* are potent aphrodisiacs (68).

In Malaysia, tongkat Ali has also gained notoriety as a male aphrodisiac and this has caused rampant, excessive, and uncontrolled encroachments into forest reserves. The raids have become so frequent and massive that the

Forestry Department in Malaysia is worried that the plant species may become extinct if immediate steps are not taken to stop the wanton uprooting (69).

Numerous scientific investigations pertaining to the aphrodisiac property of this plant have been exhaustively carried out using both the in vivo and in vitro animal models. However, the definitive criteria used to establish the aphrodisiac value of a compound still remain elusive. Nevertheless, it was found that higher erectile function observed in a treated animal provides evidence for responses and an increase in sexual pleasure (70).

Male sexual activity evaluation of the effect of this plant showed that in the absence of receptive females, sexually normal male rodents treated with various extracts of this plant did not exhibit any homosexuality during the observation period (71), unlike PCPA (*p*-chlorophenylalanine ester), which did lead to homosexuality (72). In addition, the treated male rodents exhibited increase in the penile erection index (71), using the methods previously described (73,74), in an observation cage (75).

In addition, the effects of this plant on the *pendiculation activities* (act of yawning and stretching) in the male rodents were studied following the method previously described (74), since it is pertinent that yawning, alone or associated with stretching, is considered to be an ancestral vestige surviving throughout evolution, which subserves the purpose of sexual arousal (76). Results showed that the extracts enhanced pendiculation activities in sexually normal male rodents (77) as well as in middle-aged, 9-month-old, retired breeder male rodents, but to a smaller degree (78). Thus, these results provided further evidence of erectile responses and increase in sexual pleasure (70).

The above interesting results led to further investigations on the *masculine copulatory behavior* of treated sexually normal (79) and middle-aged (80) male rodents in the presence of receptive females (81,82). Results showed that treated sexually normal male rodents exhibited increase in ejaculation latencies-1, -2, and -3 (79), thus suggesting that these extracts increased the sexual performance of the male rodents by extending the duration of coitus (83,84). In addition, the increase in the above three parameters and also decrease in both postejaculatory intervals -1 and -2 (79) led to the conclusion that these extracts intensified the sexual activity of the male rodents in a sustained manner by decreasing the refractory period between the different series of copulation. This was also observed in middle-aged rodents but to a smaller degree (80).

Further investigations were also carried out pertaining to the effect of this plant on the *libido* of sexually experienced male rodents. Sexual arousal or motivation with mount tests following penile anesthetization is a reliable index of pure libido unaffected by the reinforcing effect of genital sensation (85,86). Results showed that these extracts enhanced the libido of sexually experienced male rodents, providing evidence that this plant is a potent stimulator of sexual arousal in intact, sexually vigorous male rodents in the absence of feedback from genital sensation (87).

Further studies were also carried out pertaining to the *orientation activities* of the treated sexually experienced male rodents using the methods previously described (88,89) because modification of orientation activities is one of the criteria in determining male sexual behavior (88,90). Results showed that this plant enhanced the orientation activities of treated males toward receptive females by causing them to display vigorous anogenital investigatory behavior, and further intensified self-orientation as evidenced by increased grooming of their own genitalia (91). These improved the sexual performance of treated sexually experienced male rodents (84,92).

In addition, there was an *enhancement of the sexual motivation* in the treated sexually naïve male mice (93), middle-aged male rats (94), and noncopulator male rats (95).

Similarly, there was also a slow and transient reduction in the hesitation time before the treated sexually naïve male mice crossed the electrical grid (maintained at 0.12 mA) in the copulation cage to reach the goal cage, besides an increase in the percentage of sexually naïve male mice scoring "right choice" (goal cage with an estrous female mouse) throughout the investigation period (96). An electrical grid was used as an obstruction in the copulation cage to determine how much a negative stimulus (crossing an electrical grid) a male mouse was willing to overcome to reach the sexual contact. Similar results were obtained in sexually naïve male rats (97) and noncopulator male rats (98). *Longitudinal study* showed that these extracts were able to maintain sexual activity in aging rats (99).

Further results also indicated that these extracts promoted the *growth of accessory sexual organs*, viz. ventral prostate and seminal vesicles in the inexperienced castrated male rats (100), penis in the sexually experienced castrated male rats (101), levator ani muscle in both the uncastrated and testosterone-stimulated castrated intact male rats (102).

Potency activity of the aphrodisiac property was also evaluated in male rats treated with these extracts. Results showed that these extracts produced a dose-dependent, recurrent, and significant increase in the episodes of penile reflexes as evidenced by increase in quick flips, long flips, and erections during the observation period (103).

Other scientific investigators pursued the study of the aphrodisiac effects of aqueous extract of the roots in male rodents and found that they showed intense copulatory behavior and a 480% increase in the serum testosterone (104,105).

In addition, the *sperm quality and parameters* were also investigated after the rodents were dosed with extracts from this plant (106,107). Results showed that there was a significant increase in the total sperm count, motility, forward velocity, and fructose concentration in the cauda epididymal semen, which were probably due to an increase of androgen, caused by the proandrogenic effect of these extracts, which enhanced the physiological maturation of sperms (107).

The total sperm count and motility were calculated using the method previously described (108) and the forward velocity was calculated using the method previously described (109). Fructose concentration in the cauda epididymal semen was analyzed according to the method previously described (110).

In conclusion, the above studies clearly showed that various extracts from *E. longifolia* Jack had aphrodisiac property and this may be attributed to the presence of the active compounds in more than one fraction.

Although these studies lend further support for the use of this plant by the indigenous population as a traditional aphrodisiac, it is suggested that a detailed toxicological study should also be carried.

REFERENCES

1. Traditional medicines now a global worry. The Sun, Friday, May 17, 2002, 5.
2. Herbal products enjoying growing demand: Dr. Lim. The New Straits Times, Wednesday, August 21, 2002, B6.
3. Melchior H. Engler's Syllabus der Pflauzenfamilien. Vol. 2. Berlin: Gebruder Borntrager, 1964.
4. Nooteboom HP. Flora Malesiana 1962; 6(ser. 1):193.
5. Cronquist A. An Integrated System of Classification of Flowering Plants. New York: Columbia University Press, 1981.
6. Corner EJH. Wayside Trees of Malaya. Kuala Lumpur: Government Printing Office, 1952.
7. Jack W. Description of Malayan Plants III. Leiden: Boerhaave Press, 1977.
8. Steenis V. Flora Malesiana 1972; 6:203.
9. Malaysian Herbal Monograph. Vol 1. Kuala Lumpur: Malaysian Monograph Committee, 1999.
10. http://www.bogor.indo.net.id/kri/eurycoma.htm (verified on November 1, 2002).
11. Goh SH, Chuah CH, Mok JSL, Soepadmo E. Malaysian Medicinal Plants for the Treatment of Cardiovascular Diseases. Selangor: Pelanduk Publication Sdn Bhd, 1995.
12. Nooteboom L. Simaroubaceae. In: Steenis JV ed. Flora Malesiana. 6th ed. Groningen: Wolters-Woordhoff Publishing, 1972:205.
13. Gimlette JD, Thomson HW, eds. A Dictionary of Malayan Medicine. Kuala Lumpur: Oxford University Press, 1977:183.
14. Standard of ASEAN Herbal Medicine. Vol. 1. Jakarta: ASEAN Countries, 1993.

15. Perry LM, ed. Medicinal Plants of East and Southeast Asia. Attributed Properties and Uses. Boston: MIT Press, 1980:389.
16. Thoi LV, Suong NN. Constituents of *Eurycoma longifolia* Jack. J Org Chem 1970; 35:1104–1109.
17. Burkill IH, Haniff M. Gard Bull Straits Settl, 1930; 182.
18. Gimlette JD, Burkill IH. Gard Bull Straits Settl, 1930; 6:329.
19. Marziah M. Tanaman Perubatan Tradisional. Serdang: Universiti Pertanian Malaysia, 1987.
20. Burkill IH. A Dictionary of the Economic Products of the Malay Peninsula. Vol. 1 and 2. Malaysia: Ministry of Agriculture, 1966.
21. Jagananth JB, Ng LT. Herbs The Green Pharmacy of Malaysia. Kuala Lumpur: Vinpress Sdn. Bhd. and Malaysian Research And Development Institute, 2000.
22. Research: Tongkat Ali may be effective against cancer and HIV. The New Sunday Times, Sunday, July 21, 2002; 1–2.
23. Ensuring steady supply. The STAR, Thursday, July 4, 2002; 13.
24. Darise M, Kohda H, Mitzutani K, Tanaka O. Eurycomanone and eurycomanol, quassinoids from the roots of *Eurycoma longifolia*. Jack. Phytochemistry 1982; 21:2091–2093.
25. Suong NN, Bhatnagar S, Polonsky J, Vuilhorgne M, Prange T, Pascard C. Structure of laurycolactone A and B, new C_{18}-quassinoids from *Eurycoma longifolia* and revised structure of eurycomalactone (X-ray analysis). Tetrahedron Lett 1982; 23:5159–5162.
26. Darise M, Kodha H, Mitzutani K, Tanaka O. Revision of configuration of the 12-hydroxyl group of eurycomanone and eurycomanol, quassinoids from *Eurycoma longifolia*. Phytochemistry 1983; 22:1514.
27. Bates RB, Linz GS, Tempesta MS. Structures of eurycomalactone and related terpenoids. J Org Chem 1984; 49:2820–2821.
28. Chan KL, O'Neill MJ, Phillipson JD, Warhurst DC. Plants as sources of antimalarial drugs. Part 3. *Eurycoma longifolia* Jack. Planta Med 1986; 52:105–107.
29. Chan KL, Lee SP, Sam TW, Han BH, Isolation and structural elucidation of eurycomanol-2-*O*-β-D-glucopyranoside from *Eurycoma longifolia* Jack. UNESCO subregional seminar/workshop on the systematic identification of natural products, Bangi, Malaysia, June 13–17, 1988.
30. Chan KL, Lee SP, Sam TW, Han BH. A quassinoid glycoside from the roots of *Eurycoma longifolia*. Phytochemistry 1989; 28:2857–2859.
31. Morita H, Kishi E, Takeya K, Itokawa H, Tanaka O. New quassinoids from the roots of *Eurycoma longifolia*. Chem Lett 1990; 749–752.
32. Chan KL, Lee SP, Sam TW, Tan SC, Noguchi H, Sankawa U. 13β, 18-Dihydroeurycomanol, a quassinoid from *Eurycoma longifolia*. Phytochemistry 1991; 30:3138–3141.
33. Kardono LBS, Angerhofer CK, Tsauri S, Padmawinata K, Pezzuto JM, Kinghorn AD. Cytotoxic and antimalarial constituents of the roots of *Eurycoma longifolia*. J Nat Prod 1991; 54:1360–1367.

34. Tada H, Yasuda F, Otani K, Doteuchi M, Ishihara Y, Shiro M. New antiulcer quassinoids from *Eurycoma longifolia*. Eur J Med Chem 1991; 26:345–349.
35. Chan KL, Iitaka Y, Noguchi H, Sugiyama H, Saito I, Sankawa U. 6α-Hydroxyeurycomalactone, a quassinoid from *Eurycoma longifolia*. Phytochemistry 1992; 31:4295–4298.
36. Itokawa H, Kishi E, Morita H, Takeya K. Cytotoxic quassinoids and tirucallane-type triterpenes from the woods of *Eurycoma longifolia*. Chem Pharm Bull 1992; 40:1053–1055.
37. Morita H, Kishi E, Takeya K, Itokawa H, Iitaka Y. Highly oxygenated quassinoids from *Eurycoma longifolia*. Phytochemistry 1993; 33:691–696.
38. Itokawa H, Qin XR, Morita H, Takeya K, Iitaka Y. Novel quassinoids from *Eurycoma longifolia*. Chem Pharm Bull 1993; 41:403–405.
39. Itokawa H, Qin XR, Morita H, Takeya K. C_{18} and C_{19} quassinoids from *Eurycoma longifolia*. J Nat Prod 1993; 56:1766–1771.
40. Chan KL, Lee,SP, Yuen KH, Antipyretic Activity of Quassinoids from *Eurycoma longifolia* Jack. 11th Chemical Seminar on Natural Products, UNIMAS, Sarawak, Malaysia, June 25–28, 1995.
41. Ang HH, Chan KL, Mak JW. In vitro antimalarial activity of quassinoids from *Eurycoma longifolia* against Malaysian chloroquine-resistant *Plasmodium falciparum* Isolates. Planta Med 1995; 61:177–178.
42. Ang HH, Hitotsuyanagi Y, Takeya K. Eurycolactones A–C, novel quassinoids from *Eurycoma longifolia*. Tetrahedron Lett 2000; 41:6849–6853.
43. Jiwajinda S, Santisopasri V, Murakami A, Hirai N, Ohigashi H. Quassinoids from *Eurycoma longifolia* Jack as plant growth inhibitors. Phytochemistry 2001; 58:959–962.
44. Ang HH, Hitotsuyanagi Y, Fukaya H, Takeya K. Quassinoids from *Eurycoma longifolia*. Phytochemistry 2002; 59:833–837.
45. Jiwajinda S, Santisopasri V, Murakami A, Kawanaka M, Kawanaka H, Gasquet M, Eilas R, Balansard G, Ohigashi H. In vitro anti-tumor promoting and anti-parasitic activities of the quassinoids from *Eurycoma longifolia*, a medicinal plant in Southeast Asia. J Ethnopharmacol 2002; 82:55–58.
46. Itokawa H, Kishi E, Morita H, Takeya K, Iitaka Y. Eurylene, a new squalene-type triterpene from *Eurycoma longifolia*. Tetrahedron Lett 1991; 32:1803–1804.
47. Itokawa H, Kishi E, Morita H, Takeya K, Iitaka Y. A new squalene-type triterpene from the woods of *Eurycoma longifolia*. Chem Lett 1991; 2221–2222.
48. Morita H, Kishi E, Takeya K, Itokawa H, Iitaka Y. Squalene derivatives from *Eurycoma longifolia*. Phytochemistry 1993; 34:765–771.
49. Morita H, Kishi E, Takeya K, Itokawa H. Biphenylneolignans from wood of *Eurycoma longifolia*. Phytochemistry 1992; 31:3993–3995.
50. Mitsunaga K, Koike K, Tanaka T, Ohkawa Y, Kobayashi Y, Sawaguchi T, Ohmoto T. Canthin-6-one alkaloids from *Eurycoma longifolia*. Phytochemistry 1994; 35:799–802.
51. Ang HH, Characterisation of local *Plasmodium falciparum* isolates by cloning and susceptibility studies against antimalarial drugs. Ph.D dissertation, University Science Malaysia, Penang, Malaysia, 1992.

52. Okano M, Fukamiya N, Lee KH. Biologically active compounds from simaroubaceous plants. In: Rahman Atta-ur-, ed. Studies in Natural Products Chemistry. Vol. 7. Amsterdam: Elsevier Science Publishers, 1990:369–404.
53. Trager W, Jensen JB. Human malaria parasites in continuous culture. Science 1976; 193:673–675.
54. Trager W, Jensen JB. Cultivation of erythrocyte stage. Bull WHO 1997; 5:363–365.
55. Taberner PV. Aphrodisiacs: The Science and the Myth. London: Croom Helm, 1985.
56. http://www.santesson.com/aphrodis/animal.htm (verified on November 1, 2002).
57. Inagaki I, Oida N, Nagoya Shiritsu Daigaku, Yakugakuba Kenkyu Nempo, 1970; 57.
58. Taberner PV. Sex and drugs–Aphrodite's legacy. Trends Pharmacol Sci 1985; 6:49–54.
59. Ramachandran KK, Easa PS, Vijayakumaran P. Nair, Management of Periya Tiger Reserve—problems and perspective. Tigerpaper 1987; 14:25–33.
60. Animal rights? Wrong. Asia Mag April 4–6, 1997; 30.
61. Farnsworth NR, Bingel AS, Cordell GA, Crane FA, Fong HHS. Potential value of plants as sources of new antifertility agents II. J Pharm Sci 1975; 64:717–753.
62. Johanson DN, Diamond M. Yohimbine and sexual stimulation in the male rats. Physiol Behav 1968; 4:411–413.
63. Reid K, Surridge DH, Morales A. Double-blind trial of yohimbine in treatment of psychogenic impotence. Lancet 1987; 2:241–243.
64. Morales A, Condra M, Owen JA, Surridge DH, Fenemore J, Harris C. Is yohimbine effective in the treatment of organic impotence? J Urol 1987; 137:1168–1172.
65. Susset JG, Tessier CD, Wineze J. Effect of yohimbine in the treatment of erectile impotence: a double-blind study. J Urol 1989; 141:1360–1363.
66. Sonda LP, Mazo R, Chancellor MB. The role of yohimbine in the treatment of erectile dysfunction. J Sex Marital Ther 1990; 16:15–21.
67. Messegne M. Man and Plants. New York: Macmillan, 1973.
68. Puri HS. Vegetable aphrodisiacs of India. Q J Crude Drug Res 1971; 11:1742–1748.
69. Dept to root out problem of "tongkat Ali" pilferage. The STAR, Tuesday January 30, 2001; 6.
70. Argiolas AM, Melis MR, Gessa GL. Yawning and penile erection: central dopamine-oxytocin-adrenocorticotropin connection. Ann NY Acad Sci 1988; 525:330–337.
71. Ang HH, Sim MK. Effects of *Eurycoma longifolia* Jack on penile erection index and homosexual mountings in rats. Pharm Sci 1997; 3:117–119.
72. Whalen RE, Luttge WG. *p*-Chlorophenylalanine methyl ester: an aphrodisiac? Science 1970; 169:1000–1001.
73. Benassi Benelli A, Ferrari F, Pellegrini Quarantotti B. Penile erection induced

by apomorphine and N-*n*-propylnorapomorphine in rats. Arch Int Pharmacodyn 1979; 242:241–247.
74. Baggio G, Ferrari F. The role of dopaminergic receptors in the behavioral effects induced by lisuride in male rats. Psychopharmacology 1983; 80:38–42.
75. Mendelson SD, Gorzalka BB. An improved chamber for the observation and analysis of the sexual behavior of the female rat. Physiol Behav 1987; 39:67–71.
76. Ferrari W, Gessa GL, Vargiu L. Behavioural effects induced by intracisternally injected ACTH and MSH. Ann NY Acad Sci 1963; 104:330–345.
77. Ang HH, Sim MK. Evaluation of pendiculation activities in male rats after oral administration of *Eurycoma longifolia* Jack. Pharm Biol 1998; 36:144–146.
78. Ang HH, Lee KL. *Eurycoma longifolia* intensifies sexual arousal in middle aged male rats. The Science Conference, Yemeni Scientific Research Foundation, Sana'a, Republic of Yemen, Oct 11–13, 2001.
79. Ang HH, Sim MK. Effects of *Eurycoma longifolia* Jack on sexual behaviour of male rats. Arch Pharm Res 1997; 20:656–658.
80. Ang HH, Lee KL. Effects of *Eurycoma longifolia* Jack on masculine copulatory behaviour in middle aged male rats—a comparison study. Nat Prod Sci 2002; 8:44–47.
81. Meyerson BJ, Lindstrom L, In: James VHT, Martini L, eds. Hormonal Steroids. Excerpta Medical International Congress, 1971; serial no. 219.
82. Meyerson BJ, Lindstrom L. Sexual motivation in the female rat. Acta Physiol Scand 1973; 389(suppl):1–80.
83. Beach EA, Whalen RE. Effect of ejaculation on sexual behaviour in the male rat. J Comp Physiol Psychol 1959; 52:249–252.
84. Ferrari F, Baggio G, Mangiafico V. The dopamine autoreceptor agonist B-HT 920 markedly stimulates sexual behaviour in male rats. Experientia 1985; 41:636–638.
85. Alder N, Bermant G. Sexual behaviour of male rats: effects of reduced sensory feedback. J Comp Physiol Psychol 1966; 61:240–243.
86. Davidson JM, Gray GD, Smith ER. Animal models in the endocrinology of reproductive behaviour. In: Alexander NJ, ed. Animal Models for Research on Contraception and Fertility. New York: Harper & Row, 1978:61–62.
87. Ang HH, Sim MK. *Eurycoma longifolia* Jack enhances libido in sexually experienced male rats. Exp Anim 1997; 46:287–290.
88. Malminas CO. Monoaminergic influence on testosterone activated copulatory behaviour in the male rats. Acta Physiol Scand 1973; 89:1–128.
89. Hull EM, Nishita JK, Bitran D. Perinatal dopamine-related drugs demasculinized rats. Science 1984; 9:1011–1013.
90. Morales A, Surridge DHC, Marshall PG, Fenemote J. Non-hormonal pharmacological treatment of organic impotence. J Urol 1982; 128:45–47.
91. Ang HH, Sim MK. *Eurycoma longifolia* Jack and orientation activities in sexually experienced male rats. Biol Pharm Bull 1998; 21:153–155.
92. Doherty PC, Baum MJ, Todd RB. Effects of chronic hypoprolactinemia on sexual arousal and erectile function in male rats. Neuroendocrinology 1986; 42:368–375.

93. Ang HH, Chan KL, Gan EK, Yuen KH. Enhancement of sexual motivation in sexually naïve male mice by *Eurycoma longifolia* Jack. Int J Pharmacog 1997; 35:144–146.
94. Ang HH, Cheang HS. Effects of chronic administration of *Eurycoma longifolia* Jack on the copulatory behavior in middle aged male rats. J Herbs Species Med Plants 2002; 9:109–114.
95. Ang HH, Sim MK. Aphrodisiac effect of *Eurycoma longifolia* Jack in non-copulator male rats. Fitoter 1998; 69:445–447.
96. Ang HH, Sim MK. Aphrodisiac evaluation in sexually naïve male mice after chronic administration of *Eurycoma longifolia* Jack (tongkat Ali). Nat Prod Sci 1998; 4:58–61.
97. Ang HH, Sim MK. *Eurycoma longifolia* Jack increases sexual motivation in sexually naïve male rats. Arch Pharm Res 1998; 21:779–781.
98. Ang HH, Ngai TH. Aphrodisiac evaluation in non-copulator male rats after chronic administration of *Eurycoma longifolia* Jack. Fund Clin Pharmacol 2001; 15:265–268.
99. Ang HH, Cheang HS. Promotion of sexual activity in rats with *Eurycoma longifolia* Jack. J Herbs Spices Med Plants 1999; 6:23–28.
100. Ang HH, Cheang HS, Yusof APM. Effects of *Eurycoma longifolia* Jack (tongkat Ali) on the initiation of sexual performance of inexperienced castrated male rats. Exp Anim 2000; 49:35–38.
101. Ang HH, Cheang HS. Effects of *Eurycoma longifolia* Jack in maintaining mating behavior of sexually experienced castrated male rats. Nat Prod Sci 1999; 5:138–141.
102. Ang HH, Cheang HS. Effects of *Eurycoma longifolia* Jack on laevator ani muscle in both uncastrated and testosterone-stimulated castrated intact male rats. Arch Pharm Res 2001; 24:437–440.
103. Ang HH, Ikeda S, Gan EK. Evaluation of the potency activity of *Eurycoma longifolia* Jack. Phytother Res 2001; 15:435–436.
104. Kwan TK, Saad JM, Farizaturradiah O, Koh BH, The effect of *Eurycoma longifolia* on rat and human testicular steroidogenesis. National Medicinal Plants Convention, Kuala Lumpur, Malaysia, Oct 13–15, 1995.
105. Thambi MIM, Update on current tongkat Ali research. 11th Malaysian Urological Conference, Kuantan, Pahang, Malaysia, Nov 7–11, 2001.
106. Mahanem MN, Lukman CH, The effects of *Eurycoma longifolia* Jack (tongkat Ali) on sexual behaviour of male rats and its sperm quality. MPS Pharmacy Scientific Conference, Penang, Malaysia, Oct 31–Nov 2, 2002.
107. Ang HH, Lee KL, Matsumoto K, Sperm parameters changes induced by *Eurycoma longifolia* Jack. 19th Congress of FAPA, Seoul, Korea, Oct 5–8, 2002.
108. Besley MA, Eliarson R, Gallegos AJ, Moghissi KS, Paulsen CA, Prasad MRN. Laboratory Manual for the Examination of Human Semen and Semen Cervical Mucus Interaction. Singapore: WHO Press, 1980.
109. Ratnasoorya WD. Effect of atropine on fertility of female rat and sperm motility. Indian J Exp Biol 1984; 22:463–466.
110. Bauer JD, Ackerman PG, Toro G. Clinical Laboratory Methods. St. Louis: Mosby Co., 1974.

31

The Biological and Pharmacological Properties of *Cordyceps sinensis*, a Traditional Chinese Medicine That Has Broad Clinical Applications

Shaoping Li
University of Macau
Macau, China

Karl W. K. Tsim
Hong Kong University of Science and Technology
Hong Kong, China

I. INTRODUCTION

Cordyceps sinensis is the complex of fungus *Cordyceps sinensis* (Berk.) Sacc. (Clavicipitaceae) growing on the larva of *Hepialus armoricanus* Oberthur, which lives a few inches underground. It is also commonly known as *Cordyceps*, or "Dong Chong Xia Cao" (summer-grass and winter-worm) in Chinese, because of its appearance during different seasons. *Cordyceps* has been known and used in China for medication for more than 300 years (Fig. 1). *Cordyceps* is first recorded in *Ben Cao Cong Xin* by Wu Yiluo in A.D. 1757. Later it was revealed that the original description of *Cordyceps* was in *Ben Cao Bei Yao* by Wang Ang in A.D. 1694, who wrote: "*Cordyceps* is sweet in taste

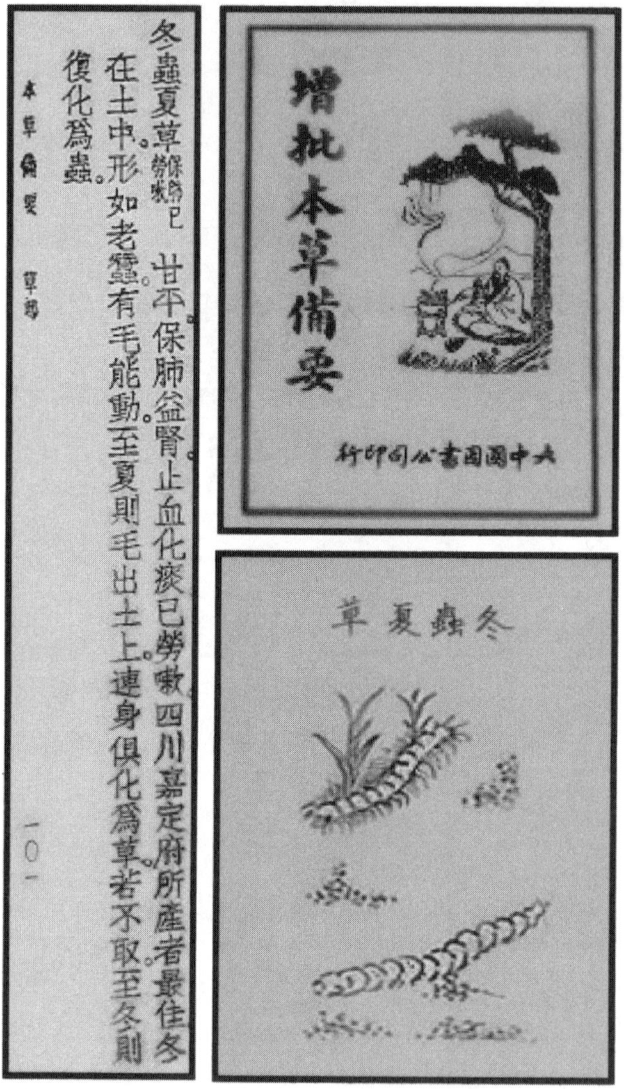

FIGURE 1 *Cordyceps* is first recorded in *Ben Cao Bei Yao* by Wang Ang in A.D. 1694. As shown here in Chinese writing, the clinical usages of *Cordyceps* are described, and *Cordyceps* derived from Jiading of Sichuan is the highest quality.

and neutral in nature, and replenishing the kidney and soothing the lung, arresting bleeding, resolving phlegm, and killing the cough. *Cordyceps* derived from Jiading of Sichuan, shows the highest quality. In winter, it appears as an old silk worm in soil, and moves with hair. In summer, hairs grow out of soil, and turn into grass. They have to be collected in summer, if not they will turn into worm again."

Cordyceps became known to the West in the seventeenth century. In A.D. 1723, *Cordyceps* was brought from Tibet to France as materia medica and shown at the conference of the Paris Science Academic Institute. *Cordyceps* was considered a precious medical material and was recorded in the memo of the conference in A.D. 1727. In 1878, the Italian scholar Saccardo named *Cordyceps* derived from China officially as *Cordyceps sinensis* (Berk.) Sacc.; this nomenclature was adopted and is used today. *Cordyceps* is known to regulate and ensure the normal functioning of various parts of the body, to strengthen the immune system and promote overall vitality and longevity, and it is commonly used in hospitals in China and as a household remedy. However, more than 350 types of so-called *Cordyceps* or its substitutes have been found worldwide today. Thus, authentication of *Cordyceps* is a serious problem on the market.

Review of the clinical usages of *Cordyceps* has been published (1,2). Here, we discuss the biological character, chemical composition, pharmacological activity, fermentation of culture mycelia as substitutes, and quality control of *Cordyceps*.

II. LIFE CYCLE OF *CORDYCEPS*

Cordyceps is composed of a fungus fruiting body and larva of the host, and its distribution is closely related to the distribution of the host. Many *Cordyceps*-related species have been found, which are based on different fungi growing on different insect hosts; however, most of them are not considered as *Cordyceps* for clinical usage except *C. sinensis*, which is listed in the Chinese *Pharmacopoeia* (3). China is the major producer of *Cordyceps* (4). In China, the parasitic complex of the fungus and the caterpillar is found in the soil of a prairie at an elevation of 3500–5000 meters, mainly in the provinces of Qinghai, Tibet, Sichuan, Yunnan, and Gansu (Fig. 2).

Cordyceps can grow on only a few species of insect hosts. At present, possible hosts of *C. sinensis* have been identified (5–19); they are listed in Table 1. An effective dispersal method of *C. sinensis* is important for the fungus to find the right host and to survive in nature; the fungus can be dispersed on a large scale through air, rain, and insects (Fig. 3). The host can be invaded in the larval state by *C. sinensis* that infects through the body wall, stoma, oral cavity, and/or orifices of the host. Another route of infection is

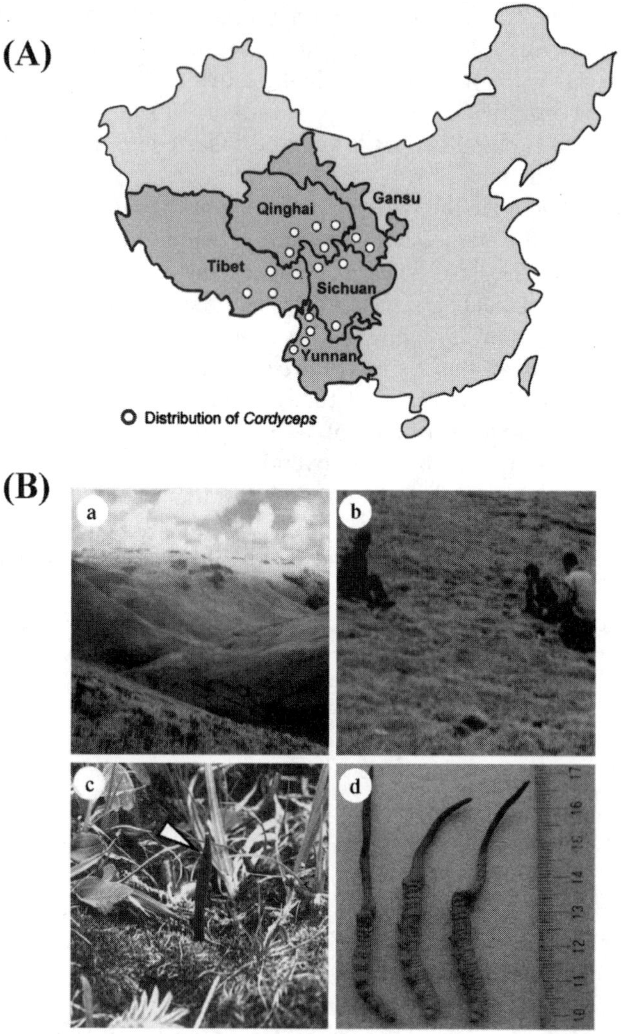

FIGURE 2 (A) The distribution of *Cordyceps* in China. (B) The parasitic complex of the fungus and the caterpillar is found in the soil of a prairie at an elevation of 3500–5000 meters, mainly in the provinces of Qinghai, Tibet, Sichuan, Yunnan, and Gansu (a and b). Freshly collected *Cordyceps* is shown in (c) and (d). Arrowhead in (c) indicates a living *Cordyceps*.

Table 1 Insect Hosts of *C. sinensis*

Species	Ref.	Species	Ref.	Species	Ref.
Hepialus armoricanus	5	*H. devidi*	6	*H. ganna*	6
H. kangdingensis	6	*H. varians*	6	*H. nebulosua*	6
H. yushuensis	6	*H. zhangmoensis*	6	*H. yunlongensis*	6
H. oblifurcus	6	*H. zhayuensis*	6	*H. lijiangensis*	6
H. menyuanicus	6	*H. kangdingroides*	6	*H. macilentus*	6
H. sichuanus	6	*H. yulongensis*	7	*H. meiliensis*	7
H. baimaensis	7	*H. deqinensis*	7	*H. renzhiensis*	8
H. pratensis	9	*H. yunnanensis*	9	*H. markamensis*	9
H. ferrugineus	10	*H. jinshaensis*	11	*H. albipictus*	11
H. jialangensis	12	*H. jianchuanensis*	12	*H. zaliensis*	12
H. anomopterus	12	*H. zhongzhiensis*	13	*H. cingulatus*	14
H. luquensis	14	*H. xunhuaensis*	14	*H. gonggaensis*	15
H. damxungensis	16	*H. bagingensis*	16	*H. latitegumenus*	17
H. bibelteus	17	*Hepialiscus nepalensis*	6	*Hepialiscus flavus*	6
Hepialiscus sylvinus	18	*Bipectilus yunnanensis*	6	*Forkalus xizangensis*	6
Phassus giganodus	6	*Napialus humanesis*	6	*Magnificus jiuzhiensis*	19
Magnificus zhiduoensis	19				

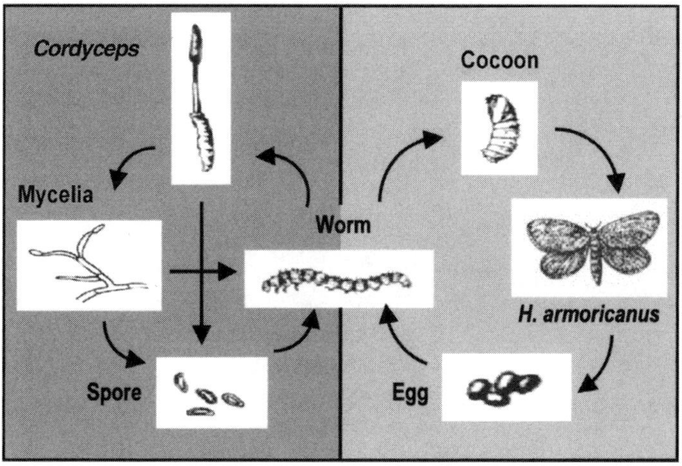

Figure 3 Host (*H. armoricanus*) can be invaded at the state of larva by *C. sinensis*. After the infection, *Cordyceps* fungus uses the bowels of the host as nutrient and starts to grow. After the host has died, the coarse mycelia will form a hard tissue. If the condition is suitable, the mycelia in the host will grow out through the oral cavity, and form the fruiting body, forming *Cordyceps*.

through food that is contaminated by *C. sinensis* mycelia or spores. After ingestion of contaminated food, *C. sinensis* invades the host through the digestive tract. The host body surface is also a route of fungus invasion. The insect body wall is composed of chitin, which can be hydrolyzed by an enzyme secreted by *C. sinensis* fungus, and thus the damaged body surface is available for fungus invasion. Penetration by mechanical pressure is another mechanism for fungal invasion (4).

Formation of *Cordyceps* can be divided into three stages: infection, parasitism (development of the fungus before insect death), and saprophyte (growth of the fungus after insect death). After infection, *Cordyceps* fungus makes use of the bowels of the host as nutrient and starts to grow. The mycelia creep over the insect body while the host is still alive. Subsequently, the color of the host body surface (shell) will fade in a few days from dark brown-yellow

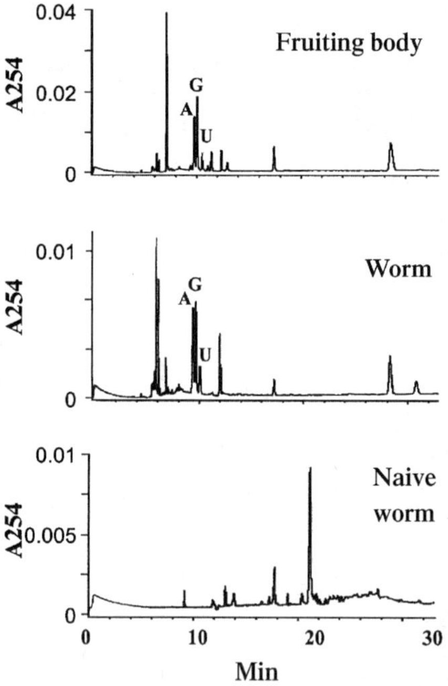

FIGURE 4 Capillary electrophoresis profiles of water-soluble constituents from fruiting body and worm of natural *Cordyceps*. Condition: pressure injection 586 kPa for 5 secs, 57 cm × 75 μm ID column, running buffer 200 mM boric acid-sodium hydroxide (pH 8.5). The profile was monitored online at 254 nm, 0.100 AU at a data collection rate of 5 Hz for 40 mins. (A) Adenosine, (G) guanosine, (U) uridine. (Data modified from Ref. 20.)

and turn into light yellow; then the entire body is covered by gray mycelia. After the host has died, the coarse mycelia will form a hard tissue. If conditions are suitable, the mycelia in the host will grow out through the oral cavity and form the fruiting body, thus forming *Cordyceps*. The host loses its own biological and chemical characteristics, and eventually is invaded by *C. sinensis* mycelia. The collected *Cordyceps* have to be dried before they are sold on the market.

To determine the nature of the worm in *Cordyceps*, the biological activity and the main constituents of the fruiting body and the worm were investigated (20). The water extracts of the individual parts were analyzed by capillary electrophoresis and the content of nucleosides was determined. The fruiting body and the worm showed a close resemblance in their nucleoside peaks and overall profiles, while the dry naïve worm with no *Cordyceps* mycelia showed a very distinct profile (Fig. 4). The nucleoside contents of the fruiting body and worm of *Cordyceps* were very similar. In addition, similar amounts of polysaccharides were found in the fruiting body and worm. The antioxidation activity of *Cordyceps*, from either the fruiting body or worm, was determined; the water extracts of the fruiting body and worm from *Cordyceps* had similar IC_{50} values in their inhibition of free-radical formation. On the other hand, the naïve worm did not show any antioxidation activity in the range of mg/mL. These results suggest that the function of the worm in *Cordyceps* is to provide a growth medium for the fruiting body, and eventually, the worm is totally invaded by *C. sinensis* mycelia (20).

III. CHEMICAL CONSTITUENTS OF *CORDYCEPS*

The chemical composition of *C. sinensis*, first described in 1947 (4), includes 25% crude protein, 8.4% fat, 18.5% crude fiber, 29% carbohydrate, and 4.1% ash. In 1957, cordycepic acid, which was identified as D-mannitol, was isolated from *C. sinensis*, and subsequently it has been used as a marker of quality control of *Cordyceps* for a number of years (21). In 1964, 3′-deoxyadenosine, namely cordycepin, was isolated from cultured *Cordyceps militaris* (4), a related species of *C. sinensis* commonly used as a substitute; however, its existence in *C. sinensis* is controversial. To date, cordycepin has never been identified from *C. sinensis*. In 1981, uracil, adenine, adenosine, trehalose, mannitol, ergosterol, and stearic acid were identified from *C. sinensis* (22). At present, *C. sinensis* is known to contain steroids, nucleosides, carbohydrates, and amino acids.

Sterols and their derivatives have been isolated from natural and cultured *Cordyceps*. They are ergosterol, Δ^3 ergosterol, ergosterol peroxide, ergosteryl-3-*O*-β-D-glucopyranoside, 22,23-dihydroergosteryl-3-*O*-β-D-glucopyranoside, β-sitosterol, daucosterol, cholesterol, cholesteryl palmitate, campesterol, and dihydrobrassicasterol. Based on the activity-guided fractionation, two antitumor compounds, 5α, 8α-epidioxy-24(R)-methylcholesta-6,22-dien-3β-D-glucopyranoside and 5,6-epoxy-24(R)-methylcholesta-7,22-dien-3β-ol (Fig. 5), were isolated from the methanol extract of *C. sinensis* (23). H1-A (Fig. 5), which suppresses the activated human mesangial cells and alleviates immunoglobulin A nephropathy (Berger's disease) with clinical and histological improvement, is a purified compound from the fruiting body of *C. sinensis* (24).

Nucleosides in *Cordyceps* have been a focus since the isolation of cordycepin from cultured *C. militaris*, which was shown to have antitumor activity. More than 10 nucleosides and related compounds have been isolated from *Cordyceps*, including adenine, adenosine, uracil, uridine, guanidine,

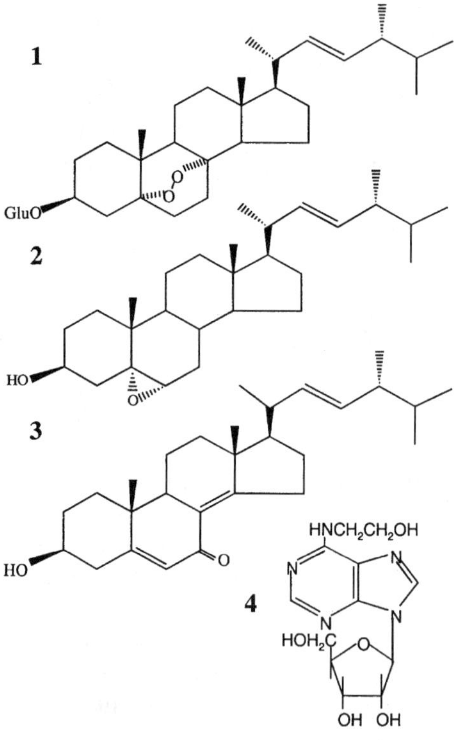

FIGURE 5 Structures of sterols and nucleoside isolated from *Cordyceps*. (1) 5α, 8α-Epidioxy-24(R)- methylcholesta-6,22-dien-3β-D-glucopyranoside; (2) 5,6-epoxy-24(R)-methylcholesta-7,22-dien-3β-ol; (3) H1-A; (4) N^6-(2-hydroxyethyl)-adenosine.

guanosine, hypoxanthin, inosine, thymine, thymidine, and deoxyuridine (25,26). In addition, N^6-(2-hydroxyethyl)- adenosine (Fig. 5), which behaves as a Ca^{2+} antagonist and an ionotropic agent, was isolated from cultured mycelia of *Cordyceps* (27).

D-Mannitol is one of the major compounds in natural *Cordyceps*, and contributes over 3.4% of the total dry weight (28). *Cordyceps* contains a large amount of polysaccharides, ranging from 3 to 8% of the total dry weight (29). A water-soluble, protein-containing galactomannan was isolated from the sodium carbonate extract of *Cordyceps*, and its molecular weight was estimated by gel filtration to be ~23 kDa. The isolated compound was composed of D-mannose and D-galactose in a molar ratio of 3:5, and contained a small proportion of protein. It is a highly branched structure composed of (1→6)-and (1→2)-linked α-D-mannopyranosyl residues in the main chain (30). Another polysaccharide with hypoglycemic activity, purified from a hot-water extract of the cultured mycelium of *C. sinensis*, was a combination of galactose, glucose, and mannose in a molar ratio of 43:33:24; its molecular weight was estimated to be about 15 kDa. The results of chemical and spectroscopic investigations suggest that the polysaccharide has a comb-type structure (31).

More than 20% of amino acid is found in *Cordyceps*, which could be responsible for its tonic and immunopotentiating activity (32). Six cyclo-dipeptides were isolated from cultured *Cordyceps*, and one of them, cyclo-(L-glycyl-L-prolyl), had antitumor and immunopotentiation activity (33).

In addition, *Cordyceps* contains about 0.18% dry weight of phospholipid, including eight phospholipids; the major constituents are phosphatidylcholine, phophatidylinositol, phosphatidylserine, phosphatidylethanolamine, and phosphatidic acid (34). Some organic acids, such as palmitic acid, stearic acid, oleic acid, and linoleic acid, and vitamin B_{12} and C were also identified in *Cordyceps*.

IV. *CORDYCEPS* ACTS ON THE IMMUNE SYSTEM

Effects of *Cordyceps* on the immune system have been reported; however, the experimental results are controversial and show that *Cordyceps* possesses both potentiation and/or inhibition effects on the immunoresponse. Thus, it is assumed that *Cordyceps* is a bidirectional modulator of the immune system.

The spleen weight of mice was significantly increased by oral administration of water extract derived from *Cordyceps*; the extract increased the synthesis of DNA and protein, which promoted the proliferation of spleen lymphocytes. The active ingredients that caused the elevation of spleen weight subsequently were identified and partially purified from the fruiting body of *Cordyceps*.

The immune system in tumor-bearing mice was greatly enhanced by treatment with *Cordyceps*. C57BL/6 mice implanted subcutaneously with EL-4 lymphoma cells were employed as the experimental targets. Oral administration of the extract led to a reduction of tumor size in the tumor-bearing mice and prolonged the survival rate of the host. Phagocytic activity of macrophages was decreased in the tumor-bearing mice treated with cyclophophamide (100 mg/kg); however, administration of *Cordyceps* extract restored the activity to higher than the normal level (35).

In animal studies, *Cordyceps* was shown to stimulate the function of mononuclear phagocytes and the expansion of adhesion cells in the abdominal cavity, phagocytes in the spleen, and Kupffer's cells in the liver (36). A polysaccharide with a size of ~43 kDa, namely CS-81002, was purified from the polysaccharide-enriched cultured medium, where the *Cordyceps* was fermented. CS-81002, when injected into the mice at a dosage of 5 mg/kg, stimulated the function of phagocytes; however, CS-81002 did not increase the number of plaque-forming cells in the spleen. In addition, CS-81002 could be hydrolyzed by acid to smaller molecules and fewer branches; the size of hydrolyzed molecules ranged from 12 to 41 kDa depending on the acid concentration. Higher molecular weight of hydrolyzed CS-81002 retained the immunoactivity, while the smallest molecule at 12 kDa lost the activity completely (37). Moreover, the function of Kupffer's cell is stimulated by *Cordyceps*. Rats were administered daily the water extract derived from *Cordyceps* p.o. at a dose of 200 mg/kg for 25 days until the day before the injection of colloidal carbon. According to the rate of carbon clearance in the blood, the *Cordyceps*-treated rats showed a shorter half-life of 36% than that of the control (38).

In contrast to the above-mentioned different lines of evidence, *Cordyceps* was shown to suppress immunity function. In cultured T lymphocytes, the application of either natural or cultured *Cordyceps* onto the cultures inhibited the lymphocyte blastogenesis stimulated by concanavalin A (Con A), and that effect was in a dose-dependent manner. Cultured *Cordyceps* also significantly inhibited E-rosette formation in humans and prolonged the survival of skin allografts and cardiac tissue transplantation in mice (39,40). Systemic lupus erythematosus is an important autoimmune disease, characterized by the presence of multiple autoantibodies in serum, of which antinuclear antibodies are the predominant species and anti-dsDNA antibodies are the disease-specific species. Female NZB/NZW F1 mice, a typical lupus animal model, were fed with *Cordyceps* at dosages of 0.025, 0.05, and 0.10 g/day from the time they were 6 weeks old. Mice treated with *C. sinensis* at 0.1 g/day had a longer survival time than controls. After a few months of *Cordyceps* treatment, the level of antinuclear antibodies remained the same as that of the controls; however, the titer of anti-dsDNA antibodies was reduced

(41). Furthermore, fractions of methanol extracts from the fruiting bodies of *Cordyceps* had positive effects on the lymphoproliferative response, natural killer cell activity, and phytohemagglutinin (PHA) stimulated interleukin-2 (IL-2) and tumor necrosis factor-α (TNF-α) production on human mononuclear cells. Further characterization of the fractions indicated that 2 of the 15 isolated fractions (CS-36-39 and CS-48–51) significantly inhibited the blastogenesis response (IC_{50}, 71.0 ± 3.0 and 21.7 ± 2.0 μg/mL, respectively), natural killer cell activity (IC_{50}, 25.0 ± 2.5 and 12.9 ± 5.8 μg/mL, respectively), and IL-2 production in PHA-treated human mononuclear cells (IC_{50}, 9.6 ± 2.3 and 5.5 ± 1.6 μg/mL, respectively). Moreover, the production of TNF-α in human mononuclear cells was blocked by CS-36-39 and CS-48-51 (IC_{50}, 2.7 ± 1.0 and 12.5 ± 3.8 μg/mL, respectively). Neither CS-36-39 nor CS-48-51 had a cytotoxic effect on mononuclear cells in culture (42).

V. *CORDYCEPS* HAS ANTITUMOR ACTIVITY

Antitumor activity of *Cordyceps* has been domonstrated both in vitro and in vivo. In mice inoculated i.p. with 1×10^6 Ehrlich carcinoma or 1×10^5 Meth A fibrosarcoma, water extract prepared from dried *Cordyceps* (1 mg protein/mouse), when injected i.p. to mice, increased the median survival time of the Ehrlich carcinoma–injected mice to 316% and Meth A fibrosarcoma–injected mice to 312% of the control. On the other hand, a cytotoxic effect of *Cordyceps* was not found on both tumor cells in vitro. The antitumor effect of *Cordyceps* on Ehrlich carcinoma inoculated in mice was significantly reduced when the mice received X-ray irradiation before the carcinoma injection, which suggested that the antitumor effect of *Cordyceps* could be mediated by potentiating the immunoresponse of the mice (43).

Cordycepin (3′-deoxyadenosine), a nucleoside isolated from *C. militaris* (a substitute of *C. sinensis*), was demonstrated to have antitumor activity. Cordycepin inhibited the proliferation of L5178Y mouse lymphoma cells with an IC_{50} of 0.27 μmol/L (44). Cordycepin also induced the apoptosis of leukemia cells and prolonged the S and G_2 phases during mitosis (45). In addition, the extract from *Cordyceps* showed a strong cytotoxicity effect on Lewis lung carcinoma and B16 melanoma although cordycepin showed no cytotoxic effect against these cells in vitro. Thus, the antimetastatic activity of *Cordyceps* is probably due to a component other than cordycepin (46). Cordycepin has not been found so far in *C. sinensis*.

The conditioned medium from *Cordyceps* polysaccharide-stimulated blood mononuclear cells significantly inhibited the proliferation of human leukemic U937 cells by 78–83%. Furthermore, the same conditioned medium from the stimulated mononuclear cells induced the differentiation of monocytes/macrophages by over 50%. However, *Cordyceps* polysaccharide alone or normal conditioned medium from blood mononuclear cells had no such effects. In addition, the secretion of interferon-γ, TNF-α, and IL-1 in cultured mononuclear cells was greatly increased by the application of *Cordyceps* polysaccharide, and the elevation of these cytokines, therefore, could explain the antitumor activity of the polysaccharide enriched from *Cordyceps* (47).

Methanol extract of *Cordyceps* inhibited the growth of K562, Vero, Wish, Calu-1, and Raji tumor cell lines; the inhibitory activities could not be due to polysaccharide, which was depleted during the extraction. Therefore, it is believed that antitumor inhibitors other than polysaccharide have to be considered (48). Based on the activity-guided fractionation, two antitumor sterols, 5α,8α-epidioxy-24(R)-methylcholesta-6,22-dien-3β-D-glucopyranoside and 5,6-epoxy-24(R)-methylcholesta-7,22- dien-3β-ol, were isolated from the methanol extract of *Cordyceps*. Both forms of sterols were found to have a strong inhibition on the proliferation of K562, Jurkat, WM-1341, HL-60, and RPMI-8226 tumor cell lines at 10 μg/mL (23).

The antitumor activity of *Cordyceps* could be due to two mechanisms: (1) *Cordyceps* inhibits tumor growth through inhibition of the synthesis of nucleic acid, protein, and/or glucose permeability through the cell membrane; (2) the balance between tumor cells and the host's immune responses is critical in the process of carcinogenesis or the progression of tumor cells. *Cordyceps* polysaccharides are capable of stimulating the proliferation and the secretion of cytokines in immune cells, which subsequently enhance the immune system and exert antitumor activity. In support of these concepts, *Cordyceps* was found to increase the expression of major histocompatibility complex (MHC) class II antigen on hepatoma cell line HA22T/VGH. This induced MHC could enhance host immune surveillance more effectively against tumor cells (49). Thus, *Cordyceps* has been used in China as adjuvant treatment of cancer, in particular, serving as a supplementary therapy for terminal cancers in combination with radiotherapy or chemotherapy.

VI. EFFECTS OF *CORDYCEPS* ON THE KIDNEY

Cordyceps has been used extensively to improve kidney function and to protect against the damage caused by certain nephrotoxic chemicals (50,51). In kidney-transplanted recipients, *Cordyceps* protected the kidney from cyclosporine-mediated nephrotoxicity. Sixty-nine kidney-transplanted recipients, who had stable transplant renal function at least 3 months after grafting, were divided into two groups at random. Each recipient was given cyclosporine at the dose of 5 mg/kg/day for 15 days. Group A (control, n = 39) was administered as placebo (glucose) 3 g while group B (n = 30) was administered 3 g of *Cordyceps* simultaneously. In both groups, the levels of blood creatine, urea, and urine *N*-acetyl-glucosaminidase were determined; these clinical parameters demonstrated that the *Cordyceps*-treated group developed less prominent nephrotoxicity as compared with the placebo group. The longer the administration time, the more significant was the difference of tested clinical results between the two groups. Thus, these findings suggested that *Cordyceps* exerts a protective effect against cyclosporine-induced nephrotoxicity (52).

F2, a fraction isolated from the methanol extract of *Cordyceps*, significantly inhibited the proliferation of human mesangial cells in cultures that were activated by IL-1 and IL-6. The immunoglobulin A nephropathy (IgAN) mice (a mouse model for Berger's disease) when fed with 1% F-2 in diet showed a reduction of hematuria and proteinuria together with histopathological improvement. The F2 fraction was then further purified by silica gel column chromatography and high-performance liquid chromatography (HPLC), and a purified compound H1-A (Fig. 5) was achieved, which suppressed the activated mesangial cells and alleviated the immunoglobulin A nephropathy in mice with clinical and histological improvement (24). Histological analysis of the kidney indicated that H1-A could inhibit the proliferation of mesangial cells that was evident in lupus nephritis (53).

VII. *CORDYCEPS* RESTORES LIVER FUNCTION

Cordyceps could be used for the treatment of chronic hepatitis and related disease conditions (54). The protective effect of *Cordyceps* on bacille Calmette Guérin (BCG)- and lipopolysaccharide-induced liver injury was determined in mice; *Cordyceps* markedly inhibited the activities of serum alanine and aspartate aminotransferases, decreased the liver- and spleen-enlarged index, reduced the level of lipid peroxide in serum and hepatic tissue in mice, and reduced the level of serum TNF-α (55). In the same liver injury model, the polysaccharides enriched with *Cordyceps* increased the activities of serum transaminase and liver superoxide dismutase. In addition, the concentration of liver malondialdehyde, the weighting index of liver, and the liver pathology were significantly improved by treatment with *Cordyceps* (56).

The upregulation of intercellular adhesion molecule-I (ICAM-I), a member of the immunoglobulin supergene family, in liver is an index of liver fibrogenesis (57). For determining the expression of ICAM, human fibroblasts were cultured together with *Cordyceps*, the level of ICAM-1 and CD126 assessed by using flow cytometry, were markedly reduced compared to the positive rate $86.63 \pm 5.94\%$ and $77.95 \pm 4.68\%$ in the control fibroblasts, respectively. The effect was in a dose-dependent manner, which could explain the antifibrotic effect in liver (58). Moreover, the effects of *Cordyceps* on carbon-tetrachloride-induced liver fibrosis were investigated in rats. The high levels of collagen I, III, and IV in liver and procollagen type III in serum of liver-damaged rats were restored by treatment with *Cordyceps* (59).

VIII. ANTIOXIDATION ACTIVITY OF *CORDYCEPS*

In China, there is a long history of using *Cordyceps* to ameliorate conditions associated with aging and senescence. Today, scientific findings reveal that *Cordyceps* has strong antioxidation activity in animals. The antioxidation activities were compared between natural and cultured *Cordyceps* by determining their effects on the levels of superoxide dismutase, glutathione peroxidase, and lipid peroxide in mouse liver. It was found that natural and cultured *Cordyceps* (0.3 g/L) markedly increased the content of these free-radical-scavenging enzymes, while both of *Cordyceps* inhibited the formation of lipid peroxide in the livers (60).

Hydroxyl radical has been shown to react with salicylic acid in forming two hydroxylation products, 2, 5- and 2,3-dihydroxybenzic acids. By using HPLC, the levels of 2, 5- and 2,3-dihydroxybenzic acids in coronary effluent and in heart tissue were identified in isolated heart that was perfused with the free-radical-inducer Adriamycin. The enzymatic activity of lactic dehydrogenase was also determined as the referent index of membrane damage. Perfusion of ethanol extract of *Cordyceps* at a dose of 0.4 g/L markedly decreased the level of dihyroxybenzic acids and the activity of lactic dehydrogenase in the Adriamycin-perfused heart (61), which suggested that *Cordyceps* could inhibit, or scavenge, the formation of hydroxyl radical.

In cultured rat myocardial cells, the level of malondialdehyde was significantly increased, and superoxide dismutase activity as well as membrane fluidity were markedly decreased during ischemic treatment. Application of *Cordyceps* to the ischemic cultures markedly decreased the level of malondialdehyde, but increased the enzymatic activity of superoxide dismutase and the membrane fluidity in a dose-dependent manner. These results suggested that *Cordyceps* could suppress lipid peroxidation during ischemia (62); however, the exact mechanism of the antilipid peroxidation of *Cordyceps* was not determined. Nevertheless, it was proposed that *Cordyceps* could reduce the damage of the lysosome and restore the decreased enzymatic activity of Na^+-K^+-ATPase during ischemia (63).

The antioxidation activity of *Cordyceps* was compared by using different methods, including inhibition of xanthine oxidase, induction of hemolysis in erythrocytes, and prevention of lipid peroxidation in the liver microsome (64). Water extract from natural or cultured *Cordyceps* significantly inhibited the formation of free radicals. In the same study, the antioxidation activities of different cultured or natural products of *Cordyceps* were compared (Table 2). Natural *Cordyceps* from Tibet had the strongest scavenging activity of free radical with an IC_{50} of 0.08 mg/mL, while *Cordyceps* from Yunnan had an IC_{50} of 0.24 mg/mL; the difference was ~3-fold between the two sources of *Cordyceps*. A similar difference could be observed in cultured *Cordyceps* that was fermented from various producers. In contrast, different sources of *Cordyceps*, either natural or cultured, showed close inhibition of the free-radical-induced hemolysis of erythrocytes; their IC_{50} varied from 1.5 to 2.0 mg/mL. Furthermore, *Cordyceps* could be enriched by ~15-fold in the polysaccharide-enriched fraction after ion exchange column. When the partially purified polysaccharide was used in the antioxidation assays, the increment of inhibition activity was ~25-fold in the xanthine oxidase assay, ~11-fold in the hemolysis assay, and ~32-fold in the lipid peroxidation assay. The results indicated that polysaccharide could be one of the active constituents of antioxidation activity in *Cordyceps* (64). In determination of the pharmacological efficiency of different parts of *Cordyceps*, the fruiting body showed a similar potency in antioxidation activity compared to the worm (caterpillar); these results were in line with the identical chemical compositions between the fruiting body and the worm, which suggested that the function of the worm is to provide nutrient for *C. sinensis* to grow (20).

TABLE 2 Inhibition of Water Extracts from Different Types of Natural and Cultured *Cordyceps* on Peroxide Anion Formation, Hemolysis, and Lipid Peroxidation

Sample	Peroxide anion formation[a]	Hemolysis[b]	Lipid peroxidation[c]
Natural *Cordyceps*			
Qinghai	0.20[d]	0.20	0.66
Xizang	0.08	0.23	0.52
Sichuan	0.08	0.17	0.39
Yunnan	0.24	0.30	0.71
Cultured *Cordyceps*			
Jiangxi	0.09	0.15	0.53
Huadong	0.21	0.18	0.68
Wanfong	0.34	0.18	0.57
Hebei	0.91	0.19	0.63

[a,b,c] Refer to Ref. 64.

[d] The mean values of five determinations are presented. The SEM is less than 5% of the mean, which is not shown for clarity.

IX. EFFECTS OF *CORDYCEPS* ON THE CARDIOVASCULAR SYSTEM

The antiarrhythmic effects of different extracts including petroleum extract from cultured *Cordyceps* were tested by using experimental arrhythmia in rats induced by aconitine and barium chloride. Pretreatment of petroleum extract of *Cordyceps* at the dose of 200 mg/kg by oral administration significantly antagonized the drug-induced arrhythmia, and prolonged the onset time of arrhythmia (85.0 $\pm$ 12.3 sec vs. 25.0 $\pm$ 19.8 sec, control), decreased the duration of persistence (19.8 $\pm$ 15.3 min vs. 40.8 $\pm$ 17.2 min, control), and diminished the degree of severity (50.0 $\pm$ 16.7 score vs. 80.0 $\pm$ 17.9 score, control) (65). In another study, water extract from *Cordyceps*, which was dialyzed overnight against buffer using a membrane cutoff size of 3.5 kDa, was assayed in anesthetized rats for hypotensive effects and in isolated aorta for vasorelaxant effects. Intravenous injection of *Cordyceps* extract suppressed the mean arterial pressure in a dose-dependent manner. In aortic rings precontracted with phenylephrine, the extract induced relaxation; the *Cordyceps*-induced vasorelaxation possibility could be mediated by release of nitric oxide and endothelium-derived hyperpolarizing factor in stimulated endothelium (66). In the atherosclerosis mouse model, *Cordyceps* suppressed the increased levels of serum lipid peroxide and aortic cholesteryl ester in a dose-dependent manner. Thus, the prevention of cholesterol deposition in the aorta by *Cordyceps* could be mediated by free radicals rather than by the reduction in serum lipid level (67).

X. HYPOGLYCEMIC ACTIVITY OF *CORDYCEPS*

Polysaccharide fraction obtained from hot-water extract of *Cordyceps*, when injected into mice intraperitoneally, showed significant hypoglycemic activity in normal and streptozotocin-induced diabetic mice; the glucose level in plasma was reduced by the extract (68). Administration of the polysaccharide to normal mice significantly increased the activities of hepatic glucokinase, hexokinase, and glucose-6-phosphate dehydrogenase, although the glycogen content in the liver was reduced. Furthermore, the polysaccharide reduced the levels of triglyceride and cholesterol in plasma of *Cordyceps*-treated mice (69). *Cordyceps* polysaccharide also increased the activity of hepatic glucokinase and decreased the protein content of facilitative glucose transporter in rat liver, which therefore could contribute to the hypoglycemic activity (31).

XI. FERMENTATION OF *CORDYCEPS*

C. sinensis has a very restricted habitat, and the yield is decreasing every year. In 2001, only a few thousand kilograms of *Cordyceps* were collected in China.

This represents a decrease of more than 70% compared to 1978. Because of environmental concerns, the Ordinance of Resources Protection on Wild Herbal Medicine was issued in 1987, and the collection of *Cordyceps* was highly restricted. The price of *Cordyceps* was US$5000/kg in 2002, which is about 100-fold higher than in the 1980s.

Scientists in China have extensively developed substitutes by using mycelial fermentation derived from natural *Cordyceps*. To date, more than nine genera including 31 species of fungus strain have been isolated from natural *C. sinensis*. Mycelia or fruiting bodies of 16 species have been produced in large quantities. More than 20 fermented products are commonly sold as health food products in China and South East Asia, and the annual production value is more than US$100 million.

The strain Cs-4, a fungus isolated from *C. sinensis*, is cultivated aseptically. Cs-4 is known as *Paecilomyces hepiali*, and its fermented products has been studied intensively in China. The fermentation methodology, chemical composition, therapeutic function, basic biology, and toxicity of Cs-4 have been thoroughly investigated. JinShuiBao capsule, the commercial product derived from Cs-4, has been sold and used in clinics throughout China. This product generates more than several million U.S. dollars of sales per year. In addition to Cs-4, several mycelial strains have been isolated from natural *Cordyceps* and some of them are manufactured, by fermentation (70). For instance, *Synnematum sinensis*, *Cephalosporium sinensis*, *Gliocladium roseum*, and *Mortierella hepiali* are the nonsexual phase strains of *Cordyceps*; their commercial names in China are BaiLing, NingXinBao, XinGanBao, and ZhiLing, respectively. In addition, *Paecilomyces sinensis*, *Scytalidium hepiali*, *Tolypocladimn sinensis*, *Hirsutella sinensis*, *Chrysosporium sinensis*, and others have been isolated from natural *Cordyceps* and manufactured in large quantities by fermentation (1,4,71). Thus, the cultivated products of *Cordyceps* as health food and medical products are very popular in China, and their marketable values are extremely high; however, adulterants of *Cordyceps* are commonly found on the market.

The biological activities of different types of mycelial fermentation products have been compared (64). The results showed that there was a great variation in their antioxidation effect in inhibiting the formation of free radicals. The lowest inhibition (IC_{50} = 0.91 mg/mL) was ~10-fold lower than the highest (IC_{50} = 0.09 mg/mL). In addition, the chemical composition of different cultivated products of *Cordyceps* has been determined. All showed a great variation in having different amounts of ergosterol, nucleoside, polysaccharide, and mannitol (Table 3). In addition, the true identity of these cultured fungus strains is not known, and whether they are the anamorphs of *C. sinensis* is uncertain. This is a common problem with these cultured *Cordyceps*.

TABLE 3 The Amounts of Major Chemical Constituents in Different Cultured *Cordyceps*

	Natural *Cordyceps*	JinShuiBao[a]	BaiLing[b]	NingXinBao[c]	XinGanBao[d]
Ergosterol	1.07[e]	0.14	0.11	0.04	0.10
Adenosine	0.01	0.26	0.07	0.32	0.27
Guanosine	0.01	0.15	0.03	0.25	0.16
Uridine	0.06	0.44	0.08	0.53	0.15
Polysaccharide	8.2	5.8	7.5	5.9	3.8
Mannitol	3.54	1.02	1.28	1.34	1.12

Fungus of fermented products:
[a] *Pacilomyces hepiali*.
[b] *Synnematum sinensis*.
[c] *Cephalosporium sinensis*.
[d] *Gliocladium roseum*.
[e] The mean values of five determinations are presented. The SEM is less than 5% of the mean, which is not shown for clarity.
Source: Data are adapted from Refs. 26,28,29,72.

Targeting the above-mentioned authentication problem, a strain named UST2000 was isolated from the fruiting body of *C. sinensis* collected in Qinghai. Molecular evidence by sequencing the spacer domain of 5S-rRNA DNA proved that the strain of UST2000 was identical to that of *C. sinensis*. Fruiting body could grow when UST2000 was cultured on artifical media or inoculated on the larva of different worms (Fig. 6). Chemical analysis and pharmacological assay showed that the fruiting body of cultured UST2000 was similar to that of natural *Cordyceps*. The level of ergosterol, an important primer of vitamin D_2 and a specific component in fungi, represents the maturation of *Cordyceps*. By using ergosterol as a marker, the growth rate of UST2000 was calibrated during the culture and the formation of fruiting body. The amount of ergosterol was increased during the beginning of growth, and reached to a plateau after 40 days of culture. The amounts of nucleosides, carbohydrates, and polysaccharides in UST2000 shared a great similarity with natural *Cordyceps*. The pharmacological properties of UST2000 were also investigated. Oral administration of UST2000 in mice at a dose of 2.0 g/kg for 10 days significantly increased the phagocytosis of macrocytes. The induced phagocytic index of mice treated with UST2000 was ~3-fold that of normal and ~4-fold that of cyclophosphamide-treated mice. The transformated lymphocytes in UST2000-treated mice was about double those of cyclophosphamide-treated mice.

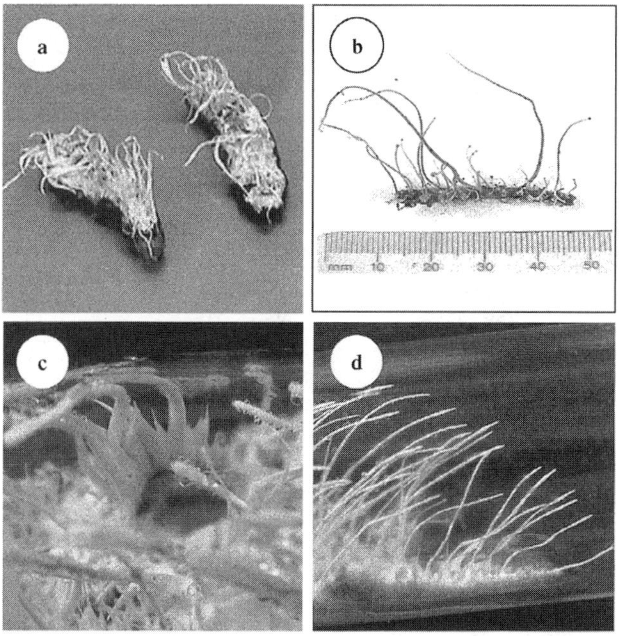

Figure 6 UST2000 grows on different worms and media. UST2000 was isolated from the fruiting body of *C. sinensis* collected in Qinghai. Molecular evidence obtained by sequencing the spacer domain of 5S-rRNA DNA proved that the strain of UST2000 is identical to that of *C. sinensis*. Fruiting body of UST2000 grows well on silkworm (a), authentic host *H. armoricanus* (b), and artificial media (c and d).

The identity of *C. sinensis* as a fungal strain is not established. By using PCR, the DNA sequences of internal transcribed spacer region (ITS) were compared in three fungal strains, *Hirsutella sinensis*, *Paecilomyces sinensis*, and *Paecilomyces gunin*, which were isolated from natural *C. sinensis*. The results indicate that *C. sinensis* and *H. sinensis* share the highest homology (97.8%), while *C. sinensis* has much less homology with the other two species (less than 70%), which suggests that the anamorph of *C. sinensis* could be *H. sinensis* (73). The same result was obtained by RAPD-PCR using eight random primers and showed 96% similarity between *C. sinensis* and *H. sinensis* (74).

In the health food market, *C. militaris* is a common substitute of *C. sinensis* (4,75). The chemical components and pharmacological activities of *C. militaris* and *C. sinensis* have been compared. The contents of protein, amino acid, organic acid, carbohydrate, alkaloid, and sterol of *C. militaris* are

TABLE 4 Pharmacological Activities of *C. sinensis* and *C. militaris*

Activity	*C. sinensis*	*C. militaris*
Immunomodulation	Yes	—
Cardiovascular	Yes	—
Renal protection	Yes	—
Liver protection	Yes	—
Antisenescence	Yes	—
Antitumor	Yes	Yes
Hormonal	Yes	Yes
Antifibrotic	Yes	Yes
Anti-inflammatory	Yes	Yes
Antimutagenic	Yes	Yes
Hypoglycemic	Yes	—
Antioxidation	Yes	—

—, very low or undetectable activity.
Source: Data adapted from Ref. 76.

similar to those of *C. sinensis*. As shown in Table 4, the pharmacological effects, including sedative, antianoxia, and anti-inflammatory, of *C. militaris* and *C. sinensis* are comparable (76).

Cordycepin (3′-deoxyadenosine) is a unique chemical from natural or cultured *C. militaris*. This compound revealed potent growth-inhibiting activity toward *Clostridium paraputrificum* and *Clostridium perfringens* without adverse effects on the growth of *Bifidobacterium bifidum*, *Bifidobacterium breve*, *Bifidobacterium longum*, *Bifidobacterium adolescentis*, *Lactobacillus acidophilus*, or *Lactobacillus casei*. Thus, cordycepin derived from *C. militaris* could serve as a naturally occurring antibacterial agent, which could be useful as a new preventive agent against various diseases caused by clostridia (77).

XII. QUALITY CONTROL OF *CORDYCEPS*

Quality control of *Cordyceps* is important for its clinical application. *Ben Cao Bei Yao* in A.D. 1694 recorded that *Cordyceps* derived from Jiading of Sichuan had the best quality. In the current health food market, *Cordyceps* from Sichuan, Qinghai, and Tibet is considered the top quality. At present, natural *Cordyceps* is rare and expensive. In addition, cultured *Cordyceps* is very popular; however, the quality of these products is a question of concern to consumers.

At present, nucleoside is believed to be the active component in *Cordyceps*. Indeed, *Cordyceps* contains a high concentration of adenosine, guanosine, and uridine (25,26). Among these nucleosides, adenosine is believed to play a key role in many pharmacological effects of *Cordyceps*. Adenosine has widespread effects on coronary and cerebral circulation, in prevention of cardiar arrhythmias, and on nerve tissue functions such as inhibition of neurotransmitter release and modulation of adenylate cyclase activity. In many circumstances, adenosine has been used as a marker for quality control of natural *Cordyceps* and culture *Cordyceps* mycelia (3).

However, the amount of nucleoside within *Cordyceps* has changed according to environmental conditions. Our study showed that fresh natural *Cordyceps* contains very little nucleoside, as compared to dry and processed *Cordyceps* (26). Furthermore, humidity and heat significantly increased the amount of nucleoside in natural *Cordyceps*. After storage of *Cordyceps* at 75% relative humidity and 40°C for 10 days, the nucleoside content in natural *Cordyceps* markedly increased about fourfold. However, the effect of humidity and heat in altering the content of nucleotide could not be determined in cultured *Cordyceps* mycelia (78). Therefore, it is believed that nucleoside in natural *Cordyceps* may be derived from the degradation of nucleic acids. Thus, using adenosine as a marker for good quality of *Cordyceps* may not be indicative.

Polysaccharide is another active component in *Cordyceps* that processes the activities of antioxidation (64), immunopotentiation, and hypoglycemia. Indeed, the pharmacological profile of *Cordyceps* correlates very well with the quality of polysaccharide (79). Based on the binding to Mono Q column, four fractions of polysaccharides were isolated from different types of natural and culture *Cordyceps*; however, the ratios of these four polysaccharide fractions varied in different cultured products of *Cordyceps* (29). The molecular weights of polysaccharides isolated from *Cordyceps* were also compared by gel filtration. The polysaccharides in natural *Cordyceps* were predominantly (>50%) high-molecular-weight molecules of over 150 kDa, which were distinct as compared to the cultured products. Thus, the use of polysaccharide in determining the quality of *Cordyceps* should be promoted.

Ergosterol is a specific component in fungi, and it is also another choice of chemical marker for *Cordyceps*. Ergosterol exists in *Cordyceps* as free and combined forms. The content of free ergosterol is high in natural *Cordyceps*, and the level of ergosterol could reflect the amount of *Cordyceps* mycelia (72). Ergosterol analogs have multiple pharmacological activities, such as cytotoxic activity (23,80), antiviral activity (81); these activities are in line with the quality of *Cordyceps* in both natural and cultured products. Therefore, ergosterol may be a useful marker for quality control of *Cordyceps*, especially the cultured product. In summary, multiple markers such as ergosterol, nucleoside, polysaccharide, and mannitol should be considered as a group for quality control of *Cordyceps* and mycelial fermentation; the active constituents within *Cordyceps* are still not certain.

XIII. CONCLUSION

Cordyceps, one of the most valued traditional Chinese medicines, consists of the dried fungus *C. sinensis* growing on the larva of the caterpillar. Animal and clinical studies suggest that it has multiple pharmacological activities, including immunomodulation, antitumor activity, protection of kidney, liver, and cardiovascular function, and hypoglycemic activity. Although many so-called active constituents have been identified, the exact roles of these chemicals in the functions of *Cordyceps* are not known. Because of the decreasing supply of natural *Cordyceps*, isolation of the mycelial strain of *Cordyceps* is being studied by many scientists in China to achieve large-scale production of *Cordyceps* by fermentation. Indeed, the current health food market is full of fermented products of *Cordyceps*; however, many of them are adulterants. Thus, the authentication of these products has to be defined, and chemical markers are needed for quality control. At present, multiple markers such as ergosterol, nucleoside, polysaccharide, and mannitol are being used for quality control of *Cordyceps* in both natural and cultured products. Unfortunately, these markers are far from optimization, and extensive work is needed to define the pharmacological efficiency of these markers.

ACKNOWLEDGMENTS

We are grateful to C. Keung Lo of our laboratory for expert technical assistance. We thank Drs. Tina Dong and K. J. Zhao for their critical suggestions during the study. The research was supported by grants from Research Grants Council of Hong Kong (AoE/B-10/01) and HKUST (DAG 01/02.SC05) to KWKT. SPL is supported by PDF matching fund from HKUST.

REFERENCES

1. Zhu JS, Halpern GM, Johns K. The scientific rediscovery of an ancient Chinese herbal medicine: *Cordyceps sinensis*: Part I. J Alt Comp Med 1998; 4:289–303.
2. Zhu JS, Halpern GM, Johns K. The scientific rediscovery of an ancient Chinese herbal medicine: *Cordyceps sinensis*: Part II. J Alt Comp Med 1998; 4:429–457.
3. The Pharmacopoiea Commission of PRC. Pharmacopoiea of the People's Republic of China. Vol. I. Chemical Industry Publishing House, 2000.

4. Wang GD. *Cordyceps*: Ecology, Culture and Application. 1st ed. Beijing: Science & Technology Documents Publishing House, 1995.
5. Zhu HF. *Hepialus armoricanus* Oberthur, host insect of *Cordyceps sinensis*. Acta Entomol Sin 1965;14:620–621.
6. Zhu HF, Wang LY. *Cordyceps sinensis* and Hepialidae. Sinozoologia 1985; 3:121–134.
7. Liang XC, Yang DR, Shen FR, Long YC, Yan YX. Four new species of the genus *Hepialus* (ghost moth) from Yunnan. China. Zool Res 1988; 9:419–425.
8. Yang DR, Shen FR, Yang YX, Liang XC, Dong DZ, Chun S, Lu Z, Sina DJ. Biological studies and notes on a new species of the genus *Hepialus* from Yunnan, China. Acta Entomol Sin 1991; 34:218–224.
9. Yang DR, Li SD, Shen FR. Three new species of the genus *Hepialus* from Yunnan and Xizang, China (Lepidoptera: Hepialidae). Zool Res 1992; 13:245–250.
10. Li CD, Yang DR, Shen FR. A new species of the genus *Hepialus* from Yunnan, China (Lepidoptera: Hepialidae). Acta Entomol Sin 1993; 36:495–496.
11. Yang DR. Two new species of the genus *Hepialus* from Yunnan, China (Lepidoptera: Hepialidae). Acta Zootaxon Sin 1993; 18:184–187.
12. Yang DR. Four new species of the genus *Hepialus* from Yunnan and Xizang, China (Lepidoptera: Hepialidae). Zool Res 1994; 15:5–11.
13. Dong YC, Luo DQ. Research of *Cordyceps sinensis* in China. Territory Natural Resources Study 1996; 3:47–51.
14. Yang DR, Yang YX, Zhang SY. Three new species of the genus *Hepialus* from Qinghai and Gansu, China (Lepidoptera: Hepialidae). Acta Entomol Sin 1995; 38:359–362.
15. Fu SQ, Huang TF. A new species of the genus *Hepialus*. Acta Zootaxon Sin 1991; 34:362–363.
16. Yang DR, Jiang CP. Two new species of the genus *Hepialus* (Lepidoptera: Hepialidae) from north Xizang, China. Entomotaxonomia 1995; 17:15–218.
17. Shen FR, Zhou YS. Two new species of the genus *Hepialus* from Yunnan, China (Lepidoptera: Hepialidae). Acta Zootaxon Sin 1997; 40:198–201.
18. Chen SJ, Jing SY. Research review on host insect of *Cordyceps sinensis* in China. Lishizhen Med Materia Med Res 1992; 3:37–39.
19. Yan L. A new genus and two new species of the Hepialidae (Lepidoptera) from Qinghai, China. J Qinghai Univ 2000; 18:1–5.
20. Li SP, Su ZR, Dong TTX, Tsim KWK. The fruiting body and its caterpillar host of *Cordyceps sinensis* show close resemblance in main constituents and anti-oxidation activity. Phytomedicine 2002; 9:319–324.
21. Yue DC, Feng XZ, Liu HY, Bao TT. *Cordyceps sinensis*. In: Institute of Materia Medica, ed. Advanced Study for Traditional Chinese Herbal Medicine. Vol. 1. Beijing: Beijing Medical University and China Peking Union Medical University Press, 1995:91–113.
22. Yu RM, Yang YC, Yang YP, Wang SF. Study of chemical components in *Cordyceps sinensis*. Pharm Bull 1981; 16:55–57.

23. Bok JW, Lermer L, Chilton J, Klingeman GH, Towers N. Antitumor sterols from the mycelia of *Cordyceps sinensis*. Phytochemistry 1999; 51:891–898.
24. Lin CY, Ku FM, Kuo YC, Chen CF, Chen WP, Chen A, Shiao MS. Inhibition of activated human mesangial cell proliferation by the natural product of *Cordyceps sinensis* (H1-A): an implication for treatment of IgA mesangial nephropathy. J Lab Clin Med 1999; 133:55–63.
25. Shiao MS, Wang ZN, Lin LJ, Lien JY, Wang JJ. Profiles of nucleosides and nitrogen bases in Chinese medicinal fungus *Cordyceps sinensis* and related species. Bot Bull Acad Sin 1994; 35:261–267.
26. Li SP, Li P, Dong TTX, Tsim KWK. Determination of nucleosides in natural *Cordyceps sinensis* and cultured *Cordyceps* mycelia by capillary electrophoresis. Electrophoresis 2001; 22:144–150.
27. Furuya T, Hirotani M, Matsuzawa M. N^6-(2-Hydroxyethyl)-adenosine, a biologically active compound from cultured mycelia of *Cordyceps* and *Isaria* species. Phytochemistry 1983; 22:2509–2512.
28. Li SP, Dong TX, Su ZR, Zhu Q, Tsim WKK. Analysis of Carbohydrates from Natural *Cardyceps sinensis* and Cultured *Cordyceps* Mycelia by HPLC. In: China Pharmaceutical Association, ed. Forum of Modern Pharmaceutical Analysis. Beijing: Xinhua Press, 2001:149–151.
29. Li SP, Li P, Ji H, Zeng Q, Wu ZB. Comparison of polysaccharides in natural and cultured *Cordyceps*. Chin J Wild Plant Resource 1999; 6:47–48.
30. Kiho T, Tabata H, Ukai S, Hara G. A minor, protein-containing galactomannan from a sodium carbonate extract of *Cordyceps sinensis*. Carbohydr Res 1986; 156:189–197.
31. Kiho T, Ookubo K, Usui S, Ukai S, Hirano K. Structural features and hypoglycemic activity of a polysaccharide (CS-F10) from the cultured mycelium of *Cordyceps sinensis*. Biol Pharm Bull 1999; 22:966–970.
32. Yang YX, Yang DR, Dong DZ, Shen FR, Zhang JR. Comparision of chemical constituents in several *Cordyceps*. Yunnan J TCM 1988; 9:33–35.
33. Feng XZ. Chemical study on active components of *Cordyceps sinensis*. In: Editorial Board of J Chin Acad Med Sci, ed. Annual review of Chinese Academy of Medical Science & Peking Union Medical College. Beijing: Peking Union Medical College Publishing House, 1990:41.
34. Xu YM, Li XN. Studies on the composition of phospholipids content in *Cordyceps sinensis*. Res Dev Nat Prod 1992; 4:29–33.
35. Yamaguchi N, Yoshida J, Ren LJ, Chen H, Miyazawa Y, Fujii Y, Huang YX, Takamura S, Suzuki S, Koshimura S, Zeng FD. Augmentation of various immune reactivities of tumor-bearing hosts with an extract of *Cordyceps sinensis*. Biotherapy 1990; 2:199–205.
36. Zhang CK, Yuan SR. Advance on immunological pharmacology of *Cordyceps sinensis* and cultured *Cordyceps* mycelia. J Capital Univ Med Sci 1997; 18:287–290.
37. Gong M, Zhu Q, Wang T, Wang XL, Ma JX, Zhang WJ. Molecular structure and immunoactivity of the polysaccharide from *Cordyceps sinensis* (Berk) Sacc. Chin Biochem J 1990; 6:486–492.

38. Nakamura K, Yamaguchi Y, Kagota S, Shinozuka K, Kunitomo M. Activation of in vivo Kupffer cell function by oral administration of *Cordyceps sinensis* in rats. Jpn J Pharmacol 1999; 79:505–508.
39. Huang MM, Zhang JF, Pang L, Jiang Z, Wang DW. Study on immunological pharmacology of *Cordyceps*. IV. Immunosuppression of fermentation *Cordyceps sinensis*. J Tongji Med Univ 1988; 17:329–331.
40. Wang DW, Huang MM. Study on immunological pharmacology of *Cordyceps*. V. Effects of fermentation *Cordyceps sinensis*. J Tongji Med Univ 1988; 17:332–334.
41. Chen JR, Yen JH, Lin CC, Tsai WJ, Liu WJ, Tsai JJ, Lin SF, Liu HW. The effects of Chinese herbs on improving survival and inhibiting anti-ds DNA antibody production in lupus mice. Am J Chin Med 1993; 21:257–262.
42. Kuo YC, Tsai WJ, Shiao MS, Chen CF, Lin CY. *Cordyceps sinensis* as an immunomodulatory agent. Am J Chin Med 1996; 24:111–125.
43. Yoshida J, Takamura S, Yamaguchi N, Ren LJ, Chen H, Koshimura S, Suzuki S. Antitumor activity of an extract of *Cordyceps sinensis* (Berk) Sacc. against murine tumor cell lines. Jpn J Exp Med 1989; 59:157–161.
44. Muller WEG, Seibert G, Beyer R, Breter HJ, Maidhof A, Zahn RK. Effect of cordycepin on nucleic acid metabolism in L5178Y cells and on nucleic acid-synthesizing enzyme systems. Cancer Res 1977; 37:3824–3833.
45. Koc Y, Urbano AG, Sweeney EB, McCaffrey R. Induction of apoptosis by cordycepin in ADA-inhibited TdT-positive leukemia cells. Leukemia 1996; 10:1019–1024.
46. Nakamura K, Yamaguchi Y, Kagota S, Kwon YM, Shinozuka K, Kunitomo M. Inhibitory effect of *Cordyceps sinensis* on spontaneous liver metastasis of Lewis lung carcinoma and B16 melanoma cells in syngeneic mice. Jpn J Pharmacol 1999; 79:335–341.
47. Chen YJ, Shiao MS, Lee SS, Wang SY. Effect of *Cordyceps sinensis* on the proliferation and differentiation of human leukemic U937 cells. Life Sci 1997; 60:2349–2359.
48. Kuo YC, Lin CY, Tsai WJ, Wu CL, Chen CF, Shiao MS. Growth inhibitors against tumor cells in *Cordyceps sinensis* other than cordycepin and polysaccharides. Cancer Invest 1994; 12:611–615.
49. Chiu JH, Ju CH, Wu LH, Lui WY, Wu CW, Shiao MS, Hong CY. *Cordyceps sinensis* increases the expression of major histocompatibility complex class II antigens on human hepatoma cell line HA22T/VGH cells. Am J Chin Med 1998; 26:159–170.
50. Wang GD. Advance of nephroprotective effects for *Cordyceps*. Liaoning J Trad Chin Med 1995; 22:93–95.
51. Liu HW, Lin YZ. Advance of experimental research on renal diseases treatment for *Cordyceps*. J Trad Chin Med 1997; 38:563–565.
52. Xu F, Huang JB, Jiang L, Xu J, Mi J. Amelioration of cyclosporin nephrotoxicity by *Cordyceps sinensis* in kidney-transplanted recipients. Nephrol Dial Transplant 1995; 10:142–143.
53. Yang LY, Chen A, Kuo YC, Lin CY. Efficacy of a pure compound H1-A

extracted from *Cordyceps sinensis* on autoimmune disease of MRL lpr/lpr mice. J Lab Clin Med 1999; 134:492–500.
54. Zhao SL. Advance of treatment for *Cordyceps* on chronic hepatic diseases. Shanxi J TCM 2000; 16:59–60.
55. Zeng XK, Tang Y, Yuan SR. The protective effects of CS and CN80-2 against the immunological liver injury in mice. Chin Pharm J 2001; 36:161–164.
56. Xu JM, Ding CH, Li LD, Mei Q, Li CR, Fan MZ. Evaluation for the protective effect of *Cordyceps* polysaccharides on immunological liver injury in mice. Acta Univ Med Anhui 1999; 34:173–175.
57. Lu LG, Zeng MD, Fan JG, Li JQ, Liu Y, Ren WP, Dai N. Intercellular adhesion molecule-1 expression in experimental liver fibrosis. Chin J Intern Med 1999; 38:37–39.
58. Wang YJ, Quan QZ, Sun ZQ, Qi F, Jiang XL. Effects of *Cordyceps sinensis* on ICAM-1 and CD126 expression in human fibroblasts. J Binzhou Med Coll 1999; 22:316–317.
59. Wang YJ, Sun ZQ, Quan QZ, Zhang XL, Qi F. Effects of *Cordyceps sinensis* on morphology and intercellular matrix synthesis of human fetal lung fibroblasts. J Binzhou Med Coll 1999; 22:226–227.
60. Yang JH, Ling YS. The antioxidation of *Cordyceps sinensis* preparation. Acad J Guangdong Coll Pharm 1997; 13:35–37.
61. Zheng X, Xu CQ, Liu FZ, Lou YP, Wang XM, Bi YF, Wang GL. Change of hydroxyl radical content in isolated rat heart perfused with adriamycin and the influence of *Cordyceps sinensis* alcohol extraction. J Harbin Med Univ 1996; 30:519–523.
62. Yu Z, He JX. The effect of *Cordyceps sinensis* on lipid peroxidation of cultured neonatal rat myocardial cells induced by anoxia-reoxygenation. J First Mil Med Univ 1998; 18:100–111.
63. Yang JW, Li LS. *Cordyceps sinensis* and the study on damage of renal anoxia-reoxygenation. Chin J Nephrol Dialy Transplant 1994; 3:37–39.
64. Li SP, Li P, Dong TTX, Tsim KWK. Anti-oxidation activity of different types of natural *Cordyceps sinensis* and cultured *Cordyceps* mycelia. Phytomedicine 2001; 8:207–212.
65. Gong XJ, Ji H, Cao Q, Li SP, Li P. Antagonistic effects of extracts from cultural mycelium of *Cordyceps sinensis* on arrhythmia. J Chin Pharm Univ 2001; 32:221–223.
66. Chiou WF, Chang PC, Chou CJ, Chen CF. Protein constituent contributes to the hypotensive and vasorelaxant activities of *Cordyceps sinensis*. Life Sci 2000; 66:1369–1376.
67. Yamaguchi Y, Kagota S, Nakamura K, Shinozuka K, Kunitomo M. Inhibitory effects of water extracts from fruiting bodies of cultured *Cordyceps sinensis* on raised serum lipid peroxide levels and aortic cholesterol deposition in atherosclerotic mice. Phytother Res 2000; 14:650–652.
68. Kiho T, Ji H, Yamane A, Ukai S. Polysaccharides in fungi. XXXII. Hypoglycemic activity and chemical properties of a polysaccharide from the cultural mycelium of *Cordyceps sinensis*. Biol Pharm Bull 1993; 16:1291–1293.

69. Kiho T, Yamane A, Ji H, Usui S, Ukai S. Polysaccharides in fungi. XXXVI. Hypoglycemic activity of a polysaccharide (CS-F30) from the cultural mycelium of *Cordyceps sinensis* and its effect on glucose metabolism in mouse liver. Biol Pharm Bull 1996; 19:294–296.
70. Yin DH, Tang XM. Advances in the study on artificial cultivation of *Cordyceps sinensis*. Chin J Chin Mat Med 1995; 20:707–709.
71. Chen SJ, Yin DH, Li L. Studies on anamorph of *Cordyceps sinensis* (Berk) from Naqu Tibet. Chin J Chin Mat Med 2001; 26:453–454.
72. Li SP, Li P, Ji H, Zhang P. RP-HPLC determination of ergosterol in natural and cultured *Cordyceps*. Chin J Mod Appl Pharm 2001; 18:297–299.
73. Zhao J, Wang N, Chen YQ, Li TH, Qu LH. Molecular identification for the asexual stage of *Cordyceps sinensis*. Acta Sci Nat Univ Sunyatseni 1999; 38:121–123.
74. Li ZZ, Huang B, Li CR, Fan MZ. Molecular evidence for anamorph determination of *Cordyceps sinensis* (Berk) Sacc. I. Relation between *Hirsutella sinensis* and *Cordyceps sinensis*. Mycosystema 2000; 19:60–64.
75. Chen SZ. Advances of study on *Cordyceps sinensis* and *Cordyceps militaris*. Chin J Biochem Pharm 1995; 16:242–245.
76. Chen BG, Luo MC, Liu SJ, Chen HH, Sun MY. Studies on the pharmacological effects of *Cordyceps militaris*. Chin Trad Herbal Drugs 1997; 28:415–417.
77. Ahn YJ, Park SJ, Lee SG, Shin SC, Choi DH. Cordycepin: selective growth inhibtor derived from liquid culture of *Cordyceps militaris* against *Clostridium* spp. J Agric Food Chem 2000; 48:2744–2748.
78. Li SP, Li P, Ji H, Zhang P, Dong TTX, Tsim KWK. The contents and their change of nucleosides from natural *Cordyceps sinensis* and cultured *Cordyceps* mycelia. Acta Pharm Sini 2001; 36:436–439.
79. Ohmori T, Tamura K, Ohgane N. The correlation between molecular weight and antitumor activity of galactosaminoglycan (CO-N) from *Cordyceps ophioglossoides*. Chem Pharm Bull (Tokyo) 1989; 37:1337–1340.
80. Nam KS, Jo YS, Kim YH, Hyun JW, Kim HW. Cytotoxic activities of acetoxyscirpenediol and ergosterol peroxide from *Paecilomyces tenuipes*. Life Sci 2001; 69:229–237.
81. Lindequist U, Lesnau A, Teuscher E, Pilgrim H. The antiviral action of ergosterol peroxide. Pharmazie 1989; 44:579–580.

32

Phytochemistry, Pharmacology, and Health Effects of *Brandisia hancei*

Ren Xiang Tan and Ling Dong Kong
Nanjing University
Nanjing, Jiangsu, People's Republic of China

I. INTRODUCTION

The folk medicinal herb *Brandisia hancei* Hook. f. (Scrophulariaceae) is mainly distributed throughout southwestern China. The whole plant has been frequently prescribed for centuries in Bai, Hani, and Yu minority areas of China to treat chronic and acute osteomyelitis, rheumatoid arthritis, chronic hepatitis, hyperlipemia, and hypercholesterolemia, while the roots and leaves are used to cure hepatitis, hematuria, enterorrhagia, and metritis (1,2). Reports dealing with *B. hancei* have shown that this plant in general appears to have a reproducible profile regarding its phytochemistry and pharmacology, which is quite consistent with its use in folk medicine. The species is commonly prepared as a main component drug in several decoctions. As this herb is so clinically important, the plant has received much chemical and biological attention to obtain a better understanding of its phytochemistry and pharmacology. This chapter is dedicated to the chemical composition, pharmacological aspects, and health effects of *B. hancei* reported so far in the literature.

II. CHEMISTRY PROFILE

The phytochemicals of *B. hancei* have been investigated by chromatographic (CC, TLC, HPLC, LC-UV, LC-MS) and spectroscopic methods (IR, ^{1}H, and ^{13}C NMR) as well as by various 2D NMR techniques such as COSY, HMBC, HMQC, and NOESY). A wide variety of caffeoylated phenylpropanoid glycosides have been characterized from the species (Fig. 1). A specific procedure for the extraction and isolation of phenylpropanoid glycosides is as follows: The whole herb (2620 g) is extracted with methanol three times, and the extract is concentrated in vacuo until 282 g methanol extract is achieved. The extract is subjected to percolation over D-101 macroresin successively with H_2O, 60% EtOH, and 90% EtOH. The 60% EtOH–eluted fraction is repeatedly chromatographed on silica gel columns using $CHCl_3$-MeOH-H_2O or $CHCl_3$-MeOH gradients to yield phenylpropanoid glycosides acteoside (= verbascoside,), 2′-*O*-acetylacteoside, and poliumoside (3). The structure of brandioside, an additional new antioxidative phenylpropanoid glycoside, has been determined on the basis of extensive spectrometric analyses (4). Furthermore, phenylethanoids arenarioside and isoaceteoside

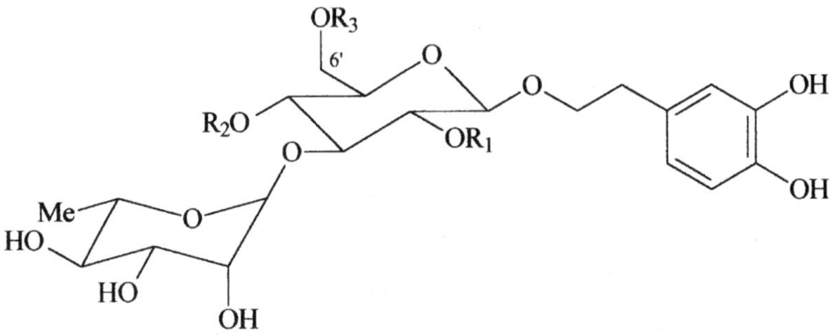

Phenylethanoids	R_1	R_2	R_3
Acteoside	H	caffeoyl	H
Isoacteoside	H	H	caffeoyl
2'-*O*-acetylacteoside	Ac	caffeoyl	H
Brandioside	Ac	caffeoyl	rha
Arenarioside	H	caffeoyl	xyl
Poliumoside	H	caffeoyl	rha

FIGURE 1 Structures of phenylethanoids isolated from the extract of *Brandisia hancei*.

were characterized in the *n*-butanol fraction of water extract of the twigs and leaves of *B. hancei* (5).

Flavonoids and iridoid glycosides are also quite common in the Scrophulariaceae family, but only flavone luteolin and iridoid glycoside mussaenoside have been detected to date from the *n*-butanol fraction of *B. hancei*. Luteolin is one of the main active principles in medicinal herbs and diets, with many pharmacological activities. Other phytochemicals reported from the species are dulcitol and mannitol as well as two β-sitosterol glycosides, daucosterol and β-sitosterol gentiobioside (3–5).

III. PHARMACOLOGY

A. Antioxidative Activity

Oxidative stress leading to the formation of free radicals has been implicated in many biological processes, damaging the cell membrane and biological molecules. Free radicals are also responsible for the development of many diseases such as arteriosclerosis, cancer, inflammation, cardiovascular disorder, ischemia, arthritis, and liver diseases. Lipid peroxidation is initiated by very potent free radicals including superoxide (O_2^-) and hydroxyl radicals (OH^-). Most of free radicals can be scavenged by the endogenous antioxidant defense systems such as superoxide dismutase (SOD), the glutathione peroxidase/glutathione system, catalase, and peroxidase. But these systems are not always completely efficient, making it imperative to receive exogenous antioxidants originally from the medicinal herbs and diet. Oxidative modification of low-density lipoprotein (LDL) has been suggested to play an important role in the development of human atherosclerosis. Accordingly, protection of LDL from oxidation can retard or effectively prevent the progression of the disease.

There has been an interest over the years in the pronounced free-radical-scavenging activity of phenylethanoid glycosides ascertained both in vitro and in vivo in the stable free-radical systems. An earlier report claimed that phenylethanoid glycoside acteoside showed its antioxidant activity both as a scavenger of superoxide anions generated in a phenazin methosulfate-NADH system and as an inhibitor of lipid peroxidation in mouse liver microsomes (6). In addition, acteoside was found to significantly repair the oxidized OH adducts of 2′-deoxyadenosine-5′-monophosphate acid (dAMP) and 2′-deoxyguanosine-5′-monophosphate acid (dGMP). This implies that it has potent antioxidant activity for reducing the oxidized OH adducts (7–9).

Another group reported that acteoside and its isomer isoacteoside, both having four phenolic hydroxy groups, could strongly protect red blood cells from oxidation-induced hemolysis (10). In antioxidative assays based on 1,1-

diphenyl-2-dipicrylhydrazyl free-radical (DPPH) scavenging and on Trolox equivalent antioxidant activity (TEAC), acteoside and isoacteoside were shown to have free-radical-scavenging effects (11,12).

Furthermore, it was observed that acteoside and isoacteoside had antioxidative effects on lipid peroxidation induced by $FeSO_4$-edetic acid in linoleic acid and on the chelating activity for Fe^{2+}. The chelating activity for Fe^{2+} of isoacteoside was twofold stronger than that of acteoside. The inhibitory effects of the two compounds with phenolic hydroxy groups on lipid peroxidation are due to the chelating property. Under physiological logical conditions the phenylethanoid glycoside-Fe^{2+} chelates are confirmed to be sufficiently stable. Thus the phenylethanoid glycosides are able to inhibit Fe^{2+}-dependent lipid peroxidation by chelating Fe^{2+}, and their therapeutic potentials are thought to be based on the same mechanism (13).

In addition, antioxidative effects have been observed for 2′-acetylacteoside, poliumoside, and brandioside isolated from *B. hancei*. They were shown to have inhibitory effects on free-radical-induced hemolysis of red blood cells and free-radical-scavenging activities in vitro. Brandioside and poliumoside exhibited stronger antioxidant effect than acteoside, 2′-acetylacteoside, and Trolox (14). On the other hand, acteoside, isoacteoside, and 2′-acetylacteoside had stronger free-radical-scavenging activities than α-tocopherol on DPPH radical and xanthine/xanthine oxidase (XOD)-generated superoxide anion radical. Among the three compounds, isoacteoside with its caffeoyl moiety at the 6′-position of the glucose chain showed an inhibitory effect on XOD. Further studies disclosed that each of them exhibited significant inhibition of both ascorbic acid/Fe^{2+}- and ADP/NADPH/Fe^{3+}-induced lipid peroxidation in rat liver microsomes (5,15). Acteoside and isoacteoside had strong protective effects against the oxidation of human LDL from Cu^{2+}-mediated oxidation. They were also effective in preventing the peroxyl free-radical-induced oxidation of α-tocopherol in human LDL. Inhibition of these phenylethanoid glycosides on the oxidation of human LDL and α-tocopherol is dose-dependent in the concentration range of 5–40 μM (16).

Interestingly, the observed antioxidative effects of phenylethanoid glycosides were found to be dependent of the number of phenolic hydroxyl groups they have. Those with four phenolic hydroxy groups have stronger antioxidative effects than those with only two or less. As to the antioxidative mechanism, these compounds were shown to have at least two mechanisms of scavenging free radicals: they are able to suppress free-radical processes at two stages: the formation of superoxide anions and the production of lipid peroxides. The antioxidative effects would offer a plausible explanation for the observed therapeutic effects for arteriosclerosis. On the other hand, phenylethanoid glycosides in *B. hancei* may partly account for its ethnomedicinal application for the relief of hyperlipemia and hypercholesterolemia.

In addition, acteoside was shown to decrease significantly the concentration of oxygen free radicals (OFR) and lipid peroxidation in skeletal muscle resulting from exhaustive exercise. The effect of reducing oxidative stress is attributable to decreasing the concentration of free radicals and the level of lipid peroxidation (17). Other investigation demonstrated that acteoside at 20.0 μM resisted significantly Bufo gastrocnemius muscle fatigue allowed electrically. This observation was attributed to the antioxidative activity of the glycoside, which is in agreement with the role of reactive oxygen species (ROS) in promoting fatigue in skeletal muscle (18).

B. Anti-Inflammatory Activity

The use of nonsteroidal antiinflammatory drugs (NSAIDs) is the main therapeutic approach for the treatment of inflammatory diseases, in spite of their renal and gastric side effects. Accordingly, there is a growing need for new anti-inflammatory compounds. Several research groups have particularly focused on searching for anti-inflammatory natural compounds.

Some phenylethanoids have been previously shown to be anti-inflammatory. Acteoside had inhibitory effects on arachidonic-acid-induced mouse ear and carrageenin-induced rat ankle edema when administered orally to the test animals (19,20). Acteoside also inhibits histamine- and bradykinin-induced contractions of guinea pig ileum. These results indicate that acteoside has anti-inflammatory properties that seem to be due, at least partly, to its action on histamine and bradykinin.

Pathogenically, inflammation is a complex process characterized by the involvement of several mediators, including prostaglandins (PGs) and nitric oxide (NO). The pivotal role of PGs in inflammation was firmly established with the discovery that the anti-inflammatory action of drugs was mediated by inhibition of the enzyme cyclooxygenase (COX), which converts arachidonic acid to PGs. Biochemically COX has two isoforms, COX-1 and COX-2. COX-1 is expressed constitutively in most mammalian cells and regulates many physiological functions through the release of PGs, while COX-2 is expressed at a very low level in most tissues, but much higher at the inflammation site. COX-2 contributes to the development of inflammation, suggesting that selective inhibition of the COX-2 isoform could be relevant to the discovery of anti-inflammatory drugs devoid of the typical side effects of most of the traditional NSAIDs (21). NO is a free radical produced in mammalian cells constitutively or induced by various cell activators through the oxidation of L-arginine by a family of isoenzymes known as nitric oxide synthases (NOS). Inhibition of NOS is effective in reducing NO generation and therefore helpful in the treatment of inflammation.

In vitro screening for anti-inflammatory phenylpropanoid glycosides as inhibitors of COX-2 and NO biosynthesis demonstrated that acteoside and arenarioside exert their anti-inflammatory action through the inhibition of COX-2 enzyme to prevent proinflammatory PG generation, as they have greater inhibitory potency on COX-2 than on Cox-1 (22).

In the same experimental model, isoacteoside, acteoside, and 2′-*O*-acetylacteoside were also found to be inhibitors of NO production. They substantially reduced nitrite accumulation in lipopolysaccharide (0.1 μg/mL)-stimulated J774.1 cells at the concentration of 100–200 μM. Specically, they inhibited at 200 μM by 32.2–72.4% nitrite accumulation induced by lipopolysaccharide (0.1 μg/mL)/interferon-γ (100 U/mL) in mouse peritoneal exudates macrophages. However, these compounds did not affect the expression of inducible nitric oxide (iNOS) mRNA, the iNOS protein level, or the iNOS activity in lipopolysaccharide-stimulated J774.1 cells. Instead, they had a clear scavenging effect (6.9–43.9%) even at low concentrations (2–10 μM) on nitrite generated from an NO donor, 1-propanamine-3-hydroxy-2-nitroso-1-propylhydrazino (PAPA NONOate). These results indicate that the phenylethanoids have NO radical-scavenging activity, which possibly contributes to their anti-inflammatory effects (23).

Acteoside was also found to be able to induce proinflammatory cytokines interleukin (IL)-1, IL-6, and tumor necrosis factor-α (TNF-α) in macrophage-like cell line J774.A1 at 1–100 ng/mL. Moreover, the stimulatory action of acteoside was studied using the bovine glomerular endothelial cell line GEN-T and it was found that it can stimulate IL-6 production. These stimulatory activities cannot be abolished by treating with polymyxin B, which is capable of inactivating lipopolysaccharide (LPS), indicating thereby that the action was not a contamination of LPS (24).

C. Anticancer Activity

Antioxidants have been shown to inhibit both initiation and promotion in carcinogenesis and counteract cell immortalization and transformation. Caffeoylated phenylethanoid glycosides acteoside and isoacteoside were cytotoxic and cytostatic, displaying in vivo anticancer activity against murine P-388 (PS) lymphocytic leukemia. The ED_{50} values were found to be 2.6 μg/mL for the former and 10 μg/mL for the latter (25). Acteoside had cytotoxic and cytostatic activity against several kinds of cancer cells. However, they did not affect the growth and viability of primary-cultured rat hepatocytes. Attention to the structure-activity relationship demonstrated that the effects of the compounds appear to be due to their *ortho*-dihydroxylated aromatic systems (26). They also selectively inhibited the growth of murine melanoma B16F10 cells with the same IC_{50} value of 8 μM. Comparison of the action with inhibitory activities of their methanolysis products showed that the 3,4-dihydroxyphenethyl alcohol group in acteoside and isoacteoside might be more essential for the activity than the caffeoyl group (27).

Acteoside remarkably decreased the growth curve and mitotic index of human gastric adenocarcinoma MGc80-3 cells and delayed the cell-doubling time in vitro. There was a 75% decrease of the tumorigenicity of the treated cells compared to the untreated cells inoculated subcutaneously in BALB/C nude mice. Scanning electron microscopy revealed that the microvilli on the surface of treated cells had been reduced. It has been confirmed that acteoside could reverse MGc80-3 cells' malignant phenotypic characteristics and induced redifferentiation of MGc80-3 cells (28).

Lung cancer is the third most common cancer in the United States and the leading cause of cancer death. The mortality is high because systemic therapies do not cure metastatic disease. The side effects and the development of drug resistance colimit the use of conventional cytotoxic chemotherapeutic agents for treating patients with lung cancer. An increase in the expression of COX-2 may play a significant role in carcinogenesis in addition to its well-known involvement in the inflammatory reaction (29,30) that is also frequently noted in a specific type of lung cancer. Acteoside, with COX-2 inhibitory and cytotoxic activities, had suppressive effect on lung metastasis of B16 melanoma cells. At a dose of 50 mg/kg acteoside was administered intraperitoneally every other day from 13 days before B16 melanoma cell injection until all mice had succumbed to the lung metastatic tumor burden in the lung. Administration of acteoside significantly prolonged survival time; the average survival time was 63.3 ± 3.4 days compared with 52.1 ± 2.5 days in control mice. The results suggest that effects of acteoside may be involved in the therapeutic effect on lung cancer (31).

Apoptosis is closely related to the development and homeostasis of normal tissues. It has become evident that alterations in the apoptotic pathways are intimately involved in a variety of cancer processes. The mechanism of cell death mediated by cytotoxic chemotherapy was once thought to be through irreversible DNA damage with subsequent mitotic failure. The spectrum of chemotherapeutic agents stimulating apoptosis suggests that the programmed cell death pathway is a central mechanism of the cytotoxic effects of current therapy. Acteoside can induce cell death in promyelocytic leukemia HL-60 cells with an IC_{50} value of 26.7/μM. Analysis of extracted DNA on agarose gel electrophoresis revealed that acteoside induced the internucleosomal breakdown of chromatin DNA characteristic of apoptosis. Apoptosis-specific DNA fragmentation was clearly detectable 4 hr after treatment with acteoside and was independent of the cell cycle phase. These data indicate that acteoside induces apoptosis in HL-60 cells (32).

Protein kinase C (PKC) represents a family of more than 11 phospholipid-dependent ser/thr kinases that are involved in a variety of pathways. They regulate various celluar processes including mitogenesis, cell adhesion, apoptosis, angiogenesis, invasion, and metastasis (33–36). PKCs are the major cellular targets that can be activated by tumor-promoting phorbol ester, and consequently are thought to play an important role in carcinogenesis (37). Thus PKCs may be important for both oxidant-mediated tumor promotion and antioxidant-mediated chemoprevention. Conceivably consistent with the generalization that diverse tumor promoters are oxidants, a variety of structurally related chemopreventive agents are antioxidants. These facts demonstrate the functional significance of antioxidant activity in cancer prevention and inhibition. Acteoside, with antioxidant activity, is a potent inhibitor of PKC from the rat brain. Biochemically acteoside, interacting with the catalytic domain of PKC, is a competitive inhibitor with the substrate ATP and a noncompetitive inhibitor with respect to the phosphate acceptor (histone IIIS). This effect was further evidenced by the fact that acteoside inhibited native PKC with an identical catalytic fragment. However, it did not affect (^{3}H)-phorbol-12,13-dibutyrate binding to PKC (38). In accordance with the above finding, it was observed that acteoside, and poliumoside showed inhibitory activity against PKC-α with IC_{50} values of 9.3 and 24.4 μM, respectively (39). These results suggested that phenolic antioxidants, being easily converted to their oxidized state, may be inhibitory against tumor promotion.

Acteoside and arenarioside are capable of scavenging reactive oxygen species such as superoxide anion, peroxide hydrogen, hypochlorous acid, and hydroxyl radical. Moreover, the use of different stimuli having various pathways of action on polymorphonuclear neutrophils (PMN) oxidative metabolism permits the establishment of the hypothesis that each phenylpropanoid ester has its own particular mechanism of action through protein kinase C or phospholipase C pathways (40).

In recent years, telomerase has emerged as a highly promising novel target for therapeutic intervention in the treatment of cancer. In approximately 85% of human cancers, however, telomerase is reactivated and acts to maintain telomere length. Acteoside has been identified as a potent inhibitor of telomerase in the human gastric carcinoma cells MKN45. Modeling and biophysical studies suggest that acteoside-mediated cell differentiation and apoptosis may be based on telomere-telomerase-cell-cycle-dependent modulation. Thus, the antitumor mechanism of acteoside is demonstrated once more to be due to its inhibition of telomerase in tumor cells (41).

D. Hepatoprotective Activity

Chemicals such as CCl_4-catabolized radicals induce lipid peroxidation, damage the membranes of liver cells and organelles, cause the swelling and necrosis of hepatocytes, and result in the release of cytosolic enzymes such as AST, ALT, and LDH into the blood. Therefore, CCl_4-induced liver injury has been employed as a convenient model for investigating radical-induced damage and its prevention in animals.

Acteoside, 2′-*O*-acetylacteoside, and isoacteoside inhibited both hepatocyte lipid peroxidation and AST release to the medium, alleviating the CCl_4-induced cell death. Furthermore, acteoside efficiently suppressed ALT release into blood circulation induced by CCl_4. At the dose of 30 or 100 mg/kg, it gave almost the same protective potency as 100 mg/kg of glycyrrhizin, a positive control substance. These results demonstrated that the compounds were potent hepatoprotective agents against CCl_4 intoxication. The anti-CCl_4-toxicant activity of phenylethanoids was believed to be partly based on their free-radical-scavenging activity and antilipid peroxidative effect. They could prevent hepatocyte damage by scavenging radicals such as those involved in the process of lipid peroxidation on the cell membrane and subcellular organelle-like microsome. The phenylethanoids affected CCl_4-induced lipid oxidation in hepatocytes to an extent equivalent to that of silybin. Addition of them to cultured rat hepatocytes efficiently prevented cell damage induced by exposure to CCl_4 or D-galactosamine (D-GalN). Moreover acteoside had pronounced antihepatotoxic activity against CCl_4 intoxication in vivo (42).

Preadministration of acteoside at 10 or 50 mg/kg subcutaneously at 12 and 1 hr prior to D-galactosamine and lipopolysaccharide (D-GalN/LPS) intoxication significantly inhibited hepatic apoptosis, hepatitis, and lethality. Tumor necrosis factor-α (TNF-α) secreted from LPS-stimulated macrophages is an important mediator for apoptosis in this model. Acteoside showed no apparent effect on the marked elevation of serum TNF-α, but it partly prevented in vitro TNF-α-induced cell death in D-GalN-sensitized hepatocytes at the concentrations of 50, 100, and 200 μM. These results indicate that D-GalN/LPS-induced hepatic apoptosis could be blocked by an exogenous antioxidant, suggesting the involvement of reactive oxygen intermediates (ROIs) in TNF-α-dependent hepatic apoptosis (43).

E. Antinephritic Activity

It has been postulated that leukocytes play an important role in the pathogenesis of nephritic disease. Acteoside given p.o. at a dose of 30 mg/kg once a day for 15 consecutive days after treatment with antiglomerular basement membrane (GBM) serum markedly suppressed the urinary protein as well as glomerular histological changes. Acteoside administered p.o. for 5 or 15 consecutive days remarkably retarded accumulation of total leukocytes as well as ED1-positive, CD4-positive, CD8-positive, interleukin-2-receptor-positive, and Ia-positive cells in the glomeruli. However, acteoside, unlike cyclosporin A, did not significantly suppress plasma antibody level against rabbit γ-globulin at this dose. Thus, acetoside may exert its antinephritic action by suppressing the accumulation of leukocytes in the glomeruli (44).

Further researches were carried out. Aceteoside, given from the first day after i.v. injection of anti-GBM serum, inhibits protein excretion into urine on crescentic-type anti-GBM nephritis in rats. In the acteoside-treated rats, cholesterol and creatine contents and antibody production against rabbit γ-globulin in the plasmas were lower than those of the nephritic control rats. Histological observation demonstrated that this agent suppresses hypercellularity and crescent formation, adhesion of capillary wall to Bowman's capsule, and fibrinoid necrosis in the glomeruli. Furthermore, rat IgG and C3 deposits on the GBM were significantly less in the acteoside-treated group than in the control nephritic group. When the treatment was started from the twentieth day after i.v. injection of anti-GBM serum, by which time the disease had been established, aceteoside resulted in a similar effect on the nephritic rats as stated above. These results suggest that aceteoside may be a useful medication against rapidly progressive glomerulonephritis, which is characterized by severe glomerular lesions with diffuse crescents (45).

It is known that adhesion molecules play a crucial role in the development of glomerulonephritis. Aceteoside treatment significantly decreased the upregulation of intercellular adhesion molecule-1 (ICAM-1) expression in nephritic glomeruli as well as in human umbilical vein endothelial cells (HUVECs) and rat mesangial cells, mediated by inflammatory cytokines or phorbol 12-myristate 13-acetate. Adhesion of neutrophils and macrophages to acteoside-treated HUVECs was suppressed to one-half of that in untreated HUVECs. Additionally, it is suggested that the antinephritic action of acteoside is due to the inhibition of intraglomerular accumulation of leukocytes through prevention of the upregulation of ICAM-1 (46).

The development of new antinephritic agents on the basis of inhibiting mesangial matrix expansion and mesangial cell proliferation in mesangioproliferative anti-Thy 1 nephritis may open new options for treatment of the disease. Acteoside treatment performed in either the early or late period significantly reduced proteinuria, mesangial matrix expansion, and mesangial proliferation. Acteoside also reduce glomerular macrophage infiltration and ICAM-1 expression in glomeruli of anti-Thy 1 nephritic rats. Furthermore, acteoside treatment markedly increased the activities of matrix metaloproteinases (MMP) in glomeruli. These results suggest that acteoside can inhibit mesangial cell proliferation and extracellular matrix overproduction by either inhibiting ICAM-1 expression or increasing activities of MMP (47).

F. Cardioactive Effects

It has been confirmed that acteoside has cardioactive effects (48). Intravenous administration of acteoside resulted in a significant decrease in blood pressure in Wistar rats (49). In the Langendorff rat heart preparation, acteoside induces a significant dose-dependent increment in chronotropism, inotropism, and coronary perfusion (50). These cardioactive effects appear to be associated with a striking increase in the level of intracellular cyclic 3,5-adenosine monophosphate (cAMP) (51).

Acteoside also significantly increased chronotropism, inotropism, and CPR when tested against the competitive α-adrenergic blocker phentolamine. It was found that acteoside induced significant increases in the levels of 6-keto-PGF1a, a rapidly formed by-product of postacyclin (PGI-2) widely used as an index of prostacyclin production. Acteoside can significantly increase prostacyclin levels (142%) (52). An increase in the prostacyclin level in Langendorff rat hearts may be responsible for stimulating cAMP production and thus account for the positive cardioactive effects mediated by acteoside.

The four purified *B. hancei* phenylethanoids exerted antiproliferative effect on cultured A7r5 rat aortic smooth-muscle cells. The rank order of effectiveness for inhibition of the cell proliferation was: brandioside ≥ poliumoside > 2′-acetylacteoside ≥ acteoside in the presence of 2% or 5% fetal bovine serum. Either brandioside or poliumoside has one additional rhamnose molecule attached to position 6′ of the glucose chain, thereby enhancing its hydrophilic property. This may partially explain why both agents were threefold more effective in the inhibition of cell proliferation. The 2′-*O*-acetyl group in those molecules is unlikely to be involved in the antipoliferative activity since acteoside and 2′-*O*-acetylacteoside (with acetyl group) or poliumoside and brandioside (with acetyl group) exhibited the same potency. The hydroxy groups on the aromatic rings seem to play a role in the inhibitory effects of the four glycosides on cell proliferation (53). These results indicate that *B. hancei* phenylethanoids may have a potential for prevention of vascular-wall-thickening-related pathological processes such as arteriosclerosis.

As described in another report, acteoside can relax rat aortic rings preconstricted by 9,11-dideoxy-11α,9α-epoxymethanoprostaglandin $F_{2\alpha}$ (U46619) with IC_{50} value of 0.22 ± 0.01 mg/mL, but it causes an increase in K + -induced tone. Removal of endothelium enhanced the relaxing effect of acteoside. In addition, pretreatment with acteoside inhibited endothelium/nitric-oxide-mediated relaxation induced by acetylcholine. Acteoside relaxed the preconstricted aortic rings probably through multiple mechanisms by acting on smooth-muscle cells (54). The cardioactive effects of phenylethanoids may be partly mediated through suppression of vascular smooth-muscle-cell proliferation.

G. Microbiological Effects

There has been interest over the years in the effects of phenylethanoid glycosides on microorganisms. Although acteoside exerted weak antibacterial effects on *Escherichia coli*, it had antiplasmid effects, including F′lac plasmid elimination, and inhibited kanamycin resistance transfer in *E. coli* (55). Similar results were observed with its isomer isoacteoside (56,57). In addition, acteoside and arenarioside exhibited a moderate antimicrobial activity against *Proteus mirabilis* and *Staphylococcus aureus* including one methicillin-resistant strain (58,59). The mode of action of acteoside toward *Staph. aureus* is related to the inhibition of leucine incorporation required for its protein synthesis. With regard to the killing kinetics, it is recognized that acteoside affects several important sites in some metabolic or structural targets on the bacterial cell (60).

Antiviral activity is a topic of wide interest, especially activity against human immunodeficient virus type 1 (HIV), which is receiving worldwide attention. Acteoside had potent inhibitory activity against HIV-1 integrase with IC_{50} values of 7.8 ± 3.6 μM (61).

Acteoside was tested in vitro against herpes simplex type I (HSV-1), vesicular stomatitis virus (VSV), and poliovirus type 1, and it had antiviral activity only against VSV. At 500 μg/mL the percentage of cellular viability at the nontoxic limit concentrations of acteoside was found to be 53.6%. However, it did not inhibit poliovirus in this survey (62).

H. Other Effects

Xanthine oxidase (XO, EC 1.2.3.2) is a key enzyme associated with the incidence of hyperuricemia-related disorders. Among the five phenylethanoids arenarioside, brandioside, acteoside, 2′-*O*-acetylacteoside, and isoacteoside, only isoacteoside competitively inhibited xanthine oxidase and substantially decreased the formation of uric acid. The IC_{50} and Ki values are 45.48 and 10.08 μM, respectively. Furthermore, it was suggested that caffeoylation of the 6′-hydroxyl group of the phenylethanoids was essential for the enzyme inhibitory action (5).

Acteoside has a significant inhibitory effect on toxicity or lethality in the KCN-induced anoxia model (63). Acteoside showed very strong inhibition of rabbit lens aldose reductase (AR), being about 2.5 times more potent than baicalein, a known natural inhibitor of AR ($IC_{50} = 9.8 \times 10^{-7}$ M) (64).

Acteoside and arenarioside are able to bind to benzodiazepine, dopaminergic, and morphine receptors. The corresponding EC_{50} values were determined and ranged from 0.4 to 4.7 mg/mL. This action may be related to the neurosedative activities, rationalizing the traditional use of the herb as a neurosedative drug (65,66).

IV. HEALTH EFFECTS

A detailed clinical trial took place in 1998 with use of crude extract prepared from whole herb of *B. hancei* against chronic hepatitis (67). A total of 174 patients with chronic hepatitis B were treated thrice daily with 5 g of the extract at Yunnan Nanjiang Hospital, Yunnan Province, China. All patients were diagnosed with chronic hepatitis B based on the clinical criteria. Of 174 patients aged 7–65 years, 116, 73, and 29 patients have had the disease for 6–12, 18–24, and more than 24 months, respectively. A total of 146 patients were successfully treated (67%), 70 felt better, but 2 showed no therapeutic effect. It was demonstrated that the extract could significantly inhibit HBV replication and decrease HBsAg, HBeAg, HBV DNA, and IgM anti-HBc levels by 32.6%, 38.5%, 61.0%, and 48.4%, respectively. The extract also significantly reduced SGPT and modulated the immunological function of the treated patients. Moreover, the extract was confirmed to have anti-inflammatory, anti-infective, immunomodulatory, and antivirus activities in animal models. No toxic effect was observed in the patients and animals treated with the *B. hancei* extract at the same doses.

V. CONCLUSION AND COMMENT

Modern physical and chemical analyses as well as in vitro and in vivo bioassays provide powerful tools for a better understanding of the chemical and biological aspects of *B. hancei*. Phenylpropanoid glycosides are the major constituents of *B. hancei* and are believed to be responsible for the various actions of this herbal medicine. Although acteoside is a representative main constituent of the phenylethanoids present in the species, the efficacy of *B. hancei* is ascribable to a complex mixture of phytochemicals in the herb.

In follow-up biomedical research of *B. hancei* aimed at finding new drug(s), the following fundamental issues must be considered:

1. Source materials: Each batch of *B. hancei* must be properly identified by botanically well-trained personnel; it is important to set up quality standards for the herb including morphological inspection, microscopic examination, chemical and physical analyses

as well as quantification of major and preferably activity-related component(s).

2. Standardization: *B. hancei* contains many phytochemicals, some of which such as phenylpropanoid glycosides are known to be associated with activities of the herb extract. However, some minor constituents of the species remain to be characterized. It is thus recommended that the levels of active or key components such as acteoside, preferably along with a chemical fingerprint, be used as indicators of the herb extract for quality and consistency controls.
3. Biological assays: The chemical profile derived from the species by itself is insufficient for the understanding of its efficacy. This is where biochemistry, molecular biology, and cell biology are invaluable in establishing quantifiable and reproducible assays. Moreover, the chemical fingerprint is important to link these biological assays and provide assurance of efficacy and consistency. In addition, it must be kept in mind that the in vitro and in vivo assays may not be consistent with the clinical results.
4. Clinical studies: It is important that clinical trials for the herb be designed in a manner that reflects the above requirements. The acceptable standard for clinical tests recommends a randomized and double-blind placebo trial with clinical indicators showing statistically significant differences between treatment and placebo groups.

REFERENCES

1. Kunming Department of Health. Yunnan Zhongcaoyao Xuan, Kunming: Kunming Press, 1970:659–660.
2. Jiangsu College of New Medicine. The Dictionary of the Traditional Chinese Medicine. 1st ed. Shanghai: Shanghai Press of Science & Technology, 1977: 2204–2205.
3. He ZD, Wang DZ, Yang CR. Phenylpropanoid glycosides from *Brandisia hancei*. Acta Botan Yunnan 1990; 12:439–446.
4. He ZD, Yang CR. Brandioside, a phenylpropanoid glycoside from *Brandisia hancei*. Phytochemistry 1991; 30:701–702.
5. Kong LD, Wolfender JL, Cheng CH, Hostettmann K, Tan RX. Xanthine oxidase inhibitors from *Brandisia hancei*. Planta Med 1999; 65:744–746.
6. Zhou YC, Zheng RL. Phenolic compounds and an analog as superoxide anion scavengers and antioxidants. Biochem Pharmacol 1991; 42:1177–1179.
7. Shi Y, Wang W, Fan B, Jia Z, Yao S, Zheng R. Fast repair of dAMP radical anions by phenylpropanoid glycosides and their analogs. Biochim Biophys Acta 2000; 1474:383–389.

8. Li YM, Han ZH, Jiang SH, Jiang Y, Yao SD, Zhu DY. Fast repairing of oxidized OH radical adducts of dAMP and dGMP by phenylpropanoid glycosides from *Scrophularia ningpoensis* Hemsl. Acta Pharmacol Sin 2000; 21:1125–1128.
9. Li W, Zheng R, Su B, Jia Z, Li H, Jiang Y, Yao S, Lin N. Repair of dGMP hydroxyl radical adducts by verbascoside via electron transfer: a pulse radiolysis study. Int J Radiat Biol 1996; 69:481–485.
10. Li J, Wang PF, Zheng R, Liu ZM, Jia Z. Protection of phenylpropanoid glycosides from *Pedicularis* against oxidative hemolysis in vitro. Planta Med 1993; 59:315–317.
11. Braca A, De Tommasi N, Di Bari L, Pizza C, Politi M, Morelli I. Antioxidant principles from *Bauhinia tarapotensis*. J Nat Prod 2001; 64:892–895.
12. Harput US, Saracoglu I, Inoue M, Ogihara Y. Phenylethanoid and iridoid glycosides from *Veronica persica*. Chem Pharm Bull (Tokyo) 2002; 50:869–871.
13. Li J, Ge RC, Zheng RL, Liu ZM, Jia ZJ. Antioxidative and chelating activities of phenylpropanoid glycosides from *Pedicularis striata*. Zhongguo Yaoli Xuebao 1997; 18:77–80.
14. He ZD, Lau KM, Xu HX, Li PC, Pui-Hay But P. Antioxidant activity of phenylethanoid glycosides from *Brandisia hancei*. J Ethnopharmacol 2000; 71:483–486.
15. Xiong Q, Kadota S, Tani T, Namba T. Antioxidative effects of phenylethanoids from *Cistanche deserticola*. Biol Pharm Bull 1996; 19:1580–1585.
16. Wong IY, He ZD, Huang Y, Chen ZY. Antioxidative activities of phenylethanoid glycosides from *Ligustrum purpurascens*. J Agric Food Chem 2001; 49:3113–3119.
17. Li JX, Xin D, Li H, Lu JF, Tong CW, Gao JN, Chan KM. Effect of verbascoside on decreasing concentration of oxygen free radicals and lipid peroxidation in skeletal muscle. Zhongguo Yaoli Xuebao 1999; 20:126–130.
18. Liao F, Zheng RL, Gao JJ, Jia ZJ. Retardation of skeletal muscle fatigue by the two phenylpropanoid glycosides: verbascoside and martynoside from *Pedicularis plicata* maxim. Phytother Res 1999; 13:621–623.
19. Murai M, Tamayama Y, Nishibe S. Phenylethanoids in the herb of *Plantago lanceolata* and inhibitory effect on arachidonic acid-induced mouse ear edema. Planta Med 1995; 61:479–480.
20. Schapoval EE, Vargas MR, Chaves CG, Bridi R, Zuanazzi JA, Henriques AT. Antiinflammatory and antinociceptive activities of extracts and isolated compounds from *Stachytarpheta cayennensis*. J Ethnopharmacol 1998; 60:53–59.
21. Vane JR. Nature 1994; 367:215.
22. Sahpaz S, Garbacki N, Tits M, Bailleul F. Isolation and pharmacological activity of phenylpropanoid esters from *Marrubium vulgare*. J Ethnopharmacol 2002; 79:389–392.
23. Xiong Q, Tezuka Y, Kaneko T, Li H, Tran LQ, Hase K, Namba T, Kadota S. Inhibition of nitric oxide by phenylethanoids in activated macrophages. Eur J Pharmacol 2000; 400:137–144.
24. Inoue M, Ueda M, Ogihara Y, Saracoglu I. Induction of cytokines by a phenylpropanoid glycoside acteoside. Biol Pharm Bull 1998; 21:1394–1395.

25. Pettit GR, Numata A, Takemura T, Ode RH, Narula AS, Schmidt JM, Cragg GM, Pase CP. Antineoplastic agents. 107. Isolation of acteoside and isoacteoside from *Castilleja linariaefolia*. J Nat Prod 1990; 53:456–458.
26. Saracoglu I, Inoue M, Cali I, Ogihara Y. Studies on constituents with cytotoxic and cytostatic activity of two Turkish medicinal plants *Phlomis armeniaca* and *Scutellaria salviifolia*. Biol Pharm Bull 1995; 18:1396–1400.
27. Nagao T, Abe F, Okabe H. Antiproliferative constituents in the plants. 7. Leaves of *Clerodendron bungei* and leaves and bark of *C trichotomum*. Biol Pharm Bull 2001; 24:1338–1341.
28. Li J, Zheng Y, Zhou H, Su B, Zheng R. Differentiation of human gastric adenocarcinoma cell line MGc80-3 induced by verbascoside. Planta Med 1997; 63:499–502.
29. Taketo MM. Cyclooxygenase-2 inhibitors in tumorigenesis (part I). J Natl Cancer Inst 1998; 90:1529–1536.
30. Taketo MM. Cyclooxygenase-2 inhibitors in tumorigenesis (part II). J Natl Cancer Inst 1998; 90:1609–1620.
31. Ohno T, Inoue M, Ogihara Y, Saracoglu I. Antimetastatic activity of acteoside, a phenylethanoid glycoside. Biol Pharm Bull 2002; 25:666–668.
32. Inoue M, Sakuma Z, Ogihara Y, Saracoglu I. Induction of apoptotic cell death in HL-60 cells by acteoside, a phenylpropanoid glycoside. Biol Pharm Bull 1998; 21:81–83.
33. Nishizuka Y. Intracellular signaling by hydrolysis of phospholipids and activation of protein kinase C. Science 1992; 258:607–614.
34. Jaken S. Protein kinase C and tumor promoters. Curr Opin Cell Biol 1990; 2:192–197.
35. Kiley SC, Clark KJ, Duddy SK, Welch DR, Jaken S. Increased protein kinase C in mammary tumor cells: relationship to transformation and metastatic progression. Oncogene 1999; 18:6748–6757.
36. Liu B, Honn KV. Protein kinase C inhibitor calphostin C inhibitor B16 melanoma metastasis. Int J Cancer Res 1992; 52:147–153.
37. Boscoboinik D, Szewczyk A, Hensey C, Azzi A. Inhibition of cell proliferation by a-tocopherol: role of protein kinase C. J Biol Chem 1991; 266:6188–6194.
38. Herbert JM, Maffrand JP, Taoubi K, Augereau JM, Fouraste I, Gleye J. Verbascoside isolated from *Lantana camara*, an inhibitor of protein kinase C. J Nat Prod 1991; 54:1595–1600.
39. Zhou BN, Bahler BD, Hofmann GA, Mattern MR, Johnson RK, Kingston DG. Phenylethanoid glycosides from *Digitalis purpurea* and *Penstemon linarioides* with PKCalpha-inhibitory activity. J Nat Prod 1998; 61:1410–1412.
40. Daels-Rakotoarison DA, Seidel V, Gressier B, Brunet C, Tillequin F, Bailleul F, Luyckx M, Dine T, Cazin M, Cazin JC. Neurosedative and antioxidant activities of phenylpropanoids from *Ballota nigra*. Arzneimittelforschung 2000; 50:16–23.
41. Zhang F, Jia Z, Deng Z, Wei Y, Zheng R, Yu L. In vitro modulation of telomerase activity, telomere length and cell cycle in MKN45 cells by verbascoside. Planta Med 2002; 68:115–118.

42. Xiong Q, Hase K, Tezuka Y, Tani T, Namba T, Kadota S. Hepatoprotective acti vity of phenylethanoids from *Cistanche deserticola*. Planta Med 1998; 64: 120–125.
43. Xiong Q, Has K, Tezuka Y, Namba T, Kadota S. Acteoside inhibits apoptosis in D-galactosamine and lipopolysaccharide-induced liver injury. Life Sci 1999; 65:421–430.
44. Hayashi K, Nagamatsu T, Ito M, Hattori T, Suzuki Y. Acteoside, a component of *Stachys sieboldii* MIQ, may be a promising antinephritic agent. 2. Effect of acteoside on leukocyte accumulation in the glomeruli of nephritic rats. Jpn J Pharmacol 1994; 66:47–52.
45. Hayashi K, Nagamatsu T, Ito M, Hattori T, Suzuki Y. Acetoside, a component of *Stachys sieboldii* MIQ, may be a promising antinephritic agent: effect of acteoside on crescentic-type anti-GBM nephritis in rats. Jpn J Pharmacol 1994; 65:143–151.
46. Hayashi K, Nagamatsu T, Ito M, Yagita H, Suzuki Y. Acteoside, a component of *Stachys sieboldii* MIQ, may be a promising antinephritic agent. 3. Effect of aceteoside on expression of intercellular adhesion molecule-1 in experimental nephritic glomeruli in rats and cultured endothelial cells. Jpn J Pharmacol 1996; 70:157–168.
47. Hattori T, Fujitsuka N, Shindo S. Effect of acteoside on mesangial proliferation in rat anti-Thy 1 nephritis. Nippon Jinzo Gakkai Shi 1996; 38:202–212.
48. Pennacchio M, Alexander E, Chisalberti EL, Richmond GS. Cardioactive effects of *Eremophila alternifolia* extracts. J Ethnopharmacol 1995; 47:91–95.
49. Ahmad M, Rizwni GH, Aftab K, Ahmad VU, Gilani AH, Ahmad SP. Acteoside: a new antihypertensive. Phytother Res 1995; 9:525–527.
50. Pennacchio M, Syah YM, Ghisalberti EL, Alexander E. Cardioactive compounds from *Eremophila* species. J Ethnopharmacol 1996; 53:21–27.
51. Pennacchio M, Alexander E, Syah YM, Ghisalberti EL. The effect of verbascoside on cyclic 3′,5′-adenosine monophosphate levels in isolated rat heart. Eur J Pharmacol 1996; 305:169–171.
52. Pennacchio M, Syah YM, Alexander E, Ghisalberti EL. Mechanism of action of verbascoside on the isolated rat heart: increases in level of prostacyclin. Phytother Res 1999; 13:254–255.
53. He ZD, Huang Y, Yao X, Lau CW, Law WI, Chen ZY. Purification of phenylethanoids from *Brandisia hancei* and the antiproliferative effects on aortic smooth muscle. Planta Med 2001; 67:520–522.
54. Wong IY, Huang Y, He ZD, Lau CW, Chen ZY. Relaxing effects of *Ligstrum purpurascens* extract and purified acteoside in rat aortic rings. Planta Med 2001; 67:317–321.
55. Molnar J, Gunics G, Musci I, Koltai M, Petri I, Shoyama Y, Matsumoto M, Nishioka I. Antimicrobial and immunomodulating effects of some phenolic glycosides. Acta Microbiol Hung 1989; 36:425–432.
56. Li J, Zhao Y, Wang B, Cui J. Phenylethanoid glucosides from *flos Buddlejae*. Zhongguo Zhongyao Zazhi 1997; 22:613–615, 640.
57. Pardo F, Perich F, Villarroel L, Torres R. Isolation of verbascoside, an

antimicrobial constituent of *Buddleja globosa* leaves. J Ethnopharmacol 1993; 39:221–222.
58. Didry N, Seidel V, Dubreuil L, Tillequin F, Bailleul F. Isolation and antibacterial activity of phenylpropanoid derivatives from *Ballota nigra*. J Ethnopharmacol 1999; 67:197–202.
59. Arciniegas A, Avendaño A, Pérez-Castorena AL, Romo de Vivar A. Flavonoids from *Buddleja pariflora*. Biochem Syst Ecol 1997; 25:185–186.
60. Avila JG, de Liverant JG, Martinez A, Martinez G, Munoz JL, Arciniegas A, Romo de Vivar A. Mode of action of *Buddleja cordata* verbascoside against *Staphylococcus aureus*. J Ethnopharmacol 1999; 66:75–78.
61. Kim HJ, Woo ER, Shin CG, Hwang DJ, Park H, Lee YS. HIV-1 integrase inhibitory phenylpropanoid glycosides from *Clerodendron trichotomum*. Arch Pharm Res 2001; 24:286–291.
62. Bermejo P, Abad MJ, Diaz AM, Fernandez L, Santos JD, Sanchez S, Villaescusa L, Carrasco L, Irurzun A. Antiviral activity of seven iridoids, three saikosaponins and one phenylpropanoid glycoside extracted from *Bupleurum rigidum* and *Scrophularia scorodonia*. Planta Med 2002; 68:106–110.
63. Yamahara J, Kitani T, Kobayashi H, Kawahara Y. Studies on *Stachys sieboldii* MIQ II: anti-anoxia action and the active constituents. Yakugaku Zasshi 1990; 110:932–935.
64. Kohda H, Tanaka S, Yamaoka Y, Yahara S, Nohara T, Tanimoto T, Tanaka A. Studies on lens-aldose-reductase inhibitor in medicinal plants. II Active constituents of *Monochasma savatierii* Franch. et Maxim. Chem Pharm Bull (Tokyo) 1989; 37:3153–3154.
65. Daels-Rakotoarison DA, Seidel V, Gressier B, Brunet C, Tillequin F, Bailleul F, Luyckx M, Dine T, Cazin M, Cazin JC. Neurosedative and antioxidant activities of phenylpropanoids from *Ballota nigra*. Arzneimittelforschung 2000; 50:16–23.
66. Seidel V, Bailleul F, Tillequin F. Diterpene and phenylpropanoid heteroside esters from *Ballota nigra* L. Ann Pharm Fr 1998; 56:31–35.
67. Huang CG, Shi TR. Efficacy of Baogan Keli (the extract of *Brandisia hancei*) observed in 218 patients with HBV. Zhongguo Minzu Minjian Zazhi 1998; 34:19–20.

33

Ephedra

Christine A. Haller
University of California, San Francisco
and San Francisco General Hospital
San Francisco, California, U.S.A.

I. INTRODUCTION

Ephedra may be the herbal medicine that best illustrates the challenges faced today in incorporating traditional remedies, used for thousands of years in Eastern cultures, into modern Western societies in which the context of use may be very different. *Ephedra* is a common plant genus that grows worldwide in temperate climates. The Chinese herbal medicine ma huang is derived from the dried above-ground parts of several *Ephedra* species found in China, primarily *E. sinica*, *E. equisetina*, and *E. intermedia* (1–5). *E. gerardiana* is the species utilized as a traditional medicine in India and Pakistan (3). Ma huang has been traditionally used in Chinese medicine for the short-term treatment of bronchospasm, cough, and nasal congestion associated with colds, allergies, and asthma (1,3,5). *Ephedra* has also been used medicinally for its diaphoretic, vasopressant, antipyretic, and antitussive properties (3,5). Because of the risk of development of tachyphylaxis and dependence, long-term use of ma huang has not been traditionally advocated (2,4,5).

Ma huang is primarily available today in the United States in the form of dietary supplements that contain concentrated extracts of *E. sinica*. It is rarely found as a single formulation, but is most commonly marketed as a primary active ingredient in multicomponent dietary supplements promoted for weight reduction and athletic and energy enhancement. Ma huang is most commonly combined with botanical sources of caffeine, such as guarana, yerba mate, or kola nut, and other herbal constituents intended to intensify the desired effects of *Ephedra*. There are few published data on the potential pharmacological interactions between *Ephedra* and the various herbal constituents in multicomponent dietary supplements.

II. CHEMISTRY

The medicinal effects of the *Ephedra* species are attributed to the stimulant and vasoconstrictive properties of (−)ephedrine and several related alkaloids. Three diastereoisomeric pairs of β-phenylethylamines are found in *Ephedra*, collectively referred to as ephedra alkaloids. (−)-Ephedrine is the alkaloid found in greatest concentration, followed by (+)-pseudoephedrine and lesser quantities of their structural relatives, including (−)-norephedrine, (+)-norpseudoephedrine, (−)-methylephedrine, and (+)-methylpseudoephedrine (Fig. 1) (6,7). The alkaloids differ only in the number of methyl groups

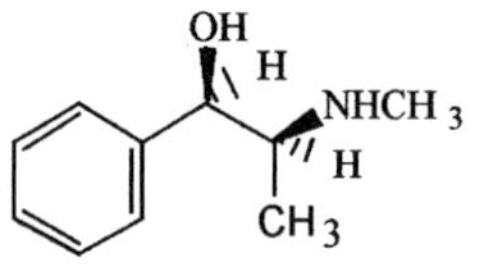

(1R,2S)-(-)-Ephedrine

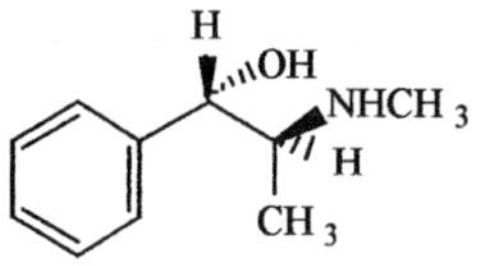

(1S,2S)-(+)-Pseudoephedrine

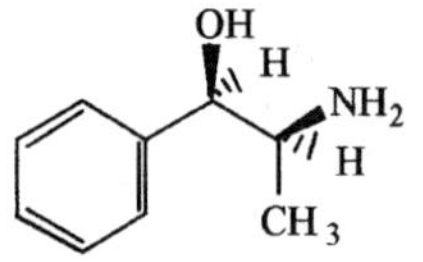

(1R,2S)-(-)-Norephedrine

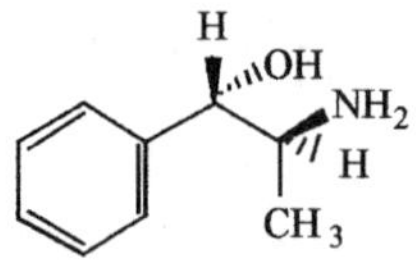

(1S,2S)-(+)-Norpseudoephedrine

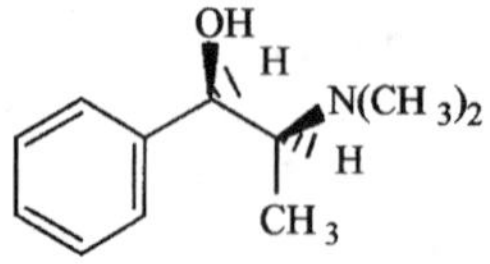

(1R,2S)-(-)-Methylephedrine

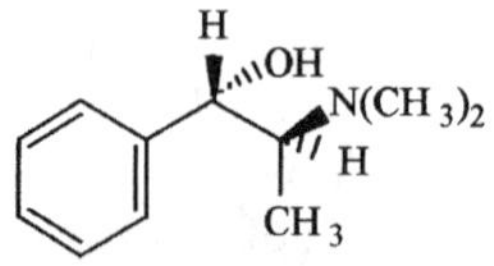

(1S,2S)-(+)-Methylpseudoephedrine

FIGURE 1 Chemical structures of ephedra alkaloids.

attached to the amine terminal, with one methyl group on ephedrine and two methyl groups on methylephedrine. Norephedrine lacks any methyl group on the amine terminal, with the prefix "nor" meaning "no methyl." The "pseudo" alkaloids differ from their isomeric partners only in the stereochemical configuration of the chiral β-carbon.

The content and concentration of the ephedra alkaloids varies between plant species, and also depends on growing conditions and plant processing. For ma huang derived from *E. sinica*, the dried, unprocessed herb contains 1–2% total alkaloids consisting of approximately 60–80% ephedrine and 10–20% pseudoephedrine (8,9). Concentrated extracts, however, may contain as much as 4–8% total ephedra alkaloids (9). Most commercially available dietary supplements contain extracts of *E. sinica* with an average of 6% total alkaloids. (−) Ephedrine and (+)-pseudoephedrine are FDA-approved drugs for the treatment of nasal congestion, bronchoconstriction, and cough due to colds, allergies, and asthma. The racemic form of norephedrine was formally available as the over-the-counter drug phenylpropanolamine (PPA) for nasal decongestion and as a weight loss aid. PPA-containing products were voluntarily withdrawn from the market in November 2000 because of a reported increased risk of hemorrhagic stroke (10). Norpseudoephedrine and methylephedrine are not approved drugs in the United States. In fact, (+)norpseudoephedrine, also known as cathine, is a constituent of khat (*Catha edulis*), a plant abused in eastern Africa for its psychoactive effects. It is classified as Schedule IV controlled substance in the United States because of its potent central nervous system effects and high abuse potential (11).

III. PHARMACOLOGY

Ephedrine and its related alkaloids have similar pharmacokinetic properties, which are summarized in Table 1 (12–15). The ephedra alkaloids are well absorbed orally with an average time to maximum plasma concentration of 1–2 hr. The duration of action of the ephedra alkaloids is approximately 3–5 hr after oral administration. Recent studies have found that the pharmacokinetics of the alkaloids in the form of ephedra extracts are similar to those of pharmaceutical forms (16–18). One study showed a slower rate of absorption and longer time to maximum plasma concentration (t_{max}) of ephedrine derived from powdered ma huang compared to synthetic ephedrine or ma huang extract (18).

The ephedra alkaloids are largely excreted unchanged in the urine, and may accumulate to toxic levels in cases of significant renal insufficiency (19). Because they are weak bases, the rate of elimination depends on the degree of ionization, which is a function of urine pH. In an alkaline urine environment, the alkaloids are largely un-ionized, and are easily reabsorbed across the

TABLE 1 Pharmacology of Major Alkaloid Constituents in Ephedra

Drug	Primary receptor site(s)	Onset of action	Duration of action	Plasma half-life	Elimination/metabolism	pKa
Ephedrine	α β_{11} β_2	15–60 min	3–5 hr	3–6 hr depending on urine pH	Mostly excreted unchanged in urine; 8–20% undergoes hepatic biotransformation to norephedrine	9.58
Pseudoephedrine	α_1	15–30 min	3–4 hr	3–6 hr depending on urine pH	Mostly excreted unchanged in urine; <1% undergoes hepatic biotransformation to norpseudoephedrine	9.4
Norephedrine	α_1 β_1	15–30 min	3 hr	4–5 hr	Mostly excreted unchanged in urine; 4% biotransformed to 4-hydroxynorephedrine and hippuric acid	9.44

cellular membranes in the distal renal tubule. Previous work shows that the elimination half-life of ephedrine is 3 hr at a urine pH of 5, but increases to 6.3 hr at a urine pH of about 6 (13,20). In one study, the half-life of pseudoephedrine was as long as 21 hr at a urine pH of 7.8 (19). This study also showed that when the urine pH is higher than 7, the elimination half-life depends on the urine flow rate. At high flow rates, the time for reabsorption in the renal tubule is diminished and the rate of clearance of pseudoephedrine is increased. Therefore, in the setting of high urine pH and low urine output, the half-life of the ephedrine alkaloids may be significantly prolonged. This could be clinically important in the setting of dehydration related to fever or strenuous exercise.

A minor elimination pathway for ephedrine and pseudoephedrine is by *N*-demethylation in the liver. Approximately 8–20% of ephedrine is metabolized to norephedrine, which is then primarily eliminated in the urine (14). About 4% of norephedrine is metabolized to 4-hydroxynorephedrine and hippuric acid (14). Less than 1% of pseudoephedrine is metabolized to norpseudoephedrine (21). (−)-Methylephedrine is more extensively metabolized than the other alkaloids, partly by *N*-demethylation to ephedrine, and then to norephedrine (20). In alkaline urine when reabsorption is high, (−) methyephedrine appears to be nearly completely metabolized (20).

IV. PHYSIOLOGICAL ACTIONS

Ephedrine and the other alkaloids are sympathomimetic amines that have both direct and indirect actions at α- and β-adrenergic receptors in the brain and peripheral nervous system (12). The physiological actions of the ephedra alkaloids depend on their relative affinities for these receptors, which provide a molecular basis to explain their different profiles of action and adverse effects. For example, (−)-ephedrine appears to have relatively more direct agonist effects and greater central nervous system affinity than either pseudoephedrine or norephedrine (22–24).

The primary action of the ephedra alkaloids is as indirect sympathetic nervous system stimulants acting to increase release of stored norepinephrine in sympathetic nerve terminals, which then diffuses into the synapse and binds to postsynaptic α- and β-adrenergic receptors (Fig. 2). These agents also can have direct agonist actions at both central and peripheral α_1, β_1, and β_2 postsynaptic receptors (22–24). Their α_1-adrenergic agonist activity produces vascular smooth-muscle contraction that results in vasoconstriction and increased peripheral vascular resistance. Stimulation of α_1 receptors in the radial pupillary muscle of the eye results in mydriasis. There are also α_1 receptors in the urethral sphincter, bladder base, and prostate that promote urinary continence. Stimulation of α_1-adrenergic receptors in the appetite

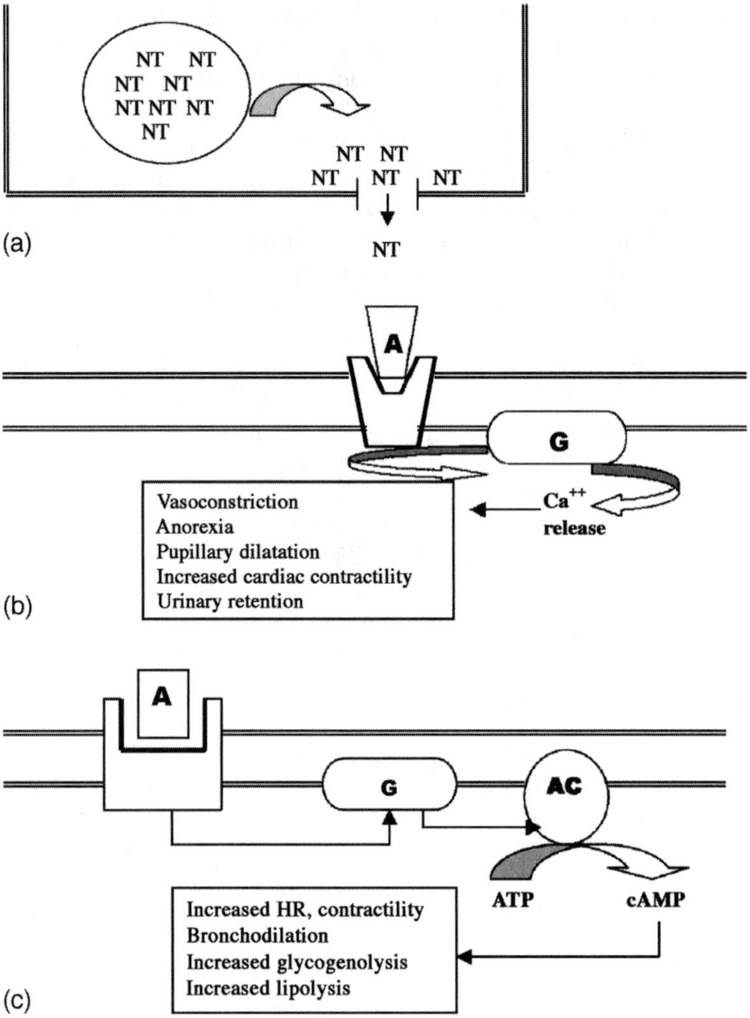

FIGURE 2 Schematic of molecular mechanisms of action of ephedra alkaloids. (a) Indirect release of stored neurotransmitters, primarily norepinephrine. (b) Direct action at postsynaptic α_1-adrenergic receptors in the brain and peripheral nervous system. (c) Direct action at postsynaptic β_1-, β_2-, and β_3-adrenergic receptors in the heart, smooth muscle, liver, and adipose tissue. NT = neurotransmitter, including norepinephrine, dopamine, and serotonin. A = agonist. G = membrane-bound G protein. AC = membrane-bound adenyl cyclase enzyme. cAMP = cyclic adenosine monophosphate. ATP = adenosine triphosphate.

center of the hypothalamus is believed to be responsible for the anorexigenic effects of the centrally acting ephedra alkaloids (25).

Stimulation of β_1-adrenergic receptors, found mostly in the heart, results in increased rate and force of contraction, leading to greater cardiac output. To a lesser extent, stimulation of α_1-receptors in the heart contributes to increased cardiac contractility. Stimulation of β_2-adrenergic receptors relaxes vascular, respiratory, and uterine smooth muscle, and increases liver glycogenolysis. β_3-Adrenergic receptors are located primarily in white adipose tissue, liver, and skeletal muscle, and activation of these receptors will increase lipid oxidation (26).

Agents with both α- and β-adrenergic stimulant actions will generally have a net effect of increasing blood pressure because the α_1 vasoconstrictive action typically supersedes β_2-mediated vascular relaxation. However, β_2-mediated bronchial smooth-muscle relaxation is not opposed by α_1-agonist activity, and therefore, ephedra alkaloids with β_2 activity will relieve bronchoconstriction.

V. CLINICAL USES

Discovery of the sympathomimetic effects of the phenethylamines led to pharmaceutical development of (−)-ephedrine, (+)-pseudoephedrine, and (+) norephedrine as nasal decongestants for allergic rhinitis. The vasoconstrictive actions of ephedrine have also been employed in the treatment of shock due to vascular collapse. Ephedrine has been used to treat hypotension and bradycardia following epidural anesthesia, particularly in obstetrics. Ephedrine has been employed as a bronchodilator because of its β_2-receptor-mediated relaxation of bronchial smooth muscle. Ephedrine has also been used to treat nocturnal enuresis due either to its relaxation effect on the detrusor muscle of the bladder or to its tendency to cause nighttime awakening (22). The racemic form of (+)-norephedrine has also previously been formulated as an over-the-counter weight loss aid, and its anorexigenic effects are theorized to be due to α_1-receptor activity in the hypothalamus (25).

Ephedra is currently marketed and used primarily in slimming regimens and athletic-performance-enhancing supplements. Under the Dietary Supplement Health and Education. Act of 1994, ephedra was classified as a dietary supplement, and therefore is not subject to the same stringent regulatory requirements as drugs. Use of ephedra has grown dramatically in the United States with sales figures and market surveys estimating that as many as 12 million Americans have used ephedra-containing products (27,28). One recent survey of patients scheduled for elective surgery found that 11% reported current use of ephedra (29).

VI. EFFECTS ON THE CARDIOVASCULAR SYSTEM

Only a few small clinical investigations have been published that describe the cardiovascular effects of ma huang, with some studies showing significant increases in heart rate and blood pressure after oral administration (17,18), and other studies showing that tolerance develops to these effects (30,31). In general, the cardiovascular response of combinations of sympathomimetic stimulants would be expected to be additive or synergistic. Because ephedrine and pseudoephedrine are present in greatest concentration in *Ephedra*, and ephedrine has relatively greater hemodynamic potency than pseudoephedrine (23), the pharmacodynamic response of ephedra supplements would be anticipated to be closest to the effects of ephedrine.

All of the ephedra alkaloids are pressor agents through their actions at α_1-adrenergic receptors on vascular smooth muscle. Experimental evidence shows that ephedrine has 4–5 times greater pressor potency and chronotropic effect on the heart than pseudoephedrine (23,24). In addition, dog studies have shown that at equipressor doses, ephedrine exhibits less tachyphylaxis than pseudoephedrine, with only minimal diminution of the pressor response after 10 repeated doses of ephedrine compared to complete tachyphylaxis after just two doses of pseudoephedrine (23). In a human investigation of the cardiovascular responses of pseudoephedrine, tachyphylaxis was observed to the pressor effect, but the heart rate remained significantly elevated after 14 days of treatment (32).

Ephedrine has been shown in a number of studies to produce clinically significant increases in heart rate, systolic and diastolic blood pressure, and cardiac output (23,24). In one study of 11 patients after major vascular surgery, ephedrine was infused at a rate of 2–6 μg/kg/min and produced means changes of 18.1 mmHg in systolic blood pressure, 8.1 mmHg in diastolic blood pressure, heart rate increase of 9 beats per minute, with no change in systemic vascular resistance (33).

Hypertension due to α_1-adrenergic activity is believed to be the mechanism for cases of subarachnoid and intracerebral hemorrhage reported with ephedrine and phenylpropanolamine (PPA) (34). In some cases, this might involve rupture of a preexisting aneurysm. Intracerebral hemorrhage related to cerebral vasculitis has been reported with a variety of sympathomimetic drugs, including amphetamine, ephedrine, and PPA (35,36). A recent case-control study linked the use of appetite suppressants and cough or cold remedies containing PPA to a higher risk of hemorrhagic stroke in women, resulting in a voluntary recall of all PPA-containing products in November 2000 (10).

Ephedrine and related alkaloids are capable of inducing arterial vasospasm, similar to other sympathomimetic agents such as cocaine. This mechanism may cause or contribute to acute ischemic injury in some individuals. There are several reported cases of myocardial infarction and ischemic strokes in users of ephedra-containing supplements (37–39). This may be due to severe vasospasm alone, or the result of the additive effects of reduced blood flow and preexisting atherosclerosis in the setting of increased tissue oxygen demands. In addition, sympathomimetics such as ephedrine appear to promote thrombus formation via vasocontriction with stasis, and through their platelet stimulant actions (40). Cases of myocarditis related to ephedra alkaloids are most likely due to small-coronary-artery vasoconstriction producing myocyte necrosis, although there is also a report of hypersensitivity myocarditis (41).

Compensatory mechanisms are active in opposing the hemodynamic effects of ephedrine and related alkaloids. An increase in systolic blood pressure is accompanied by decreased central sympathetic outflow, and baroreceptor-mediated reflex slowing in heart rate. These mechanisms serve to normalize hemodynamic function, without which dramatic increases in blood pressure and heart rate would result. However, parasympathetic activity not only suppresses heart rate, but also shortens the atrial refractory period, facilitating reentrant arrhythmias. With the added β_1-adrenergic stimulation from ephedrine, the arrhythmogenic potential is increased, and may be further exacerbated by additional demands on the heart such as myocardial ischemia, strenuous exercise, or coronary vasospasm. This may explain why adverse cardiac events such as sudden death occur on rare occasions in apparently healthy individuals taking ephedra alkaloids (42).

VII. CENTRAL-NERVOUS-SYSTEM EFFECTS

The actions of the ephedra alkaloids on the central nervous system depend on their ability to penetrate the blood-brain barrier. Ephedrine, similar to amphetamine, readily crosses the blood-brain barrier, and produces a range of central nervous system effects from increased alertness and mood elevation to euphoria, insomnia, and even psychosis. Studies in humans and animals have shown that (−)-ephedrine is a more potent central nervous system stimulant than (+)-pseudoephedrine (24,43). The anorexigenic effects of ephedrine and norephedrine are believed to be related to α_1 activity in the satiety center of the hypothalamus. The mechanism of action of the other central nervous system effects is not entirely clear, but may be related to indirect release of brain norepinephrine and dopamine (44).

Insomnia is a well-known side effect of ephedrine taken by patients with asthma. Chronic use and misuse of ephedrine to "get high" has also been associated with addictive behavior (45), and cases of mania and psychosis similar to amphetamine-related psychotic syndromes have been described (46,47). Several cases of acute psychosis have recently been reported in persons taking "herbal ecstasy," a term coined for ephedra-containing products that were formally marketed as legal stimulants (48). Herbal products labeled, marketed, and sold under this name or for the purpose of getting high are now illegal. The use of ephedra for weight loss and athletic performance enhancement may also result in significant central-nervous-system effects, possibly associated with long-term use. A recent study of 36 female weight lifters found that 19% displayed signs of ephedrine dependence (49).

Ephedrine has also been reported to cause seizures in apparently healthy persons (50). This would be an expected adverse outcome of any central-nervous-system-stimulant drug, particularly if taken in high doses.

VIII. METABOLIC/THERMOGENIC EFFECTS

Ephedra is promoted as a "fat burner" or thermogenic agent because of its reported effectiveness in increasing basal metabolic rate and contributing to weight loss. Several small studies have documented that the combination of ephedrine and caffeine increases oxygen consumption and lipid oxidation, raises resting energy expenditure (REE), and promotes weight loss (51–54). In contrast, there is no experimental evidence that caffeine or ephedrine alone is more effective than placebo in producing weight loss, despite demonstrated increased thermogenesis of the individual agents (55,56). Studies involving ephedra- and caffeine-containing dietary supplements have also shown modest weight loss compared to placebo (30,31).

Some published data show that the basal metabolic rate remains elevated by an average of 10% with chronic treatment, suggesting a sustained thermogenic effect of ephedrine without development of tolerance (57,58). However, persistent long-term weight reduction maintenance after ephedra is stopped would not be anticipated without adjuvant dietary/lifestyle modification.

Astrup has proposed that the thermogenic response induced by ephedrine is a result of increased energy expenditure in resting skeletal muscle. (59) The mechanism is hypothesized to be a result of indirect norepinephrine release in peripheral sites and β_2-adrenergic-mediated increased blood flow that raises the resting energy expenditure of skeletal muscle (59). Thermogenic responsiveness in brown and white adipose tissue, splanchnic organs, and cardiac and respiratory tissue appears to account for only a small portion of the increased resting energy expenditure. Ephedrine increases plasma insulin and glucose, but consistent effects on plasma lactate, glycerol, or nonesterified fatty acids (NEFA) have not been seen (51,60). This raises the question about the significance of the metabolic effects of ephedrine in contributing to weight loss.

It appears that, through several mechanisms, including metabolic actions, increased peripheral sympathetic tone, and centrally mediated effects on appetite, ephedrine and caffeine interact synergistically to produce weight loss.

IX. ERGOGENIC EFFECTS

Substances that increase the time to exhaustion during strenuous exercise are termed ergogenic, which means "energy-producing." One of the major purported claims of ephedra-containing dietary supplements is their ability to boost energy and increase exercise tolerance, thereby improving athletic performance. These effects would theoretically be of benefit in sports that rely on stamina such as running, cycling, and swimming. Athletes involved in sports that require specialized skill, physical strength, or agility would not be expected to benefit from ephedra use. Ephedra alkaloid use is currently banned by the National Football League, the National Collegiate Athletic Association, and the International Olympic Committee. However, ephedra is still a frequently used performance-enhancing supplement, as reported in surveys of amateur athletes from the junior high school to the collegiate level (61–63).

To date, there have been no published trials investigating the effects of ephedra-containing dietary supplements as ergogenic aids, but there are several reported exercise studies involving pharmaceutical ephedrine (63–66). Studies of healthy individuals have shown that oral ephedrine use decreases the run time in 5-km and 10-km distance events, and increases the time to exhaustion after cycling at maximal effort in a controlled laboratory setting (63,64,66). However, the mean decrease in 10-km run time between ephedrine and placebo groups was 48 secs, which represents only a 1.75% reduction in total run time. Pseudoephedrine used in modest doses prior to 40-km cycling trials has not been found to have the same ergogenic effect as ephedrine (67). Caffeine appears to enhance the ergogenic effect of ephedrine in short-duration exercise tests lasting 10–20 mins, but not in activities of longer duration (64,65).

The mechanism for the ergogenic action of ephedrine is thought to be related either to CNS stimulation or to favorable alterations in peripheral substrate utilization (65). It has been postulated that the ergogenic effect may depend on the type of exercise activity (65). For example, in tests that involve strenuous exertion to the point of exhaustion, increased motivation may be the ergogenic effect mediated through heightened CNS arousal. Favorable changes in skeletal muscle metabolism may be the ergogenic effect in tests of short-duration, intense exercise lasting 10–20 min. The finding that pseudoephedrine, with less CNS activity than ephedrine, has no demonstrated ergogenic effect in endurance cycling supports the hypothesis that the mechanism is primarily centrally mediated (67). In addition, most exercise studies have shown that blood levels of lactate, glucose, and NEFA do not differ significantly between ephedrine and placebo groups. Thus, it appears that the mechanism of ephedrine's ergogenic effect is primarily CNS stimulation rather than alterations in substrate utilization.

X. REGULATORY/POLICY ISSUES

The increasing number of adverse events reported in association with use of ephedra-containing dietary supplements has raised some concerns among health care professionals (68,69) about the accessibility and widespread use of these products by the general population. In addition, highly publicized reports of catastrophic adverse outcomes associated with ephedra use have drawn the attention of concerned lawmakers at the state and national levels. Indeed, several states, including Texas, New York, Hawaii, Florida, and California, have passed laws restricting the use of ephedra, required warning statements on product labels, and mandated an adverse-event reporting system. And, more recently, the FDA has announced a ban on all dietary supplements that contain ephedra alkaloids. Ephedra will remain legal as a traditional Chinese herbal medicine.

Inarguably, ephedra is a drug with pharamacological actions that mirror the clinical effects of pharmaceutical grades of ephedrine, pseudoephedrine, and phenylpropanolamine. The prior classification of ephedra as a nutritional product was inappropriate and potentially dangerous to consumers who view such products as the same as multivitamin or mineral supplements. Because of their easy availability on health food and drugstore shelves and via the Internet, many ephedra products were used without consultation with a physician or pharmacist. Some consumers may have underlying diseases, whether known or unknown, that can be exacerbated by the sympathomimetic actions of ephedra alkaloids, such as the relatively common conditions of hypertension, diabetes, hyperthyroidism, psychiatric and seizure disorders, coronary and cerebral artery disease, renal dysfunction, glaucoma, and prostatic hypertrophy. In fact, many of these conditions are comorbidities of obesity, which is one of the principal uses for which ephedra-containing supplements were promoted.

A key challenge for regulators is to enact change that will adequately protect consumers from preventable adverse outcomes, without restricting free access to alternative therapies that have been clearly mandated by the public. Perhaps an appropriate approach would be to classify natural products with established pharmacological actions and acceptable evidence of safety and efficacy as neither food nor drugs, but as a third category of "traditional or alternative medicines," with regulatory requirements that are intermediate between drugs and nutritional supplements. This approach could be modeled after alternative medicine regulatory frameworks in other countries such as Germany and Japan, where herbal medicines are commonly prescribed and used.

REFERENCES

1. Schulz V, Hansel R, Tyler VE. Rational Phytotherapy: A Physician's Guide to Herbal Medicine. 4th ed. Heidelberg, Germany: Springer-Verlag, 2001.
2. Blumenthal M, et al., eds. The Complete German Commission E Monographs. Boston, MA: Integrative Medicine Communications, 1998.
3. Fleming T, ed. Physician's Desk Reference for Herbal Medicines. 2d ed. Montvale, NJ: Medical Economics Company, 2000.
4. McGuffin M, Hobbs C, Upton R, Goldberg A, eds. American Herbal Products Association's Botanical Safety Handbook. Boca Raton, FL: CRC Press, 1997.
5. Jellin JM, Gregory PJ, Batz F, Hitchens K, et al. Pharmacist's Letter/Prescriber's Letter Natural Medicines Comprehensive Database. 4th ed. Stockton, CA: Therapeutic Research Faculty, 2002.
6. Zhang JS, Tian Z, Lou ZC. Quality evaluation of twelve species of Chinese ephedra (ma huang). Acta Pharm Sin 1989; 24(11):865–871.
7. Liu YM, Sheu SJ, Chiou SH, Chang HC, Chen YP. A comparative study on commercial samples of ephedrae herba. Planta Med 1993; 59:376–378.
8. Betz JM, Gay ML, Mossoba MM, Adams S. Chiral gas chromatographic determination of ephedrine-type alkaloids in dietary supplements containing ma huang. J AOAC Int 1997; 80(2):303–315.
9. Hurlbut JA, Carr JR, Singleton ER, Faul KC, Madson MR, Storey JM, et al. Solid-phase extraction cleanup and liquid chromatography with ultraviolet detection of ephedrine alkaloids in herbal products. J AOAC Int 1998; 81(6):1121–1127.
10. Kernan WN, Viscoli CM, Brass LM, Broderic JP, Brott T, et al. Phenylpropanolamine and the risk of hemorrhagic stroke. N Engl J Med 2000; 343:1826–1832.
11. Kalix P. The pharmacology of psychoactive alkaloids from *Ephedra* and *Catha*. J Ethnopharmacol 1991; 32:201–208.
12. Hardman JG, Limbird LE, Molinoff PB, Ruddon RW, Gilman AG, eds. Goodman and Gilman's The Pharmacological Basis of Therapeutics. 9th ed. New York: McGraw-Hill, 1995.
13. USP DI Volume I - Drug Information for the Health Care Professional. 21st ed. Englewood, CO: Micromedex, 2001.

14. Kanfer I, Dowse R, Vuma V. Pharmacokinetics of oral decongestants. Pharmacotherapy 1993; 13(6):116S–128S.
15. Sinsheimer JE, Dring LG, Williams RT. Species differences in the metabolism of norephedrine in man, rabbit, and rat. Biochem J 1973; 136:763–771.
16. Gurley BJ, Gardner SF, White LM, Wang PL. Ephedrine pharmacokinetics after the ingestion of nutritional supplements containing *Ephedra sinica* (ma huang). Ther Drug Monit 1998; 20(4):439–445.
17. Haller CA, Jacob P, Benowitz NL. Pharmacology of ephedra alkaloids and caffeine after single dose dietary supplement use. Clin Pharmacol Ther 2002; 71(6):421–432.
18. White LM, Gardner SF, Gurley BJ, Marx MA, Wang PL, Estes M. Pharmacokinetics and cardiovascular effects of ma huang (*Ephedra sinica*) in normotensive adults. J Clin Pharmacol 1997; 37:116–122.
19. Brater DC, Kaojarern S, Benet LZ, Lin ET, Lockwood T, Morris RC, McSherry EJ, Melmon KL. Renal excretion of pseudoephedrine. Clin Pharmacol Ther 1980; 28(5):690–694.
20. Wilkinson GR, Beckett AH. Absorption, metabolism, and excretion of the ephedrines in man. I. The Influence of urinary pH and urine volume output. J Pharmacol Exp Ther 1968; 162(1):139–147.
21. Benezra SA, McRae JW. Pseudoephedrine hydrochloride. In: Florey K, ed. Analytical Profiles of Drug Substances. New York: Academic Press, 1979:489–507.
22. Bowman WC, Rand MJ, eds. Textbook of Pharmacology. 2d ed. London: Blackwell Scientific Publications, 1980.
23. Patil PN, Tye A, Lapidus M. A pharmacological study of the ephedrine isomers. J Pharmacol Exp Ther 1965; 148(2):158–168.
24. Bye C, Dewsbury D, Peck AW. Effects on the human central nervous system of two isomers of ephedrine and triprolidine and their interaction. Br J Clin Pharmacol 1974; 1:71–78.
25. Bray GA. A concise review on the therapeutics of obesity. Nutrition 2000; 16:953–960.
26. Weyer C, Gautier JF, Danforth E. Development of beta 3-adrenoceptor agonists for the treatment of obesity and diabetes—an update. Diabetes Metab 1999; 25(1):11–21.
27. Kanayama G, Gruber AJ, Pope HG, Borowiecki JJ, Hudson JI. Over-the-counter drug use in gymnasiums: an underrecognized substance abuse problem? Psychother Psychosom 2001; 70:137–140.
28. Dietary Supplement Market View. Chevy Chase, Md: FDC Reports, August 2000.
29. Kaye AD, Clarke RC, Sabar R, Vig S, Dhawan P, Hofbauer R, Kaye AM. Herbal medicines: current trends in anesthesiology practice—a hospital survey. J Clin Anesthesiol 2000; 12:468–471.
30. Boozer CN, Nasser JA, Heymsfield SB, Wang V, Chen G, Solomon JL. An herbal supplement containing ma huang-guarana for weight loss: a randomized, double-blind trial. Int J Obesity 2001; 25:316–324.

31. Boozer CN, Daly PA, Blanchard D, Nasser JA, Solomon JL, Homel. Herbal ephedra/caffeine for weight loss: a 6-month trial [abstr]. FASEB J 2001; 15(4):A403A403.
32. Bye C, Hill HM, Hughes DTD, Peck AW. A comparison of plasma levels of L(+)pseudoephedrine following different formulations, and their relation to cardiovascular and subjective effects in man. Eur J Clin Pharmacol 1975; 8:47–53.
33. Westman L, Hamberger B, Jarnberg PO. Effects of ephedrine on renal function in patients after major vascular surgery. Acta Anaesthesiol Scand 1988; 32:271–277.
34. Bruno A, Nolte K, Chapin J. Stroke associated with ephedrine use. Neurology 1993; 43:1313–1316.
35. Fallis RJ, Fisher M. Cerebral vasculitis and hemorrhage associated with phenylpropanolamine. Neurology 1985; 35:405–407.
36. Wooten MR, Khangure MS, Murphy MJ. Intracerebral hemorrhage and vasculitis related to ephedrine use. Ann Neurol 1983; 13:337–340.
37. Traub SJ, Hoyek W, Hoffman RS. Dietary supplements containing ephedra alkaloids [letter]. N Engl J Med 2001; 344(14):1095–1096.
38. Vahedi K, Domigo V, Amarenco R, Bousser MG. Ischaemic stroke in a sportsman who consumed mahuang extract and creatine monohydrate for body building. J Neurol Neurosurg Psychiatry 2000; 68:112–113.
39. Zahn KA, Li RL, Purssell RA. Cardiovascular toxicity after ingestion of "herbal ecstasy". J Emerg Med 1999; 17:289–291.
40. Schnetzer GW. Platelets and thrombogenesis—current concepts. Am Heart J 1972; 83:552–564.
41. Zaacks SM, Klein L, Tan CD, Rodriquez ER, Leikim JB. Hypersensitivity myocarditis associated with ephedra use. J Toxicol Clin Toxicol 1999; 37(4):485–489.
42. Theoharides TC. Sudden death of a healthy college student related to ephedrine toxicity from a ma-huang containing drink. J Clin Psychopharmacol 1997; 17(5):437–439.
43. Lanciault G, Wolf HH. Some neuropharmacological properties of the ephedrine isomers. J Pharm Sci 1965; 54:841–844.
44. Goldfrank LR, Flomenbaum NE, Lewin NA, Weisman RS, Howland MA, Hoffman RS, eds. Goldfrank's Toxicologic Emergencies. 6th ed. Stamford, CT: Appleton and Lange, 1998.
45. Martin WR, Sloan JW, Sapira JD, Jasinski DR. Physiologic, subjective, and behavioral effects of amphetamine, methamphetamine, ephedrine, phenmetrazine, and methyphenidate in men. Clin Pharmacol Ther 1971; 12(2):245–258.
46. Herridge CF, A'Brook MF. Ephedrine psychosis. Br Med J 1968; 2:160.
47. Bartoszewski J, Majewska E. A case of mental disorder due to chronic ephedrine abuse. Psychiatr Pol 1972; 6:671–674.
48. Doyle H, Kargin M. Herbal stimulant containing ephedrine has also caused psychosis. Br Med J 1996; 313:756.
49. Gruber AJ, Pope JG. Ephedrine abuse among 36 female weightlifters. Am J Addict 1998; 7(4):256–261.

50. Kockler DR, McCarthy MW, Lawson CL. Seizure activity and unresponsiveness after hydroxycut ingestion. Pharmacotherapy 2001; 21(5):647–651.
51. Astrup A, Toubro S, Cannon S, Hein P, Madsen J. Thermogenic synergism between ephedrine and caffeine in healthy volunteers: a double-blind, placebo-controlled study. Metabolism 1991; 40(3):323–329.
52. Horton TJ, Geissler CA. Post-prandial thermogenesis with ephedrine, caffeine, and aspirin in lean, pre-disposed obese and obese women. Int J Obesity 1996; 20:91–97.
53. Dulloo AG, Miller DS. The thermogenic properties of ephedrine/methylxanthine mixtures: human studies. Int J Obesity 1986; 10:467–481.
54. Greenway FL, Raum WJ, DeLany JP. The effect of an herbal dietary supplement containing ephedrine and caffeine on oxygen consumption in humans. J Alt Comp Med 2000; 6(6):553–555.
55. Pasquali R, Baraldi G, Cesari MP, Melchondia N, Zamboni M, Stefanini C, Raitano A. A controlled trial using ephedrine in the treatment of obesity. Int J Obesity 1985; 9:93–98.
56. Astrup A, Breum L, Toubro S, Hein P, Quaade F. The effect and safety of an ephedrine/caffeine compound compared to ephedrine, caffeine and placebo in obese subjects on an energy restricted diet: a double blind trial. Int J Obesity 1992; 16:269–277.
57. Astrup A, Lundsgaard C, Madsen J, Christensen NJ. Enhanced thermogenic responsiveness during chronic ephedrine treatment in man. Am J Clin Nutr 1985; 42:83–94.
58. Astrup A, Madsen J, Holst JJ, Christensen NJ. The effect of chronic ephedrine treatment on substrate utilization, the sympathoadrenal activity, and energy expenditure during glucose-induced thermogenesis in man. Metabolism 1986; 35(3):260–265.
59. Astrup A. Thermogenesis in human brown adipose tissue and skeletal muscle induced by sympathomimetic stimulation. Acta Endocrinol 1986; 112:1–32.
60. Ramsey JJ, Colman RJ, Swick AG, Kemnitz JW. Energy expenditure, body composition, and glucose metabolism in lean and obese rhesus monkeys treated with ephedrine and cafeeine. Am J Clin Nutr 1998; 68:42–51.
61. Green GA, Uryasz FD, Petr TA, Bray CD. NCAA study of substance use and abuse habits of college student-athletes. Clin J Sports Med 2001; 11:51–56.
62. Blue Cross Blue Shield National Performance-Enhancing Drug Study. Chicago, IL: C&R Research Inc, 2001.
63. Bell DG, Jacobs I. Combined caffeine and ephedrine ingestion improves run times of Canadian Forces Warrior Test. Aviat Space Environ Med 1999; 70:325–329.
64. Bell DG, Jacobs I, Zamecnik J. Effects of caffeine, ephedrine, and their combination on time to exhaustion during high-intensity exercise. Eur J Appl Physiol Occup Physiol 1998; 77:427–433.
65. Bell DG, McLellan TM, Sabiston CM. Effect of ingesting caffeine and ephedrine on 10-km run performance. Med Sci Sports Exer 2002; 344–349.
66. Bell DG, Jacobs I, Ellerington. Effect of caffeine and ephedrine ingestion on anaerobic exercise performance. Med Sci Sports Exer 2001; 33:1399–1403.

67. Gillies H, Derman WE, Noakes TD, Smith P, Evans A, Gabriels G. Pseudoephedrine is without ergogenic effects during prolonged exercise. J Appl Physiol 1996; 81:2611–2617.
68. Wolfe SM, Ardati A, Woolsley R. Petition to the FDA requesting the ban of production and sale of dietary supplements containing ephedrine alkaloids. Public Citizen Health Research Group Publication #1590. Available at http://www.citizen.org/publications/release.cfm?ID = 7053.
69. Association of Food and Drug Officials letter to Food and Drug Administration, 9/18/01. Available at http://www.afdo.org/posstatements.asp.

34

Echinacea and Immunostimulation

Lester A. Mitscher
The University of Kansas
Lawrence, Kansas, U.S.A.

Raymond Cooper
Pharmanex, LLC
Provo, Utah, U.S.A.

I. INTRODUCTION

A comparatively ancient folk remedy, echinacea preparations are among the most widely used herbal preparations. Nevertheless the evidentiary basis for the use of these materials as immunostimulants and for wound healing is inconsistent. Although many studies have been performed, the results are divided between those supporting significant activity and those that suggest inactivity. No completely convincing evidence is yet in hand identifying any active constituent. The problem is compounded by a collection of factors decreasing confidence in the literature available: poor species identification, adulteration, uncertain quality control, failure to indicate how the preparations have been processed and stored, unclear end points, and poorly controlled clinical trials characterize many of the studies.

Evidence is accumulating in favor of the assertion that the primary immunostimulant activity is associated with water-soluble polysaccharide fractions. There is, however, significant evidence supporting activity among some of the solvent soluble low-molecular-weight components also. It seems likely that activity lies in both classes but few data are available that compare the potency of these preparations side by side. More research is required to resolve this issue with confidence.

II. HISTORICAL ASPECTS

Use of echinacea for medicinal purposes by native cultures in the high plains region of midcontinental North America long predates European contact. Whereas echinacea readily flourishes in many countries when planted in temperate climates, it is native only to the trans-Mississippian high plains region of the United States. Native Americans belonging to at least 14 different tribes chewed the roots for toothaches and sore gums and employed the juice and teas prepared from the leaves and roots to treat colds, stomach problems, and a number of other health complaints. Poultices were also used for treatment of arthritis, rheumatism, snakebite, and venereal diseases. Early settlers of European origin following initial contact quickly took up medicinal use of echinacea and the plant was highly valued. European botanists became aware of the genus in the 1700s and Moench named the genus *Echinacea* (in 1794) based on its spiny cone (1). Medicinal preparations (patent medicines) containing echinacea, often mixed with other plant products, were introduced by 1870 and by 1890 their use was common. Unruh apparently was the first to describe its immune stimulatory properties (1915) (2). Its use in homeopathic medicine dates from about 1902. Popular use in Germany dates from about 1930. It was officially recognized in the *National Formulary, USA*, from the fourth to the eighth editions finally disappearing after 1950 along with many other natural remedies. Despite fading official support, echinacea use has remained popular with the domestic laity, especially in Europe. The early history of the use of echinacea has been reviewed frequently (3–14).

Today the German Commission E approves echinacea preparations for supportive treatment of flu symptoms and also for urinary tract infections. External use of the juice for treatment of superficial wounds that heal slowly is also supported. Canadian health authorities recognize its use for colds. The World Health Organization monograph contains dosage recommendations for it. No less than 17 books devoted to echinacea and its properties are available (8,15–34). A number of more general monographs also provide valuable background and insights (25,34–42). Nonetheless none of the official medicinal compendia of the United States recognize echinacea at this time. Consequently there is no consensus about what standards would be most useful for quality assurance.

Echinacea is the most popular herbal immunostimulant in Europe and in the United States today (43). It is widely employed in oral form for the treatment and/or prevention of the common cold as well as for upper- and lower-respiratory-tract infections, and to a lesser extent, topically for skin irritations and for the treatment of wounds and vulvovaginal candidiasis. The market value of echinacea preparations is estimated to lie between \$5 and \$10 billion per year representing 12% of herbal supplement sales in herbal stores in 1997, and sales are rapidly increasing. Including homeopathic preparations, more than 800 echinacea-containing drugs are currently on the market in Germany. A recent survey by the FDA found that 16 million Americans currently use botanical supplements and the industry has consistently grown at a rate of 25% annually since 1990 (43). Supplements containing echinacea are particularly popular based on a recent survey published in *USA Today* indicating that 19% of adult Americans have used it for the treatment of cold and flu symptoms.

Despite this level of popularity, the scientific support for these uses is weak. Conclusions based on the technical literature fail to allow a convincing choice of the best species, the best plant part, the best dosage forms, the most appropriate dosing and schedule, and the best means of preparation (44,45).

Reliable scientific research into the purported medicinal uses of echinacea is comparatively recent and mostly centered in a few German laboratories. Clinical studies are scattered, often poorly performed, and the results are contradictory. In the early studies there is significant confusion about which plant was being used, what part was involved, and how the preparation was made. There is still no recognized method of therapeutic standardization and experts differ on what active constituent, if any, is responsible for utility. Adding to the confusion, the plant has been adulterated classically with *Eryngium praealtum* and more recently with *Parthenium integrifolium* ("Missouri snakeroot"), whose cut and sifted roots can easily be confused with echinacea upon visual inspection (8,19,46). These adulterations are even more troublesome to detect when the material is commercialized in the form of hydroalcoholic tinctures. In addition, laboratory examination reveals all too often that commercial preparations consist of mixtures of *Echinacea pallida* and *E. angustifolia*. Early preparations frequently used more than one species of echinacea and often the species under use was apparently misnamed. A review of this early literature led to the conclusion that chemical analyses were done with *E. angustifolia*, particularly the earliest ones, whereas the biological activity was tested with *E. purpurea* (47). Even when particular constituents are chosen against which to standardize, the results vary greatly from medicament to medicament or even with different batches of the same product. For example, analysis for cichoric acid and dodeca-2E,4E,8Z,10E/Z-tetraenoic acid isobutylamide in 25 echinacea-containing commercial products revealed dramatic variations in quantity ranging from rich to zero (48)! Thus the literature is hard to reconcile.

A wide range of natural products has been identified in the plants. Opinion is divided as to whether any of these materials are immunostimulant in the clinic and, if so, whether the active constituents are the solvent solubles, the water solubles, or some combination thereof. Given this level of confusion, it is not possible at present to devise suitable analytical means of standardizing echinacea preparations to ensure purity, consistency, potency, and stability. It seems probable that the confused state of the clinical literature results from a combination of these causes.

Considering the widespread use of echinacea and the unsatisfactory state of the scientific and clinical literature, additional and much more systematic scientific examination is clearly needed.

III. SOME BOTANICAL CONSIDERATIONS

Botanically, the North American *Echinacea* genus consists of nine species and multiple varieties with *E. purpurea*, *E. angustifolia*, and *E. pallida* finding most use medicinally. The genus belongs to the Heliantheae, the largest tribe within the family Compositae (Asteraceae). Various authorities have described this genus and the presently accepted scheme is based on the comparative morphological and anatomical studies of McGreggor (3,49). *E. angustifolia* (*Braumeria angustifolia*), *E. atrorubens* (*Rudbeckia atrorubens*), *E. laevigata* (*B. laevigata*), *E. pallida* (*R. pallida*, *B. pallida*), *E. paradoxa* (*B. paradoxa*), *E. purpurea* (*R. purpurea*, *R. hispida*, *R. serotina*, *E. speciosa*, *E. intermedia*), *E. simulata* (*E. speciosa*), *E. sanguinea*, and *E. tennesseensis* (*B. tennesseensis*) are recognized. The genus is indigenous to Arkansas, Oklahoma, Missouri, and Kansas although it grows well in a variety of temperate climates. While the species are, in general, relatively distinct from one another, specific differences are based on subtle morphological features and are often hard to discern in the field. All taxa will hybridize when brought together and considerable natural hybridization occurs (49). *E. angustifolia* and *E. atrorubens* show geographic introaggression and exhibit considerable overlap in stem and petiole structures. Hybrids of *E. simulata* and *E. sanguinea* appear very similar to the Arkansas race of *E. pallida*, and *E. simula* has been confused with *E. pallida*. Further studies between *E. simulata* and *E. pallida* show differences in pollen size and morphology. Fortunately natural hybrids are sterile (49). Thus studies performed in industrial laboratories find frequent confusion and substitution of species.

The material used in commerce is often of uncertain provenance in part because of field hybridizations producing plants whose external appearance is often intermediate between *E. pallida* and *E. angustifolia*. Further, adulteration with *Parthenium integrifolium* and other unrelated plants has often occurred (4,50,51).

IV. CULTIVATION

Expanding global demand for echinacea threatens to result in unsustainable levels of wild harvest, and significant habitat destruction contributes to these concerns. Worries about the presence of undesirable agricultural residues such as herbicides, fertilizers, heavy metals, and pesticides also must be dealt with. This suggests that cultivation under carefully controlled conditions should be investigated to produce sustainable quantities of safe material of high potency, yields, and purity. Cultivation is, in fact, easy from seeds, and the perennial nature of the plant suggests that this should be economical.

Echinacea grows well under a variety of temperate conditions supporting the notion that cultivation in suitable regions of the Southern Hemisphere would provide a continuous supply of plant material year-round.

Cultivation appears to be preferable to field collection to relieve pressure on wild populations as long as the material can be shown to be fundamentally equivalent. There is a vogue for natural materials, however, and this results in a premium price to collectors for field-collected wild material. Conservation concerns have been raised for nearly a century. It is estimated that 50 tons have been harvested and shipped overseas for many years and domestic demand is escalating. No systematic study of echinacea availability over its range has been performed. Two species, *E. tennesseensis* and *E. sanguinea*, are already protected under the Federal Endangered Species Act partly owing to their overharvest for medicinal purposes. Fortunately *E. purpurea* is relatively easy to cultivate. *E. angustifolia* appears to be increasingly threatened but the evidence is at present anecdotal (9,52).

Study is required before one can establish with reasonable certainty whether wild or cultivated material is to be preferred. The identification of an active component and its quantitation is a necessary prerequisite before this could be done. Failing this, bioassay should be performed. This is well within technical capability now and can draw upon experience with antibiotics for historical precedence and experience.

V. CHEMICAL CONSTITUENTS OF ECHINACEA

A. Lower-Molecular-Weight Components

At present the literature is divided as to whether the low-molecular-weight alcohol-extractable materials or the high-molecular-weight oligosaccharides of echinacea are responsible for the species' immunostimulatory properties.

There is evidence to support both views and it is quite possible that both classes contribute. It is not clear, however, which may contribute the most or whether they are additive or even synergistic.

The lower-molecular-weight secondary constituents of echinacea belong to several classes: caffeic acid analogs, phenolics, phenolic glycosides, terpenes, polyunsaturated amides, polyunsaturated acetylenes, and alkaloids.

Chemical work on echinacea and its constituents began in the 1890s (53) and the results reflect the comparatively crude methods available at that time. For example, sugars, volatile oils, alkaloids, and such general plant constituents were quantified but not identified at the molecular level. Much of the early work is somewhat doubtful because of confusion about the identity of the plant material employed.

Solid modern work that connects specific echinacea compounds with biological activity can be dated from the efforts of Stoll, who identified echinacoside as a weak antibiotic (54), but the chemical structure of this compound required three decades more to be settled (55). Echinacoside is present in many species of echinacea but apparently not in *E. angustifolia*, so it is not a reliable genus marker. Verbascoside is an echinacoside analog lacking a glucosyl residue (56). Descaffeoylechinacoside and desrhamnosylverbascoside have also been isolated from *E. pallida* (57). One also finds in echinacea species a variety of caffeoyl cyclitol analogs including chlorogenic acid and cynarin (58). Of the various caffeoyl-substituted tartrates, cichoric acid is characteristic of *E. purpurea* but less so of *E. angustifolia* (59). Cichoric acid occurs in several different plant species in which the optical isomer of the tartaric acid component varies. That in *Echinacea* species appears to be (2R,3R)-(+)-tartrate. Caftaric acid and a variety of other analogs of cichoric acid have also been found in various echinacea species (56,57). (Formula Charts 1 and 2).

Echinacea species are rich in flavonoids and flavonoid glycosides. Luteolin, kaempferol, quercetin, quercetagetin-7-glucoside, luteolin-7-glucoside, kaempferol-3-glucoside, quercetin-3-arabinoside, quercetin-3-galactoside, quercetin-3-xyloside, quercetin-3-glucoside, kaempferol-3-rutinoside, rutoside, isorhamnetic-3-rutinoside, and others have been found in the leaves of *E. angustifolia* (3,60,61). Likewise, the leaves of *E. purpurea* were found to contain quercetin, quercetin-7-glucoside, kaempferol-3-rutinoside, quercetin-3-glucoside, rutin, quercetin-3-robinobioside, quercetin-3-xylosylgalactoside (or an isomer thereof), and others.

Clearly quercetin and its glycosides are plentiful in these leaves. In addition to these, *Echinacea* species were also found to contain cyanidin-3-*O*-(β-D-glucopyranoside) and cyanidin-3-*O*-(6-*O*-malonyl-β-D-glucopyranoside (62).

Echinacea contains a variety of essential oils in quantities ranging from 0.1 to 4% depending on the plant part and the season. Notable among these

Caffeoyl glycosides

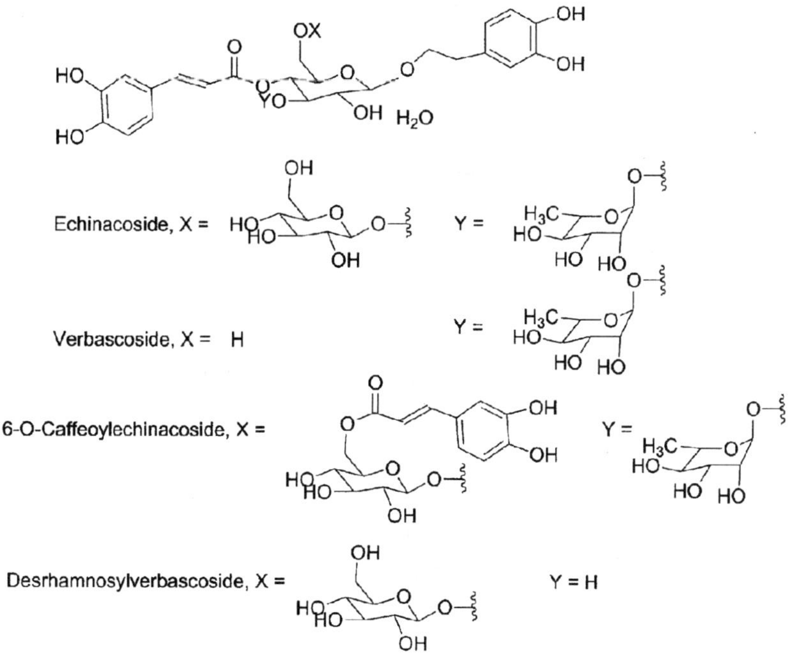

Caffeoyl cyclitols

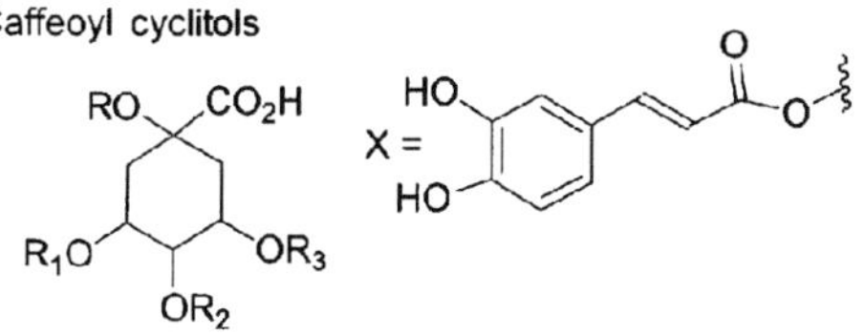

	R	R1	R2	R3
Chlorogenic acid	H	X	H	H
An isochlorogenic acid	H	X	X	H
An isochlorogenic acid	H	X	H	X
An isochlorogenic acid	H	H	X	X
Cynarin	X	H	H	X

FORMULA CHART NO. 1 Caffeoyl glycosides and cyclitols.

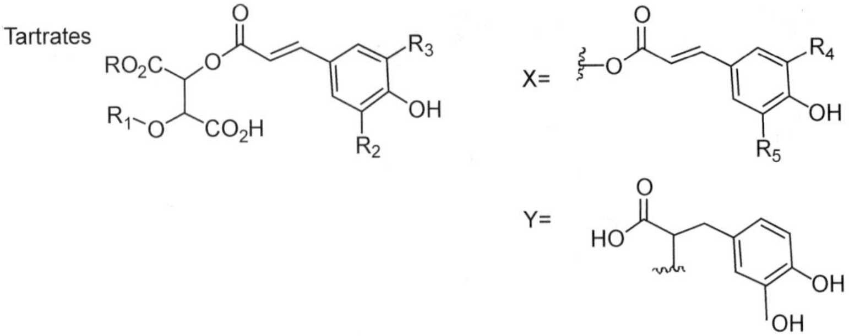

	R	R1	R2	R3	R4	R5
Caftaric acid	H	H	H	OH	-	-
Cichoric acid	H	X	OH	H	OH	H
Cichoric acid methyl ester	Me	X	OH	H	OH	H
2-O-Feruloyltartaric acid	H	H	OMe	H	-	-
2-O-Caffeoyl-3-O-coumeroyl-tartaric acid	H	X	OH	H	H	H
2-O-Caffeoul-3-O-feruloyl-tartaric acid	H	X	OH	H	OMe	H
2,3-O-Di[5-alphacarboxy-beta-(3,4-dihydroxyphenyl)-ethyl)-caffeoyl]tartaric acid	H	Y	OH	Y	OH	H
2-O-Caffeoyl-3-O-[5-alpha-carboxy-beta-(3,4-dihydroxyphenyl)-ethyl)-caffeoyl]tartaric acid	H	Y	OH	H	OH	H

Formula Chart No. 2 Cichoric acid analogs.

are pentadeca-(1,8Z)-diene, 1-pentadecene diene (63) and echinolone ((*E*)-10-hydroxy-4,10-dimethyl-4,11-dodecadien-2-one) (64). Among the nonvolatile sesquiterpenes, four cinnamoyl esters of the germacrane and guaiane skeletal types have been isolated from *E. purpurea* roots (65). Many other terpenes have been found in echinacea oils (3). (Formula Chart 3).

Polyacetylenes are frequently found in the Compositae and the Asteraceae are not exceptional in this. These compounds are not stable, readily undergoing air oxidation on standing, so it is doubtful that commercial echinacea dosage forms contain much of them in native form. Schulte et al. (66) determined the total and partial structures of 15 such compounds. The first two of these were among those present in significant quantity and these

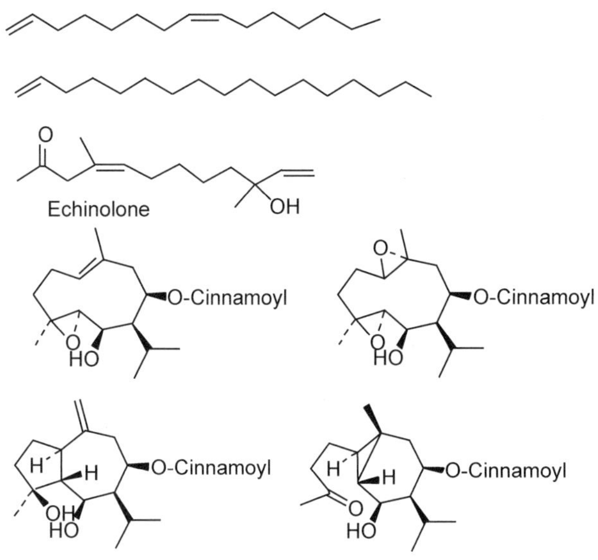

FORMULA CHART NO. 3 Miscellaneous terpenes from echinacea.

showed mild antibacterial and antifungal activity. Many of the remaining analogs were present in very small quantities allowing only partial characterization. Later Bauer et al. (67) investigated the roots of *E. pallida* and determined the structures of eight ketones and three hydroxylated analogs that did not occur in *E. angustifolia*. In a similar work (68), two additional hydroxylated acetylenes were characterized. Subsequently, many papers have appeared that describe qualitative and quantitative investigation of these analogs. (Formula Charts 4 and 5).

1. Unsaturated Alkyl Amides

Secondary substituents of this type have a somewhat restricted distribution in higher plants. They are, however, fairly common in *Echinacea* species and are

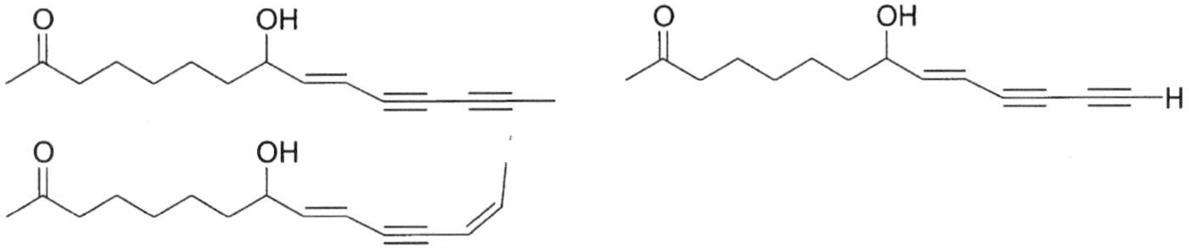

FORMULA CHART NO. 4 Unsaturated keto alcohols of echinacea.

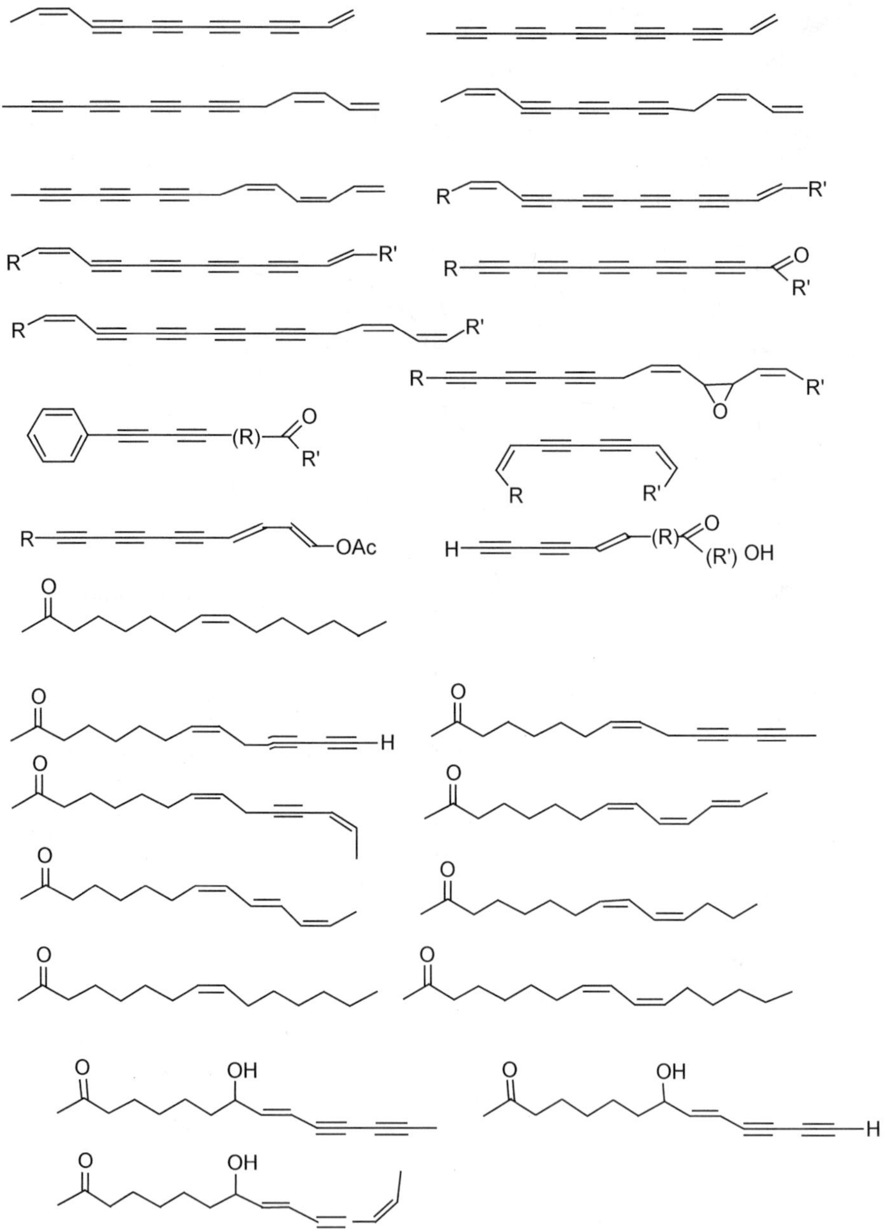

Formula Chart No. 5 Unsaturated polyenes and acetylenes of echinacea.

believed to be primarily responsible for the tingling and local anesthetic effects observed on the tongue when these materials and plants are placed in the mouth. Herbalists often use this effect as an indication that the plants are mature enough to harvest. Interestingly, these kinds of compound are present in spicy plants as well and a number of such species (pepper, containing piperine and chavacine, for example, but not *Echinacea* species) are used in cooking. Despite their evident ability to undergo Michael-type addition reactions, they are apparently not especially toxic to humans in the doses normally applied. The first of these to be characterized chemically from echinacea is echinacein (69). It was shown to be toxic to houseflies. Subsequently a large number of other polyunsaturated amides of echinacea have been characterized. Because they have excellent ultraviolet (UV) chromophores and their specific distribution among the *Echinacea* species is characteristic, they have been popular HPLC fingerprinting substances to demonstrate which species of *Echinacea* is present (70). (Formula Charts 6 and 7).

2. Alkaloids

Early reports suggested the presence of alkaloids in *Echinacea* species but several subsequent workers were unable to verify this. The common plant

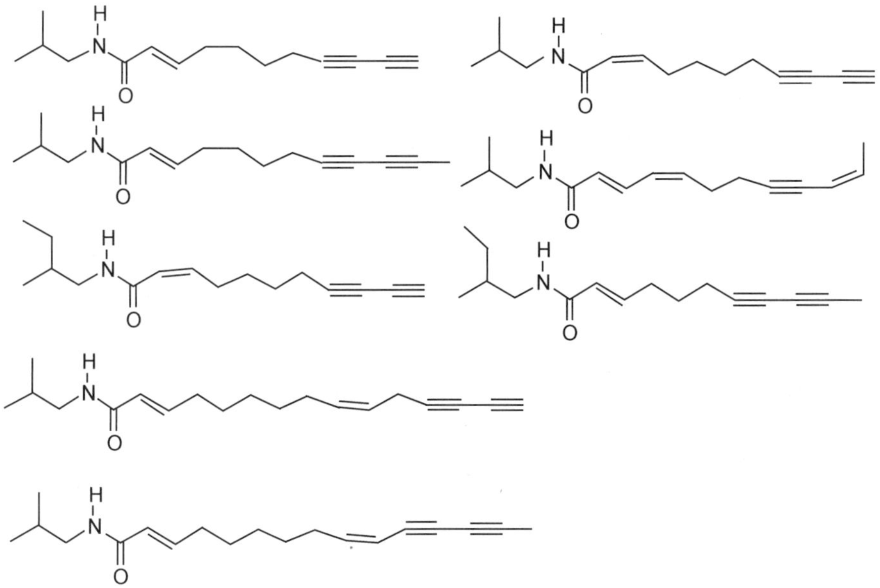

FORMULA CHART NO. 6 Unsaturated alkyl amides of echinacea.

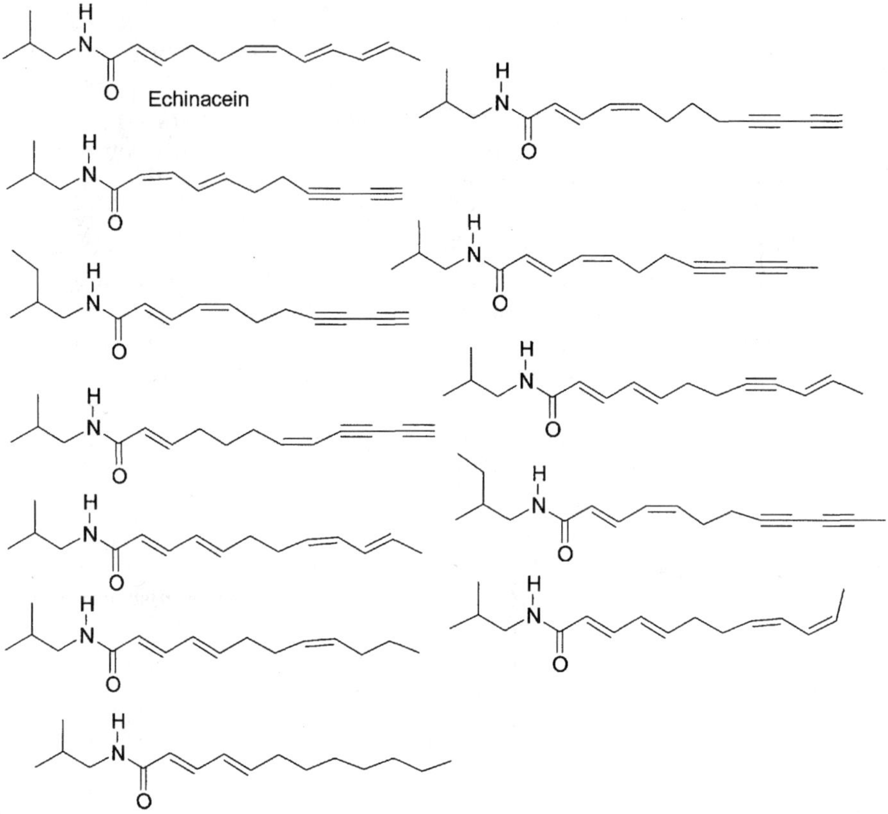

FORMULA CHART NO. 7 Additional unsaturated alkyl amides of echinacea.

constituent glycine betaine, however, has been definitely identified as present. Subsequently the pyrrolizidine alkaloids tussilagine and isotussilagine were detected in *E. purpurea* and *E. angustifolia* (71). Some pyrrolizidine alkaloids are known to produce oxidative metabolites following ingestion that are carcinogenic. At present, however, there is no evidence of carcinogenicity for the echinacea alkaloids. (Formula Chart 8).

B. Plant Identification via Analysis of Solvent Soluble Components

Identification of echinacea material can be done conveniently even in powdered form and in extracts by HPLC and TLC examination of the

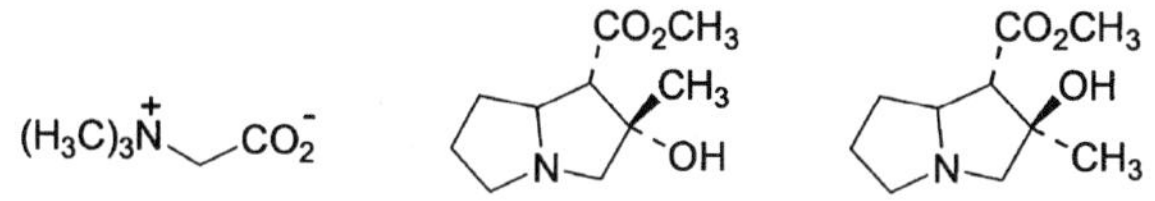

Glycine betaine Tussillagine Isotussilagine

FORMULA CHART NO. 8 Echinacea alkaloids.

organic-soluble materials because they are easily separated and detected by UV. Alcoholic tinctures of echinacea contain caffeic acid derivatives and polyacetylenes (72). In particular, the roots of *E. angustifolia* and *E. pallida* contain 0.3–1.7% echinacoside (65,73) while extracts of the two plants can be distinguished in that 1,3- and 1,5-*O*-dicaffeoylquinic acids are present only in the roots of *E. angustifolia* (67). Cichoric acid and caftaric acid are significant *E. purpurea* root constituents but echinacoside is not present. Cichoric acid is a prominent constituent in the aerial parts of most echinacea species (57,75,76). The aerial parts of *E. angustifolia* and *E. pallida* also contain verbascoside (57). Des-rhamnosylverbascoside and 6-*O*-caffeoylechinacoside have been isolated from *E. pallida* (57). *E. purpurea* leaves also contain cichoric acid methyl ester, 2-*O*-caffeoyl-3-*O*-feruloyltartaric acid and 2-*O*-caffeoyl-3-*O*-cumaroyltartaric acid (54). Other work showed the presence of 2-*O*-caffeoyl-3-*O*-feruloyltartaric acid, 2,3-*O*-*di*-5-[α-carboxyl-β-(3,4-dihydroxyphenyl)ethylcaffeoyl] tartaric acid, and 2-*O*-caffeoyl-3-*O*-[5-{α-carboxy-β-(3,4-dihydroxyphenyl) ethyl}caffeoyll]tartaric acid in *E. pallida* (57). These variations in the levels of caffeic acid derived constituents are not regarded as being particularly meaningful in terms of immunostimulation but they clearly have excellent potential value in distinguishing among the various plants that might be commercialized under the name echinacea.

Numerous flavonoids, such as rutoside, have been identified in echinacea leaves (59,67,77). The general flavonoid content is about 0.38–0.48%.

Cichoric acid is especially abundant in the flowers of all *Echinacea* species examined (1.2–3.1%) and in the roots of *E. purpurea* (0.6–2.1%). Much less is present in the other aboveground parts (67). The content of cichoric acid is quite variable based on the season and the state of development of the plant. Quantitation is further complicated in that it is not stable during preparation of alcoholic tinctures and in expressed juices (73,75). Analysis of cichoric and caftaric acids by a micellar electrokinetic chromatographic method (MECK) apparently works well for extracts of *E. purpurea* (78). In this methodology a surfactant is used to produce micelles to facilitate the separations.

The major 2-ketoalkenes and 2-ketoalkynes of *E. pallida* roots are tetradeca-8Z-ene-11,13-diyn-2-one, pentadeca-8Z-11,13-diyn-2-one, pentadeca-8Z,13Z-diene-11-yn-2-one, pentadeca-8Z-,13Z-diene-11-yn-2-one, pentadeca-8Z,11E,13Z-triene-2-one, and pentadeca-8Z-11Z-diene-2-one (4,67). These are found only in traces in *E. angustifolia* and *E. purpurea.* These unsaturated compounds readily autooxidize on storage to β-hydroxylated analogs even in root powder form (4). The differing concentration of these auto-oxidation products would provide a suitable means of distinguishing between *E. pallida* and *E. angustifolia* but their specific amounts would be time-dependent.

As detailed above, many alkamides are present in *E. angustifolia* roots where they are particularly abundant in quantity. Their structures are derived from undeca- and dodecanoic acid and differ from one another in the degree of unsaturation and the configuration of the double bonds (66). In *E. purpurea* roots there are characteristic differences in that most of the 11 alkamides possess a 2,4-diene moiety. This makes a convenient marker for distinguishing the source of the material (4,75). The aerial parts contain similar constituents (67,68). The concentration of most of these compounds is significantly less than 1% (0.001–0.151%). Alkamide levels in various parts of *E. purpurea* differ sufficiently to suggest that measurements of their distribution could be used to determine the origin of extracts (79). The photochemical instability of such compounds would require considerable caution in sample preparation and handling (80).

Pyrrolizidine alkaloids (tussilagine and isotussilagine) have been isolated from *Echinacea* species (81) but these seem to be of little interest from a chemotaxonomic viewpoint since they do not have a convenient UV chromophore.

A gas chromatographic method has been published that detects the presence of uracil herbicides in the roots of *E. angustifolia.* This would be useful in characterizing either cultivated or wild-picked echinacea materials (82). The gas chromatographic–mass spectroscopic methodology has also been applied to the analysis of echinacea mixtures themselves (83).

The variations in the kinds and amounts of solvent-soluble constituents from plant to plant part make identification and standardization of commercial preparations possible but their number and variation make this a complex undertaking. A recent study has analyzed the effect of some processing variables on the content of solvent-soluble constituents. Chopping altered the level of some alkamides slightly in *E. purpurea* roots but drying had no significant effect on the amounts detected. Levels of all alkamides fell by over 80% on storage at room temperature for 16 months and also fell significantly even when the plant material was stored at 18°C (82).

Adulteration by *Parthenium* can also be detected readily by chromatographic methods based on the presence of sesquiterpene esters that are not present in echinacea (46,65,68).

In summary, despite the complexity of extracts, they are readily assayed and such assays can serve as surrogate markers for species verification. The lack of strong evidence supporting a causal relationship between an individual constituent and its presence in extracts reduces the value of such determinations. It seems prudent for the time being to perform biological assays as well.

C. Higher-Molecular-Weight Components

The presence of oligosaccharides in higher plants is common. Early studies confirmed their presence in *Echinacea* species but, other than assigning molecular weights of approximately 50 kDa to these, structural information was limited (3). Pharmacological studies suggested that they possessed weak antihyaluronidase activity (84, as synopsized in Ref. 3).

Studies of particular relevance to immunostimulation were reported by the Wagner group starting in 1981 (85–87). Two immunostimulatory polysaccharides were isolated from the aboveground parts of *E. purpurea*, one with an apparent molecular weight of 35 kDa and the other of 50 kDa. The first, named PS 1, was a methylated polymer of glucuronic acid and arabinose and the second, named PS 2, was an acidic polymer of galactose, arabinose, and xylose. Partial structures of the repeating units of these materials were assigned. A third polysaccharide of apparent molecular weight of about 80,000 kDa was shown to contain xylose and glucose. The expressed juice contained a pectinoid that, however, had very weak immunostimulatory power. The primary assay used in these studies was stimulation of macrophage ingestion of carbon particles. This method primarily measures the speed and efficiency of macrophages in engulfing carbon particles. It is convenient but does not allow easy determination of all participating cells in the immune system nor does it allow quantitative examination of the maturation process and intercellular signaling between participating cells. The carbon clearance tests present convincing evidence that the solvent-soluble constituents, including cichoric acid, of echinacea, stimulate nonspecific immune capacity (3,67,69,73,88,89). Echinacoside is not immunostimulatory (56,90–92). These constituents would be present in hydroalcoholic extracts and in juice preparations and indeed are routinely analyzed in marketed products. (Formula Chart 9).

In later work, successful large-scale tissue culture work using *E. purpurea* resulted in isolation of three homogeneous polysaccharides whose structures differ from those of the whole plants. Two of these are neutral polymers of fucose, galactose, and glucose (of 10 kDa and 25 kDa, respectively) and the third an acidic arabinogalactan of molecular weight about 75 kDa. Partial structures have been assigned to these as well (74,93,94). The arabinogalactan was subsequently shown to activate macrophages against

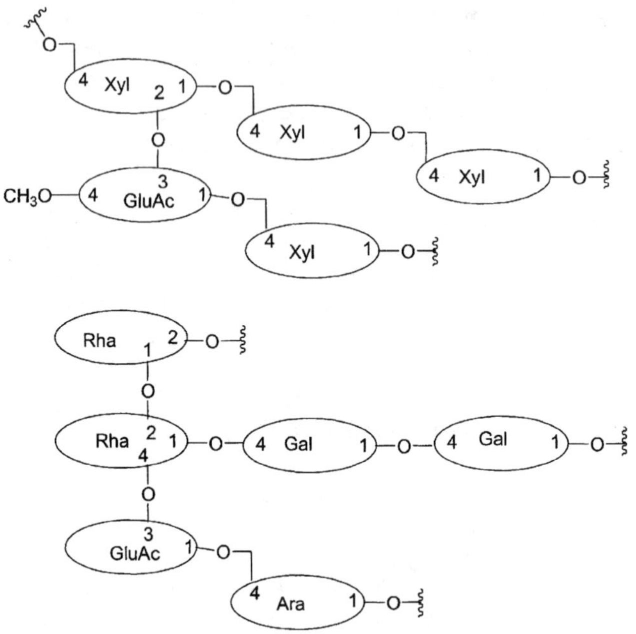

FORMULA CHART NO. 9 Echinacea polysaccharides.

tumor cells and microorganisms. The material did slightly increase T-cell but not B-cell proliferation. The macrophages were shown to produce IL-2, IFN-β, and TNF-α (95). (Formula Charts 10 and 11).

D. Analysis of High-Molecular-Weight Constituents of Echinacea

From the immediately preceding account, it can be seen that characteristic water-soluble polysaccharides with immunostimulatory properties (a 4-*O*-methyl-glucuronylarabinoxylan of average MW 35,000, an acidic arabinorhamnogalactan of MW 45,000 from the aerial parts of *E. purpurea*, xyloglucan, MW 79,500, from the leaves and stems, and a pectin-like polysaccharide from the expressed juice) are present in echinacea but these are more difficult to analyze chemically than the low-molecular-weight organics because of their complexity and their lack of a suitable chromophore. On the other hand, bioassay can be performed readily (4,85,88,92). The bioassays have the virtue of reflecting the intended end product use of echinacea preparations. The carbon clearance assays covered briefly above have greatly

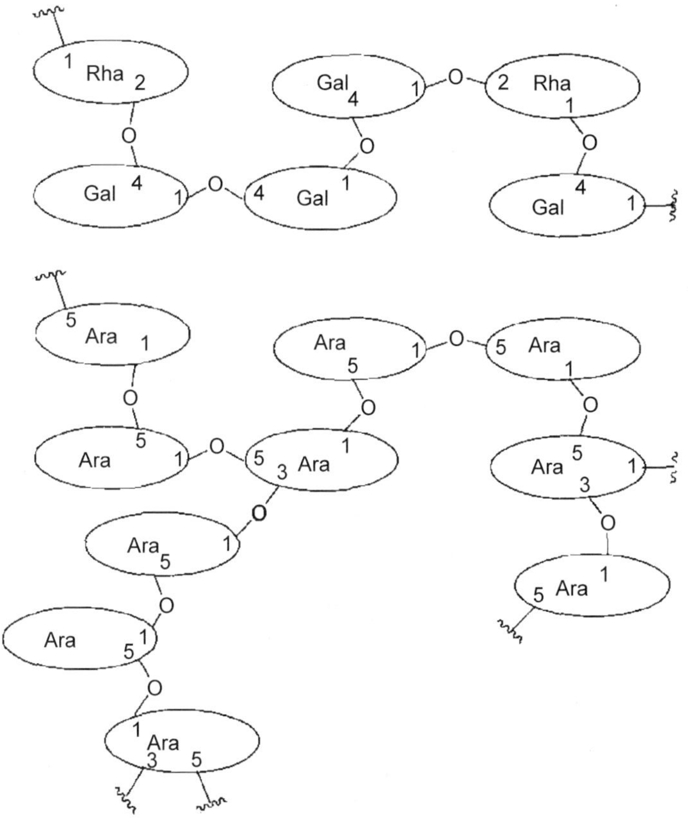

FORMULA CHART NO. 10 Echinacea polysaccharides continued.

clarified the situation. The three glycoproteins (MW 17,000, 21,000, and 30,000; approximately 3% protein content) that have been isolated from *E. angustifolia* and *E. purpurea* roots contain arabinose (64–84%), galactose (1.9–5.3%), and glucosamine (6%) as well as large amounts of aspartate, glycine, glutamate, and alanine (93) and an ELISA assay has been developed for the glycoproteins (94,95). An arabinogalactan protein was isolated from pressed juice of *E. purpurea* and shown to have a molecular weight of about 1,200,000 and to contain about 83% polysaccharide and about 7% protein. The core saccharides are highly branched (92). Polysaccharides have also been isolated and characterized from cell culture material but these are chemically significantly different from those isolated from the field-grown plants because of the intrinsic characteristics of plants grown in tissue culture (74,89).

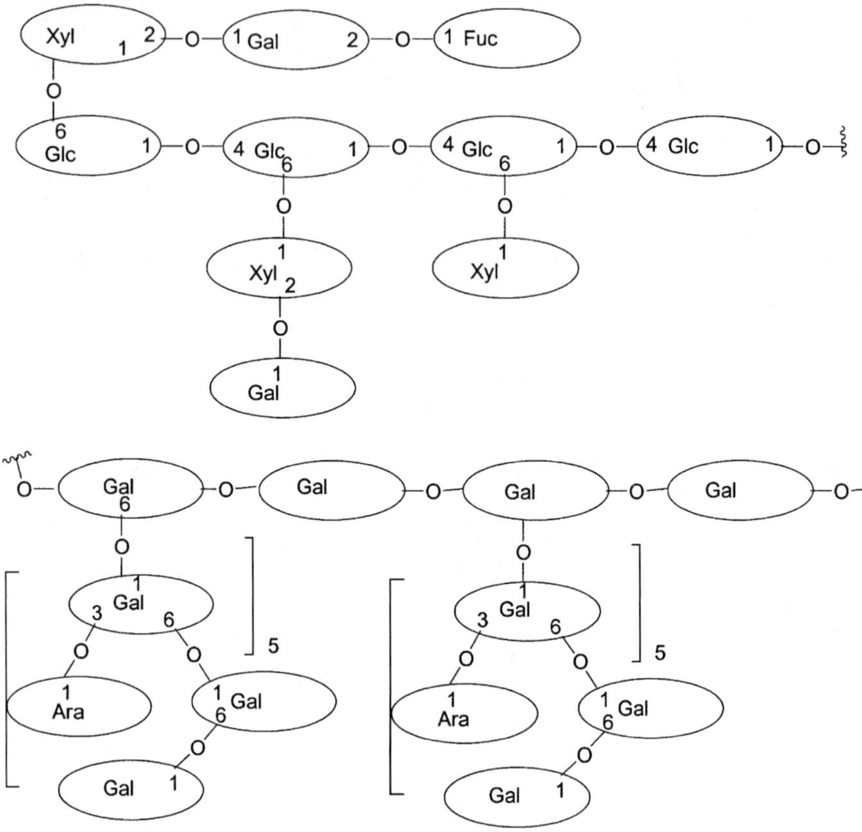

FORMULA CHART NO. 11 Echinacea polysaccharides continued.

Capillary electrophoresis has been used for the analysis of *Echinacea* species (96,97). The technique is particularly valuable for the analysis of high-molecular-weight polysaccharides and glycoproteins (98,99).

1. In Vitro, Ex Vivo, and Animal Tests

Early pharmacological tests of echinacea preparations are not particularly relevant to the question of immune stimulation as this activity was not suspected before about 1960. Suitable pharmacological assays are asserted to have been underdeveloped at that time and there is considerable doubt about the specific plant material used. This work primarily focused on wound healing, anti-inflammatory activity, and direct antimicrobial and antiviral activity and has been reviewed (3). This summary will focus on the immunological work. The available literature is now vast—amounting to about 200 papers. Most frequently used has been echinacin, an injectable commercial product containing an extract of the juice of the aerial portions of *E. purpurea* along with 22% of alcohol for preservative purposes. Oral versions are also used. Esberitox has also been studied. This material contains extract of *E. purpurea* along with *Thuja orientalis* and *Baptisia tinctoria* extracts.

The earliest study appears to have been the observation that use of a commercial preparation led to an increase in properdin (the normal serum globulin that stimulates the alternative complement pathway) levels following i.v. use in rabbits (100). Similar findings were reported with spleen tissue experiments (101) but the results of both studies were criticized because of methodological flaws, and other explanations for the findings were advanced. More recently, however, a study of healthy female volunteers (ranging from 22 to 51 years of age) who were administered standardized extracts in a double-blind, placebo-controlled trial showed that the subjects had their complement properdin increased by about 20% when a mixed *E. purpurea/angustifolia* preparation was given orally for 4 weeks (102). Thus the original work may have been valid after all.

Using isolated, perfused rat liver, an *E. purpurea* extract produced a positive effect on phagocytosis. Several species, plant parts, and extracts were involved in this study with the best phagocytosis enhancement being demonstrated by ethanolic root extracts (73,103). Interestingly, chloroform extracts prepared from the hydroethanolic extracts were more active than the aqueous portions. A later study using chemiluminescence as an indicator for phagocytic activity of granulocytes induced by zymosan in whole blood gave results that depended on the dose and methods of application. No clear conclusions were drawn from this work (104). When the alcoholic extracts were administered orally to mice, a marked increase in phagocytosis was observed. These data have been reviewed subsequently and it is concluded that both the aqueous and the lipid fractions are active but that the lipid materials are more active (3,105). A direct test of the purified alkamides and cichoric acid demonstrated activity in the carbon clearance test but ecinacoside was not active (73). The various fractions in this study contained only small amounts of the polysaccharides. In another study, the alcoholic extracts from the aerial parts and the roots of *Echinacea* species were tested for phagocyte-stimulating activity with the result that the lipophilic components showed the highest activity (69,73). The ethanolic extracts of the aerial parts of *E. angustifolia* and *E. purpurea* demonstrated immunomodulating activity on the phagocytic, metabolic, and bactericidal activities of peritoneal macrophages in mice (67,73,106). Commercial preparations of *E. purpurea* containing fresh pressed or dried juice produced cytokines in the macrophages as measured by ELISA.

After 18 hr of incubation IL-1 secretion increased. After 36 hr TNF-α, IL-6 and IL-10, were also secreted in increased amounts (107). The alkyl amides of *E. purpurea* have been demonstrated to engender a significant stimulation of phagocytic activity in alveolar macrophages when given orally by gavage to rats. These results were measured by the carbon clearance method (108,119). TNF-α and NO were both produced in increased quantity by these macrophages. This appeared to be superior to the effect of similar administration of cichoric acid and the polysaccharides (120). Echinacoside has low antibacterial and antiviral activity but does not have immunostimulatory activity (109,110). Cichoric acid shows stimulation of phagocytosis in vitro and in vivo but echinacoside, verbascoside, and 2-caffeoyltartaric acid do not (4). Cichoric acid also inhibits hyaluronidase (111) and protects collagen III from free-radical-induced damage (112). Purified alkamide fractions from *E. angustifolia* and *E. purpurea* roots enhanced phagocytosis in carbon clearance tests. The main component, dodecatetraenoic acid isobutylamide, showed only weak activity, however. This finding suggests that the substances are unstable or that other compounds are responsible for the bulk of this action. The mixed alkamides also inhibited 5-lipoxygenase activity in porcine leukocytes and cyclooxygenase in ram seminal vesicle microsomes (73).

Thus there is substantial evidence that the low-molecular-weight solvent extractables enhance phagocytosis. Side-by-side comparisions with the polysaccharides in the water-soluble portions are, unfortunately, largely lacking.

Recently it was shown that a 14-day dietary intake of echinacea preparations in aging mice stimulated the production of natural killer cells as well as enhancing their function against tumors and virus-mediated infections (113). Later it was shown that purpurea root extract was capable of enhancing the number and activity of NK cells and prolonging the survival time of leukemic mice (114). A study of the question of whether echinacea preparations could produce antigen-specific in vivo immunomodulatory action was made using rats exposed to antigen keyhole limpet hemocyanin over time. The product was active suggesting that echinacea can enhance immune function by increasing antigen-specific immunoglobulin production (115).

The polysaccharides have been demonstrated to stimulate phagocytosis and to enhance the production of oxygen radicals by macrophages in mouse cells (85,87,94,96,116). Studies of the polysaccharides derived from the aerial parts provide the strongest support for a useful immunostimulant action of echinacea at present. The immunostimulatory action of the polysaccharides is attributed to binding to cell surface receptors on the cell surface of macrophages and T lymphocytes (although some of the latter may be due to contamination with proteinaceous materials) (3). Later, more purified materials were shown to be active but at somewhat lower potency. Other workers have shown that the macrophages stimulated by the polysaccharides from tissue culture release TNF-α, interleukins-1, -6, -10, and interferon-β2 (117,118). Stimulation of the T cells is said to be nonspecific and result in transformation, production of interferon, and secretion of lymphokines leading to enhanced T-cell mitogenesis, macrophage phagocytosis, antibody binding, natural killer cell activity, and increased numbers of circulating PMS cells (3,36). There seems to be no toxicity to macrophages even at comparatively high doses of polysaccharide preparations (3). These preparations did not stimulate proliferation of T lymphocytes and had a small effect on B cells. Mice infected with *Candida albicans* 24 hr after i.v. administration of echinacea polysaccharides revealed lower levels of the yeast in their kidney cells upon surgical removal. In addition, polysaccharides enhanced the survival rate of mice against otherwise lethal *C. albicans* and *Listeria* infections (118, 119). The polysaccharides from *E. angustifolia* were shown to have anti-inflammatory activity as well (120,121). Purified extracts containing the glycoprotein-polysaccharide complex exhibited B-cell stimulation and induced the release of IL-1, TNF-α, and IFN-α,β. This effect was also seen in murine studies (96,97,122). The mitogenic activity of crude polysaccharide mixtures on T lymphocytes is thought probably to be due to nitrogenous impurities as later work with purified polysaccharides failed to show this activity (88, 116,117).

Inulin is a major constituent in the roots of *E. angustifolia* and it activates the alternative complement pathway and thus promotes chemotaxis of neutrophils, monocytes, and eosinophils, solubilization of immune complexes, neutralization of viruses, and bacteriolysis (3).

An ex vivo study has been reported using culture supernatants of stimulated whole blood cells derived from 23 tumor patients treated over a 4-week period orally with a spagyric extract from a three-herb preparation that included *E. angustifolia* (and *Thuja orientalis* plus *Eupatorium perfoliatum*). A wide range of cytokines was found in the treated and the control group. After therapy with the herbal mixture, no significant alteration in the production of the cytokines was observed and the leukocyte populations remained constant (123). This result is considered to be negative.

In normal mice, administration of a commercial preparation of echinacea root (not further identified) in the diet for 7–14 days resulted in numerically increased NK cells and monocytes (both mediators of nonspecific immunity) in the bone marrow and the spleen about 1 week after treatment was begun. Other hemopoietic and immune cell populations in bone marrow and spleen remained essentially unchanged. These data would support a prophylactic role for echinacea (124).

Despite the weight of all these mainly positive studies, there are contrary reports. In a recent study rats were fed a commercial echinacea product and two extemporaneous tinctures marketed by local herbalists. No evidence of altered NK cell activity, T-cell-mediated delayed-type hypersensitivity, or specific antibody formation was seen at high doses over a 6-week period (125). Uncertainty over the composition of these preparations lessens the impact of this work.

Glycoproteins isolated from *E. purpurea* and *E. angustifolia* increase the production of IL-1 and interferons (100,126) as demonstrated by an antiviral action against vesicular stomatitis virus. Insufficient research was done to determine whether differences exist between immunostimulation by polysaccharides and by glycoproteins.

In a brief recent report using flow cytometric measurements of human leukocytes ex vivo and gene expression arrays, Wagner and Bauer's results with the water-soluble polysaccharides were confirmed and extended to maturation of B, T, and NK cells. This work demonstrated that the water-soluble extracts of plant material had pronounced immunostimulatory activity. The activity of the low-molecular-weight organic constituents was considerably weaker (127).

The general conclusion derived from these studies is that no single echinacea constituent is responsible for the immunostimulant activity of expressed juice or of extracts. Both the lipophilic constituents and the aqueous-soluble constituents have demonstrated activity in immunostimulant tests although it is difficult to decide based on the evidence available which fraction is the more important. The methodologies employed differ from study to study, complicating analysis. No single constituent stands forth from all this work as predominantly active. There is also no decisive information favoring the use of one particular plant or plant part over another.

The most supportable conclusion is that certain echinacea products promote nonspecific T-cell activation in the form of transformation, production of interferon, and secretion of certain lymphokines. This results in enhanced T-cell mitogenesis, macrophage phagocytosis, antibody binding, natural-killer-cell activity, and increased numbers of circulating polymorphonuclear cells. This action is more closely tied to the polysaccharides than to the other constituents (85,86,88,89,118). Comparatively few of the studies involve purified components and combinations of these have never been studied.

The predominantly active components of echinacea are complex polysaccharide functional moieties that make up the cell wall building blocks in plant tissues or as the carbohydrate functional groups associated with glycoproteins. Oral activity of such high-molecular-weight materials is generally attributed to contact with mucosa-associated lymphoid tissue of the gut (GALT) because they are unlikely to be absorbed without digestion. Transportation intact via M cells of the intestinal lumen would result in direct contact with lymphocytes and macrophages in the Peyer's patches. T lymphocytes are motile throughout the lymphatic system and can recruit other cells through excretion of lymphokines. A transient tendency toward a decrease in the ratio of T-helper cells to suppressor/cytotoxic T cells immediately after treatment of human subjects with echinacea-expressed juice has been attributed to emigration and redistribution of T cells throughout the body (128).

VI. CLINICAL TESTS

Traditionally echinacea has been administered orally in the form of a tea or fluid extract. The majority of the clinical data in the United States were recorded between 1895 and 1930 although the topic has recently been taken up again in a number of laboratories. The early studies more closely resemble testimonials rather than careful scientific work and are not generally acceptable by current standards. Indeed, they were strongly criticized at the time. Studies in Germany date primarily from 1940 and continue to this date (3). In recent years a number of North American and Australian studies have appeared. Although, as has been seen, many laboratory studies have been carried out on root-derived materials, in the clinic the most convincing results have come with the expressed juice of the aerial parts. Most of the earlier German studies represent therapeutic rather than prophylactic applications.

The review that follows places primary emphasis on clinical studies completed in the last 10 years but includes a few earlier studies that produced particularly informative results. Much of this information represents use by injection. The most consistently positive clinical results involving echinacea preparations are those using the expressed juices, particularly using a commercial product named Echinacin, which contains an extract of the juice of the aerial portion of *E. purpurea* preserved by the addition of 22% of ethanol (4). An adjuvant study of the use of expressed juice of *E. purpurea* over 6 months on recurrent vaginal *Candida* infections showed that a 6-day local treatment with Econazol led to a 60% recurrence rate contrasted with a 5–16% rate with the expressed echinacea juice (128).

A retrospective study of 1280 children with acute bronchitis demonstrated that treatment with the expressed juice led to faster healing than in the cohort treated with an antibiotic (129). It is speculated that viral infections partly account for this difference, for an antibiotic would not be expected to be useful in such cases.

In a placebo-controlled, double-blind study of 108 patients given 2–4 mL of expressed juice orally over 8 weeks, fewer and less severe infections were noted and the duration of infection was decreased slightly (5.34 vs. 7.54 days) (130). The intensity of symptoms and the end point in such a study are rather subjective.

A study in terminal cancer patients given Echinacin i.m., produced a decrease in the absolute numbers of CD8+ cells whereas the CD4+ cells increased in number. The number of natural-killer cells and peripheral polymorphs increased (131). This degree of immunostimulation could have been of some value at least in preventing opportunistic infections accompanying the usual immunosuppression associated with cancer chemotherapy.

In another double-blind, placebo-controlled study including 180 volunteers, it was found that 2 dropperfuls of unstandardized *E. purpurea* herb hydroalcoholic extract was only as effective as a placebo preparation in relieving the symptoms of and duration of flu-like infections. The improvement with 4 dropperfuls was statistically better than placebo (132). The uncertain description of the medication provided significantly decreases confidence in this result.

Recently a study of 95 patients with the symptoms of an early flu infection were treated in a double-blind, placebo-controlled manner with 5 daily cups of an echinacea compound herbal tea preparation (Echinacea Plus) for 1–5 days. The patients reported improvement in their symptoms and a shorter duration of discomfort with no reported adverse effects (133). The testimonial-like character of the responses and the possibility of the operation of a significant placebo effect diminish the value of this study.

In a randomized, double-blind, placebo-controlled study of 80 persons with early cold symptoms, administration of Echinacein resulted in a shortening of symptoms from 9 to 6 days as compared to the placebo group (134).

In a multicenter (15) study of 263 patients who already exhibited cold symptoms, three different echinacea-containing medicaments were used resulting in definite shortening of the duration and intensity of symptoms (135). A smaller study (of 32 subjects) came to a similar conclusion but the nature of the echinacea preparation was only vaguely described (136).

In a study involving triathletes, daily oral treatments for 28 days using pressed juice of *E. purpurea* or magnesium supplements and flow cytometry measurements revealed slight changes in peripheral T lymphocytes but enhanced exercise-induced increases in urinary IL-6 and serum cortisol. None of the treated athletes developed upper-respiratory infections in contrast to the control group (136). Interestingly, strenuous prolonged exertion and heavy training by athletes are associated with depressed immune function. Administration of vitamins laced with echinacea is undertaken to prevent this problem but the evidence supporting this action is unconvincing (137). The use of flow cytometry to measure the increase in immune system cells enhances confidence in this work.

In healthy volunteers, a commercial echinacea preparation was administered i.m. on 4 successive days to 12 healthy men. Phagocytosis by granulocytes against *C. albicans* and the activity of natural-killer cells were measured and correlated with echinacea administration. A definite increase in cellular activity was seen and this declined when administration stopped (138). The results of this study are encouraging but the comparatively small number of patients involved weakens its value.

A second study with healthy volunteers involved use of an alcoholic extract of *E. purpurea* roots whose constituents had been determined by HPLC. This was given orally to 24 healthy men daily for 5 days. Phagocytosis was stimulated and this decreased when administration stopped. These preparations were well tolerated (139). Interestingly, oral administration appeared to produce a greater rate of increase than did injection. This study is one of the few chemically controlled clinical trials. As noted above, the HPLC measurements of compounds of unestablished immunostimulant properties is not particularly helpful but at least an attempt was made to ascertain the identity and quality of the material used.

In an interesting recent study, 117 healthy volunteers were divided into control and disease subjects and then subjected to deliberate infection with rhinovirus type 23 or placebo and then treated with 900 mg daily of an echinacea preparation shown by analysis to contain 0.16% cichoric acid and almost no echinacosides or alkamides. This echinacea preparation (which was not defined further) failed to decrease the incidence or severity of the infection (140). The strength of this study lies in the use of a known pathogen and an echinacea preparation that was standardized. The result casts doubt that cichoric acid is of value as an immunostimulant but leaves the value of other, largely unmeasured, components to be established.

In patients with acute viral and bacterial infections that had produced inflammations, white cells proliferated while T-4 cells decreased whereas T-8 cells did not. This study did involve pretreatment of controls with phytohemagglutinin A and pokeweed mitogen but time courses were not measured, so this study has been criticized. Comparable results were obtained in another study involving patients with contact eczema, neurodermatitis, herpes simplex, and *Candida* infection. Leukocytosis and granulocytosis were recorded and the percentage of T-helper cells slightly decreased. After 7 days of treatment, the percent of T-helper cells was down and helper-suppressor-cell ratios were decreased. After 8 days, overall lymphocytosis was recorded (141).

In a study on patients with viral infections accompanied by leukopenia. i.m. treatment once a day on 3 successive days improved significantly the initial low leukocyte count in over half of the patients (142). On the other hand, a study of 50 patients with genital herpes over a 1-year period revealed no statistically significant benefit with respect to the frequency or severity of outbreaks associated with treatment with Echinaforce (143).

In a trial involving 108 patients having a history of susceptibility to colds, treatment with a fluid extract of *E. purpurea* twice daily by mouth failed to be effective in decreasing the incidence, duration, or severity of colds (144).

A Swedish study of various fresh plant preparations of *Echinacea* species against colds involved 246 patients. The results were generally positive with respect to relief of symptoms and freedom from adverse effects (145).

In a Phase I clinical trial of the polysaccharide fraction isolated from *E. purpurea* tissue culture, injection at 1 mg and 5 mg produced an increase in the number of leukocytes, segmented granulocytes, and TNF-α production (146). A recent clinical trial by this same group of investigators using ethanolic extracts from *E. purpurea* and *E. angustifolia* roots in four military institutions and one industrial plant failed to reveal a useful prophylactic effect (148). An ethanolic extract, depending on the concentration of the ethanol, might not contain significant concentrations of the polysaccharides.

Extracts of *E. purpurea* were shown to enhance cellular immune function of peripheral blood mononuclear cells from normal individuals and patients with depressed cellular immunity (based on diagnosis of chronic fatigue syndrome and AIDS) (147).

Treatment of advanced gastric cancer with etoposide, leucovorin, and 5-fluorouracil usually produces a decrease in white blood cells. Treatment of a group of such patients i.v. with a polysaccharide preparation isolated from tissue cultures of *E. purpurea* resulted in a significant increase in leukocytes 14–16 days after chemotherapy (3630 cells/μL compared with the control level of 2370 cells). This suggests that the polysaccharides might be a useful adjunct to chemotherapy in reducing chemotherapy-induced leukopenia and certainly supports a positive immune-enhancing effect (148).

A placebo-controlled, double-blind study of the equivalent of 900 mg/day in the form of an alcoholic extract of *E. purpurea* roots involving 180 patients with common cold symptoms led to a significant decrease in symptoms with the extract as compared with placebo and a lower dosage (equivalent to 450 mg/day) (149). A similar study on 160 patients with a hydroalcoholic extract of *E. pallida* roots showed slightly quicker recovery from an upper-respiratory-tract infection as compared to the placebo group (150).

Homeopathic preparations are on the market also but there are no comparative studies that could be used to decide which preparations, if any, can be supported (3).

Clinical studies involving echinacea herbals combined with other herbals have been performed but these are difficult to evaluate given the complexities of judging the utility of echinacea by itself let alone what its clinical contribution might be when mixed with other complex substances. Two examples of recent studies of this type claiming utility are available (150,151).

A recent review of clinical studies of the use of echinacea in medicine concludes that the available work does not convincingly establish the value of echinacea in immunostimulation or the prevention/relief of colds. The review suggests that a major source of the confusion stems from uncertain identity of the material being evaluated and little information being provided that could bear on the mechanism of action if a positive result were obtained. Some preparations are definitely of value in reducing the severity of symptoms but only some preparations. These appear to include mainly fresh juice and isolated polysaccharides (152).

Another recent review evaluated clinical studies published between 1961 and 1997. These authors concluded that all of the studies had methodological deficiencies ranging from too few participants to unknown sources of medication. Twelve studies reported efficacy for treating the common cold. Of five studies published since 1997, two showed lack of efficacy in upper-respiratory-tract infections (URTI), and three reported utility. These studies also were judged to have procedural inadequacies (153).

Another extensive recent review of clinical studies involving 3396 patients in eight prevention and eight treatment trials concluded that variations in preparations and the poor methodological quality of the trials prevented drawing definitive conclusions (158).

A review of about 100 publications dealing with echinacea and its putative value in preventing or treating URTI concludes that most of the trials have deficiencies but that echinacea may indeed have value in early treatment of URTI, but firm recommendations could not be made from the data and little support for long-term ingestion for the prevention of URTI exists (159).

Wagner has recently commented that more than 300 German clinical trials have taken place utilizing various herbals that include echinacea intended for immunostimulation. These studies have at least demonstrated safety (25).

Most recent reviews are consistent with these conclusions (152,154–157,160–164).

Despite lack of clear-cut evidence of efficacy, the apparent lack of adverse effects suggests that the lay use of echinacea is probably harmless and should not necessarily be discouraged (165).

Overall, some echinacea preparations appear to be helpful but no strong recommendation can be made from the data available with respect to the preparation whose use can be supported in the treatment or prevention of common colds (166).

VII. TOXICITY

There is comparatively little information in print about the side effects and toxicity of echinacea preparations. The clinical studies rarely report side effects or intolerance following oral use in ordinary doses although a number of patients do not like the taste (160). This generally agrees with historic data. Parenteral administration is comparatively less common but shivering and other flu-like symptoms have been reported (perhaps resulting from macrophage stimulation resulting in release of interferon and interleukin I?). On occasion, acute allergic reactions can be seen (160).

The LD_{-50} of intravenous Echinacin is 50 mL/kg in mice and rats. In mice, LD_{-50} values of >2500 and >5000 mg/kg were found indicating very low acute toxicity (163,167). A later study showed that oral administration to rats and mice in single large doses or chronically in doses proportionally many times those used in humans showed no significant toxicity even after necropsy.

The polysaccharides in *E. purpurea* aerial parts have an LD_{50} of 1000–2500 mg/kg interperitoneally in rats. These doses are many multiples of those intended for humans (163).

There is a report of a woman who took a variety of medications and who developed an anaphylactic reaction while taking echinacea. Subsequent skinprick and RAST testing revealed hypersensitivity (164). Later studies also report hypersensitive reactions to echinacea preparations, including anaphylaxis (165). Clearly one should be cautious in the use of echinacea in individuals prone to allergy.

One also supposes that the use of echinacea preparations should be avoided in cases where autoimmune diseases are likely. In those cases, an effectively immunostimulent treatment would likely be harmful.

Mutagenicity studies failed to reveal any problem (162,166,167).

The question of the safety of using echinacea preparations during pregnancy often comes up. As a general rule, ingestion of novel materials during pregnancy should be minimized or avoided as a precaution against birth defects. Furthermore, among other considerations, experience indicates that a significant number of pregnancies are unplanned, so many instances of coincidental echinacea use in the first trimester are likely. Examination of data gathered from 112 women who used echinacea early in their pregnancies revealed no obvious defects statistically significant over the control group (168). This is comforting. There is no significant evidence that echinacea use in pregnancy is harmful but not much direct study has been done as yet (169,170).

In a recent study of antibiotic susceptibilities following neutraceutical use, garlic, zinc salts, and echinacea were all reported to decrease the action of antibiotics against ampicillin-resistant strains (171). The clinical meaning of this is unclear.

VIII. CHRONIC USE

One unanswered question that also requires more study relates to whether echinacea should be used on a continual basis. Work in healthy individuals indicates that a period of initial stimulation (typically 1–7 days) is followed by a period (typically after about 11 days) when the immune system no longer responds as before (3,8). Accordingly, echinacea is often prescribed in 10-day treatment periods followed by 2 weeks of no administration. This appears to be prudent but the evidence underlying this is flimsy.

A recent study evaluated the ability of *E. angustifolia* root preparations to inhibit the action of cytochrome P450 isozyme CYP3A4 in vitro. Suppression of this important isoenzyme at high dilution indicates the potential for significant drug-drug interactions that should, therefore, be guarded against (173). Despite this potential concern, however, a review of the literature failed to reveal any clear-cut cases of interactions between echinacea and other drugs (174).

Mutagenicity tests in bacteria and in mice were negative, as were carcinogenicity studies in hamster embryo cells (175).

IX. SUMMARY

In evaluating the literature on a herbal remedy one normally considers eight questions.

1. Is there a history of human use? Clearly echinacea qualifies based on written records extending back for 300 years and there is anecdotal evidence considerably predating this.
2. What claims are made? Modern claims for the efficacy of echinacea center about its purported immunostimulatory activity. In particular, it is claimed that consumption of various preparations prevents or at least shortens the symptoms associated with colds and influenza. Topical use is claimed to be of benefit in wound healing.
3. What science backs these claims? Many in vitro, in vivo, ex vivo, and clinical studies have been published on this topic.
4. Is the evidence credible? Does it link the claims and the results? Here the evidence is contradictory owing to the often comparatively poor quality of some of the studies.
5. Are there reliable sources of material? Botanical authentication is not difficult although there are instances of adulteration and contamination from time to time. Biological validation is possible but the methodologies have yet to be perfected. Chemical validation is only of value at present for species confirmation.

6. Are the active constituents known? No. There is evidence for immunostimulatory properties for some of the low-molecular-weight organic components but no single pure components have yet been validated. There is evidence for immunostimulatory properties for some of the high-molecular-weight water-soluble carbohydrates. A consensus is presently lacking.
7. Are there suitable assays? Partially. Bioassays are presently possible and these would reflect the end product uses intended. Chemical, chromatographic, and spectroscopic assays are potentially available, but without knowledge of the active component(s) these cannot be relied upon at present.
8. Is it safe? Generally, yes. Aside from allergy and bad taste, side effects or toxic reactions have not been documented. Drug-drug interactions based on competing metabolism are likely but as yet this has not been satisfactorily delineated.

Thus a great deal of experimental evidence is now available bearing on the question of whether echinacea preparations have immunostimulatory properties and, if so, what constituents are primarily responsible. Unfortunately no clear answer emerges from a study of these works. The weight of evidence supports the notion that a positive effect is present and that the polymeric carbohydrates possess the bulk of the activity. The clinical findings are more equivocal primarily as a result of lack of standardization of materials being marketed. More work is clearly called for using adequately described materials before the use of echinacea for immunostimulation can be recommended without reservations.

ACKNOWLEDGMENTS

This work was supported in part by grants from the Pharmanex Corporation (a division of the NuSkin Corporation) and by funds from the NICAM.

REFERENCES

1. Moench K. Meth Plant 1794.
2. Unruh V. Nat Eclec Med Assoc Q 1915; 7:63.
3. Bauer R, Wagner H. *Echinacea*-species as potential immunostimulatory drugs. In: Farnsworth NR, Wagner H, eds. Phytomedicines of Europe: Chemistry and Biologic Activity. New York: Academic Press, 1991.
4. Bauer R. Echinacea: biological effects and active principles. In: Lawson L, Bauer R, eds. Phytomedicines of Europe: Chemistry and Biological Activity. ACS Symposium Series 691, 1998:140–157.

5. Gilmore MR. Coll Nebraska State Hist Soc 1913; 17:314.
6. Gilmore MR. Coll Nebraska State Hist Soc 1913; 17:358.
7. Gilmore MR. Annual Report No. 33. Smithsonian Institution Bureau of American Ethnology, 1919.
8. Hobbs CR. The Echinacea Handbook. Portland: Eclectic Medical Publications, 1989.
9. Kindscher K. Econ Bot 1989; 43:498.
10. Moerman DE. Medicinal Plants of Native America, Research Report on Ethnobotany, Contribution 2. Technical report No. 19. University of Michigan Museum of Anthropology, 1986.
11. Shemluck M. J Ethnopharmacol 1982; 5:303.
12. Smith HH. Bull Pub Museum Milwaukee 1928; 4:175.
13. Vogel VJ. American Indian Medicine. University of Oklahoma Press, Norman: Rev. ed., 1990
14. Borchers AT, Keen CL, Stern JS, Gershwin ME. Am J Clin Nutr 2000; 72: 339.
15. Elkins R. Echinacea. London: Woodland Publishing, Inc., 1996.
16. Upton R. Echinacea. New York: McGraw-Hill, 1996.
17. Berkoff N, Collins E. Echinacea and Immunity. Roseville, CA: Prima Publ, 2000.
18. Davies JR. Echinacea. Boston: Element Books, 1999.
19. Foster S. Echinacea: Nature's Immune Enhancer, Inner Traditions Interanaion. Rochester, VT: Healing Arts Press, 1991.
20. Stengler M. Echinacea: Supercharge Your Immune System. Green Bay, WI: IMPAKT Communications, Inc., 1999.
21. Miovic M, Baugh B, eds. Echinacea: The Immune Herb. Johannesburg, S. A.: Botanica Press, 1996.
22. Schar D. Echinacea: The Plant That Boosts Your Immune System. Berkeley, CA: North Atlantic Books, 2000.
23. Bergner P. The Healing Power of Echinacea and Goldenseal and Other Immune System Herbs. Roseville, CA: Prima Publishing, 1997.
24. Hobbs C. Herbal Remedies for Dummies. New York: John Wiley & Sons, Inc., 1998.
25. Wagner H. Immunomodulatory Agents from Plants. Boston: Birkhauser, 1999.
26. Roundtree R, Colman C. Immunotics. New York: Berkley Publishing Group, 2001.
27. Conkling W. Secrets of Echinacea. New York: St. Martin's Press, 1999.
28. Thomas L, Johansen K. Ten Essential Herbs: Everyone's Handbook to Health. Prescott, AZ: Hohm Press, 1996.
29. Brody JE, Grady D. The New York Tiems Guide to Alternative Health: A Consumer Reference. New York: Holt & Co, 2001.
30. Mowrey DB. Echinacea. New York: McGraw-Hill, 1993.
31. Pedersen S. Echinacea: Amazing Immunity. New York: Dorling Kindersley Pub., Inc., 2000.
32. Tyler V. Herbs of Choice. Binghamton, N. Y.: Pharmaceutical Products Press, 1994.

33. Johnson M, Foster S, Hobbs C. Echinacea: The Immune Herb. Johannesburg, S. A.: Botanica Press, 1996.
34. Bauer R, Wagner H. Echinacea—Ein Handbuch fuer Aerzte, Apotheker und andere Naturwissenschaftler. Stuttgart: Wissenschaftlich Verlagsgesellschaft, 1990.
35. Wagner H. Pure Appl Chem 1990; 62:1217.
36. Wagner H, Proksch A. Immunostimulatory drugs of fungi and higher plants. In: Farnsworth N, Wagner H, eds. Economic and Medicinal Plant Research. Vol. 1. London: Academic Press, 1985.
37. Anon. Echinacea. Austin, TX: Am Herbal Council, 2000.
38. World Health OrganizationHerba Echinaceae Purpureae Radix Echinacea and Radix EchinaceaWHO Monographs on Selected Medicinal Plants. Vol. 1. Geneva: World Health Organization, 1999:125–135, 136–144.
39. Hobbs C. Echinacea: a literature review: botany, history, chemistry, pharmacology, toxicology and clinical uses. HerbalGram, Special supplement #30, 1994.
40. Blumenthal M, Busse WR, Goldberg A, Gruenwald J, Hall T, Riggins CW, Rister RS. The Complete German Commission E Monographs: Therapeutic Guide to Herbal Medicines. Austin, TX: American Botanical Council, 1998.
41. American Botanical Council. *Echinacea purpurea* (L.) Moench [Fam. Asteraceae], Austin, TX.
42. Wagner H. Environ Health Perspect 1999; 107:779.
43. Brevoort P. The booming U. S. botanical market. HerbalGram 1998; 44:33–46.
44. Melchert D, Linde K, Worku F, Sarkady L, Holzmann M, Jurcic K, Wagner H. J Altern Complement Med 1995; 1:145.
45. Reichling H. Deutsch Med Wochenschr 1998; 123:58.
46. Bauer R, Khan I, Wagner H. Planta Med 1985; 10:426.
47. Schumacher A, Friedberg KD. Arzneimittelforschung 1991; 42:141.
48. Osowski S, Rostock M, Bartsch HH, Massig U. Forsch Komplementarmed Klass Naturheilkd 2000; 7:294.
49. McGreggor RL. University of Kansas Sci Bull 1968; 48:132.
50. Bauer R, Khan I, Wagner H. Deutsche Apotheker Zeitung 1987; 18:1325.
51. Bauer R. Echinacea: Biological effects and active principles. In: Lawson L, Bauer R, eds. Phytomedicines of Europe: Chemistry and Biological Activity. ACS Symposium Series 691, 1998:140–157.
52. Kindscher K. Econ Bot 1989; 43:498.
53. Lloyd JU. Eccl Med J 1897; 57:28.
54. Stoll A, Renz J, Brak A. Helv chim Acta 1950; 33:1877.
55. Becker H, Hsieh WC, Wylde R, Lafitte C, Andary C. Z Naturforsch Teil c 1982; 37:351.
56. Bauer R, Remiger P, Wagner H. Deutsch Apoth Ztg 1988; 128:174.
57. Cheminat A, Zawatzky R, Becker H, Brouillard R. Phytochemistry 1988; 27:2787.
58. Bauer R, Alstat E. Planta Med 1990; 56:533.
59. Becker H, Hsieh WC. Z Naturforsch Teil e 1985; 40:585.

60. Malonga-Makosi. Quoted in Ref. 3, 1983.
61. Malonga-Makosi JP. Dissertation, Un. Heidelberg, 1991.
62. Cheminat A, Brouillard R, Guerne P, Bergmann P, Rether B. Phytochemistry 1989; 28:3246.
63. Voaden DJ, Jacobson M. J Med Chem 1972; 15:619.
64. Jacobson M, Redfern RF, Mills GD Jr. Lloydia 1975; 38:473.
65. Bauer RFX, Khan IA, Lotter H, Wagner H. Helv chim Acta 1985; 68:2355.
66. Schulte KE, Ruecker G, Perlick J. Arzneim Forsch 1967; 17:825.
67. Bauer R, Khan IA, Wagner H. Planta Med 1988; 54:426.
68. Bauer R, Khan IA, Wray V, Wagner H. Phytochemistry 1987; 26:1198.
69. Jacobson AI. J Org Chem 1967; 32:1646.
70. Sloley BD, Urichuk LJ, Tywin C, Coutts RT, Pang PK, Shan JJ. J Pharm Pharmacol 2001; 53:849.
71. Roeder E, Wiedenfeld H, Hille T, Britz-Kirstgen R. Deutsch Apoth Ztg 1984; 124:2316.
72. Bauer R, Foster S. Planta Med 1991; 57:447.
73. Bauer R, Remiger P. Planta Med 1989; 55:367.
74. Wagner H, Stuppner H, Pohlmann J, Jurcic K, Zenk MA, Lohmann-Matthes ML. Z Phytother 1987; 8:125.
75. Bauer R. J Herbs, Spices Medicinal Plants 1999; 6:51.
76. Egert D, Beuscher N. Planta Med 1991; 58:163.
77. Christ B, Muller KH. Arch Pharm 1960; 293:1033.
78. Pomponio R, Gotti R, Hudalb M, Cavrini V. J Chromatogr A 2002; 945:239.
79. Perry NB, vanKlink JW, Burgess EJ, Parmentier GA. Planta Med 1997; 63:58.
80. Perry NB, vanKlink JW, Burgess EJ, Parmentier GA. Planta Med 2000; 66:54.
81. Roder E, Wiedenfeld H, Hille T, Britz-Kistgen R. Pyrrolizidine in *Echinacea angustifolia*, DC, *Echinacea purpurea* MOENSCH—Isolierung und Analytik. Deutsch Apoth Ztg 1984; 124:16.
82. Tekel J, Tahotna S, Vaverkova S. J Pharm Biomed Anal 1998; 16:753.
83. Lienert D, Anklam E, Panne U. Phytochem Anal 1998; 9:88.
84. Bonadeo I, Bottazzi G, Lavazza M. Riv. Ital. Essente-Profumi-Piante officin.-aromi-saponi-Cosmetici-Aerosol 1971; 53:281.
85. Wagner H, Proksch A. Z angew Phytother 1981; 2:166.
86. Wagner H, Proksch A, Riess-Maurer I, Vollmar A, Odenthal S, Stuppner H, et al. Arzneim Forsch 1984; 34:659.
87. Proksch A, Wagner H. Phytochemistry 1987; 26:1989.
88. Stimpel M, Proksch A, Wagner H, Lohmann-Mathes M-L. Infect Immun 1984; 46:845.
89. Wagner H, Stuppner H, Schaefer W, Zenk MA. Phytochemistry 1988; 27:119.
90. Wagner H, Stuppner H, Puhlmann J, Bruemmer B, Deppe K, Zenk MA. Z Phytother 1989; 10:35.
91. Leuttig B, Steinmuller C, Gifford GE, Wagner H, Lohmann-Matthes ML. J Natl Cancer Inst 1989; 81:669.
92. Classen B, Witthohn K, Blaschek W. Carbohydr Res 2000; 327:497.
93. Beuscher KH, Kopanski L, Erwein G. Adv Biosci 1987; 68:329.

94. Beuscher KH, Bodinet C, Willigmann I, Egert D. Z Phytother 1995; 16:157.
95. Egert D, Beuscher H. Planta Medi 1992; 58:163.
96. Issaq H. Electrophoresis 1997; 18:2438.
97. Issaq H. Electrophoresis 1999; 20:3190.
98. Chiesa C, Horvath C. J Chromatogr 1993; 645:337.
99. Ristolainen M. J Chromatogr 1998; 832:203.
100. Buesing KH. Arzneim-Forsch 1952; 2:467.
101. Taennerhoff FK, Schwabe JK. Arzneim-Forsch 1956; 6:330.
102. Kim LS, Waters RF, Burkholder PM. Altern Med Rev 2002; 7:138.
103. Voemel Th. Arzneim-Forsch 1985; 35:1437.
104. Bauer R, Remiger P, Jurcic K, Wagner H. Ztschr Phytother 1989; 10:43–48.
105. Gaisbauer M, Schleich T, Stickl HA, Wilczek I. Arzneimittelforschung 1990; 40:594.
106. Bohlmann F, Grenz M. Chem Ber 1966; 99:3197.
107. Burger RA, Torres AR, Warren RP, Caldwell VD, Hughes BG. Int J Immunopharmacol 1997; 19:371.
108. Goel V, Chang C, Slama JV, Barton R, Bauer R, Gahler R, Basu TK. Int Immunopharmacol 2002; 2:381.
109. Beuscher N, Beuscher HN, Bodinet C. Planta Medi 1989; 55:660.
110. Bodinet C, Beuscher N. Planta Med 1991; 57s2:A33.
111. Soicke H, Al-Hassan G, Goerler K. Planta Med 1988; 54:175.
112. Sicha J, Hubik J, Dusek J. Cesk Farm 1989; 38:124.
113. Currier NL, Miller SC. Exp Gerontol 2000; 35:627.
114. Currier NL, Miller SC. J Altern Complement Med 2001; 7:241.
115. Rehman J, Dillow JM, Carter SM, Chou J, Le B, Maisel AS. Immunol Lett 1999; 68:391.
116. Lohman-Matthes M-L, Wagner H. Z Phytother 1989; 10:52.
117. Luettig B, Steinmueller C, Gifford GE, Wagner H, Lohmann-Matthes M-L. J Natl Cancer Inst 1989; 81:669.
118. Roesler J, Steinmueller C, Kiderlein A, Emmendoerffer A, Wagner H, Lohmann-Matthes M-L. Int J Immunopharmacol 1991; 13:27; Bodinet C, Beuscher N. Planta Med 1991; 57s2:A33; Roesler J, Emmendoerffer A, Steinmueller C, Luestig B, Wagner H, Lohmann-Mathes M-L. Int J Immunopharmacol 1991; 13:931.
119. Steinmuller C, Roesler J, Grottrup E, Franke G, Wagner H, Lohmann-Mathes ML. Int J Immunopharmacol 1993; 15:605.
120. Tubaro A, Tragni E, Del Negro P, Galli CL, Della Logia R. J Pharm Pharmacol 1987; 39:567.
121. Tragni E, Galli CL, Tubaro A, Del Negro P, Della Logia R. Pharmacol Res Commun 1988; 20(S20 V):87.
122. Beuscher N, Beuscher HN, Bodinet C. Planta Med 1989; 55:660.
123. Elsaesser-Beile U, Willenbacher W, Bartsch HH, Gallati H, Schulte J, vonKleist S. J Clin Lab Anal 1996; 10:441.
124. Sun LZ, Currier NL, Miller SC. J Altern Complement Med 1999; 5:437.
125. South EH, Exon JH. Immunopharmacol Immunotoxicol 2001; 23:411.

126. Beuscher H, Bodinet C, Neumann-Haefelin D, Marston A, Hostetmann K. J Ethnopharmacol 1994; 42:101.
127. Mitscher LA, Pillai S. Abstr. 43rd Annual Meeting. Am Soc Pharmacog New Brunswick, NJ, July 27–31, 2002.
128. Coeugniet E, Elek E. Onkologie 1987; 10:S27.
129. Coeugniet EG, Kuehnast R. Therapiewoch 1986; 36:3352.
130. Baetgen D. Therapiewoche Paediatr 1988; 1:66.
131. Schoeneberger D. Forum Immunol 1992; 2:18.
132. Lersch C, Zeuner M, Bauer A, Siebenrock K, Hart R, Wagner F, Fink U, Dancygier H, Classen M. Arch Geschwulstforsch 1990; 60:379.
133. Braeunig B, Dorn M, Limburg E, Knick B. Z Phytother 1992; 13:7.
134. Lindenmuth GF, Lindenmuth EB. J Altern Complement Med 2000; 6:327.
135. Schulten B, Bulitta M, Ballering-Bruhl B, Koster U, Schafer M. Arzneimittelforschung 2001; 51:563.
136. Barrett B. Phytomedicine 2003; 10:66.
137. Berg A, Northoff H, Koenig D, Weinstock C, Grathwohl D, Parnham MJ, Stuhlfauth I, Keul J. J Clin Res 1998; 1:367.
138. Gleeson M, Lancaster GI, Bishop NC. Can J Appl Physiol 2001; 26:S23–S35.
139. Moese JR. Medwelt 1983; 34:1463.
140. Jurcic K, Melchart D, Holzmann M, Martin P, Bauer R, Doernicke A, Wagner H. Z Phytother 1989; 10:67.
141. Turner RB, Riker DB, Gangemi JD. Antimicrob Agents Chemother 2000; 44:1708.
142. Moeller H, Naumann H. Therapeutikon 1987; 1:56.
143. Vonau B, Chard S, Mandalla S, Wilkinson D, Barton SE. Int J Stud AIDS 2001; 12:154.
144. Grimm W, Muller HH. Am J Med 1999; 106:138.
145. Brinkeborn RM, Shah DV, Degearing FH. Phytomedicine 1999; 6:1.
146. Melchart D, Linde K, Worku F, Bauer R, Wagner H. Phytomedicine 1994; 1:245.
147. Melchart D, Walther E, Linde K, Brandmaier R, Lersch C. Arch Fam Med 1998; 7:541.
148. See DM, Broumand N, Sahl L, Tilles JG. Immunopharmacology 1997; 35:229.
149. Melchart D, Clemm C, Weber B, Draczynski T, Worku F, Linde K, et al. Phytother Res 2002; 16:138.
150. Braeunig B, Knick E. Naturheilpraxis 1993; 1:72.
151. Henneicke-von Zepelin H, Hentschel C, Schnitker J, Kohnen R, Kohler G, Wustenberg P. Curr Med Res Opin 1999; 15:214.
152. Wustenberg P, Henneicke-von Zepelin HH, Kohler G, Stammwitz U. Adv Ther 1999; 16:51.
153. Percival SS. Biochem Pharmacol 2000; 15:155.
154. Giles JT, Palat CT IIIrd, Chien SH, Chang ZG, Kennedy DT. Pharmacotherapy 2000; 20:690.
155. Ernst E. Ann Intern Med 2002; 136:42.
156. Ness J, Sherman FT, Pan CX. Geriatrics 1999; 54:33.

157. Dorsch W. Z Arztl Fortbild 1996; 90:117.
158. Pinn G. Aust Fam Physician 2001; 30:1154.
159. Melchart D, Linde K, Fischer P, Kaesmayr J. Echinacea for preventing and treating the common cold. Cochrane Database Syst Rev, 2000.
160. Barrett B, Vohmann M, Calabrese C. Echinacea for upper respiratory infection. J Fam Pract 1999; 48:628.
161. Lersch C, Zeuner M, Bauer A, Siemens M, Hart R, Drescher M, Fink U, Dancygier H, Classen M. Cancer Invest 1992; 10:343.
162. Lenk M. Z Phytother 1989; 10:49.
163. Schimmer O, Abel G, Behninger C. Z Phytother 1989; 10:39.
164. Mengs U, Clare CB, Poiley JA. Arzneimittelforschung 1991; 41:1076.
165. Mullins RJ. Med J Aust 1998; 168:170.
166. Mullins RJ, Heddle R. Ann Allergy Asthma Immunol 2002; 88:42.
167. Parnham MJ. Phytomedicine 1996; 3:95.
168. Shohan J. TIPS 1985; 6:178.
169. Gallo M, Sarkar M, Au W, Pietrzak K, Comas B, Smith M, Jaeger TV, Einarson A, Koren G. Arch Intern Med 2000; 13:160.
170. Gallo M, Koren G. Can Fam Physician 2001; 47:1727.
171. Tsui B, Dennehy CE, Tsourounis C. Am J Obstet Gynecol 2001; 185:433.
172. Ward P, Fasitsas S, Katz SE. J Food Prot 2002; 65:528.
173. Budzinski JW, Foster BC, Vandenhoek S, Arnason JT. Phytomedicine 2000; 7:273.
174. Izzo AA, Ernst E. Drugs 2001; 61:2163.
175. Mengs U, Clare CB, Poiley JA. Arzneimittelforschung 1991; 41:1076.

35

Medical Attributes of St. John's Wort (*Hypericum perforatum*)

Kenneth M. Klemow, Emily Bilbow, David Grasso, Kristen Jones, Jason McDermott, and Eric Pape
Wilkes University
Wilkes-Barre, Pennsylvania, U.S.A.

I. INTRODUCTION

St. John's wort, known botanically as *Hypericum perforatum*, is a sprawling, leafy herb that grows in open, disturbed areas throughout much of temperate North America and Australia. St. John's wort has been used as an herbal remedy to treat a variety of internal and external ailments since ancient Greek times. Since then, it has remained a popular treatment for anxiety, depression, cuts, and burns. Sales of products made from St. John's wort presently exceed several billion dollars each year.

St. John's wort produces dozens of biologically active substances, two being the most clinically effective. Hypericin and its naphthodianthrone analogs are produced by small, dark glands on the surfaces of the yellow petals, constituting 0.1–0.3% of the dry mass of the foliage. Hyperforin is a lipophilic phloroglucinol derivative derived from the buds and flowers, constituting 2–4.5% of the mass of the foliage.

H. perforatum has been intensively studied on isolated tissue samples, using animal models, and through human clinical trials. The effectiveness of St. John's wort as an antidepressive agent has been particularly well studied. At the cellular level, hypericin and hyperforin both inhibit uptake of key neurotransmitters like serotonin (5-HT), dopamine, noradrenaline, GABA, and L-glutamate at the synaptic cleft in the brain. Hyperforin may also increase the density of 5-HT receptors, thus providing potential long-term benefits.

Meta-analyses of clinical trials conducted in Europe since the 1980s indicated that St. John's wort was more effective in alleviating depression than placebo. Moreover, St. John's wort was shown to be as effective in treating depression as standard tricyclic synthetic drugs—with fewer adverse effects. However, two multicenter studies conducted in the United States between 1998 and 2001 did not find any difference between St. John's wort and placebo, especially in patients with moderate to severe depression. Taken together the studies indicate that St. John's wort appears to have some efficacy in treating mild to moderate depression, but no proven value in treating moderate to severe depression.

St. John's wort has value as an antibacterial and antiviral agent. Hyperforin is particularly active against gram-positive bacteria, including meticillin-resistant and penicillin-resistant *Staphylococcus aureus*. Extracts have been shown to be active against enveloped viruses, especially when activated by light. In the 1990s, St. John's wort was examined as a therapy for HIV, though a Phase I clinical trial published in 1999 indicated no discernible effect coupled with low tolerability.

Both hyperforin and hypericin show potential as anticancer therapies. Hyperforin inhibits tumor cell growth in vitro by induction of apoptosis through the activation of caspases. In the presence of light and oxygen, hypericin kills tumors by generating superoxide radicals that yield cytotoxic species. Hypericin has potential to be used in photodynamic therapy (PDT) against a variety of neoplastic tissues. However, St. John's wort extracts may interfere with the success of treatments involving the anticancer agent irinotecan.

Though generally well tolerated, especially at typically recommended doses, St. John's wort may produce adverse effects including gastrointestinal symptoms, dizziness, confusion, restlessness, and lethargy. More significantly, St. John's wort can interact adversely with a wide range of prescription and over-the-counter medications, as well as with other herbal remedies. Especially noteworthy are adverse interactions with standard antidepressants, and with drugs that are metabolized by hepatic cytochrome enzymes. Individuals taking other medications or suffering from moderate to severe psychological or physical ailments should consult with their physician before taking extracts of St. John's wort.

II. SPECIES DESCRIPTION

H. perforatum, commonly called the common St. John's wort, klamathweed, tiptonweed, goatweed, and enolaweed (1), is a native of Europe, but has spread to temperate locations in Asia, Africa, North and South America, and Australia (2,3). It thrives in poor soils, and is commonly found in meadows, fields, waste areas, roadsides, and abandoned mines and quarries (1,2,4).

Individuals of St. John's wort are freely branching perennials that typically range from 40 to 80 cm tall (Fig. 1) (1,2). The stems are herbaceous, though the bases are somewhat woody. The stems and branches are densely covered by oblong, smooth-margined leaves that range from 1 to 3 cm long and 0.3 to 1.0 cm wide. The leaves are interrupted by minute translucent spots that are evident when held up to the light. The upper portions of mature plants can produce several dozen five-petaled yellow flowers that are typically 1.0–

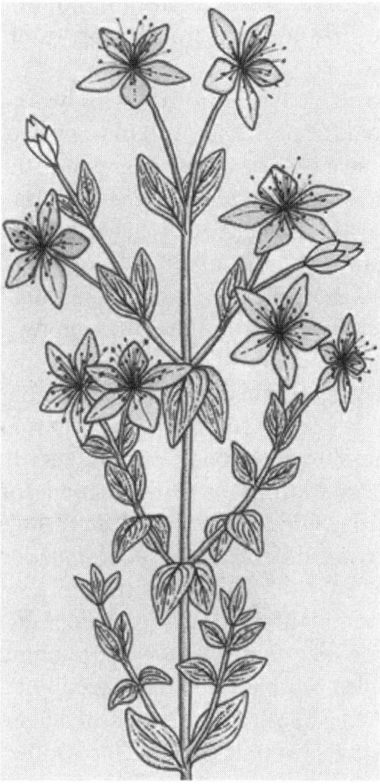

FIGURE 1 Diagram of St. John's wort, *Hypericum perforatum*. (Image from http://www.thorne.com/altmedrev/hypericum.jpg.)

2.0 cm wide. The edges of the petals are usually black-dotted. Crushed flowers produce a blood-red pigment. By late summer, the flowers produce capsules that contain dozens of tiny dark-brown seeds. St. John's wort reproduces both by seed and by ground-level rhizomes.

Because of concerns over phototoxicity to livestock, *H. perforatum* is listed as a noxious weed in seven western states in the United States. Programs promoting its eradication are underway in Canada, California, and Australia. Some of those measures include use of the *Chysolina* beetle, which is a natural predator (3).

III. HERBOLOGY

St. John's wort was been considered to be a medicinally valuable plant for over 2000 years. The first-century Greek physicians Galen, Dioscorides, and Hippocrates recommended it as a diuretic, wound-healing herb, as a treatment for menstrual disorders, and as a cure for intestinal worms (3,5). In the sixteenth century, the Swiss herbalist Paracelsus used St. John's wort externally to treat wounds and alleviate pain (3).

The species gained a reputation during the Middle Ages as having mystical properties, and plants were collected for use as a talisman to protect one from demons and to drive away evil spirits. According to legend, the greatest effect was obtained when the plant was harvested on St. John's day (June 24th), which is often the time of peak blooming (3). The generic name *Hypericum* originated from the Greek name for the plant "hyperikon." Literally translated, the name is an amalgamation of the root words "hyper" (meaning "over") and "eikon" (meaning "image") (3), though its meaning is less clear.

St. John's wort's use as a medicinal herb continued in Europe throughout the nineteenth and twentieth centuries. It was commonly made into teas and tinctures for treatment of anxiety, depression, insomnia, water retention, and gastritis. Externally, vegetable oil preparations have been used for treatment of hemorrhoids and inflammation. Others have used St. John's wort extracts to treat sores, cuts, minor burns, and abrasions, especially those involving nerve damage (3,6,7).

St. John's wort enjoys a worldwide reputation as having therapeutic value for treating depression and other mood disorders. Products containing St. John's wort in the form of tablets, capsules, teas, and tinctures accounted for $400 million in sales in 1998 in the United States (8) and an estimated $6 billion in Europe (8,9).

As noted by Barnes et al. (10), St. John's wort has been the subject of several pharmacopoeias and monographs, including the *British Herbal Pharmacopoeia* (11); *European Scientific Cooperative on Phytotherapy*

(ESCOP) (12); *American Herbal Pharmacopoea* (13); Parfitt (14); Barnes et al. (15); and the *European Pharmacopoeia* (16).

Pharmaceutical-grade preparations of St. John's wort are typically comprised of dried aerial parts. One widely available extract that is commonly used in clinical trials, LI 160, is produced by Lichtwer Pharma. It is standardized to contain 0.3% hypericin derivatives, and normally comes in 300-mg capsules (17). A second preparation, Ze 117 (Zeller AG, Switzerland), is a 50% ethanolic extract with an herb to extract ratio of 4–7:1. The hyperforin content of Ze 117 is 0.2%, lower than that of LI 160, whose hyperforin content ranges between 1 and 4%. The dosage of Ze 117 is 500 mg/day (18). The German Commission E and ESCOP monographs recommend 900 mg of standardized extract per day (7,12). Clinical trials using various *H. perforatum* preparations have typical dosages in the range of 300–1800 mg/day (10).

In the United States, St. John's wort (like all herbal remedies) is listed as a dietary supplement by the U.S. Food and Drug Administration (FDA). Therefore, it is not subject to strict scrutiny for safety and efficacy that standard pharmaceutical drugs must pass. The FDA mandates that all herbal remedies must contain a disclaimer informing the consumer that any claims about therapeutic value have not been evaluated by that agency.

IV. CHEMICAL CONSTITUENTS

Chemical investigations into the constituents of *H. perforatum* have detected several classes of compounds. The most common classes include naphthodianthrones, flavonoids, phloroglucinols, and essential oils (10,19–21). The major active constituents are considered to be hypericin (a naphtodianthrone; Fig. 2a), hyperforin (a phloroglucinol; Fig. 2b), rutin and other flavonoids, and tannins (10). Approximately 20% of extractable compounds are considered biologically active, according to standard bioanalytical techniques (22–24).

A. Naphthodianthrones

The most researched class of compounds isolated from *H. perforatum* is the naphthodianthrones, which occur in concentrations ranging from 0.1% up to 0.3% (9,25,26). The most common naphthodianthrones include hypericin, pseudohypericin, isohypericin, and protohypericin (10,21). Of those, hypericin is the best known and, to date, the most studied. Hypericin is a reddish pigment that is responsible for the red color of St. John's wort oils. Hypericin is found in greatest abundance in the flowers, particularly in the black dots that are located on the petals of St. John's wort flowers (3).

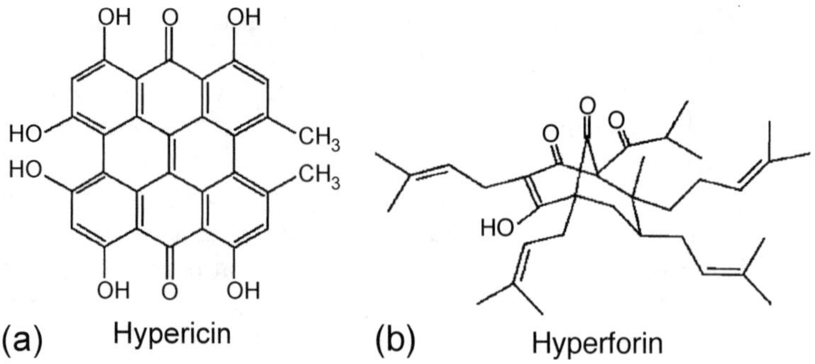

FIGURE 2 Structures of chemically active constituents of St. John's wort, *Hypericum perforatum*. (a) Hypericin—a naphtodianthrone found primarily in the black dots on the flower petals. (b) Hyperforin—an acylated phloroglucinol typically derived from buds and flowers.

Hypericin is highly photoreactive, owing to its chemical structure. Biochemically, hypericin is a polycyclic quinone, having four hydroxyl groups that lie adjacent to two carbonyl groups (Fig. 2a). Owing to resonance of the molecule and the relatively short distance between oxygens (~2.5 angstroms), the hydroxyl hydrogen is able to transfer back and forth from the hydroxyl oxygen to the carbonyl oxygen when in the presence of fluorescent light (27). Therefore, the hydrogen is in constant flux between both oxygens when under fluorescent light (28). Studies examining the fluorescence spectrum of hypericin and its analogs have demonstrated the existence of a "protonated" carbonyl group, therefore proving the H-atom transition (27). This hydrogen transfer causes acidification of the surrounding environment (29,30).

B. Flavonoids

Flavonoids found in *H. perforatum* range from 7% in stems to 12% in flowers (21) and leaves (9). Flavonoids include flavonols (kaempferol, quercetin), flavones (luteolin), glycosides (hyperside, isoquercitrin, rutin), biflavonoids (biapigenin), amentoflavone, myricetin, hyperin, proanthocyanidins, and miquelianin (10,20). Rutin concentration is reported at 1.6% (10).

C. Lipophilic Compounds

Extracts of St. John's wort contain several classes of lipophilic compounds, including phloroglucinol derivatives and oils, that have potential or demonstrated therapeutic value. Acylated phloroglucinols are typically derived from buds and flowers of *H. perforatum* (16). Hyperforin, found in concentrations of 2–4.5% (9,31), consists of phloroglucinol expanded into a bicyclo (2,1) nonaendionol, substituted with several lipophilic isoprene chains. Other phloroglucinols include adhyperforin (0.2–1.9%), furohyperforin, and other hyperforin analogs (9,10,21,32).

Essential oils are found in concentrations ranging from 0.05% to 0.9% (9). They consist mainly of mono and sesquiterpines, mainly 2-methyl-octane, n-nonane, α- and β-pinene, α-terpineol, geranil, and trace amounts of myrecene, limonene, caryophyllene, and others (20,32).

D. Additional Compounds

Other compounds of various classes have been determined to occur in *H. perforatum*. These include tannins (concentrations vary from 3% to 16%), xanthones (1.28 mg/100 g), phenolic compounds (caffic acid, chlorogenic acid, and *p*-coumaric acid), and hyperfolin. Other compounds include acids (nicotinic, myristic, palmitic, stearic), carotenoids, choline, pectin, hydrocarbons, and long-chain alcohols (21). Amino acids that occur include cysteine, GABA (γ-aminobutyric acid), glutamine, leucine, lysine, and others (9,19,32).

V. THERAPEUTIC USES OF ST. JOHN'S WORT

The widespread popularity of St. John's wort's use as an herbal remedy results from studies that appear to verify its efficacy, especially in treating mild to moderate depression. In return, its use has generated widespread interest among scientists seeking to firmly evaluate its effectiveness. Such studies have included in vitro analyses on the effects of St. John's wort extracts on isolated tissue samples, studies using animal models, and clinical analyses and meta-analyses of humans given St. John's wort extracts. Comprehensive reviews of the research on St. John's wort have been recently prepared by Greeson et al. (9) and Barnes et al. (10).

A. St. John's Wort and Depression

Mood disorders are common illnesses that force individuals to seek relief by physicians and other health care providers. Worldwide, 3–5% of the world's population requires treatment for depression (33). The disorder brings with it a series of symptoms such as strong feelings of sadness and guilt, a loss of interest or pleasure, irregular sleeping patterns, a loss of energy, the decreased ability to concentrate, and an increase or decrease of appetite. Even more serious symptoms are repeating thoughts of suicide and death (34).

Depression is often viewed as originating from a disruption of the normal brain neurochemistry. A primary cause is a deficiency of amine neurotransmitters like acetylcholine, norepinephrine, dopamine, and serotonin [5-hydroxytryptamine (5-HT)]. Drugs used to treat depression typically raise the levels of those neurotransmitters, especially in nerve-nerve synapses (34).

Synthetic antidepressants widely used today fall into two categories: tricyclics and selective serotonin reuptake inhibitors (SSRIs). Tricyclics include amitriptyline (Elavil), desipramine (Norpramin), imipramine (Tofranil), nortriptyline (Aventyl, Pamelor), and trimipramine (Surmentil). Commonly prescribed SSRIs include citalopram (Celexa), fluoxetine (Prozac), paroxetine (Paxil), and sertraline (Zoloft). A third category of antidepressants, not as commonly used as the tricyclics and SSRIs, are the monoamine oxidase inhibitors (MAOI) such as phenelzine (Nardil) and tranylcypromine (Parnate) (35).

1. Active Principles—In Vitro Studies

Early research suggested that hypericin was the main antidepressant constituent of *H. perforatum*. Those studies attributed hypericin's mode of action as increasing capillary blood flow (21). Later, studies on rat brain mitochondria found hypericin to be a strong inhibitor of the enzyme of monoamine oxidase (MAO) A and B (10,25,36). MAO is involved in the degradation of amine neurotransmitters, and inhibiting their degradation boosts their levels in the synapse. However, further studies determined that the ability of hypericin to act as an inhibitor of MAO was not as high as originally estimated. Moreover, the levels of hypericin necessary to obtain significant MAO inhibition were far greater than those likely to be found in human brain tissue at normal doses (36,37). Hypericin has been shown to have a strong affinity for sigma receptors, which regulate dopamine levels. It also acts as a receptor antagonist at adenosine, benzodiazepine, GABA-A, GABA-B, and inositol triphosphate receptors, which regulate action potentials caused by neurotransmitters (37,38). While hypericin has been shown to have antidepressant properties, current thought is that hypericin alone cannot completely account for the antidepressant activity of St. John's wort.

Much recent research has focused on hyperforin as an active compound in the antidepression pharmacology (39). Hyperforin has been demonstrated to be a potent reuptake inhibitor of serotonin, dopamine, noradrenaline, GABA, and L-glutamate from the synaptic cleft (21,40–43). IC_{50} values (concentration resulting in 50% inhibition) of about 0.05–0.1 μg/mL for neurotransmitters were reported in synaptosomal preparations (44). Blocking reuptake of serotonin (5-HT) from the synaptic cleft would alleviate symptoms of depression by allowing the serotonin to bind 5-HT receptors and elicit a greater response (45,46). Studies show that hyperforin inhibits serotonin reuptake by elevating intracellular Na^+ levels (47,48). This is the first specific serotonin reuptake inhibitor (SSRI) known to do this. More recently, Müller et al. (42) found that hyperforin is associated with changes of ionic conductance pathways.

Hyperforin has a second, and possibly additive, effect, by increasing the number of 5-HT receptors, as demonstrated in studies on the brains of rats (49). Studies have shown that the density of 5-HT receptors increased by 50% over controls in the brains of rats treated with St. John's wort extract (49). This suggests a possible long-term therapeutic benefit of St. John's wort treatment. Results of clinical trials also demonstrated that the level of therapeutic effects of St. John's wort extract is directly dependent on the concentration of hyperforin (50). Despite those findings, therapeutic effects of St. John's wort extracts may depend on other constituents besides hypericin or hyperforin (31). This is still a topic of debate among St. John's wort advocates.

2. Clinical Studies

Clinical studies of the effectiveness of St. John's wort have been conducted since the 1980s. Some of the studies have compared populations receiving St. John's wort to controls. Others have compared populations receiving St. John's wort to those receiving standard antidepressants. Other studies are three-legged, comparing populations receiving St. John's wort to a second population receiving a standard antidepressant and a third receiving a placebo. Excellent reviews of the clinical literature through 2001 have been provided by Greeson et al. (9) and Barnes et al. (10).

Several meta-analyses, integrating the results of numerous studies mostly performed in Germany, have been conducted to help gain a broader perspective on the efficacy of St. John's wort (51–53). A study prepared by Linde and Mulrow (53) was published as a Cochrane Review, and has received considerable attention from individuals researching St. John's wort. Using computerized searches of several databases, Linde and Mulrow investigated whether extracts of *Hypericum* were more effective than placebo and as effective as standard antidepressants in the treatment of depressive disorders in adults, and whether they have fewer side effects than standard antidepressant drugs. To be included in their analysis, trials had to be randomized; include patients with depressive disorders; compare preparations that included St. John's wort with placebos or other antidepressants; and include an objective clinical assessment of symptoms. The Linde and Mulrow analysis included 27 trials containing a total of 2291 patients who met inclusion criteria. Seventeen trials with 1168 patients were placebo-controlled, while 10 with 1123 patients compared *Hypericum* with other antidepressant or sedative drugs. Most trials were 4–6 weeks long. Participants usually had "neurotic depression" or "mild to moderate severe depressive disorders." Linde and Mulrow (53) found that preparations containing *H.*

perforatum extracts were significantly superior to placebo and as effective as standard antidepressants. Only 26.6% of the patients taking *Hypericum* single preparations reported side effects, compared to 44.7% given standard antidepressants. Based on that evidence, the authors concluded that extracts of *Hypericum* are more effective than placebo for the short-term treatment of mild to moderately severe depressive disorders. However, they felt that the evidence was inadequate to establish whether *Hypericum* is as effective as other antidepressants, and suggested that additional studies be done (53).

Barnes et al. (10) reported on seven additional clinical studies examining mono-preparations of St. John's wort. Two compared St. John's wort against a placebo. Three studies compared St. John's wort against each of one standard antidepressant including fluoxetine, sertraline, and imipramine. One study compared St. John's wort to both a placebo and imipramine. St. John's wort extracts were standard preparations, including LI 160, ZE 117, WS 5572, WS 5573, and LoHyp-57. Dosages varied from 500 to 900 mg/day, and typically ran for 6 weeks. Outcomes were assessed by objective criteria, typically through a Hamilton Depression Scale. In general, patients receiving St. John's wort extracts reported a higher reduction in depression scores than those taking the placebo. Likewise, studies comparing St. John's wort to standard antidepressants found little difference between the two. Fewer side effects were reported among the St. John's wort group than the group taking the synthetic antidepressants. One of the studies, conducted by Laakmann et al. (50), found that individuals receiving preparations containing 5% hyperforin responded better than those receiving 0.5% hyperforin or a placebo. Reports of adverse events were similar among the three groups, however.

Barnes et al. (10) note that the trials comparing St. John's wort to synthetic antidepressants have been criticized because the dosages of the latter were unrealistically low (54). Other criticisms [e.g., Spira (55)] point to the study's usage of somewhat outdated tricyclics and a short (6-week) duration of the analysis. Barnes et al. (10) acknowledged that trials comparing St. John's wort to more modern SSI antidepressants were also needed.

Two recent studies conducted in the United States did not support the idea that St. John's wort is effective in treating moderate to major depression. The first was conducted between 1998 and 2000 by Shelton et al. (56). Their study included 200 adult outpatients diagnosed as having major depression [defined as having a baseline Hamilton Rating Scale for Depression (HAM-D) score of at least 20] in 11 academic medical centers in the United States. After a 1-week, single-blind run-in of placebo, participants were randomly assigned to receive either St John's wort extract ($n = 98$; 900 mg/day for 4 weeks, increased to 1200 mg/day in the absence of an adequate response thereafter) or placebo ($n = 102$) for 8 weeks. Outcomes measured included rates of change on the HAM-D over the treatment period, and four other tests as secondary determinants. The study found that significantly more patients administered St. John's wort reached remission of illness than those taking placebo ($p = .02$). Unfortunately, the rates were very low in the full-intention-to-treat analysis 14.3% vs. 4.9%, respectively. Shelton et al. (56) agreed that St. John's wort was safe and well tolerated, with headache being the only adverse reaction that was higher than with the placebo. The authors concluded, however, that St. John's wort was not effective for treatment of major depression, and even called into question its efficacy for treating moderate depression (56). The Shelton et al. study was critiqued by Hawley and Gale (57), who expressed concern that the methodology did not use a three-arm approach in which St. John's wort would have been compared against both a placebo and a reference agent of known efficacy.

A second study, conducted by the *Hypericum* Depression Trial Study Group (58), was a double-blind multicenter investigation aimed at determining whether St. John's wort (LI-160) was useful in treating major depression. Their study had the benefit of being three-armed, involving comparisons against a control group receiving a placebo and a second receiving the SSRI sertraline. The study involved 340 adult outpatients at 12 academic and community psychiatric research clinics in the United States. Patients were randomly assigned daily doses of *H. perforatum* that ranged from 900 to 1500 mg, sertraline from 50 to 100 mg, or a placebo for 8 weeks. The study found that the overall response rates of patients receiving the St. John's wort were 38.1%, actually lower than those receiving the placebo (43.1%) and the sertraline (48.6%). Perhaps most noteworthy was the finding that neither *H. perforatum* nor sertraline yielded response rates higher than the placebo. The authors concluded that the findings failed to support any claims for efficacy of *H. perforatum* in treating moderately severe major depression. They admitted that their results might have been due to low assay sensitivity of the trial. However, the three-armed design of the test was significant, because without a placebo group, one might conclude that St. John's wort was as effective as an established synthetic antidepressant.

The lack of statistical difference between *Hypericum* and placebo contrasted markedly with findings of previous studies that did find such a difference (53). Likewise, the lack of difference between the sertraline and placebo was also striking. Rather than showing a lack of efficacy for either the St. John's wort or the sertraline, Kupfer and Frank (59) attributed the lack of statistical difference to an unusually high placebo response. They expressed concerns that variability in placebo response from trial to trial may obscure interpretation of controlled experiments on natural and synthetic antidepressants alike.

Other critiques of the *Hypericum* Depression Trial Study Group suggested that the study included individuals with untreatable, long-term depression (60,61), that an inappropriate placebo was selected because it did not mimic the side effects of the treatments (especially the sertraline) (61), and that bias on the part of clinicians confounded results (62). Linde et al. (63) speculated that the difference between the U.S. and German studies may be due to the latter's focus on patients with mild to moderately severe depression. They suggested studies may be needed to determine whether St. John's wort appears to be particularly effective in Germany, but not elsewhere.

The research evidence to date indicates that the application of *H. perforatum* for the treatment of depression can be helpful in cases that are mild to moderate; however, it is still uncertain if using it to treat major depression is appropriate. The consequences that may result from inadequate therapies of major depression, like suicide, are too dangerous to risk. In the case of severe depression, patients should stay with the traditional treatments of synthetically derived prescription antidepressants.

B. Antibacterial and Antiviral Activities

As noted, extracts of *H. perforatum* have been used for millennia to treat cuts, abrasions, and other wounds. Its usefulness in reducing inflammation is well known, and appears related, at least in part, to its ability to serve as an antibacterial agent. Recent research also suggests that it is useful in combating viruses.

1. Antibacterial

Antibacterial properties of *H. perforatum* extracts were reported by Russian scientists in 1959 (64). The main antibacterial principle was determined to be hyperforin and its chemical structure was elucidated in 1975 (65). Recent studies have shown that hyperforin inhibited growth of certain types of microorganisms. Growth inhibition occurred for all gram-positive bacteria that were tested, though no growth-inhibitory effects were seen in the gram-negative bacteria tested (65). Meticillin-resistant (MRSA) and penicillin-resistant (PRSA) *Staphylococcus aureus* were especially susceptible to hyperforin. The MRSA strain was shown to be resistant to several types of penicillins, ofloxacin, clindamycin, erythromycin, cephalosporins, and gentamicin (65). Little toxicity of purified hyperforin in vitro has been observed in peripheral blood mononuclear cells (65). Oral administration of hyperforin-containing extract of St. John's wort was well tolerated and this supports the potential systemic use of hyperforin (66).

In Russia, acetone extracts of St. John's wort have been used to treat bacterial infections. This extract, novoimanine, is commonly used as an antibiotic preparation for treatment of gram-positive bacteria (67). Various teas showed antibacterial effects against gram-positive bacteria, especially toward MRSA *Staph. aureus* (67). These results provide a rationale for topical treatment of wounds and skin lesions with preparations of St. John's wort.

2. Antiviral

Extracts of St. John's wort have long been regarded as being effective against various classes of viruses. Studies by Mishenkova et al. (68) indicated that flavonoid- and catechin-containing fractions of St. John's wort were active against influenza virus. Since 1988, the virucidal activities of hypericin extract have been investigated against many other forms of viruses (69). Two common characteristics have been established for the antiviral activities of hypericin compounds. First, these compounds are effective against enveloped viruses, but have no effect against nonenveloped viruses (69). Second, the virucidal potential of hypericin is greatly enhanced by light against certain enveloped viruses (70–72). Studies have shown that hypericin inactivates enveloped viruses at different points in the viral life cycle (73). Degar et al. (74) suggested that the inactivation of enveloped viruses by hypericin was attributed to alterations in viral proteins. This form of inactivation contrasts to the antiviral nucleoside treatments that target viral nucleic acids (74). Other studies suggest that the inactivation of enveloped viruses by hypericin is due to the inhibition of fusion. Fusion is a membrane-specific process that all enveloped viruses must perform and loss of the ability to fuse to may be a direct result of hypericin (73,74). Lack of the fusion function may be the reason that hypericin inactivates enveloped viruses rather than nonenveloped.

These promising in vitro results have begun to promote various in vivo studies of certain viruses in mice. These include: LP-BMS murine immunodeficiency viruses, murine cytomegalovirus (MCMV), Sindbis virus, Friend virus, and Ranscher leukemia virus (75–77). Hypericin has also shown in vitro activity against influenza and herpes viruses (78), vesiculostomatitis and Sendai viruses (73), and duck hepatitis B virus (79).

Hypericin has been used to inactivate several enveloped viruses present in human blood and to treat AIDS patients (76,80). AIDS is a retrovirus that uses reverse transcriptasc activity to replicate. Degar et al. (74) observed changes in the p24 protein and the p24-containing *gag* precursor, p55, by Western blot analysis. They also observed that a recombinant p24 formed an anti-p24 immunoreactive material. This indicated that alterations of p24 occurred, and such alterations may be able to inhibit the release of reverse transcriptase activity (74).

Gulick et al. (81) conducted a Phase I clinical trial of 30 HIV-infected patients with CD4 counts less than 350 cells/mm^3. Hypericin was administered intravenously at doses of 0.25 or 0.5 mg/kg of body weight twice weekly, or 0.25 mg/kg three times weekly, or orally at 0.5 mg/kg daily. Sixteen of the thirty patients who were enrolled discontinued treatment early because of toxic effects, often due to severe cutaneous phototoxicity. None of the parameters examined, including HIV p24 antigen level, HIV titer, HIV RNA copies, and CD4 cell counts, showed improvement significant to warrant hypericin as being effective in treating HIV, even for those patients who could tolerate the side effects at the doses given.

Hypericin impacts other viruses. It completely inactivated bovine diarrhea virus (BVDV) in vitro in the presence of light (82). BVDV, a pestivirus, has structural similarities to hepatitis C virus (HCV) (83,84). Jacobson et al. (85) examined the effects of hypericin on HCV, and found that in the doses studied, hypericin demonstrated no detectable anti-HCV activity. Plasma HCV levels were not lowered in HCV-infected patients nor was any effect seen on improving serum liver enzyme levels in the patients studied (85). These results provide significant evidence that, in the doses administered, hypericin is not an effective treatment of HCV (85). While some studies have shown that hyperforin and hypericin may be effective in treating various microbial or viral infections, one should consult a physician before taking these extracts to treat pathogen-induced disease.

C. Anticancer Properties

In addition to their use as antidepressants and antimicrobial compounds, hyperforin and hypericin have been examined for their anticancer properties. According to Schempp et al. (86), hyperforin inhibits tumor cell growth in vitro by induction of apoptosis (programmed cell death) through the activation of caspases. Caspases are cysteine proteases that play a central role in the apoptotic process and trigger a cascade of proteolytic cleavage occurrences in mammalian cells. Hyperforin also causes the release of cytochrome c from isolated mitochondria. Mitochondrial activation is an early event during hyperforin-mediated apoptosis and hyperforin inhibits tumor growth in vivo (86). Schempp and his colleagues agree that since hyperforin has significant antitumor activity, is readily available in high quantities (since it is naturally occurring in abundance), and has a low toxicity in vivo, hyperforin holds "promise of being an interesting novel antineoplastic agent."

Hypericin has also been investigated as an anticancer agent, owing mainly to its photodynamic properties. In the presence of light and oxygen, hypericin acts as a powerful natural photosensitizer, generating superoxide radicals. In turn, those superoxide radicals often form peroxide or hydroxyl radicals, or singlet oxygen molecules that kill tumor cells.

Photodynamic therapy (PDT) consists of systemic administration of a photosensitizer and targeted delivery of light to tumor lesions. At first this therapy was only used for skin lesions, but is becoming increasingly accepted as treatment for many types of tumors. Reactive oxygen species lead to tumor destruction, as well as extreme changes in the vasculature of the tumor (87). Since hypericin is photodynamic, its application as a potential photosensitizer and cancer therapeutic agent has been investigated (87). Agostinis et al. recommend that it be introduced into clinical trials because it has powerful photosensitizing and tumor-seeking characteristics, as well as having minimal dark toxicity.

Fox et al. (88) found that hypericin inhibits the growth of cells derived from a variety of neoplastic tissues including glioma, neuroblastoma, adenoma, mesothelioma, melanoma, carcinoma, sarcoma, and leukemia. Photoactivation of hypericin with white light and/or ultraviolet light promotes its antiproliferative effect (88). Hypericin could induce near-complete apoptosis (94%) in malignant cutaneous T cells and lymphoma T cells when photoactivated with white or ultraviolet light (88).

Exposing tumors cells to hypericin in conjunction with laser irradiation led to toxic effects on human prostatic cancer cell lines (89), human urinary bladder carcinoma cells (90), and pancreatic cancer cell lines (91) in in vitro systems. Experiments using nude mice receiving implants of pancreatic cancer cells and human squamous carcinoma cells showed reductions in cancer proliferation following laser photodynamic therapy using hypericin (10,91,92).

In contrast, extracts of St. John's wort, when given in conjunction with the anticancer drug irinotecan, reduces the plasma levels of the active metabolite SN-38—a derivative of irinotecan (93). Reduction in the plasma levels of SN-38 may have an adverse effect on irinotecan-based cancer treatments. Treatments based on compounds similar to irinotecan may be similarly compromised if St. John's wort compounds are included.

While hyperforin and hypericin both show promise as anticancer agents, more research is clearly needed to evaluate their efficacy, mode of action, and deleterious interactions.

VI. ADVERSE EFFECTS/INTERACTIONS

As with any pharmacologically active substance, treatments involving St. John's wort may lead to adverse effects, either when used alone or in conjunction with other medications.

A. Adverse Effects

As noted earlier, normal dosages of St. John's wort have relatively few side effects. Indeed many of the clinical trials indicated that rates of adverse effects were lower than for patients using synthetic tricyclic or SSRI antidepressants.

Reviews of adverse drug reactions (ADR) were presented by Greeson et al. (9) and Barnes et al. (10), and readers seeking a detailed account are referred to those sources. In general, the most common adverse effects include gastrointestinal symptoms, dizziness, confusion, restlessness, and lethargy. Woelk et al. (94) reported ADR rates of 2.4% for 3250 patients taking St. John's wort for mild depression. An analysis by Lemmer et al. (95) reported an ADR rate of 0.125% among 6382 patients. Isolated instances of subacute toxic neuropathy and induced mania have also been reported (96,97).

Extracts of St. John's wort have been found to lack genotoxic potential and mutagenic activity, based on in vivo and in vitro studies (10).

Hypericin has a unique phototoxic effect when taken in high doses. The toxic effects are attributed to an acidification of the surrounding environment caused by the transfer of hydrogen between hydroxyl groups upon receiving light energy (98,99). A growing body of literature states that this drop in pH affects viral replication (27). However, while phototoxicity is being studied for its possible therapeutic benefits, excessive phototoxicity can result in photodermatitis. Excessive phototoxicity is usually observed only with high doses of hypericin (0.5 mg/kg of body weight) such as those associated with AIDS treatments. As noted, clinical trials on high-dose hypericin AIDS treatments resulted in 48% of the participants displaying severe cutaneous phototoxicity (81). Normal doses of St. John's wort taken for mild depression (300 mg extract containing 0.3% hypericin taken 3 times daily) do not have any significant associated phototoxic effects (21,38).

B. Drug Interactions

While adverse drug reactions are relatively rare for individuals taking St. John's wort extracts alone, interactions with other drugs are more commonly reported, and should be a source of concern for those taking St. John's wort along with other medications. Greeson et al. (9) and Barnes et al. (10) provide excellent reviews of drug interactions. The herb in some cases can increase the effectiveness of other compounds when taken together. This increase may be helpful to the individual or may increase the reaction of the compound to the point of toxicity. Conversely, the herb may decrease or even cancel the effectiveness of another compound (100).

The compounds thought to be effective in the treatment of depression are believed to act similar to selective serotonin reuptake inhibitors as well as monoamine oxidase inhibitors. The use of St. John's wort in association with other antidepressants containing the active ingredients sertraline or nefazodone, clorgyline, clomipramine, lithium, carbamazepine, benzodiazepine, bromocriptine, L-dopa/carbidopa, levothyroxine, and others can create potential serotonin syndrome (100). Typical symptoms include changes in mental state and autonomic changes, as well as neuromuscular changes. Clinical studies have shown an increased rate of hypersensitivity, nausea, vomiting, anxiety, confusion, dizziness, hyperactivity, lethargy, and diaphoresis when St. John's wort is taken concomitantly with synthetic antidepressants (101).

St. John's wort extracts may lead to an increase in hair loss when taken in conjunction with other tricyclic antidepressants as well as selective SSRIs (38). Microscopic examination of patients showing hair loss revealed a mixed telogen and normal anagen morphology that suggests drug interaction (100).

St. John's wort extracts apparently induce some cytochrome (CYP)-drug-metabolizing enzymes in the liver, while inhibiting others. Those changes may lead to alterations in serum levels of a variety of drugs such as calcium blockers, chemotherapeutic agents, antifungal agents, glucocorticoids, cisapride, fentanyl, losartan, midazolam, omeprazole, ondansetron, and fexofenadine (38). Extracts of the herb have also been shown to induce intestinal P-glycoprotein drug transporter, which would decrease oral bioavailability of cyclosporine. The concomitant use can decrease plasma cyclosporine levels by up to 61%. This decrease can cause the rejection of organs during a transplant. Stopping St. John's wort treatment and starting antithymocyte globulin (ATG) will lead to a resolution of the rejection episode (102).

St. John's wort when taken with non-nucleoside reverse transcriptase inhibitors (NNRTIs) can decrease serum levels of the NNRTIs, which in turn decreases the plasma concentrations of the protease inhibitor indiavir. This is associated with therapeutic failure, development of viral resistance, and development of drug class resistance (38). St. John's wort causes this to happen by inducing intestinal and hepatic cytochrome 3A4 and intestinal P-glycoprotein/MDR-1, a drug transporter (38).

Use of St. John's wort concomitantly with other herbs taken as dietary supplements may lead to other interactions. The documented cases of concomitant use of St. John's wort with herbs that have sedative properties where the combination may have enhanced both the therapeutic and the adverse effects include interactions with calamus, canendula, California poppy, catnip, capsicum, celery, couch grass, elecampane, Siberian ginseng, German chamomile, goldenseal, gotu kola, hops, Jamaican dogwood, kava, lemon balm, sage, sassafras, scullcap, shepherd's purse, stinging nettle, valerian, wild carrot, wild lettuce, ashwaganda root, and yerba mensa (38). Another herb known to show side effects when used in conjunction with St. John's wort is foxglove or members of the digitalis family of herbs. Concomitant use has been shown to decrease the therapeutic effects of the digitalis by about 25% (38).

St. John's wort usage along with oral contraceptive may decrease steroid concentrations and induce the cytochrome P450 3A4 enzymes. This can result in breakthrough bleeding and irregular menstrual bleeding. When use of the herb was discontinued, the menstrual cycles returned to normal although alternate forms of birth control are suggested if the use of St. John's wort is continued (38).

St. John's wort taken in conjunction with barbiturates and narcotics may enhance sleep time. Likewise, when taken with foods containing trymaine, hypertensive crisis may occur (38).

VII. CONCLUSIONS

St. John's wort has a long history of use as an herbal treatment for a variety of ailments. During the past 20 years, it has become a mainstream alternative treatment for depression, as well as holding promise as a therapy for cancer, bacterial and viral infections, and other disorders.

Thanks to its popularity, the effectiveness of St. John's wort has been intensively studied since the mid-1980s. Those studies have focused on the pharmacology of its constituents, and on clinical trials. Pharmacological investigations show that extracts of St. John's wort do have neuroactive properties. Interestingly, those properties appear to derive primarily from the constituent hyperforin, rather than hypericin, which has been investigated for a longer period of time.

A large number of studies conducted in Germany in the 1990s indicate that individuals showing mild to moderate depression who take St. John's wort show improvement in mood at rates higher than those taking placebo. Moreover, rates of improvement were seen as being similar to those experienced by individuals taking synthetic antidepressants. Those clinical studies comparing the effects of St. John's wort against synthetics have been criticized, however, on the basis of their short duration and a claim that the dosage of the synthetics was below typical dosage. Two recent studies, conducted in the United States, failed to show a clear benefit of St. John's wort over a synthetic antidepressant and a placebo. At least the latter study was criticized because the response rate of the placebo seemed abnormally high.

Therefore, while a substantial body of literature points toward the efficacy of St. John's wort toward treating mild to moderate depression, more recent studies argue that the case is far from conclusive. It is interesting to note that the greatest clinical success for the herbal remedy was achieved in Europe, where the use of herbal therapies is standard, compared to the findings for the United States, where reliance on synthetic medicines is highest.

St. John's wort does appear to be an effective treatment for other disorders, particularly some skin ailments and possibly cancer. However, its once-promising use as an anti-HIV therapy has not been borne out by clinical studies.

The preponderance of clinical studies point toward St. John's wort as being relatively safe, especially at typical dosages. However, high dosages might lead to phototoxicity in susceptible individuals. Extracts of St. John's wort do appear to interact with other medications, especially owing to impact on liver enzyme function. Therefore, individuals taking St. John's wort along with other medications should be cognizant of such potential drug interactions.

As with any herbal remedy, any individual using St. John's wort is advised to consult with his or her physician to ascertain that is the best course of action when seeking the most efficacious remedy for any condition.

REFERENCES

1. Muenscher WC. Weeds. New York: Macmillan, 1946.
2. Gleason HA, Cronquist A. Manual of Vascular Plants of Northeastern United States and Adjacent Canada. 2d ed. Bronx, NY: New York Botanical Garden, 1991.
3. Foster S. St. John's wort. http://www.stevenfoster.com/education/monograph/hypericum.html. 2000.
4. Klemow KM, Raynal DJ. Population biology of an annual plant in a temporally variable habitat. J Ecol 1983; 71:691–703.
5. Redvers A, Laugharne R, Kanagaratnam G, Srinivasan G. How many patients self-medicate with St. John's wort? Psychiatr Bulll 2001; 25:254–256.
6. Foster S, Duke JA. Eastern/Central Medicinal Plants and Herbs. Peterson Field Guides. Boston: Houghton Mifflin, 2000.
7. Blumenthal M, Busse WR, Goldberg A, Gruenwald J, Hall T, Riggins CW, Rister RD, eds. The Complete German Commission E Monographs; Therapeutic Guide to Herbal Medicines. Boston: American Botanical Council, 1998.
8. Ernst E. Second thoughts about the safety of St. Johns wort. Lancet 1999; 354:2014–2015.
9. Greeson JM, Sanford B, Monti DA. St. John's wort (*Hypericum perforatum*): a review of the current pharmacological, toxicological, and clinical literature. Psychoparmacology 2001; 153:402–414.
10. Barnes J, Anderson L, Phillipson JD. St. John's wort (*Hypericum perforatum* L.): a review of its chemistry, pharmacology, and clinical properties. J Pharm Pharmacol. 2001; 53:583–600.
11. British Herbal Pharmacopoeia. Bournemouth, UK: British Herbal Medicine Association, 1996.
12. European Scientific Cooperative on Phytotherapy. St. John's wort. Monographs on the medicinal use of plant drugs. Fascicule 1. Hyperici herba. 1996.
13. American Herbal Pharmacopeia. St. John's Wort. *Hypericum perforatum*. Quality Control, Analytical and Therapeutic Monograph. Austin, Texas: American Botanical Council, 1997.
14. Parfitt K, ed. Martindale: The Complete Drug Reference. 32d ed. London: Pharmaceutical Press, 1999.

15. Barnes J, Anderson LA, Phillipson JD. Herbal medicines: a guide for health care professionals. CD-ROM Complementary and Alternative Medicine Microdex Series, 2000.
16. European Pharmacopoeia 2000 (suppl). Strasbourg: Masionneuve. 2000.
17. Bloomfield HH, Nordfors M, McWilliams P. *Hypericum* and Depression. Los Angeles, CA: Prelude Press, 1996.
18. Marquez LR. Update on research of *Hypericum perforatum* as an antidepressant. Methods Findings Exp Clin Pharmacol 2002; 24(suppl A):55–56.
19. Bombardelli E, Morazzoni P. *Hypericum perforatum*. Fitoterapia 1995; 66:43–68.
20. Reuter H. Chemistry and biology of *Hypericum perforatum* (St. John's wort). ACS Symp Ser 1998; 691:287–298.
21. DerMarderosian A, Beutler J. The Natural Review of Products. St. Louis, MO: Facts and Comparisons, 2002.
22. Nahrstedt A, Butterwick V. Biologically active and other chemical constituents of the herb *Hypericum perforatum* L. Pharmacopsychiatry 1997; 30:129–134.
23. Erdelmeier C. Hyperforin, possibly the major non-nitrogenous secondary metabolite of *Hypericum perforatum* L. Pharmocopsychiatry 1998; 31:2–6.
24. Staffeldt B, Kerb R, Brockmoller J, Ploch M, Roots I. Pharmacokinetics of hypericin and pseudohypericin after oral intake of *Hypericum* extract LI 160 in healthy volunteers. J Geriatr Neurol 1994; 7:S47–S53.
25. Robbers J, Tyler VE. Tyler's Herbs of Choice: The Therapeutic Use of Phytomedicinals. New York: Haworth Press, 1999.
26. Grainger-Bisset N, Wichtl M. Herbal Drugs and Phytopharmaceuticals. 2d ed. Stuttgart, Germany: Medpharm GmbH Scientific Publishers, 2001.
27. Petrich JW. Excited-state intramolecular H-atom transfer in nearly symmetrical perylene quinones: hypericin, hypocrellin, and their analogues. Int Rev Phys Chem 2000; 19:479–500.
28. Smirnov A, Fulton DB. Exploring ground-state heterogeneity of hypericin and hypocrellin A and B. J Am Chem Soc 1999; 121:7979–7989.
29. Fehr M, McCloskey MA, Petrich JW. Light-induced acidification by the antiviral agent hypericin. J Am Chem Soc 1995; 117:1833–1837.
30. Sureau F, Miskovsky P, Chinsky L, Turpin P. Hypericin-induced cell photosensitization involves an intracellular pH decrease. J Am Chem Soc 1996; 118:9484–9488.
31. Chatterjee S, Noldner M, Koch E, Erdelmeier C. Antidepressant activity of *Hypericum perforatum* and hyperforin: the neglected possibility. Pharmacophychiatry 1998; 31(suppl 1):7–15.
32. Hahn G. *Hypericum perforatum* (St. John's wort): a medicinal herb used in antiquity and still of interest today. J Naturopath Med 1992; 3:94–96.
33. Lieberman S. Evidence-based natural medicine: nutriceutical review of St. John's wort (*Hypericum perforatum*) for the treatment of depression. J Women's Health 1998; 7:177–182.
34. Remick RA. Diagnosis and management of depression in primary care: a clinical update and review. Can Med Assoc J 2002; 167:1253–1260.

35. American Academy of Family Physicians. http://familydoctor.org/handouts/012.html, 2000.
36. Suzuki O, Oya M, Bladt S, Wagner H. Inhibition of monoamine oxidase by hypericin. Planta Med 1984; 2:272.
37. Chavez ML, Chavez PI. Saint John's wort. Hosp Parm 1997; 32(12):1621–1632.
38. Jellin JM, Gregory PJ, Batz F, Hitchen K. Pharmacist's Letter/Prescriber's Letter Natural Medicines Comprehensive Database. 4th ed. Stockton, CA: Therapeutic Research Faculty, 2002.
39. Cervo L, Rozio M, Ekalle-Soppo CB, Guiso G, Morazzoni P, Caccia S. Role of hyperforin in the antidepressant-like activity of *Hypericum perforatum* extracts. Psychopharmacology (Berl) 2002; 164:423–428.
40. Calapai G, Crupi A, Firenzuoli F, Constantino G, Inferrera G, Campo GM, Caputi AP. Effects of *Hypericum perforatum* on levels of 5-hydroxytrytamine, noradrenaline, and dopamine in the cortex, diencephalon, and brainstem of the rat. J Pharm Pharmacol 1999; 51(6):723–726.
41. Laakman G, Schule C, Dienel A. Effects of *Hypericum* extract on adenohypophysial hormone secretion and catecholamine metabolism [abstr]. Biocenter Symposium on Drug Therapy/Pharmacology of St. John's Wort (*Hypericum perforatum* L.) and Its Constituents, Frankfurt, Germany, 2000.
42. Müller WE, Singer A, Wonnemann M. Hyperforin—antidepressant activity by a novel mechanism of action. Pharmacopsychiatry 2001; 34:S98–S102.
43. Vormfelde S. Hyperforin in extracts of St. John's wort (*Hypericum perforatum*) for depression. JAMA 2000; 160:2548.
44. Chatterjee S, Bhattacharya SK, Wonnemann M, Singer A, Muller WE. Hyperforin as possible antidepressant component of *Hypericum* extracts. Life Sci 1998; 63:499–510.
45. Jones BJ, Blackburn TP. The medical benefit of 5-HT research. Pharmacol Biochem Behav 2002; 71:555–681.
46. Molderings GJ. Physiological and therapeutic relevance of serotonin and the serotonergic system. Arzneim-Forsch 2002; 52:145–154.
47. Singer A, Wonnemann M, Muller WE. Hyperforin, a major antidepressant constituent of St. John's wort, inhibits serotonin uptake by elevating free intracellular Na^{+1}. J Parmacol Exp Ther 1999; 290:1363–1368.
48. Muller WE. Current St. John's wort research from mode of action to clinical efficacy. Pharmacol Res 2003; 47:101–109.
49. Teufel-Meyer R, Gleitz J. Effects of long-term administration of *Hypericum* extracts on the affinity and density of the central serotonergic 5-HT1 A and 5-HT2 A receptors. Pharmacopsychiatry 1997; 30:113–116.
50. Laakmann G, Schule C, Baghai T, Keiser M. St. John's wort in mild to moderate depression: the relevance of hyperforin for the clinical efficacy. Pharmacopsychiatry 1998; 31(suppl):54–59.
51. Linde K, Ramirez G, Mulrow CD, Pauls A, Weidenhammer W, Melchart D. St. John's wort for depression—an overview and meta-analysis of randomized clinical trials. Br Med J 1996; 313:253–258.

52. Kim HL, Streltzer J, Goebert D. St. John's wort for depression: a meta-analysis of well-defined clinical trials. J Nerv Ment Dis 1999; 187:532–539.
53. Linde K, Mulrow CD. St. John's Wort for Depression (Cochrane Review). The Cochrane Library. Issue 1. Oxford: Update Software, 2001.
54. Linde K, Berner M. Commentary: Has *Hypericum* found its place in antidepressant treatment? Br Med J 1999; 319:1539.
55. Spira JL. Study design casts doubt on value of St. John's wort in treating depression. Br Med J 2001; 322:493.
56. Shelton RC, Keller MB, Gelenberg A, Dunner DL, Hirschfeld R, Thase ME, Russell J, Lydiard RB, Crits-Cristoph P, Gallop R, Todd L, Hellerstein D, Goodnick P, Keitner G, Stahl SM, Halbreich U. Effectiveness of St. John's wort in major depression: a randomized controlled trial. JAMA 2001; 285:1978–1986.
57. Hawley C, Gale T. Commentary. St. John's wort was no better than placebo for reducing depression scores. Evidence-Based Med 2001; 6:185.
58. *Hypericum* Depression Trial Study Group. Effect of *Hypericum perforatum* (St. John's wort) in major depressive disorder: a randomized controlled trial. JAMA 2002; 287:1807–1814.
59. Kupfer DJ, Frank E. Placebo in clinical trials for depression: complexity and necessity. JAMA 2002; 287:1853–1854.
60. Wheatley D. St. John's wort and depression. JAMA 2002; 288:446.
61. Jonas W. St. John's wort and depression. JAMA 2002; 288:446.
62. Speilmans GI. St. John's wort and depression. JAMA 2002; 288:446–447.
63. Linde K, Melchart D, Mulrow C, Berner M. St. John's wort and depression. JAMA 2002; 288:447–448.
64. Schempp CM, Pelz K, Wittmer A, Schopf E, Simon JC. Antibacterial activity of hyperforin from St. John's wort, against multiresistant *Staphylococcus aureus* and gram-positive bacteria. T Lancet 1999; 353:2129.
65. Bystrov NS, Chernov BK, Dobrynin VN, Kolosov MN. The structure of hyperforin. Tetrahedron Lett 1975; 32:2791–2794.
66. Biber A, Fischer H, Romer A, Chatterjee SS. Oral bioavailability of hyperforin from *Hypericum* extracts in rats and human volunteers. Pharmacopsychiatry 1998; 31(suppl):36–43.
67. Reichling J, Weseler A, Saller R. A current review of the antimicrobial activity of *Hypericum perforatum* L. Pharmacopsychiatry 2001; 34(suppl 1):S116–S118.
68. Mishenkova EL, Derbentseva NA, Garagulya AD, Litvin LN. Antiviral properties of St. John's wort and preparations produced from it. Tr. S'ezda Mikrobiol Ukr 1975; 222–223.
69. Diwu Z. Novel therapeutic and diagnostic applications of hypocrellins and hypericins. Photochem Photobiol 1995; 61:529–539.
70. Hudson JB, Harris L, Towers GH. The importance of light in the anti-HIV effect of hypericin. Antiviral Res 1993; 20:173–178.
71. Hudson JB, Graham EA, Towers GH. Antiviral assays on phytochemicals: the influence of reaction parameters. Planta Med 1994; 60:329–332.

72. Carpenter S, Kraus GA. Photosensitization is required for inactivation of equine infectious anemia virus by hypericin. Photochem Photobiol 1991; 53:169–174.
73. Lenard J, Rabson A, Vanderoef R. Photodynamic inactivation of infectivity of human immunodeficiency virus and other envelope viruses using hypericin and rose bengal: inhibition of fusion and synctia formation. Proc Natl Acad Sci USA 1993; 90:158–162.
74. Degar S, Prince AM, Pascual D, Lavie G, Levin B, Mazur Y, Lavie D, Ehrlich LS, Carter C, Meruelo D. Inactivation of the human immunodeficiency virus by hypericin: evidence for photochemical alterations of p24 and a block in uncoating. AIDS Res Hum Retroviruses 1992; 8:1929–1936.
75. Stevenson NR, Lenard J. Antiviral activities of hypericin and rose bengal: photodynamic effects on Friend leukemia virus-infection of mice. Antiviral Res 1993; 21:119–127.
76. Meruelo D. The potential use of hypericin as inactivator of retroviruses and other viruses in blood products. Blood 1993; 82:205A.
77. Hudson JB, Lopez-Bazzocchi I, Towers GH. Antiviral activities of hypericin. Antiviral Res 1991; 15:101–112.
78. Tang J, Colacino JM, Larsen SH, Spitzer W. Virucidal activity of hypericin against enveloped and non-enveloped DNA and RNA viruses. Antiviral Res 1990; 13:313–326.
79. Moraleda G, Wu TT, Jilbert AR, Aldrich CE, Condreay LD, Larsen SH, Tang JC, Colacino JM, Mason WS. Inhibition of duck hepatitis B virus replication by hypericin. Antiviral Res 1993; 20:235–247.
80. Holden C. Treating AIDS with worts. Science 1991; 254:522.
81. Gulick RM, McAuliffe V, Holden-Wiltse J, Crumpacker C, Liebes L, Stein DS, Meehan P, Hussey S, Forcht J, Valentine FT. Phase I studies of hypericin, the active compound in St. John's wort, as an antiretroviral agent in HIV-infected adults. AIDS Clinical Trials Group Protocols 150 and 258. Ann Intern Med 1999; 130:510–514.
82. Prince AM, Pascual D, Meruelo D, Liebes L, Mazur Y, Dubovi E, Mandel M, Lavie G. Strategies for evaluation of enveloped virus inactivation in red cell concentrates using hypericin. Photochem Photobiol 2000; 71:188–195.
83. Le SY, Siddiqui A, Maizel JV Jr, A common structural core in the internal ribosome entry sites of picornavirus, hepatitis C virus, and pestivirus. Virus Genes 1996; 12:135–147.
84. Ohba K, Mizokami M, Lau JY, Orito E, Ikeo K, Gojobori T. Evolutionary relationship of hepatitis C, pesti-, flavi-, plant viruses, and newly discovered GB hepatitis agents. FEBS Lett 1996; 378:232–234.
85. Jacobson JM, Feinman L, Liebes L, Ostrow N, Koslowski V, Tobia A, Cabana BE, Lee D, Spritzler J, Prince AM. Pharmacokinetics, safety, and antiviral effects of hypericin, a derivative of St. John's wort plant, in patients with chronic hepatitis C virus infection. Antimicrob Agents Chemother 2001; 45:517–524.
86. Schempp CM, Kirkin V, Simon-Haarhaus B, Kersten A, Kiss J, Termeer CC, Gilb B, Kaufmann T, Borner C, Sleeman JP, Simon JC. Inhibition of tumour

cell growth by hyperforin, a novel anticancer drug from St. John's wort that acts by induction of apoptosis. Oncogene 2002; 21:1242–1250.

87. Agostinis P, Vantieghem A, Merlevede W, de Witte PAM. Hypericin in cancer treatment: more light on the way. Int J Biochem Cell Biol 2002; 34:221–241.
88. Fox FE, Niu Z, Tobia A, Rook AH. Photoactivated hypericin is an antiproliferative agent that induces a high rate of apoptotic death of normal, transformed, and malignant T-lymphocytes: implications for the treatment of cutaneous lymphoproliferative and inflammatory disorders. J Invest Dermatol 1998; 111:327–332.
89. Colasanti A, Kisslinger A, Liuzzi R, Quarto M, Riccio P, Roberti G, Tramontano D, Villani F. Hypericin photosensitization of tumor and metastatic cell lines of human prostate. J Photochem Photobiol B 2000; 54:103–107.
90. Kamuhabwa AR, Agostinis P, D'Hallewin MA, Kasran A, de Witte PA. Photodynamic activity of hypericin in human urinary bladder carcinoma cells. Anticancer Res 2000; 20:2579–2584.
91. Liu CD, Kwan D, Saxton RE, McFadden DW. Hypericin and photodynamic therapy decreases human pancreatic cancer in vitro and vivo. J Surg Res 2000; 93:137–143.
92. Chung PS, Rhee CK, Kim KH, Paek W, Chung J, Paiva MB, Eshraghi AA, Castro DJ, Saxton RE. Intratumoral hypericin and KTP laser therapy for transplanted squamous cell carcinoma. Laryngoscope 2000; 110:1312–1316.
93. Mathijssen RH, Verweij J, de Bruijn P, Loos WJ, Sparreboom A. Effects of St. John's wort on irinotecan metabolism. J Natl Cancer Inst 2002; 94:1247–1249.
94. Woelk H, Burkard G, Grunwald J. Benefits and risks of the *Hypericum* extract LI 160: drug monitoring study with 3250 patients. J Geriatr Psychiatry Neurol 1994; 7(suppl 1):34–38.
95. Lemmer W, von den Driesch V, Klieser E. Wirksamkeit im Alter und bei chronischen Verlaufsformen. Munch Med Wschr Fortschr Med 1999; 141:43.
96. Bove GM. Acute neuropathy after exposure to sun in a patient treated with St. John's wort. Lancet 1998; 352:1121–1122.
97. Nierenberg AA, Burt T, Matthews J, Weiss AP. Mania associated with St. John's wort. Biol Psychiatry 1999; 46:1707–1708.
98. Fehr M, McCloskey MA, Petrich JW. Light-induced acidification by the antiviral agent hypericin. J Am Chem Soc 1995; 117:1833–1837.
99. Sureau F, Miskovsky P, Chinsky L, Turpin P. Hypericin-induced cell photosensitization involves an intracellular pH decrease. J Am Chem Soc 1996; 118:9484–9488.
100. Parker V, Wong A, Boon H, Seeman M. Adverse reactions to St. John's wort. Can J Psychiatry 2001; 46:77–79.
101. Cupp M. Herbal remedies: adverse effects and drug interactions. Am Fam Physician 1999; 59:1239–1245.
102. Ruschitzka F, Meier P, Turina M, Luscher T, Noll G. Acute heart transplant rejection due to Saint John's wort. Lancet 2000; 355:548–549.

36

Therapeutic Potential of Curcumin Derived from Turmeric (*Curcuma longa*)

Bharat B. Aggarwal and Anushree Kumar
The University of Texas M. D. Anderson Cancer Center
Houston, Texas, U.S.A.

Alok Chandra Bharti
Institute of Cytology and Preventive Oncology (ICMR)
Uttar Pradesh, India

I. INTRODUCTION

Curcumin is a diferuloylmethane present in turmeric (*Curcuma longa*). This nonnutritive phytochemical is pharmacologically safe, considering that it has been consumed as a dietary spice, at doses up to 100 mg/day, for centuries (1). Recent Phase I clinical trials indicate that people tolerate a dose as high as 8 g/day (2,3). In the United States, curcumin is used as a coloring agent in cheese, spices, mustard, cereals, pickles, potato flakes, soups, ice creams, and yogurts (www.kalsec.com). Curcumin is not water-soluble but is soluble in ethanol or in dimethylsulfoxide. Numerous studies indicate that this polyphenol has antioxidant and anti-inflammatory properties.

II. ANTICANCER PROPERTIES OF CURCUMIN

A. Curcumin Inhibits Tumorigenesis

Curcumin blocks tumor initiation induced by benzo[a]pyrene and 7, 12-dimethylbenz [a]anthracene (4) and suppresses phorbol-ester-induced tumor promotion (5,6). In vivo, curcumin was found to suppress carcinogenesis of the skin (6–10), the forestomach (11,12), the colon (13–15), and the liver (16) in mice. Curcumin also suppresses mammary carcinogenesis (17,18).

B. Curcumin Exhibits Antiproliferative Effects Against Cancer Cells

Compounds that block or suppress the proliferation of tumor cells have potential as anticancer agents. Curcumin has been shown to inhibit the proliferation of a wide variety of tumor cells, including B-cell and T-cell leukemia (19–22), colon carcinoma (23), and epidermoid carcinoma (24). It has also been shown to suppress the proliferation of various breast carcinoma cell lines in culture (25–27). We showed that the growth of the breast tumor cell lines BT20, SKBR3, MCF-7, T47D, and ZR75-1 is completely inhibited by curcumin as indicated by MTT dye uptake, [^{3}H]-thymidine incorporation, and clonogenic assay (25). We also showed that curcumin can overcome adriamycin resistance in MCF-7 cells (25). Recently, we have shown that curcumin can activate caspase-8, which leads to cleavage of Bid, thus resulting in sequential release of mitochondrial cytochrome C and activation of caspase-9 and caspase-3 (28).

C. Curcumin Downregulates the Activity of Epidermal Growth Factor Receptor (EGFR) and Expression of HER2/neu

HER2/neu and EGFR activity represent one possible mechanism by which curcumin suppresses the growth of breast cancer cells. Almost 30% of the breast cancer cases have been shown to overexpress the HER2/neu proto-oncogene (29), and both HER2 and EGF receptors stimulate proliferation of breast cancer cells. Overexpression of these two proteins correlates with progression of human breast cancer and poor patient prognosis (for references see Ref. 29). Curcumin has been shown to downregulate the activity of EGFR (24,30) and HER2/neu (24,30) and to deplete the cells of HER2/neu protein (31). Additionally, we have recently found that curcumin can down-regulate bcl-2 expression, which may contribute to its antiproliferative activity (32).

D. Curcumin Downregulates the Activation of Nuclear Factor-κB (NF-κB)

Curcumin may also operate through NF-κB. NF-κB is a nuclear transcription factor required for the expression of genes involved in cell proliferation, cell invasion, metastasis, angiogenesis, and resistance to chemotherapy (33). This factor is activated in response to inflammatory stimuli, carcinogens, tumor promoters, and hypoxia, which is frequently encountered in tumor cells (34). Several groups, including ours, have shown that activated NF-κB suppresses apoptosis in a wide variety of tumor cells (35–37), and it has been implicated in chemoresistance (35). We have shown that cells that overexpress NF-κB are resistant to paclitaxel-induced apoptosis (38). Furthermore, the constitutively active form of NF-κB has been reported in human breast cancer cell lines in culture (39), carcinogen-induced mouse mammary tumors (40), and biopsies from patients with breast cancer (41). Our laboratory has shown that various tumor promoters, including phorbol ester, TNF, and H_2O_2, activate NF-κB and that curcumin downregulates the activation (42). Subsequently, others showed that curcumin-induced downregulation of NF-κB is mediated through suppression of IκBα kinase activation (43,44).

E. Curcumin Downregulates the Activation of Activator Protein-1 (AP-1) and c-Jun N-Terminal Kinase (JNK)

AP-1 is another transcription factor that has been closely linked with proliferation and transformation of tumor cells (45). The activation of AP-1 requires the phosphorylation of c-jun through activation of stress-activated kinase JNK (46). The activation of JNK is also involved in cellular transformation (47). Curcumin has been shown to inhibit the activation of AP-1 induced by tumor promoters (48) and JNK activation induced by carcinogens (49).

F. Curcumin Suppresses the Induction of Adhesion Molecules

The expression of various cell surface adhesion molecules, such as intercellular cell adhesion molecule-1, vascular cell adhesion molecule-1, and endothelial leukocyte adhesion molecule-1, on endothelial cells is absolutely critical for tumor metastasis (50). The expression of these molecules is in part regulated by nuclear factor NF-κB (51). We have shown that treatment of endothelial cells with curcumin blocks the cell surface expression of adhesion molecules and this accompanies the suppression of tumor cell adhesion to endothelial cells (52). We have demonstrated that downregulation of these adhesion molecules is mediated through the downregulation of NF-κB activation (52).

G. Curcumin Downregulates Cyclooxygenase-2 (COX-2) Expression

Overexpression of COX-2 has been shown to be associated with a wide variety of cancers, including colon (53), lung (54), and breast (55) cancers. The role of COX-2 in suppression of apoptosis and tumor cell proliferation has been demonstrated (56). Furthermore, celebrex, a specific inhibitor of COX-2, has been shown to suppress mammary carcinogenesis in animals (57). Several groups have shown that curcumin downregulates the expression of COX-2 protein in different tumor cells (44,58) most likely through the downregulation of NF-κB activation (44), which is needed for COX-2 expression.

H. Curcumin Inhibits Angiogenesis

For most solid tumors, including breast cancer, angiogenesis (blood vessel formation) is essential for tumor growth and metastasis (59). The precise mechanism that leads to angiogenesis is not fully understood, but growth factors that cause proliferation of endothelial cells have been shown to play a critical role in this process. Curcumin has been shown to suppress the proliferation of human vascular endothelial cells in vitro (60) and abrogate the fibroblast growth-factor-2-induced angiogenic response in vivo (61), thus suggesting curcumin is also an antiangiogenic factor. Indeed curcumin has been shown to suppress angiogenesis in vivo (62).

I. Curcumin Suppresses the Expression of Matrix Metalloproteinase (MMP)-9 and Inducible Nitric Oxide Synthase (iNOS)

MMPs make up a family of proteases that play a critical role in tumor metastasis (for references see Ref. 63). MMP-9 is one of the proteases that has been shown to be regulated by NF-κB activation (64), and curcumin has been shown to suppress its expression (64). Curcumin has also been demonstrated to downregulate iNOS expression, also regulated by NF-κB and involved in tumor metastasis (65). All these observations suggest that curcumin must have antimetastatic activity. Indeed, there is a report suggesting that curcumin can inhibit tumor metastasis (66).

J. Curcumin Downregulates Cyclin D1 Expression

Cyclin D1, a component subunit of cyclin-dependent kinase (Cdk)-4 and Cdk6, is a rate-limiting factor in progression of cells through the first-gap (G1) phase of the cell cycle (67). Cyclin D1 has been shown to be overexpressed in many cancers including breast, esophagus, head and neck, and prostate (68–73). It is possible that the antiproliferative effects of curcumin are due to inhibition of cyclin D1 expression. We found that curcumin can

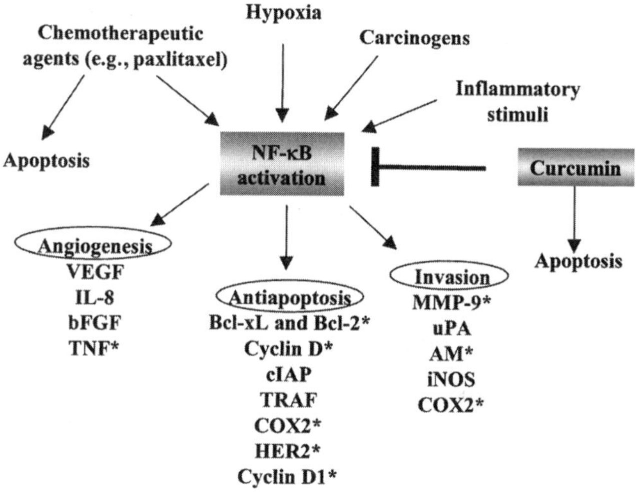

FIGURE 1 Role of curcumin in prevention and therapy of cancer. Curcumin downregulates multiple pathways involved in tumor growth and metastasis. *Gene expression inhibited by curcumin.

indeed downregulate cyclin D1 expression (32,74,75), and this downregulation occurs at the transcriptional and posttranscriptional level.

Overall, numerous mechanisms, as indicated above, could account for the tumor-suppressive effects of curcumin (Fig. 1). Curcumin also has modulatory effects in diseases besides cancer (Fig. 2). These effects are described below.

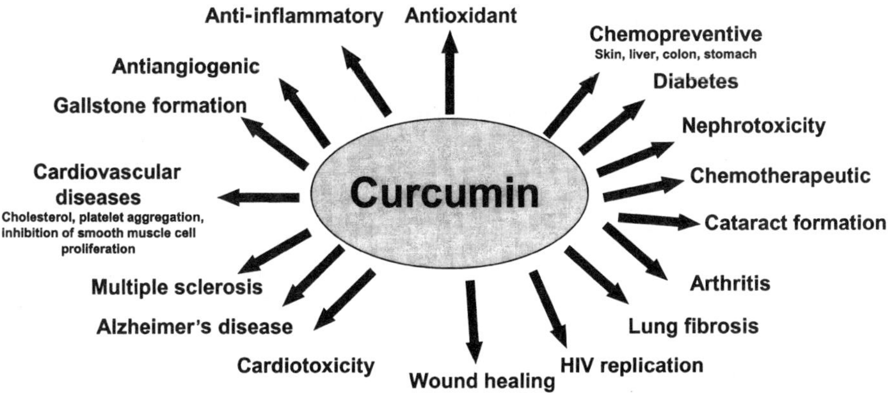

FIGURE 2 Effect of curcumin on various diseases.

III. EFFECT OF CURCUMIN ON ATHEROSCLEROSIS AND MYOCARDIAL INFARCTION

A. Curcumin Inhibits the Proliferation of Vascular Smooth-Muscle Cells

The proliferation of peripheral blood mononuclear cells (PBMC) and vascular smooth-muscle cells (VSMC) is a hallmark feature of atherosclerosis. Huang et al. investigated the effects of curcumin on the proliferation of PBMC and VSMC (76). Proliferative responses were determined from the uptake of [^{3}H]-thymidine. In human PBMC, curcumin dose-dependently inhibited the response to phytohemagglutinin and the mixed lymphocyte reaction at dose ranges of 1–30 μM and 3–30 μM, respectively. Curcumin (1–100 μM) dose-dependently inhibited the proliferation of rabbit VSMC stimulated by fetal calf serum. Curcumin had a greater inhibitory effect on platelet-derived, growth-factor-stimulated proliferation than on serum-stimulated proliferation. Analogs of curcumin (cinnamic acid, coumaric acid, and ferulic acid) were much less effective than curcumin as inhibitors of serum-induced smooth-muscle-cell proliferation. This suggested that curcumin may be useful for the prevention of the pathological changes associated with atherosclerosis and restenosis.

Chen and Huang examined the possible mechanisms underlying curcumin's antiproliferative and apoptotic effects using the rat VSMC cell line A7r5 (77). Curcumin (1–100 μM) inhibited serum-stimulated [^{3}H]-thymidine incorporation of both A7r5 cells and rabbit cultured VSMC. Cell viability, as determined by the trypan blue dye exclusion method, was unaffected by curcumin at the concentration range 1–10 μM in A7r5 cells. However, the number of viable cells after 100 μM curcumin treatment was less than the basal value. Following curcumin (1–100 μM) treatment, cell cycle analysis revealed a G0/G1 arrest and a reduction in the percentage of cells in S phase. Curcumin at 100 μM also induced cell apoptosis as demonstrated by hematoxylin-eosin staining, TdT-mediated dUTP nick end labeling, DNA laddering, cell shrinkage, chromatin condensation, and DNA fragmentation. The membranous protein tyrosine kinase activity stimulated by serum in A7r5 cells was significantly reduced by curcumin (10–100 μM). On the other hand, phorbol-myristate-acetate–stimulated cytosolic protein kinase C (PKC) activity was reduced by 100 μM curcumin. The level of c-myc mRNA and bcl-2 mRNA was significantly reduced by curcumin but it had little effect on the p53 mRNA level. These results demonstrate that curcumin inhibited cell proliferation, arrested cell cycle progression, and induced cell apoptosis in VSMC. These results may explain how curcumin prevents the pathological changes of atherosclerosis and postangioplasty restenosis.

B. Curcumin Lowers Serum Cholesterol Levels

Numerous studies suggest that curcumin lowers serum cholesterol levels (78–84). Soudamini et al. investigated the effect of oral administration of curcumin on serum cholesterol levels and on lipid peroxidation in the liver, lung, kidney, and brain of mice treated with carbon tetrachloride, paraquat, and cyclophosphamide (81). Oral administration of curcumin significantly lowered the increased peroxidation of lipids in these tissues produced by these chemicals. Administration of curcumin also significantly lowered the serum and tissue cholesterol levels in these animals, indicating that the use of curcumin helps in conditions associated with peroxide-induced injury such as liver damage and arterial diseases. Soni and Kuttan examined the effect of curcumin administration in reducing the serum levels of cholesterol and lipid peroxides in 10 healthy human volunteers receiving 500 mg of curcumin per day for 7 days (82). A significant decrease in the level of serum lipid peroxides (33%), an increase in high-density-lipoproteins (HDL) cholesterol (29%), and a decrease in total serum cholesterol (12%) were noted. As curcumin reduced serum lipid peroxides and serum cholesterol, the study of curcumin as a chemopreventive substance against arterial diseases was suggested.

Curcuma xanthorrhiza Roxb., a medicinal plant used in Indonesia (known as temu lawak, or Javanese turmeric), has been shown to have diverse physiological functions. However, little attention has been paid to its effect on lipid metabolism. Yasni et al. investigated the effects of *C. xanthorrhiza* on serum and liver lipids, serum HDL cholesterol, apolipoprotein, and liver lipogenic enzymes in rats. In rats given a cholesterol-free diet, *C. xanthorrhiza* decreased the concentrations of serum triglycerides, phospholipids, and liver cholesterol and increased serum HDL cholesterol and apolipoproteins (85). The activity of liver fatty acid synthase, but not glycerophosphate dehydrogenase, was decreased by the medicinal plant. In rats on a high-cholesterol diet, *C. xanthorrhiza* did not suppress the elevation of serum cholesterol, although it did decrease liver cholesterol. Curcuminoids prepared from *C. xanthorrhiza* had no significant effects on the serum and liver lipids. These studies, therefore, indicate that *C. xanthorrhiza* contains an active principle other than the curcuminoids that can modify the metabolism of lipids and lipoproteins.

In later studies Yasni et al. identified the major component (approx. 65%) of the essential oil as α-curcumene. Addition of essential oils (0.02%), prepared by steam distillation, to a purified diet lowered hepatic triglyceride concentration without influencing serum triglyceride levels, whereas addition of the hexane-soluble fraction (0.5%) lowered the concentration of serum and hepatic triglycerides (86). Rats fed the essential oil and hexane-soluble fraction had lower hepatic fatty acid synthase activity. The fraction containing α-curcumene, prepared from the hexane-soluble fraction by silica gel column chromatography, suppressed the synthesis of fatty acids from [^{14}C] acetate in primary cultured rat hepatocytes. Thus, α-curcumene is one of the active principles exerting triglyceride-lowering activity in *C. xanthorrhiza*.

C. Curcumin Inhibits LDL Oxidation

The oxidation of low-density lipoproteins (LDL) plays an important role in the development of atherosclerosis. Atherosclerosis is characterized by oxidative damage, which affects lipoproteins, the walls of blood vessels, and subcellular membranes. Several studies suggest that curcumin inhibits oxidation of LDL (87–90). Naidu and Thippeswamy examined the effect of curcumin on copper-ion-induced lipid peroxidation of human LDL by measuring the formation of thiobarbituric acid reactive substance (TBARS) and relative electrophoretic mobility of LDL on agarose gel. Curcumin inhibited the formation of TBARS effectively throughout the incubation period of 12 h and decreased the relative electrophoretic mobility of LDL (90). Curcumin at 10 μM produced 40–85% inhibition of LDL oxidation. The inhibitory effect of curcumin was comparable to that of BHA but more potent than ascorbic acid. Further, curcumin significantly inhibited both the initiation and propagation phases of LDL oxidation.

Ramirez-Tortosa et al. evaluated the effect of curcumin on LDL oxidation susceptibility and plasma lipids in atherosclerotic rabbits (88). A total of 18 rabbits were fed for 7 weeks on a diet containing 95.7% standard chow, 3% lard, and 1.3% cholesterol, to induce atherosclerosis. The rabbits were divided into groups, two of which were also orally treated with turmeric extract at doses of 1.66 (group A) and 3.2 (group B) mg/kg body weight. A third group (group C) acted as a control. Plasma and LDL lipid composition, plasma α-tocopherol, plasma retinol, LDL TBARS, and LDL lipid hydroperoxides were assayed and aortic atherosclerotic lesions were evaluated. The low but not the high dosage of turmeric extracts decreased the susceptibility of rabbit LDL to lipid peroxidation. Both doses produced lower levels of total plasma cholesterol than the control group. Moreover, the lower dosage group had lower levels of cholesterol, phospholipids, and triglycerides than the 3.2-mg-dosage group.

Quiles et al. evaluated the antioxidant capacity of a *C. longa* extract on the lipid peroxidation of liver mitochondria and microsome membranes in atherosclerotic rabbits (87). Male rabbits fed a 3% (w/w) lard and 1.3% (w/w) cholesterol diet were randomly assigned to three groups. Two groups were treated with different dosages of a turmeric extract (A and B) and the third group (control) with a curcumin-free solution. Basal and in vitro 2,2′-azobis

(2-amidinopropane) dihydrochloride-induced hydroperoxide and TBARS production in liver mitochondria and microsomes was analyzed. Group A had the lowest concentration of mitochondrial hydroperoxides. In microsomes, the basal hydroperoxide levels were similar in all groups but after the induction of oxidation, group C registered the highest value; TBARS production followed the same trend in mitochondria. These findings suggest that active compounds in curcuma extract may be protective against lipoperoxidation of subcellular membranes in a dosage-dependent manner.

Asai and Miyazawa examined the effect of curcumin on lipid metabolism in rats fed a control, moderately high-fat diet (15 g soybean oil/100 g diet) and those given supplements of 0.2 g curcuminoids/100 g diet. Liver triacylglycerol and cholesterol concentrations were significantly lower in rats fed curcumin than in control rats (89). Plasma triacylglycerols in the very-low-density lipoproteins fraction were also lower in curcumin-fed rats than in control rats ($p < .05$). Hepatic acyl-CoA oxidase activity of the curcumin group was significantly higher than that of the controls. Furthermore, epididymal adipose tissue weight was significantly reduced with curcuminoid intake in a dose-dependent manner. These results indicated that dietary curcuminoids have lipid-lowering potency in vivo, probably due to alterations in fatty acid metabolism.

D. Curcumin Inhibits Platelet Aggregation

Platelet aggregation contributes to the pathway resulting in atherosclerosis. There are reports that suggest that curcumin can inhibit platelet aggregation (91–93). Srivastava et al. examined the effect of curcumin on platelet aggregation and vascular prostacyclin synthesis (92). In vitro and ex vivo effects of curcumin and acetylsalicylic acid (ASA) on the synthesis of prostacyclin (PGI_2) and on platelet aggregation have been studied in rat. Both drugs inhibited adenosine diphosphate-epinephrine (adrenaline)- and collagen-induced platelet aggregation in monkey plasma. Pretreatment with ASA (25–100 mg/kg), but not curcumin (100–300 mg/kg), inhibited PGI_2 synthesis in rat aorta. In the in vitro system, too, curcumin caused a slight increase in the synthesis of PGI_2, while ASA inhibited it. Curcumin may, therefore, be preferable in patients prone to vascular thrombosis and requiring antiarthritic therapy. Srivastava et al. showed that curcumin inhibited platelet aggregation induced by arachidonate, adrenaline, and collagen (93). This compound inhibited thromboxane B_2 production from exogenous [^{14}C] arachidonate (AA) in washed platelets and concomitantly increased the formation of 12 lipoxygenase products. Moreover, curcumin inhibited the incorporation of [^{14}C] AA into platelet phospholipids and inhibited the deacylation of AA-labeled phospholipids (liberation of free AA) on stimulation with calcium ionophore A23187. Curcumin's anti-inflammatory property may, in part, be explained by its effects on eicosanoid biosynthesis.

E. Curcumin Inhibits Myocardial Infarction

The effect of curcumin on myocardial infarction (MI) in the cat and the rat has been investigated (94–97). Dikshit et al. examined the prevention of ischemia-induced biochemical changes by curcumin in the cat heart (94). Myocardial ischemia was induced by ligation of the left descending coronary artery. Curcumin (100 mg/kg, i.p.) was given 30 min before ligation. Hearts were removed 4 hr after coronary artery ligation. Levels of glutathione (GSH), malonaldelhyde (MDA), myeloperoxidase (MPO), superoxide dismutase (SOD), catalase, and lactate dehydrogenase (LDH) were estimated in the ischemic and nonischemic zones. Curcumin protected the animals against decrease in the heart rate and blood pressure following ischemia. In the ischemic zone, after 4 h of ligation, an increase in the level of MDA and activities of MPO and SOD (cytosolic fraction) were observed. Curcumin pretreatment prevented the ischemia-induced elevation in MDA contents and LDH release but did not affect the increase in MPO activity. Thus curcumin prevented ischemia-induced changes in the cat heart.

Nirmala and Puvanakrishnan investigated the effect of curcumin on lysosomal hydrolases (β-glucuronidase, β-*N*-acetylglucosaminidase, cathepsin B, cathepsin D, and acid phosphatase) in serum and heart after isoproterenol (ISO)-induced MI (95). Rats treated with ISO (30 mg/100 g body weight) showed a significant increase in serum lysosomal hydrolase activities, which were found to decrease after curcumin treatment. ISO administration to rats resulted in decreased stability of the membranes, which was reflected by the lowered activity of cathepsin D in mitochondrial, lysosomal, and microsomal fractions. Curcumin treatment returned the activity levels almost to normal, showing that curcumin restored the normal function of the membrane. Histopathological studies of the infarcted rat heart also showed a decreased degree of necrosis after curcumin treatment. Nirmala and Puvanakrishnan also examined the effect of curcumin on the biochemical changes induced by ISO administration in rats (96). ISO caused a decrease in body weight and an increase in heart weight and water content as well as in the levels of serum marker enzymes, viz. creatine kinase (CK), LDH, and LDH1 isozyme. It also produced electrocardiographic changes such as an increased heart rate, reduced R amplitude, and elevated ST. Curcumin at a concentration of 200 mg/kg, when administered orally, decreased serum enzyme levels, and the electrocardiographic changes were restored toward normalcy. MI was accompanied by the disintegration of membrane polyunsaturated fatty acids expressed by an increase in TBARS, a measure of lipid peroxides, and by the impairment of natural scavenging, characterized by a decrease in the levels of SOD, catalase, glutathione peroxidase, ceruloplasmin, α-tocopherol, GSH, and ascorbic acid. Oral pretreatment with curcumin 2 days before and during ISO administration decreased the effect of lipid peroxidation. Curcumin has a membrane-stabilizing action by inhibiting the release of β-glucuronidase from nuclei, mitochondria, lysosome, and microsomes. Curcumin given before and during treatment decreased the severity of pathological changes and thus could have a protective effect against the damage caused by MI.

Nirmala et al. showed that curcumin treatment modulates collagen metabolism in ISO-induced myocardial necrosis in rats (97). This study evaluated whether curcumin had any specific role in the synthesis and degradation of collagen in rat heart with myocardial necrosis induced by ISO. The effect of curcumin (200 mg/kg) was examined on ISO-induced myocardial necrosis and collagen metabolism. The incorporation of [^{14}C] proline into collagen was studied as an index of collagen synthesis. The heart weight/body weight ratio, heart RNA/DNA ratio, and protein were found to increase significantly in ISO-treated animals. Curcumin given before and during treatment with ISO reversed these changes and attenuated the development of cardiac hypertrophy 2 weeks after the second dose of ISO. Increased fractional synthesis rate and enhanced degradation of newly synthesized collagen were observed in ISO-treated animals. Curcumin before and during treatment with ISO decreased the degree of degradation of the existing collagen matrix and collagen synthesis, 2 weeks after the second dose of ISO. The observed effects could have been due to free-radical-scavenging capacity and inhibition of lysosomal enzyme release by curcumin.

The SOD family of enzymes are key regulators of cellular oxidant stress caused by ischemia-reperfusion. In particular, the mitochondrial-associated Mn-SOD enzyme has been implicated in protection from ischemia-reperfusion injury. Shahed et al. investigated the effect of curcumin compounds on expression of antioxidant enzymes mRNA in vivo in rat kidney after ureteral obstruction or ischemia/reperfusion injury (98). Curcumin exhibited renoprotective properties by modulating the expression of Mn-SOD.

IV. CURCUMIN SUPPRESSES DIABETES

Arun and Nalini investigated the efficacy of turmeric and curcumin on blood sugar and polyol pathway in diabetic albino rats (99). Alloxan was used to induce diabetes. Administration of turmeric or curcumin reduced the blood sugar, hemoglobin, and glycosylated hemoglobin levels significantly. Turmeric and curcumin supplementation also reduced the oxidative stress encountered by the diabetic rats, as demonstrated by lower levels of TBARS, which may have been due to the decreased influx of glucose into the polyol pathway leading to an increased NADPH/NADP ratio and elevated activity of the potent antioxdiant enzyme GPx. Moreover, the activity of sorbitol dehydrogenase, which catalyzes the conversion of sorbitol to fructose, was lowered significantly by treatment with turmeric or curcumin. These results also appeared to reveal that curcumin was more effective in attenuating diabetes-mellitus-related changes than turmeric. Srinivasan investigated the effect of curcumin on blood sugar in a diabetic subject (100).

Babu and Srinivasan also examined the influence of dietary curcumin on the progression of experimentally induced diabetes induced by cholesterol feeding in the albino rat (101). A 0.5% curcumin diet or 1% cholesterol diet was given to albino rats that were rendered diabetic with streptozotocin injection. Diabetic rats maintained on curcumin diet for 8 weeks excreted less albumin, urea, creatinine, and inorganic phosphorus. Urinary excretion of the electrolytes sodium and potassium was also significantly lowered under curcumin treatment. Dietary curcumin also partially reversed the abnormalities in plasma albumin, urea, creatine, and inorganic phosphorus in diabetic animals. On the other hand, glucose excretion or the fasting-sugar level was unaffected by dietary curcumin, so also the body weights were not improved to any significant extent. The curcumin diet lowered liver weight and lowered lipid peroxidation in plasma and urine at the end of the study compared to controls. The extent of lipid peroxidation was still higher in cholesterol-fed diabetic groups compared to diabetic rats fed with control diet. Thus, the study reveals that curcumin feeding improves the metabolic status in diabetic conditions, despite having no effect on hyperglycemic status or body weight. The mechanism by which curcumin improves this situation is probably by virtue of its hypocholesterolemic influence and its antioxidant and free-radical-scavenging properties.

In another study, Babu and Srinivasan showed the hypolipidemic action of curcumin in rats with streptozotocin-induced diabetes (102). Rats were maintained on 0.5% curcumin-containing diet for 8 weeks. The diet lowered blood cholesterol significantly exclusively by decreasing the LDL-VLDL fraction. A significant decrease in blood triglyceride and phospholipids was also brought about by dietary curcumin. In a parallel study, wherein diabetic animals were maintained on a high-cholesterol diet, the extents of hypercholesterolemia and phospholipidemia were higher than in those maintained on the control diet. Curcumin lowered cholesterol and phospholipid levels in these animals also. Liver cholesterol and triglyceride and phospholipid contents were elevated under diabetic conditions. Dietary curcumin showed a distinct tendency to counter these changes in lipid fractions of liver. This effect of curcumin was also seen in diabetic animals maintained on a high-cholesterol diet. Dietary curcumin significantly countered renal cholesterol and triglyceride elevation in diabetic rats. To understand the mechanism of hypocholesterolemic action of dietary curcumin, activities of hepatic cholesterol-7α-hydroxylase and HMG-CoA reductase were measured. Hepatic cholesterol-7α-hydroxylase activity was markedly higher in curcumin-fed diabetic animals, suggesting a higher rate of cholesterol catabolism.

Suresh and Srinivasan showed amelioration of renal lesions associated with diabetes by dietary curcumin in Wistar rats with streptozotocin-induced diabetes (103). For these studies, curcumin was fed at 0.5% in the diet for 8 weeks. Renal damage was assessed by the amount of proteins excreted in the urine and the extent of leaching of the renal tubular enzymes NAG, LDH, AsAT, A1AT, and alkaline and acid phosphatases. The integrity of the kidney was assessed by measuring the activities of several key enzymes of the renal tissue: glucose-6-phosphate dehydrogenase, glucose-6-phosphatase, and LDH (carbohydrate metabolism); aldose reductase and sorbitol dehydrogenase (polyol pathway); and transaminases, ATPases, and membrane polyunsaturated/saturated fatty acid ratio (membrane integrity). Data on enzymuria, albuminuria, activity of kidney ATPases, and fatty acid composition of renal membranes suggested that dietary curcumin significantly inhibited the progression of renal lesions in diabetes. These findings were corroborated by histological examination of kidney sections. This beneficial influence was possibly mediated through curcumin's ability to lower blood cholesterol levels.

V. CURCUMIN STIMULATES MUSCLE REGENERATION

Skeletal muscle is often the site of tissue injury due to trauma, disease, developmental defects, or surgery. Yet to date no effective treatment is available to stimulate the repair of skeletal muscle. Thaloor et al. investigated the kinetics and extent of muscle regeneration in vivo after trauma following systemic administration of curcumin to mice (104). Biochemical and histological analyses indicated a faster restoration of normal tissue architecture in mice treated with curcumin after only 4 days of daily intraperitoneal injection, whereas controls required >2 weeks to restore normal tissue architecture. Curcumin acted directly on cultured muscle precursor cells to stimulate both cell proliferation and differentiation under appropriate conditions. The authors suggested that this effect of curcumin was mediated through suppression of NF-κB; inhibition of NF-κB-mediated transcription was confirmed using reporter gene assays. The authors concluded that NF-κB exerts a role in regulating myogenesis and that modulation of NF-κB activity within muscle tissue is beneficial for muscle repair. The striking effects of curcumin on myogenesis suggest therapeutic applications for treating muscle injuries.

VI. CURCUMIN ENHANCES WOUND HEALING

Tissue repair and wound healing are complex processes that involve inflammation, granulation, and remodeling of the tissue. Sidhu et al. examined the wound-healing capacity of curcumin in rats and guinea pigs (105). Punch wounds in curcumin-treated animals closed faster in treated than in untreated animals. Biopsies of the wound showed reepithelialization of the epidermis and increased migration of various cells including myofibroblasts, fibroblasts, and macrophages in the wound bed. Multiple areas within the dermis showed extensive neovascularization, and Masson's trichrome staining showed greater collagen deposition in curcumin-treated wounds. Immunohistochemical localization showed an increase of transforming growth factor $beta_1$ (TGF-β_1) in curcumin-treated wounds as compared with untreated wounds. In situ hybridization and polymerase chain reaction analysis also showed an increase in the mRNA transcripts of TGF-β_1 and fibronectin in curcumin-treated wounds. Because TGF-β_1 is known to enhance wound healing, it possible that curcumin modulates TGF-β_1 activity.

To further understand its therapeutic effect on wound healing, the antioxidant effects of curcumin on hydrogen peroxide (H_2O_2) and hypoxanthine-xanthine-oxidase–induced damage to cultured human keratinocytes and fibroblasts were investigated by Phan et al. (106). Cell viability was assessed by colorimetric assay and quantification of LDH release. Exposure of human keratinocytes to curcumin at 10 μg/mL significantly protected the keratinocytes from hydrogen-peroxide-induced oxidative damage. Interestingly, exposure of human dermal fibroblasts to curcumin at 2.5 μg/mL showed significant protective effects against hydrogen peroxide. No protective effects of curcumin on either fibroblasts or keratinocytes against hypoxanthine-xanthine-oxidase–induced damage were found. These investigators thus concluded that curcumin indeed possessed powerful inhibitory capacity against hydrogen-peroxide-induced damage in human keratinocytes and fibroblasts and this protection may contribute to wound healing.

VII. CURCUMIN SUPPRESSES SYMPTOMS ASSOCIATED WITH ARTHRITIS

Deodhar et al. were the first to report on the antirheumatic activity of curcumin in human subjects (107). They performed a short-term, double-blind, crossover study in 18 patients with "definite" rheumatoid arthritis to compare the antirheumatic activity of curcumin (1200 mg/day) with that of phenylbutazone (300 mg/day). Subjective and objective assessment in patients who were taking corticosteroids just prior to the study showed significant ($p < 0.05$) improvements in morning stiffness, walking time, and joint swelling, after 2 weeks of curcumin therapy.

Liacini et al. examined the effect of curcumin in articular chondrocytes. Interleukin-1 (IL-1), the main cytokine instigator of cartilage degeneration in arthritis, induces matrix metalloproteinase-3 (MMP-3) and MMP-13 mRNA and protein in chondrocytes through activation of mitogen-activated protein kinase (MAPK), AP-1, and NF-κB transcription factors (108). Curcumin achieved 48–99% suppression of MMP-3 and 45–97% of MMP-13 in human and 8–100% (MMP-3) and 32–100% (MMP-13) in bovine chondrocytes. Inhibition of IL-1 signal transduction by these agents could be useful for reducing cartilage resorption by MMPs in arthritis.

VIII. CURCUMIN REDUCES THE INCIDENCE OF CHOLESTEROL GALLSTONE FORMATION

Hussain and Chandrasekhara studied the efficacy of curcumin in reducing the incidence of cholesterol gallstones induced by feeding a lithogenic diet in young male mice (83). Feeding a lithogenic diet supplemented with 0.5% curcumin for 10 weeks reduced the incidence of gallstone formation to 26%, as compared to 100% incidence in the group fed with the lithogenic diet alone. Biliary cholesterol concentration was also significantly reduced by curcumin feeding. The lithogenic index, which was 1.09 in the cholesterol-fed group, was reduced to 0.43 in the 0.5% curcumin-supplemented group. Further, the cholesterol:phospholipid ratio of bile was also reduced significantly when 0.5% curcumin-supplemented diet was fed. A dose-response study with 0.2%, 0.5%, and 1% curcumin-supplemented lithogenic diets showed that 0.5% curcumin was more effective than a diet with 0.2% or 1% curcumin. How curcumin mediates antilithogenic effects in mice was further investigated by this group (84). For this purpose, the hepatic bile of rats was fractionated by gel filtration chromatography, and the low-molecular-weight (LMW) protein fractions were tested for their ability to influence cholesterol crystal growth in model bile. The LMW protein fraction from the lithogenic-agent-fed control group's bile shortened the nucleation time and increased the crystal growth rate and final crystal concentration. But with the LMW protein fractions from the bile of rats given curcumin, the nucleation times were prolonged and the crystal growth rates and final crystal concentrations were decreased. The LMW fractions were further purified into three different sugar-specific proteins by affinity chromatography. A higher proportion of LMW proteins from the control group bile was bound to Con-A, whereas higher proportions of LMW proteins from the groups fed with curcumin were bound to wheat germ agglutinin and Helix pomatia lectin. The Con-A-bound fraction obtained from the control group showed a pronucleating effect. In contrast, the WGA-bound fraction obtained from curcumin group showed a potent antinucleating activity.

IX. CURCUMIN MODULATES MULTIPLE SCLEROSIS

Multiple sclerosis (MS) is an inflammatory disease of the central nervous system (CNS) that afflicts more than 1 million people worldwide. The destruction of oligodendrocytes and myelin sheath in the CNS is the pathological hallmark of MS. MS is an inflammatory autoimmune disease of the CNS resulting from myelin antigen-sensitized T cells in the CNS. Experimental allergic encephalomyelitis (EAE), a $CD4^+$ Th1-cell-mediated inflammatory demyelinating autoimmune disease of the CNS, serves as an animal model for MS. IL-12 plays a crucial proinflammatory role in the induction of neural-antigen-specific Th1 differentiation and pathogenesis of CNS demyelination in EAE and MS.

Natarajan and Bright investigated the effect of curcumin on the pathogenesis of CNS demyelination in EAE (109). In vivo treatment of SJL/J mice with curcumin significantly reduced the duration and clinical severity of active immunization and adoptive transfer EAE (109). Curcumin inhibited EAE in association with a decrease in IL-12 production from macrophage/microglial cells and differentiation of neural-antigen-specific Th1 cells. In vitro treatment of activated T cells with curcumin inhibited IL-12-induced tyrosine phosphorylation of Janus kinase 2, tyrosine kinase 2, and STAT3 and STAT4 transcription factors. The inhibition of Janus kinase-STAT pathway by curcumin resulted in a decrease in IL-12-induced T-cell proliferation and Th1 differentiation. These findings show that curcumin inhibits EAE by blocking IL-12 signaling in T cells and suggest its use in the treatment of MS and other Th1-cell-mediated inflammatory diseases.

X. CURCUMIN BLOCKS THE REPLICATION OF HIV

Transcription of type 1 human immunodeficiency virus (HIV-1) provirus is governed by the viral long terminal repeat (LTR). Drugs can block HIV-1 replication by inhibiting the activity of its LTR. Li et al. examined the effect of curcumin on HIV-1 LTR-directed gene expression and virus replication (110). Curcumin was found to be a potent and selective inhibitor of HIV-1 LTR-directed gene expression, at concentrations that have minor effects on cells. At the studied concentrations, curcumin inhibited p24 antigen production in cells either acutely or chronically infected with HIV-1 through transcriptional repression of the LTR. Sui et al. examined the effect of the HIV-1 and HIV-2 proteases by curcumin and curcumin boron complexes (111). Curcumin is a modest inhibitor of the HIV-1 (IC_{50} = 100 μM) and

HIV-2 (IC_{50} = 250 μM) proteases. Simple modifications of the curcumin structure raise the IC_{50} value, but complexes of the central dihydroxy groups of curcumin with boron lower the IC_{50} to a value as low as 6 μM. The boron complexes are also time-dependent inactivators of the HIV proteases. The increased affinity of the boron complexes may reflect binding of the orthogonal domains of the inhibitor in interesecting sites within the substrate-binding cavity of the enzyme, while activation of the α,β-unsaturated carbonyl group of curcumin by chelation to boron probably accounts for time-dependent inhibition of the enzyme.

Mazumder et al. examined the effect of curcumin analogs with altered potencies against HIV-1 integrase (112). They reported the inhibitory activity of curcumin against HIV-1 integrase. They also synthesized and tested analogs of curcumin to explore the structure-activity relationships and mechanism of action of this family of compounds in more detail. They found that two curcumin analogs, dicaffeoylmethane and rosmarinic acid, inhibited both activities of integrase with IC_{50} values below 10 μM. They demonstrated that lysine 136 may play a role in viral DNA binding. They showed equivalent potencies of the two curcumin analogs against both this integrase mutant and wild-type integrase, suggesting that the curcumin-binding site and the substrate-binding site may not overlap. Combining one curcumin analog with the recently described integrase inhibitor NSC 158393 resulted in integrase inhibition that was synergistic, again suggesting that drug-binding sites may not overlap. These authors also determined that these analogs could inhibit binding of the enzyme to the viral DNA but that this inhibition is independent of divalent metal ion. Furthermore, kinetic studies of these analogs suggest that they bind to the enzyme at a slow rate. These studies can provide mechanistic and structural information to guide the future design of integrase inhibitors.

The transcription of HIV-1 provirus is regulated by both cellular and viral factors. Various pieces of evidence suggest that Tat protein secreted by HIV1-infected cells may have additional activity in the pathogenesis of AIDS because of its ability to also be taken up by noninfected cells. Barthelemy et al. showed that curcumin used at 10–100 nM inhibited Tat transactivation of HIV1-LTR lacZ by 70–80% in HeLa cells (113). To develop more efficient curcumin derivatives, they synthesized and tested in the same experimental system the inhibitory activity of reduced curcumin (C1), which lacks the spatial structure of curcumin; allyl-curcumin (C2), which possesses a condensed allyl derivative on curcumin that plays the role of metal chelator; and tocopheryl-curcumin (C3), which enhances the antioxidant activity of the molecule. Results obtained with the C1, C2, and C3 curcumin derivatives showed a significant inhibition (70–85%) of Tat transactivation. Despite the fact that tocopheryl-curcumin (C3) failed to scavenge O^2, this curcumin derivative exhibited the most activity; 70% inhibition was obtained at 1 nM, while only 35% inhibition was obtained with the curcumin.

XI. CURCUMIN AFFECTS ALZHEIMER'S DISEASE

Inflammation in Alzheimer's disease (AD) patients is characterized by increased cytokines and activated microglia. Epidemiological studies suggest reduced AD risk is associated with long-term use of nonsteroidal anti-inflammatory drugs (NSAIDs). Whereas chronic ibuprofen suppressed inflammation and plaque-related pathology in an Alzheimer transgenic APPSw mouse model (Tg2576), excessive use of NSAIDs targeting cyclooxygenase can cause gastrointestinal, liver, and renal toxicity. One alternative NSAID is curcumin, which has an extensive history as a food additive and herbal medicine in India and is also a potent polyphenolic antioxidant. Lim et al. found that curcumin reduces oxidative damage and amyloid pathology in an Alzheimer transgenic mouse model (114). To evaluate whether it could affect Alzheimer-like pathology in the APPSw mice, they tested the effect of a low (160 ppm) and a high dose of dietary curcumin (5000 ppm) on inflammation, oxidative damage, and plaque pathology. Low and high doses significantly lowered oxidized proteins and IL-1β, a proinflammatory cytokine elevated in the brains of these mice. With low-dose, but not high-dose, curcumin treatment, the astrocytic marker glial fibrillary acidic protein was reduced, and insoluble β-amyloid (Aβ), soluble Aβ, and plaque burden were significantly decreased, by 43–50%. However, levels of amyloid precursor in the membrane fraction were not reduced. Microgliosis was also suppressed in neuronal layers but not adjacent to plaques. In view of its efficacy and apparent low toxicity, this Indian spice component showed promise for the prevention of Alzheimer's disease.

XII. CURCUMIN PROTECTS AGAINST CATARACT FORMATION

Age-related cataractogenesis is a significant health problem worldwide. Oxidative stress has been suggested to be a common underlying mechanism of cataractogenesis, and augmentation of the antioxidant defenses of the ocular lens has been shown to prevent or delay cataractogenesis. Awasthi et al. tested the efficacy of curcumin in preventing cataractogenesis in an in vitro rat model (115). Rats were maintained on an AIN-76 diet for 2 weeks, after which they were given a daily dose of corn oil alone or 75 mg curcumin/kg in corn oil for 14 days. Their lenses were removed and cultured for 72 hr in vitro in the presence or absence of 100 μmol 4-hydroxy-2-nonenal (4-HNE)/L, a highly electrophilic product of lipid peroxidation. The results of these studies showed that 4-HNE led to opacification of cultured lenses as indicated by the measurements of transmitted light intensity using digital image analysis. However, the lenses from curcumin-treated rats were resistant to 4-HNE-induced opacification. Curcumin treatment significantly inducted the glutathione S-transferase (GST) isozyme rGST8-8 in rat lens epithelium. Because rGST8-8 utilizes 4-HNE as a preferred substrate, we suggest that the protective effect of curcumin may be mediated through the induction of this GST isozyme. These studies suggest that curcumin may be an effective protective agent against cataractogenesis induced by lipid peroxidation.

XIII. CURCUMIN PROTECTS FROM DRUG-INDUCED MYOCARDIAL TOXICITY

Cardiotoxicity is one of the major problems associated with administration of most chemotherapeutic agents. Venkatesan examined the protective effect of curcumin on acute Adriamycin (ADR) myocardial toxicity in rats (116). ADR toxicity, induced by a single intraperitoneal injection (30 mg/kg), was revealed by elevated serum creatine kinase (CK) and LDH. The level of the lipid peroxidation products, conjugated dienes and malondialdehyde, was markedly elevated by ADR. ADR caused a decrease in myocardial glutathione content and glutathione peroxidase activity and an increase in cardiac catalase activity. Curcumin treatment (200 mg/kg) 7 days before and 2 days (after administration of) ADR significantly ameliorated the early manifestation of cardiotoxicity (ST-segment elevation and an increase in heart rate) and prevented the rise in serum CK and LDH exerted by ADR. ADR-treated rats that received curcumin displayed a significant inhibition of lipid peroxidation and augmentation of endogenous antioxidants. These results suggest that curcumin inhibits ADR cardiotoxicity and might serve as novel combination chemotherapeutic agent with ADR to limit free-radical-mediated organ injury.

XIV. CURCUMIN PROTECTS FROM DRUG-INDUCED LUNG INJURY

Cyclophosphamide causes lung injury in rats through its ability to generate free radicals with subsequent endothelial and epithelial cell damage. Venkatesan and Chandrakasan examined the effect of curcumin on cyclophosphamide-induced early lung injury (117). To observe the protective effects of curcumin on cyclophosphamide-induced early lung injury, healthy, pathogen-free male Wistar rats were exposed to 20 mg/100 g body weight of cyclophosphamide, given intraperitoneally as a single injection. Prior to cyclophosphamide intoxication, curcumin was administered orallydaily for 7 days. At various times (2, 3, 5, and 7 days postinsult) serum and lung samples were analyzed for angiotensin-converting enzyme (ACE), lipid peroxidation, reduced glutathione, and ascorbic acid. Bronchoalveolar lavage fluid was analyzed for biochemical constituents. The lavage cells were examined for lipid peroxidation and glutathione content. Excised lungs were analyzed for antioxidant enzyme levels. Biochemical analyses revealed increased lavage fluid total protein, albumin, ACE, LDH, *N*-acetyl-β-D-glucosaminidase, alkaline phosphatase, acid phosphatase, lipid peroxide, GSH, and ascorbic acid levels 2, 3, 5, and 7 days after cyclophosphamide intoxication. Increased levels of lipid peroxidation and decreased levels of GSH and ascorbic acid were seen in serum, lung tissue, and lavage cells of cyclophosphamide-treated groups. Serum ACE activity increased, coinciding with the decrease in lung tissue levels. Activities of antioxidant enzymes were reduced with time in the lungs of cyclophosphamide-treated group, whereas a significant reduction in the lavage fluid biochemical constituents and lipid peroxidation products in the serum, lung, and lavage cells, with concomitant increase in antioxidant defense mechanisms, occurred in curcumin-fed cyclophosphamide rats. Therefore, the study indicated curcumin as an effective agent in moderating the cyclophosphamide-induced early lung injury.

In another study, Venkatesan et al. investigated the effect of curcumin on bleomycin (BLM)-induced lung injury (118). The data indicated that BLM-mediated lung injury resulted in increases in lung lavage fluid biomarkers such as total protein, ACE, LDH, *N*-acetyl-β-D-glucosaminidase, lipid peroxidation (LPO) products, SOD, and catalase. BLM administration also resulted in increased levels of malondialdehyde in bronchoalveolar lavage fluid and bronchoalveolar lavage (BAL) cells and greater amounts of alveolar macrophage (AM) superoxide dismutase activity. By contrast, lower levels of reduced GSH were observed in lung lavage fluid, BAL cell, and AM. Stimulated superoxide anion and H_2O_2 release by AM from BLM-treated rats were higher. Curcumin treatment significantly reduced lavage fluid biomarkers. In addition, it restorated the antioxidant status in BLM rats. These data suggested that curcumin treatment reduces the development of BLM-induced inflammatory and oxidant activity. Therefore, curcumin offers the potential for a novel pharmacological approach in the suppression of drug- or chemical-induced lung injury.

Punithavathi et al. also evaluated the ability of curcumin to suppress BLM-induced pulmonary fibrosis in rats (119). A single intratracheal instillation of BLM (0.75 U/100 g, sacrificed 3, 5, 7, 14, and 28 days post-BLM) resulted in significant increases in total cell numbers, total protein, and ACE and in alkaline phosphatase activities in bronchoalveolar lavage fluid. Animals with fibrosis had a significant increase in lung hydroxyproline content. AM from BLM-treated rats elaborated significant increases in

TNF-α release, and superoxide anion and nitric oxide production in culture medium. Interestingly, oral administration of curcumin (300 mg/kg) 10 days before and daily thereafter throughout the experimental time period inhibited BLM-induced increases in total cell counts and biomarkers of inflammatory responses in BALF. In addition, curcumin significantly reduced the total lung hydroxyproline in BLM-treated rats. Furthermore, curcumin remarkably suppressed the BLM-induced AM production of TNF-α, superoxide anion, and nitric oxide. These findings suggest curcumin as a potent anti-inflammatory and antifibrotic agent against BLM-induced pulmonary fibrosis in rats.

Paraquat (PQ), a broad-spectrum herbicide, can cause lung injury in humans and animals. An early feature of PQ toxicity is the influx of inflammatory cells, releasing proteolytic enzymes and oxygen free radicals, which can destroy the lung epithelium and result in pulmonary fibrosis. Therefore, suppressing early lung injury before the development of irreversible fibrosis would be an appropriate therapeutic goal. Venkatesan showed that curcumin confers remarkable protection against PQ-induced lung injury (120). A single intraperitoneal injection of PQ (50 mg/kg) significantly increased the levels of protein, ACE, alkaline phosphatase, *N*-acetyl-β-D-glucosaminidase (NAG), TBARS, and neutrophils in the BALF, while it decreased GSH levels. In PQ-treated rats BAL cells, TBARS concentration was increased with a simultaneous decrease in glutathione content. In addition, the data demonstrated that PQ caused a decrease in ACE and glutathione levels and an increase in levels of TBARS and myeloperoxidase activity in the lung. Interestingly, curcumin prevented the general toxicity and mortality induced by PQ and blocked the rise in BALF protein, ACE, alkaline phophatase, *N*-acetyl glucosaminidase, TBARS, and neutrophils. Similarly, curcumin prevented the rise in TBARS content in both BAL cell and lung tissue and MPO activity of the lung. In addition, PQ induced reduction in lung ACE, and BAL cell and lung glutathione levels were abolished by curcumin treatment. These findings indicate that curcumin has important therapeutic implications in facilitating the early suppression of PQ lung injury.

XV. CURCUMIN PREVENTS ADRIAMYCIN-INDUCED NEPHROTOXICITY

Nephroxicity is another problem observed in patients who are administered chemotherapeutic agents. Venkatesan et al. showed that curcumin prevents ADR-induced nephrotoxicity in rats (116,121). Treatment with curcumin markedly protected against ADR-induced proteinuria, albuminuria, hypoalbuminemia, and hyperlipidemia. Similarly, curcumin inhibited ADR-induced increase in urinary excretion of *N*-acetyl-β-D-glucosaminidase (a marker of renal tubular injury), fibronectin, glycosaminoglycan, and plasma cholesterol. Curcumin restored renal function in ADR-treated rats, as judged by the increase in GFR. The data also demonstrated that curcumin protected against ADR-induced renal injury by suppressing oxidative stress and increasing kidney glutathione content and glutathione peroxidase activity. In like manner, curcumin abolished ADR-stimulated kidney microsomal and mitochondrial lipid peroxidation. These data suggest that administration of curcumin is a promising approach in the treatment of nephrosis caused by ADR.

XVI. CONCLUSION

From all these studies, it is clear that curcumin exhibits activities against cancer, cardiovascular diseases, and diabetes, the major ailments in the United States. This drug has also shown therapeutic effects against Alzheimer's disease, MS, cataract formation, HIV, and drug-induced nonspecific toxicity in the heart, lung, and kidney. Several of the studies establishing curcumin's potential were carried out in animals. Further testing of curcumin in human is required to confirm these observations. A clinical development plan for using curcumin to treat cancer was recently described by the National Cancer Institute (3).

How curcumin produces its therapeutic effects is not fully understood, but they are probably mediated in part through the antioxidant and anti-inflammatory action of curcumin. It is quite likely that curcumin mediates its effects through other mechanisms as well. More than a dozen different cellular proteins and enzymes have been identified to which curcumin binds. High-throughput, ligand-interacting technology can reveal more molecular targets of curcumin. Microarray gene chip technology may in the future indicate which genes are regulated by curcumin.

ACKNOWLEDGMENT

This research was supported by the Clayton Foundation for Research (to BBA), by Department of Defense of the U.S. Army Breast Cancer Research Program BC010610 (to BBA), and by P50 Head and Neck SPORE grant from National Institute of Health (to BBA). We would like to thank Walter Pagel for a careful review of the manuscript.

ABBREVIATIONS

EGF, epidermal growth factor; EGFR, EGF receptor; NF-κB, nuclear factor-κB; TNF, tumor necrosis factor; H_2O_2, hydrogen peroxide; AP-1, activating protein-1; JNK, c-jun N-terminal kinase; MMP, matrix metalloprotease; COX, cyclooxygenase; iNOS, inducible nitric oxide synthase; PBMC, peripheral blood mononuclear cells; VSMC, vascular smooth muscle cells; HDL, high-density lipoprotein; TBARS, thiobarbituric acid reactive substance; LDL, low-density lipoprotein; VLDL, very-low density lipoprotein; ASA, acetylsalicylic acid; PGI_2, prostacyclin I_2; AA, arachidonic acid; GSH, glutathione; MDA, malondialdehyde; SOD, superoxide dismutase; LDH, lactate dehydrogenase; ISO, isoproterenol; NAG, *N*-acetyl glucosaminidase; TGF-β_1 transforming growth factor beta_1; IL, interleukin; MS, multiple sclerosis; CNS, central nervous system; EAE, experimental allergic encephalomyelitis; STAT, signal transducers and activators of transcription; HIV, human immunodeficiency virus; LTR, long terminal repeat; LMW proteins, low-molecular-weight proteins; NSAIDs, nonsteroidal anti-inflammatory drugs; APP, amyloid precursor; 4-HNE, 4-hydroxy-2-nonenal; GST, gluthathione S-transferase; ADR, Adriamycin; LDH, lactate dehydrogenase; BLM, bleomycin; BAL, bronchoalveolar lavage; ACE, angiotensin-converting enzyme; PQ, paraquat.

REFERENCES

1. Ammon HP, Wahl MA. Pharmacology of *Curcuma longa*. Planta Med 1991; 57:1–7.
2. Cheng AL, Hsu CH, Lin JK, et al. Phase I clinical trial of curcumin, a chemopreventive agent, in patients with high-risk or pre-malignant lesions. Anticancer Res 2001; 21:2895–2900.
3. Clinical development plan: curcumin. J Cell Biochem 1996; 26(suppl):72–85.
4. Huang MT, Wang ZY, Georgiadis CA, Laskin JD, Conney AH. Inhibitory effects of curcumin on tumor initiation by benzo[a]pyrene and 7,12-dimethylbenz[a]anthracene. Carcinogenesis 1992; 13:2183–2186.
5. Huang MT, Lou YR, Xie JG, et al. Effect of dietary curcumin and dibenzoylmethane on formation of 7,12-dimethylbenz[a]anthracene-induced mammary tumors and lymphomas/leukemias in Sencar mice. Carcinogenesis 1998; 19:1697–1700.
6. Conney AH, Lysz T, Ferraro T, et al. Inhibitory effect of curcumin and some related dietary compounds on tumor promotion and arachidonic acid metabolism in mouse skin. Adv Enzyme Regul 1991; 31:385–396.
7. Huang MT, Lysz T, Ferraro T, Abidi TF, Laskin JD, Conney AH. Inhibitory effects of curcumin on in vitro lipoxygenase and cyclooxygenase activities in mouse epidermis. Cancer Res 1991; 51:813–819.
8. Lu YP, Chang RL, Lou YR, et al. Effect of curcumin on 12-*O*-tetradecanoylphorbol-13-acetate- and ultraviolet B light-induced expression of c-Jun and c-Fos in JB6 cells and in mouse epidermis. Carcinogenesis 1994; 15:2363–2370.

9. Limtrakul P, Lipigorngoson S, Namwong O, Apisariyakul A, Dunn FW. Inhibitory effect of dietary curcumin on skin carcinogenesis in mice. Cancer Lett 1997; 116:197–203.
10. Huang MT, Ma W, Yen P, et al. Inhibitory effects of topical application of low doses of curcumin on 12-*O*-tetradecanoylphorbol-13-acetate-induced tumor promotion and oxidized DNA bases in mouse epidermis. Carcinogenesis 1997; 18:83–88.
11. Huang MT, Lou YR, Ma W, Newmark HL, Reuhl KR, Conney AH. Inhibitory effects of dietary curcumin on forestomach, duodenal, and colon carcinogenesis in mice. Cancer Res 1994; 54:5841–5847.
12. Singh SV, Hu X, Srivastava SK, et al. Mechanism of inhibition of benzo[a]pyrene-induced forestomach cancer in mice by dietary curcumin. Carcinogenesis 1998; 19:1357–1360.
13. Rao CV, Rivenson A, Simi B, Reddy BS. Chemoprevention of colon carcinogenesis by dietary curcumin, a naturally occurring plant phenolic compound. Cancer Res 1995; 55:259–266.
14. Kim JM, Araki S, Kim DJ, et al. Chemopreventive effects of carotenoids and curcumins on mouse colon carcinogenesis after 1,2-dimethylhydrazine initiation. Carcinogenesis 1998; 19:81–85.
15. Kawamori T, Lubet R, Steele VE, et al. Chemopreventive effect of curcumin, a naturally occurring anti-inflammatory agent, during the promotion/progression stages of colon cancer. Cancer Res 1999; 59:597–601.
16. Chuang SE, Kuo ML, Hsu CH, et al. Curcumin-containing diet inhibits diethylnitrosamine-induced murine hepatocarcinogenesis. Carcinogenesis 2000; 21:331–335.
17. Singletary K, MacDonald C, Wallig M, Fisher C. Inhibition of 7,12-dimethylbenz[a]anthracene (DMBA)-induced mammary tumorigenesis and DMBA-DNA adduct formation by curcumin. Cancer Lett 1996; 103:137–141.
18. Inano H, Onoda M, Inafuku N, et al. Chemoprevention by curcumin during the promotion stage of tumorigenesis of mammary gland in rats irradiated with gamma-rays. Carcinogenesis 1999; 20:1011–1018.
19. Kuo ML, Huang TS, Lin JK. Curcumin, an antioxidant and anti-tumor promoter, induces apoptosis in human leukemia cells. Biochim Biophys Acta 1996; 1317:95–100.
20. Ranjan D, Johnston TD, Reddy KS, Wu G, Bondada S, Chen C. Enhanced apoptosis mediates inhibition of EBV-transformed lymphoblastoid cell line proliferation by curcumin. J Surg Res 1999; 87:1–5.
21. Piwocka K, Zablocki K, Wieckowski MR, et al. A novel apoptosis-like pathway, independent of mitochondria and caspases, induced by curcumin in human lymphoblastoid T (Jurkat) cells. Exp Cell Res 1999; 249:299–307.
22. Han SS, Chung ST, Robertson DA, Ranjan D, Bondada S. Curcumin causes the growth arrest and apoptosis of B cell lymphoma by downregulation of egr-1, c-myc, bcl-XL, NF-kappa B, and p53. Clin Immunol 1999; 93:152–161.
23. Chen H, Zhang ZS, Zhang YL, Zhou DY. Curcumin inhibits cell proliferation

by interfering with the cell cycle and inducing apoptosis in colon carcinoma cells. Anticancer Res 1999; 19:3675–3680.
24. Korutla L, Kumar R. Inhibitory effect of curcumin on epidermal growth factor receptor kinase activity in A431 cells. Biochim Biophys Acta 1994; 1224:597–600.
25. Mehta K, Pantazis P, McQueen T, Aggarwal BB. Antiproliferative effect of curcumin (diferuloylmethane) against human breast tumor cell lines. Anticancer Drugs 1997; 8:470–481.
26. Ramachandran C, You W. Differential sensitivity of human mammary epithelial and breast carcinoma cell lines to curcumin. Breast Cancer Res Treat 1999; 54:269–278.
27. Simon A, Allais DP, Duroux JL, Basly JP, Durand-Fontanier S, Delage C. Inhibitory effect of curcuminoids on MCF-7 cell proliferation and structure-activity relationships. Cancer Lett 1998; 129:111–116.
28. Anto RJ, Mukhopadhyay A, Denning K, Aggarwal BB. Curcumin (diferuloylmethane) induces apoptosis through activation of caspase-8, BID cleavage and cytochrome c release: its suppression by ectopic expression of Bcl-2 and Bcl-xl. Carcinogenesis 2002; 23:143–150.
29. Slamon DJ, Clark GM, Wong SG, Levin WJ, Ullrich A, McGuire WL. Human breast cancer: correlation of relapse and survival with amplification of the HER-2/neu oncogene. Science 1987; 235:177–182.
30. Korutla L, Cheung JY, Mendelsohn J, Kumar R. Inhibition of ligand-induced activation of epidermal growth factor receptor tyrosine phosphorylation by curcumin. Carcinogenesis 1995; 16:1741–1745.
31. Hong RL, Spohn WH, Hung MC. Curcumin inhibits tyrosine kinase activity of p185neu and also depletes p185neu. Clin Cancer Res 1999; 5:1884–1891.
32. Mukhopadhyay A, Bueso-Ramos C, Chatterjee D, Pantazis P, Aggarwal BB. Curcumin downregulates cell survival mechanisms in human prostate cancer cell lines. Oncogene 2001; 20:7597–7609.
33. Baldwin AS. Control of oncogenesis and cancer therapy resistance by the transcription factor NF-kappaB. J Clin Invest 2001; 107:241–246.
34. Pahl HL. Activators and target genes of Rel/NF-kappaB transcription factors. Oncogene 1999; 18:6853–6866.
35. Wang CY, Mayo MW, Baldwin AS Jr, TNF- and cancer therapy-induced apoptosis: potentiation by inhibition of NF-kappaB. Science 1996; 274:784–787.
36. Lee H, Arsura M, Wu M, Duyao M, Buckler AJ, Sonenshein GE. Role of Rel-related factors in control of c-myc gene transcription in receptor-mediated apoptosis of the murine B cell WEHI 231 line. J Exp Med 1995; 181:1169–1177.
37. Giri DK, Aggarwal BB. Constitutive activation of NF-kappaB causes resistance to apoptosis in human cutaneous T cell lymphoma HuT-78 cells. Autocrine role of tumor necrosis factor and reactive oxygen intermediates. J Biol Chem 1998; 273:14008–14014.
38. Manna SK, Aggarwal BB. Lipopolysaccharide inhibits TNF-induced apopto-

sis: role of nuclear factor-kappaB activation and reactive oxygen intermediates. J Immunol 1999; 162:1510–1518.
39. Nakshatri H, Bhat-Nakshatri P, Martin DA, Goulet RJ Jr, Sledge GW Jr, Constitutive activation of NF-kappaB during progression of breast cancer to hormone-independent growth. Mol Cell Biol 1997; 17:3629–3639.
40. Kim DW, Sovak MA, Zanieski G, et al. Activation of NF-kappaB/Rel occurs early during neoplastic transformation of mammary cells. Carcinogenesis 2000; 21:871–879.
41. Sovak MA, Bellas RE, Kim DW, et al. Aberrant nuclear factor-kappaB/Rel expression and the pathogenesis of breast cancer. J Clin Invest 1997; 100:2952–2960.
42. Singh S, Aggarwal BB. Activation of transcription factor NF-kappa B is suppressed by curcumin (diferuloylmethane) [corrected]. J Biol Chem 1995; 270:24995–25000.
43. Jobin C, Bradham CA, Russo MP, et al. Curcumin blocks cytokine-mediated NF-kappa B activation and proinflammatory gene expression by inhibiting inhibitory factor I-kappa B kinase activity. J Immunol 1999; 163:3474–3483.
44. Plummer SM, Holloway KA, Manson MM, et al. Inhibition of cyclo-oxygenase 2 expression in colon cells by the chemopreventive agent curcumin involves inhibition of NF-kappaB activation via the NIK/IKK signalling complex. Oncogene 1999; 18:6013–6020.
45. Karin M, Liu Z, Zandi E. AP-1 function and regulation. Curr Opin Cell Biol 1997; 9:240–246.
46. Xia Y, Makris C, Su B, et al. MEK kinase 1 is critically required for c-Jun N-terminal kinase activation by proinflammatory stimuli and growth factor-induced cell migration. Proc Natl Acad Sci USA 2000; 97:5243–5248.
47. Huang C, Li J, Ma WY, Dong Z. JNK activation is required for JB6 cell transformation induced by tumor necrosis factor-alpha but not by 12-*O*-tetradecanoylphorbol-13-acetate. J Biol Chem 1999; 274:29672–29676.
48. Huang TS, Lee SC, Lin JK. Suppression of c-Jun/AP-1 activation by an inhibitor of tumor promotion in mouse fibroblast cells. Proc Natl Acad Sci USA 1991; 88:5292–5296.
49. Chen YR, Tan TH. Inhibition of the c-Jun N-terminal kinase (JNK) signaling pathway by curcumin. Oncogene 1998; 17:173–178.
50. Ohene-Abuakwa Y, Pignatelli M. Adhesion molecules in cancer biology. Adv Exp Med Biol 2000; 465:115–126.
51. Iademarco MF, Barks JL, Dean DC. Regulation of vascular cell adhesion molecule-1 expression by IL-4 and TNF-alpha in cultured endothelial cells. J Clin Invest 1995; 95:264–271.
52. Kumar A, Dhawan S, Hardegen NJ, Aggarwal BB. Curcumin (diferuloylmethane) inhibition of tumor necrosis factor (TNF)-mediated adhesion of monocytes to endothelial cells by suppression of cell surface expression of adhesion molecules and of nuclear factor-kappaB activation. Biochem Pharmacol 1998; 55:775–783.

53. Fournier DB, Gordon GB. COX-2 and colon cancer: potential targets for chemoprevention. J Cell Biochem 2000; 77:97–102.
54. Hida T, Yatabe Y, Achiwa H, et al. Increased expression of cyclooxygenase 2 occurs frequently in human lung cancers, specifically in adenocarcinomas. Cancer Res 1998; 58:3761–3764.
55. Harris RE, Alshafie GA, Abou-Issa H, Seibert K. Chemoprevention of breast cancer in rats by celecoxib, a cyclooxygenase 2 inhibitor. Cancer Res 2000; 60:2101–2103.
56. Williams CS, Mann M, DuBois RN. The role of cyclooxygenases in inflammation, cancer, and development. Oncogene 1999; 18:7908–7916.
57. Reddy BS, Hirose Y, Lubet R, et al. Chemoprevention of colon cancer by specific cyclooxygenase-2 inhibitor, celecoxib, administered during different stages of carcinogenesis. Cancer Res 2000; 60:293–297.
58. Zhang F, Altorki NK, Mestre JR, Subbaramaiah K, Dannenberg AJ. Curcumin inhibits cyclooxygenase-2 transcription in bile acid– and phorbol ester–treated human gastrointestinal epithelial cells. Carcinogenesis 1999; 20:445–451.
59. Folkman J. Can mosaic tumor vessels facilitate molecular diagnosis of cancer? Proc Natl Acad Sci USA 2001; 98:398–400.
60. Singh AK, Sidhu GS, Deepa T, Maheshwari RK. Curcumin inhibits the proliferation and cell cycle progression of human umbilical vein endothelial cell. Cancer Lett 1996; 107:109–115.
61. Mohan R, Sivak J, Ashton P, et al. Curcuminoids inhibit the angiogenic response stimulated by fibroblast growth factor-2, including expression of matrix metalloproteinase gelatinase B. J Biol Chem 2000; 275:10405–10412.
62. Arbiser JL, Klauber N, Rohan R, et al. Curcumin is an in vivo inhibitor of angiogenesis. Mol Med 1998; 4:376–383.
63. Kumar A, Dhawan S, Mukhopadhyay A, Aggarwal BB. Human immunodeficiency virus-1-tat induces matrix metalloproteinase-9 in monocytes through protein tyrosine phosphatase-mediated activation of nuclear transcription factor NF-kappaB. FEBS Lett 1999; 462:140–144.
64. Lin LI, Ke YF, Ko YC, Lin JK. Curcumin inhibits SK-Hep-1 hepatocellular carcinoma cell invasion in vitro and suppresses matrix metalloproteinase-9 secretion. Oncology 1998; 55:349–353.
65. Pan MH, Lin-Shiau SY, Lin JK. Comparative studies on the suppression of nitric oxide synthase by curcumin and its hydrogenated metabolites through down-regulation of IkappaB kinase and NFkappaB activation in macrophages. Biochem Pharmacol 2000; 60:1665–1676.
66. Menon LG, Kuttan R, Kuttan G. Anti-metastatic activity of curcumin and catechin. Cancer Lett 1999; 141:159–165.
67. Baldin V, Lukas J, Marcote MJ, Pagano M, Draetta G. Cyclin D1 is a nuclear protein required for cell cycle progression in G1. Genes Dev 1993; 7:812–821.
68. Bartkova J, Lukas J, Muller H, Lutzhoft D, Strauss M, Bartek J. Cyclin D1 protein expression and function in human breast cancer. Int J Cancer 1994; 57:353–361.

69. Adelaide J, Monges G, Derderian C, Seitz JF, Birnbaum D. Oesophageal cancer and amplification of the human cyclin D gene CCND1/PRAD1. Br J Cancer 1995; 71:64–68.
70. Caputi M, Groeger AM, Esposito V, et al. Prognostic role of cyclin D1 in lung cancer: relationship to proliferating cell nuclear antigen. Am J Respir Cell Mol Biol 1999; 20:746–750.
71. Nishida N, Fukuda Y, Komeda T, et al. Amplification and overexpression of the cyclin D1 gene in aggressive human hepatocellular carcinoma. Cancer Res 1994; 54:3107–3110.
72. Gumbiner LM, Gumerlock PH, Mack PC, et al. Overexpression of cyclin D1 is rare in human prostate carcinoma. Prostate 1999; 38:40–45.
73. Drobnjak M, Osman I, Scher HI, Fazzari M, Cordon-Cardo C. Overexpression of cyclin D1 is associated with metastatic prostate cancer to bone. Clin Cancer Res 2000; 6:1891–1895.
74. Bharti AC, Donato N, Singh S, Aggarwal BB. Curcumin (diferuloylmethane) downregulates the constitutive activation of nuclear factor-kappaB and I kappa B alpha kinase in human multiple myeloma cells leading to suppression of proliferation and induction of apoptosis. Blood 2003; 101:1053–1062.
75. Mukhopadhyay A, Banerjee S, Stafford LJ, Xia CX, Liu M, Aggarwal BB. Curcumin-induced suppression of cell proliferation correlates with donregulation of cyclin D1 expression and CDK4-mediated retinoblastoma protein phosphorylation. Oncogene 2002; 21:8852–8861.
76. Huang HC, Jan TR, Yeh SF. Inhibitory effect of curcumin, an anti-inflammatory agent, on vascular smooth muscle cell proliferation. Eur J Pharmacol 1992; 221:381–384.
77. Chen HW, Huang HC. Effect of curcumin on cell cycle progression and apoptosis in vascular smooth muscle cells. Br J Pharmacol 1998; 124:1029–1040.
78. Rao DS, Sekhara NC, Satyanarayana MN, Srinivasan M. Effect of curcumin on serum and liver cholesterol levels in the rat. J Nutr 1970; 100:1307–1315.
79. Patil TN, Srinivasan M. Hypocholesteremic effect of curcumin in induced hypercholesteremic rats. Indian J Exp Biol 1971; 9:167–169.
80. Keshavarz K. The influence of turmeric and curcumin on cholesterol concentration of eggs and tissues. Poult Sci 1976; 55:1077–1083.
81. Soudamini KK, Unnikrishnan MC, Soni KB, Kuttan R. Inhibition of lipid peroxidation and cholesterol levels in mice by curcumin. Indian J Physiol Pharmacol 1992; 36:239–243.
82. Soni KB, Kuttan R. Effect of oral curcumin administration on serum peroxides and cholesterol levels in human volunteers. Indian J Physiol Pharmacol 1992; 36:273–275.
83. Hussain MS, Chandrasekhara N. Effect on curcumin on cholesterol gall-stone induction in mice. Indian J Med Res 1992; 96:288–291.
84. Hussain MS, Chandrasekhara N. Biliary proteins from hepatic bile of rats fed curcumin or capsaicin inhibit cholesterol crystal nucleation in supersaturated model bile. Indian J Biochem Biophys 1994; 31:407–412.
85. Yasni S, Imaizumi K, Nakamura M, Aimoto J, Sugano M. Effects of *Curcuma*

xanthorrhiza Roxb. and curcuminoids on the level of serum and liver lipids, serum apolipoprotein A-I and lipogenic enzymes in rats. Food Chem Toxicol 1993; 31:213–218.
86. Yasni S, Imaizumi K, Sin K, Sugano M, Nonaka G, Sidik. Identification of an active principle in essential oils and hexane-soluble fractions of *Curcuma xanthorrhiza* Roxb. showing triglyceride-lowering action in rats. Food Chem Toxicol 1994; 32:273–278.
87. Quiles JL, Aguilera C, Mesa MD, Ramirez-Tortosa MC, Baro L, Gil A. An ethanolic-aqueous extract of *Curcuma longa* decreases the susceptibility of liver microsomes and mitochondria to lipid peroxidation in atherosclerotic rabbits. Biofactors 1998; 8:51–57.
88. Ramirez-Tortosa MC, Mesa MD, Aguilera MC, et al. Oral administration of a turmeric extract inhibits LDL oxidation and has hypocholesterolemic effects in rabbits with experimental atherosclerosis. Atherosclerosis 1999; 147:371–378.
89. Asai A, Miyazawa T. Dietary curcuminoids prevent high-fat diet-induced lipid accumulation in rat liver and epididymal adipose tissue. J Nutr 2001; 131:2932–2935.
90. Naidu KA, Thippeswamy NB. Inhibition of human low density lipoprotein oxidation by active principles from spices. Mol Cell Biochem 2002; 229:19–23.
91. Srivastava R, Dikshit M, Srimal RC, Dhawan BN. Anti-thrombotic effect of curcumin. Thromb Res 1985; 40:413–417.
92. Srivastava R, Puri V, Srimal RC, Dhawan BN. Effect of curcumin on platelet aggregation and vascular prostacyclin synthesis. Arzneimittelforschung 1986; 36:715–717.
93. Srivastava KC, Bordia A, Verma SK. Curcumin, a major component of food spice turmeric (*Curcuma longa*) inhibits aggregation and alters eicosanoid metabolism in human blood platelets. Prostaglandins Leukot Essent Fatty Acids 1995; 52:223–227.
94. Dikshit M, Rastogi L, Shukla R, Srimal RC. Prevention of ischaemia-induced biochemical changes by curcumin and quinidine in the cat heart. Indian J Med Res 1995; 101:31–35.
95. Nirmala C, Puvanakrishnan R. Effect of curcumin on certain lysosomal hydrolases in isoproterenol-induced myocardial infarction in rats. Biochem Pharmacol 1996; 51:47–51.
96. Nirmala C, Puvanakrishnan R. Protective role of curcumin against isoproterenol induced myocardial infarction in rats. Mol Cell Biochem 1996; 159:85–93.
97. Nirmala C, Anand S, Puvanakrishnan R. Curcumin treatment modulates collagen metabolism in isoproterenol induced myocardial necrosis in rats. Mol Cell Biochem 1999; 197:31–37.
98. Shahed AR, Jones E, Shoskes D. Quercetin and curcumin up-regulate antioxidant gene expression in rat kidney after ureteral obstruction or ischemia/reperfusion injury. Transplant Proc 2001; 33:2988.
99. Arun N, Nalini N. Efficacy of turmeric on blood sugar and polyol pathway in diabetic albino rats. Plant Foods Hum Nutr 2002; 57:41–52.

100. Srinivasan M. Effect of curcumin on blood sugar as seen in a diabetic subject. Indian J Med Sci 1972; 26:269–270.
101. Babu PS, Srinivasan K. Influence of dietary curcumin and cholesterol on the progression of experimentally induced diabetes in albino rat. Mol Cell Biochem 1995; 152:13–21.
102. Babu PS, Srinivasan K. Hypolipidemic action of curcumin, the active principle of turmeric (*Curcuma longa*) in streptozotocin induced diabetic rats. Mol Cell Biochem 1997; 166:169–175.
103. Suresh Babu P, Srinivasan K. Amelioration of renal lesions associated with diabetes by dietary curcumin in streptozotocin diabetic rats. Mol Cell Biochem 1998; 181:87–96.
104. Thaloor D, Miller KJ, Gephart J, Mitchell PO, Pavlath GK. Systemic administration of the NF-kappaB inhibitor curcumin stimulates muscle regeneration after traumatic injury. Am J Physiol 1999; 277:C320–C329.
105. Sidhu GS, Singh AK, Thaloor D, et al. Enhancement of wound healing by curcumin in animals. Wound Repair Regen 1998; 6:167–177.
106. Phan TT, See P, Lee ST, Chan SY. Protective effects of curcumin against oxidative damage on skin cells in vitro: its implication for wound healing. J Trauma 2001; 51:927–931.
107. Deodhar SD, Sethi R, Srimal RC. Preliminary study on antirheumatic activity of curcumin (diferuloyl methane). Indian J Med Res 1980; 71:632–634.
108. Liacini A, Sylvester J, Li WQ, Zafarullah M. Inhibition of interleukin-1-stimulated MAP kinases, activating protein-1 (AP-1) and nuclear factor kappa B (NF-kappaB) transcription factors down-regulates matrix metalloproteinase gene expression in articular chondrocytes. Matrix Biol 2002; 21:251–262.
109. Natarajan C, Bright JJ. Curcumin inhibits experimental allergic encephalomyelitis by blocking IL-12 signaling through Janus kinase-STAT pathway in T lymphocytes. J Immunol 2002; 168:6506–6513.
110. Li CJ, Zhang LJ, Dezube BJ, Crumpacker CS, Pardee AB. Three inhibitors of type 1 human immunodeficiency virus long terminal repeat-directed gene expression and virus replication. Proc Natl Acad Sci USA 1993; 90:1839–1842.
111. Sui Z, Salto R, Li J, Craik C, Ortiz de Montellano PR. Inhibition of the HIV-1 and HIV-2 proteases by curcumin and curcumin boron complexes. Bioorg Med Chem 1993; 1:415–422.
112. Mazumder A, Neamati N, Sunder S, et al. Curcumin analogs with altered potencies against HIV-1 integrase as probes for biochemical mechanisms of drug action. J Med Chem 1997; 40:3057–3063.
113. Barthelemy S, Vergnes L, Moynier M, Guyot D, Labidalle S, Bahraoui E. Curcumin and curcumin derivatives inhibit Tat-mediated transactivation of type 1 human immunodeficiency virus long terminal repeat. Res Virol 1998; 149:43–52.
114. Lim GP, Chu T, Yang F, Beech W, Frautschy SA, Cole GM. The curry spice curcumin reduces oxidative damage and amyloid pathology in an Alzheimer transgenic mouse. J Neurosci 2001; 21:8370–8377.
115. Awasthi S, Srivatava SK, Piper JT, Singhal SS, Chaubey M, Awasthi YC.

Curcumin protects against 4-hydroxy-2-trans-nonenal-induced cataract formation in rat lenses. Am J Clin Nutr 1996; 64:761–766.
116. Venkatesan N. Curcumin attenuation of acute Adriamycin myocardial toxicity in rats. Br J Pharmacol 1998; 124:425–427.
117. Venkatesan N, Chandrakasan G. Modulation of cyclophosphamide-induced early lung injury by curcumin, an anti-inflammatory antioxidant. Mol Cell Biochem 1995; 142:79–87.
118. Venkatesan N, Punithavathi V, Chandrakasan G. Curcumin protects bleomycin-induced lung injury in rats. Life Sci 1997; 61:PL51–PL58.
119. Punithavathi D, Venkatesan N, Babu M. Curcumin inhibition of bleomycin-induced pulmonary fibrosis in rats. Br J Pharmacol 2000; 131:169–172.
120. Venkatesan N. Pulmonary protective effects of curcumin against paraquat toxicity. Life Sci 2000; 66:PL21–PL28.
121. Venkatesan N, Punithavathi D, Arumugam V. Curcumin prevents Adriamycin nephrotoxicity in rats. Br J Pharmacol 2000; 129:231–234.

37

Extracts from the Leaves of *Chromolaena odorata*
A Potential Agent for Wound Healing

Thang T. Phan and Seng-Teik Lee
National University of Singapore
and Singapore General Hospital
Singapore, Republic of Singapore

Sui-Yung Chan
National University of Singapore
Singapore, Republic of Singapore

Margaret A. Hughes and George W. Cherry
Oxford Wound Healing Institute
and Churchill Hospital
Oxford, England

Renée J. Grayer
Jodrell Laboratory, Royal Botanic Gardens
Kew, Richmond, Surrey, England

The-Trung Le and Manh-Hung Pham
Military Academy of Medicine
Hanoi, Vietnam

I. INTRODUCTION

Chromolaena odorata (L.) R. King and H. Robinson (formerly *Eupatorium odoratum* L.), a perennial belonging to the plant family Asteraceae (= Compositae), is a diffuse, scrambling shrub that is mainly a weed of plantation crops and pastures of southern Asia and western Africa. It forms a bush 3–7 meters in height when growing in the open (Fig. 1). Native to Mexico, the West Indies, and tropical South America, it was spread widely by early navigators. It is a weed of 13 crops in 23 countries (Holm, 1977).

Traditionally, fresh leaves and a decoction of *C. odorata* have been used throughout Vietnam for many years as well as in other tropical countries for the treatment of leech bites, soft-tissue wounds, burn wounds, skin infection, and dentoalveolitis (Le, 1995). A number of studies demonstrated that the extract of the leaves of *C. odorata* inhibited the growth of bacteria (*Pseudomonas aeroginosa*, *Escherichia coli*, *Staphylococcus aureus*, and *Neisseria gonorrhoeae*) (Le, 1995; Akah, 1990; Irobi, 1992; Caceres, 1995). Enhancement of hemostasis and blood coagulation with use of *C. odorata* extract has also been reported (Akah, 1990; Triaratana et al., 1991). A clinical trial of *C. odorata* extract was conducted in the National Institute of Burns in Hanoi, Vietnam between 1987 and 1991 on 136 patients with full-thickness wounds and an average wound size of 79.9 cm^2. The stimulatory effects of a *C. odorata* extract on the formation of granulation tissue and wound reepithelialization were demonstrated clinically and histologically (Le, 1995).

Experiments were conducted to investigate the effects of the *C. odorata* extract on wound healing using different methodologies. This work illustrates that plant-based medicines that are used by folk practitioners to improve wound healing can be examined via scientific methods using cell culture technology and in vitro wound-healing models.

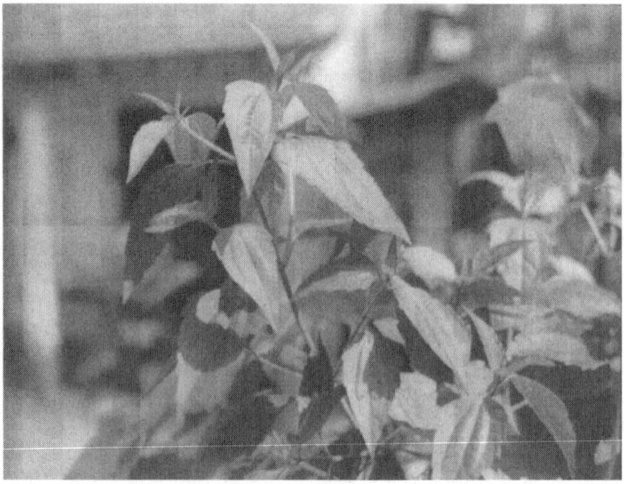

FIGURE 1 The *C. odorata* plant.

II. METHODOLOGY

A. Preparation of Crude Total Ethanol Extract

Fresh leaves of *C. odorata* (10 kg) were collected, washed, and dried in the sun for 5 days and then in a 45°C incubator for another 3 days. A 1-kg amount of clean, dried leaves was powdered, divided into three batches, and then extracted with 4000 mL of absolute ethanol in a Soxhlet apparatus for 12 hr per batch. Twelve liters of the ethanol fraction was evaporated under vacuum using a Rotary Vacuum Evaporator, RE 100, Bibby, UK Chlorophyll, resin, and lipids were removed by Whatman paper filtration and by extraction of the residue with petroleum ether in a Pyrex separating funnel. This yielded 50 g, considered as the total ethanol extract, which was lyophilized until the weight did not change using Hetotrap FD. 1.060-e, Heto Lab Equipment, Denmark. The extract was then dissolved in 1000 mL of distilled water. The aqueous portion was shaken with five portions of diethyl ether to extract lipophilic substances. The diethyl ether was evaporated under vacuum to yield 5 g of a thick yellow solution. For cell culture experiments, the lipophilic extract was reconstituted in dimethylsulfoxide (DMSO; Sigma, USA) (Fig. 2), which was adjusted to a final volume in culture medium $< 0.1\%$ (v/v). Various dilutions of the extract in the medium were prepared on the day of the experiment.

B. Fractionation by Column Chromatography

The dry residue obtained from the diethyl ether extraction was fractionated by column chromatography on silica gel 60 (Merck), using different proportions of ethyl acetate/methanol as eluting solvents (Fig. 2). Three of four fractions were found to be strongly antioxidant when tested on the cell culture system.

C. Component Separation by Semipreparative High-Performance Liquid Chromatography

The three antioxidant fractions obtained by column chromatographic fractionation were labeled A, B, and C. Further separation of these fractions was performed by high-performance liquid chromatography (HPLC) (Fig. 2). Hewlett-Packard HPLC equipment with Diode Array Detection was used (HP-1100). Separation was carried out using a C18 semipreparative column (Hewlett-Packard) at room temperature. A mixture of methanol and water was used as the mobile phase with a flow-rate of 2 mL/min. Detection took place at the wavelengths of 254, 290, and 335 nm, and for the separations, 100 μL of each fraction was injected. Different fractions were collected and

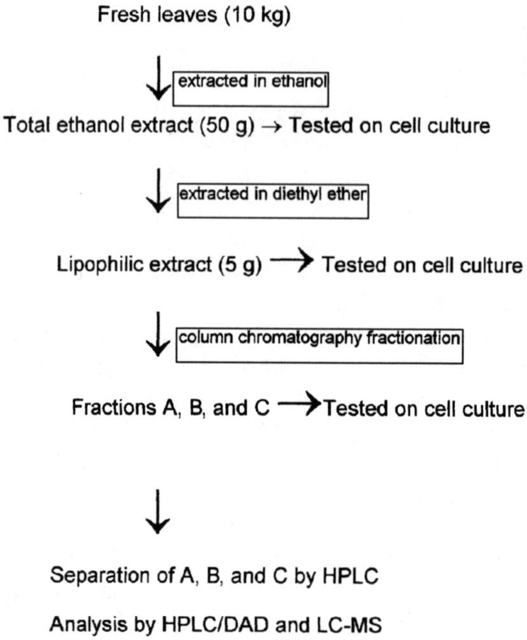

FIGURE 2 Overview of the fraction and identification of the *C. odorata* plant extract.

lyophilized for chemical analysis by analytical HPLC coupled with a diode array detection (DAD) and atmospheric pressure chemical ionization mass spectrometry (APCI-MS).

D. Cell Proliferation Assay

Fibroblasts, endothelial cell, or keratinocytes were seeded in growth media in 96-multiwell plates at a density of 1×10^3 cells/well for fibroblasts and endothelial cells or 2×10^3 cells/well for keratinocytes and incubated at 37°C in a 5% CO_2/95% air atmosphere for 24 hr or 48 hr. In these conditions, cells recover from trypsinization subculture. After 24 hr, cells were switched to basal media for another 48 hr. Then various concentrations of the plant extract diluted in basal media were added to the cells. Two sets of cells fed with basal or growth media without addition of the extract were considered as negative or positive control, respectively. Cell growth was estimated by MTT or cell-counting assays at different time intervals.

E. Antioxidant Assay

Cultured fibroblasts and keratinocytes were employed in the in vitro experiments to assess the protective effects of the extracts on cells against oxidative-induced damage. Commercial hydrogen peroxide (H_2O_2) or hypoxanthine-xanthine oxidase (HX/XO), strong oxidant agents, were prepared for addition to cells. Cells were seeded in growth media in 96-well plates at high densities of 6000 cells/well or 10,000 cells/well and incubated at 37°C in a 5% CO_2/95% air atmosphere. Cells were grown to confluence. To investigate the protective or scavenging activities of plant extracts, cells were washed with a buffer solution and the different concentrations of the extracts and hydrogen peroxide (H_2O_2) or hypoxanthine-xanthine oxidase in serum-free media were simultaneously added to the cells. The controls were normal cell cultures without addition of extracts or oxidant agents and cells exposed to oxidative damage without the presence of extracts. Cells were then incubated for another 3 hr, washed twice with buffer solution, and fresh serum-free media were dispensed to the wells. The MTT and LDH assays were used for the assessment of both cell damage and the effects of the extracts on the extent of oxidative damage.

F. In Vitro Wound Assay

This assay was carried out as previously described (Phan et al., 2000a). Briefly, human keratinocytes, either second or third passage (P2 or P3), were trypsinised, seeded into 32-mm tissue culture dishes at densities from 5×10^5 to 8×10^5 cells/dish in KGM, and fed every 2 days until they reached 100% confluence. Medium was then replaced with RPMI/10% FCS. After 4 hr a scratch was made with a micropipette tip and cells were washed with PBS to remove loosened debris. RPMI/2%FCS medium with or without the extract (1–300 μg/mL) was added to sets of two dishes per dose. Each dish was oriented on the bottom of a six-well plate lid and fixed using Super Glue 3. For each scratch four consecutive fields were selected using the following criteria: relatively little cell debris within the scratch; even scratch, with straight edges; both edges visible under a single field using the ×10 objective; fields not too close to either end of the scratch, where distortions uncharacteristic of the main part of the scratch could be seen to occur during the "healing" process. The coordinates on the vernier scales of the microscope stage were noted for every field.

A fiber optic camera linked to a VDU monitor and a video recorder were attached to the inverted microscope (Leitz Diavert) using a C mount with a 0.63 lens so that size of image on the monitor corresponded to that in the field of the microscope. The condition of each field was recorded on videotape at various intervals over periods up to 72 hr, as long as there was still a denuded area. Photographs of each field were also taken at the same time points.

Analysis of the videoed fields was carried out using the Microscan system (Fibre Optics Research). The average percentage of the initial area still denuded was calculated for each treatment set for the total of eight fields per set.

G. In Vitro Study of Effects of the Extract on Adhesion Molecule and Matrix Production by Keratinocytes

First- or second-passage keratinocytes were seeded onto 12-well slides at a density of 2×10^3 cells/well in keratinocyte growth medium (KGM). After 48 hr the medium was replaced by keratinocyte basal medium (KBM) containing various concentrations of the extract, with one set being maintained in KGM as a control. At 70–80% confluence, the slides were washed three times in PBS, air-dried, and stored at −70°C until required for indirect immunofluorescence. A standard indirect immunofluorescent technique was used to determine the expression of the adhesion complex components and fibronectin by cultured human kearinocytes maintained in KBM and treated with the extract. A rhodamine counterstain used at a 1:40 dilution was added to the fluorescent-labeled antimouse secondary antibody to reduce the nonspecific green fluorescent background staining. Using this counterstain, cells not expressing the antigen were a dull orange-brown color, while cells expressing the protein of interest fluoresced green. Monoclonal antibodies were used to detect the expression of laminin 1, laminin 5, collagen IV, fibronectin, integrin $\alpha 6$, $\beta 1$, $\beta 4$, and tenascin. The negative controls were L15 tissue culture medium and nonimmune ascites control fluid. Eight-micrometer cryostat sections of normal human skin served as the tissue control for the specificity of the monoclonal antibodies.

III. RESULTS AND DISCUSSION

A. *C. odorata* Extract Enhances Proliferation of Fibroblasts, Keratinocytes, and Endothelial Cells (Phan et al., 1998, 2001b)

This study showed that the extract from the leaves of *C. odorata* at concentrations of 10 μg/mL and 100 μg/mL enhanced the growth of fibroblasts and endothelial cells. The extract at concentrations from 0.1 to 5 μg/mL significantly stimulated the expansion of human keratinocyte colonies in monolayer in basal medium as it did in growth medium (Fig. 3). With increasing doses of the extract, from 50 to 300 μg/mL, colonies did not further expand,

(a) (b) (c) (d)

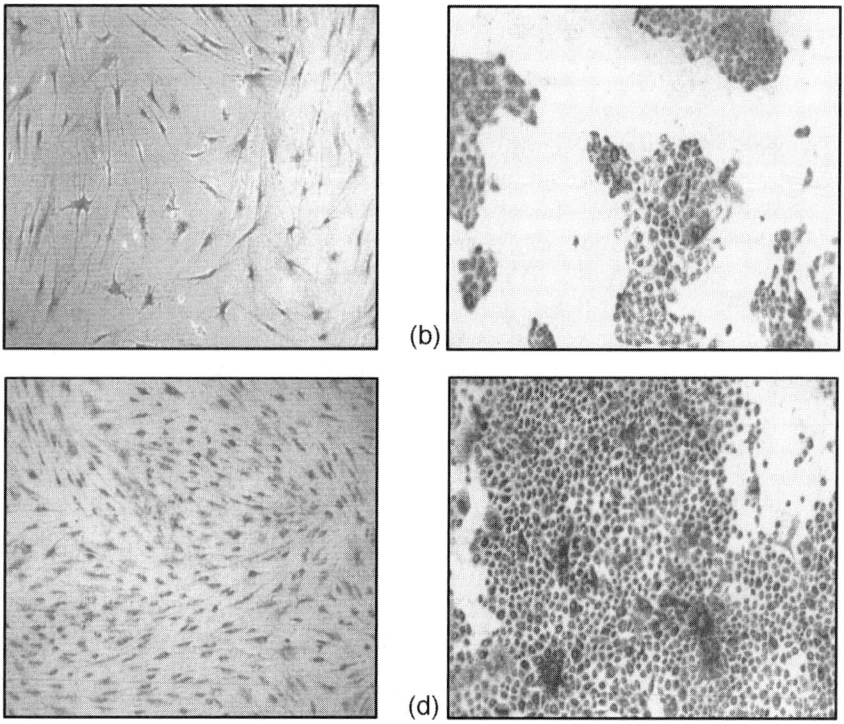

FIGURE 3 Growth of human dermal fibroblasts (a, c) and epidermal keratinocytes (b, d) in monolayer by *C. odorata* extract, monitored under the light microscope in basal medium with or without *C. odorata* extract (100×) on day 5 (a, c) or day 2 (b, d). Cells were stained with MTT to visualize living cells. Fibroblasts in basal medium (a) and basal medium plus 100 μg/mL extract (c). Keratinocytes in basal medium (b) and basal medium plus 1 μg/mL extract (d). (With permission for reprint from *Wound Repair and Regeneration* and *Plastic and Reconstructive Surgery*.)

but cells tended to differentiate and form layers. Fibroblasts, endothelial cells, and keratinocytes are indispensable in cutaneous tissue repair. Fibroblasts and endothelial cells play very important roles in the initial phase of wound healing. Fibroblasts migrate into the wound site 24 hr after injury. During this phase of healing (4–21 days), fibroblasts are activated and undergo a burst of proliferative and synthetic activity, producing high amounts of fibronectin, and then synthesizing the other protein components of the extracellular matrix, including collagen, elastin, and glycosaminoglycans. Fibroblasts also contribute to the contraction of the wound (Cherry et al., 1994; Singer and

Clark, 1999). Endothelial cells play a key role in angiogenesis and are critical mediators of the repair reaction. Their proliferation and organization into a vascular network at the wound site, as well as their biosynthetic capacity, are essential for the successful completion of tissue repair (Cherry et al., 1994; Amenta et al., 1996). Keratinocytes are very important in reepithelialization and wound closure. Keratinocytes are also known to produce a vast array of cytokines and growth factors as well as adhesion molecules that regulate fibroblast proliferation, angiogenesis, and formation of the basement membrane zone (Cherry et al., 1994; Singer and Clark, 1999).

The results of these studies demonstrated that the *C. odorata* extract promoted fibroblast, keratinocyte, and endothelial cell growth, and this could explain in part the beneficial effects that have been observed.

B. *C. odorata* Extract Enhances Keratinocyte Migration in an In Vitro Model of Wound Reepithelialization (Phan et al., 2001b)

In this study, the effect of *C. odorata* extract on keratinocyte migration, an important phenomenon in wound healing, was investigated in vitro. It was shown that concentrations of extract from 5 to 60 μg/mL always led to faster migration of keratinocytes and closure of the scratch although there was not a clear dose-dependent relationship (Fig. 4).

Until the wound is resurfaced by epithelium and the protective stratum corneum is reestablished, the patient remains at risk of infection, and continues to suffer loss of water, heat, nutrients, and others components from the wound surface. Understanding the way in which reepithelialization occurs is therefore obviously one of the most important aspects of wound healing science. Reepithelialization involves both locomotion and proliferation of keratinocytes remaining in or around the wound site. The most important sources of keratinocytes are the remaining hair follicles, sebaceous and sweat glands, or the wound edge (Woodley, 1996). The increased migration of human keratinocytes demonstrated in vitro might explain in part the reepithelialization and closure enhancement of wounds treated with *C. odorata* extract.

C. *C. odorata* Extract Upregulates Adhesion Complex Proteins and Fibronectin Production by Human Keratinocytes (Phan et al., 2000b)

This study demonstrated that the *C. odorata* extract increased the expression of several components of the adhesion complex and of fibronectin by human keratinocytes. Using indirect immunofluorescence, an increased expression (dose-dependent) of laminin 1, laminin 5, collagen IV, and fibronectin was

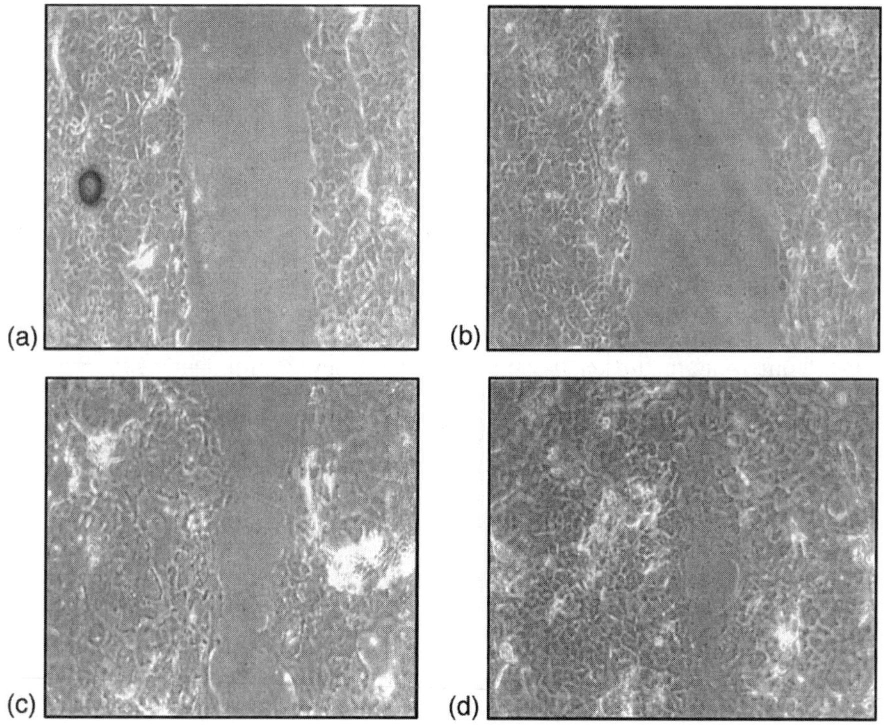

FIGURE 4 Reepithelialization of in vitro scratch wounds by *C. odorata* extract. Phase-contrast micrographs of a single representative field immediately after wounding. (a) and (b) Control and *C. odorata* extract treatment at 0 hr. (c) and (d) Control and *C. odorata* extract treatment at 34 hr after wounding. Wound reepithelialization was faster in the group treated with 10 μg/mL extract (d). (With permission for reprint from *Wound Repair and Regeneration*.)

found (Fig. 5). The expression of the β1 and β4 integrins was upregulated by the extract at low concentrations (0.1 and 1 μg/mL), but the expression was decreased at higher doses of the extract (10–150 μg/mL) (Fig. 5).

Extracellular matrix (ECM) and basement membrane zone (BMZ) components as "adhesion" molecules serve several critical functions for effective wound repair and are crucial to basal cell regeneration and wound reepithelialization. BMZ components serve as a scaffold for tissue organization and as a template for tissue repair. These components are produced and regulated by keratinocytes, fibroblasts, and cytokines (Uitto et al., 1996).

The adhesion complex proteins are essential to wound healing, especially to stabilized epithelium, and this effect of the *C. odorata* extract could contribute to the clinical efficacy of the extract used for the treatment of burns and wounds.

D. Investigation of Antioxidant Effects of *C. odorata* Extract on Cultured Skin Cells from Oxidative Damage: Identification of the Extract Active Compounds (Phan et al., 2001a,d)

Oxidants are involved in burn injury and tissue repair. Oxygen free radicals may contribute to further tissue damage in the events following skin injury and an overabundance is known to impair the healing process. Antioxidants, on the other hand, significantly prevent tissue damage and stimulate wound healing. H_2O_2 and HX/XO were applied to a skin cell culture to serve as an in vitro wound-healing model for oxidative damage and the protective antioxidant effects of *C. odorata* were tested on this model. With the use of total crude extract, the concentrations at 400 μg/mL and 800 μg/mL showed maximum and consistent protective effects against the oxidant toxification

FIGURE 5 Enhanced expression and secretion of adhesion complex proteins and fibronectin by human epidermal keratinocytes treated with *C. odorata* extract. Magnification is at 400×. In vivo skin localization (indicated by arrows; e = epidermis, d = dermis, e-d j = epidermal-dermal junction) of laminin 1 (a), laminin 5 (d), collagen IV (g), fibronectin (j), β1 integrin (m), and β4 integrin (p). There was no expression of laminin 1 in keratinocytes maintained in basal medium (b). There was expression of laminin 1 in cells treated with 50 μg/mL extract (c). A little extracellular secretion of laminin 5 was maintained in basal medium (e), this extracellular secretion increased and became more dense and extensive with 50μg/mL of *C. odorata* extract in culture medium (f). Collagen IV, a structural protein of the epiderm-dermal junction, was only weakly expressed by keratinocytes maintained in basal medium (h), but there was increased expression and extracellular secretion by cells treated with 50 μg/mL extract (i). Only a few keratinocytes expressed fibronectin when maintained in the basal medium (k), but there was a high increase in the expression and extracellular secretion of fibronectin by keratinocytes treated with 50 μg/mL extract (l). There was very weak expression of the β1 integrin in keratinocytes cultured in basal medium (m), but it was stimulated by *C. odorata* extract at 0.1 μg/mL (p). β4 integrin, an important component of epidemal-dermal junction, was expressed by keratinocytes in basal medium (q), but increased by cells treated with 0.1 μg/ml *C. odorata* extract. (With permission for reprint from the *European Journal of Dermatology*.)

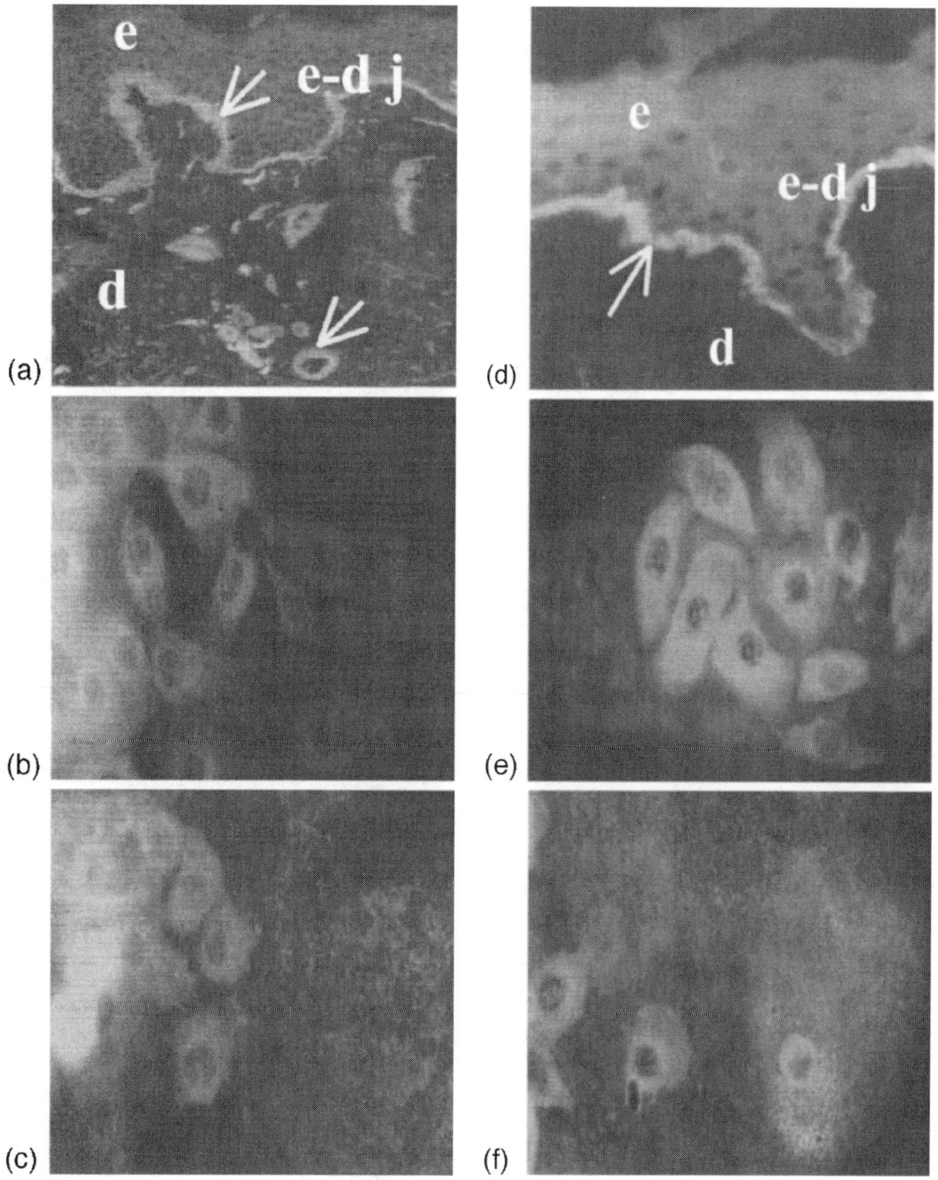
e
e-d j
d
(a)
(b)
(c)
e
e-d j
d
(d)
(e)
(f)

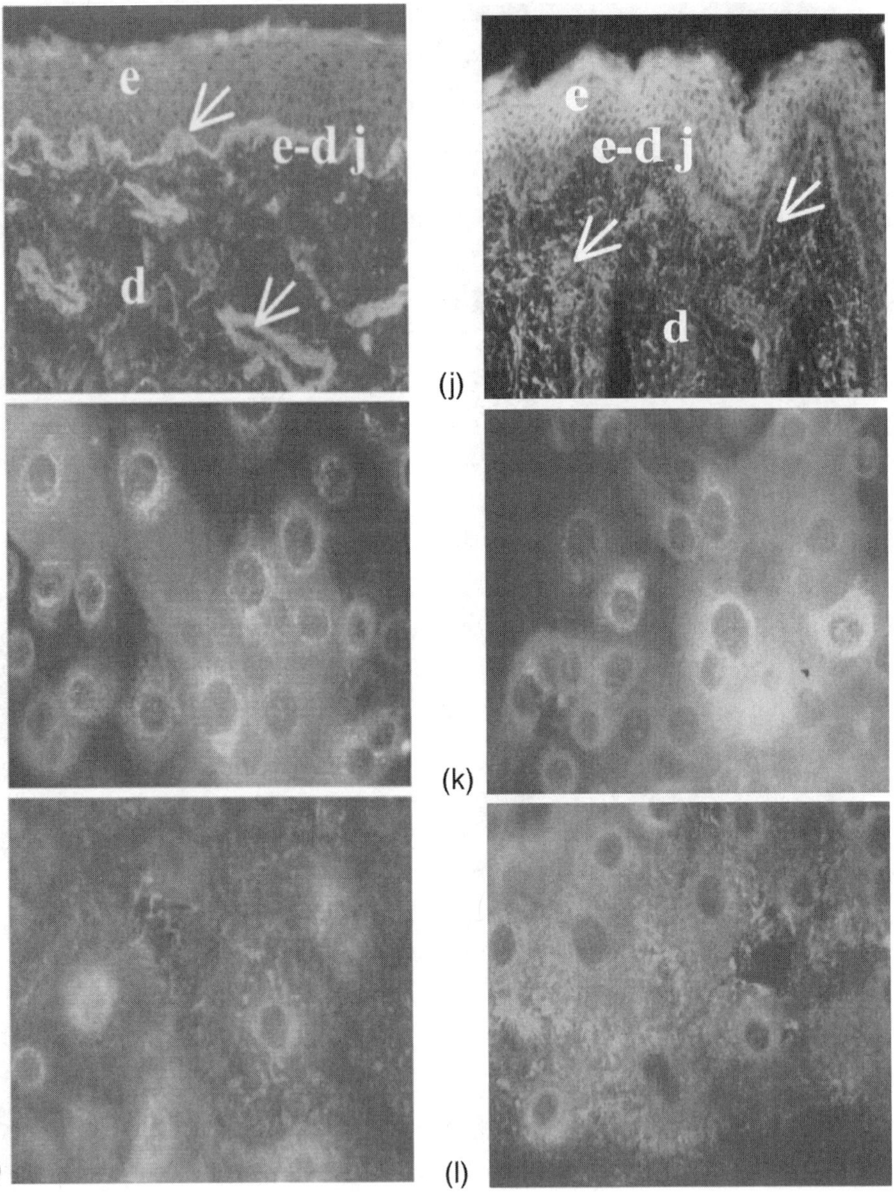

(g) (h) (i) (j) (k) (l)

FIGURE 5 Continued.

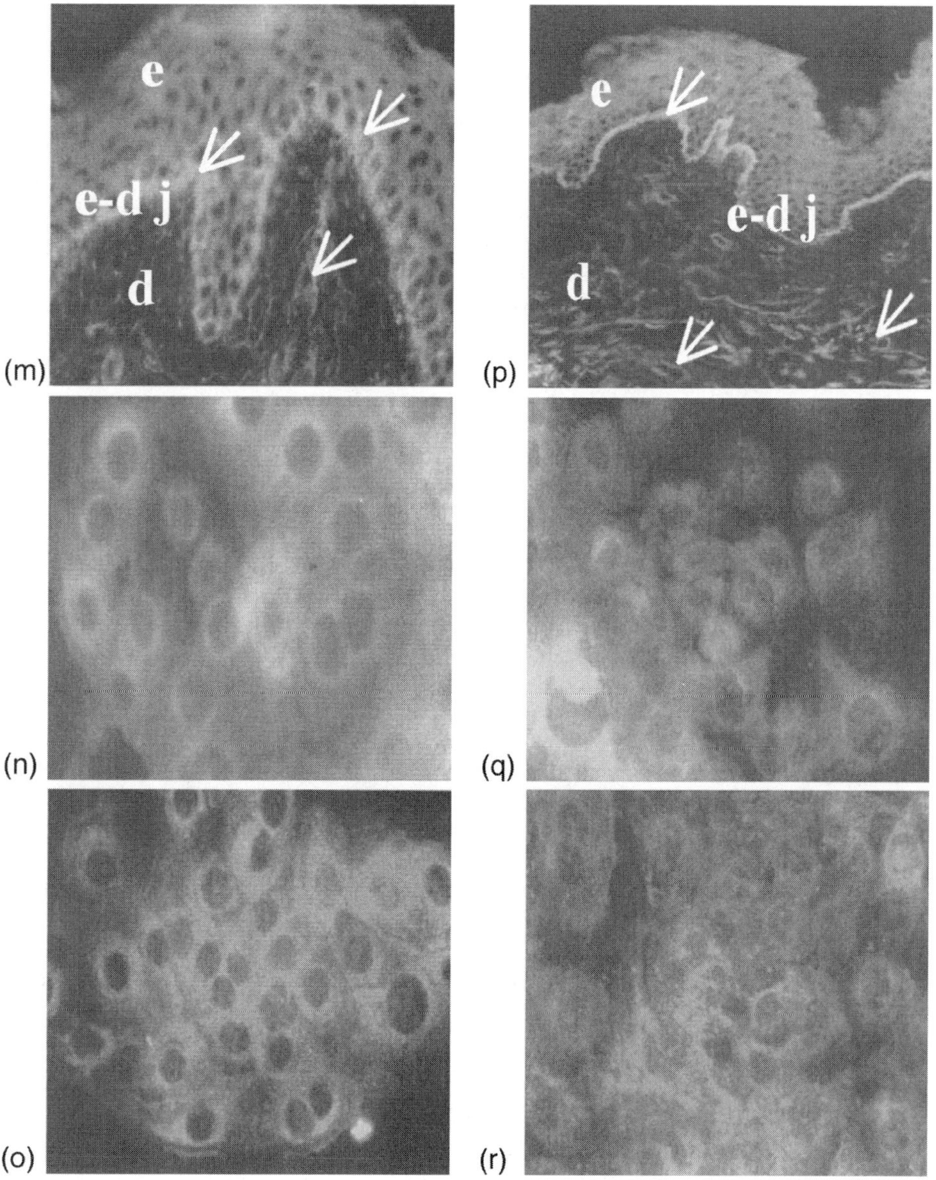

FIGURE 5 Continued.

of cells in low or high doses of oxidants. The 50-μg/mL concentration also had significant and slightly protective effects on fibroblasts against both H_2O_2- and HX/XO-induced damage. For keratinocytes, the dose-dependent relationship of oxidant toxicity was seen only in H_2O_2 but the protective strength of the extract correlated with the oxidant dosage. The extract at 400 μg/mL and 800 μg/mL showed dose-dependent effects on both low and high concentrations of oxidants. The concentration at 50 μg/mL had no effect on keratinocytes (Phan et al., 2001a).

In this study, H_2O_2- and HX/XO- generated superoxides (O^{2-}) were employed as an in vitro model to cause cultured skin cell injury, on which the protective effects of the *C. odorata* extract fractions were assessed.

The effects of column fractions from the extract on human dermal fibroblasts and epidermal keratinocytes, which are pivotal and crucial in cutaneous wound repair, were further evaluated. Hydrogen peroxide and superoxide radicals generated by the HX/XO reactions were employed to induce oxidative stress to in vitro cell cultures. The cytotoxicity of the oxidants and the protective effects of the extracts were indirectly assessed via cell viability. The most active antioxidant compounds were also identified using HPLC and LC-MS technology. Fractions B and C consistently showed the most protective effects on skin cell cultures injured by hydrogen peroxide

---

FIGURE 6 Protective effect of the column fractions of *C. odorata* extract on H_2O_2 and xanthine-oxidase-induced damage to human dermal fibroblasts. Cells were incubated for 3 hr at 37°C with 2×10^{-4} mol/L H_2O_2 (6A) or 2×10^{-2} units/mL xanthine oxidase (b) with or without fractions. Cells were then washed and assayed by the MTT assay. Bars represent mean ± SEM of seven wells. Comparison with cells exposed to generated oxidants with or without fractions is indicated ($p < .001$). Fractions B and C show perfect protection on fibroblasts injured by oxidants.

Protective effect of the column fractions of *C. odorata* extract on H_2O_2 and xanthine-oxidase-induced damage to human epidermal keratinocytes. Cells were incubated for 3 hr at 37°C with 2×10^{-4} mol/L H_2O_2 (c) or 2×10^{-2} units/ml xanthine oxidase (d) with or without fractions. Cells were then washed and assayed by the MTT assay. Bars represent mean ± SEM of seven wells. Comparison with cells exposed to generated oxidants with or without fractions is indicated. Fractions A, B, and C show good or almost complete protection on keratinocytes injured by oxidants ($p < .001$, .05, respectively).

Human keratinocytes exposed to hydrogen peroxide damage without (e) or with (f) *C. odorata* protection. (e) Keratinocytes were killed under toxicity of hydrogen peroxide. (f) Keratinocytes were protected by *C. odorata* extract fraction. (With permission for reprint from the Biological and Pharmacological Bulletin.)

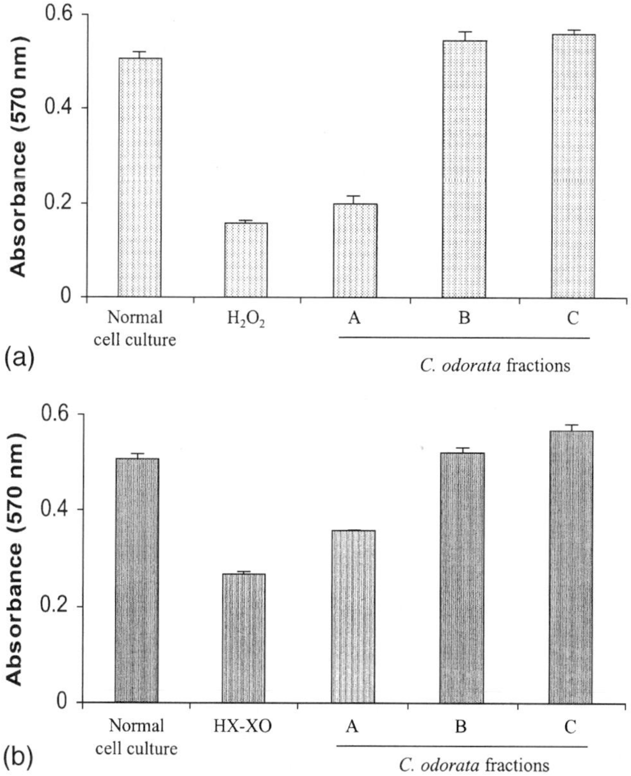

and superoxide radicals in vitro (Fig. 6). Chemical analysis of these fractions (see Table 1) indicated that the major constituents in fraction B were *p*-coumaric acid (*p*-CA = 4-hydroxycinnamic acid) and *p*-hydroxybenzoic acid (*p*-HBA = 4-hydroxybenzoic acid) and that the major compound in fraction C was protocatechuic acid (PCA = 3,4-dihydroxybenzoic acid). Minor compounds in fraction B were ferulic acid (FA = 4-hydroxy-3-methoxycinnamic acid) and vanillic acid (VA = 4-hydroxy-3-methoxybenzoic acid) and a tetrahydroxy-monomethoxyflavanone. The same flavanone, VA and *p*-CA, were minor constituents in fraction C. *p*-HBA is an important natural antioxidant. It is well established as an in vitro effective hydroxyl radical scavenger and has Trolox equivalent antioxidant activity (TEAC) (Rice-Evans et al., 1996; Ohsugi et al., 1999). Other published pharmacological characteristics of *p*-HBA are antibacterial and hypoglycemic properties (Orjala et al., 1993; Cho et al., 1998). The presence of *p*-HBA in the extract can account for its bacterial-growth inhibition in human wounds observed previously by clinical researchers.

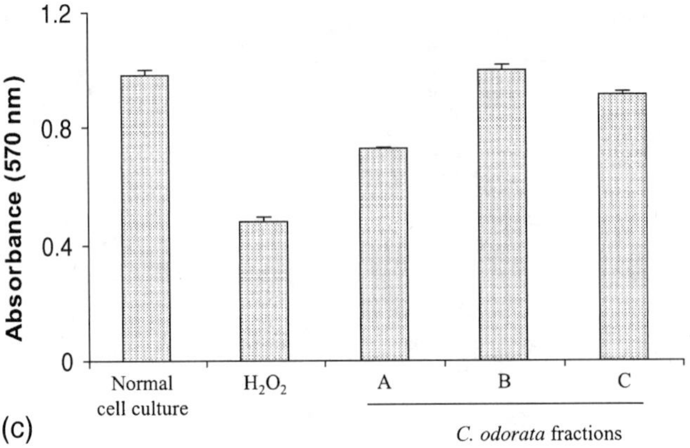

(c)

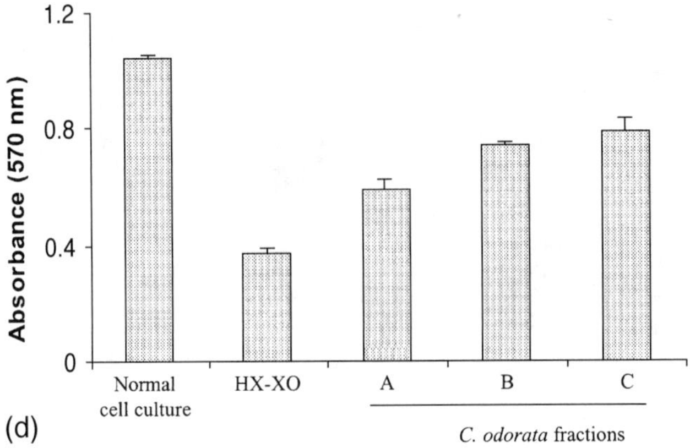

(d)

Figure 6 Continued.

Another hydroxybenzoic acid, protocatechuic acid (PCA), was detected in fraction C of the extract as a major compound. PCA also is a strongly antioxidant phenolic acid. A number of reports described PCA as a potential chemopreventive agent against carcinogenesis and tumor promotions (Tanaka et al., 1995). PCA isolated from traditional herbal medicines showed strong inhibitory activity against superoxide anion radical (O^{2-}) (Ohsugi et al., 1999). PCA was also found to have similar protective effects as caffeic acid in terms of exhibition of potent protection on cultured endothelial cells against oxidized low-density lipoproteins (Vieira et al., 1998). In the studies of a polyphenolic extract from *Cudrania cochinchinesis*, another medicinal plant

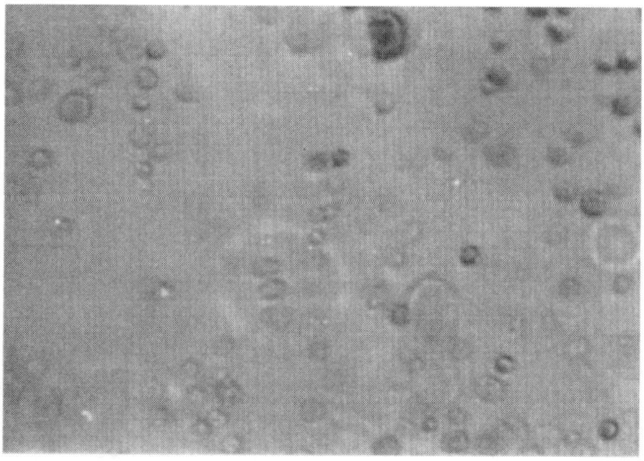

(e)

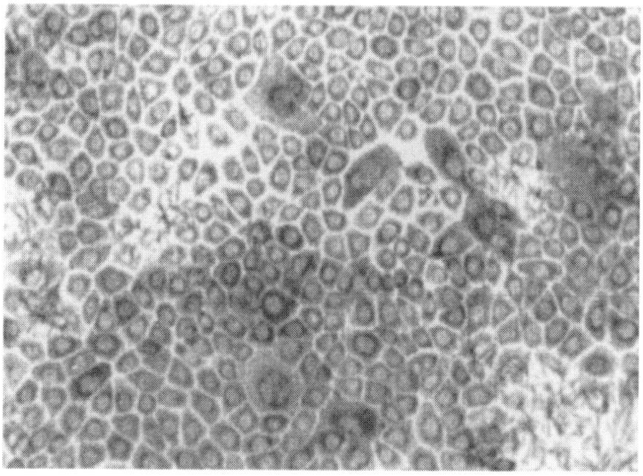

(f)

FIGURE 6 Continued.

for wound healing, PCA was the major constituent and was speculated to be responsible for protection of fibroblasts and endothelial cells against hydrogen peroxide– and HX/XO-induced damage and to be a stimulator of fibroblast proliferation (Tran et al., 1997). A third hydroxybenzoic acid, vanillic acid (VA), was found in both fractions B and C. This compound has anti-inflammatory activity in vitro (Harborne et al., 1999).

The *C. odorata* extract also contains two hydroxycinnamic acid derivatives, *p*-coumaric acid (*p*-CA) and ferulic acid (FA). *p*-CA is a major constituent in fraction B and a minor one in fraction C. Hydroxycinnamic acids such as *p*-CA, FA, and caffeic and chlorogenic acids are among the

TABLE 1 Major and Minor Constituents of Fractions A, B, and C

Purified fraction	Constituents	Compound class	Retention time (min)	UV spectrum (nm)	Molecular mass (m/z)
A	Tamarixetin[a]	Flavonol	19.8	254, 369	316
	Trihydroxy-monomethoxy-flavanone[a]	Flavanone	19.1	290, 330sh	302
	Pentamethoxy-flavanone[a]	Flavanone	19.3	290, 330sh	374
	Dihydroxy-trimethoxy-chalcone[a]	Chalcone	23.1	237, 373	330
	Eupatilin[a]	Flavone	21.4	269, 342	344
	5,6,7,4′-Tetramethoxy-flavone	Flavone	22.4	265, 322	342
	5-Hydroxy-6,7,3′,4′-tetramethoxyflavone	Flavone	22.2	275, 341	358
	Kaempferide	Flavonol	23.2	264, 362	300
	Protocatechuic acid	Hydroxybenzoic acid	4.4	259, 294	154
B	*p*-Coumaric acid[a]	Hydroxycinnamic acid	11.7	290sh, 309	164

	p-Hydroxybenzoic acid[a]	Hydroxybenzoic acid	7.1	255	138
	Ferulic acid	Hydroxycinnamic acid	12.3	300sh, 322	194
	Vanillic acid	Hydroxybenzoic acid	8.1	259, 292	168
	Tetrahydroxy-monomethoxy-flavanone[a]	Flavanone	17.3	290, 340sh	318
C	Protocatechuic acid[a]	Hydroxybenzoic acid	4.4	259, 294	154
	Vanillic acid	Hydroxybenzoic acid	8.1	258, 293	168
	p-Coumaric acid	Hydroxycinnamic acid	11.7	290sh, 309	164
	Tetrahydroxy-monomethoxy-flavanone	Flavanone	17.3	290, 340sh	318
	Sinensetin	Flavone	20.7	240, 266sh, 331	372
	Rhamnetin	Flavonol	21.4	255, 371	316

sh, shoulder or inflection.
[a] Major constituents.

most widely distributed phenylpropanoids in plant tissues (Rice-Evans et al., 1996) and their biological activities have been widely investigated. They are potential chemopreventive agents against carcinogenesis and tumor growth (Rice-Evans et al., 1996) and they are also recognized to be strong free-radical scavengers to hydroxyl radicals (Rice-Evans et al., 1996; Zang et al., 2000).

Hydroxycinnamic acid derivatives were also found to be effective inhibitors of xanthine oxidase. The phenolic OH group, present in their molecules, displays an important contribution to the XO-inhibitory activities. The absence of this group in the molecule induces the reduction of the inhibition on XO (Chang et al., 1994; Chan et al., 1995). Other antioxidant activities of hydroxycinnamic acid derivatives have been reported. They were able to scavenge reactive species of oxygen and nitrogen (Nakayama, 1994; Harborne et al., 1999). The presence of representatives of two groups of antioxidant phenolic acids (hydroxybenzoic and hydroxycinnamic acids) in fractions B and C can account for their strong inhibition of the cytotoxicity of superoxide radicals and hydrogen peroxide (H_2O_2).

To investigate the synergistic effect of the *C. odorata* lipophilic fractions on skin cells, solutions of pure *p*-HBA, PCA, *p*-CA, and FA (Sigma) in similar concentrations to those of *C. odorata* fractions were applied on fibroblasts and keratinocytes injured by H_2O_2 or HX/XO. No protection was observed in these experiments, suggesting that the single compounds provided less effect than the mixture of compounds in the *C. odorata* fractions. On the other hand, phenolic compounds in the extract worked in a synergistic manner to protect skin cells from oxidative damage, leading to enhanced healing.

Two well-known antioxidant compounds, α-tocopherol and curcumin (Sigma), were also tested in comparison with *C. odorata* fractions. The α-tocopherol solution, at the same concentrations as the extract fractions, showed about 50% less protective effects on skin cells than fractions B and C. Curcumin has strong protective effect on fibroblasts and keratinocytes against H_2O_2 damage. But there was no effect on HX/XO-induced damage (Phan et al., 2001c).

Fraction A contained mostly methoxylated flavonoids (flavonols, flavanones, flavones, and a chalcone, see Table 1). Although a variety of different flavonoids had already been reported from *C. odorata* (Barua et al., 1978; Triaratana et al., 1991), our present investigations revealed that many more are present in the plant, especially flavanones. Some of the compounds have been demonstrated earlier to be responsible for the hemostatic effect of the *C. odorata* extract (Triaratana et al., 1991). The presence in fraction A of tamarixetin and kaempferide, which are the 4′-methyl ethers of the well-known antioxidant and anti-inflammatory flavonols quercetin and kaempferol, and of small amounts of protocatechuic acid can explain some of the protective effects on keratinocytes injured by superoxide radicals and H_2O_2. These mixtures of phenolic compounds in the lipophilic fractions of *C. odorata* are likely to be the major contributors to the antioxidant properties of this plant species. In addition, kaempferide has been reported to inhibit inflammation induced by tumor-promoting phorbol esters, and the flavone eupatilin, which is also present in fraction A, selectively inhibits 5-lipoxygenase of cultured mastocytoma cells (Harborne et al., 1999).

It has been scientifically demonstrated that the extract of *C. odorata* has therapeutic properties in some aspects of wound healing. The results of this study suggest that one of the possible mechanisms by which *C. odorata* contributes to wound healing could be the antioxidant effect of the phenolics present. PCA, *p*-HBA, also the *p*-CA, FA, and VA, the major constituents of fractions B and C, are also the main active compounds of many medicinal plants including plants for wound healing, and many biological activities and potential therapeutic applications of these compounds have been reported. Although these compounds are not new, this is the first time, to our knowledge, that these acids were identified in an extract of *C. odorata* and demonstrated to be responsible for the protection of cultured skin cells against oxidative damage. The flavonoids identified in the various fractions are likely to have a synergistic effect.

IV. CONCLUSION

Crude extract of *C. odorata* has been used successfully for treating wounds. In this study, the therapeutic properties of the *C. odorata* extract were demonstrated scientifically with:

- enhanced proliferation of fibroblasts, endothelial cell, and keratinocytes;
- stimulation of keratinocyte migration;
- upregulation of keratinocyte production of extracellular matrix proteins and basement membrane components;
- protection of skin cells against oxidative damage;
- antioxidant effects of a mixture of phenolic compounds found in the extract

The activities shown in this study provide an important scientific basis for understanding how the *C. odorata* extract could have benefited wound healing in vivo and leads to further speculation that these properties could explain the observed enhancement of wound healing. These findings also provide a rationale for the wide use of *C. odorata* preparations in tropical countries to treat burns and wounds, regardless of income and status, with the potential to improve the quality of life of patients at low cost.

The clinical efficacy of this plant extract or its preparations should be further investigated by prospective, randomized, controlled trials. Perhaps a new potent agent for wound healing could be developed from this plant extract.

ABBREVIATIONS

APCI-MS	Atmospheric pressure chemical ionization mass spectrometry
ChA	Chlorogenic acid
CID	Collision induced dissociation
DAD	Diode array detection
DMF	*N,N*-Dimethyformamide
DMEM	Dulbecco's modified eagle medium
FA	Ferulic acid
FCS	Fetal calf serum
HBSS	Hanks' balanced salt solution
HPLC	High-performance liquid chromatography
H_2O_2	Hydrogen peroxide
HX-XO	Hypoxanthine-xanthine oxidase
KBM	Keratinocyte basal medium
KGM	Keratinocyte growth medium
MTT	[3-(4,5-Dimethylthiazol-2-yl)2,5-diphenyltetrazolium bromide]
PBS	Phosphate-buffered saline
PCA	Protocatechuic acid
p-CA	*para*-Coumaric acid
p-HBA	*para*-Hydroxybenzoic acid

REFERENCES

Akah PA. Mechanism of hemostatic activity of *Eupatorium odoratum*. J Crude Drug Res 1990; 28:235–253.

Amenta PS, Martinez-Hernandez A, Trelstad R. Repair and regeneration. In: Damjanov I, Linder J, eds. Anderson's Pathology. Vol. 1. St. Louis: Mosby-Year Book, 1996.

Barua RN, Sharma RP, Thyagarajan G, Herz W. Flavonoids from *Chromolaena odorata*. Phytochemistry 1978; 17:1807–1808.

Caceres A. Antigonorrhoeal activity of plant used in Guatemala for the treatment of sexually transmitted diseases. J Ethnopharmacol 1995; 48:85–88.

Chan WS, Wen PC, Chiang HC. Structure-activity relationship of caffeic acid analogues on xanthine oxidase inhibition. Anticancer Res 1995; 15:703–708.

Chang WS, Chang YH, Lu FJ, Chiang HC. Inhibitory effects of phenolics on xanthine oxidase. Anticancer Res 1994; 14:501–506.

Cherry GW, Hughes MA, Kingsnorth AN, Arnold FW. Wound healing. In: Morris PJ, Malt RA, eds. Oxford Textbook of Surgery. Vol. 1. Oxford: Oxford University Press, 1994.

Cho JY, Moon JH, Seong KY, Park KH. Antimicrobial activity of 4-hydroxybenzoic acid and *trans* 4-hydroxycinnamic acid isolated and identified from rice hull. Biosci Biotechnol Biochem 1998; 62:2273–2276.

Harborne JB, Baxter H, Moss GP. Phytochemical Dictionary. London: Taylor & Francis, 1999.

Holm GLR. *Chromolaena odorata*. In: Holm GLR, Plucknet DL, Pancho JV, Herberger JP, eds. The World's Worst Weeds: Distribution and Biology. Honolulu: University Press of Hawaii, 1977.

Irobi ON. Activities of *Chromolaena odorata* (Compositae) leaf extract against *Pseudomonas aeroginosa* and *Streptococcus faecalis*. J Ethnopharmacol 1992; 37:81–83.

Le TT. The use of Eupolin prepared from *Eupatorium odoratum* to treat soft tissue wounds. T 5th European Tissue Repair Society Annual Meeting, Padova, Italy, 1995.

Nakayama T. Suppression of hydroperoxide-induced cytotoxicity by polyphenols. Cancer Res 1994; 54:1991s–1993s.

Ohsugi M, Fan W, Hase K, Xiong Q, Tezuka Y. Active-oxygen scavenging activity of traditional nourishing-tonic herbal medicines and active constituents of *Rhodiola sacra*. J Ethnopharmacol 1999; 67:111–119.

Orjala J, Erdelmeier CA, Wright AD, Rali T, Sticher O. Five new prenylated *p*-hydroxybenzoic acid derivatives with antimicrobial and molluscicidal activity from *Piper aduncum* leaves. Planta Med 1993; 59:546–551.

Phan TT, Hughes MA, Cherry GW. Enhanced proliferation of fibroblasts and endothelial cells treated with an aqueous extract from the leaves of *Chromoleana odorata* (Eupolin), a herbal remedy for treating wounds. Plast Reconstruct Surg 1998; 101:756–765.

Phan TT, Lee ST, Chan SY, Hughes MA, Cherry GW. Investigating plant-based medicines for wound healing with the use of cell culture technologies and in vitro models: a review. Ann Acad Med Singapore 2000a; 29:27–36.

Phan TT, Allen J, Hughes MA, Cherry GW, Wojnarowska F. Upregulation of the epidermal basement membrane and extracellular matrix proteins by human keratinocytes treated with an aqueous extract from the leaves of *Chromolaena odorata* (Eupolin). Eu J Dermatol 2000b; 10(7):522–527.

Phan TT, See J, Lee ST, Chan SY. Antioxidant effects of the extracts from the leaves of *Chromolaena odorata* on human dermal fibroblasts and epidermal keratinocytes against hydrogen peroxide and hypoxanthine-xanthine oxidase induced damage. Burns 2001a; 27(4):319–327.

Phan TT, Hughes MA, Cherry GW. Effects of an aqueous extract from the leaves of *Chromoleana odorata* (Eupolin) on human keratinocytes proliferation and migration in an in vitro model of wound re-epithelialization. Wound Repair Regen 2001b; 9(4):305–313.

Phan TT, See P, Lee ST, Chan SY. Protective effect of curcumin on skin cells in vitro against oxidative damage: its implication for wound healing. Trauma 2001c; 51(5):927–931.

Phan TT, Wang LZ, See P, Grayer RJ, Chan SY, Lee ST. Phenolic compounds of *Chromoleana odorata* protect cultured skin cells from oxidative damage: implication for cutaneous wound healing. Biol Pharmacol Bull 2001d; 24(12):1373–1379.

Rice-Evans CA, Miller NJ, Paganga G. Structure-antioxidant activity relationships of flavonoids and phenolic acids. Free Rad Biol Med 1996; 20:933–956.

Singer AJ, Clark RAF. Cutaneous wound healing. N Engl J Med 1999; 341:738–746.

Tanaka T, Kojima T, Kawamori T, Mori H. Chemoprevention of digestive organs carcinogenesis by natural product protocatechuic acid. Cancer 1995; 75:1433–1439.

Tran VH, Hughes MA, Cherry GW. In vitro studies on the antioxidant and growth stimulatory activities of a polyphenolic extract from *Cudrania cochichinensis* used in the treatment of wounds in Vietnam. Wound Repair Regen 1997; 5:159–167.

Triaratana T, Suwannuraks R, Naengchomnong W. Effect of *Eupatorium odoratum* on blood coagulation. J Med Assoc Thailand 1991; 74(5 suppl):283–286.

Uitto J, Mauviel A, McGrath J. The derma-epidermal basement membrane zones in cutaneous wound healing. In: Clark RAF, ed. The Molecular and Cellular Biology of Wound Repair. New York: Plenum Press, 1996.

Vieira O, Escargueil-Blanc I, Meihac O, Basile JB. Effect of dietary phenolic compounds on apoptosis of human cultured endothelial cells induced by oxidized LDL. Br J Pharmacol 1998; 123:565–573.

Woodley D. Re-epithelialization. In: Clark RAF, ed. The Molecular and Cellular Biology of Wound Repair. New York: Plenum Press, 1996.

Zang LY, Cosma G, Gardner H, Shi XL, Castranova V, Vallyathan V. Effect of antioxidant protection by *p*-coumaric acid on low-density lipoprotein cholesterol oxidation. Am J Physiol 2000; 279:C954–C960.

38

Medicinal Properties of Eucommia Bark and Leaves

Eu Leong Yong
National University of Singapore
Republic of Singapore

I. INTRODUCTION

Eucommia ulmoides Oliver (Du-Zhong) (EU), of the family Eucommiacaea, is a large deciduous tree originating in China. The bark of the tree (commonly referred to as cortex eucommiae) has been used as a natural medicine since ancient times in China (1,2). Currently, the herb is widely used as decoctions or commercially manufactured pills, essences, and extracts in Chinese communities worldwide especially in mainland China, Taiwan, Hong Kong, and Singapore. In Japan, dried eucommia leaves are consumed commonly as Tochu tea. The trunk bark of *E. ulcommia ulmoides* Oli is produced mainly in the Sichuan, Yunnan, Guizhou, Hubei, and Shanxi provinces of China. The bark is stripped off between April and June. After the coarse outer corky layer is scraped off, the bark pieces are piled up until the inner surface becomes purplish-brown and then dried in the sun. The large bark is cut into segments and stir-baked with salt. This herb is called fried "eucommia bark" or "eucommia bark charcoal." The herb appears as flattened pieces that are 3–7 mm thick. The outer surface of the bark is fissured longitudinally. Pieces are easily broken from the bark and such pieces are linked by fine, dense silvery and elastic rubber bands. The tree has been cultivated for its rubber.

II. CLASSIC ACTION AND USES

In ancient pharmacopoeia, the herb is used to tonify the liver and kidney, to strengthen bones and tendons, and to prevent miscarriage (1,2). Decoctions of eucommia bark have been used for, among other things, the relief of back pain, to increase strength, to make bones and muscles strong, to increase recovery from fatigue, to increase ability to remember, and to induce an antiaging effect. It is prepared as Du-Zhong tincture (5 or 100%), 1–5 mL taken orally thrice daily. It is frequently formulated with ginseng, *Cordyceps*, angelica root, and many other herbs (3). Ingestion of EU bark and leaves and their extracts has not been reported to induce any known side effects.

A. Formulation

A synergistic effect by using the leaves of *E. ulmoides* Oliver, Eucomiaceae (Du-Zhong leaf) and the roots of *Panax ginseng* C. A. Meyer (Ginseng) has been reported (4). The formula consists of amounts that exert no effect when used individually. Several formula ratios of ginseng and Du-Zhong leaf, 1:1, 1:2, 1:3, and 1:4, were tested. It was demonstrated that the formula ratio of ginseng to Du-Zhong leaf of 1:3 was the most effective for stimulation of collagen synthesis and prevention of decreased protein metabolism in aging (4).

III. CHEMISTRY

The herb contains irridoids, phenols (pyrogallol, protocatechuic acid, and *p-trans*-coumaric acid), tannins, coumarin, lactones and their glycosides, alkaloids, triterpenes, saponins, (+)-pinoresinol-di-*O*-β-D-glucopyranoside, catechol, 3-(3-hydroxyphenyl)propionic acid, dihydrocaffeic acid, guiacyglycerol, *trans*-4-hydroxycyclohexane-1-carboxylic acid resins, long-chain poly-*trans* prenols (>9 mers), ajugoside, reptoside, harpagide acetate ($C_{26}H_{32}O_{12}$), other organic acids, and some alkaloids (5–9). Among the constituents, irridoids are considered to be bioactive; these include geniposidic acid, geniposide, asperulosidic acid, deacetyl asperulosidic acid, asperuloside, and their glycoxylated derivatives such as encommiol ($C_9H_{16}O_4$) and 1-deoxyeucommiol and aucubin ($C_{15}H_{22}O_9$). Three percent of the leaf contains cholorogenic acid. The biological actions of many of these compounds have not been investigated.

A. Effect of Processing

Processing affects the chemical composition of the herb. Concentrations of compounds in eucommia are influenced by the area where it is produced, harvest time, and treatment after harvesting. Thus the content of pinoresinol diglucoside in postprocessed bark is higher than that in preprocessed bark (10). Leaves collected from June to September had an aucubin content that was 2.5% higher than at other times (11). On the other hand, geniposidic acid concentration was 5.5% higher in June and July. Since leaves are usually harvested in October and November, the levels of the suspected bioactives, aucubin and geniposidic acid, are actually lowest in marketed Tochu leaves.

IV. TOXICITY AND DRUG METABOLISM

When the dose of geniposide was higher than 50 mg/kg/day, toxicity was encountered in rat models (12). Eucommia leaf extracts also increased the activities of cytochrome P450 and carboxylesterase and accelerated detoxification of an organophosphorus insecticide, chlorpyrifos, in the livers of mice pretreated with the herbal extract (13). This increase in liver metabolism may have implications for other ingested drugs that are metabolized in the liver.

V. BIOLOGICAL ACTIONS

Modern research on the mode of action of eucommia has been performed in only limited number of laboratories, most notably from the group at Nihon University, Chiba, Japan (4,5,12,14–18). Efforts have focused on verifying the basis of the herb's traditional use to strengthen bone and muscles. More modern approaches include studies on its potential applications as an antimutagenic agent, as an antioxidant, antihypertensive, hypocholesterolemic agent, and also as an antibiotic against bacteria, fungi, and viruses.

A. Muscle Strength, Stamina, Collagen Metabolism

It has been noted that the muscles of eels fed Tochu leaf powder were 1.8 times harder than those of the controls (19). Although the component analysis showed no difference in moisture, lipid, or protein content between the muscles of control and Tochu-fed eels, there was a great difference in the amount of muscle protein stroma fraction that consisted of collagen. The perimysium and endomysium of the muscle was observed microscopically to be firm and thick compared to control. The administration of *E. ulmoides* Oliver leaf along with light intensity training was reported to enhance the ability of a muscle to resist fatigue in rat studies (16). Mechanical training and the use of EU leaf extracts cooperatively can increase the ability of rats to avoid lactate accumulation in skeletal muscle, and the administration of the EU leaf along with light intensity training enhances the ability of a muscle to resist fatigue. EU leaves contain compounds similar to the bark and are reported to have similar pharmacological effects. Since irridoid monoglycosides, such as geniposidic acid and aucubin, in EU can stimulate collagen synthesis in aged model rats (15), it is thought that the active compounds are actually geniposidic acid or aucubin (17).

Granuloma maturation and deposition of collagen in the granuloma of rats were also reported to be improved by the oral administration of *E. ulmoides* Oliver leaf (12). Granuloma formation, induced by the formalin-soaked filter-paper-pellet method, was significantly increased owing to ingestion of the dried leaf at a dose of 1.8 g/kg of body weight/day. The collagen content in the granuloma was also significantly increased. In the case of the collagen profile, the pepsin-solubilized collagen content and its relative percentage of the total collagen were significantly higher than in the control. Histochemical examination showed that the granuloma tissues were well developed and displayed many newly synthesized capillary vessels and a greater quantity of fibroblasts and monocytes in the 1.8-g-leaf group. High-density-lipoprotein (HDL) cholesterol and triglyceride content in the blood plasma were significantly higher than in the control. These results suggest that granuloma maturation was accelerated and the energy was supplied from fatty acid metabolism. Eucommiol, a main component in the water fraction of the methanol extract, was found to be the effective compound and geniposidic acid and aucubin were the main effective compounds in the leaf for collagen synthesis. The administration of geniposidic acid or aucubin stimulated collagen synthesis in aged model rats (18) Thus administration of *E. ulmoides* Oliver leaf may be effective in speeding up the wound-healing process.

B. Antimutagenic Activity

Crude extracts of Tochu tea were able to suppress the induction of chromosome aberrations in CHO cells and mice (7). When CHO cells were treated with Tochu tea crude extract after MMC treatment, the frequency of chromosome aberrations was reduced. Of 17 Tochu tea components, five irridoids (geniposidic acid, geniposide, asperulosidic acid, deacetyl asperulosidic acid, and asperuloside) and three phenols (pyrogallol, protocatechuic acid, and *p-trans*-coumaric acid) were found to have anticlastogenic activity. Since the anticlastogenic irridoids had an α-unsaturated carbonyl group, this structure was considered to play an important role in the anticlastogenicity (protective effect against chromosomal aberrations). The mutagenic potential of eucommia was studied with the Ames test (20). *E. ulmoides* Oliver was found to significantly induce His^+ revertants in *Salmonella typhimurium*

TA98 and/or TA100. The mutagenicity of Tochu tea in the urine before and after ingestion of raw fish and cooked beef had been studied using *S. typhimurium* YG1024 (21). Urine samples were examined from seven healthy, nonsmoking Japanese women before and after ingestion of raw fish and cooked beef. The mutagenicity of urine from the Tochu-tea-drinking group was much lower. Similar results were observed when the women switched groups; the tea-drinking group became the control group, and the control group became the Tochu-tea-drinking group. Again, the mutagenicity of urine collected from the Tochu-tea-drinking group was much lower. These results suggest that the decrease in the mutagenicity of the urine from the Tochu-tea-drinking group was due to the intake of Tochu tea, suggesting that the ingestion of Tochu tea may reduce human exposure to dietary mutagens.

C. Antioxidant Action

The molecular mechanism of this antimutagenic activity may be related to its reported antioxidant properties. Leaf extract of Du-Zhong had an inhibitory effect on oxidative damage in biomolecules such as deoxyribose, DNA, and 2′-deoxyguanosine (2′-dG) as induced by the Fenton reaction (22). All of the Du-Zhong extract inhibited the oxidation of deoxyribose induced by $Fe^{(3+)}$-EDTA/H_2O_2/ascorbic acid in a concentration-dependent manner. At a concentration of 1.14 mg/mL, the inhibitory effect of the extracts of leaves, roasted cortex, and raw cortex was 85.2%, 68.0%, and 49.3%, respectively. The extract of leaves inhibited the strand breaking of DNA induced by the Fenton reaction at concentrations of 5 and 10 μg/μL. The leaf extract had a marked inhibitory effect on Fenton-reaction-induced oxidative damage in biomolecules. The extract of roasted cortex exhibited modest inhibition while the extract of raw cortex had the least inhibitory effect on oxidative damage in biomolecules. This is in contrast to gallic acid in the same reaction system, whose higher reducing power and weaker chelating ability may contribute to its pro-oxidant effect. Biologically active compounds from Du-Zhong leaves, raw cortex, and roasted cortex demonstrated free-radical or reactive oxygen species (ROS)-scavenging effect (23). The hot-water extract of Du-Zhong leaves showed marked activity as a ROS scavenger, and the scavenging effect was concentration-dependent. The extract of roasted cortex exhibited a modest scavenging effect on ROS, while the extract of raw cortex had the weakest scavenging effect. The scavenging activity of Du-Zhong extract on ROS was correlated to its protocatechuic acid (PCA) content. The content of PCA in Du-Zhong determined by HPLC followed the order of leaves (17.17 mg/g) > roasted cortex (2.99 mg/g) > raw cortex (1.16 mg/g). The inhibitory activity of leaf extract of Du-Zhong was stronger than that of PCA on the peroxidation of linoleic acid at the same concentration of 0.1 mg/mL. The results indicate that extract of Du-Zhong could possibly act as a prophylactic agent to prevent free-radical-related diseases. Therefore, drinking of Du-Zhong tea over a long period of time may have anticancer potential because of this antioxidant activity.

D. Lipid Metabolism

Du-Zhong leaf extract can suppress significantly the high-fat-diet-induced increases in serum cholesterol and serum triacyglyerol in animal models. The herb was able to suppress diet-induced increases in VLDL and LDL lipolproteins, suggesting the leaf extract may be beneficial for the regulation of hyperlipedimia (14). In another study, administration of 5% Tochu leaf powder was reported to markedly prevent the elevation of serum total cholesterol in a stroke-prone, spontaneously hypertensive rat fed a high-fat-and-high-cholesterol diet (24). High-density lipoprotein (HDL) cholesterol and triglyceride content in the blood plasma were significantly higher than in the control.

E. Antihypertensive Effect

The herb has reported antihypertensive effects that are mild but long in duration (25). It acts centrally and its effects can be reduced by atropine or vagotomy. In low doses it can dilate the peripheral vessels while in high doses it causes vasoconstriction. The herb also has a diuretic effect. The major antihypertensive principle was thought to be pinoresinol diglucoside (26).

F. Antiviral

The alkaline extract of Du-Zhong tea leaves was reported to suppress HIV-induced cytopathicity using HIV (HTLV-III)-infected MT-4 cells, having extremely low cytotoxicity (27). Its 50% effective concentration (EC_{50}) was 12–67 μg/mL, while 50% cytotoxic concentration (CC_{50}) was higher than 1.0 mg/mL. The authors suggest that HIV infection may be suppressed by daily intake of the alkaline extract of Du-Zhong tea.

G. Antifungal Activity

Antifungal peptides have been purified from the bark of *E. ulmoides* Oliver (28). Their primary structures consists of 41 residues with a N-terminal blockage by pyroglutamic acid and all contain 10 cysteines, which are cross-linked to form five disulfide bridges with a pairing pattern (C1–C5, C2–C9, C3–C6, C4–C7, C8–C10). They exhibit relatively broad spectra of antifungal activities against eight pathogenic fungi from cotton, wheat, potato, tomato, and tobacco. Their inhibition activity can be effective on both chitin-containing and chitin-free fungi. The values of IC_{50} range from 35 to 155 μg/mL for EAFP1 and from 18 to 109 μg/mL for EAFP2. Their antifungal effects are strongly antagonized by calcium ions. Five active principles against yeast enzyme were isolated and characterized. Among them, quercetin was considered to contribute mostly to the activity of the Tochu leaves (29).

H. Other Effects

α-Glucosidase inhibitory activity was found in aqueous methanol extracts of Tochu-cha, (29) and anticomplementary activities of its constituents have been described (30). Inhibition of adenosine 3′,5′-cyclic monophosphate phosphodiesterase by lignan glucosides of eucommia bark had been reported (31).

VI. SUMMARY

Although Du-Zhong and Tochu tea have been used for millennia alone, and as part of complex formulations with other herbs, no clinical studies on their effects have been conducted using modern scientific methods. Some of their chemical constituents have been characterized, and a limited number of cell and animal studies have been performed to establish their physiological effects. These animal models suggest that crude extracts of these herbs may increase muscle bulk and stamina and improve collagen deposition and maturation. Antimutagenic, antioxidant, antihypertensive, antiviral, and antifungal properties have been reported in cell and animal studies. The lack of modern human studies makes it difficult to comment on the safety and efficacy of these herbs when used as medicinal drugs.

REFERENCES

1. Herbal Classic of the Divine Ploughman [Shen Nong Ben Cao Chien] circa 100 B.C. Authors unknown.
2. Li SC. [Ben Cao Kong Mu] 1580.
3. Long Zhixian. Beijing University of Traditional Chinese Medicine. Formulas of Traditional Chinese Medicine. Beijing: Academy Press, 1998.
4. Metori K, Furutsu M, Takahashi S. The preventive effect of ginseng with Du-Zhong leaf on protein metabolism in aging. Biol Pharm Bull 1997; 20:237–242.
5. Li JS. Related Articles [Chemical analysis of duzhong (*Eucommia ulmoides*) bark and leaves]. Zhong Yao Tong Bao. 1986; 11:41–42.
6. Hattori M, Che QM, Cewali MB, Yasuyuki T, Kikuchi T, Namba T. 1988 Studies on Du Zhong leaves: constituents of the leaves of *Eucommia ulmoides*. Shoyakugaku Zasshi 1988; 42:76–80.

7. Nakamura T, Nakazawa Y, Onizuka S, Satoh S, Chiba A, Sekihashi K, Miura A, Yasugahira N, Sasaki YF. Antimutagenicity of Tochu tea (an aqueous extract of *Eucommia ulmoides* leaves): 1. The clastogen-suppressing effects of Tochu tea in CHO cells and mice. Mutat Res 1997; 388:7–20.
8. Qi X, Zhang S. [A reversed-phase high performance liquid chromatographic method for the determination of pinoresinol diglucopyranoside in *Eucommia ulmoides* Oliv]. Se Pu. 1998; 16:161–163. Chinese.
9. Bamba T, Fukusaki E, Kajiyama S, Ute K, Kitayama T, Kobayashi A. The occurrence of geometric polyprenol isomers in the rubber-producing plant, *Eucommia ulmoides* Oliver. Lipids 2001; 36:727–732.
10. Hao W, Zhu Z, Zhu Y. Effect of processing on the contents of pinorescinol diglucoside in cortex eucommiae. Zhong Guo Zhong Yao Zazhi 1996; 21:410–411.
11. Koike K, Nakamura H, Takahashi S. The seasonal changes of aucubin and geniposidic acid concentrations in *Eucommia ulmoides* Oliver leaves. Wakan Iyaku Gakkai 1998; 15:225–227. Japanese.
12. Li Y, Metori K, Koike K, Kita F, Che QM, Sato T, Shirai W, Takahashi S. Granuloma maturation in the rat is advanced by the oral administration of *Eucommia ulmoides* Oliver leaf. Biol Pharm Bull 2000; 23:60–65.
13. Furutsu M, Koyama Y, Kusakabe M, Takahashi S. Preventive effect of Du Chong leaves and ginseng root on acute toxicity of chloritos. Jpn J Toxicol Environ Health 1997; 43:92–100.
14. Metori K, Obashi S, Takahasi S, Tamura T. Effect of Du Zhong leaf extract on serum and hepatic lipids in rats fed a high fat diet. Biol Pharm Bull 1994; 17:917–920.
15. Li Y, Kamo S, Metori K, Koike K, Che QM, Takahashi S. The promoting effect of eucommiol from eucommiae cortex on collagen synthesis. Biol Pharm Bull 2000; 23:54–59.
16. Li Y, Koike K, Che Q, Yamaguchi M, Takahashi S. Changes in lactate dehydrogenase and 3-hydroxyacetyl-CoA dehydrogenase activities in rat skeletal muscle by the administration of *Eucommia ulmoides* Oliver leaf with spontaneous running-training. Biol Pharm Bull 1999; 22:941–946.
17. Li Y, Metori K, Koike K, Che QM, Takahashi S. Improvement in the turnover rate of the stratum corneum in false aged model rats by the administration of geniposidic acid in *Eucommia ulmoides* Oliver leaf Biol Pharm Bull 1999; 22:582–585.
18. Li Y, Sato T, Metori K, Koike K, Che QM, Takahashi S. The promoting effects of geniposidic acid and aucubin in *Eucommia ulmoides* Oliver leaves on collagen synthesis. Biol Pharm Bull 1998; 21:1306–1310.
19. Tanimoto S, Ikuma K, Takahashi S. 1993 Studies on the efficacy of Tochu leaf on muscle protein. Part I. Improvement in raw meat texture of cultured eel by feeding of tochu leaf powder. Biosci Biotechnol Biochem 1993; 57:205–208.
20. Yin XJ, Liu DX, Wang HC, Zhou Y. A study on the mutagenicity of 102 raw pharmaceuticals used in Chinese traditional medicine. Mutat Res 1991; 260:73–82.

21. Sasaki YF, Chiba A, Murakami M, Sekihashi K, Tanaka M, Takahoko M, Moribayashi S, Kudou C, Hara Y, Nakazawa Y, Nakamura T, Onizuka S. Antimutagenicity of Tochu tea (an aqueous extract of *Eucommia ulmoides* leaves). 2. Suppressing effect of Tochu tea on the urine mutagenicity after ingestion of raw fish and cooked beef. Mutat Res 1996; 371:203–214.
22. Hsieh CL, Yen GC. Antioxidant actions of Du-Zhong (*Eucommia ulmoides* Oliv.) toward oxidative damage in biomolecules. Life Sci 2000; 66:1387–1400.
23. Yen GC, Hsieh CL. Reactive oxygen species scavenging activity of Du-Zhong (*Eucommia ulmoides* Oliv.) and its active compounds. J Agric Food Chem 2000; 48:3431–3436.
24. Ogawa H, Tasak M, Meguro T, Sasagawa S. Effect of Tochu leaf powder on lipid metabolism in hypercholesterolemic stroke prone spontaneously hypertensive rats. Nippon Kiyo, Shokuryo Gakkaishi 1998; 4:301–306. Japanese.
25. Huang Kee Chang. The Pharmacology of Chinese Herbs. New York: CRC Press, 1999:82.
26. Sih CJ, Ravikumar PR, Huang FC, Buckner C, Whitlock H Jr, Letter: Isolation and synthesis of pinoresinol diglucoside, a major antihypertensive principle of Tu-Chung (*Eucommia ulmoides*, Oliver). J Am Chem Soc 1976; 98:5412–5413.
27. Nakano M, Nakashima H, Itoh Y. Anti-human immunodeficiency virus activity of oligosaccharides from rooibos tea (*Aspalathus linearis*) extracts in vitro. Leukemia 1997; 11(suppl 3):128–130.
28. Huang RH, Xiang Y, Liu XZ, Zhang Y, Hu Z, Wang DC. Two novel antifungal peptides distinct with a five-disulfide motif from the bark of *Eucommia ulmoides* Oliv. FEBS Lett 2002; 521:87–90.
29. Watanabe J, Kawabata J, Kurihara H, Niki R. Isolation and identification of alpha-glucosidase inhibitors from Tochu-cha (*Eucommia ulmoides*). Biosci Biotechnol Biochem 1997; 61:177–178.
30. Oshima Y, Takata S, Hikino H, Deyama T, Kinoshita G. Anticomplementary activity of the constituents of *Eucommia ulmoides* bark. J Ethnopharmacol 1988; 23:159–164.
31. Deyama T, Nishibe S, Kitagawa S, Ogihara Y, Takeda T, Ohmoto T, Nikaido T, Sankawa U. Inhibition of adenosine 3′,5′-cyclic monophosphate phosphodiesterase by lignan glucosides of eucommia bark. Chem Pharm Bull (Tokyo) 1988; 36:435–439.

39

Systematic Reviews of Herbal Medicinal Products
Doing More Good Than Harm?

Edzard Ernst
Peninsula Medical School
Universities of Exeter & Plymouth
Devon, England

I. INTRODUCTION

Herbal medicinal products (HMPs) are medicines that exclusively contain plant material. Single chemicals isolated from plants (e.g., morphine) are not considered to be HMPs. HMPs usually contain several pharmacologically active constituents, and most herbalists believe that they act synergistically to achieve healing. With many HMPs it is not known what these constituents are.

Between 1990 and 1997, the usage of HMPs by the general U.S. population increased by 380%—in 1990 the 1-year prevalence was 2.5% and in 1997 it had risen to 12.1% (1). According to these survey data, HMPs were most commonly employed for allergies, insomnia as well as respiratory and digestive problems. In 1997, the out-of-pocket expenditure in the United States was estimated at $5.1 billion (1). In 1999, the North American market for supplements amounted to $14.5 billion and the global market for HMPs was around $19 billion (2). In England, medical herbalism is one of the most popular forms of all complementary medicine (3), and in Germany some 65% of the general population use HMPs each year (4).

These data clearly show that the acceptance of herbal medicine is again high. But acceptance must not be confused with evidence of efficacy or safety. Herbalists sometimes assume that no scientific evidence is required and claim that the remarkable popularity of HMPs is sufficient proof of their effectiveness and safety. The public is often led to believe that "the test of time" has proven HMPs to be effective and safe: could the use of HMPs otherwise have survived for hundreds, even thousands, of years? Yet we know that the "test of time" is less than reliable (5):

- A treatment might have changed over time (e.g., a change in the source of raw material or production process can impact on the pharmacological properties of an HMP).
- New routes of administration may be associated with new risks.
- Interactions could exist with new conventional treatments.
- A given HMP may have been used safely for one indication but current use for other conditions may not necessarily be risk-free.
- Today's users of HMPs may have different characteristics than people hundreds of years ago (e.g., different lifestyles, diets, or concomitant diseases).

Proof of efficacy should come from (placebo-controlled, double-blind) randomized clinical trials (RCTs). Many such tests of HMPs are now available. Unfortunately, their results are rarely totally uniform. The best way to generate an unbiased overall finding is to conduct systematic reviews and meta-analyses of RCTs, an approach that minimizes both random and selection biases.

This chapter is an attempt to conduct risk-benefit assessments based on such evidence. It will be confined to a selection of HMPs only. For more extensive analyses, the reader is referred to other sources (6,7).

II. ECHINACEA (*E. PURPUREA, E. PALLIDA, E. AUGUSTIFOLIA*)

Today oral HMPs of echinacea are used predominantly for the prevention and treatment of the common cold. A systematic review (8) included 16 RCTs with a total of 3396 participants. Five of the RCTs were placebo-controlled. Their methodological quality was variable but, on average, satisfactory. Results suggested that some echinacea preparations have an effect over and above that of placebo. Unfortunately, the trials were highly heterogeneous in many respects. No clear evidence emerged for one echinacea species being superior to another. The authors of the systematic review concluded that "there is, to date, insufficient evidence to recommend a specific Echinacea product, or Echinacea preparation, in the treatment or prevention of the common cold" (8).

No systematic review of the safety of echinacea has yet been published. Few adverse effects are on record. The most frequent ones relate to allergic reactions, which can occasionally be severe (anaphylactic shock) but are probably rare. As an immunostimulant, echinacea could theoretically decrease the effects of immunosuppressants (7), but no case reports have been published where this has resulted in clinical problems.

Weighing the known risks against the benefits, it is concluded that some encouraging, albeit not compelling, evidence supports the use of echinacea HMPs for the treatment and prevention of the common cold. Its use seems most promising in the very early stages of the condition. In view of its apparent safety, echinacea seems worthy of further research. To date the evidence is, however, not strong enough to recommend any echinacea HMP for routine use.

III. GARLIC (*ALLIUM SATIVUM*)

Traditionally garlic has been used for a wide range of conditions, e.g., the common cold and other infections. Today, the main indication for garlic is hypercholesterolemia. A recent meta-analysis (9) included 13 placebo-controlled, double-blind RCTs with a total of 806 patients with hypercholesterolemia. The methodological quality of these studies was good (Jadad score 3–5). The results of the meta-analysis demonstrated a weighted mean difference of −15.7 mg/dL (95% CI = −25.6 to −5.7). For the most rigorous RCTs, the effect size was only −9.4 mg/dL and not any longer statistically significant. Our overall conclusion therefore was "garlic is superior to placebo...but the effect is modest and of debatable clinical relevance" (9).

No systematic review of the safety of garlic is currently available. The most frequent adverse effects are mild and transient; they include body odor, allergic reactions, nausea, heartburn, and flatulence. Garlic has antiplatelet activity and can therefore increase the effect of anticoagulants, which, in rare cases, has been associated with bleeding. For the same reason, it seems prudent to discontinue garlic medication several days before major surgery (7).

Despite the relatively small effect on total cholesterol the benefits of garlic may well outweigh its risk. This is true particularly because garlic has a range of further beneficial actions on the cardiovascular system, including effects on blood pressure, coagulation factors, and arterial compliance (7).

IV. GINKGO (*GINKGO BILOBA*)

Ginkgo is used for a range of indications, most importantly perhaps for vascular dementia and Alzheimer's disease. A systematic review (10) included nine double-blind RCTs with a total of 606 patients suffering from dementia. The methodological quality of these studies was on average good (Jadad score 3–5). The dosage regimen varied by more than 100%. All but one of the nine trials yielded positive findings, and our overall judgment was therefore optimistic: "findings are encouraging and warrant independent, large scale confirmatory and comparative trials" (10). The question whether ginkgo enhances cognitive function in healthy subjects where it is not impaired, is still controversial. Both positive and negative answers have so far been provided by RCTs.

No systematic review of the safety of ginkgo has yet been published. Adverse effects are rare, usually transient, and mild; they include gastrointestinal disturbances, diarrhea, vomiting, allergic reactions, pruritus, headache, dizziness, and nosebleeds. Ginkgo also has antiplatelet effects and therefore the same cautions apply as for garlic (7).

On balance, this collective evidence suggests that the risk-benefit profile of ginkgo is encouraging. There are few risks with proper use and the potential benefit for dementia patients is substantial.

V. HAWTHORN (*CRATAEGUS*)

A recent meta-analysis pooled data from 13 placebo-controlled, double-blind RCTs of hawthorn as a treatment of congestive heart failure (CHF) (11). Eight trials could be submitted to a meta-analysis. They included a total of 632 patients suffering from CHF, NYHA Class I–III. A significant differential effect was found for maximal workload in favor of hawthorn compared to placebo (weighted mean difference 6.9 WaH, 95% confidence interval = 2.6–11.1). The pressure–heart rate product and subjective symptoms showed similar positive effects. Our conclusion therefore was that "the best evidence available to date suggests significant positive effects compared with placebo in patients receiving hawthorn extract as an adjunctive treatment for CHF."

No systematic review of the risks of hawthorn is currently available. The adverse effects include nausea, dizziness, fatigue, and sweating. Hawthorn contains cardiac glycosides; thus it may cause problems when combined with other such drugs, e.g., digitalis. In high doses sedation, hypotension, or arrhythmias can occur. With excessive doses respiratory failure may develop (7).

On balance, hawthorn is a powerful medicinal herb that can both benefit and harm patients. CHF is a serious condition that is not normally self-diagnosable. Hawthorn extracts should therefore be prescribed only by doctors experienced in using this herbal medicine.

VI. HORSE CHESTNUT SEED EXTRACT (*AESCULUS HIPPOCASTANUM*)

Horse chestnut seed extracts are often used for chronic venous insufficiency (CVI). A systematic review (12) included eight placebo-controlled trials and five trials conducted against reference treatments. They included a total of 1083 patients with CVI of moderate severity. The methodological quality of these trials was on average good (Jadad score = 3–5). The overall results indicated that active treatment is significantly more effective than placebo and equivalent to reference treatments. Both objective signs and subjective symptoms responded to treatment. On the basis of these findings we concluded that "horse chestnut seed extract is superior to placebo and as effective as reference medications in alleviating the objective signs and subjective symptoms of CVI" (12).

To date no systematic review has addressed the safety of horse chestnut seed extract. Adverse effects include pruritus, nausea, gastrointestinal upset, bleeding, nephropathy, and allergic reactions. Horse chestnut seed extract may increase the effects of anticoagulants and should therefore be discontinued before major surgery (7).

On balance, the benefits of horse chestnut seed extracts seem to outweigh its risks, which are rare and usually minor. The standard treatment for CVI is, of course, external compression (i.e., compression stockings). Compliance with this treatment is, however, notoriously poor. Thus horse chestnut seed extracts could play an important role in the treatment of this condition.

VII. KAVA (*PIPER METHYSTICUM* FORST)

Kava is used mostly for the symptomatic treatment of anxiety. A systematic review (13) included seven placebo-controlled, double-blind RCTs with a total of 477 patients. The methodological quality of these studies was on average good (Jadad score = 2–5). All trials yielded positive results (weighted mean difference was 9.69, 95% CI = 3.54–15.83). Comparative trials suggest therapeutic equivalence with synthetic anxiolytics. Our overall conclusion was that "kava extract is superior to placebo as a symptomatic treatment for anxiety" (13).

A systematic review of the safety of kava has been published (14). It revealed a range of mild and transient adverse effects. However, the suspicion has recently arisen that kava might cause liver damage. As of August 2002, 68 such cases had been reported worldwide. Some of these cases were serious, but causality is difficult to establish on the basis of such (mostly incomplete) reports. Based on this evidence, kava has been taken off the market in several European countries (15). Until further data become available, the use of kava should not be recommended.

VIII. SAW PALMETTO (*SERENOA REPENS*)

Saw palmetto is used for benign prostate hyperplasia (BPH). A meta-analysis (16) of 18 RCTs included 2939 patients with this condition. The methodological quality of these studies was variable but some were of the highest standard. The results of the meta-analysis revealed a weighted mean difference in symptom score of −1.41 points (95% CI = −2.52–0.30). This corresponds to a statistically significant and clinically relevant improvement of BPH symptoms compared to placebo. One important caveat is the lack of long-term data, particularly as the treatment of BPH is by definition long-term. The authors of this meta-analysis concluded that "*Serenoa repens* improves urologic symptoms and flow measures" (16).

No systematic review of the safety of saw palmetto is available at present. Adverse effects include breast tenderness, gastrointestinal complaints, constipation, diarrhea, dysuria, and decreased libido (7). Saw palmetto has hormonal effects and could therefore interact with hormone therapies.

One can conclude from this collective evidence that the risk-benefit profile of saw palmetto is encouraging. Its adverse effects are rare and usually mild; its therapeutic potential to relieve the symptoms of BPH is considerable. It can therefore be recommended for BPH patients who prefer a herbal to a synthetic drug treatment.

IX. ST. JOHN'S WORT (*HYPERICUM PERFORATUM*)

St. John's wort is used mostly for mild to moderate depression. There are numerous systematic reviews of St. John's wort. The first meta-analysis (17) included 23 RCTs with a total of 1757 patients. The methodological quality of trials was variable but some were excellent. The results of the meta-analysis clearly showed that St. John's wort is more effective than placebo or as effective as synthetic antidepressants. This finding has been confirmed by several subsequent systematic reviews. The evidence comparing St. John's wort with conventional antidepressants is, however, still relatively weak. Recently, several RCTs have produced negative results. It is important to note that these related to severe rather than mild to moderate depression. The authors of the original meta-analysis (17) concluded that "extracts of *Hyper-*

icum are more effective than placebo in the treatment of mild to moderate depression." This conclusion still holds and is corroborated by new trial data that have become available since then (18).

A systematic review of the safety of St. John's wort (19) pooled all relevant data from case reports, clinical trials, postmarketing surveillance, and drug-monitoring studies. Collectively this evidence suggested that St. John's wort is well tolerated with an incidence of adverse effects similar to that of placebo. The most common adverse effects were gastrointestinal symptoms, dizziness/confusion, and tiredness/sedation. A potentially serious adverse effect is photosensitivity, but this appears to occur extremely rarely. Since the publication of this review we have learned much about the interactions between St. John's wort and other drugs (20). Extracts of St. John's wort activate enzymes of the cytochrome P450 system, namely CYP3A4. It can therefore lower the plasma levels of a range of drugs given concomitantly; cyclosporin, oral contraceptives, phenoprocoumon, warfarin, amitriptyline, indinavir, and digoxin. When used with other SSRIs it can cause a serotonin syndrome.

On balance, the benefits of St. John's wort as a symptomatic treatment of mild to moderate depression outweigh its risks—provided, of course, that these risks are managed adequately. Essentially St. John's wort should not be combined with drugs metabolized via the cytochrome P450 enzyme system.

X. DISCUSSION

Systematic reviews (including meta-analyses) represent the most conclusive evidence for or against efficacy and safety. This holds for all medical interventions, and HMPs are no exception. However, this approach is not totally free of limitations. For instance, if one submits flawed RCTs to a systematic review, the result will necessarily be flawed as well. Publication bias is another important problem. We know that negative trials tend to remain unpublished (21). Thus the published evidence might, in some cases, be biased toward a false-positive overall result.

The English medical literature is demonstrably biased toward positive results, and negative trials thus tend to emerge in journals published in other languages (22). It is therefore important to not restrict systematic reviews to the English literature. In herbal medicine this is perhaps more important than in other areas since much of the primary trial data used to be published in German.

Further problems with systematic reviews of HMPs relate to the (lack of) standardization of extracts. If one preparation of a given herb is shown to be effective, this does not necessarily apply to another preparation of the same herb. Systematic reviews are therefore at risk of generating a misleading overall result. There is no easy way around this problem except insisting that all HMPs, particularly those used in clinical trials, are adequately standardized.

The evidence summarized in this chapter clearly shows that not all HMPs have been demonstrated to do more good than harm. It is simply not possible to generalize across different HMPs, and every set of data has to be evaluated on its own merit. On the other hand, the evidence also clearly demonstrates that not all HMPs are clinically useless. In fact, most of the HMPs discussed above are powerful drugs. It is therefore obvious that they should be adequately regulated. In many countries (e.g., United States and England), HMPs are marketed as dietary supplements, a status that invites suboptimal quality as well as multiple other problems and therefore does not provide a regulatory framework for the adequate protection of the consumer.

In conclusion, some HMPs have been investigated in sufficient depth to allow tentative risk-benefit assessments. In doing this, each HMP has to be judged on its own merit—generalizations about the risks or benefits of HMPs are counterproductive.

REFERENCES

1. Eisenberg D, David RB, Ettner SL, Appel S, Wilkey S, Van Rompay M, Kessler RC. Trends in alternative medicine use in the United States; 1990–1997. JAMA 1998; 280: 1569–1575.
2. Gruenwald J. The supplement markets in the US and Europe. Nutraceuti World 2000 July/August; 36–37.
3. Ernst E, White AR. The BBC survey of complementary medicine use in the UK. Complement Ther Med 2000; 8:32–36.
4. Häusermann D, Heptinstall S, Groenewegen WA, Spangenberg P, Loesche W. Wachsendes Vertrauen in Naturheilmittel. Extracts of feverfew may inhibit platelet behavior via neutralization of sulphydryl groups. Dtsch Ärzteblatt 1997; 94:1857–1858.
5. Ernst E, De Smet PAGM, Shaw D, Murray V. Traditional remedies and the "test of time." Eur J Clin Pharmacol 1998; 54:99–100.
6. Ernst E. Herbal medicinal products: an overview of systematic reviews and meta-analyses. Perfusion 2001; 14:398–404.
7. Ernst E, Pittler MH, Stevinson C, White AR, Eisenberg D. The Desktop Guide to Complementary and Alternative Medicine. Edinburgh: Mosby, 2001.
8. Melchart D, Linde K, Fischer P, Kaesmayr J. Echinacea for the prevention and treatment of the common cold. The Cochrane Library, 1999. Oxford. Update software.
9. Stevinson C, Pittler MH, Ernst E. Garlic for treating hypercholesterolemia. Ann Intern Med 2000; 133:420–429.
10. Ernst E, Pittler MH. Ginkgo biloba for dementia: a systematic review of double-blind placebo-controlled trials. Clin Drug Invest 1999; 17:301–308.

11. Pittler MH, Schmidt K, Ernst E. Hawthorn extract for treating chronic heart failure: a meta-analysis of randomised trials. Am J Med 2003; 114:665–674.
12. Pittler MH, Ernst E. Horse-chestnut seed extract for chronic venous insufficiency: a criteria-based systematic review. Arch Dermatol 1998; 134:1356–1360.
13. Pittler MH, Ernst E. Efficacy of kava extract for treating anxiety: systematic review and meta-analysis. J Clin Psychopharmacol 2000; 20:84–89.
14. Stevinson C, Huntley A, Ernst E. A systematic review of the safety of kava extract in the treatment of anxiety. Drug Safety 2002; 25:251–261.
15. Ernst E. Safety concerns about kava. Lancet 2002; 359:1865.
16. Wilt TJ, Ishani A, Stark G, MacDonald R, Lau J, Mulrow C. Saw palmetto extracts for treatment of benign prostatic hyperplasia: a systematic review. JAMA 1998; 280:1576.
17. Linde K, Ramirez G, Mulrow CD, Paul A, Weidenhammer W, Melchart D. St. John's wort for depression—an overview and meta-analysis of randomised clinical trials. Br Med J 1996; 313:253–258.
18. Stevinson C, Ernst E. *Hypericum* for depression: an update of the clinical evidence. Eur Neuropsychopharmacol 1999; 9:501–505.
19. Ernst E, Rand JI, Barnes J, Stevinson C. Adverse effects profile of the herbal antidepressant St. John's wort (*Hypericum perforatum* L.). Eur J Clin Pharmacol 1998; 54:589–594.
20. Izzo AA, Ernst E. Interactions between herbal medicines and prescribed drugs: a systematic review. Drugs 2001; 15:2163–2175.
21. Easterbrook PJ, Berlin JA, Gopalan R, Mathews DR. Publication bias in clinical research. Lancet 1991; 337:867–872.
22. Egger M, Zellweger-Zähner T, Schneider M, Junker C, Lengeler C, Antes G. Language bias in randomised controlled trials published in English and German. Lancet 1997; 350:326–329.

40

Use of Silicon-Based Oligonucleotide Chip in Authentication of Toxic Chinese Medicine

Maria C. Carles
The Scripps Research Institute
La Jolla, California, U.S.A.

Nancy Y. Ip
Hong Kong University of Science and Technology
Hong Kong, China

I. INTRODUCTION

Traditional Chinese medicine (TCM) is widely used in Asia, especially in China, and plays an important part in the health care of overseas Chinese worldwide. Their methods, processing, and formulations have been worked out over the last 2000 years (1). TCM prescriptions and preparations are derived from natural sources; about 80% of the total is derived from plants, and the rest includes minerals or animal parts. Even though the effectiveness and safety of TCM have been documented by controlled clinical studies, several cases of severe or even fatal poisoning are reported every year. Most of the poisoning cases are reported after ingestion of Chinese medicine preparations that contain aconitine, anticholinergics, or podophyllin (2–4). The preparations commonly used to treat chronic illnesses such as rheumatism or arthritis, as well as for bruises, fractures, and cardiac complaints, may contain species of *Aconitum* (*A. carmicaelli*, *A. kusnezofii*, *A. brachypodum*, *A. pendulum*, *A. nagarum*, or *A. coreanum*), which are considered highly toxic (4–6). Species of the genus *Datura* (*D. innoxia*, *D. metel*) are regularly used for treatment of bronchial asthma, chronic bronchitis, pains, and flu symptoms (7). Moreover, there are reports on poisoning caused by adulterants or erroneous substitutes involving species of *Podophyllum emodi* (7) and by the ingestion of dried venom from *Bufo gargarizans* or *Bufo melanostictus* used as an aphrodisiac (8).

Occasionally there may be cases of acute poisoning with other Chinese medicines such as *Huechys sanguinea*, *Lytta caraganae*, *Mylabris phalerata*, *Mylabris chicorii*, *Rhododendron molle*, *Croton tiglium*, *Euphorbia fischeriana*, *Stellera chamaejasme*, *Euphorbia kansui*, *Dyosma versipellis*, *Dyosma pleiantha*, *Sophora tokinensis*, *Garcinia morella*, *Arisaema amurense*, *Pinellia ternate*, *Pinellia cordata*, *Pinellia pedatisecta*, *Typhonium giganteum*, *Allocasia macrorrhizos*, *Euphorbia lathyris*, *Hyoscyamus niger*, *Strychnos nux-vomica*, and *Strychnos pierriana*. This situation prompted the Hong Kong Special Administrative Region (HKSAR) to implement legal controls for dispensing and use of Chinese medicines as described in the "HKSAR in Ordinance No. 47, 1999" (9). Table 1 lists the regulated TCM used. These regulations will be useful not only for Hong Kong physicians, but for anyone who practices TCM. When dealing with natural resources from either animal or plant origin, it is crucial to perform an accurate identification of the material in used. Today the identification of TCM depends largely on expert morphological and chemical characterization. After collection and identification of the fresh medicinal products, these medicines are highly processed, making their identification a challenge for the untrained eye.

This chapter describes the fabrication and characterization of a silicon (Si)-based chip as an alternative solid support for the fabrication of novel DNA microarrays used for identification of toxic Chinese medicinal herbs. Briefly, genomic DNA is extracted from TCM material. The spacer domain of the 5S-rRNA gene is amplified by the polymerase chain reaction (PCR), cloned, and sequenced. The sequences obtained are then analyzed and used to identify species-specific variable regions of the gene. Based on these sequences three types of oligonucleotides are designed and synthesized: (1) disulfide-modified probes for immobilization, (2) sense PCR primers, and (3) fluorescent-labeled antisense primers used in subsequent asymmetrical PCR reactions. Self-assembled layers of MPTS (3-mercaptopropyl)trimethoxysilane were formed as a bifunctional linker on the surface of 1 cm^2 silicon chips and 5′-thiol-modified oligonucleotides were deposited on the surface in a microarray. Asymmetrical PCR is performed and products obtained are then

TABLE 1 HKSAR-Regulated Chinese Medicines

Chinese name	Scientific name	Action
山豆根	*Sophora tonkinensis*	Remove toxic heat, promote subsidence of swelling, soothe sore throat, antipyretic
生千金子	*Euphorbia lathyris*	Drastic purgation for treating edema, eliminate blood stasis for treating masses
生川烏	*Aconitum carmicaelli*	Relieve rheumatic conditions and alleviate pain by warming the channels
生附子	*Aconitum carmicaelli*	Relieve rheumatic conditions and alleviate pain by warming the channels
雪上一枝蒿	*Aconitum pendulum*	Relieve rheumatic conditions and alleviate pain by warming the channels
鬼臼 (小葉蓮)	*Podophyllum emodi*	Regulate menstruation and promote the flow of blood
鬼臼 (八角蓮)	*Dysosma versipellis*	Regulate menstruation and promote the flow of blood
鬼臼 (八角蓮)	*Dysosma pleiantha*	Regulate menstruation and promote the flow of blood
生馬錢子	*Strychnos nux-vomica*	Promote flow of qi and blood in the collaterals, relieve pain, subsidence of swelling
生天仙子	*Hyoscyamus niger*	Relieve spasm and pain, cause tranquilization
生天南星	*Arisaema amurense*	Remove swelling, damp phlem, dispel wind, and arrest convulsions.
生巴豆	*Croton tiglium*	Cauterization by external use
生甘遂	*Euphorbia kansui*	Drastic purgation and expel retained water
生白附子	*Typhonium giganteum*	Eliminate blood stasis, promote the flow of qi, remove undigested food, relieve pain
生半夏 (半夏)	*Pinellia ternata*	Remove damp, phlegm, nausea, vomiting, stuffiness in chest and epigastrium
(滴水珠)	*Pinellia cordata*	Remove damp, phlegm, nausea, vomiting, stuffiness in chest and epigastrium

TABLE 1 Continued

Chinese name	Scientific name	Action
(虎掌)	*Pinellia pedatisecta*	Remove damp, phlegm, nausea, vomiting, stuffiness in chest and epigastrium
鬧羊花	*Rhododendron molle*	Relieve rheumatic conditions, eliminate blood stasis, alleviate pain
生草烏	*Aconitum kusnezoffi*	Relieve rheumatic conditions, warm the channels, alleviate pain
洋金花 (曼陀羅花)	*Datura metel*	Relieve asthma and cough, alleviate pain, and arrest spasm
洋金花 (毛曼陀羅)	*Datura innoxia*	Relieve asthma and cough, alleviate pain, and arrest spasm
洋金花 (紫花曼陀羅)	*Datura tatula*	Relieve asthma and cough, alleviate pain, and arrest spasm
蟾酥	*Bufo gargarizans*	Counteract toxicity, relieve pain, restore consciousiness, aphrodisiac
蟾酥	*Bufo melanoctictus*	Counteract toxicity, relieve pain, restore consciousiness, aphrodisiac

used for hybridization with the immobilized species-specific probes. Contact-angle measurements, XPS, VASE, and AFM were used to characterize and optimize the process and fabrication of TCM microarrays. Si-based TCM microarrays provide fast, economical, and reliable methods for identification of toxic Chinese medicines, as described elsewhere (10).

II. FABRICATION OF Si-BASED TOXIC TCM MICROARRAYS

There are currently two main types of microarrays: c-DNA- and oligonucleotide-based arrays. These arrays may be made using different surfaces as solid supports. Glass and nitrocellulose are the still the most commonly used owing to their low cost and general availability (11–13), but they lack the versatility of Si surfaces such as the possibility of integration with other Si-based components such as micro PCR reactors (14), microfluidic transport, micro-capillary electrophoresis (15) and detection systems (16), uniformity of DNA deposition, and low signal-to-noise ratio (17,18).

A. Methods

The reagents used were of analytical grade purchased from Fluka and Sigma-Aldrich (Milwaukee, WI, USA). Modified oligonucleotides were purchased from Synthetic Genetics (San Diego, CA, USA). PCR primers were made in-house in a PE 8909 nucleic acid system. Experts in the field from different provinces of China collected and identified all TCM material used for this project.

1. Extraction of Genomic DNA

Plant DNA was extracted as described previously (19,20) with slight modifications. Briefly, about 0.2 g of fresh leaves from TCM was frozen in liquid nitrogen and ground into a fine powder using a mortar and pestle (Table 1). The powder was mixed with extraction buffer (25 mM Tris-HCl, pH 8.0, 50 mM EDTA, 0.5% SDS, 10 μg/mL RNA A, 0.2% β-mercaptoethanol), and then incubated at 58°C for 1 hr, then centrifuged at 10,000 g for 10 min. The supernatant was recovered, mixed with equal volume of phenol:chloroform: isoamyl alcohol (1:24:1) by inversion, and centrifuged at 14,000 g for 10 min, 2 times. The supernatant was transferred to a new tube, mixed with chloroform:isoamyl alcohol, and centrifuged as above. The supernatant was recovered, mixed with 1/10 of 3M sodium acetate, pH 5.2 and 2.5 volumes of 95% ethanol, placed at −20°C for 1hr and centrifuged for 10 min at 14,000 g. The DNA pellet was washed twice with 70% ethanol and resuspended in double-distilled autoclaved water.

2. Design and Fabrication of Probes

Species-Specific Oligonucleotide Probes. DNA-polymorphism-based analyses have been successfully used for the identification of herbal medicines (19,21,22). We chose the 5S-rRNA gene as our probe normally used as marker for phylogenetic analysis (23) because of its dual properties: it is widely conserved throughout prokaryotes and eukaryotes, but it is also highly variable at the internal transcribed spacer region within species (24). The 5S-rRNA gene from the TCM plants was amplified by PCR. The primers used for the amplification of the 5S- rRNA gene were: sense primer: 5′ GGA TCC GTG CTT GGG CGA GAG TAG TA 3′ and antisense: 5′ GGA TCC TTA GTG CTG GTA TGA TCG CA 3′ (19). PCR products were subcloned using the TA Cloning Kit (Invitrogen) and electroporated into *Escherichia coli* XL-1 blue. Plasmid DNA from positive clones was extracted by alkaline lysis, digested with restriction enzymes, analyzed by gel electrophoresis, and subjected to DNA sequencing using the AutoRead Sequencing Kit (Amersham Pharmacia Biotech). Oligonucleotide probes used for the microarrays described here were designed and fabricated based on the variable sequences obtained from the internal transcribed spacer (ITS) domain of the gene. The probes used for immobilization had a 5′ disulfide modification, a carbon spacer (6–18 carbons), and 20–26 base sequences.

3. Development of Toxic TCM DNA Microarrays

Silicon surface modifications included a methodical cleaning procedure, a thermal oxidation process, and the self-assembly of thiol layers used as heterofunctional linkers for immobilization of disulfide-modified probes. Initial cleaning, as well as thermal oxidation procedures, was performed in a class 1000 clean room using CMOS-compatible processing. Briefly, all n-type Si(100) wafers were immersed in a "piranha" bath (90% H_2SO_4, 10% H_2O_2; 125°C) for 10 min followed by 1-min treatment with 2% solution of hydrofluoric acid (HF). Then the wafers were rinsed 10 times with double-distilled water and blow-dried. A 1000-Å layer of dry silicon dioxide was grown in an oxidation furnace at 1100°C, followed by 4000 Å of wet oxide (Fig. 1). The wafers were cut into 1-cm^2 chips using a Disco automatic dicing saw DAD341.

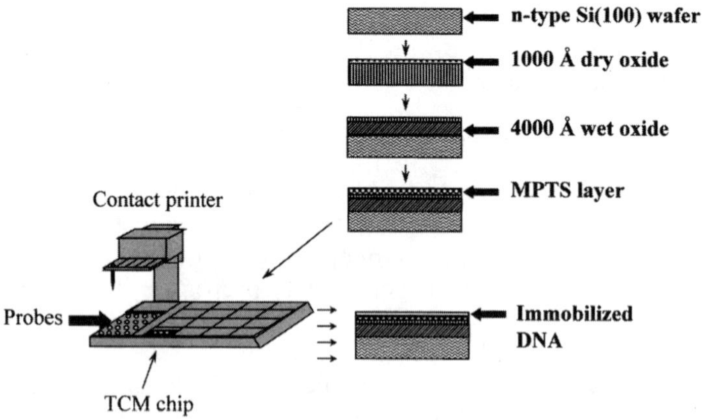

FIGURE 1 Fabrication of TCM chip. Schematic diagram showing the steps followed during fabrication of the Si-based TCM chip.

4. Hydroxylation of the Surface and Formation of Self-Assembled MPTS Layer

Organic contaminants were removed by immersing the 1-cm^2 chips in a potassium permanganate–sulfuric acid solution (0.5 g $KMNO_4$ in 15 mL H_2SO_4) for 30 sec, then rinsed with copious amounts of water. The cleaned chips were incubated for 35 min in 3.3% of ammonium hydroxide solution at 60°C to restore the OH groups in the surface, rinsed with isopropanol, and dried under nitrogen gas. The chips were placed in a heat-resistant container with a solution consisting of 100 mL isopropanol p.a., 800 μL (3-mercapto-propyl)trimethoxysilane (MPTS), and 200 μL H_2O, then placed in the oven at 80°C for 35 min. The chips were then rinsed first with isopropanol, then with water, and blow-dried with N_2 gas. Finally, the chips were heated at 115°C for 30 min to remove H_2O traces.

5. Printing the Arrays

Species-specific thiol-modified oligonucleotide probes were diluted with sodium chloride/sodium citrate buffer (SSC; 3 M NaCl, 0.3 M Na citrate·2 H_2O, pH 4.5) and 5% DMSO to a final concentration of 20 μM and spotted (100-μm diameter) in 5 × 25 arrays onto the silicon surface to form disulfide bonds with the free thiol groups of the MPTS layer on the surface (Fig. 1). The microarrays were incubated overnight at room temperature in a humidified chamber, then washed in washing solution (2X SSC, 1% SDS) for 10 min on a shaker and rinsed 3 times with water. They were blow-dried with nitrogen gas. The tip was rinsed 3 times with station washing buffer (10 mM Tris-HCl pH 7.0, 0.5% Tween 20) between samples. DNA microarrays were printed using a Cartesian PixSys 7500 arrayer (Fig. 1).

6. Asymmetrical PCR Reactions, Hybridization and Detection

A 50-μL total asymmetrical PCR reaction consisted of 20–100 ng DNA template, PCR buffer to a final concentration of 1.5 mM magnesium chloride, 2.5 units of Taq Polymerase (GIBCO/BRL), 0.4 μM dNTPs (GIBCO/BRL), 0.4 μM antisense Texas Red–labeled primer, and 0.004 μM sense primer. The reactions were performed using the following profile: 94°C/4 min (94°C/1 min; 53°C/30 sec; 72°C/30 sec) × 45 cycles. Asymmetrical PCR products were speed-vacuumed for 2 hr and resuspended in 12 μL of hybridization buffer [6x SSC pH 7, 5x Denhardt's solution (1% BSA (bovine serum albumin), 2% Ficoll 400, 2% polyvinylpyrollidone (PVP)], 0.5 % sodium dodecylsulfate (SDS), sheared salmon sperm DNA (5 μg/mL)). A schematic drawing of the hybridization procedure is shown in Figure 2. The arrays were covered with a cleaned microscope slide cover glass, filled with the PCR reaction by capillary force, and incubated in a hybridization

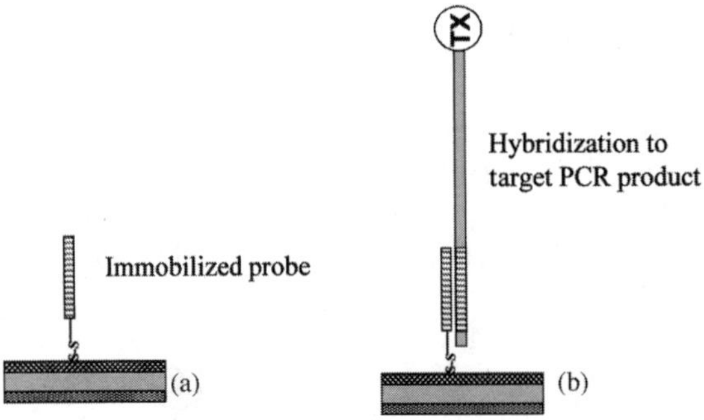

FIGURE 2 Schematic representation of hybridization assays used to identify regulated TCMs. The immobilized probe is 20–26 bases long and contains a 5′-thiol modification and an 18-carbon chain between the thiol group and the first base. This physical separation is needed for successful hybridization.

chamber at 53°C overnight. Then the chips were washed 3 times with washing solution in a shaker for 10 min, then with water, and blow-dried with nitrogen gas. Hybridization was detected using a GSI Lumonics scanner 5000 and its software was used for detection and analysis of the data acquired from the microarrays.

III. CHARACTERIZATION OF Si AS SOLID SUPPORT FOR DNA MICROARRAYS

The characterization of Si as support for TCM microarrays included several physical measurements performed after every step in the process, from cleaning to immobilization of oligonucleotides.

A. Contact Angle Measurements, XPS, VASE, and AFM

A Kruss Contact Angle Measuring System, Model G-10 was used for all contact angle measurements. A mass of approximately 20 mg H_2O was deposited onto the surface; the readings were taken 30 sec after deposition at room temperature. X-ray photoelectron spectroscopy (XPS) spectra were acquired using Physical Electronics 5600 multitechnique system with monochromatic Al Kα X-ray source (1486.6 eV). The radiation was focused on the sample at an electron takeoff angle (TOA) of 45 $\pm$ 3° relative to the substrate surface. The spectra for sulfur, S (2p); oxygen, O (1s); carbon, C (1s); and silica, Si (2p) were acquired using the respective Physical Electronics software. An electron flood gun was used to compensate for the insulating properties of the sample. The Si (2p) peak was chosen as the reference binding energy (103.3 eV). Variable-angle spectroscopic ellipsometry (VASE) measurements were acquired using Variable Angle Ellipsometry System H-VASE GE005 (Woollam). The optical constant for the MPTS layer was set to 1.4420 (25°C) (25). Scanning Probe Microscope-NanoScope (Digital Instruments) was used for atomic force microscopy (AFM). Data were acquired in tapping mode using a resolution of 512 pixels per line and analyzed using Digital Instrument software.

IV. RESULTS AND DISCUSSION

A. Surface Characterization of the Si-Based TCM Chip

Initial experiments showed the need for a thorough cleaning pretreatment as well as rehydroxylation of the Si surface before the formation of the MPTS layer and deposition of the DNA. It has been shown that adequate substrate rehydration is crucial for self-assembly of MPTS layer (26). The surface characteristics were monitored during processing of the Si surface by goniometry, XPS, VASE, and AFM. The information obtained included: thickness of the layers deposited on the surface, their arrangement, and their possible orientation.

B. Contact Angle Measurements

Changes in contact angle measurements were monitored during the processing of the silicon chips. The mean values are listed in Table 2. A contact angle of 3° after the treatment of the chips in NH_4OH indicated almost complete hydroxylation of the surface (27). After formation of the self-assembled layer of MPTS, the contact angle increased from 3° to 81.13°. The hydrophobicity imparted to the surface facilitated the deposition of the

TABLE 2 Physical Measurements Taken During Fabrication of the TCM Chip

Surface	Treatment	Contact angle (°)	VASE (thickness)	AFM (particle size)
Native Si	n/a	69.35	0.5 mm	n/a
SiO_2 5000 Å	Piranha and HF	58.43	4972.1 Å	44 nm^2
SiO_2 5000 Å	Re-OH	3.00	n/a	n/a
SiO_2 5000 Å	Roughness layer	n/a	16.8 Å	n/a
SiO_2 5000 Å	MPTS layer	81.13	38.8 Å	89 nm^2
SiO_2 5000 Å	MPTS-DNA layer	42.90		250 nm^2
SiO_2 5000 Å	DNA-DNA layer	n/a	29.0 Å	1500 nm^2

n/a: measurements were not taken or they do not apply to the instrument used; Re-OH: rehydroxylated.

oligonucleotide while printing the array. After immobilization of DNA the contact angle decreased to 42.90° as expected owing to the hydrophilic properties of the DNA itself.

C. X-ray Photoelectron Spectroscopy (XPS)

The XPS spectrum based on the unique electron binding energies allowed us to analyze the elements present in the surface during cleaning rehydroxylation and self-assembly of the thiol layer used as heterofunctional linker to immobilize the DNA to the Si surface of the TCM chip. The XPS spectrum taken immediately after cleaning indicated a low carbon content of 4.08% on the surface. The amount of carbon recorded on the surface was likely due to the deposition of contaminants present in the ambient air. This indicated that it is preferable to deposit the MPTS layer immediately after cleaning. The XPS spectra of the MPTS layer of the sulfur peak (S 2p) was detected at 163.7 eV, which indicated that all of the sulfur was present as thiol or disulfide (28) and ready for immobilization of the oligonucleotide probes.

D. Atomic Force Microscopy (AFM)

Surface changes that occur during the processing of the chips were also evaluated by AFM. During the cleaning and rehydroxylation process some material appeared to be removed by desorption of $Si(OH)_4$ into the solution, leading to an increase in roughness of the surface (data not shown). The formation of MPTS layers led to an increase in the grain size from 44 nm^2 to 89 nm^2 and a small change in the topography (Fig. 3a). The AFM image of the immobilized oligonucleotide layer (Fig. 3b) showed a controlled pattern on the arrangement of the molecules on the surface. A dense coverage may cause steric hindrance during hybridization (29). AFM data obtained after hybridization revealed that big clusters of hybridized oligonucleotides were distributed over the surface. The mean grain size of these spots as calculated from AFM data increased from 250 nm^2 (immobilized oligonucleotide layer) to 1500 nm^2 (hybridized layer), as shown in Figure 3c. A summary of the values obtained is shown in Table 2.

E. Variable-Angle Ellypsometry (VASE)

VASE measurements generated estimated thickness values for the layers formed on the chip surface during processing. A summary of the values obtained is shown in Table 2. Based on the topography detected by AFM, a roughness layer was calculated (16.8 Å) and included in the calculated spectra. The thickness of the MPTS layer, 38.8 $\pm$ 7 Å was larger than expected for a monolayer, suggesting the formation of multiple layers of MPTS during the

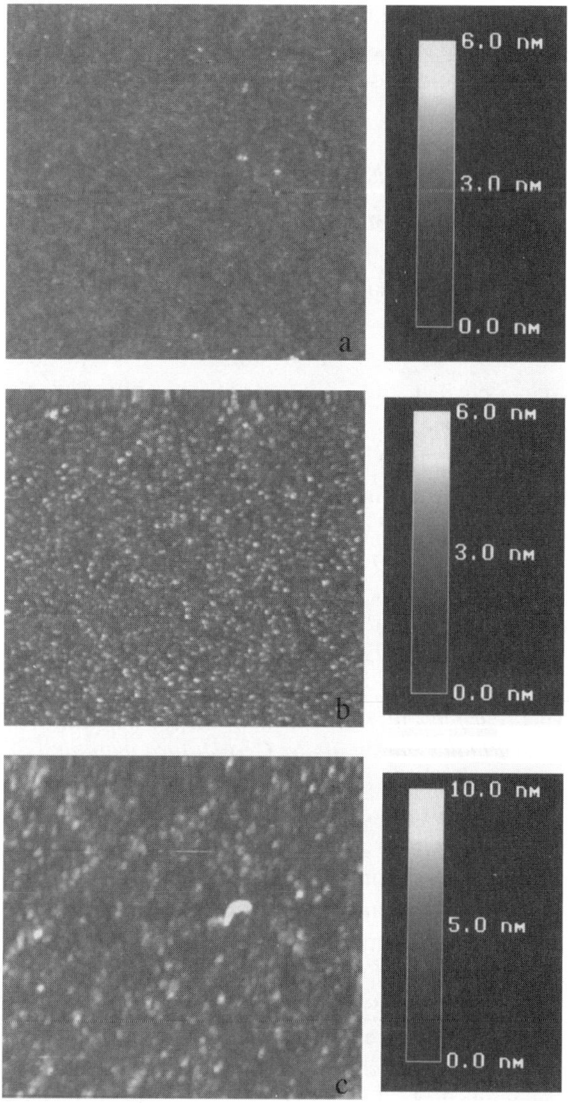

FIGURE 3 AFM images of Si-based TCM microarray. (a) MPTS, (b) immobilized oligo, (c) hybridized oligo.

self-assembly process owing to the amount of water present in the reaction. The hybridization layer was not uniform and yielded a thickness of 29.0 ± 5 Å, suggesting that the oligonucleotides do not stand at 90° angle to the surface.

F. Immobilization and Analysis of TCM Oligonucleotide Probes

Dithiol bonds formed during immobilization are heat-stable at least to 95°C (17,30). The 5′-thiol-modified oligonucleotide probes were covalently bound to the MPTS layer by direct disulfide bond formation.

G. Regulated TCM Microarray

Species-specific probes derived from the intragenic spacer domain of the 5S rRNA, 12S rRNA, chloroplast t-RNA genes were designed for 24 species listed in the HKSAR Ordinance 47, 1999. The oligonucleotide probes were immobilized via disulfide bond to the silicon oxide surface of the chip in arrays of 5 x 25. These arrays were printed in the following order: (1) positive immobilization control; (2) *Bufo melanostictus*; (3) *B. gargarizans*; (4) *Strychnos nux-vomica*; (5) *Hyoscyamus niger*; (6) *Typhonium diverticatum*; (7) *T. giganteum*; (8) *Pinellia pedatisecta*; (9) *P. cordata*; (10) *P. ternate*; (11) *Arisaema amurense*; (12) *Dysosma pleiantha*; (13) *D. versipellis*; (14) *Euphorbia kansui*; (15) *Allocasia macrorrhiza*; (16) *Stellera chamaejasme*; (17) *Aconitum carmicaelli*; (18) *A. carmicaelli*; (19) *A. kusnezoffii*; (20) *A. pendulum*; (21) *Croton tiglium*; (22) *Rhododendron molle*; (23) *Datura innoxia*; (24) *D. tatula*; (25) *D. metel*. Each of the species-specific probes had five replicas in each array. There were 25 arrays in total and each of them was hybridized with their respective asymmetrical PCR product. Figure 4 shows a representative example for successful dentification of regulated TCMs. Figure 4 contains three microarrays. Each of them was hybridized individually to an asymmetrical PCR product from three species of the genus *Datura*; *Datura metel*, *Datura tatula*, *Datura anoxia*. Figure 4 shows low cross-reactivity between species from the same genus and in some cases from a different genus, but the signal is strong enough to differentiate a positive identification to the species level. The Si chip shows almost no background fluorescence, allowing an effective and reliable method for the identification of toxic TCM material.

V. SUMMARY

We have developed a CMOS-compatible (complementary metal oxide semiconductor processes) Si-based chip for authentication and identification of regulated Chinese medicines. The Si-based chip was characterized using

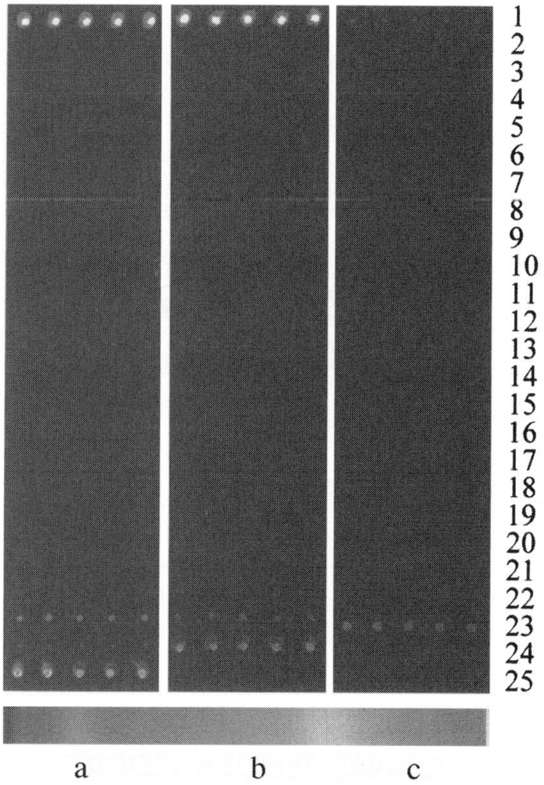

FIGURE 4 Regulated TCM microarrays corresponding to 24 species of toxic traditional Chinese medicines. The chip was hybridized to the symmetrical PCR product of (a) *Datura metel*, (b) *Datura tatula*, (c) *Datura innoxia*. The order of the array was as follows: (1) positive immobilization control; (2) *Bufo melanostictus*; (3) *B. gargarizans*; (4) *Strychnos nux-vomica*; (5) *Hyoscyamus niger*; (6) *Typhonium diverticatum*; (7) *T. giganteum*; (8) *Pinellia pedatisecta*; (9) *P. cordata*; (10) *P. ternate*; (11) *Arisaema amurense*; (12) *Dysosma pleiantha*; (13) *D. versipellis*; (14) *Euphorbia kansui*; (15) *Allocasia macrorrhiza*; (16) *Stellera chamaejasme*; (17) *Aconitum carmicaelli*; (18) *A. carmicaelli*; (19) *A. kusnezoffii*; (20) *A. pendulum*; (21) *Croton tiglium*; (22) *Rhododendron molle*; (23) *Datura innoxia*; (24) *D. tatula*; (25) *D. metel*. Each of the species-specific probes had five replicas in each array. PMT/laser gain for (a, b) is 70/70 and for (c) it is 60/60.

physical methods allowing us to optimize the conditions used during the manufacturing of the regulated TCM chip. Species-specific probes were immobilized via disulfide bonds making a sturdy, heat-stable, reusable, and economical chip and can be incorporated into many other applications. Regulated Chinese medicines listed in Table 1 were successfully identified using the regulated TCM chip. This method proves useful as a first step in the authentication of TCM material. It should not replace chemical fingerprinting or any other traditional characterization methods. Keep in mind that using this method one can only certify that toxic species are present in the sample, not the toxins produced by specific species. Additional efforts should be directed to obtaining sequence information for the major TCM used and sold to make a comprehensive database and ease their initial identification.

REFERENCES

1. Hu Shiu Ying. Sixty-three years with Chinese herbal medicines; memoir of a botanist. Am J Chin Med 1998; 26(3–4):383–389.
2. Chan TY, Chan JC, Tomlinson B, Critchley JA. Chinese herbal medicines revisited: a Hong Kong perspective. Lancet 1993; 342(8886–8887):1532–1534.
3. Chan TY, Critchley JA. Usage and adverse effects of Chinese herbal medicines. Hum Exp Toxicol 1996; 1:5–12.
4. Chan TY, Tomlinson B, Critchley JA, Cockram CS. Herb-induced aconitine poisoning presenting as tetraplegia. Vet Hum Toxicol 1994; 36(2):133–134.
5. Bisset NG. Arrow poisons in China. Part II. Aconitum-botany, chemistry, and pharmacology. J Ethnopharmacol 1981; 4(3):247–336.
6. Chan TY. Anticholinergic poisoning due to Chinese herbal medicines. Vet Hum Toxicol 1995; 37(2):156–157.
7. But PP. Herbal poisoning caused by adulterants or erroneous substitutes. J Trop Med Hyg 1994; 97(6):371–374.
8. Brubacher JR, Lachmanen D, Ravikumar PR, Hoffman RS. Efficacy of digoxin specific Fab fragments (Digibind) in the treatment of toad venom poisoning. Toxicon 1999; 37(6):931–942.
9. The Hong Kong Special Administrative Region, Ordinance No. 47 1999; A1273–A1277.
10. Carles M, Lee T, Moganti S, Lenigk R, Tsim WK, Ip N, Hsing I-M, Sucher N. Chips and qi: microcomponent based analysis in traditional Chinese medicine. Fresenius J Anal Chem 2001; 371:190–194.
11. Zammatteo N, Jeanmart L, Hamels S, Courtois S, Louette P, Hevesi L, Remacle J. Comparison between different strategies of covalent attachment of DNA to glass surfaces to build DNA microarrays. Anal Biochem 2000; 280(1):143–150.
12. Rogers YH, Jiang-Baucom P, Huang ZJ, Bogdanov V, Anderson S, Boyce-Jacino MT. Immobilization of oligonucleotides onto a glass support via disulfide bonds: a method for preparation of DNA microarrays. Anal Biochem 1999; 266(1):23–30.

13. Stillman BA, Tonkinson JL. FAST slides: a novel surface for microarrays. Biotechniques 2000; 29(3):630–635.
14. Lee TM, Hsing IM, Lao AL, Carles MC. A miniaturized DNA amplifier: its application in traditional Chinese medicine. Anal Chem 2000; 72(17):4242–4247.
15. Chan YC, Lenigk R, Carles M, Sucher NJ, Wong M, Zohar Y. Glass-silicon bonding technology with feed-through electrodes for micro capillary electrophoresis. Transducers'01 2000; 1166 1169.
16. Xu W, Li J, Xue M, Carles M, Trau DW, Lenigk R, Sucher NJ, Ip NY, Chan M. Surface characterization of DNA microarray on silicon dioxide and compatible silicon materials. MRS Proc 2001; 711:299–302.
17. Lenigk R, Carles M, Ip NY, Sucher N. Surface characterization of silicon-chip based DNA microarray. Langmuir 2001; 17(8):2497–2501.
18. Trau D, Lee TMH, Lao AIK, Lenigk R, Hsing I-M, Ip NY, Carles MC, Sucher NJ. Genotyping on a CMOS silicon PCR chip with integrated DNA microarray. Anal Chem 2002; 74:3168–3173.
19. Cai ZH, Li P, Dong TX, Tsim KWK. Molecular diversity of 5S-rRNA spacer domain in *Fritillaria* species revealed by PCR analysis. Planta Med 1999; 65:360–364.
20. Sambrook J, Fritsch EF, Maniatis T. Molecular Cloning, a Laboratory Manual. 2d ed. Cold Spring Harbor, NY: Cold Spring Harbor Laboratory Press, 1989.
21. Shaw PC, But PPH. Authentication of *Panax* species and their adulterants by random-primed polymerase chain reaction. Planta Med 1995; 61:466–469.
22. Ha WY, Yau FC, But PP, Wang J, Shaw PC. Direct amplification of length polymorphism analysis differentiates *Panax ginseng* from *Panax guinquefolius*. Planta Med 2001; 67(6):587–589.
23. Suzuki H, Moriwaki K, Sakura S. Sequences and evolutionary analysis of mouse 5S-rDNAs. Mol Biol Evol 1994; 11(4):704–710.
24. Lau DT, Shaw PC, Wang J, But PP. Authentication of medicinal *Dendrobium* species by the internal transcribed spacer of ribosomal DNA. Planta Med 2001; 67(5):456–460.
25. Handbook of Data on Organic Compounds. Boca Raton, FL: CRC Press, 1989.
26. Iler RK. The Chemistry of Silica. New York: John Wiley & Sons, 1979.
27. Legrange JD. Effects of surface hydroxylation on the deposition of silane monolayers in silica. Langmuir 1993; 9:1749–1753.
28. Moulder JF, Stickle WF, Sobol PE, Bomben KD. Handbook of X-ray Photoelectron Spectroscopy. Eden Prairie, MN: Perkin-Elmer Corporation, 1992.
29. Shchepinov MS, Case-Green SC, Southern EM. Steric factors influencing hybridization of nucleic acids to ligonucleotide arrays. Nucl Acids Res 1997; 25(6): 1155–1161.
30. National Research Development Corporation. Immobilised Polynucleotides. Patent WO 91/00868, 1991.

41

Traditional Chinese Medicine
Problems and Drawbacks

Barry Halliwell
National University of Singapore
Singapore, Republic of Singapore

I. INTRODUCTION

Traditional Chinese medicine (TCM) is one of a range of complementary treatments that are widely used in Asia, but are also becomingly increasingly popular in Western countries. This popularity is growing even in countries such as England where conventional medical treatment is free to the end-user, whereas TCM rarely is (1). Annual sales of herbal remedies in the United States exceed US$350 million (2) and the global market for all herbal and homoeopathic remedies has been estimated at over US$4 billion in the United States, over US$6 billion in Europe (3), and over US$2 billion in Asia (4). TCM encompasses several different treatments, including acupuncture, moxibustion, medicinal food, herbs, traditional massage, and qigong, but I will concern myself here only with herbal therapies. These "natural" remedies are widely perceived as safer than pharmaceutical company drugs, more "natural," "gentle," and less likely to cause side effects. In fact, just because a product is natural does not mean it is safe: examples of plant-produced toxins include cyanide (5), many carcinogens, a prime example being the powerful carcinogen aflatoxin (6), digitalis, ergot, and belladonna. Indeed the use of selected plant extracts to eliminate enemies and induce abortion has been widespread throughout the centuries. In general also, the more effective a drug, the more side effects might be predicted. Thus by reasoning from first principles, the safest medicine might be homoeopathic, although its effectiveness is as yet uncertain.

Despite the rising popularity of TCM and the setting up of a Center for Alternative Medicine (CAM) at the prestigious National Institutes of Health in the United States, TCM is still regarded skeptically by the Western medical profession, because in general its effectiveness has not been proved by rigorous clinical trials. However, the same is true for several commonly used medical and surgical procedures, and the impact of some "trial-confirmed" procedures such as chemotherapy on the patient's quality of life can be devastating (7). The fact that TCM practitioners often tailor treatment (or claim to do this) to each patient makes it difficult to do conventional controlled clinical trials. However there is growing evidence that conventional treatments developed for, for example, white European or American men (on whom the majority of published trials have been done) are not optimal for other races (8).

In approaching the area of TCM, there seem to be several different standpoints taken by various parties:

1. Accept TCM as a "given," known to be effective and useful, popularize it and set up courses to teach it in the West
2. Take a skeptical view and attempt to used evidence-based medicine to establish whether or not TCM is effective
3. Take TCM that are thought to be effective for a particular condition and use conventional pharmacology to isolate effective ingredients. For example, the cholinesterase inhibitor huperzine was isolated from a plant thought to improve memory (9). The antimalarial artemisinin was evolved from *Artemisia annua*, an ancient Chinese herb (quinghao) used to treat fevers (10). Plants have been the origin of some of our most helpful medicines, including taxol, vincristine, aspirin, and morphine.

However, several other key issues must be addressed (Table 1), most of them focused around the issue of quality control. To quote Lee (1), "As TCM is winning support, it must demonstrate that its products are both safe and of high quality... and safe from contaminants." This is rarely the case today. Indeed the U.S. Alpha–National Association Newsletter recommends, "Don't use herbal remedies for serious illnesses, don't give herbs to children and don't use them if you are pregnant or trying to get pregnant. Also, tell your doctor about all products that you take."

Let us examine these issues in turn.

TABLE 1 Problems with TCM

Toxicity of the product (just because it is natural does not mean it is safe).
Is it what it is supposed to be?
Often no established quality control tests.
When established tests exist, they are rarely simple to use.
Variable potency (part of plant, stage in growth cycle, time of year, year to year, different soil composition in different areas).
Contamination with toxins (microbial, chemical, e.g., pesticides, metal from containers, elements from soil, e.g., selenium).
Deliberate adulteration.
Deterioration on storage.
Perception of safety encourages excessive use.
Coprescription of several products, possibility of interactions with other TCM ingredients or conventional drugs.
Placental transport, excretion into breast milk, possible teratogenicity.
Toxicity to growing children?

II. PROBLEM 1: THE PRODUCT IS TOXIC

As Paracelsus said, "The right dose differentiates a poison from a remedy." For example, the balance of clinical evidence favors the view that *Hypericum perforatum* (St. John's Wort) is effective in treating mild to moderate depression (2,3), although not all studies support this (11). Its mechanism of action appears to involve monoamine oxidase inhibition (2) and so excessive doses, or coadministration with synthetic MAO inhibitor antidepressants, are likely to cause side effects. Absinthe was a popular emerald green liqueur in the nineteenth and early-twentieth centuries in Europe, but was eventually banned because of its dose-dependent and progressive toxicity, due to constituents of the wormwood oil used to make it (12). Wormwood extracts were used in antiquity to kill intestinal worms, and are still used now for gastrointestinal and liver problems in some countries (12,13).

Several problems have arisen with various herbal products that induce hepatotoxicity. Herbal teas from germander (*Teucrium chamaedrys*) have been widely used throughout antiquity, but several cases of germander-induced hepatitis with periportal inflammation and centrilobular necrosis associated with consumption of capsules containing germander extract led to the banning of all germander products in France (14). Jin bu huan (JBH) has been used in TCM as a sedative, analgesic, and decongestant, but chronic consumption of some products can cause hepatotoxicity (14). One problem is that a variety of herbs are marketed as JBH, although the offending one was labeled as an extract of *Polygala chinensis* (14). Indeed it is common in TCM for one name to apply to a group of botanically unrelated materials. Other organ damage can also occur. In Taiwan, consumption of extracts from leaves of *Sauropus androgynus* as a slimming aid produced lung damage resembling bronchiolitis obliterans (15). Whereas hepatotoxicity often resolves on discontinuing the offending product (14), the lung damage induced by *S. androgynus* appeared to be permanent (15).

The gallbladders of animals are used in TCM in some countries, but bile constituents can be variably toxic: the grass carp bile appears especially so and cases of human hemolysis and renal failure have been reported (16). On a related topic, a case of parasitic infestation after consumption of snake bile and blood has occurred (17).

III. PROBLEM 2: THE PRODUCT IS NOT WHAT IT IS SUPPOSED TO BE

The essential basic requirement for any herbal product is that the correct plant(s) are used. Even then there can be differences: the chemical composition of plants varies enormously depending on developmental stage, soil composition, amount of water and sunlight, etc. (Table 1). Nevertheless, occasionally the wrong plant is used and sometimes the same name in TCM can encompass several different plants (see above). Two patients consuming a range of herbal products "to cleanse the body" presented with digitalis poisoning, due to the use of *Digitalis lanata* instead of plantain in the formulation. Investigation revealed that approximately 2700 kg of this product had been imported into the United States, and only vigorous action by the Food and Drug Administration in recalling supplies prevented more problems (18).

In Belgium, over 40 patients consuming products allegedly containing the Chinese herbs *Stephania tetrandra* and *Magnolia officinalis* developed interstitial fibrosis and progressive renal failure. Chemical analysis revealed that a nephrotoxic herb, *Aristolochia fangchi*, had, apparently accidentally, been substituted for *S. tetrandra*. *Aristolochia* species contain powerful carcinogens and indeed patients with the above "Chinese herb nephropathy" are at high risk of urothelial carcinoma (19). Cases have also been reported in England and a local British newspaper (20) commented: "There are now more than 3000 clinics prescribing 400 unlicensed Chinese herbal treatments and no-one really knows what's being prescribed."

Ginkgo biloba leaf extract is widely consumed to improve mental function (11), but of 14 products tested by the Hong Kong Consumer Council, none of them met the specifications recommended by the World Health Organization (WHO). Eleven had insufficient active ingredients overall, and 13 had an excess content of gingkolic acid (21). In the United

States, analysis of commercial ginseng preparations showed that 25% contained no ginseng at all (22).

In fact, authentication of the starting plant material is a key problem. Detailed reference standards (e.g., herbarium-authenticated specimens, descriptive illustrated monographs) are not available for the majority of plants used in TCM. DNA fingerprinting of plant material may make some contribution, but once powders and extracts have been generated it becomes difficult. NMR-, HPLC-, and LC-MS-based analysis of chemical composition is a valuable tool, as illustrated by its use in the digitalis poisoning cases (18), examination of the authenticity of *Ginkgo* and ginseng preparations (21,22), identification of toxic components of grass carp bile (16), and investigation of JBH-induced hepatotoxicity (14). However, in the frequent absence of official standards and given the natural variation in chemical composition of even the same plant at different times (Table 1), the use of analytical techniques can be limited. Examples of their value include the HPLC method specified by the British Pharmacopeia for the evaluation of the active constituents of licorice (22), a common ingredient in herbal preparations. Much more work is yet to be done.

IV. PROBLEM 3: THE PRODUCT MAY HAVE DETERIORATED OR BECOME CONTAMINATED

A pharmaceutical product is described as stable if it meets the five elements of stability: physical, chemical, microbial, toxicological, and therapeutic. Many natural compounds readily oxidize and degrade, giving products with different properties. For example, the carotenoids β-carotene and lycopene may have antioxidant properties as intact molecules, yet their degradation products can be cytotoxic in cell cultures (23). Flavonoids and other plant polyphenolics are also easily oxidizable (24). Plant materials contain enzymes that affect their constituents; for example, the difference between green tea and black tea is the inactivation of an enzyme that oxidizes phenols during the preparation of the former but not the latter (25). Drying of plant material can cause loss of thermolabile constituents and further loss can occur on storage, especially if storage conditions are moist or too hot. However, shelf lives of TCM are rarely given on the packaging.

Microbial contamination from soil and during handling of plants, or bacterial and fungal infection during storage, is a potential problem. Plant materials are especially susceptible because of their organic nature, being good substrates for bacterial/fungal growth, especially if the moisture level in the environment is high. Aflatoxins are among the noxious products that can be generated (6,26). Medicinal plant materials can also contain pesticide residues (27) and sometimes toxic elements from the soil including arsenic, cadmium, and selenium (11,28,29). Metals can also be introduced during processing, e.g., by the preparation of medicines in lead containers (28,29).

V. PROBLEM 4: THE PRODUCT MAY HAVE BEEN DELIBERATELY ADULTERATED

The deliberate addition of compounds to herbal preparations is an even more worrisome problem. Adulterants include phenylbutazone, indomethacin, dexamethasone, prednisolone, acetaminophen, fenfluramine, and aminopyrine (11,22,30). Phenylbutazone can cause severe agranulocytosis, which is why its use as a drug is now very limited, but several cases of damage by herbs containing it as an adulterant have been reported (22,31,32). In 2002 in Singapore the Health Sciences Authority identified phenylbutazone in the herbal remedy serbuk jarem (encok), used to treat rheumatism and "body aches." In England, herbal creams prescribed by TCM practitioners to treat facial and other eczema were analyzed and eight were found to be adulterated with dexamethasone, in some cases at a level that should not be used on the face (33). Yet another example is PC-SPES (see below).

VI. PROBLEM 5: THE PRODUCTS MAY PRODUCE HARM BY INTERACTING WITH EACH OTHER OR WITH PHARMACEUTICALS TAKEN CONCURRENTLY

TCM prescriptions may contain multiple different products whose ingredients can interact with each other in unexpected ways, or can influence the effects of Western drugs taken concurrently. TCM is often used by subjects with chronic diseases, who are likely to take Western drugs at the same time. For example, PC-SPES is allegedly a combination of eight herbs sometimes used by patients with prostate cancer. It was found to have potent oestrogenic activity (34). Coadministration of PC-SPES with estrogens might thus cause overdose problems, and PC-SPES in high doses may itself produce side effects such as breast tenderness and loss of libido (34). PC-SPES was banned in 2002 in the United States after chemical analysis showed it to be adulterated with diethylstilbestrol (a known carcinogen) indomethacin and warfarin (35). The action of St. John's wort in inhibiting monoamine oxidase can potentiate the effects of serotonin-reuptake inhibitors (3,36). It also induces hepatic enzymes, accelerating the clearance of several drugs including theophylline, cyclosporin, and warfarin and decreasing their plasma levels (36). Garlic extracts affect the metabolism of paracetamol and warfarin, and kava can interact with drugs used in the treatment of Parkinson's disease (3). The Lancet recently discussed the need for surgeons to monitor intake of herbal products and to recommend that ingestion of such products as ginseng, kava, St. John's wort, and valerian should stop several days before surgery (37). It is well known that grapefruit juice contains agents that inhibit intestinal cytochrome P450 (CYP3A4) and result in higher blood levels of certain drugs (e.g., amiodarone, cyclosporin, benzodiazepines, nifedipine, lovastatin, saquinavir), possibly to a toxic level (38). It seems likely that many similar phenomena involving ingredients in TCM remain to be discovered.

VII. CONCLUSION: THE WAY FORWARD

The data reviewed above show that TCM cannot at present be taken as an acceptable given body of knowledge. Practitioners need to be licensed and subject to quality control checks on their prescriptions to deter adulteration. They should participate in national or international adverse-event-reporting networks. They should be monitored by a disciplinary body. Better monitoring of prescribed and "over-the-counter" TCM products for adulterants and contaminants is needed. Products should be registered and evidence that the manufacturer complies with GMP should be available. The labels should specify the composition of the product, both active and "inactive" ingredients, the supplier, and the country of origin. Data on stability should be obtained and used to provide "sell by" and "use by" dates. Much more work needs to go into genetic and chemical methods to identify and quality-control TCM, and standards need to be established. Finally, the public needs to be educated to be prudent in what they take, not to overdose, to buy from reputable suppliers, to patronize only licensed TCM practitioners, and to alert their doctors to any TCM that they are taking. The use of TCM in infants, pregnant women, and nursing mothers cannot be considered safe, since present data are insufficient to establish or rule out teratogenic actions or adverse effects on children. Work to address some of the above problems is already underway (4,39–42).

REFERENCES

1. Lee H. The challenges facing TCM in the West. Asia Pacific Biotech News 2001; 5:3–11.
2. Ernst E. Herbal medications for common ailments in the elderly. Drugs Aging 1999; 15:423–428.
3. Izzo AA, Ernst E. Interactions between herbal medicines and prescribed drugs: a systematic review. Drugs 2001; 6:2163–2175.
4. Fung SKW. Commercial development of TCM in Hong Kong. Asia-Pacific Biotech News 2000; 4:488–510.
5. Engler HS, Spencer KC, Gilbert LE. Preventing cyanide release from leaves. Nature 2000; 406:144–145.

6. Ames BW, Gold LS. Paracelsus to parascience: the environmental cancer distribution. Mutat Res 2000; 447:3–13.
7. Gearin-Tosh M. Living Proof: A Medical Mutiny. London, UK: Scribner Press, 2002.
8. Goh BC, Lee SC, Wang LZ, Fan L, Guo JY, Lamba J, Schuetz E, Lim R, Lim HL, Ong AB, Lee HS. Explaining inter-individual variability of docetaxel pharmacokinetics and pharmacodynamics in Asians through phenotyping and genotyping strategies. J Clin Oncol 2002; 20:3683–3690.
9. Gao W, Jiang S, Zhu D. Three lycopodium alkaloid *N*-oxides from *Huperzia serrata*. Planta Med 2000; 66:644–667.
10. Klayman DL. Qinghaosu (artemisinin): an antimalarial drug from China. Science 1985; 228:1049–1055.
11. DeSmet AGMP. Herbal remedies. N Engl J Med 2002; 347:2046–2056.
12. Höld KM, Sirisoma N, Ikeda T, Narahashi T, Casida JE. α-Thuione (the active component of absinthe): γ-aminobutyric acid type A receptor modulation and metabolic detoxification. Proc Natl Acad Sci USA 2000; 97:3826–3831.
13. Woolf A. Essential oil poisoning. Clin Toxicol 1999; 37:721–727.
14. Brent J. Three new herbal hepatotoxic syndromes. Clin Toxicol 1999; 37:715–719.
15. Lai RS, Chiang AA, Wu MT, Wang JS, Lai NS, Lu JY, Ger LP, Roggli V. Outbreak of bronchiolitis obliterans associated with consumption of *Sauropus androgynus* in Taiwan. Lancet 1996; 348:83–85.
16. Yeh YH, Wang DY, Deng JF, Chen SK, Huang DF. Short-term toxicity of grass carp bile powder, 5α-cyprinol and 5α-cyprinol sulfate in rats. Comp Biochem Physiol 2002; C131:1–8.
17. Yu ZQ, Fu WB, Hua HM, Feng CT. Viper's blood and bile. Lancet 1997; 349: 250.
18. Slifman WR, Obermeyer WR, Aloi BK, Musser SM, Correl WA Jr, Cichowicz SM, Betz JM, Love LA. Contamination of botanical dietary supplement by *Digitalis lanata*. N Engl J Med 1998; 339:806–811.
19. Nortier JL, Martinez MCM, Schmeiser HH, Aret VM, Bieler CA, Petein M, Depierreux MF, De Pauw L, Abramowicz D, Vereerstraeten P, Vanherweghem JL. Urothelial carcinoma associated with use of a Chinese herb (*Aristolochia fangchi*). N Engl J Med 2000; 342:1686–1692.
20. Task force searches for herbal killers. News of the World, August 12, 2001: 41.
21. Anon. Gingko products fail WHO criteria. Asia Pacific Biotech News 2000; 4: 452.
22. El-Masry S, Mrssa JB, Khalial SAH. A critical approach to the quality control testing of herbal medicines. Saudi Pharm J 1995; 3:143–155.
23. Yeh SL, Hu ML. Induction of oxidative DNA damage in human foreskin fibroblast Hs68 cells by oxidised β-carotene and lycopene. Free Rad Res 2001; 35:203–213.
24. Long LH, Clement MV, Halliwell B. Artifacts in cell culture: rapid generation of hydrogen peroxide on addition of (−)-epigallocatechin, (−)-epigallocatechin gallate, (+)-catechin, and quercetin to commonly used cell culture media. Biochem Biophys Res Commun 2000; 273:50–53.

25. Dufresne CJ, Farnworth ER. A review of latest research findings on the health promotion properties of tea. J Nutr Biochem 2001; 12:404–421.
26. Roy AK, Sinha KK, Chourasia HK. Aflatoxin contamination of some common drug plants. Appl Environ Microbiol 1988; 54:842–843.
27. Xu H, Zhang N, Casida JE. Insecticides in Chinese medicinal plants; survey leading to jacaranone, a neurotoxicant and glutathione-reactive quinol. J Agr Food Chem 2003; 51:2544 2547.
28. Chi YW, Chen SL, Yang MH, Hwang RC, Chu ML. Heavy metals in traditional Chinese medicine: ba-pao-neu-hwang-san. Zhonghua Min Guo Xiao Er Ke Yi Xue Hui Za Zhi 1993; 34:181–190.
29. Ong ES, Yong YL, Woo SO. Determination of arsenic in traditional Chinese medicine by microwave digestion with flow injection-inductively coupled plasma mass spectrometry (FI-ICP-MS). J Am Oil Assoc Chem Int 1999; 82:903–937.
30. Metcalfe K, Corns C, Fahie-Wilson M, Mackenzie P. Chinese medicines for slimming still cause health problems. Br Med J 2002; 324:679.
31. Ries CA, Sakud MA. Agranulocytosis caused by Chinese herbal medicines: dangers of medication containing aminopyrine and phenylbutazone. JAMA 1975; 231:352–355.
32. Brooks PM, Lowenthal RM. Chinese herbal arthritis care and agranulocytosis. Med J Aust 1977; 2:860–861.
33. Keane FM, Munn SE, du Vivier AWP, Taylor WF, Higgins EM. Analysis of Chinese herbal creams prescribed for dermatological conditions. Br Med J 1999; 318:563–564.
34. Di Paola RS, Zhang H, Lambert GH, Meeker R, Licitra E, Rafi MM, Zhu BT, Spaulding H, Goodin S, Toledano MB, Haut WW, Gallo MA. Clinical and biologic activity of an estrogenic herbal combination (PC-SPES) in prostate cancer. N Engl J Med 1998; 339:785–791.
35. Marcus DM, Grollman AP. Botanical medicines—the need for new regulations. N Engl J Med 2002; 347:2073–2076.
36. Ernst E. Second thoughts about safety of St. John's wort. Lancet 1999; 354:2014–2016.
37. Larkin M. Safe use of herbal products before surgery proposed. Lancet 2001; 358:128.
38. Ho PC, Saville DJ, Wanwimolruk S. Inhibitation of human CYP3A4 activity by grapefruit flavonoids, furanocoumarins and related compounds. J Pharm Pharm Sci 2001; 4:217–227.
39. Man RYK. Traditional Chinese medicine research at the University of Hong Kong. Asia-Pacific Biotech News 2000; 4:484–485.
40. Ong CN. Research on TCM at the National University of Singapore. Asia-Pacific Biotech News 2000; 4:486–487.
41. Fung SKW. Commercial development of TCM in Hong Kong. Asia-Pacific Biotech News 2000; 4:488–510.
42. Ko KM. Traditional Chinese medicine research at the Hong Kong University of Science and Technology. Asia-Pacific Biotech News 2000; 4:482–483.

42

Review of Adverse Effects of Chinese Herbal Medicine and Herb-Drug Interactions

Brian Tomlinson, Henry Hin-Chung Chu, and Paul Pui-Hay But
Chinese University of Hong Kong
Shatin, Hong Kong, China

G. Neil Thomas
University of Hong Kong
Pokfulam, Hong Kong, China

Wei Lan
Roche Hong Kong Limited
Tsuen Wan, Hong Kong, China

I. INTRODUCTION

In recent years herbal medicines and other forms of complementary or alternative medicine (CAM) are being chosen with increasing frequency in Western countries (1,2). Conversely, in many parts of developing countries, traditional medicines may be the only form of health care readily available or affordable to the majority of the population. Chinese herbal medicine (CHM) is a major component of traditional Chinese medicine (TCM), which has a history in China of several thousand years and is a highly developed, well-documented system with its own theoretical background. Neighboring countries, such as Japan, Korea, Vietnam, and Taiwan, have developed their own variants of TCM and TCM is readily available throughout the world in Chinese communities and is now also used by many other ethnic groups.

One of the perceived advantages of these forms of therapy is an apparent lack of side effects compared with the drug therapies used in allopathic medicine (3). While it is true in most circumstances that side effects are infrequent, there are a number of situations in which adverse effects occur. The safety of the materials employed in CHM or the other herbal medicine systems has generally been established by their empirical usage over many centuries, but they have not been studied in the systematic way that is applied to modern pharmaceutical drugs. This review will draw on examples from experience of adverse effects of CHM from Hong Kong. Similar problems have been encountered in mainland China and other Asian countries but these are generally less well documented in the English-language literature.

Most of the ingredients in CHM have a high therapeutic index and are unlikely to cause toxicity even if used in considerable excess, but a few materials with well-recognized toxicity are still in common usage or may be given erroneously (4–7). In CHM, the raw materials are commonly used in combinations, which may allow the use of smaller doses of herbs with synergistic beneficial effects, and some materials may counteract the potential toxicity of others. Some herbal combinations that may potentiate toxicity have been recognized and can usually be avoided but interactions between herbal materials and standard drug treatments have not been widely studied and represent an area of increasing concern. Also, some forms of TCM, particularly Chinese proprietary medicines, have been implicated in causing toxicity because of adulteration with heavy metals or Western drugs.

Serious side effects from herbal medicines are still relatively rare in Western countries, especially compared with those from pharmaceutical drugs. In fact, many cases of herbal adverse reactions have been the result of inexperience or negligence. Herbal medicines contain an array of chemicals, the relative concentration of which varies considerably depending on the genetics of the plant, the growing conditions, the plant parts used, the time of harvesting, the technique of preparation, and the storage (8). Lack of standardization and differences in composition between products or even between different batches of the same product lead to difficulty in making generalizations about both efficacy and safety. In TCM if contraindications are ignored, processing procedures inadequately completed, dosages liberally assigned, combinations of herbs ill-conceived, dispensing carelessly handled, decoctions improperly prepared, and diagnosis erroneously made, adverse reactions might easily occur (9).

When a case of adverse reaction to CHM is suspected, the difficulty in establishing the diagnosis is well recognized. Each preparation (herbs or compound medicines) typically is made up of a number of ingredients that in turn consist of many different chemicals. Very often, the chemical nature and pharmacological actions of these ingredients and their constituents are largely unknown. If the actual prescription cannot be traced, chemical analysis of each ingredient is not possible. On the other hand, success in making the diagnosis to some extent will also depend on the clinician's suspicion and an awareness of particular patterns of clinical features that may suggest CHM toxicity rather than being features of the underlying disease or being related to toxic effects of pharmaceutical drugs (10).

CHM involves the prescription of combinations of herbs for topical application or ingestion. Topical applications appear more likely to result in allergic reactions than those ingested. Toxicity from ingestion of herbs can occur for a variety of different reasons or sometimes a combination of reasons. The examples described are grouped under the most common reasons for toxicity occurring with that material.

II. MISIDENTIFICATION, SUBSTITUTION, OR CONTAMINATION

Misidentification or mislabeling of herbs may result in unexpected adverse clinical effects. One problem in the identification of herbal ingredients is that the plant materials can be named in four different ways—the common English name, the transliterated name, the Latinized pharmaceutical name, and the scientific name. The Chinese names of different substances are sometimes similar and a raw material may have several Chinese proprietary names. It is desirable that plants are referred to by their binomial Latin names for genus and species; misidentification is more likely to occur when other names are used. Furthermore, plant material can be misidentified when wild plants are harvested or at the time of the manufacturer's bulk purchase.

A. Guijiu

One tragic example occurred in Hong Kong when the toxic herb guijiu, which is derived from the root and rhizome of *Podophyllum hexandrum* (*P. emodi*), was found as an adulterant of the herb longdancao (*Gentiana rigescens*) in 1989, which led to two cases of serious and permanent neuropathy and encephalopathy (11). Subsequent investigations revealed that the adulteration was made by the supplier in mainland China, but no one in the supply chain noticed the error until the occurrence of the adverse event. This same toxic herb also appeared as a contaminant in samples of the herb weilingxian

(*Clemetis* sp.) resulting in miniepidemics of three and nine cases of neuropathy in 1995 and 1996, respectively (12).

The products of the rootstock of *P. emodi* are generally too toxic to be used other than for external application. The toxic constituent of guijiu is podophyllotoxin, which is predominantly a neurotoxin but it can also damage the liver, intestine, and pancreas. It appears to inhibit protein synthesis and mitosis (13). The symptoms of toxicity include nausea, vomiting, diarrhea, and abdominal pain and in severe cases neuropathy and encephalopathy may develop and result in permanent neurological damage. Abnormal liver function tests, thrombocytopenia, and leukopenia may also occur. Bajiaolian, the root of *Dysosma pleianthum*, one of the species in the mayapple family, has been widely used in mainland China and Taiwan as a TCM remedy for snakebites, general weakness, poisoning, condyloma acuminatum, lymphadenopathy, and certain tumors. Toxic effects have resulted from accidental ingestion or topical application and some cases occurred when some people took what they thought were therapeutic doses, resulting in podophyllotoxin toxicity (14).

B. Anticholinergic Toxicity

Likewise, the erroneous dispensing of yangjinhua (the flowers of *Datura metel* L.) instead of the prescribed lingxiaohua (flower of *Campsis grandiflora*) has led to four cases of drowsiness or acute confusion due to the anticholinergic effects of this herb (15). Herbs such as yangjinhua or naoyanghua (flowers of *Rhododendron molle*) may be used for upper-respiratory problems such as chronic bronchitis or asthma or various painful conditions but in excessive dosage they may result in an acute confusional state with signs of central nervous system and peripheral anticholinergic toxicity (16). The typical features include confusion or coma, fever, tachycardia, flushed dry skin, dilated pupils, dry mouth, and urinary retention. The herbs contain scopolamine, hyoscyamine, and atropine. *Datura* species were the most common cause of plant poisonings in a series of TCM poisoning cases from Taiwan (17).

C. Aristolochic Acid

Another case of erroneous substitution occurred in Belgium when guangfangji (*Aristolochia fangchi*) was used instead of fangji (*Stephania tetrandra*) in a combined slimming regimen that included some Western medications (18). *A. fangchi* contains the nephrotoxin aristolochic acid; this resulted in a number of cases of renal toxicity with rapidly progressive fibrosing interstitial nephritis and some patients developed irreversible end-stage renal failure or carcinoma in the urinary tract (19,20). The toxic effect could have been potentiated by the other drugs used such as acetazolamide (18,19).

D. Chansu

Chansu, or toad cake, is made from the dried venom of the toad *Bufo bufo gargarizans* or *B. melanostictus*. This is prepared from the skin and venom glands of the toad. It is stored in a disc shape of dry material, which has been mistaken for another innocuous material prepared from the hide of the ass. Chansu is used for its anti-inflammatory analgesic and anesthetic properties. It contains bufotoxins, which have a digoxin-like effect, and excessive doses may cause cardiac arrhythmias that may be fatal. Chansu was the most common cause of fatal toxicity due to TCM in a series reported from Taiwan where over 14 years there were 7 deaths related to this of a total of 43 (17). It is also found in the proprietary Chinese medicine lushenwan, which is a popular remedy for upper-respiratory symptoms or used as a topical preparation for skin infections. Overdosage of lushenwan pills can cause cardiac glycoside toxicity in children and topical applications may cause local skin inflammation.

E. Ginseng

In TCM ginseng is considered a panacea and has been attributed with many activities, including as an adaptogen, antistress, antifatigue, anticancer, antiaging, immunomodulating, as well as a performance enhancer, and aphrodisiac, although scientific evidence to support such claims is limited (21–23). Ginseng is generally regarded as safe but a number of adverse effects have been reported with ginseng products including central-nervous-system excitatory effects, hypertension, insomnia, tachycardia, and hormonal effects resulting from corticosteroid-, estrogen-, or androgen-like actions (21,22,24–26). Some of the adverse effects attributed to ginseng preparations may have been due to misidentification or substitution and there is a great variation in the quality of different products (27). Ginseng historically refers to the products from the *Panax* species. Chinese and Korean ginsengs come from *Panax ginseng* C.A. Meyer whereas American ginseng is prepared from *Panax quinquefolius* L. These have different combinations of chemical components and different uses but all the *Panax* species products should contain ginsenosides, the steroidal saponins with a 4-*trans*-ring steroid skeleton that are associated with pharmacological activities and are used as markers of quality control (28).

Siberian ginseng is prepared from the roots of *Eleutherococcus senticosus*, which is from the same family (Araliaceae) but a different genus than the *Panax* species. It does not contain ginsenosides but has eleutherosides, which are used as quality control markers for these products. These are chemically related to cardiac glycosides and may interact with some digoxin assays. This may have been responsible for a case of apparent elevation of serum digoxin levels with no signs of toxicity when Siberian ginseng and digoxin were taken together (29) although it was also suggested that the herb may have been misidentified (30). Another case involving neonatal androgenization associated with maternal use of Siberian ginseng (31) appears to have been due to misidentification of the herb involved as it was later identified as Chinese silk vine (*Periploca sepium*) (24). Studies in rats showed Siberian ginseng was not associated with androgenicity (32).

Estrogenic effects have been attributed to ginseng in both oral and topical preparations resulting in postmenopausal bleeding (25,33) or mastalgia (34) but the source and purity of the products involved were not specified. Likewise, the "ginseng abuse syndrome," which involved elevation of mood, hypertension, nervousness, sleeplessness, skin eruptions, diarrhea, and edema, was attributed to long-term usage of ginseng with other stimulants such as coffee but the origin, composition, and dosages of the products involved were not specified (35).

Interactions with other drugs have been reported with ginseng therapy. Ginseng has been reported to interact with phenelzine and other MAOIs to have a stimulatory effect on the central nervous system inducing headache and tremor (36,37) An interaction with warfarin was apparent as the International Normalised Ratio (INR) clotting index fell from 3.1 to 1.5 while the combination was taken and normalized after withdrawal of the ginseng (38). This interaction has not been confirmed by other studies and one study in rats showed no significant impact of ginseng on the pharmacokinetics or pharmacodynamics of warfarin given in single or multiple doses (39). In healthy human subjects *P. ginseng* acute or 28-day supplementation had no significant effect on the activity of CYP1A2, CYP2D6, CYP2E1, or CYP3A4 measured by a cocktail of probe drugs (40). Studies in rabbit platelets showed that some components of ginseng had antiplatelet activity (41).

III. LACK OF STANDARDIZATION OR INADEQUATE PROCESSING

Poor quality of herbs that require proper curing and of proprietary medicines is also found to be a major cause of herbal poisoning. The relative proportions of therapeutic and toxic components of plants vary depending on the part of the plant used, stage of ripeness, geographic area where the plant is grown, and storage conditions. Therefore, batch-to-batch reproducibility of active chemical ingredients should ideally be assessed in the production of marketed products, but in practice the active ingredients are often not known and most herbal suppliers and practitioners do not have the facilities or training to undertake chemical standardization, so product variation in herbal medicines can be significant.

A. Aconites

One of the major causes of serious and sometimes fatal toxicity in Hong Kong has been the use of aconites from the dried rootstocks of *Aconitum carmichaeli* and *A. kusnezoffii* (5–7). These preparations are commonly used in TCM for their anti-inflammatory analgesic effects. They contain C_{19}-diterpenoid esters, aconitine, mesaconitine, hypaconitine, and other derivatives, which activate sodium channels resulting in neurological and cardiac toxicity. Aconitine was previously popular in Western medicine but fell into disrepute toward the end of the nineteenth century when cases of toxicity were recognized, and its only role in Western medicine now is in experimental pharmacology to induce arrhythmias in animal preparations.

The initial symptoms of toxicity include paresthesias in the mouth and tongue with progression to involve the extremeties. Nausea and vomiting are common and there may be muscle weakness, hypotension, and dizziness (42–44). The most serious effects are arrhythmias, which include both bradycardia and tachyarrhythmias such as ventricular flutter or fibrillation (45–48). A number of deaths have occurred from these ventricular arrhythmias (49).

Toxicity was often related to the use of excessive doses of these herbs or to inadequate processing. Like most herbs in CHM the aconites are subjected to a process of "curing," which in this case involves steaming or boiling in water to reduce the toxicity by converting aconitine alkaloids to aconines and benzoylaconitines. The processed herb is supplied to the patient with a combination of other herbs and the patient is instructed to prepare a decoction by boiling the herbs for a certain period of time. This will further reduce the toxicity of the aconites. Thus there are a number of stages in this process where variations in technique may lead to excessive amounts of the toxic ingredients remaining in the preparation that the patient ingests. In some cases the dosage prescribed was too high. The recommended dosage in the *Pharmacopoeia of the People's Republic of China* is 1.5–3 g for both caowu (main root of *A. kusnezoffii*) and for chuanwu (main root of *A. carmichaeli*) and 3–5 g for fuzi (lateral root of *A. carmichaeli*). Some prescriptions have included 6 g or more of each of the first two aconite preparations. Other factors that may contribute to toxicity include differences in the amount of alkaloids present in the plant roots at the time of harvest and the use of inappropriate combinations with other herbs.

IV. HEAVY METAL CONTAMINATION

Heavy metals have been used over the centuries for their medicinal effects although they have largely been replaced in allopathic medicine by less toxic pharmaceuticals. In the theory of TCM heavy metals may be used as active ingredients of some herbal prescriptions and Chinese proprietary medicines often contain cinnabar (mercuric sulfide), realgar (arsenic sulfide), or litharge (lead oxide) as part of the traditional formula. Furthermore, during growth and storage, crude plant material can become contaminated by pesticide residues, microorganisms, aflatoxins, radioactive substances, and heavy metals; lead, cadmium, mercury, arsenic, and thallium have been reported as contaminants of some herbal preparations (50). In a case series of five patients in England with lead poisoning from Asian traditional remedies, the preparations implicated contained 6–60% by weight of lead (51).

A proprietary medicine, "Niuhuang Jiedu Pian," was incriminated in a fatal case in Macau (52). The patient, a 13-year-old girl had taken a high dosage of this proprietary medicine and developed an illness involving multiorgan failure, which was considered to be compatible with arsenic toxicity. When the tablets were analyzed they were found to contain excessive amounts of arsenic and this product and other similar ones were withdrawn from the market in Macau until they were proven to free of arsenic contamination. A number of cases of acute or chronic arsenic poisoning were reported from Singapore in children and adults taking "Sin Lak Pill", "Lu Shen Wan," and other "antiasthma" preparations (53). These proprietary medicines, which were manufactured in China, Hong Kong, and other Asian countries, were found to contain levels of inorganic arsenic ranging from 25 to 107,000 ppm. In Taiwan, heavy-metal poisoning of newborn infants fed "Ba Pao Neu Hwang San" is reported annually (54). In 1983, the death of a 5-month-old female infant resulted from consumption of the drug, which was found to have contained lead at 44,000 ppm. Despite such cases this TCM is still widely used. In 1992, a survey revealed mercury contamination of this product ranging from 34,500 to 65,700 ppm (54).

V. ADULTERATION WITH WESTERN DRUGS

Data from Taiwan have highlighted the widespread use of adulterants in TCM preparations. Examination of 2,609 products found 23.7% were adulterated and of these 52.8% contained two or more adulterants (55). Of the adulterants 34.5% contained caffeine, 27.0% paracetamol, 24.6% indomethacin, 20.6% hydrochlorothiazide, and 14.8% prednisolone (55). TCM hospitals had the lowest rates of adulteration (9.0%) with herbalists providing the least authentic preparations, with 34.6% containing adulterants (55). Ginseng preparations in the United States were found to be adulterated with a number of different components including *Mandragora officinarum* (scopolamine), *Rauwolfia serpentia* (reserpine), and *Cola* species.

VI. HERB-DRUG INTERACTIONS

Interactions between herbs and drugs have been the subject of a number of reviews (21,22,26,56–60). However, data regarding interactions with CHM are relatively few and the subject has not been studied systematically although attempts are being made to remedy this (40). The study of some of these interactions has provided insights into the mechanisms involved and helps to predict what other problems may occur. Problems are most likely to be encountered with drugs that have a narrow therapeutic window such as warfarin, digoxin, or cyclosporin. Much of the evidence of interactions of CHM with such drugs comes from anecdotal reports and the true risk is difficult to assess (61).

A. Grapefruit Juice

Drug interactions with grapefruit juice serve as a good example of how an apparently innocuous dietary constituent can interact with potent drugs, which could result in serious toxicity. A number of Chinese herbal medicines are derived from citrus fruits such as chen pi (rind of *Citrus reticulata*) or zhi shi (unripe fruits of *Citrus aurantium*) and these could have similar effects although it has been suggested that the interaction is specific for grapefruit products and in vitro findings suggested the flavonoid, naringenin, or the furanocoumarin, 6′,7′-dihydroxybergamottin, were the active components causing drug interactions (62).

The serendipitous finding that grapefruit juice increased the oral bioavailability of felodipine and to a lesser extent nifedipine provided the instigation for a series of investigations to explore the mechanism of this effect (63). Lown and colleagues reported that grapefruit juice decreased small-bowel epithelial cell CYP3A4 concentration by 62%, but did not alter CYP3A4 mRNA levels or the concentrations of small-bowel CYP1A1, CYP2D6, or *P*-glycoprotein, or colonic CYP3A5, or the activity of hepatic CYP3A4 (64). They concluded that grapefruit juice caused selective post-translational downregulation of CYP3A4 expression in the intestinal wall. This interaction is likely to have the greatest effect in individuals with the highest inherent baseline enteric CYP3A4 and with drugs with innately low oral bioavailability because of substantial presystemic metabolism mediated by CYP3A4 (62). Clinically relevant interactions are likely with cyclosporin, terfenadine, saquinavir, some HMG CoA reductase inhibitors, and a number of other drugs. Understanding this mechanism should help to limit possible adverse drug interactions and might also be useful to develop possible beneficial drug combinations that could lower treatment costs or increase efficacy.

B. St. John's Wort

St. John's wort, derived from the flowering tips of *Hypericum perforatum*, provides another example where a herbal drug that has gained considerable popularity in Western countries proved to be capable of causing important herb-drug interactions. It appeared to be a safe alternative antidepressant with an efficacy similar to low-dose tricyclic antidepressants or selective serotonin reuptake inhibitors (65–69) apart from the risk that it might interact with the serotonin reuptake inhibitors to produce a mild serotonin syndrome (26,56,70,71). However, in 1999 reports started to appear of interactions between St. John's wort and a variety of drugs and it was shown to reduce the plasma concentrations of digoxin (72) and theophylline (73) and to result in breakthrough bleeding during oral contraceptive use (74). Case reports then emerged suggesting interactions with cyclosporin could reduce the immunosuppressive effect resulting in rejection of transplanted organs including heart (75,76), liver (77), and renal (78–80) transplants. It was also shown to decrease plasma levels of the HIV protease inhibitors indinavir (81) and nevirapine (82), as well as amitriptyline (83) and some HMG CoA reductase inhibitors (84).

Studies examining the mechanism of these interactions showed that administration of St. John's wort extract to rats for 14 days resulted in a 3.8-fold increase in expression of the intestinal drug efflux transporter *P*-glycoprotein, the product of the multidrug resistance (MDR) gene 1, and in a 2.5-fold increase in hepatic CYP3A2 expression (85). In healthy volunteers administration of St. John's wort extract for 14 days resulted in 1.4- and 1.5-fold increased expressions of duodenal *P*-glycoprotein/MDR1 and CYP3A4, respectively, and in a 1.4-fold increase in the functional activity of hepatic CYP3A4 assessed by 14C-erythromycin breath test (85). Likewise, St. John's wort given for 16 days produced a 4.2-fold increase in expression of *P*-glycoprotein and enhanced the *P*-glycoprotein-mediated drug efflux function in peripheral blood lymphocytes of healthy volunteers (86).

Another study using an in vivo probe drug cocktail approach showed that short-term administration of St. John's wort had no effect on CYP activities whereas long-term (2 weeks) administration decreased the bioavailability of oral midazolam by >50% but when midazolam was given intravenously there was only a 20% decrease, indicating relatively selective induction of CYP3A activity in the intestinal wall (87). There was no change in CYP1A2, CYP2C9, or CYP2D6 activities as a result of St. John's wort administration (87). However, in the LS180 intestinal cell model St. John's wort increased the expression of CYP1A2 in a concentration- and time-dependent manner (88). Conversely, incubation of St. John's wort in vitro with a panel of recombinant human CYP isoforms showed inhibition of the 1A2, the 2C6, and especially the 2C19 isoforms (89).

A molecular mechanism for the interaction was demonstrated as hyperforin, a constituent of St. John's wort with antidepressant activity, was found to be a potent ligand for the pregnane X receptor, an orphan nuclear receptor that regulates expression of the cytochrome P450 (CYP) 3A4 (90). Treatment of primary human hepatocytes with hypericum extracts or hyperforin results in a marked induction of CYP3A4 expression. Activation of this nuclear receptor would lead to upregulation of the expression of *P*-glycoprotein/MDRI and CYP3A4 expression in the intestinal wall and to a lesser extent CYP3A4 in the liver.

C. Danshen

Danshen, the root of *Salvia miltiorrhiza*, is a herb commonly used in TCM for the treatment of atherosclerotic cardio- and cerebrovascular diseases. It has been reported to have a number of anticoagulatory effects, including inhibition of platelet aggregation, antithrombin III–like activity, antagonism of extrinsic blood coagulation, and profibrinolytic properties (91). One study showed some components may have scavenging effects on free radicals (92). When taken in combination with the anticoagulant warfarin, excessive anticoagulation has been reported in a number of cases (93–96). This could represent a pharmacodynamic interaction on different coagulation mechanisms, but as danshen does not usually affect the PT directly the increases seen in prothrombin time suggests a pharmacokinetic effect and danshen has also been reported to increase plasma concentrations of both *R*- and *S*-warfarin and decrease clearance in a rat model (97). Much of the activity of danshen has been attributed to the tanshionone components that can be identified following hydrophobic extraction, and include tanshionone IIA and sodium tanshionone sulfonate. Recently, the sulfonate has been reported to be a noncompetitive inhibitor of CYP2C9 in human hepatic microsomes (98).

D. Dong Quai

Dong quai, or danggui, is the Chinese herb prepared from the dried root of *Angelica sinensis*. It is used as an antispasmodic, a "blood purifier," and a tonic and as a treatment for various gynecological disorders including menstrual cramping, irregular menses, and menopausal symptoms. Phytochemical analyses showed it contains coumarin derivatives and other constituents possessing antithrombotic and antiarrhythmic effects (99) and it is recommended to avoid using it in patients with coagulation disorders (100). Some of the pharmacological effects may be related to the phytoestrogen content and gynecomastia has been reported in a man taking a dong quai preparation (101) although no evidence of an estrogen effect was seen in a study in postmenopausal women (102), and in an in vitro study it did not have an estrogen effect but it did increase the growth of a human breast cancer cell line (103). A case was described of a patient stabilized on warfarin who showed an increase in prothrombin time and INR after taking dong quai (104). The exact mechanism of the interaction is not known although one study showed that dong quai affected the pharmacodynamics but not the pharmacokinetics of warfarin in rabbits (105).

E. Ginkgo (*Ginkgo biloba*)

The fruits and seeds of ginkgo have been used in TCM for thousands of years and leaf extracts are one of the most commonly used European herbal extracts (22,106). The active components have been attributed with a number of activities that promote small-vessel blood flow, including that in the cerebral arteries, as well as antiplatelet and other hemorrheological actions, antihypoxic, neuroprotective, membrane-stabilizing, and capillary-fragility-decreasing effects (21,22,106). Ginkgo has been reported to provide moderate improvements in symptoms of intermittent claudication (107) and a standardized form of the leaf extract (EGb761) has been approved in Germany for the treatment of dementia (21,22).

Ginkgo appears to be relatively safe with side effects that are usually mild and limited to gastrointestinal complaints, headache, nausea, and vomiting (22,106). However, a small number of serious bleeding problems have been reported for subjects taking ginkgo preparations, who in most cases were receiving concurrent anticoagulant drugs. These have included two subdural hematomas (108,109), one in a patient who was taking paracetamol and an ergotamine-caffeine preparation (109), one intracerebral hemorrhage when ginkgo was taken with warfarin (110), one subarachnoid hemorrhage (111), and a case of hyphema resulting from combination with aspirin (112). The significance of these reports is uncertain but it seems advisable for patients taking anticoagulants or antiplatelet drugs not to take ginkgo (22). A study using probe drugs for CYP1A2, CYP2D6, CYP2E1, and CYP3A4 activity showed no significant effect on CYP activity with 28-day supplementation with a *G. biloba* preparation (40).

F. Other Herbs

Garlic or dasuan, the tuber of *Allium sativum* L., is used in TCM both orally and topically for various effects including as an anthelmintic, antiseptic, antidote, and tonic. Various preparations of garlic exhibited an inhibitory effect on human CYP-mediated metabolism of marker substrates for 2C9*1,

2C19, 3A4, 3A5, and 3A7 but not 2D6, whereas extracts of fresh garlic stimulated CYP2C9*2 metabolism of the marker substrate in an in vitro system (113). Using the probe drug approach, in vivo garlic oil reduced CYP2E1 activity after 28 days but had no effect on CYP1A2, CYP2D6, or CYP3A4 activity (40).

Piperine, a major component of black pepper, inhibited *P*-glycoprotein-mediated digoxin and cyclosporin A transport in Caco-2 cells and CYP3A4-mediated verapamil metabolism in human liver microsomes, so it could affect plasma concentrations of drugs subject to first-pass elimination by these mechanisms (114).

VII. CONCLUSIONS

When used as monotherapy or in appropriate combinations recommended by an experienced TCM practitioner, most of the herbal preparations used in CHM obtained from reliable sources are relatively safe with minor adverse effects. However, when obtained from unscrupulous sources there is an increased chance of misidentification, adulteration, or contamination that may be associated with serious adverse events. Additionally, concomitant use of pharmaceutical drugs may lead to herb-drug interactions that may be potentially fatal. Studies with grapefruit juice and St. John's wort have demonstrated some mechanisms by which pharmacokinetic interactions may occur. However, despite clear evidence that herbal preparations may lead to severe interactions, information regarding possible and proven interactions is very limited. Care should be taken when herbal preparations are given with pharmaceutical drugs and physicians must identify the use of such herbal preparations to reduce the chances of these interactions occurring.

REFERENCES

1. Eisenberg DM, Kessler RC, Foster C, Norlock FE, Calkins DR, Delbanco TL. Unconventional medicine in the United States: Prevalence, costs, and patterns of use. N Engl J Med 1993; 328:246–252.
2. Eisenberg DM, Davis RB, Ettner SL, Appel S, Wilkey S, Van Rompay M, Kessler RC. Trends in alternative medicine use in the United States, 1990–1997: results of a follow-up national survey. JAMA 1998; 280:1569–1575.
3. Ernst E. Harmless herbs? A review of the recent literature. Am J Med 1998; 104:170–178.
4. Tai YT, But PH, Tomlinson B. Adverse effects from traditional Chinese medicine: a critical reappraisal. J Hong Kong Med Assoc 1993; 45:197–201.
5. Chan TY, Chan JC, Tomlinson B, Critchley JA. Chinese herbal medicines revisited: a Hong Kong perspective. Lancet 1993; 342:1532–1534.

6. Chan TY, Chan JC, Tomlinson B, Critchley JA. Poisoning by Chinese herbal medicines in Hong Kong: a hospital-based study. Vet Hum Toxlcol 1994; 36:546–547.
7. Tomlinson B, Chan TY, Chan JC, Critchley JA, But PP. Toxicity of complementary therapies: an Eastern perspective. J Clin Pharmacol 2000; 40:451–456.
8. O'Hara M, Kiefer D, Farrell K, Kemper K. A review of 12 commonly used medicinal herbs. Arch Fam Med 1998; 7:523–536.
9. But PPH. Attitudes and approaches of traditional chinese medicine to herbal toxicity. J Nat Toxins 1995; 4:207–217.
10. Chan TY, Chan AY, Critchley JA. Hospital admissions due to adverse reactions to Chinese herbal medicines. J Trop Med Hyg 1992; 95:296–298.
11. Ng TH, Chan YW, Yu YL, Chang CM, Ho HC, Leung SY, But PP. Encephalopathy and neuropathy following ingestion of a Chinese herbal broth containing podophyllin. J Neurol Sci 1991; 101:107–113.
12. But PP, Tomlinson B, Cheung KO, Yong SP, Szeto ML, Lee CK. Adulterants of herbal products can cause poisoning [letter]. Br Med J 1996; 313:117.
13. Yang CM, Deng JF, Chen CF, Chang LW. Experimental podophyllotoxin (bajiaolian) poisoning. III. Biochemical bases for toxic effects. Biomed Environ Sci 1994; 7:259–265.
14. Kao WF, Hung DZ, Tsai WJ, Lin KP, Deng JF. Podophyllotoxin intoxication: toxic effect of bajiaolian in herbal therapeutics. Hum Exp Toxicol 1992; 11:480–487.
15. Chan JC, Chan TY, Chan KL, Leung NW, Tomlinson B, Critchley JA. Anticholinergic poisoning from Chinese herbal medicines. Aust NZ J Med 1994; 24:317–318.
16. Chan JC, Tomlinson B, Kay R, Chan TY, Critchley JA. Acute confusion, Chinese herbal medicines and tuberculous meningitis [letter]. Aust NZ J Med 1994; 24:590–591.
17. Lin TJ, Deng JF, Tsai MS. Chinese traditional medicine poisonings in Taiwan. Int J Intens Care 2002; 9:118–127.
18. But PP. Herbal poisoning caused by adulterants or erroneous substitutes. J Trop Med Hyg 1994; 97:371–374.
19. Vanherweghem JL, Depierreux M, Tielemans C, Abramowicz D, Dratwa M, Jadoul M, Richard C, Vandervelde D, Verbeelen D, Vanhaelen-Fastre R, et al. Rapidly progressive interstitial renal fibrosis in young women: association with slimming regimen including Chinese herbs. Lancet 1993; 341:387–391.
20. Vanherweghem JL, Tielemans C, Simon J, Depierreux M. Chinese herbs nephropathy and renal pelvic carcinoma. Nephrol Dial Transplant 1995; 10:270–273.
21. Cupp MJ. Herbal remedies: adverse effects and drug interactions. Am Fam Physician 1999; 59:1239–1245.
22. Miller LG. Herbal medicinals: selected clinical considerations focusing on known or potential drug-herb interactions. Arch Intern Med 1998; 158:2200–2211.

23. Vogler BK, Pittler MH, Ernst E. The efficacy of ginseng: a systematic review of randomised clinical trials. Eur J Clin Pharmacol 1999; 55:567–575.
24. Awang DV. Maternal use of ginseng and neonatal androgenization [letter]. JAMA 1991; 266:363.
25. Hopkins MP, Androff L, Benninghoff AS. Ginseng face cream and unexplained vaginal bleeding. Am J Obstet Gynecol 1988; 159:1121–1122.
26. Izzo AA, Ernst E. Interactions between herbal medicines and prescribed drugs: a systematic review. Drugs 2001; 61:2163–2175.
27. Harkey MR, Henderson GL, Gershwin ME, Stern JS, Hackman RM. Variability in commercial ginseng products: an analysis of 25 preparations. Am J Clin Nutr 2001; 73:1101–1106.
28. Attele AS, Wu JA, Yuan CS. Ginseng pharmacology: multiple constituents and multiple actions. Biochem Pharmacol 1999; 58:1685–1693.
29. McRae S. Elevated serum digoxin levels in a patient taking digoxin and Siberian ginseng. Can Med Assoc J 1996; 155:293–295.
30. Awang DV. Siberian ginseng toxicity may be case of mistaken identity. Can Med Assoc J 1996; 155:1237.
31. Koren G, Randor S, Martin S, Danneman D. Maternal ginseng use associated with neonatal androgenization. JAMA 1990; 264:2866.
32. Waller DP, Martin AM, Farnsworth NR, Awang DV. Lack of androgenicity of Siberian ginseng [letter]. JAMA 1992; 267:2329.
33. Greenspan EM. Ginseng and vaginal bleeding. JAMA 1983; 249:2018.
34. Palmer BV, Montgomery AC, Monteiro JC. Gin seng and mastalgia. Br Med J 1978; 1:1284.
35. Siegel RK. Ginseng abuse syndrome: problems with the panacea. JAMA 1979; 241:1614–1615.
36. Jones BD, Runikis AM. Interaction of ginseng with phenelzine [letter]. J Clin Psychopharmacol 1987; 7:201–202.
37. Shader RI, Greenblatt DJ. Phenelzine and the dream machine—ramblings and reflections [editorial]. J Clin Psychopharmacol 1985; 5:65.
38. Janetzky K, Morreale AP. Probable interaction between warfarin and ginseng. Am J Health Syst Pharm 1997; 54:692–693.
39. Zhu M, Chan KW, Ng LS, Chang Q, Chang S, Li RC. Possible influences of ginseng on the pharmacokinetics and pharmacodynamics of warfarin in rats. J Pharm Pharmacol 1999; 51:175–180.
40. Gurley BJ, Gardner SF, Hubbard MA, Williams DK, Gentry WB, Cui Y, Ang CY. Cytochrome P450 phenotypic ratios for predicting herb-drug interactions in humans. Clin Pharmacol Ther 2002; 72:276–287.
41. Kuo SC, Teng CM, Lee JC, Ko FN, Chen SC, Wu TS. Antiplatelet components in *Panax ginseng*. Planta Med 1990; 56:164–167.
42. Chan TY, Tomlinson B, Critchley JA. Aconitine poisoning following the ingestion of Chinese herbal medicines: a report of eight cases. Aust NZ J Med 1993; 23:268–271.
43. Chan TY, Tomlinson B, Chan WW, Yeung VT, Tse LK. A case of acute aconitine poisoning caused by chuanwu and caowu. J Trop Med Hyg 1993; 96:62–63.

44. Chan TY, Tomlinson B, Critchley JA, Cockram CS. Herb-induced aconitine poisoning presenting as tetraplegia. Vet Hum Toxicol 1994; 36:133–134.
45. Tai YT, But PP, Young K, Lau CP. Cardiotoxicity after accidental herb-induced aconite poisoning [see comments]. Lancet 1992; 340:1254–1256.
46. Tai YT, Lau CP, But PP, Fong PC, Li JP. Bidirectional tachycardia induced by herbal aconite poisoning. Pacing Clin Electrophysiol 1992; 15:831–839.
47. Tomlinson B, Chan TY, Chan JC, Critchley JA. Herb-induced aconitine poisoning [letter]. Lancet 1993; 341:370–371.
48. Chan TY, Tomlinson B, Tse LK, Chan JC, Chan WW, Critchley JA. Aconitine poisoning due to Chinese herbal medicines: a review. Vet Hum Toxicol 1994; 36:452–455.
49. Dickens P, Tai YT, But PP, Tomlinson B, Ng HK, Yan KW. Fatal accidental aconitine poisoning following ingestion of Chinese herbal medicine: a report of two cases. Forens Sci Int 1994; 67:55–58.
50. Ernst E, Thompson CJ. Heavy metals in traditional Chinese medicines: a systematic review. Clin Pharmacol Ther 2001; 70:497–504.
51. Bayly GR, Braithwaite RA, Sheehan TMT. Lead poisoning from Asian traditional remedies in the West Midlands—report of a series of five cases. Hum Exp Toxicol 1995; 14:24–28.
52. Cunha J, Pereira L, Pun MI, Lopes V, Vong SK. Arsenic and acute lethal intoxication. Hong Kong Pharm J 1998; 7:50–53.
53. Kang-Yum E, Oransky SH. Chinese patent medicine as a potential source of mercury poisoning. Vet Hum Toxicol 1992; 34:235–238.
54. Chi YW, Chen SL, Yang MH, Hwang RC, Chu ML. [Heavy metals in traditional Chinese medicine: ba-pao-neu-hwang-san]. Zhonghua Min Guo Xiao Er Ke Yi Xue Hui Za Zhi 1993; 34:181–190.
55. Huang WF, Wen KC, Hsiao ML. Adulteration by synthetic therapeutic substances of traditional Chinese medicines in Taiwan. J Clin Pharmacol 1997; 37:344–350.
56. Fugh-Berman A. Herb-drug interactions. Lancet 2000; 355:134–138.
57. Heck AM, DeWitt BA, Lukes AL. Potential interactions between alternative therapies and warfarin. Am J Health Syst Pharm 2000; 57:1221–1227.
58. Fugh-Berman A, Ernst E. Herb-drug interactions: review and assessment of report reliability. Br J Clin Pharmacol 2001; 52:587–595.
59. Ioannides C. Pharmacokinetic interactions between herbal remedies and medicinal drugs. Xenobiotica 2002; 32:451–478.
60. Scott GN, Elmer GW. Update on natural product-drug interactions. Am J Health Syst Pharm 2002; 59:339–347.
61. Vaes LP, Chyka PA. Interactions of warfarin with garlic, ginger, ginkgo, or ginseng: nature of the evidence. Ann Pharmacother 2000; 34:1478–1482.
62. Bailey DG, Malcolm J, Arnold O, Spence JD. Grapefruit juice–drug interactions. Br J Clin Pharmacol 1998; 46:101–110.
63. Bailey DG, Spence JD, Munoz C, Arnold JM. Interaction of citrus juices with felodipine and nifedipine. Lancet 1991; 337:268–269.
64. Lown KS, Bailey DG, Fontana RJ, Janardan SK, Adair CH, Fortlage LA,

Brown MB, Guo W, Watkins PB. Grapefruit juice increases felodipine oral availability in humans by decreasing intestinal CYP3A protein expression. J Clin Invest 1997; 99:2545–2553.
65. Firenzuoli F, Luigi G. Safety of *Hypericum perforatum*. J Altern Comp Med 1999; 5:397–398.
66. Kim HL, Streltzer J, Goebert D. St. John's wort for depression: a meta-analysis of well-defined clinical trials. J Nerv Ment Dis 1999; 187:532–538.
67. Whiskey E, Werneke U, Taylor D. A systematic review and meta-analysis of *Hypericum perforatum* in depression: a comprehensive clinical review. Int Clin Psychopharmacol 2001; 16:239–252.
68. Kasper S. *Hypericum perforatum*—a review of clinical studies. Pharmacopsychiatry 2001; 34:S51–S55.
69. Di Carlo G, Borrelli F, Izzo AA, Ernst E. St. John's wort: prozac from the plant kingdom. Trends Pharmacol Sci 2001; 22:292–297.
70. Beckman SE, Sommi RW, Switzer J. Consumer use of St. John's wort: a survey on effectiveness, safety, and tolerability. Pharmacotherapy 2000; 20:568–574.
71. Barbenel DM, Yusufi B, O'Shea D, Bench CJ. Mania in a patient receiving testosterone replacement postorchidectomy taking St. John's wort and sertraline. J Psychopharmacol 2000; 14:84–86.
72. Johne A, Brockmoller J, Bauer S, Maurer A, Langheinrich M, Roots I. Pharmacokinetic interaction of digoxin with an herbal extract from St. John's wort (*Hypericum perforatum*). Clin Pharmacol Ther 1999; 66:338–345.
73. Nebel A, Schneider BJ, Baker RK, Kroll DJ. Potential metabolic interaction between St. John's wort and theophylline. Ann Pharmacother 1999; 33:502.
74. Ernst E. Second thoughts about safety of St. John's wort. Lancet 1999; 354:2014–2016.
75. Ruschitzka F, Meier PJ, Turina M, Luscher TF, Noll G. Acute heart transplant rejection due to Saint John's wort. Lancet 2000; 355:548–549.
76. Ahmed SM, Banner NR, Dubrey SW. Low cyclosporin-A level due to Saint-John's-wort in heart transplant patients. J Heart Lung Transplant 2001; 20:795.
77. Karliova M, Treichel U, Malago M, Frilling A, Gerken G, Broelsch CE. Interaction of *Hypericum perforatum* (St. John's wort) with cyclosporin A metabolism in a patient after liver transplantation. J Hepatol 2000; 33:853–855.
78. Breidenbach T, Kliem V, Burg M, Radermacher J, Hoffmann MW, Klempnauer J. Profound drop of cyclosporin A whole blood trough levels caused by St. John's wort (*Hypericum perforatum*). Transplantation 2000; 69:2229–2230.
79. Mandelbaum A, Pertzborn F, Martin-Facklam M, Wiesel M. Unexplained decrease of cyclosporin trough levels in a compliant renal transplant patient. Nephrol Dial Transplant 2000; 15:1473–1474.
80. Barone GW, Gurley BJ, Ketel BL, Abul-Ezz SR. Herbal supplements: a potential for drug interactions in transplant recipients. Transplantation 2001; 71:239–241.
81. Piscitelli SC, Burstein AH, Chaitt D, Alfaro RM, Falloon J. Indinavir concentrations and St. John's wort. Lancet 2000; 355:547–548.

82. de Maat MM, Hoetelmans RM, Math t RA, van Gorp EC, Meenhorst PL, Mulder JW, Beijnen JH. Drug interaction between St. John's wort and nevirapine. AIDS 2001; 15:420–421.
83. Johne A, Schmider J, Brockmoller J, Stadelmann AM, Stormer E, Bauer S, Scholler G, Langheinrich M, Roots I. Decreased plasma levels of amitriptyline and its metabolites on comedication with an extract from St. John's wort (*Hypericum perforatum*). J Clin Psychopharmacol 2002; 22:46–54.
84. Sugimoto K, Ohmori M, Tsuruoka S, Nishiki K, Kawaguchi A, Harada K, Arakawa M, Sakamoto K, Masada M, Miyamori I, Fujimura A. Different effects of St. John's wort on the pharmacokinetics of simvastatin and pravastatin. Clin Pharmacol Ther 2001; 70:518–524.
85. Durr D, Stieger B, Kullak-Ublick GA, Rentsch KM, Steinert HC, Meier PJ, Fattinger K. St. John's wort induces intestinal *P*-glycoprotein/MDR1 and intestinal and hepatic CYP3A4. Clin Pharmacol Ther 2000; 68:598–604.
86. Hennessy M, Kelleher D, Spiers JP, Barry M, Kavanagh P, Back D, Mulcahy F, Feely J. St. John's wort increases expression of *P*-glycoprotein: implications for drug interactions. Br J Clin Pharmacol 2002; 53:75–82.
87. Wang Z, Gorski JC, Hamman MA, Huang SM, Lesko LJ, Hall SD. The effects of St. John's wort (*Hypericum perforatum*) on human cytochrome P450 activity. Clin Pharmacol Ther 2001; 70:317–326.
88. Karyekar CS, Eddington ND, Dowling TC. Effect of St. John's wort extract on intestinal expression of cytochrome P4501A2: studies in LS180 cells. J Postgrad Med 2002; 48:97–100.
89. Zou L, Harkey MR, Henderson GL. Effects of herbal components on cDNA-expressed cytochrome P450 enzyme catalytic activity. Life Sci 2002; 71:1579–1589.
90. Moore LB, Goodwin B, Jones SA, Wisely GB, Serabjit-Singh CJ, Willson TM, Collins JL, Kliewer SA. St. John's wort induces hepatic drug metabolism through activation of the pregnane X receptor. Proc Natl Acad Sci USA 2000; 97:7500–7502.
91. Chan TY. Interaction between warfarin and danshen (*Salvia miltiorrhiza*). Ann Pharmacother 2001; 35:501–504.
92. Zhao BL, Jiang W, Zhao Y, Hou JW, Xin WJ. Scavenging effects of *Salvia miltiorrhiza* on free radicals and its protection for myocardial mitochondrial membranes from ischemia-reperfusion injury. Biochem Mol Biol Int 1996; 38:1171–1182.
93. Tam LS, Chan TY, Leung WK, Critchley JA. Warfarin interactions with Chinese traditional medicines: danshen and methyl salicylate medicated oil. Aust NZ J Med 1995; 25:258.
94. Yu CM, Chan JC, Sanderson JE. Chinese herbs and warfarin potentiation by "danshen." J Intern Med 1997; 241:337–339.
95. Izzat MB, Yim AP, El-Zufari MH. A taste of Chinese medicine! Ann Thorac Surg 1998; 66:941–942.
96. Cheng TO. Warfarin danshen interaction. Ann Thorac Surg 1999; 67:894.
97. Chan K, Lo AC, Yeung JH, Woo KS. The effects of danshen (*Salvia*

miltiorrhiza) on warfarin pharmacodynamics and pharmacokinetics of warfarin enantiomers in rats. J Pharm Pharmacol 1995; 47:402–406.
98. Takahashi K, Ran LH, Watanabe M, Hanatani T, Takahashi K, Komatsu K, Azuma J. Prediction of herb drug interaction through cytochrome P450 (CYP) by Chinese traditional medicine (danshen). 9th International Symposium of the Pacific Rim Association for Clinical Pharmacogenetics, Hong Kong, Oct. 19–20, 2001.
99. Zhu DP. Dong quai. Am J Chin Med 1987; 15:117–125.
100. Roemheld-Hamm B, Dahl NV. Herbs, menopause, and dialysis. Semin Dial 2002; 15:53–59.
101. Goh SY, Loh KC. Gynaecomastia and the herbal tonic "dong quai." Singapore Med J 2001; 42:115–116.
102. Hirata JD, Swiersz LM, Zell B, Small R, Ettinger B. Does dong quai have estrogenic effects in postmenopausal women? A double-blind, placebo-controlled trial. Fertil Steril 1997; 68:981–986.
103. Amato P, Christophe S, Mellon PL. Estrogenic activity of herbs commonly used as remedies for menopausal symptoms. Menopause 2002; 9:145–150.
104. Page RL, 2nd, Lawrence JD. Potentiation of warfarin by dong quai. Pharmacotherapy 1999; 19:870–876.
105. Lo AC, Chan K, Yeung JH, Woo KS. Danggui (*Angelica sinensis*) affects the pharmacodynamics but not the pharmacokinetics of warfarin in rabbits. Eur J Drug Metab Pharmacokin 1995; 20:55–60.
106. Ernst E. The risk-benefit profile of commonly used herbal therapies: ginkgo, St. John's wort, ginseng, echinacea, saw palmetto, and kava. Ann Intern Med 2002; 136:42–53.
107. Pittler MH, Ernst E. *Ginkgo biloba* extract for the treatment of intermittent claudication: a meta-analysis of randomized trials. Am J Med 2000; 108:276–281.
108. Gilbert GJ. *Ginkgo biloba*. Neurology 1997; 48:1137.
109. Rowin J, Lewis SL. Spontaneous bilateral subdural hematomas associated with chronic *Ginkgo biloba* ingestion. Neurology 1996; 46:1775–1776.
110. Matthews MK, Jr. Association of *Ginkgo biloba* with intracerebral hemorrhage. Neurology 1998; 50:1933–1934.
111. Vale S. Subarachnoid haemorrhage associated with *Ginkgo biloba*. Lancet, 1998; 352:36.
112. Rosenblatt M, Mindel J. Spontaneous hyphema associated with ingestion of *Ginkgo biloba* extract [letter]. N Engl J Med 1997; 336:1108.
113. Foster BC, Foster MS, Vandenhoek S, Krantis A, Budzinski JW, Arnason JT, Gallicano KD, Choudri S. An in vitro evaluation of human cytochrome P450 3A4 and *P*-glycoprotein inhibition by garlic. J Pharm Pharmaceut Sci 2001; 4:176–184.
114. Bhardwaj RK, Glaeser H, Becquemont L, Klotz U, Gupta SK, Fromm MF. Piperine, a major constituent of black pepper, inhibits human *P*-glycoprotein and CYP3A4. J Pharmacol Exp Ther 2002; 302:645–650.

Index

Page references followed by f *denote figures and page references followed by* t *denote tables.*